Sheehy's

EMERGENCY NURSING

Principles and Practice

Sheehy's
EMERGENCY NURSING
Principles and Practice

Fourth Edition

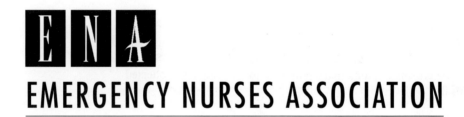

EMERGENCY NURSES ASSOCIATION

Edited by

Lorene Newberry, RN, MS, CEN
Clinical Nurse Specialist
Emergency/Trauma
Promina Northwest Health System
Marietta, Georgia

with 583 illustrations

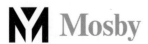 Mosby

St. Louis Baltimore Boston Carlsbad Chicago Minneapolis New York Philadelphia Portland
London Milan Sydney Tokyo Toronto

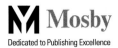

Mosby
Dedicated to Publishing Excellence

Mosby–Year Book, Inc.
11830 Westline Industrial Drive
St. Louis, Missouri 63146

Library of Congress Cataloging-in-Publication Data
Sheehy's emergency nursing : principles and practice.—4th ed. /
    edited by Lorene Newberry.
        p.   cm.
    Rev. ed. of: Emergency nursing : principles and practice / edited
by Susan Budassi Sheehy. 3rd ed. 1992.
    Includes bibliographical references and index.
    ISBN 0-8151-7678-3
    1. Emergency nursing.   I. Newberry, Lorene.   II. Sheehy, Susan
Budassi, 1948-   .
    [DNLM: 1. Emergency nursing.   WY 154 S541 1997]
RT120.E4E48   1997
610.73'61—dc21
DNLM/DLC   97-17575

        99   00   01   /   9   8   7   6   5   4   3   2

CONTRIBUTORS

Sherrilynne Almeida, RN, MSN, MEd, DrPHc
EMS Administrator
Houston Fire Department
Emergency Medical Services
Houston, Texas

Susan Barnason, PhD, RN, CEN, CCRN
Clinical Nurse Specialist
Bryan Memorial Hospital
Lincoln, Nebraska

Cynthia S. Baxter, RN, BSN, CCRN, CEN
Unit Coordinator
Critical Care Transport
Central Baptist Hospital
Lexington, Kentucky

Doreen K. Begley, RN, BS, CEN
Emergency Department Staff Nurse
Washoe Medical Center
Reno, Nevada

Lisa Marie Bernardo, RN, PhD, CEN
Assistant Professor
Health and Community Systems
University of Pittsburgh School of Nursing
Pittsburgh, Pennsylvania

Julie E. Bracken, RN, MS, CEN
Director, Nursing Education
Cook County Hospital
Chicago, Illinois

Catherine A. Chapman RN, BSN, CEN
Trauma Coordinator
Emergency Department
George Washington University Medical Center
Washington, DC

Courtney Cosby, MS, MN, CNA
Cardiology Product Line Manager
Columbia/Richmond Division
Richmond, Virginia

Laura M. Criddle, RN, MS, CEN, CCRN, CNRN, CFRN
Flight Nurse
STAR Flight
Brackenridge Hospital
Austin, Texas

Nancy Stephens Donatelli, RN, MS, CEN, CNA
Director, Ambulatory Services
St. Francis Hospital of New Castle
New Castle, Pennsylvania

Darcy Egging, RN, MS, CS-ANP, CEN
Nurse Practitioner
Delnor Community Hospital—Emergency Department
Edward Health Care Center—Family Practice
Oswego, Illinois

Lynn M. Feeman, RN, MSN, CEN, CCRN
Trauma Nurse Coordinator
Grady Health Systems
Atlanta, Georgia

Kathy Fountain, RN, MPH, MSN, CPNP
CHIPS Outreach Director
Children's Hospital of Alabama
University of Alabama at Birmingham
Birmingham, Alabama

Chris M. Gisness, RN, MSN, FNP, CEN
Staff Nurse
Grady Memorial Hospital
Emergency Care Center
Atlanta, Georgia

Jackie Gondeck, RN, BSN, MHA, CEN
Clinical Education Coordinator
Emergency Department
Brackenridge Hospital
Austin, Texas

Susan L. Hatfield, RN, MS, CEN, FNP
Family Nurse Practitioner–Certified
Internal Medicine
Cartersville, Georgia

Muriel L. Herman, RN, BSN, MSN
Assistant Professor
School of Nursing
Floyd College
Rome, Georgia

Reneé Semonin Holleran, RN, PhD, CEN, CCRN, CFRN
Chief Flight Nurse
University Air Care
University of Cincinnati
Cincinnati, Ohio

Patricia Kunz Howard, RN, MSN, CCRN, CEN
Director
Emergency Department and Critical Care Transport
Central Baptist Hospital
Lexington, Kentucky

T. Randall Huey, RN, MS, CEN
Clinical Nurse Specialist
Emergency Department
Piedmont Hospital
Atlanta, Georgia

Barbara Bennett Jacobs, RN, MPH, MS
Assistant Professor of Nursing
St. Joseph College
West Hartford, Connecticut;
Clinical Instructor in Surgery
University of Connecticut
School of Medicine
Farmington, Connecticut

Charose James, RN, BSN, CEN
Staff Nurse
Methodist Hospital–Emergency Department
Omaha, Nebraska

Kathleen M. Kearney, RN, MSN, CEN
Clinical Nurse Specialist
Beth Israel Medical Center
New York, New York

Zeb Koran, RN, MSN, CEN, CCRN
Director, Educational Services
Emergency Nurses Association
Park Ridge, Illinois

Linda L. Larson, PhD, RN, FNP, CEN
Nurse Practitioner
Internal Medicine and Geriatrics
G. Kenneth Deagman, MD
Aurora, Colorado

Susan Engman Lazear, RN, MN, CEN, CFRN
Director
Specialists in Medical Education
Woodinville, Washington;
Former Chief Flight Nurse
Airlift Northwest
Seattle, Washington

Genell Lee, RN, MSN, JD
Nurse Attorney
Birmingham, Alabama

Patricia A. Lenaghan, RN, MS, CEN
Service Executive–Emergency Department
Methodist Hospital
Omaha, Nebraska

Diana M. Lombardo, RN, BSN, CCRN
Staff Nurse, Trauma ICU
University Medical Center
Las Vegas, Nevada

John R. Lunde, RN, BSN, CEN, CCRN, TNS, EMT-P
Assistant Manager, Emergency/Trauma
The Medical Center
Columbus, Georgia

Estelle MacPhail, RN, MS, CEN, CNAA
Director, Emergency Services
Coordinator, SNHRMC Trauma Service
Southern New Hampshire Regional Medical Center
Nashua, New Hampshire

Anne Manton, RN, PhD, CEN
Assistant Professor
Fairfield University
Fairfield, Connecticut;
Staff Nurse (per diem)
Hospital of St. Raphael
New Haven, Connecticut

Sharon K. Mason, RN, CEN, CCRN
Emergency Room Staff Nurse
Cartersville, Georgia

Dell T. Miller, RN, MSN, EMTP, CCRN, CEN
Manager, Emergency/Trauma Nursing
The Medical Center
Columbus, Georgia

Susan Moore, RN, MS, CCRN, CEN
Staff Nurse
Emergency Department
Washoe Medical Center
Reno, Nevada

Joan Morris, RN, MSN, CEN
Center Manager
University of Illinois Medical Center at O'Hare
Chicago, Illinois

Catherine M. Olson, BA, RN, CEN
Staff Nurse, Emergency Department
Sherman Hospital
Elgin, Illinois

Mary Ellen McNally Pedersen, RN, BS, CPTC
New England Organ Bank
Maine Transplant Program
Bangor, Maine

Barbara Pierce, RN, MN
Divisional Director, Emergency Services
The Children's Hospital of Alabama
Birmingham, Alabama

Cherie J. Revere, RN, MSN, CRNP, CEN
Emergency Department Nurse Practitioner
South Baldwin Hospital
Foley, Alabama;
Emergency Department Clinical Nurse Specialist
University of South Alabama Medical Center
Mobile, Alabama

Suzanne Rita, RN, MSN, CEN, CNS
Clinical Specialist
Emergency Department
Sentara Norfolk General Hospital
Sentara Leigh Hospital
Sentara Bayside Hospital
Norfolk, Virginia

Tracy McIntyre Ross, RN, BSN, CEN
Staff Nurse, Emergency Department
Virginia Beach General Hospital;
Staff Nurse, Patient First
Urgent Care Clinic
Virginia Beach, Virginia

Kim M. Rouse, RN, BSN
Manager, Emergency Services
Nebraska Methodist and Children's Hospitals
Omaha, Nebraska

Anita Ruiz-Contreras, RN, MSN, CEN, MICN
Emergency Staff Developer
Santa Clara Valley Medical Center
Sexual Assault Nurse Examiner
Santa Clara County, California

Ellen E. Ruja, RN, MSN, CEN
Clinical Nurse Specialist
Emergency Services/Urgent Care
Provenant St. Anthony's Hospitals
Denver, Colorado

Carole Rush, RN, MEd, CEN
Emergency Care and Injury Prevention Educator
Irving, Texas

S. Kay Sedlak, RN, MS, CEN
Clinical Nurse Specialist
Emergency Department
St. Mary's Regional Medical Center
Reno, Nevada

Rebecca A. Steinmann, RN, MS, CEN, CCRN
Clinical Nurse Specialist
Emergency Services
University Hospitals of Cleveland
Cleveland, Ohio

Janet P. Taylor, DSN, RN
Instructor
Associate Degree Nursing
Jones County Junior College
Ellisville, Mississippi

Joe E. Taylor, Jr., PhD, RN, CEN, FNP
Family Nurse Practitioner
Family Medical Associates
Collins, Mississippi

Deborah Trautman, RN, MSN
Director of Nursing
Department of Emergency Medicine
Johns Hopkins Hospital
Baltimore, Maryland

Tener Goodwin Veenema, MS, RN, PNP
Pediatric Nurse Practitioner
Coordinator for Case Management, Emergency Services
University of Rochester Medical Center
Rochester, New York

Deborah Whelchel-Revis, RN, PhD
Director, Emergency Care Services
Grady Memorial Hospital
Atlanta, Georgia

E. Marie Wilson, RN, MPA
Chief, System Development
Office of Emergency Medical Services
Connecticut Department of Public Health
Hartford, Connecticut

Tracey J. Wood, RN, BSN, CEN
Emergency Department
Kennestone Hospital
Marietta, Georgia

Cheryl Wraa, RN, BSN, CFRN
President, National Flight Nurses Association
Clinical III Resource Nurse
University of California
Davis Medical Center Life Flight
Sacramento, California

REVIEWERS

Celeste Chamberlain, RN, BSN, MS, CEN, CCRN
Unit Director
Emergency Center/Level I Trauma Center
Medical College of Pennsylvania Hospital
Philadelphia, Pennsylvania

Linda M. Scott, RN, MSN, PhD, CEN
Associate Professor
School of Nursing
Marshall University
Huntington, West Virginia

Russell Wilshaw, RN, MS, CEN
Trauma Coordinator
Urban South Intermountain Health Care
Utah Valley Regional Medical Center
Provo, Utah;
Former Clinical Instructor
Brigham Young University
Salt Lake City, Utah

*To the thousands of emergency nurses
who have made a difference to their patients and each other.*

FOREWORD

There have been many occasions when my nursing colleagues have asked about the genesis of *Emergency Nursing: Principles and Practice*. The entire idea, in fact, happened quite serendipitously. In the mid-seventies, I took a new position as a clinical nurse specialist at UCLA's Emergency Department (now known as the Emergency Medicine Center). In my newly evolving role, I was charged with developing the clinical expertise of the nursing staff. I spent countless hours researching and developing lesson plans and handouts, mostly derived from internal medicine, surgery, and some sparse emergency medicine literature. Neither emergency nursing nor emergency medicine had yet been recognized as specialties. At that time, I had often wished that there was a textbook I could use as a foundation for my program development. I searched the library catalogs for such a book and found that there were few and none that met my needs. I called several large medical and nursing publishing companies only to find that the book I was looking for did not exist. One fortuitous phone call to Mosby led to a response from Mosby editor Wallace Hood, who wanted to know more about what it was I was looking for. When I explained, he said that Mosby, too, was interested in such a book. In fact, they were seeking an author or authors who could write such a text.

I was put in touch with Janet Barber from Indiana who had contacted Mosby about her idea for an emergency nursing textbook. Wallace believed that the book would best be written by two or more authors from different parts of the country. California seemed to be a place where emergency medicine was beginning to take root—remember Johnny Gage and Roy Desoto? And the University of Southern California had begun one of the first emergency medicine residency programs in the country. So why not an emergency nursing book written by a co-author from California? So in all of my young naivete, I accepted the offer to become a co-author of this new textbook.

I equate the development of a textbook to conceiving, bearing, and birthing a child. And as Prissy so aptly put it in *Gone With the Wind*, "Miss Scarlett, I don't know nothin' about birthin' no baby!" The idea became fertile, and the book began to grow. At first there were lots of ideas, then those ideas began to take form as chapters were written and rewritten, rewritten again, and then edited and reedited, and reedited again. Quite like preparing a nursery for the new baby, I searched for the right setting—certain illustrations and charts and tables that would make it look just right. Janet and I wrote most of the chapters back then—little did

we know how much we didn't know. We did have a few invited chapter contributors, but not very many.

Finally, the book went into production and the "last trimester" began. It was introduced at the Emergency Nurses Association Scientific Assembly (then known as The Emergency Department Nurses Association) in 1979. It was like giving birth! Was it going to have all of its fingers and toes? Would I know what to do to take care of it? What would people say? Would I be a good mother?

Over the next two decades, like a child, the book matured as the specialty of Emergency Nursing matured. It was used by many to prepare for the Certification in Emergency Nursing examination. I received much feedback from my nursing colleagues; some were general comments and some were wonderful suggestions for future editions. It was time for the "child" to go to school. The second edition was written for a specialty that was beginning to take root. Many new chapters were added and old chapters were rewritten to reflect our expanding scope of knowledge and practice. Several new chapter contributors were recruited. I was thrilled with the talented people involved in our new specialty.

By the time the third edition was due to be written (I equate it to becoming a teenager), I realized that our body of knowledge had expanded so greatly that I was no longer able to write the bulk of the text by myself. Many new chapter contributors were recruited, and a third edition was produced that far surpassed the first two editions in its depth and breadth.

Now the time has come for the fourth edition to be published. *Emergency Nursing: Principles and Practice* has grown up. And as all children who come to maturity, the time has come for the "child" to leave the nest and try its own wings. The time has come for *Emergency Nursing: Principles and Practice* to be turned over to someone who will value its development, cherish its past, and bring it into the third millennium. I have chosen the Emergency Nurses Association to take on this responsibility—and I am very grateful that they have done so. As my career has evolved, my clinical expertise has dulled just a bit around the edges as I have pursued new roles in emergency nursing. It is time to turn this beloved "child" (who is no longer a child) over to those who are now the clinical experts. I am deeply grateful to the Emergency Nurses Association for accepting the responsibility for the continuation of *Emergency Nursing: Principles and Practice* and am very proud of the Emergency Nurses Association; the editor of this text, Lorene Newberry; and the numerous chapter contributors for a wonderful fourth edition.

Susan Budassi Sheehy

PREFACE

Emergency nursing has changed dramatically since publication of the first edition of *Emergency Nursing*. Treatments are more sophisticated, and the requisite knowledge base for emergency nursing is greater. The practice of emergency nursing is no longer limited to multipurpose emergency departments but now occurs in urgent care centers, primary care centers, flight programs, prehospital programs, and specialized pediatric emergency departments. Just as emergency nursing has grown and changed, *Sheehy's Emergency Nursing: Principles and Practice* has changed to keep pace. This fourth edition has been expanded and significantly revised to meet the changing face of emergency nursing practice.

The material in this edition has been grouped into six units: Foundations of Emergency Nursing, Professional Practice, Clinical Foundations of Emergency Nursing, Major Trauma Emergencies, Medical and Surgical Emergencies, and Special Patient Situations. Chapter formats have been expanded so that anatomy, physiology, and patient assessment are addressed in each clinical chapter. Nursing diagnoses are highlighted at the end of each clinical chapter, and additional photos, illustrations, and tables are included throughout the text. Practical tips have been included in the narrative.

Existing chapters have been revised, combined, or split accordingly. Separate chapters now address Gastrointestinal Trauma, Renal and Genitourinary Trauma, Gastrointestinal Emergencies, Renal and Genitourinary Emergencies, Obstetric Emergencies, and Gynecologic Emergencies. Pediatric triage and assessment are discussed in conjunction with Pediatric Emergencies, whereas psychosocial and psychiatric emergencies are addressed in the chapter on Mental Health Emergencies. Discussion on infection control has been expanded to Infectious and Communicable Diseases.

Eleven new chapters address a variety of topics. A chapter on Cultural Dimensions provides an overview of select cultural groups, whereas the chapter on Case Management discusses use of clinical pathways in the emergency department. Trauma care in non–trauma centers is described in the chapter on Emergency Department Trauma Management. Other new chapters address Elder Trauma, Obstetric Trauma, Mechanisms of Injury, Fluids and Electrolytes, Domestic Violence, Elder Abuse and Neglect, Substance Abuse, and Sexual Assault.

Contributors to the text come from rural, suburban, and urban areas and represent a broad range of clinical positions: staff nurses, clinical specialists, nurse managers, and nursing instructors. This depth and breadth of clinical experience adds texture to the material and reflects the true nature of emergency nursing.

Susan Budassi Sheehy left an indelible mark on emergency nursing through her work in previous editions of *Emergency Nursing*. Her commitment to clinical expertise, development of a strong conceptual and theoretical knowledge base, and recognition of diverse practice areas are a legacy of which the field of emergency nursing can be proud. This distinguished heritage continues as the text moves under the auspices of the Emergency Nurses Association. You will find this same commitment throughout this newest edition of *Sheehy's Emergency Nursing: Principles and Practice*.

ACKNOWLEDGMENTS

Completion of this project like other successes in life did not occur in isolation. A number of people made it possible. I am honored to acknowledge their contributions and to say thank you—I couldn't have done it without you!

The Emergency Nurses Association had the vision to support this project and move emergency nursing into the next millennium. In addition to administrative and technical advice, the moral support was priceless. Zeb Koran was a miracle worker who always made me laugh and put everything into perspective. Members of Metro Atlanta ENA provided support and friendship throughout the project.

The chapter writers did a tremendous job, met impossible deadlines, produced terrific chapters with depth and breadth of content that left me speechless, while maintaining chaotic personal and professional lives—despite collapsed roofs, waterlogged computers, family illness, and a multitude of other challenges. Special thanks to Zeb Koran, Patti Howard, and Cyndi Baxter who came through with last minute chapter revisions.

We would not have made the publication deadline without the efforts of the Mosby–Year Book, Inc. staff who demonstrated such terrific teamwork. I want to specifically thank Sally Schrefer, Executive Editor, who removed any remaining doubts I had about doing this project; Rae Robertson, Associate Developmental Editor, who found just the right photo, table, or figure time after time and always made me feel better after we talked; and Cheryl Abbott Bozzay, Production Editor, who helped me through the final production phase. A word of appreciation for the reviewers whose critical eyes and cogent comments made this a better text.

The staff at PROMINA Kennestone Hospital Emergency Center remind me why I love emergency nursing—it is fun, challenging, rewarding, and definitely not for the faint of heart. Their support during the past year is a gift from God that I wouldn't have missed for the world. The physicians of the Kennestone Emergency Group gave me strength, knowledge, support, and countless memories. Special thanks to Doug Krug, Don Freeman, Mike Ray, Bob Gisness, and Jon Morris for more reasons than I can mention.

Thanks to Dr. David Tucker and Dr. Frank McCoy who kept me honest and healthy during the past year. I couldn't get away with anything! I always had to tell them how I really felt and what was going on with me. Their support and professionalism made a difference in my life.

My family supported me despite legitimate questions regarding my sanity. Their love, patience, faith in God, and enjoyment of life's simple pleasures helped me keep things in the middle of the road—most of the time.

Special thanks to special friends who supported me during what turned out to be a significant personal challenge that occurred in the midst of various editing crises. I cannot imagine a day without each one in my life: Shannon Sayre, Denyse Pike, Marvina Williams, Michele Wilhoit, Vicky Boys, Gwen Barnett, Nona Harris, Sharon Mason, Chris Gisness, Carol Morgan, Pat Hanks, Sheila Davenport, Anne Smith, Lisa Ray, and Marilyn and Gerald Hobbs. Finally, thanks to my favorite hedonist who always reminded me to have fun!

Lorene Newberry

Contents

FOUNDATIONS OF
EMERGENCY NURSING

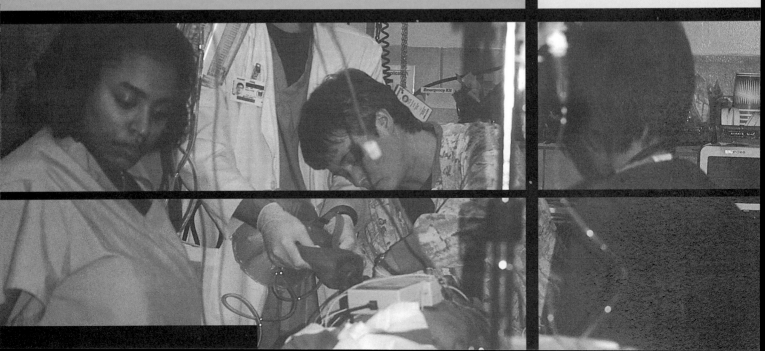

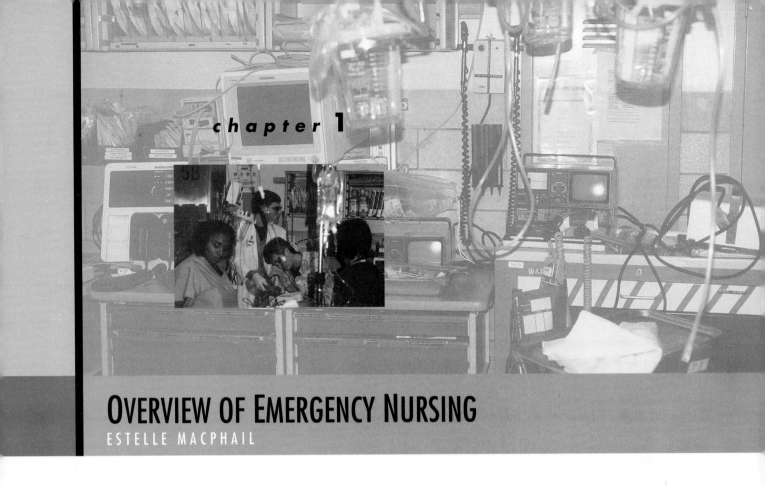

OVERVIEW OF EMERGENCY NURSING

ESTELLE MACPHAIL

Emergency nursing began during the Florence Nightingale era; however, the specialty practice of emergency nursing has evolved during the past 25 years. By definition, emergency nursing is care of individuals of all ages with perceived or actual physical or emotional alterations of health that are undiagnosed or that require further interventions. Emergency nursing care is episodic, primary, and usually acute.

Most specialty nursing groups are defined by alliance or affiliation with a specific body system, disease process, care setting, age group, or population. Conversely, emergency nursing is defined by diversity of knowledge, patients, and disease processes. Emergency nurses care for all ages and populations, over the broad spectrum of disease, injury prevention, lifesaving, and limb-saving measures. Emergency nursing practice requires a unique blend of generalized and specialized assessment, intervention, and management skills. The dimensions of emergency nursing specify roles, behaviors, and processes inherent in emergency nursing practice and delineate characteristics unique to emergency nursing. Practice area, patient populations, and variety in those who provide care are just as diverse in emergency nursing as in the nursing profession as a whole.

The scope of emergency nursing practice encompasses assessment, diagnosis, treatment, and evaluation. Problems can be perceived, actual or potential, sudden or urgent, physical or psychosocial. They are primarily episodic or acute, and occur in a variety of settings. Resolution may require minimal care or life-support measures, patient and family education, appropriate referral, and knowledge of legal implications.

Care delivery occurs where the consumer lives, works, plays, and goes to school. Box 1-1 identifies just a few practice areas for emergency nursing.

Emergency nursing is multidimensional, requiring knowledge of multiple body systems, disease processes, and age groups common to other nursing specialties. Processes unique to emergency nursing such as triage and emergency operations preparedness are discussed in later chapters. In addition to unique processes, emergency nursing is governed by a unique set of unwritten rules that have come about as a result of the environment and the patients (Box 1-2).

Nursing roles include patient care, research, management, education, consultation, and advocacy. Emergency nursing practice is defined through specific role functions as delineated in the Emergency Nurses Association's (ENA) Standards of Emergency Nursing Practice, Scope of Practice Statement, and Emergency Nursing Core Curriculum. Roles are further defined in ENA's Trauma Nursing Core Course, Emergency Nursing Pediatric Course, and Prehospital Core Curriculum. Roles are also determined by practice arena. The emergency nurse in a teaching institution may function very differently than the emergency nurse in a small rural hospital.

STANDARDS

A standard is an acknowledged measure of quantitative or qualitative value. It reflects ongoing changes in practice and clarifies the distinction between competence and excellence in practice. The minimally acceptable level of performance

---

Box 1-1   Emergency Nursing Practice Settings

Hospital Emergency Department (ED)
Prehospital Arena
Air and Ground Transport Units
Military Arena
Urgent Care Center
Health Clinic
Health Maintenance Organization
Ambulatory Services
Schools and Universities
Business/Industry
Correctional Institution

Box 1-2   Emergency Nursing Environment

Unplanned situations that require immediate intervention.
Allocation of limited resources.
Need for immediate care perceived by the patient or others.
Geographic variables.
Unpredictable numbers of patients.
Unknown patient severity, urgency, and diagnosis.

Box 1-3   Standards of Emergency Nursing Practice

Potential uses

Criterion-based job descriptions and performance evaluations
Policies and procedures
Standardized care plans
Orientation and education programs
Quality improvement programs
Research projects

Box 1-4   Emergency Nursing Foundation Purpose

Enhance emergency health care services to the public by:
Promoting emergency nursing through research and education.
Enhancing professional development through research.
Providing a means for the education of health care profession-
    als in the care and treatment of emergency patients.
Educating the general public on emergency-related subjects.
Providing research grants and educational scholarships.

---

is reflected in competency level outcomes. Excellence is practice that surpasses the competency level and, ultimately, contributes to growth and advancement of emergency nursing. Standards are a measure by which the consumer views emergency nursing performance and a measure to which nurses are held accountable.

Standards represent a philosophy. They are a compilation of recommendations and general guidelines that contain outcome criteria to measure and evaluate performance. The original Standards of Emergency Nursing Practice (1983) provided a springboard for growth of emergency nursing. Since their development, the Standards have been used for a variety of purposes (Box 1-3). In 1992 practice standards from the American Nurses Association were incorporated into the Standards. This strengthened the Standards by highlighting the depth and breadth of emergency nursing practice.

Emergency nursing practice is systematic. It includes the nursing process, nursing diagnosis, decision making, and analytic and scientific thinking and inquiry. Professional behaviors inherent in emergency nursing practice are acquisition and application of a specialized body of knowledge and skills, accountability and responsibility, communication, autonomy, and collaborative relationships with others.

RESEARCH IN EMERGENCY NURSING

Promoting research in emergency nursing adds to the knowledge of the discipline and contributes to sound clinical decisions. Collaborative research endeavors broaden the scope of emergency nursing knowledge. The ENA Code of Ethics for Emergency Nursing (1989) provides a distinctive set of ideals and standards of conduct regarding research activities. Ethical principles are the moral bond linking the professions, the patients they serve, and the public.

In 1991 ENA established the Emergency Nursing Foundation (ENF) to promote availability, quality, and effectiveness of emergency nursing through education and research. Box 1-4 clarifies the goals of ENF. Interest from monies raised and invested is distributed for scholarships, research, and special projects.

SPECIALTY PRACTICE

A characteristic inherent in emergency care is integration of the emergency health care team. In no other place in health care are teamwork and mutual respect more important. Quality of care depends on this team concept. Nurses, physicians, physician assistants, paramedics, emergency medical technicians, and first responders must function as colleagues to provide optimal patient care to the ill or injured patient.

The outcome of care in the hospital is greatly influenced by the field team's effort during initial stabilization, transfer, and by ongoing communication. Personnel needs in the emergency medical service (EMS) system vary with type of call, community protocol, and available resources. Table 1-1 describes specific emergency personnel and their responsibilities. It is beyond the scope of this text to provide a comprehensive description of each discipline. The brevity of information provided should not be construed as a reflection of the importance of each team member.

Table **1-1**	**EMS Personnel and Responsibilities**
Personnel	**Responsibilities**
First responders	Establish basic life-support procedures. Include police, fire, and civilian personnel.
EMS dispatchers	Triage, prioritize, and relay call for help. Dispatch essential personnel and equipment. Provide instructions for first responders until advanced help arrives.
Advanced responders	Include EMTs, paramedics, nurses, respiratory therapists, and physicians. Vary with type of call and community-accepted protocol. Provide advanced care at scene and during transport.

Certified Emergency Nurse

The examination for certified emergency nurses (CEN) is a mechanism by which knowledge and skills for safe and competent practice can be measured. It is administered by the Board of Certification for Emergency Nursing (BCEN) to promote health and welfare of emergency patients, advancing the science and art of emergency nursing through the certification process. A nurse with the CEN credential has demonstrated knowledge in the specialty of emergency nursing. Chapter 3 discusses certification.

Emergency Nurse Practitioner

The nurse practitioner is a professional registered nurse with advanced education in delivery of primary care to adult and pediatric patients. The emergency nurse practitioner is a nurse practitioner who specializes in emergency care through education and clinical experience. Responsibilities include care of emergency patients under the medical supervision of the attending physician. Certification for nurse practitioners is provided by professional boards such as the American Nurses Credentialing Center. Nurse practitioner programs last 44 to 72 weeks and cover acute and nonacute emergency situations. Practice areas include emergency departments open 24 hours a day, urgent care centers, and rural clinics with minimal or no physician coverage.

Clinical Nurse Specialist

The clinical nurse specialist (CNS) is a registered nurse who, through advanced study of scientific knowledge and supervised advanced clinical practice at the master's or doctoral level, has become an expert in emergency nursing. An emergency CNS demonstrates expertise through innovative, comprehensive, and high-quality performance in emergency nursing. Specific responsibilities include accountability for development and application of practice standards as well as research to enhance the quality of care for patients, their significant others, communities, and potential consumers of emergency care. Ultimately the emergency CNS strives to improve patient care and enhance treatment outcomes.

The emergency CNS exemplifies professional nursing practice through direct and indirect patient care. Specific role functions are expert clinical practitioner, educator, consultant, researcher, and leader. Within each role, the emergency CNS is a role model, patient advocate, change agent, and cost-effective practitioner. Through application of these responsibilities, the emergency CNS is in a unique position to affect the profession, the specialty, and most importantly, the patient.

Case Manager

The case manager role enhances quality patient care while promoting cost effectiveness in the hospital or clinic arena. Case managers cross departmental lines; therefore authority and ability to negotiate with multiple providers is essential to ensure optimal care in the most cost-effective manner possible. The case manager has a global focus, covering the spectrum of the patient's visit from arrival to discharge and beyond. Chapter 9 describes case management and the role of the case manager.

Specialties within Emergency Nursing

With the explosion of information and technology, nursing has become more and more specialized. Conventional wisdom that "a nurse is a nurse is a nurse" no longer applies. This is also true for emergency nursing. A subspecialty is, by definition, a group of nurses who work in a specific environment, care for special patient groups, perform special functions, or have special interests related to emergency nursing. Recognized subspecialties within emergency nursing include flight nursing, pediatric emergency nursing, trauma nursing, prehospital nursing, and mobile intensive care nursing. As emergency nursing copes with a changing world, additional subspecialties are emerging. These include groups who deal with infomatics, sexual assault, and forensics. Each subspecialty has unique needs related to education, practice, and networking. Recognition of the unique and diverse contributions of these groups strengthens the practice of all emergency nurses.

Prehospital nursing. Prehospital nursing dates back more than 100 years. In the 1970s, nurses staffed mobile advanced life support units. Today nurses in the prehospital arena are an extension of the acute and nonacute setting. In 1992, ENA published the Prehospital Core Curriculum to establish core knowledge and skills pertinent to prehospital nursing practice.

Flight nursing. Flight nursing requires a strong background in critical care and emergency nursing. Flight nurses provide a high level of care at the scene of an accident, in the referring hospital, and during transport by fixed wing or rotary wing aircraft. The flight nurse integrates knowledge of the nursing process and practice standards set forth by the National Flight Nurses Association.

HOSPITAL EMERGENCY DEPARTMENT

Dramatic changes have occurred in the ED during the past 2 decades. Emergency rooms became emergency departments, which in turn became emergency centers incorporating prehospital care, flight programs, ambulatory care, occupational health programs, observation units, fast-track treatment areas, and satellite units. The Medicare Act of 1965 and Medicaid Act of 1966 gave millions of Americans access to health care. The Vietnam war led to recognition of trauma as a leading cause of death and disability. Federal grants supported development of emergency medical systems. Special units such as the pediatric emergency department emerged across the country.

Emergency departments care for millions of people each year. Emergency medical evaluation and initial treatment are provided through a well-defined plan based on community need and the defined capabilities of each hospital. The ED is the only physician many people ever know. It serves not only as a receiving center for critically ill and injured people, but also as a 24-hour shelter for people who are frightened and have nowhere else to go. The number of individuals seen in the ED has grown steadily during the past decade. Reasons for these increases are multiple and complex (Box 1-5). Recent changes in health care and the advent of managed care may reverse this trend by diverting patients to primary care centers. Primary care centers in combination with increasingly complex reimbursement systems such as capitated contracts may significantly decrease the census in many EDs. It is too early to predict with certainty the full impact of these changes. Suffice it to say, the ED will experience dramatic change into the next century.

Urgent Care Centers

According to a Government Accounting Office study, census increased in 85% of all U.S. hospitals from 1986 to 1990. Emergency department visits increased almost 20% nationwide from 1985 to 1990. The greatest increase in census has been in those patients who fall in the urgent or non-emergent category—patients who could be seen in a primary care physician's office. Fast track and urgent care centers emerged as a way to manage these patients. Urgent care centers may be part of the existing ED or function as a separate entity outside the ED. Treating patients with minor complaints outside the ED reduces treatment time and enhances patient satisfaction.

CONCLUSION

Advances in technology may soon be overshadowed by an increasing demand for emergency care, particularly for critically ill patients. As the ED cares for more critical patients for longer periods, the need for sophisticated monitoring equipment increases. Technology previously reserved for the critical care unit is now commonplace in the ED. As these and other changes occur, emergency nursing becomes more complex and demanding.

As the population ages, health care needs of its members change and become more complex. Preventive medicine is prohibitively expensive for the indigent and most elders. Patients are discharged earlier after surgery, myocardial infarction, and many other conditions. Unfortunately, this means patients are sicker when they arrive in the ED and they stay longer. This situation is exacerbated by lack of home care and other essential community resources.

Emergency nurses serve increasingly demanding consumers. The public expects the latest technology and sophistication without loss of "high-touch" care. Insurance companies and employers are looking for the lowest health care cost available. New reimbursement rules drive decision making. In the past, hospitals received reimbursement from the government and other third-party payers based on cost. In today's health care market, reimbursement is based on a specified number of covered lives rather than actual cost of care provided. Simply put, the hospital is paid what is in its contract, regardless of how much it actually costs to do the procedure or care for the patient.

Faced with capitation, health care administrators have tightened their budgetary belts, asking fewer to do more with less. Many issues will affect nursing as the health care system undergoes radical change. The nursing profession and how it is perceived will change. As nursing becomes more active in the decision-making process and speaks with a single voice, these changes become shining opportunities. Emergency nurses must join together with a new energy, speak with a new voice, and create a new presence for emergency nursing.

Box **1-5**   **Potential Causes of Increased ED Census**
No appointment required.
Lack of accessibility to private physicians.
Convenient for those with limited resources.
Treatment regardless of ability to pay.
Open on weekends, holidays, and after hours.

SUGGESTED READING

Emergency Nurses Association: *Code of ethics,* Chicago, 1989, The Association.

Emergency Nurses Association: *Position paper: role of the clinical nurse specialist,* Chicago, 1989, The Association.

Emergency Nurses Association: Scope of practice statement, *JEN* 15(4):361, 1989.

Emergency Nurses Association: *Pre-hospital core curriculum,* Chicago, 1991, The Association.

Emergency Nurses Association: *Standards of emergency nursing practice,* ed 3, St. Louis, 1992, Mosby.

Emergency Nurses Association: *Core curriculum,* ed 4, Philadelphia, 1994, WB Saunders.

Emergency Nurses Association: Trauma nursing core course, ed 3, Chicago, 1995, The Association.

Emergency Nurses Association: Emergency nursing pediatric course, Park Ridge, Ill, 1993, the Association.

Emergency Nurses Association: *Position statement,* Park Ridge, Ill, 1995, The Association.

Emergency Nurses Association: *Triage: meeting the challenge,* Park Ridge, Ill, 1995, The Association.

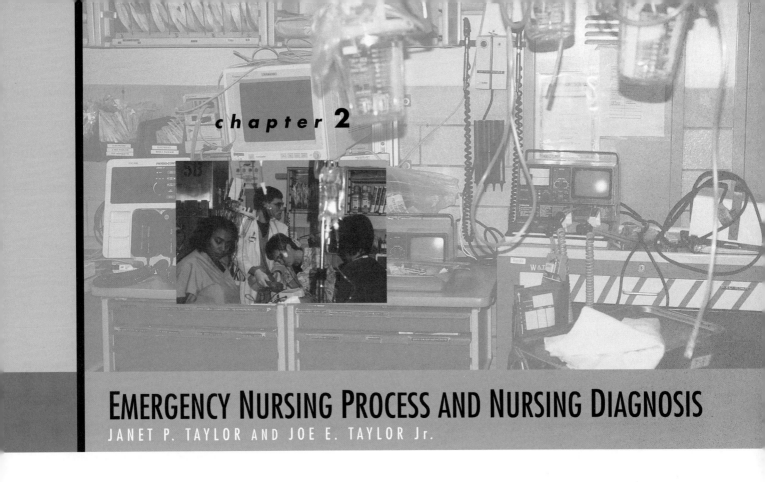

chapter 2

EMERGENCY NURSING PROCESS AND NURSING DIAGNOSIS

JANET P. TAYLOR AND JOE E. TAYLOR Jr.

Nursing is a challenging and complex profession involving more than disease processes. Nurses also deal with the patient's and family's responses to actual or potential health problems.[8] Responses that nurses encounter involve the entire spectrum of human emotions, feelings, symptoms, and manifestations. Nurses must make clinical judgments about these natural responses to disease and disease states. This clinical judgment is called a nursing diagnosis. Nursing diagnosis is part of a sophisticated problem-solving approach called the nursing process. In the emergency setting, nurses are called upon to use a problem-solving approach to make life-or-death decisions about their patients. In many cases, a problem-solving approach must be implemented and completed in a matter of minutes. The purpose of this chapter is to outline the nursing process and its applicability to the emergency nurse. Issues related to formulation of nursing diagnoses are also discussed. Case scenarios are presented with examples of how the nursing process can be applied in specific situations.

OVERVIEW OF THE NURSING PROCESS

The nursing process has evolved as a vital tool in performance of day-to-day functions of nurses in all health care arenas, providing the organizing framework for assessment, diagnosis, planning, implementation, and evaluation of patient care. Through this framework, nurses use theoretic and empiric knowledge to provide individualized and competent care to the patients they encounter. Proficient use of the nursing process provides the foundation for efficient and comprehensive care in all areas of nursing practice. In the emergency setting, nurses must assimilate essential data to formulate the plan of care for their patients in a fast-paced setting. Therefore it is imperative that the nurse in this setting be an expert clinician and diagnostician to care for the emergent patient.

Appropriate execution of the nursing process requires the nurse to have specialized skills, a vast clinical knowledge base, various psychomotor skills, critical thinking skills, creativity, and flexibility. The dynamic nature of the nursing process requires the nurse to be constantly aware of changes in the patient's status and alert to new cues that may develop in the course of care. In this discussion, each step of the nursing process is analyzed separately, however, the steps may occur simultaneously, overlap, or occur out of sequence. Flexibility to adapt to changes that take place in the emergent patient is absolutely essential for maintaining an up-to-date plan of care for the ED patient. Table 2-1 gives an overview of the nursing process.

Assessment

The nursing process begins with assessment at the onset of the nurse-patient relationship and continues throughout the encounter. In the ED, assessment begins before the patient enters the facility as the nurse processes information received from EMS personnel, family members, and previous patient encounters by hospital staff. Although

Table **2-1**	The Nursing Process
Component	Description
Assessment	Begins with the nursing history and performance of a health assessment. Ends with verification of wellness or illness. A precursor to the nursing diagnosis.
Diagnosis	A determination or conclusion reached by the nurse based on assessment data. Lists patient problem, etiology, and signs and symptoms.
Planning	Determination of action plan to assist the patient toward goal of optimal wellness. Involves priority setting. Leads to a written plan of care.
Implementation	Initiation and completion of actions necessary to accomplish the defined goal of optimal fulfillment of human needs.
Evaluation	Appraisal of changes experienced by the patient in relation to goal achievement resulting from the nurse's actions.

comprehensive data is helpful in planning long-term patient care, in an emergency situation selected assessment data may be processed to begin the patient care process. For example, when an unresponsive patient presents to the ED, a quick assessment of the patient's airway, breathing, and circulation is all that is needed to determine whether life-saving measures should be implemented.

The nurse must cluster data into groups called diagnostic cues, which provide the nurse with a direction for formulation of an appropriate nursing diagnosis. In the example above, airway, breathing, and circulation are factors necessary to sustain life. Absence of these factors leads the nurse to form a diagnostic cue related to the diagnosis *altered tissue perfusion*. Once this diagnosis is made, the nurse determines that implementation of cardiopulmonary resuscitation (CPR) is the best approach to meet the identified needs. This scenario provides a rather simplistic view of the diagnostic process while emphasizing the assessment phase of the nursing process.

During the patient care encounter, the nurse continuously assesses the patient to determine whether interventions are effective, if further problems are developing, or more intervention is needed. Assessment data are fed back into the nursing process, making the process cyclic. Through experience, nurses are able to gather and process data quickly, almost unconsciously, when providing care to their patients.

Diagnosis

The diagnosis phase of the nursing process seems to be the most difficult for many nurses. In 1967, Yura and Walsh

published the first edition of *The Nursing Process.* At that time, it did not contain nursing diagnosis. In 1973, the American Nurses Association (ANA) published its *Standards of Nursing Practice,* which led Yura and Walsh[11] to add nursing diagnosis as an integral part of the nursing process in their third edition. The ANA[1] formally brought nursing diagnosis into practice by stating that "nursing diagnoses are derived from health status data" and that "the plan of nursing care includes goals derived from the nursing diagnosis."

The ANA Standards formed the foundation of the National Conferences on the Classification of Nursing Diagnoses. The goal was to "initiate the process of preparing an organized, logical, comprehensive system for classifying those health problems or health states diagnosed by nurses and treated by means of nursing interventions."[3] Later conferences emphasized refinement and review of approved diagnoses; use of nursing diagnoses in clinical practice, education, and research; and examination of proposed theoretic frameworks for the nursing diagnosis as a part of the nursing process.[2]

Since the first mention of nursing diagnosis as a concept, many definitions have been formulated. Gordon[8] provided the most widely accepted definition, "Nursing diagnosis, or clinical diagnosis made by professional nurses, describes actual or potential health problems which nurses, by virtue of their education and experience, are capable and licensed to treat."

Formulating a correct diagnosis requires diagnostic reasoning for data collection, analyses, and interpretation. Application of diagnostic reasoning is also necessary to accurately formulate the nursing diagnosis. To make an accurate diagnosis, the nurse must consider data within the context of the individualized patient situation. Cues either support or eliminate the diagnosis in question. An accurate diagnosis has been formulated when all cues have been considered and nonrelevant cues have been eliminated. Writing the diagnostic statement involves use of knowledge from behavioral and biologic sciences, critical thinking skills, and the art of interpretation. This step is considered the most difficult part of the nursing process.

Planning

The third step of the nursing process involves development of a plan to meet needs identified in the previous phases. By reviewing possible nursing actions, the nurse can decide which actions will be most beneficial for the patient in this situation. In the ED, there is little room for trial and error. The nurse must depend on expertise gained from prior experience and an extensive repertoire of skills to plan the most effective strategy.

Setting priorities is one of the most important components of the planning phase. The nurse may identify a number of problems that need to be addressed for the patient; however, all the problems do not have equal significance in the patient care scenario. Establishing a list of priorities is as important as identification of the problems themselves. To the inexperienced nurse, all patient problems may have top priority; however, keen assessment skills and accurate clustering of data cues enable the nurse to address multiple problems with subtle distinctions in acuteness.

When plans have been constructed to meet patient care needs, goals and outcome criteria are necessary to determine progress toward achievement of desired results. Goals are simple, unifocal, stated in clear, concise terms, and indicate the desired result of nursing actions. Outcome criteria are specific measurable components of the goals and are stated in terms that can be objectively evaluated throughout implementation of patient care. When writing the goal and outcome criteria for each diagnosis, the two are written as one statement with the goal separated from outcome criteria with the phrase *as evidenced by.* For example, the diagnosis *ineffective airway clearance* related to retained thickened mucus has been identified for the patient with an upper respiratory infection. The goal for this patient is to achieve maximum airway clearance. Criteria needed for objective assessment of goal attainment include no adventitious breath sounds on auscultation, effective cough with expectoration of mucus, and respiratory rate of 12 to 20 breaths per minute. Appropriately written in the plan of care, the entire statement reads "*ineffective airway clearance* related to retained thickened mucus; goal/outcome criteria: The patient will achieve maximum airway clearance as evidenced by: no adventitious breath sounds on auscultation; effective cough with expectoration of mucus; and respiratory rate of 12 to 20 breaths per minute." This entire statement enables all nurses who care for this patient throughout the ED visit and subsequent hospitalization to evaluate goal achievement without the need for subjective interpretation. Avoid vague outcome criteria or stating outcome criteria in the form of a nursing intervention. For example, using the example above, stating "the patient will not experience shortness of breath" is subjective and open for judgment by each nurse participating in the patient's care. Shortness of breath is a subjective patient symptom and not easily verified by observation. Moreover, stating in the outcome criteria that "the patient will participate in deep breathing exercises" is not appropriate since this is an intervention and does not provide information about the patient's airway clearance. With these points in mind, the nurse can write a concise, accurate plan of care that can be utilized throughout the patient's hospital experience, thus providing continuity and ensuring quality patient care.

Planning does not end when the initial plan is formulated. Planning continues throughout the nurse-patient interaction. As interventions are implemented, continued planning is needed as the patient advances toward goal achievement. As new problems develop and old problems are solved, revi-

sions in the plan are necessary to provide continued, up-to-date care.

Implementation

The fourth step of the nursing process is implementation, which involves putting the plan into action. The nurse must possess a variety of psychomotor skills to carry out required interventions as well as a variety of psychosocial skills to meet the ED patient's emotional needs. The implementation phase of the nursing process includes actual nursing procedures and other patient interactions.

Evaluation

Although evaluation is the fifth and final step of the nursing process, it occurs throughout the nursing process. Progress toward goal achievement through effectiveness of interventions is evaluated. During this phase, it becomes apparent that carefully constructed goals and outcome criteria make the evaluation process more efficient. In the previous example, the goal was for the patient to achieve maximum airway clearance. Outcome criteria for this goal were no adventitious breath sounds on auscultation, effective cough with expectoration of mucus, and respiratory rate of 12 to 20 breaths per minute. As the nurse evaluates progress toward goal achievement, he or she notes some crackles in the upper lobes of both lungs, a productive cough, and a respiratory rate of 16 breaths per minute. With this objective information, the nurse can easily determine that the patient is progressing positively toward the goal of maximum airway clearance because two of the three outcome criteria are met. The nurse then evaluates which interventions were effective and should be continued and what interventions should be added to clear the crackles in the upper lobes.

To effectively carry out the evaluation process, the nurse must collect additional data, then determine which diagnoses are appropriate, which goals have been met, and if additional diagnoses are needed to meet newly discovered patient needs. Throughout the evaluation process the nursing diagnosis, goals, outcome criteria, interventions, and prioritized needs are evaluated and revised as necessary to provide effective patient care.

PUTTING THE NURSING PROCESS INTO ACTION

Nursing is a complex set of actions performed to meet a variety of patient care needs. With complex technologic advances in health care, the nurse is faced with multifaceted challenges that must be met to effectively provide care necessary to help restore and maintain health. Critical thinking skills are absolutely essential for putting the nursing process into action in the clinical setting. Critical thinking is differentiated from random thinking in that critical thinking is goal-oriented, scientifically based, and involves diagnostic reasoning. Collier, McCash, and Bartram[6] describe several important aspects necessary to make accurate clinical judgments.

Relevant information must be identified. The nurse must identify relevant information from assessment of a variety of sources. Data are categorized into critical clusters, then irrelevant data are eliminated. A good starting point for determining relevant data is the patient's chief complaint.

Alternative diagnoses must be considered. To avoid premature data closure and formulation of an incorrect diagnosis, the nurse must explore all possible diagnoses. Using data clusters, the nurse can rule out differential diagnoses and validate the presence of other diagnoses. If data clusters are inaccurate, the entire nursing process is built on an irrelevant nursing diagnosis and is ineffective in meeting patient care needs.

Accurate diagnoses must be formulated. Data cues collected during assessment must support the nursing diagnosis identified. When patient-reported data and objective data conflict, the nurse should obtain additional data to formulate an accurate diagnosis.

Individualized plans of care are developed. Although commonalities exist among data clusters, defining characteristics of the nursing diagnoses, and interventions to meet identified needs, the nurse must consider each patient individually. Each patient is unique; therefore a variety of interventions may be necessary to meet the same goals in different patients. The need to provide individualized care underscores the importance of including the patient in the plan of care.

Interventions must be timely. The emergency nurse must be able to make decisions rapidly and effectively. Priorities must be set and continual evaluation must occur throughout the process. Critical thinking skills enable the nurse to achieve a balance between speed and accuracy.

Care is continually evaluated. While providing care, nurses must make judgments about the effectiveness of the care. Through evaluation of goal achievement, the nurse can determine which interventions are effective and which ones should be revised. Careful assessment is the basis for effectively carrying out the nursing process. Implementation of creative interventions and constant evaluation of all activities help the nurse ensure the patient's needs are met.

The benefits of establishing a unified taxonomy for nursing affect the entire profession. Using nursing diagnoses in the clinical setting enhances and streamlines patient care planning. All phases must be worked through; however, the most important time related to development of the diagnostic statement is the diagnosis part of the process phase. A major consideration when developing the diagnostic statement is consistency. All diagnoses should be written uniformly for clarity and continuity. Several formats have been suggested to enhance uniformity. One such format called PES is based on problem, etiology, signs, and symptoms. Box 2-1 illustrates the PES format. Patient acuity levels are more readily evaluated when nursing diagnoses are written for each patient. Use of nursing diagnoses helps nursing service "parcel out" that which is uniquely nursing. This facili-

---

Box 2-1 PES Format for Nursing Diagnoses

Problem

Usually a diagnosis accepted by the North American Nursing Diagnosis Association (NANDA)

Behavior that can be improved through nursing assistance and intervention

Statement may have qualifying or quantifying adjectives to identify stages, phases, or levels of a problem, e.g., acute, chronic, mild, severe

An anatomic site may also be specified

The problem represents a state of the patient, not a nursing activity, e.g., write *"ineffective airway clearance,"* rather than "needs suctioning"

Etiology

This consists of physiologic, situational, and maturational factors that cause the problem or influence its development

The cause of the patient's problem influences the nursing action

Preceded by the phrase "related to" in a diagnostic statement

Signs and symptoms

Signs are objective

Symptoms are subjective

Used in a diagnostic statement to clarify and justify

May or may not be incorporated into the statement

---

tates "costing out" nursing services. Finally, a unified taxonomy aids computerized documentation of nursing services, which in turn assists with implementation of various health care services.

ISSUES SURROUNDING NURSING DIAGNOSIS

Hagey and McDonough[9] suggested the term *nursing diagnosis* conveys the erroneous message that nurses are primarily concerned with deviate or pathologic problems rather than promoting health and the patient's potential. Hagey and McDonough further postulated that nursing diagnoses may simplify and even obliterate the perception of the patient's importance while in the nurse's care. The authors were concerned the nurse might associate the patient with the diagnosis rather than the patient's holistic nature. Including the patient in planning care ensures the nurse's care remains patient centered.

Other authors such as Bircher[3] also weighed negative points associated with nursing diagnosis against positive aspects. Negative factors included lack of agreement about nursing diagnosis between clinicians, lack of appropriate labeling, lack of uniformity, vagueness of definition, misuse of diagnoses, premature labeling, and stereotyping of patients. On the positive side Bircher stated that nursing diagnosis is a convenient shorthand system, a guide for the nurse, easily remembered, and a ready point of reference for the clinician in daily interaction with the patient and family. Overall, Bircher's pros outweigh the cons.

Some confusion still surrounds the difference between medical and nursing diagnoses. Bockrath[4] differentiated the two by stating that unlike the medical diagnosis, which focuses on a disease process, nursing diagnosis focuses on a response to the problem. Unlike medical diagnoses, most nursing diagnoses change continually as the patient progresses through various stages of illness to health. Another unique characteristic of the nursing diagnosis is identification of potential health problems. Bockrath argued that nursing diagnosis documents what nursing is and does and therefore distinguishes nursing from any other profession.

Lash[10] also advocated the process by stating that nursing diagnosis is a route to accountability. Nurses have long been concerned about accountability. Recording nursing diagnoses should overcome the anonymity that has been a major obstacle to true accountability. Lash also stated that nursing started as a basically dependent profession, but eventually autonomy and independent decision making became major issues. Nursing diagnosis was viewed as a process that facilitates autonomy and independent decision making by providing deliberate analysis of functions, developing knowledge unique to nursing practice, and changing the nursing educational system to perpetuate autonomy.

Another issue affecting nursing diagnosis is the legal implications of making diagnoses. Fortin and Rabinow[7] cited two legal problems that could arise, the first being failure to diagnose. The case cited involved a nurse who failed to recognize cancerous skin changes in a postinjury patient. The court ruled the nurse should have been able to recognize and diagnose such a problem. The second major legal problem is misdiagnosis. The cited case involved nurses who diagnosed a young patient as being feverish; however, the child later died of congestive heart failure after an attack of rheumatic fever. The court ruled that the nurse(s) should have identified the symptoms and signs correctly. The author summarized by stating, "Nurses do not diagnose because the law demands it; they diagnose because their professional responsibilities cannot be met by doing anything less."[7]

Finally, Bruce and Snyder[5] stated that nurses have the legal right and responsibility to diagnose. They wrote that the process of nursing diagnosis has become a standard, especially with the legitimate position of nursing diagnosis in the ANA practice standards. Therefore the process is part of the care duties the nurse owes the patient. Failure to diagnose adequately and intervene appropriately constitutes a breach of duty to care.

FORMULATING NURSING DIAGNOSES

Differentiating medical diagnoses from nursing diagnoses is the first important guideline when writing a nursing diagnostic statement. The medical diagnosis labels the pathology present in each individual patient. Medical diagnosis is verified by the same means as the nursing diagnosis; however, the physician is specially trained and licensed to make the medical diagnoses. Nurses are not responsible for making a medical diagnosis unless they have additional education and function in the role of a nurse practitioner. Medical diagnoses are used to define the patient's hospitalization period and amount of insurance reimbursement through the use of diagnosis-related groups (DRGs). Medical diagnoses evolved over a period of 2 centuries and have been refined and validated. Consequently, nursing diagnoses are considered young in comparison and need to evolve further before they are placed in the same position of importance. Nonetheless, nursing diagnoses are an important part of the patient's plan of care and must be made accurately and appropriately. Medical diagnoses are not included as part of the diagnostic statement; however, the patient's response to the medical pathology is the focus of the nursing diagnosis. To illustrate, recall the patient described earlier who entered the ED with an upper respiratory infection. Production of copious amounts of secretions interfered with airway clearance. As a result, the nurse chose the diagnosis *ineffective airway clearance* related to retained thickened mucus. Using the statement "*ineffective airway clearance* related to upper respiratory infection" is not correct because the nurse's actions are not directed toward the upper respiratory infection. They are directed toward retained thickened mucus—the patient's response to the medical pathology. The nurse institutes measures to thin secretions, such as increasing fluid intake, providing a humidifier, and teaching the patient to effectively cough and deep breathe. In contrast, the physician focuses on the upper respiratory infection through the administration of antibiotics and antihistamines.

Another guideline to remember when constructing the diagnostic statement is to make diagnostic statements that are legally defensible. While the diagnosis itself is standard, the "related to" portion of the statement is individualized to the patient's needs. Consider the patient who has been bedridden for several days and presents to the ED with a stage III decubitus ulcer. The diagnosis of *impaired skin integrity* is established. The "related to" part of the diagnosis could read "related to lack of turning and appropriate skin care." By making this statement, the nurse is passing judgment on the caregiver and opens up the possibility of libel. It is more appropriate for the nurse to say "*impaired skin integrity* related to prolonged bed rest." The focus of care then shifts from blaming someone for negligent care to teaching the caregiver the appropriate way to care for the bedridden patient's skin. Other statements that may be legally inadvisable or judgmental include:

- *Fear* related to frequent beatings by husband
- *Ineffective family coping* related to mother-in-law's continual harassment of daughter-in-law
- *Risk for altered parenting* related to mother's low IQ
- *Noncompliance* related to failure to return for follow-up visits

Writing the diagnostic statement to include defining characteristics or diagnostic cues for the nursing diagnosis is also

Table **2-2**	**Concepts Often Confused With a Nursing Diagnosis**
Concept	Example
Medical diagnoses	Diabetes mellitus, asthma
Medical pathology	Decreased cerebral tissue oxygenation
Diagnostic studies	Cardiac function tests, catheterization
Goals	Patient shall perform own colostomy care
Patient needs	Patient needs to walk every shift
Nursing needs	Change dressing

Box **2-2**	**Dependence Domains of Nursing Practice**	
Independent domain	Interdependent domain	Dependent domain
NURSING DIAGNOSIS	**CLINICAL NURSING PROBLEM**	**MEDICAL PROBLEM OR DIAGNOSIS**
Range of motion	Levine tube	Swan-Ganz catheter
Maintenance of skin integrity	Egg-crate mattress	Fetal monitoring
Psychosocial intervention	Oxygen therapy	Medications
	Diet therapy	
Nurse		Physician

Table **2-3**	**Patient Scenarios for the Diagnostic Process**	
Patient description	Nursing diagnoses	Goal/outcome criteria
A 76-year-old man has a medical diagnosis of acute onset congestive heart failure, moderate to severe. Initial assessment reveals bilateral rales and rhonchi, tachypnea, cough with frothy secretions, slight cyanosis, dyspnea, anxiety, confusion, restlessness, coated tongue, and oral plaque.	Ineffective airway clearance related to increased pulmonary secretions	The patient will exhibit increased airway clearance as evidenced by absence of adventitious breath sounds on auscultation, respiratory rate of 12 to 20 breaths per minute, and arterial blood gases within normal limits
	Altered oral mucous membranes related to administration of oxygen by face mask	The patient shows improvement in oral mucous membrane integrity as evidenced by intact oral membranes, verbalization of no pain in mouth, and lack of malodorous breath
A 15-year-old female is brought to the ED within 1 hour of sexual assault. She is apprehensive, fearful, and shaken. Poor eye contact and extraneous movements of her extremities are noted. Parents are unable to meet her emotional needs. She seems humiliated and engages in self-blame.	Anxiety related to fear of further injury	The patient will show reduced anxiety as evidenced by verbalization that she feels safe in her home or the hospital, discussing the rape experience without panic, stating two coping mechanisms she is willing to try, and participating in activities outside the home
	Pain related to physical injury sustained during the attack	The patient will experience a reduction in pain as evidenced by verbalization that the pain is reduced, vital signs within normal limits, and participation in activities of daily living
	Altered family processes related to withdrawal from the family unit	The patient will display more effective family relationships as evidenced by participation in family activities and talking with one or more family members about the rape experience in a functional way

inappropriate when constructing the diagnostic statement. Remember the patient who presented to the emergency department with the upper respiratory infection. The diagnosis of *ineffective airway clearance* was chosen. If the nurse continued the statement with "related to crackles and wheezes on auscultation," the nurse has not provided direction for focus-ing the care of this patient. Crackles and wheezes are signs of ineffective airway clearance and do not provide insight as to why the patient is having respiratory difficulty.

Another common error in writing the diagnostic statement is using therapeutic nursing interventions in the diagnostic statement rather than the cause of the patient's problem. Consider again the patient with the diagnosis *ineffective airway clearance*. Completing the diagnostic statement by saying "related to lack of suctioning" is inappropriate because this is a nursing intervention. Inclusion of two diagnoses in the same diagnostic statement is also inappropriate. The diagnosis *ineffective airway clearance* related to *ineffective breathing pattern* is confusing because the nurse does not know which diagnosis has priority. Also, no direction is given if an etiology is not stated.

Frequently, statement errors are made because the nurse tries to address problems located in the interdependent and dependent domains of nursing practice. These areas require intervention from someone other than the nurse, so nursing diagnoses cannot be made. Basically, three dependence domains exist in nursing. These domains are located on a continuum and are identified in Box 2-2. Consideration of these dependence domains illustrates the complexities of nursing care and may cause confusion for the inexperienced practitioner, who may erroneously identify medical diagnoses, medical pathology, and other concepts for nursing diagnosis. Table 2-2 presents concepts and examples of the concepts that are often confused with nursing diagnoses.

With a good understanding of information presented in this section, the nurse is now prepared to make diagnostic statements for patients in the real world. Patient scenarios presented in Table 2-3 show how the process can be applied to the clinical setting. Examples should serve as a guide for ED utilization of the nursing process. The examples are in no way meant to imply that the diagnoses listed are priority diagnoses for these patients or that these are the only diagnoses needed for these patients. Each patient situation should be treated individually since many other diagnoses are possible for patients presenting with similar problems.

SUMMARY

The nursing process is a valuable clinical tool for the nurse. Formulation of nursing diagnoses can assist nurses in providing uniform, consistent, and efficient care because the language is understood by all nurses. From the first mention of nursing diagnosis in the 1950s to the establishment of nursing diagnosis as the second step in the nursing process in 1980, nursing diagnosis has been surrounded by controversy. However, clinical validation mechanisms have made

nursing diagnosis more widely accepted as part of the language of nursing. Consistent use of nursing diagnoses is necessary for further development of nursing as a profession with its own unique body of knowledge and as a means of communicating to other members of the health care team that which is uniquely nursing.

The ED often serves as the patient entry point into the health care system. The emergency nurse's accurate and efficient use of the nursing process is vital to ensure continuity in concert with quality patient care. Emergency nurses require a vast repertoire of highly specialized skills and knowledge to meet the challenges they face when caring for their patients. Refinement of these skills should continue throughout the nurse's career. Growth and maturity are vital for the emergency nurse to meet the demands of this fast-paced arena of nursing.

REFERENCES

1. American Nurses Association: *Standards of nursing practice,* Kansas City, 1973, The Association.
2. American Nurses Association: *Standards of nursing practice,* Kansas City, 1980, The Association.
3. Bircher A: On the development and classification of nursing diagnosis, *Nurs Forum* 14(1):10, 1975.
4. Bockrath M: Your patient needs two diagnoses: medical and nursing, *Nurs Life* 2(2):29, 1982.
5. Bruce J, Snyder M: The right and responsibility to diagnose, *Am J Nurs* 82(4):645, 1982.
6. Collier I, McCash K, Bartram J: *Writing nursing diagnoses,* St. Louis, 1996, Mosby.
7. Fortin J, Rabinow J: Legal implications of nursing diagnosis, *Nurs Clin North Am* 14(3):553, 1979.
8. Gordon M: Nursing diagnosis and the diagnostic process, *Am J Nurs* 76(8):1298, 1976.
9. Hagey R, McDonough P: The problem of professional labeling, *Nurs Outlook* 32(3):151, 1984.
10. Lash A: A re-examination of nursing diagnosis, *Nurs Forum* 17(4):333, 1978.
11. Yura H, Walsh M: *The nursing process: assessing, planning, implementing, and evaluating,* ed 3, Norwalk, Conn, 1978, Appleton-Century-Crofts.

SUGGESTED READING

Aspinall M: Nursing diagnosis: the weak link, *Nurs Outlook* 24(7):433, 1976.
Guzzetta C, Dossey B: Nursing diagnosis, *Heart Lung* 12(3):282, 1983.

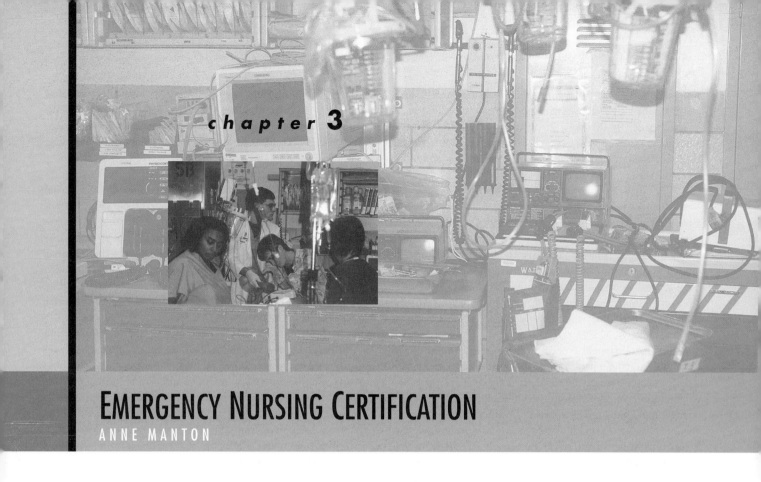

chapter 3

EMERGENCY NURSING CERTIFICATION

ANNE MANTON

The opportunity for certification in a nursing specialty dates back to 1945, when certification was first initiated by the American Association of Nurse Anesthetists. Most certifications in nursing, however, were established in the last 2 decades. Increase in the number of nursing specialty organizations has been a major factor in proliferation of nursing certifications. More than 40 certifications are available. Most specialty organizations offer only one certification; however, the American Nurses Association (ANA) offers at least 26 certifications.

OVERVIEW

What is the purpose of certification? Why do nurses participate in this process? The primary purpose of certification, whether in nursing or another discipline, is to assure the public that an individual has acquired a specific body of knowledge. Certification thus benefits both the individual nurse and the employer and also serves the public interest.

In addition to providing the public with information, certification in a nursing specialty benefits the nurse who attains certification. It provides a mechanism by which the nurse can demonstrate mastery of a specific body of knowledge. Achieving certification may also lead to greater respect from employers and colleagues, salary increases, and perhaps most important, greater self-esteem.

Employers and potential employers also benefit from nursing certification. Certification provides an objective measure of an employee's knowledge base as well as valuable information about prospective employees.

The nursing profession also benefits from certification. Because of the certification process, bodies of specialty nursing knowledge are defined and examined; certification demonstrates to other health care disciplines that nurses are able to articulate their defined body of knowledge and establish levels of specialty competence based on that knowledge.

Another way in which certification benefits nursing is through preparation for the certification examination. Certification requires thorough study of the body of knowledge of the specialty. Certification renewal encourages the practicing nurse to remain current in all aspects of specialty nursing practice.

A nurse can obtain certification in three ways. One way is certification by a state or government agency. State certification resembles a legal endorsement of a nurse's ability to function in certain expanded nursing roles. This process is different from that by which a nurse becomes registered. Certification by a state usually refers to a specific aspect of nursing practice that is beyond the level addressed in a state board examination for registration. State certification is often based on prior certification by a nurse certification body, completion of an education program, or both. In some instances, a certifying examination is administered by a state agency. Requirements for state certification vary; therefore, certification by one state may not be recognized by another.

State certification has advantages and disadvantages. Among the advantages are public recognition of specialty nursing and expanded roles in nursing practice. Perhaps most important, state certification allows the state to exercise control over those who perform in specialty or expanded roles. In this way the public is better protected from persons not competent to practice in specialty roles.

Disadvantages of state certification include additional responsibilities placed on state boards of nursing, which are usually already overburdened. The effects on other aspects of a board's responsibilities, be they neglect or delay, must be carefully considered. Another possible disadvantage is that regulations may be so narrowly interpreted they restrict dimensions of usual nursing practice. Perhaps the most obvious and ominous disadvantage is that when practice issues are placed in so public a domain, the door is opened for powerful lobbying groups (e.g., third-party payers, medical societies, and other care providers) to influence nursing practice.

Certification can also occur through an institution. The institution may be a health care facility or an educational system. This type of certification is usually based on successful completion of an educational offering, often varying in length and characteristics. Most often the state or profession does not control content or requisites for such certification. This type of certification has limited appeal outside the particular certifying institution, because consumers and professionals alike seem to value academic degrees or certifications based on national standards more highly. Some local triage, trauma nursing, or mobile intensive care nursing certifications are examples of this type of certification.

The usual way to obtain certification in a nursing specialty is through a professional organization. Many types of certifications are offered by the ANA. Most nursing practice specialty organizations have also developed, or are in the process of developing, a certification process in their specialty. These efforts are testimony to the belief that knowledge beyond the level of safe basic nursing practice is required for specialty nursing practice.

Although mechanisms for certification vary from one specialty to another, certification granted by a specialty organization is nationally and internationally recognized. Certification associated with a specialty nursing organization is also more relevant to that specialty's nursing practice and defined body of knowledge.

SPECIALTY CERTIFICATION

Many nursing organizations have various requirements for certification and renewal of certification. Requirements for nursing specialty certification fall into the following categories: education, practice, demonstration of knowledge, and renewal mechanisms.

All nursing specialty certification organizations require that candidates be registered nurses. This requirement assumes successful completion of the state board examination of nursing (NCLEX). Some specialties require or are considering requiring a bachelor's degree as the minimum for certification eligibility. Completion of a master's degree is a requirement for eligibility for some ANA advanced practice certification examinations. The ANA and other certifying organizations also require specific courses and clinical experiences for certifications such as nurse practitioner and nurse midwife.

Some certifications have practice requirements in addition to educational requirements. To be eligible to take the certification examination, the nurse must have spent a minimum number of hours in specialty practice. Often the practice component of the certification process is a strong recommendation, rather than an absolute requirement. It has been demonstrated that nurses with at least 2 years practice in a specialty are more likely to achieve a passing score on the certification examination than those with less practice time in the specialty.

All nursing specialty certifications require the applicant for certification to demonstrate mastery of the body of specialty nursing knowledge by written examination. Certification examinations vary in length and format, but all are sufficient, according to the experts within the specialty, to broadly examine the applicant's knowledge base in the specialty. Written examinations provide the most objective measure of mastery of core knowledge of the specialty. Practical or psychomotor examinations measure attainment of requisite knowledge, however, most certifying agencies find these examinations too cumbersome to conduct with the consistency, objectivity, and integrity necessary for the examination process.

The final component of the certification process that all nursing specialty certification agencies have in common is renewal of certification. In almost all instances, certification is granted for a limited time, usually 3 to 5 years. This finite period of certification recognizes the dynamic, always changing and evolving state of nursing knowledge. Thus the certified nurse's continued mastery of the knowledge base of the specialty must be verified at regular intervals. The mechanism by which certification is renewed varies with the certifying body. Many opt to require candidates to retake the examination, whereas others choose mandatory continuing education hours. Regardless of the method used, the purpose of recertification is to ensure competence. Weisfeld and Falk stated that "with the half-life of medical knowledge usually estimated at 5 years, and the pace of obsolescence even faster in some allied occupations, little justification can be found for requiring a demonstration of initial competence, while ignoring the need for continuing competence."[3]

EMERGENCY NURSING CERTIFICATION

The first emergency nursing certification examination was administered in July 1980 and the examination has been offered each July and February since that time. Originally, answers to all 250 questions of the examination were calculated into the score, and the number of correct answers necessary for a passing score and certification was consistent at 175. Since 1980, the certification examination has evolved into a more sophisticated measure of emergency nursing knowledge. All question-and-answer sets are now pretested on an exam for accuracy, clarity, and reliability prior to inclusion among those questions that determine the passing score. Currently each examination contains 50 pretest items and 200 items that are scored.

Because the degree of difficulty for each question is determined in advance through pretesting, each new version of the examination is weighted accordingly. Therefore the number of correct answers necessary for a passing score and certification varies slightly with each new examination. Because of this weighting procedure, there is no advantage in taking one examination over another.

Examination Content for Certification in Emergency Nursing

To ensure the certification examination reflects current emergency nursing practice, two role delineation studies (RDS) have been completed by the Board of Certification for Emergency Nursing (BCEN). The first RDS was conducted in 1989-1990. Analysis of that study's findings indicated considerable concurrence between content of the emergency nursing certification examination and emergency nursing practice. Changes were made so the examination closely reflects information from the RDS. A second RDS in 1994 found a high degree of consistency between emergency nursing practice and certification examination content.

Minor adjustments to the content blueprint for the certification examination have been made as a result of practice changes reflected in the analysis of responses to the latest RDS. The blueprint for the examination is two dimensional. One dimension, the areas of clinical practice, is summarized in Table 3-1. The other dimension, components of the nursing process, is summarized in Table 3-2. The certification examination is constructed according to percentages found in both these tables.

Certification Renewal

Certification in emergency nursing is granted for 4 years. Initial certification can only be accomplished by successfully passing the certification examination. Effective as of the February 1992 examination, recertification can be accomplished by reexamination or by a renewal option (CEN-RO) that includes a self-assessment test and continuing education. The renewal option **cannot** be used for two consecutive renewals. For example, a nurse who certified by testing in 1992 and exercised the renewal option for certification in 1996, must pass the certification examination in 2000 to remain a certified emergency nurse (CEN). The renewal option could be used again in 2004. Certified emergency nurses have the option to renew certification every 4 years by formal testing.

The CEN-RO program. Two important steps are required for renewal of emergency nursing certification with the CEN-RO program. The first step is completion of a self-assessment test. Approximately 2 years after initial certification, self-assessment tests are mailed automatically to all CENs several months prior to the deadline for completion. If the certified nurse chooses the CEN-RO program, a self-assessment test must be completed and returned to the testing company with the appropriate fee by the designated deadline. Deadline for completion of the self-assessment test varies according to when the certification examination was last taken. The date can be found on the individual's score report from his or her most recent CEN examination and with materials sent with the self-assessment test. Because deadlines are strictly adhered to, any questions concerning deadlines should be addressed to the BCEN.

Table **3-1**	**Content Areas by Percentage of Examination**		
Clinical practice areas			
Percentage	Content area	Percentage	Content area
5%	Abdominal Emergencies	2.5%	Ocular Emergencies
9%	Cardiovascular Emergencies	6%	Orthopedic Emergencies
2%	Emergency Operations Preparedness	9%	Patient Care Management
4%	Environmental Emergencies	9%	Respiratory Emergencies
4%	Genitourinary and Gynecologic Emergencies	7%	Shock and Multisystem Trauma Emergencies
3%	Maxillofacial Emergencies	6%	Substance Abuse and Toxicology Emergencies
8%	Medical Emergencies and Communicable Diseases	4%	Wound Management
4.5%	Mental Health Emergencies	2%	Stabilization and Transfer
7%	Neurologic Emergencies	1.5%	Patient and Community Education
2.5%	Obstetric Emergencies		
Professional issues			
2%	Legal	2%	Organizational Issues

From Newberry L, Barnason S, Carlson K et al: *CEN review manual*, ed 2, Park Ridge, Ill, 1996, Emergency Nurses Association.

Table **3-2**	**Nursing Process Classification by Percentage of Test Questions**
Percentage	Clinical practice area
32%	Assessment
16%	Analysis/Nursing Diagnosis
32%	Planning/Intervention
16%	Evaluation

From Newberry L, Barnason S, Carlson K et al: *CEN review manual*, ed 2, Park Ridge, Ill, 1996, Emergency Nurses Association.

The certified emergency nurse may choose not to renew emergency nursing certification using the CEN-RO program. In that case, the self-assessment test is disregarded and the nurse registers at the appropriate time to take the certification examination.

The second step in the CEN-RO program is obtaining 100 hours of continuing education credit. An accurate record of continuing education credit (CE Log) must be maintained and submitted for review with application and appropriate fee by the CE Log filing deadline. Of 100 continuing education credit hours, **at least** 75 of those credit hours must be in the *clinical* category, with up to 25 credits from the *other* category.

According to the BCEN, the *clinical* category for continuing education credits "includes any educational offerings that primarily contain information applicable to direct nursing practice in the clinical area. The program content must be primarily focused on the knowledge the nurse can apply in providing direct care. . ."[1]

The *other* category "includes any educational offerings related to the professional practice of nursing and the emergency care system."[1] It is the responsibility of the CEN seeking renewal of certification to ensure appropriate categorization of continuing education on the CEN-RO continuing education filing log. Questions about *clinical* versus *other* categorization should be addressed to the BCEN. Candidates should do this well in advance of their filing deadline. Materials received after the postmark deadline will be returned unprocessed. Of those materials received on time, a randomly selected number of CE Logs are selected for verification. Those selected submit documentation of all continuing education activities reflected on the log, including course materials, objectives, outlines, and certificates received. Failure to meet verification requirements of the CEN-RO program means the individuals must take and pass the CEN examination to maintain their CEN credential.

TESTING

Testing provokes anxiety in virtually everyone. It is impressive, then, that to become certified, so many nurses choose to place themselves in this situation. The number of certified nurses is a testament to the confidence nurses have in their mastery of the specialty knowledge base and to their high level of professionalism. Not surprisingly, however, many nurses resist being tested to renew their certification.

Anxiety in the testing situation is normal. Uneasiness and anxiety occur because of the significance we and others attach to our success or failure on examinations. Although a certain amount of test anxiety is normal and may even be helpful, such anxiety must be controlled. Uncontrolled test anxiety can interfere with the ability to think clearly and demonstrate knowledge effectively. The following strategies may help nurses reduce that uncomfortable feeling of anxiety.

Foremost among strategies to reduce anxiety is to prepare for the examination. Confidence in your knowledge base and your ability to respond correctly to a broad variety of questions is essential.

Developing a Study Plan

To study well, you must first determine your strengths and weaknesses in the material to be tested. Recognize that everyone has weaknesses. Once you identify your particular weaknesses, you can rectify them.

In preparing for the CEN examination, the next step is review of the content outline for the examination, described in the *Certification Examination for Emergency Nurses Handbook for Candidates.*[2] With the content outline in mind, focus on identification of your specific areas of strength and weakness. Review the *Emergency Nursing Core Curriculum* or another comprehensive emergency nursing text. As you survey each chapter, ask yourself whether you could answer questions related to that content area. Be honest with yourself. Armed with your self-assessment knowledge, look once again at the CEN examination content outline. Your studying priorities should be a combination of your relative strength or weakness in the content area and its importance, that is, percentage of questions, in the examination.

Creating a list of priorities with time lines for your study plan may be helpful. Areas of your greatest perceived weakness that are also of high importance in the examination should be studied first. Areas of increasing strength of knowledge, areas of decreasing importance in the examination, or a combination of these, should then be studied. The last content areas to be studied should be those in which your knowledge base is strong or those in which content importance in the examination is slight. When designing a successful study plan consider two components. The first consideration is that studying should occur over a period of months, not weeks or days. *Cramming does not lead to success.* The other component is that some time should be left at the conclusion of your study for a review. If you have followed the study plan and prepared well, review may not be necessary; however, reviewing during the week before the examination may increase your self-confidence, an important element of success in most endeavors.

Remember, developing a study plan is vital to your success in testing. Failing to plan may mean planning to fail.

Study Techniques

Studying from a book is different from reading a novel, the purpose is different and so is the method. Professional literature includes advice on successful strategies for studying. One common suggestion is to conduct a preliminary survey of the section to be studied. This survey includes a brief preview of the introductory paragraph, headings, definitions, rules, and summary paragraph to identify core ideas. Another suggestion in many books and articles is to develop questions related to the material being studied. Some experts suggest reading the material for ideas and questions after conducting the survey. Others suggest that, once core ideas have been identified through the preliminary survey, the learner should construct questions appropriate to the content area and proceed with reading to answer the questions. Whether you read first then formulate questions to be answered in a self-review or generate questions to be answered in subsequent reading of the content, formulation of questions is essential to studying. Although generating questions may seem to consume valuable time, asking and answering questions makes the content meaningful and, therefore, easily retained. When studying for the CEN examination, relate questions to the nursing process— 96% of the examination is nursing-process based. Box 3-1 provides examples of questions that might be formulated.

As you read each section, concentrate on the content and give attention to ideas and concepts rather than words alone. Conceptualize rather than attempt to memorize. Know and understand basic principles, and reflect on their application as you study various sections. Many principles apply in a variety of instances, for example, airway, breathing, and circulation (ABCs). Keeping these principles in mind as you study each section makes answering those questions about the nursing process easier. Significance of an assessment finding or the value of a particular intervention becomes evident as a point of logic, not as something to be recalled from memory alone.

After in-depth, concentrated reading of each section, attempt to answer questions about that section. This self-questioning often reveals areas for further review. Another strategy is use of a book such as the *CEN Review Manual* published by the Emergency Nurses Association. Use review questions in the book as a self-assessment aid after studying a particular clinical area. The 1996 edition also includes a 250-question test that can be taken to simulate the testing environment. There are a number of comparable texts available that can also serve as adjuncts for test preparation. If self-questioning identifies areas of knowledge deficits, reread those sections in the *Emergency Nursing Core Curriculum* or another emergency nursing text until understanding and recollection are achieved.

Develop "thinking skills" as you study. Establish frameworks or categories for the information rather than attempting to memorize details or isolated facts. For example, think of the actions of various drug classifications and when they would be useful rather than when they might be harmful. Rather than memorizing information about laboratory tests, think about what the abnormal values tell you about the patient. Box 3-2 contains more suggestions for effective use of texts and other study aids.

Organizing and implementing a study plan is a matter of individual study style. Some prefer to study alone at an individual pace, while others find studying in groups more beneficial because discussion can generate and answer questions, identify larger issues and principles, and facilitate understanding. To make a study group successful, some guidelines should be considered. It is important to develop a plan and structure to which all group members can agree. Each member should have a role, or responsibility, in presentation and discussion of topics. Allow time for socializing, preferably at the conclusion of each planned topical discussion. When socializing is not planned, members often use study time for this purpose. Be selective about group membership

---

Box **3-1**	**Potential Questions Related to the Nursing Process**

How is _____ related to _____ ?
What do I look for in assessment of _____ ?
What information leads me to conclude the problem is _____ _____ ?
If I see _____ in the presence of _____ , what does this tell me?
What is the most appropriate treatment for _____ ? Why?
How do I know the situation is improving? Deteriorating?

Box **3-2**	**Suggestions for Effective Use of Texts and Study Aids**

Look for clues that suggest a larger meaning, i.e., principle.
Pay close attention to diagrams, graphs, tables, and illustrations. They often summarize an important concept or idea.
Look for sentences in boldface or italics. Look closely at all sequences of numbered items.
Look for patterns of relationships. Don't just look at the trees— remember the forest!
Reduce subject matter to easily remembered divisions such as the nursing process.

and the size of the group. Remember that study groups can be an effective way to prepare for the certification examination or they can waste valuable time.

Another effective study technique is use of audio tapes. Audio tapes are flexible—you can listen in the car, on the beach, or in the health club. Audio tapes appeal more to the person who studies alone or who learns more with repetition. Selection of a specific study technique is dependent on your specific knowledge. If you have a limited knowledge base, review of texts and development of study aids may be the most effective study technique. As you gain experience, question-and-answer books may be more beneficial. Regardless of how you study, use a technique that meets your needs and your existing knowledge base.

Test-Taking Strategies

Perhaps the most influential factor in successful test taking is attitude. It is possible to thoroughly know the test material yet fail an examination because of poor attitude. Fear conditions the mind for failure. Fear and anxiety can cause tension and inability to think clearly. Fear can so overwhelm thought processes that what was known only moments before can no longer be recalled. The ability to think logically, solve problems, and determine relationship or associations can be greatly reduced because of fear. Fear can cause careless mistakes. It is imperative to address fear and determine strategies to manage it before taking a test. Test taking involves skill. The test taker must develop a positive attitude toward his or her ability to master this skill.

The person with a successful attitude anticipates the examination as an opportunity to demonstrate what he or she knows, not a negative situation with potential for failure. The attitude of challenge rather than defeat leads to constructive preparation, which in turn leads to increased self-confidence and a positive attitude toward the anticipated outcome of the examination.

Even well-prepared test takers experience some anxiety; therefore well-internalized test-taking strategies are most helpful. It may be beneficial, especially for poor test takers, to practice these skills on sample test questions. The CEN handbook for candidates includes a number of such practice questions, as does the computer software and review manual available from the ENA.

When it comes time to actually take the examination, remember that extreme fear and anxiety can influence even the

---

Box 3-3   General Test-Taking Tips

There is no penalty on the CEN examination for incorrect responses. Your computed score is based only on the number of correct responses. Answer every question, even if you have to guess.

Once you decide on an answer, don't change it without good reason. Your first response is likely to be the correct one. The temptation to change an answer is often caused by reading too much into the question or thinking of the unusual rather than the usual.

You should answer 65 to 70 questions per hour to complete the examination in approximately 4 hours. Check periodically to make sure you are using your time effectively. Don't be distracted by those who finish quickly. Speed is not an indicator of expertise. Take the time to read the questions carefully and answer them correctly.

Every 15 to 20 questions, check to make sure the number on the answer sheet corresponds to the question number on the examination. You don't want to discover you are out of sequence once the examination is completed.

After completing the answer sheet, check the entire sheet once more. Make sure each answer space has been filled. If you deferred questions, make sure these are finished.

Box 3-4   Tips for Answering the Examination Questions

Read the stem of each question carefully. Observe qualifying terms such as always, never, most, usually, not, except, first, initial, primary, next, best, most important, highest, lowest, least, and contraindicated. These words tell you what the question is really asking.

After reading the stem, formulate an answer before looking at your choices. When you think you know the answer, look to see if it is one of your choices. If not, reread the stem. Did you misinterpret what was asked? Is there a choice similar to yours with different terminology? If you are still not sure, rule out any choices you know are incorrect.

When the content is unfamiliar, think of general principles such as the ABCs or the nursing process to choose an answer or eliminate a choice. Think of answers with content that is therapeutic, ensures patient safety, promotes comfort, demonstrates respect, and communicates acceptance. Eliminate responses that are bizarre, hostile, inappropriate, or punitive. Look for terminology in the stem compatible with or suggestive of one particular option.

If the content is familiar but you don't consider any of the choices correct, don't get flustered. Reread the stem to make sure you correctly interpreted the question, then select the best choice, even if it is not the answer you prefer.

Don't skip randomly through the questions. Answer the questions sequentially. If you don't know the answer, go to the next question. Mark the question lightly in the margin of the answer sheet.

Don't read too much into the question. Don't make assumptions about information that is not given. Use only the information provided in the stem of the question. Think in terms of the usual, not the unusual.

If a choice contains a totally unfamiliar term, try to decipher its meaning by considering its roots. If the word remains a mystery, the response is probably incorrect. A totally unfamiliar term is not likely to be part of an idea that is being tested. Unfamiliar terms are often distractors, so don't be fooled.

most basic test activities. Pay attention to the instructions and follow them carefully. This often helps the test taker overcome initial nervousness. Box 3-3 discusses general test-taking tips relative to the CEN examination, whereas Box 3-4 provides specific tips for answering the examination questions. Throughout the examination, control your fear and anxiety. Periodically stretch and take breaths. It may be helpful to remind yourself that 50 questions are pretest questions and do not count toward your final score. Above all, believe in yourself and your ability to successfully pass the CEN examination or any other examination!

SUMMARY

Certification is a relatively new process in nursing. Issues related to certification concern not only emergency nursing, but all specialty nursing certification. These include educational requirements, practice requirements, certification period, renewal mechanisms, advanced certification options, costs, examination validity and reliability, potential liability, and recognition by professional colleagues and the public. The Board of Certification for Emergency Nursing (BCEN) has addressed many of these issues as they relate to the CEN exam. Validity and reliability are analyzed for each exam. The test blueprint is revised when appropriate to ensure accuracy of the content areas. Renewal options have been expanded to include a continuing education track. The BCEN is also exploring avenues for resolution of complaints.

The future of emergency nursing certification is truly promising. Certification may soon be available through a computerized testing medium. The number of new CENs and the number of CENs who renew their certification continues to increase. Certification is a significant professional accomplishment that benefits the profession, the patient, and the public.

REFERENCES

1. Board of Certification for Emergency Nursing: *CEN renewal option CEN-RO program,* Chicago, 1995, BCEN.
2. Board of Certification for Emergency Nursing: *International certification examination for emergency nurses candidate handbook 1996 examinations,* Chicago, 1996, BCEN.
3. Newberry L, Barnason S, Carlson K et al: *CEN review manual,* ed 2, Park Ridge, Ill, 1996, Emergency Nurses Association.
4. Weisfeld N, Falk D: Chasing elusive competence, *Hospitals* 57(5):68, 1983.

SUGGESTED READING

Collins HL: Certification: is the payoff worth the price? *RN* 50(7):36, 1987.
Dickenson-Hazard N: The importance of recertification, *Pediatr Nurs* 14(2):137, 1988.
Knapp JE: Assuring continuing competency: a snapshot of current practice, *Spec Nurs Forum* 2(3):1, 1990.
Kortbawi PA: Test taking skills: giving yourself an edge, *Nurs '90* 20(6):95, 1990.
Sides MB, Korchek N: *Nurses guide to successful test-taking,* ed 2, Philadelphia, 1994, JB Lippincott.

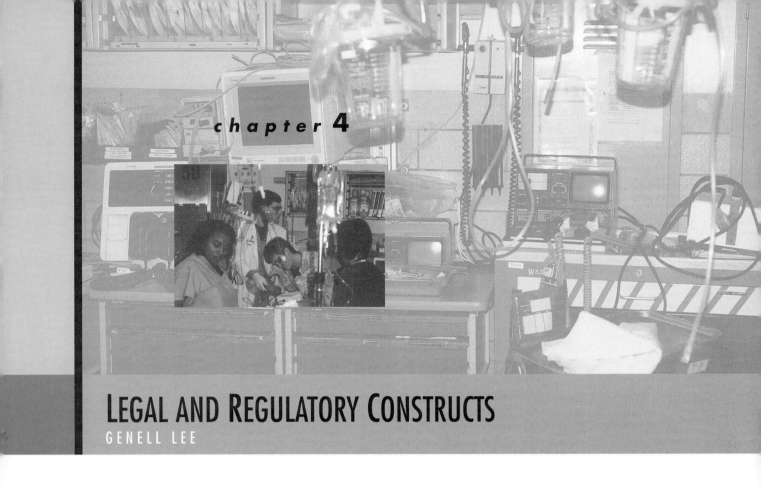

chapter **4**

LEGAL AND REGULATORY CONSTRUCTS

GENELL LEE

Emergency nursing is a complex blend of skill, experience, knowledge, and personality. In no other area of nursing is a nurse expected to know "cradle-to-grave" information about the pathophysiology of disease, the latest technologic innovations in monitoring and treatment devices, and when to contact the police or health department, all while being a patient and family advocate. The emergency department (ED) is like a minihospital, often seeing more patients per year than there are patient days on the hospital's inpatient side. The number of regulations and laws that affect emergency nursing practice is phenomenal. This chapter provides a snapshot of legal and regulatory constructs that affect the ED most. Examples of case law, statutes, and regulations are provided for illustration only, not as the definitive word on a particular situation. Hospital legal counsel should be consulted for specific concerns. Discussion covers sources of law, medical records, consent to and refusal of treatment, the Emergency Medical Treatment and Active Labor Act (EMTALA),[5] managed care, preservation and collection of evidence, and mental health issues.

SOURCES OF LAW AND REGULATION

The U.S. Constitution is the supreme law. Through the Bill of Rights, the Constitution guarantees certain individual rights that affect care in the ED. The free exercise clause of the First Amendment affects refusal of care for religious reasons, whereas the free speech clause supports employee or patient statements about care. Right to privacy is not explicitly stated in the Constitution, but has been interpreted by

the courts to encompass the right to refuse medical care. Protection against search and seizure and rights of criminal defendants indirectly affect the ED when law enforcement officers request collection of evidence. The emergency nurse is not expected to be a constitutional expert, but should remember an individual entering the ED brings all his or her individual rights and constitutional protections. Table 4-1 summarizes sources of law and regulation.

Congress is designated by the Constitution to make laws. At the state level, each state's constitution designates the state legislature as the source of state laws. A law passed by Congress or a state legislature is a statute. If a statute directly conflicts with a constitutional principle, the courts strike down the statute as unconstitutional. One example of a federal statute is EMTALA. Examples of state statutes are consent laws and licensure of medical professionals.

The Executive Branch of federal and state government enforces laws through various administrative agencies that develop rules or regulations to enforce applicable statutes. Agencies such as the Occupational Safety and Health Administration (OSHA) can enforce regulations through inspections, fines, and other procedures allowed by law. One example of a regulation established by OSHA is the occupational exposure to blood-borne pathogens regulation, which requires universal precautions if exposure to blood or body fluids is possible.[1]

The Judicial Branch interprets the law and develops common law or judge-made law as cases are decided. Various legal analyses are used by the Judicial Branch to interpret fed-

Table **4-1**   **Sources of Law and Regulation**

Type of law	Source or origin	Content or focus	Examples
Supreme Law	Constitution	Individual rights	Right to free speech Freedom of religious expression Right to privacy
Statute	Congress or state legislature	Focus varies, but cannot conflict with the Constitution	Consent laws Licensure of medical professionals Reportable events and conditions
Common Law	Judicial Branch	Judge-made laws that change as society and its laws change	Abortion laws Drunk driving laws
Regulations	Executive Branch of federal and state government	Enforce federal and state laws	Occupational Safety and Health Administration (OSHA)

eral and state laws. Common law develops over centuries and changes as society and laws change.

MEDICAL RECORDS

The requirement to maintain medical records on patients treated in the ED comes from state licensure statutes, Joint Commission on Accreditation of Healthcare Organizations (JCAHO) standards, and federal and state regulations.[34] The hospital usually retains the right to control the record, but patients generally have rights to information in the record.[40] Release of information without consent from the patient can lead to criminal and civil liability in some circumstances. Confidentiality of medical records may be covered by institutional policy, state statute, or federal law. Sensitive areas, often specified in state or federal law, include alcohol and drug treatment, mental health, acquired immunodeficiency syndrome (AIDS), and the patient's HIV status. In the absence of a legal or regulatory obligation, a moral or ethical obligation to protect the patient's privacy may exist.[33]

Computerization of medical records raises many sensitive issues. Entry of all or part of the medical record into a hospital information system (HIS) raises questions of control and access. Systems and personnel security usually limit access to authorized persons.[34] User passwords with differing levels of secured access are the minimum controls in most computerized systems. Developing technology should enhance measures to secure medical record confidentiality. In addition to computerization, transmission of medical information over modems, facsimile (fax) machines, and internal computer networks raises further issues of system and personnel security. The risk of violating patient confidentiality is greater when the communication tool uses public channels. Existing security measures include user verification, retaining transmitted data, and incorporating a confidentiality statement on the fax cover sheet.[5] Current technology allows the sender to verify the telephone number where the fax was received.

The documentation system for the medical record is important, but does not surpass the need to make entries legible, coherent, accurate, and complete. Narrative notes,

Box **4-1**   **Medical Record Documentation**

Write legibly. Use correct spelling and acceptable medical abbreviations.

Do not leave blank lines. They create the impression you will return later and fill in information.

Identify all medical personnel who care for the patient by title and a legible signature.

Document in chronologic order and as contemporaneously as possible.

Correct errors by drawing a line through the error then initialing it. Write *error, incorrect entry,* or *void* above the error. Never use correction fluid to cover errors.

Use late entries to complete documentation, never in contemplation of litigation. Identify late entries in the medical record.

Obtain physician signature on verbal orders to verify the order and its accuracy.

checklists, SOAP notes, or charting by exception are accepted methods of documentation. Box 4-1 summarizes essential rules for medical record documentation. A signature identifies the person providing care and ensures authenticity in a legal proceeding. A rubber stamp, written signature, initials, or computer keys may be used to authenticate an entry into the medical record; however, it is the individual that controls the integrity of any system. Legal implications of various forms of data authentication should be discussed with legal counsel prior to implementation.

CONSENT

Consents are obtained in the ED daily, usually through use of standardized consent forms. If the patient is not given the opportunity to read and question information in the consent form, the courts may later find the patient did not consent. Most ED consent forms used during initial registration provide consent for treatment, consent for disclosure of medical records to third-party payers, and a contractual agreement to assume financial responsibility for any charges not paid by insurance. Many also include consent to fax medical information to the primary care physician. Table 4-2 summarizes the types of consent.

Informed consent occurs when the patient has a full understanding of the risks and benefits of the proposed treatment, is not under the influence of mind-altering drugs, and has the legal capacity to consent as evidenced by age and competency. Physicians are generally responsible for obtaining informed consent. Nurses frequently witness the patient's signature and assist with treatment; however, questions regarding the treatment should be answered by the physician before the patient signs the consent form. The patient can withdraw consent at any time. Verbal withdrawal of consent supersedes written consent.

States generally recognize an emergency exception to informed consent when life- or limb-threatening conditions exist. This doctrine, called *implied consent,* is a legal device created to allow treatment in emergency situations. Implied consent is based on the premise that the patient would, if able, provide consent for lifesaving treatment.[37] Two cases stemming from the emergency exception to informed consent illustrate the difficulties encountered in consent situations.

In *Crouch v. Most,*[10] an amateur snake handler was bitten by a rattlesnake on the left index and middle fingers. Initial treatment included ice therapy and injection of antivenin into the fingers. The patient subsequently required amputation of the fingers. The patient sued the treating physician, arguing that full disclosure of risks of antivenin should have occurred before its administration. In upholding the trial court's judgement for the physician, the New Mexico Supreme Court stated, "It would indeed be most unusual for a doctor, with his patient who had just been bitten by a venomous snake, to calmly sit down and first fully discuss the various available methods of treating snakebite and the possible consequences, while the venom is being pumped through the patient's body."[17] While management of snake bites has changed since this case was decided, the principles related to consent are still valid.

Whether a patient under the influence of drugs or alcohol can provide valid consent is a constant source of concern in the ED. In the case of *Miller v. Rhode Island Hospital,*[12] an unrestrained passenger with blood alcohol content of 0.233 mg/dl, well above any state's legal limit, arrived in the ED for evaluation after a motor vehicle crash. Trauma surgeons prepared to perform diagnostic peritoneal lavage (DPL) when the patient began questioning what they were doing. After the physicians explained the procedure, the patient attempted to sit up and told the physicians not to perform the procedure. Physicians informed the patient the extent of injury needed evaluation. Since the patient had been drinking, DPL was the standard of care for this evaluation. The patient fought and was ultimately restrained. The patient maintained he was given anesthesia after restraint and woke up with an incision in his abdomen. Physicians admitted the pa-

Table **4-2**	**Types of Consent**
Type	Description
Consent for treatment	Covers evaluation and treatment such as medications, x-rays, and lab studies. Blanket consent for treatment does not cover invasive or surgical procedures.
Informed	Patient has a full understanding of risks and benefits of the proposed consent treatment, is not under the influence of mind-altering substances, and has the legal capacity to consent.
Implied consent	Allows treatment in an emergency situation. Based on presumption that a patient would, if able, provide consent for lifesaving treatment.

tient for observation. He signed out against medical advice, and brought suit against the hospital and physicians for battery. The trial court granted a judgment in the patient's favor, but the hospital and physicians appealed. Rhode Island Supreme Court found the trial court judge committed a reversible error in not allowing expert testimony regarding mechanism of injury and indications for DPL. The trial court had not allowed a hospital trauma surgeon to testify on the hospital's protocol regarding nonconsensual DPL, and also instructed the jury not to consider intoxication as a factor in their decision. Appellate court overturned the judgment of the trial court and sent the case back for retrial.[32] Whether intoxication impairs an individual's ability to consent to or refuse treatment is a matter of state law. Sheer numbers of alcohol and drug users in the ED make it essential that every ED have specific policies regarding obtaining consent from these individuals.

The age at which an individual can consent is found in state law. In cases of sexually transmitted diseases, pregnancy, alcoholism, and substance abuse, many states provide that minors below the age of majority can consent for examination and treatment without parental consent. Many states recognize emancipated minors, individuals below the statutory age of consent recognized in the same legal capacity as an adult. The emancipated minor is self-supporting or lives alone without parental supervision or involvement. When an individual who is incompetent or a nonemancipated minor presents to the ED for treatment, state law dictates who has authority to consent.

Managed care is changing health care delivery in the United States. Tension between managed care systems and other forms of health care delivery is magnified by the ED environment. Consent and payment issues become intertwined when a patient enrolled in a managed care plan presents to a nonparticipating ED. Patients in managed care plans are usually assigned a primary physician, who serves as the gatekeeper for covered services. The gatekeeper must authorize payment for treatment in a nonparticipating ED; however, consent for this treatment must come from the patient. If an emergency exists, most managed care plans will reimburse the nonparticipating ED for initial stabilization. In the absence of specific consent forms for interactions with managed care patients, the prudent approach is to do what is in the patient's best interests.[38]

Individuals in the custody of law enforcement are generally allowed to consent to or refuse treatment. One area of concern is collection of blood or urine specimens for alcohol and drug testing requested by law enforcement. State law determines whether the patient must consent for tests. The nurse or other health care provider is often released from civil or criminal liability if the specimen is obtained in a medically acceptable manner. Specific ED policies and procedures related to this issue should be approved by legal counsel. As an illustration, Indiana law allows a law enforcement officer to use "reasonable force" to assist the health care provider if the patient in custody refuses to consent and resists obtaining the specimen. Physicians, hospitals, and agents of the hospital including nurses are protected from civil and criminal liability in obtaining the sample if requested by a law enforcement officer.[26]

Consent is an important defense against intentional torts of false imprisonment, assault, and battery. *False imprisonment* occurs when a patient is intentionally held in a bounded area. Standing in the doorway of a treatment room to prevent a patient from leaving the room raises potential false imprisonment claims. Concise documentation of the patient's behavior, verbal threats or applicable statements, and therapeutic interventions can defend against false imprisonment claims if the patient is impaired and judged a danger to self or others. *Assault* occurs when an intentional threat to inflict injury is coupled with apparent ability to immediately carry out the threat. *Battery* is unconsented touching of another person that results in harmful contact. The emergency nurse who inserts an intravenous catheter despite refusal from a rational adult may be liable for battery in a civil or criminal action. If a patient initially refuses then later consents after explanation of the procedure, the nurse should document this interaction in the medical record.

Other consent issues include photographs, videotaping trauma resuscitations, disclosure of medical information, and participation in research protocols. Seek advice of legal counsel before implementing a policy covering these issues.

The patient allowed to consent is also allowed to refuse treatment. As Justice Brennan wrote in one Supreme Court opinion, "The right to be free from unwanted medical attention is a right to evaluate the potential benefit of treatment and its possible consequences according to one's own values and to make a personal decision whether to subject oneself to the intrusion."[18] It does not matter if refusal occurs in an emergency situation or is a rational decision in the presence of a terminal condition.

A rational, competent adult can refuse administration of blood even if it is deemed life-saving. Jehovah's Witnesses routinely refuse blood transfusions due to religious objections. In the case of minors and incompetent adults, hospitals usually seek a court order to allow treatment such as blood transfusions. Courts are likely to protect individuals because of the state's interest in protecting life. Waiting for the patient to lapse into unconsciousness and then providing treatment does not provide protection against liability. Proper refusal of treatment does not change because the patient's mental status changed.[38]

Right-to-die cases led Congress to pass the Patient Self-Determination Act in 1990.[4] It requires hospitals to ask patients, on admission, if the patient has an advance directive and to document this interaction in the medical record. An advance directive includes a living will and durable power of attorney for health care. The type of advance directive available is determined by state law. When the patient does have an advance directive, communication of its existence to all health care providers is often difficult. Techniques used to ensure dissemination of this information include permanent armbands, a laminated pocket-size copy of the advance directive, or including the advance directive in the medical record. Legality of photocopies of living wills should be clarified for specific practice areas.

Patients may refuse treatment by leaving the ED before evaluation, during evaluation, after evaluation but before discharge, or at the time of discharge but before completing necessary paperwork including aftercare instructions. Not every patient who leaves does so against medical advice (AMA). The patient who leaves during evaluation may not inform ED staff. When this occurs, the situation should be clearly documented. If the patient does discuss refusal of treatment and elects to leave AMA, the nurse should ensure the patient understands potential consequences prior to signing release forms. The medical record should reflect this discussion, patient response, and patient understanding of the consequences of refusing treatment.

EMERGENCY MEDICAL TREATMENT AND ACTIVE LABOR ACT

The Emergency Medical Treatment and Active Labor Act (EMTALA),[5] formerly known as COBRA/OBRA, is a federal statute originally passed by Congress to address patient dumping—transfer of unstable patients for financial reasons. Enforcement and regulation of EMTALA are the responsibility of the Health Care Financing Administration (HCFA) of the Department of Health and Human Services (DHHS). Regulations identified in EMTALA do not supersede state laws governing medical negligence or simple negligence actions, but do prevail over state law if there is a direct conflict between the provisions of EMTALA and state law. Table 4-3 summarizes specific EMTALA provisions and definitions.

Under EMTALA, all individuals presenting to the ED for examination and treatment are entitled to an appropriate medical screening to determine if an emergency medical condition exists.[6] The statute does not clearly define what constitutes an appropriate medical screening. The Sixth Circuit Court of Appeals, in *Cleland v. Bronson Health Care Group,* described *appropriate* as "one of the most wonderful weasel words in the dictionary."[16] Studying case law from appellate courts in each circuit provides some direction regarding the courts' definition of an appropriate medical screening. The Eleventh Circuit Court of Appeals said an appropriate medical screening is based on application of the same screening procedures to paying and indigent patients, rather than adequacy of the exam itself.[21]

Regional referral centers and hospitals with specialized capabilities such as trauma centers, neonatal centers, and burn units are obligated to accept all appropriate transfers of patients who require the care if they have the capacity to treat the individual.[9] An EMTALA violation can result in a civil penalty up to $50,000 per violation for hospitals and physicians. The hospital and physician may also be terminated as Medicare providers.[8] In some hospitals, the triage nurse "triages out" patients with nonurgent complaints after the initial medical screening.[30] "Triaging out" refers to the process of sending patients away from the ED after an initial nursing assessment, but before medical evaluation. This pro-

cedure could result in an EMTALA violation if an emergency medical condition exists. Protocols related to "triaging out" must have support from physicians, administration, and legal counsel to minimize potential EMTALA hazards.

Use of EMTALA to sue base station, or resource, hospitals has thus far been unsuccessful. In *Johnson v. University of Chicago Hospitals,*[14] an infant's mother sued, claiming an EMTALA violation. The infant suffered cardiopulmonary arrest. Paramedics contacted the University of Chicago Hospitals (UCH), their designated resource hospital. The "telemetry nurse" directed the paramedics to another hospital because UCH was on "partial bypass." The infant was treated at another hospital and subsequently transferred to Cook County Hospital. Some time after the transfer, the infant died and the mother sued. The appellate court upheld the trial court's dismissal of the EMTALA complaint, stating that in the plain meaning of the law, the infant never "came to" UCH or its ED. The appellate court further stated that "a hospital-operated telemetry system is distinct from that same hospital's emergency room."[28] The appellate court allowed part of the mother's claims to go forward under state law. In the interim ruling, DHHS stated that "coming to the

Table **4-3** **Key EMTALA Provisions**	
Provision	Description/definition
Medical screening	Applies to any individual who comes to the ED and requests treatment. Appropriate medical screening determines if an emergency medical condition exists.
Emergency medical condition	Medical condition manifesting acute symptoms of sufficient severity, including pain, that, absent immediate medical attention, could reasonably be expected to result in placing the health of the individual, including an unborn fetus, in serious jeopardy; serious impairment to bodily functions; or serious dysfunction of any bodily organ or part. With respect to pregnant women having contractions, there is inadequate time to effect a safe transfer to another hospital before delivery *or* transfer may pose a threat to the health or safety of the woman or unborn child.
Stabilize	Provide treatment to ensure, within reasonable medical probability, that no material deterioration is likely to result from or occur during the transfer.
Transfer	Movement, including discharge, of an individual outside a hospital's facilities at the direction of any person employed by or associated with the hospital. Does not include movement of a dead individual or an individual who leaves the facility without permission.
Patient refusal	Patients can refuse examination, treatment, and/or transfer. Reasonable steps should be taken to secure written informed consent to refuse.
Physician certification	A physician is required to certify that medical benefits outweigh the risks of the transfer. Certification must contain summary of risks and benefits upon which certification is based.
Appropriate transfer	Transfer is appropriate when the receiving facility has available space, qualified personnel, and agrees to accept the patient in transfer.
Transfer records	Refers to all medical records for the patient and for this specific visit. Includes diagnostic test results, informed written consent or certification, and, when appropriate, the name and address of any on-call physician who refused or failed to appear within a reasonable time to provide necessary stabilizing treatment.
Nondiscrimination	A participating hospital with specialized capabilities or facilities shall not refuse to accept an appropriate transfer of an individual who requires such specialized capabilities or facilities if the hospital has the capacity to treat the individual.
EMTALA claim	A claim must be brought within 2 years of the alleged violation.
Financial inquiries	A participating hospital may not delay appropriate medical screening exams in order to inquire about the individual's method of payment or insurance status.

ED" included property owned by the hospital, including hospital-based ambulance services.[3] Court interpretations of this rule are yet to come.

Regulations found in EMTALA require specific documentation and retention of transfer records. State licensure evaluations and JCAHO often incorporate a review of transfer records into site surveys. Documentation forms and documentation systems are not specified by EMTALA. The only requirement is that the information be maintained.

One goal of managed care is elimination of hospitalization in nonparticipating facilities. Whether the managed care plan is operated privately or by the state, patient transfer from the ED of a nonparticipating facility to a participating facility is definitely covered by EMTALA. The ED often finds itself caught between following managed care policies or complying with federal law. In Tennessee, Medicaid patients are stabilized in a nonparticipating facility then transferred to a participating facility for admission.[22] If the patient cannot be stabilized and the nonparticipating facility has the resources to provide care, transfer for financial reasons falls within EMTALA prohibitions. No provisions exist in EMTALA to compensate nonparticipating hospitals for medical screening exams or nonreimbursed hospitalizations of managed care patients.

Patients who require transfer must be transported with an appropriate vehicle, equipment, and qualified personnel.[7] This provision applies to every transfer. Transferring a patient who requires advanced life support in a basic life support vehicle with emergency medical technicians violates this provision of EMTALA. Appropriate vehicle and equipment is determined by factors such as time, distance, terrain, geographic considerations such as rush-hour traffic, patient needs, and availability of monitoring devices. Qualified personnel means the providers' scope of practice matches the patient's needs.[15] Scope of practice for nurses, emergency medical technicians, paramedics, and respiratory therapists is determined by state law.

The future promises increased tension between emergency care providers and regulatory constructs. A recent EMTALA case illustrates rising tensions between medical and nursing care and law. The mother of an encephalic infant demanded aggressive management, including mechanical ventilation.[27] Although the mother was advised that mechanical ventilation provided no palliative or therapeutic purpose, she insisted that everything be done to keep her baby alive. She contacted a state agency responsible for enforcing antidiscrimination laws against handicapped or disabled individuals. The agency made it clear to the hos-pital and doctors it would pursue any remedies available to Baby K. The Fourth Circuit Court of Appeals separated the treatment of acute symptoms from the underlying condition, a position in direct conflict with standard medical and nursing practice. The case has been interpreted by some critics as EMTALA requiring provision of any technologically available treatment to any patient regardless of underlying condition, even if the condition or illness is fatal.[29] The Fourth

Circuit Court's decision is not interpreted law in other circuits, but demonstrates the impending collision between legal interpretation and emergency patient care.

PRESERVATION AND COLLECTION OF EVIDENCE

Each state identifies specific considerations that must be reported to local or state authorities. These should be listed in the ED policy and procedure. Common disclosures include child abuse, elder abuse, communicable diseases, gunshot wounds, stabbings, sexual assault, burns, suspicious deaths, animal bites, and poisonings.[35] The emergency nurse is often required to collect evidence in these and other potential criminal cases. State laws govern the type of evidence needed in each situation; therefore the emergency nurse must be familiar with local and state laws that govern evidence collection. Medical examiners, local law enforcement, and district attorneys are excellent resources when developing specific policies and procedures for evidence collection and preservation. Legal counsel should be involved to ensure policies and procedures fall within the nurse's and hospital's scope of practice. Placing a forensic kit at the bedside aids in collection and preservation of evidence.[19] Kits should include applicable laws, guidelines, and telephone numbers as a handy reference.[28]

Evidence collection in sexual assault is generally standardized in each state. Rape kits contain instructions, diagrams, evidence containers, and specific documentation requirements. Most states require specific patient consent for evidentiary examination and photographs. Issues discussed in the consent section of this chapter apply to sexual assault cases.[31] Many states use specially trained sexual assault nurse examiners.[3]

As a rule, victims or perpetrators of violent crimes who enter the ED for treatment are candidates for evidence collection. General guidelines for evidence preservation and collection are described in Box 4-2.

MENTAL HEALTH PATIENTS

The psychiatric patient presents a unique challenge in the ED and deserves special mention since state and federal laws exist regarding mental health patients. Facilities that do

---

Box 4-2   Guidelines for Evidence Preservation

Do not discard clothing. Place bloody clothing in a paper bag.
Do not wash the hands of a person with a gunshot wound. Cover with paper bags until the police examine the patient.
Cut around bullet holes and knife cuts in clothing.
Document what the patient says about the incident.
Describe extent of surface wounds and amount of blood present.
Document the patient's behavior.
Delay cleaning until police examine the patient unless it is necessary for essential procedures.

not have inpatient psychiatric services are not exempt from providing emergency psychiatric care. A patient diagnosed with a mental illness is competent to consent to medical care unless a court determines legal incompetency exists. The most pressing issue for these patients is the potential for violence. Patients expressing suicidal or homicidal ideation require immediate intervention to prevent injury to self or others. Each state has laws regarding commitment procedures for psychiatric patients.[41] A psychiatric patient may be held for a time in the ED against his or her express wishes, if state law allows. Policies and procedures should address specific requirements for involuntary holding of psychiatric patients.

Restraint policies should address the decision to restrain, how restraint is accomplished, monitoring the restrained patient, and at what point restraints are removed. Documentation should reflect the patient's behavior and the reason for the intervention. A physician's order is generally necessary when a patient is restrained. If the situation requires immediate intervention, the physician signature may be obtained after the patient is restrained.

MEDICAL NEGLIGENCE

The elements of a medical negligence cause of action are duty, breach of duty, cause in fact, proximate cause, and damages (Table 4-4). Although all elements are important, breach of duty is significant in medical negligence, or malpractice, cases. With some exception, expert witnesses are

Table 4-4 Elements of Medical Negligence

Element	Description
Duty	Exists when a hospital, nurse, or physician establishes a relationship with a patient and volunteers to assume care.
Breach of duty	Occurs when commission or omission falls below established standard of care.
Cause in fact	The injury would not have occurred but for the conduct of the nurse. The conduct of the nurse was, more likely than not, a substantial factor in the patient's injury.
Proximate cause	Determined by foreseeability. The emergency nurse should have foreseen that injury would occur with this particular conduct.[36]
Damages	Compensation for medical care, lost wages, and pain and suffering. Punitive damages may be asked if the conduct reached the point of willful, wanton, or intentional injury. These damages serve to punish and deter bad conduct.

used in medical negligence actions to define the standard of care and to render an opinion regarding whether the standard of care was met in a particular case. Emergency nurses are generally required to exercise skill and judgment that a reasonably prudent emergency nurse would use under similar circumstances.[23]

Sources for the standards of emergency nurses include ED policy and procedure manuals, JCAHO standards, state nurse practice acts, and federal and state law. Professional standards, such as the Standards of Emergency Nursing Practice (ENA),[20] authoritative textbooks, and specialty courses may also be sources. Certification courses and professional standards documents frequently disclaim legal use of their material. However, attorneys and nurse expert witnesses may use the information to establish the standard of care for a particular patient situation. A word of caution is necessary regarding institutional policies and procedures. Using *all, always, never,* and *shall* turns the policy and procedure into a mandate, rather than a guideline for professional judgment in patient care decisions. If particular conduct is mandated, each nurse should be aware of the policy and follow the policy mandate. The more flexibility afforded the emergency nurse in asserting professional judgment in patient care decisions, the less the likelihood that an internal policy and procedure can be used against the nurse or institution. All ED policies and procedures should be reviewed with an eye toward maximizing clarity. If a policy exists that no one follows, the result can be devastating to the hospital or nurse in a nursing negligence action.

In *Marks v. Mandel,*[11] the ED received notice of the pending arrival of a patient with a gunshot wound to the chest. A moonlighting orthopedic resident did not follow the ED's on-call policy, which required the on-call thoracic surgeon be notified before a thoracic gunshot wound (GSW) patient arrived in the ED. A delay occurred in reaching the thoracic surgeon, and the patient died of his injuries. In the suit that followed, the trial court excluded the ED policy and procedure manual from evidence. Appellate court reversed the trial court, stating that internal policy and procedure manuals "should be admitted when they contain either (1) evidence of a general industry custom or standard, or (2) evidence that the defendant violated its own policy or an industry standard."[25] The appellate court sent the case back to the trial court for retrial with the direction that the ED policy and procedure manual should be admitted into evidence.

One of the first cases recognizing nursing negligence was *Darling v. Charleston Community Memorial Hospital.*[2] A plaster cast was applied in the ED after an 18-year-old patient broke his leg in a college football game. Shortly after cast application, the patient complained of pain and his toes became swollen and dark. The patient was admitted to the hospital but was subsequently transferred after complications developed. Ultimately the leg was amputated. The court addressed the nursing standard of care, stating that the "jury could reasonably have concluded that nurses did not test for circulation in the leg as frequently as necessary, that skilled nurses would have promptly recognized the conditions that signaled a dangerous impairment of circulation in the plaintiff's leg, and would have known that the condition would become irreversible in a matter of hours. At that point it became the nurses' duty to inform the attending physician, and if he failed to act, to advise the hospital authorities so that appropriate action might be taken."[24] Although the case is criticized in legal literature for the legal analysis of other issues, *Darling* stands for the principle that a nurse can be held liable for nursing negligence.

Managed care physicians and nurses are subject to state laws regarding medical liability or negligence. In *Hand v. Tavera,*[13] the hospital, emergency physician, and on-call managed care physician were sued for medical negligence. Hand, a member of the Humana Health Care Plan 1, arrived in the participating ED complaining of a 3-day headache. The patient had hypertension and his father had died of a brain aneurysm. The emergency physician decided to admit the patient but Dr. Tavera, the Humana physician on call for authorizing admissions, refused, stating the patient could be treated on an outpatient basis. Hand was sent home and suffered a stroke a few hours later. A claim against the hospital, emergency physician, and Dr. Tavera resulted. The hospital settled and the emergency physician was dropped from the case. Dr. Tavera, the remaining defendant, argued that no physician-patient relationship existed and he owed no duty to Hand. The trial court agreed and ruled in favor of Dr. Tavera in a pretrial motion, but the ruling was appealed. The appellate court determined that the Humana managed care plan brought Hand and Tavera together. The appellate court held, "When a patient who has enrolled in a prepaid medical plan goes to a hospital emergency room and the plan's designated doctor is consulted, the physician-patient relationship exists and the doctor owes the patient a duty of care."[13] The case was sent back to the trial court for a determination of other issues in the case. The prudent approach in the ED is for the patient to speak directly to the on-call physician for the managed care plan. Responsibility for disclosure of alternative treatment plans and specifics regarding benefit coverage rests with the managed care plan entity, not the ED.[39]

SUMMARY

The essence of liability prevention in all areas of medical and nursing practice is providing and documenting care within accepted standards. Practicing sound medical and nursing principles, including documentation, can reduce the fear of litigation. Education of ED staff on medicolegal issues with frequent review and updating of policies and procedures is essential. Quality management processes can ensure correction of deficiencies and strengthen competent practice. The ED patient expects high-quality care that meets medical and legal standards of care. The competent emergency nurse can deliver this.

REFERENCES

1. 29 CFR §1910.1030 (1995).
2. 211 NE2d 253 (Ill 1965).
3. 42 CFR 489.24(b).
4. 42 USCA §1395 (Suppl 1995).
5. 42 USCA §1395dd (Suppl 1995).
6. 42 USCA §1395dd (a) (Suppl 1995).
7. 42 USCA §1395dd (c)(2)(D) (Suppl 1995).
8. 42 USCA §1395dd (d) (Suppl 1995).
9. 42 USCA §1395dd (g) (Suppl 1995).
10. 432 P2d 250 (NM 1967).
11. 477 So 2d 1036 (Fla Ct Appl 1985).
12. 625 A2d 778 (RI 1993).
13. 864 SW2d 678 *Hand v. Tavera* (Tex Ct App 1993).
14. 982 F2d 230 (7th Cir 1992).
15. Boyko SM: Interfacility transfer guidelines: an easy reference to help hospitals decide on appropriate vehicles and staffing for transfers, *JEN* 20:18, 1994.
16. *Cleland v. Bronson Health Care Group Inc.,* 917 F2d 266, 271 (6th Cir 1990).
17. *Crouch v. Most,* 432 P2d 250, 254 (NM 1967).
18. *Cruzan v. Director, Missouri Dept Health,* 110 S Ct 2841, 111 LEd2d 224 (1990).
19. Easter CR, Muro GA: An emergency department forensic kit, *JEN* 21:440, 1995.
20. Emergency Nurses Association: *Standards of emergency nursing practice,* ed 3, St. Louis, 1995, Mosby.
21. *Holcomb v. Monahan,* 30F3d 116 (11th Cir 1994).
22. Hule KD, Beeler LM: TennCare: the impact of state health care reform on emergency patients and caregivers, *JEN* 21:282, 1995.
23. *Id.* at §2.20.
24. *Id.* at 258.
25. *Id.* at 1039.
26. Ind. Code Ann. §9-30-6-6 (Burns Suppl 1995).
27. In the Matter of Baby K, 16F3d 590 (4th Cir 1994), cert denied, US 1994.
28. *Johnson v. University of Chicago Hospitals,* 982 F2d 230, 232 (7th Cir 1992).
29. Krebs-Markrich J, Coffey JE, Korjus JLW: EMTALA: the next generation, *Health Lawyer* 8:1, 1995.
30. Kuensting LL: "Triaging out" children with minor illnesses from an emergency department by a triage nurse: where do they go? *JEN* 21:102, 1995.
31. Ledray LE: Sexual assault evidentiary exam and treatment protocol, *JEN* 21:355, 1995.
32. *Miller v. Rhode Island Hospital,* 625 A2d 778 (RI 1993).
33. Pozgar GD: *Legal aspects of health care administration,* ed 5, Gaithersburg, 1993, Aspen.
34. Roach WH Jr, Aspen Health Law Center: *Medical records and the law,* ed 2, Gaithersburg, 1994, Aspen.
35. Rothenberg MA: *§2.6, Emerg Med Malpractice,* ed 2, New York, 1994, John Wiley & Sons.
36. Rothenberg MA: *§2.10, Emerg Med Malpractice,* ed 2, New York, 1994, John Wiley & Sons.
37. Rozovsky FA: *Consent to treatment: a practical guide,* ed 2, Boston, 1990, Little, Brown.
38. Rozovsky FA: *Consent to treatment,* ed 2 (suppl), Boston, 1995, Little, Brown.
39. Rozovsky FA: *§12.13, Consent to treatment,* ed 2 (suppl), Boston, 1995, Little, Brown.
40. Tomes JP: *Healthcare records: a practical legal guide,* Dubuque, Iowa, 1990, Kendall/Hunt.
41. Wexler DB: *Therapeutic jurisprudence: the law as a therapeutic agent,* Durham, NC, 1990, Carolina Academic.

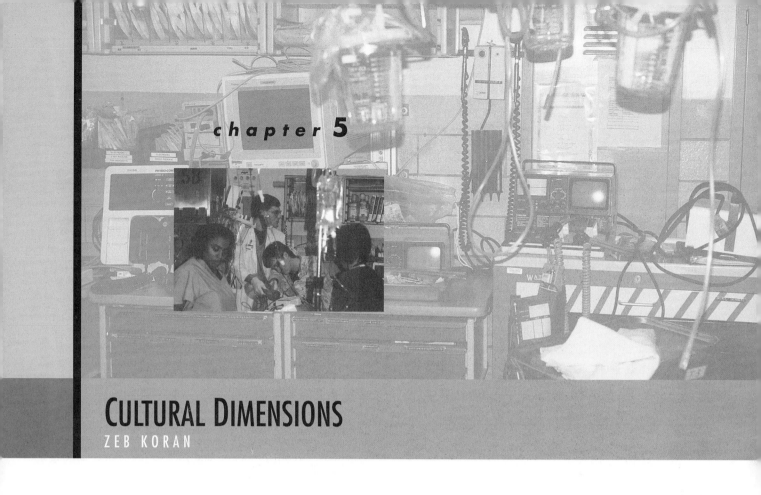

CHAPTER 5

CULTURAL DIMENSIONS

ZEB KORAN

The United States has long been called a melting pot because of the varied ethnic representation in its heritage. Increased affluence and easy global transportation have further increased cultural diversity in the United States. In 1992, the U.S. Census Bureau identified more than 30 ethnic designations individually recognized by more than 100,000 people, with numerous other ethnic designations identified by a smaller number of respondents.[1] This diversity challenges the ordinary citizen as well as the practicing health care professional.

An essential first step toward cultural harmony is understanding what constitutes culture. Culture does not mean the person's social level, racial group, or ethnic heritage. Leininger,[2] a well-known transcultural nursing theorist, defines culture as "values, beliefs, norms, and practices of a particular group that are learned and shared and that guide thinking, decisions, and actions in a patterned way." Six distinct phenomena vary among most cultures—communication, time, space, biologic variations, social organization, and environmental control (Table 5-1).

Styles of communication are a defining characteristic within each culture. Communication is the vehicle for passage of cultural beliefs from generation to generation. Verbal and nonverbal communication are a product of culture. Verbal differences between cultures include language or dialect used, definition of specific words, inflections used when speaking, and loudness with which words are spoken. Nonverbal communication such as touch, eye contact, body posture, and facial expressions also has different meaning in various cultures.

Views of time and personal space are defined by culture. Orientation to the past, present, or future determines normal pace of life within the culture as well as timing for events such as marriage and adulthood. Personal space represents security, autonomy, privacy, and self-identity and varies between cultures. How an individual responds when stopped on the street for directions or forced to share a room with someone he or she doesn't know is a product of culture.

As the world becomes more culturally diverse, emergency nurses will be confronted by many patients different from themselves and from each other. Immediacy of need inherent in emergency care requires familiarity with many cultural groups to avoid stereotyping. Comprehensive review of all recognized cultures is not possible within the confines of this chapter; readers are encouraged to seek other sources to expand knowledge of major cultures within their practice area. What follows is a brief description of cultures frequently encountered in the United States. Social, familial, and health-related information is included. Table 5-2 highlights select cultural beliefs related to the cause of illness. Brevity of information provided on some cultures is the result of limited available information rather than an opinion on importance of the culture.

SPECIFIC CULTURAL GROUPS

Names for cultures change with time and geographic relocation. The name used for each cultural group discussed in the following section reflects the current name in literature and public record.

Table 5-1 Cultural Phenomena

Phenomena	Defining characteristics
Communication	Language spoken, voice quality, use of silence, physical movements, gestures, eye contact, touch
Space	Comfort distance between self and an unknown person
Social organization	Family structure is patriarchal or matriarchal
Time	Orientation is past, present, or future; dictates when certain life events occur, i.e., marriage
Environmental control	Locus-of-control is internal or external; belief in witchcraft, voodoo, magic, or prayer; health care beliefs unique to the specific culture
Biologic variations	Illness prevalent within the specific culture

African-American

African-Americans have been subjected to discrimination in many parts of the country, so many feel angry and powerless. Most prefer being called Mr. or Mrs.; identifying them by their first name without permission is considered disrespectful and demeaning. Most speak standard English, but may use black English when conversing with others of their cultural group. Black English is a rhythmic, stylized pattern of verbal communication. Individuals may also remain silent rather than speak when they are in a strange environment.

Women are the most important element in the family and are responsible for family health. More than half of all African-American heads of household in the United States are female.

Life is viewed as a series of opposites, for example, a birth for a death, with time orientation present or future. A small personal space is accepted without anxiety. Illness is considered the result of disharmony in a person's life. Males generally postpone seeking health care; usually the need for medication is the driving force when an African-American seeks health care. Many believe in folk medicine, voodoo, witchcraft, and magic. There is a high incidence of hypertension, coronary artery disease, sickle cell disease, diabetes mellitus, keloid formation, and lactose intolerance among this population.

Table 5-2 Perceived Causes of Illness

Cause	Description	Treatment	Cultural group(s)
Imbalance between yin and yang	Yin and yang are powers from the universe that control the body. *Yin* is the female force, inactive and negative; *yang* is the male force, active and positive.	Restore the balance. Eat yin foods for illness caused by yang forces and yang foods for illness caused by yin forces. *Acupuncture*—needles inserted in areas of body to treat diseases from yang forces. *Herbal medicines*—various mixtures used for specific conditions. *Cupping*—a substance is heated in a glass to create a vacuum. The glass is immediately turned upside down onto the skin, where it remains until it can be removed easily. It leaves a circular burn. *Coining*—a coin is heated and rubbed over the body. The appearance of welts verifies the presence of illness. Also called skin scraping. *Moxibustion*—moxa plants are heated and laid near a painful area. The plants leave craters in the skin. *Massage*—used to concentrate energy on areas of illness.	Chinese Vietnamese
Evil eye	Someone with special powers admires a child, but does not touch the child.	That same person should touch the child. Egg mixed with water is laid under the child's head.	Mexican-American
Hot and cold imbalance	Exposure to something with either hot or cold properties.	Exposure to the opposite, e.g., headache is a hot condition so cold herbs are placed at the temples as treatment.	Mexican-American Vietnamese

Arabic

Individuals from Arabic countries may be Islamic or Christian, diet and death rites are determined by specific religious affiliation. Arabic culture is patriarchal, with decisions made by elder men. Extended families are common, with members subject to group censorship and pressure. Women have limited rights and must maintain an air of subservience to males. Arabic people often believe in disease-causing entities such as the evil eye. Illness or injury is seen as the will of God, so instruction on prevention is usually unsuccessful. Orientation is to the present, so Arabic persons often arrive late for appointments or not at all. Patients may withhold information because the interview is considered intrusive. Arabic persons are not expected to engage in self-care or make decisions regarding recovery, but view health care givers as personal employees. Prevalent health problems include urinary infections, cardiovascular disease, diabetes, and thalassemia. Any display of flesh, for example, an underwear advertisement, is considered pornographic. Displaying the sole of the foot to others is considered offensive.

Appalachian

Many Appalachians remain in the Appalachian mountains; however, mobility has increased migration to larger cities in the northeastern and southeastern United States. The people of Appalachia emigrated from countries such as France, Wales, Germany, and Scotland. Various dialects spoken may be difficult to understand. Appalachians are very private, use few adjectives to communicate, and consider direct eye contact rude. This makes obtaining historical information difficult, particularly information related to assessment of pain.

The nuclear and extended families are important in Appalachian culture. The family unit is patriarchal; however, health advice usually comes from the oldest woman or "grandma" of the unit. Folk medicine is important to most. Producing children demonstrates a man is really a man while ensuring the woman is fulfilled, so large families are normal.

Appalachian people tend to focus on the state of their blood (thick or thin; high or low; good or bad). Status of blood is controlled by eliminating or consuming certain foods. High blood means too much blood, as manifested by headaches or dizziness; drinking brine off pickles is an accepted cure. Appalachian people expect others to care for them and wait on them during illness or injury. There is an inherent distrust of hospitals since they are regarded as places to die. Illness is considered the will of God. Treatment should be immediate; however, any need for medication or treatments beyond this immediate need is not understood or followed. Consequently Appalachians are typically noncompliant with long-term medication and health care regimens. Common health problems include tuberculosis, diabetes mellitus, and coronary artery disease.

Chinese

Keeping face by not being embarrassed, defeated, or contradicted is extremely important to the Chinese. The culture is very formal, so the first name should not be used unless prefaced with Mr. or Mrs. Demonstrating signs of pain is considered a sign of weakness. The Chinese are very uncomfortable with any physical contact involving strangers. They utilize high-context communication, messages are sent internally and by physical context; if used, verbal communication is less important than nonverbal. Chinese believe accepting something when first offered is rude; therefore pain medication should be offered several times.

Elderly people are highly respected and recognized authority figures. Consequently grandparents and parents are involved in decisions regarding a child. Moral purity is important to the Chinese, so any public display of affection is strongly discouraged. Needs of the family take priority over individual needs. Marriage is discouraged until after college, with exchange of rings optional. Traditionally the bride retains her own name. The mother plays a more active role than the father in nurturing children. Child abuse is rare in Chinese culture. Shame and guilt are used as forms of discipline.

Hospitals are considered places to die, rather than to get well. Euthanasia and organ donation are acceptable to the Chinese. They believe blood is the source of life and may resist having blood drawn. The Chinese also believe a person's spirit may escape during surgery. The body is considered a gift from parents and ancestors. Health is a balance between the yin and the yang, illness occurs with an imbalance between the two. Yin represents the female, inactive, or negative force, while yang represents the male, active, or positive force. After birth of a child, a mother does not bathe for 7 to 30 days and is limited to eating certain foods. Soy sauce is thought to make the child's skin darker and may be avoided. Ginseng is used as a strength tonic in pregnant women. Commonly occurring health problems include hypertension, liver and stomach cancer, and lactose intolerance.

Cuban

Cubans are outgoing, friendly, love social events, and are also very hard working. Hand gestures are an important part of communication, used to reinforce emotions and ideas. Interrupting another is not considered impolite. Eye contact indicates sincerity. Marriages usually occur during the twenties, common law marriage is not common.

Cubans believe some illnesses occur because of supernatural powers such as the evil eye. Amulets worn as a necklace, bracelet, or pinned to clothing are used as protection against these powers and should not be removed without permission. Cubans believe that only magic spells and ethnic treatments can overcome illness that is the result of the evil eye. Health problems include diabetes mellitus and lactose intolerance.

Eastern Indian

Many Eastern Indians practice Hinduism, Jainism, Buddhism, or Sikhism, religions that believe in reincarnation and the caste system whereby people work their way up the caste levels with each reincarnation. Ultimately individuals reach the highest level, which renders them free from life on earth so they can continue a better existence.

The term *thanks* is not used or recognized by East Indians. Social acts are duties that do not require recognition. Nods of the head for "yes" and "no" are opposite those used in the United States. Certain gestures such as winking or whistling are considered unacceptable behaviors for women. An apology is necessary if an individual's feet or shoes touch another person. Public displays of affection are not appropriate. Men are allowed direct eye contact with each other, whereas women are expected to keep their eyes cast down when addressing men in their family.

The father is the head of the household; the elderly are held in high regard and cared for by other members of the family. Decisions are deferred to the elderly, when they are present. Marriage, many of which are still arranged by parents, is considered sacred. Divorce is unacceptable because marriage continues past death. Chastity is a virtue held in high regard, so females may refuse treatment from a man.

Terminal illness should not be discussed with a patient, but deferred to conversations with the family. Illness is thought to occur when an imbalance exists between five essential elements of the body, fire, earth, wind, space, and water. Thalassemia occurs frequently in this population.

Japanese

Japanese consider social rank very important, so those in authority are never questioned. Direct eye contact demonstrates lack of respect. Verbal communication is less important than nonverbal; however, touch as a means of communication is minimal in the Japanese population. Patting on the back is unacceptable. Answers to questions are usually vague.

Boys are taught to be assertive and competitive, whereas girls are taught to suppress thoughts and opinions. Husbands are the head of the household; however, important decisions are made by the entire family. Families are consulted before the person seeks health care.

Health is considered a balance between the universe and oneself. Illness is thought to occur because energy no longer flows through the body, so treatment focuses on returning energy flow through acupuncture, massage, moxibustion, and acupressure. There is some belief in the supernatural or the evil eye. Japanese are very stoic with regard to pain. Fevers are managed by application of warm blankets and drinking hot fluids so the person sweats the fever out. There is a high incidence of lactose intolerance, liver cancer, and stomach cancer in this population, and Japanese have one of the highest incidences of hypertension of all groups. Isoniazid is inactive in the Japanese population. Succinylcholine takes longer to be inactivated, so muscular paralysis lasts much longer in the Japanese patient.

Laotian

Direct, prolonged eye contact is viewed as lack of respect. Only parents are allowed to touch the head of a child. Three or four generations typically live together with health care decisions made by the oldest man. The family name is always written first, followed by the given name. Males are not circumcised. Women's breasts are used for infant feeding only, whereas the lower torso from waist to knees remains covered at all times. In order to avoid capture by evil spirits, the newborn is never complimented. Colostrum is considered poisonous for the newborn, so breastfeeding does not begin until the mother has a milk supply.

Laotians have a strong belief in herbal medicine, which leads to a high level of home care. Herbal medicines are considered "cool" medicines, whereas western medicines are considered "hot" medicines. Laotians believe illness is caused by "bad winds." To release these winds and regain health, the affected body area is scratched or pinched until red lines or marks appear. Loss of soul, another cause of illness, is prevented by wearing strings around the waist, neck, and ankles. Physicians are considered authority figures and are not questioned or expected to explain treatments or care. Pain is usually severe before medication is requested. Tuberculosis occurs frequently in this group.

Mexican-American

Mexican-Americans are very demonstrative; friends may fully embrace as a greeting or kiss each other on the cheek. Many believe touching while bestowing a compliment decreases power of the evil eye. Women do not expose their bodies to males or other women; men may also be extremely modest. Common law marriages are an acceptable practice within the Mexican-American community. Flattering statements to passing females are accepted behavior for Mexican-American males. Coins may be strapped to a newborn's navel to make the child attractive.

Alcohol use is a common way to celebrate life, so alcohol consumption begins at a very early age. Excessive drinking is considered manly as long as the man is able to work and support his family. Men make all family decisions except when health care is needed for a child. Pediatric health care decisions are left to the woman; however, the man signs the consent and receives all instructions.

There is a strong belief in the evil eye and hexes placed by another person. Disease is considered the result of an imbalance between hot and cold, with severity determined by presence of blood and the amount of pain. Folk healers often play an important role in the maintenance of health. Same-sex health care providers are preferred. Pain relief may be refused as a means of atonement. Colostrum is considered unhealthy, so bottled milk is used until the mother can provide breast milk. Warm blankets and hot fluid are used to treat a fever. Mexican-Americans are oriented to the present, so they often do not comply with long-term treatment regimens. Diabetes mellitus and lactose intolerance are common health problems.

Native American Indian

There are more than 200 tribes of Native American Indians in the United States, each with unique customs, languages, and beliefs. Dominant characteristics within the majority of Native American groups include orientation to the present, regard for the elderly, strong family ties, belief in herbal or folk medicine, and use of medicine men or women. Native Americans have little regard for the future. Historically, many tribes did not have a word for time. Illness is

seen as an imbalance of forces or the result of some violation of taboo or witchcraft. Germ theory is not understood, many tribes do not have a word for germ.

Navajo Indians do not shake hands, they lightly tap the extended hand. The extended family is the family norm, with elders acting as the family leader. Navajo Indians do not touch the body or belongings of a deceased person. Wisdom and tradition are very important. Good health is believed to be a balance between the spiritual and social worlds. Health care is a combination of traditional religious practices and Western health care. Explicit explanations are important. Lactose intolerance is common among Navajo Indians. There is some indication they metabolize alcohol differently, which may contribute to the incidence of alco-

Table **5-3**	**Religions, Health Practices, and Death Rites**	
Religion	Health practices	Death rites
Buddhism	May follow vegetarian diet.	Cover body with a sheet, do not touch with hand. Do not close the mouth or eyes, leave body as it is at death.
Catholicism	Abstain from meat on Friday. Contraception and abortion are condemned.	Sacrament of Anointing of the Sick is given to those suffering serious illness or infirmity and is especially important at the time of death. Organ donation supported, autopsies permitted.
Christian Science	Do not use drugs or blood transfusions and accept only those immunizations required by law.	
Church of God	Encourage observation of clean and unclean meat described in Bible.	
Church of Jesus Christ of Latter Day Saints	Do not smoke or drink alcohol, tea, or coffee. May wear special garments.	
Hare Krishna	Abstain from eating meat, fish, and eggs. Do not drink, gamble, or engage in sex outside marriage.	
Hinduism	Strict vegetarian or may not eat beef, pork, or eggs.	Prefer to die at home. Atmosphere at death must be peaceful. Body must be attended until cremation. Nuptial threads or amulets worn by married women should not be removed until just before death. Autopsy is not favored. Before 130 days, fetus treated as discarded tissue, afterwards as fully developed human being.
Islam	Do not eat pork or products made from pork. Abstain from all intoxicants. Only women should care for women. Only cotton pads should be provided after delivery.	After death, eyes gently shut, mouth closed with bandage, and arms and legs straightened.
Jehovah's Witness	Do not accept blood transfusions.	Organ donation not supported.
Judaism	May follow strict kosher diet. Amputated parts must be buried.	Burial should take place within 24 hours. Body should not be left unattended until burial. Cremation is not acceptable.
Salvation Army	Abstain from alcohol, tobacco, and nonprescription drugs.	
Seventh Day Adventist	Abstain from alcohol, tobacco, and drugs found in colas, tea, and coffee.	

From Ontario Multifaith Council on Spiritual and Religious Care (1995).

holism in this group. Common health problems include heart disease, diabetes mellitus, and cirrhosis.

Vietnamese

Vietnamese consider public display of affection inappropriate; however, members of the same sex may hold hands in public while walking. Vietnamese are uncomfortable with confrontation and may respond to questions with the term "ya," which means they heard what was said. Often mistaken for "yes," ya does not mean they understand or agree with what was said.

Three or four generations usually live in one household with health care decisions made by the oldest family member. Family name is always written first followed by given name. A woman's breasts are considered functional organs for breastfeeding; however, lower torso from waist to knees is considered extremely private and remains covered at all times. Males are not circumcised. Colostrum is considered poisonous to the newborn, so breastfeeding does not begin until the mother produces milk. Vietnamese believe the head is a spiritual pointer, so they frown upon touching the top of a child's head. Complimenting a newborn may lead to its capture by evil spirits. Dating usually begins in the late teens, but marriage is discouraged until the twenties.

Vietnamese also believe illness is caused by "bad winds." Coin rubbing and other dermal abrasive practices are used to release winds and restore health. There is a strong belief in herbal, or "cool," medicines so illness is usually managed at home. Physicians are not questioned or expected to explain treatment. Requests for pain medications are usually made only for severe pain. Tuberculosis is a common health problem.

RELIGION

Spiritual expression is often associated with culture. Major religions recognized around the world include Buddhism, Christianity, Hinduism, Islam, and Judaism, with numerous denominations and other religions also practiced. The emergency nurse cannot assess and treat the patient without consideration of the person's religious or spiritual beliefs. Each religion has specific beliefs and tenets, some of which relate to health and death. A brief review of selected health practices and death rites is offered as a superficial introduction to these issues in Table 5-3. Emergency nurses are encouraged to expand their knowledge of these and other religions practiced in their area.

SUMMARY

Cultural groups have unique communication, social, and cultural needs. Recognition of and respect for cultural differences is the first step toward acceptance and, we hope, cultural harmony. Regardless of personal views, the emergency nurse should treat each patient with respect and dignity.

REFERENCES

1. Good D: *Compton's encyclopedia,* New York, 1995, Compton's New-Media.
2. Leininger M: *Transcultural care, diversity and universality: a theory of nursing, Nurs Health Care* 6(4):209, 1985.

SUGGESTED READING

Geissler EM: *Pocket guide to cultural assessment,* St. Louis, 1994, Mosby.

Giger JN, Davidhizar RE: *Transcultural nursing: assessment and intervention,* St. Louis, 1995, Mosby.

Ontario Multifaith Council on Spiritual and Religious Care: *Multifaith information manual,* Toronto, Ontario, 1995, The Council.

Skabelund GP, Sims SM, editors: *Culturgrams,* Brigham Young University, Utah, 1995, David M Kennedy Center for International Studies.

unit II

PROFESSIONAL PRACTICE

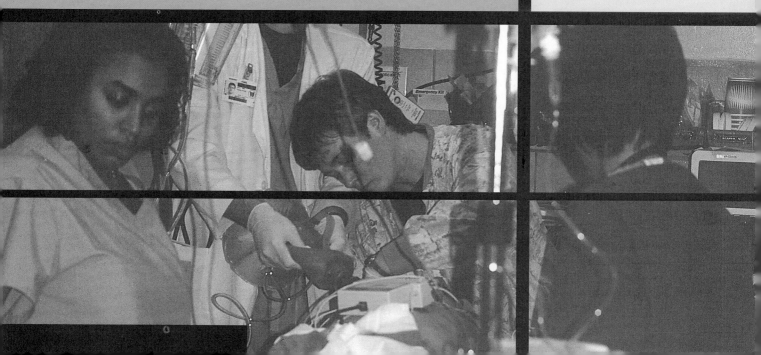

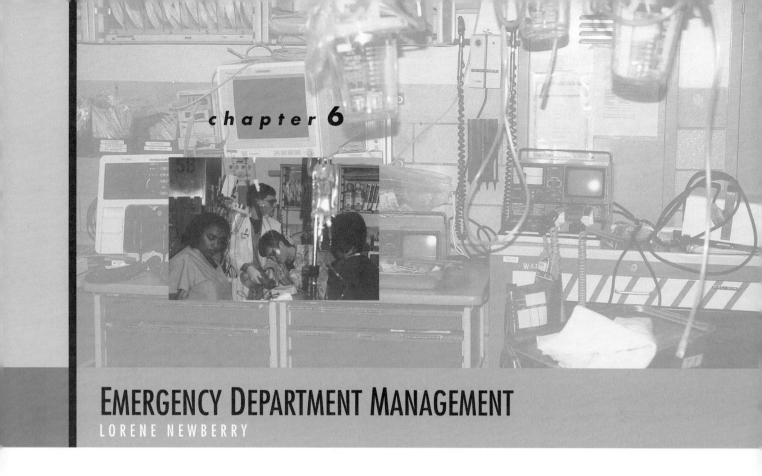

chapter **6**

EMERGENCY DEPARTMENT MANAGEMENT

LORENE NEWBERRY

Emergency department (ED) management is one of the most exciting, challenging fields in health care today. The impact of managed care on the ED is significant. Triage from the ED to another care source, visit authorization, and capitation are just a few areas the ED manager must consider in today's health care arena. Increasing need to communicate frequent changes while controlling costs affects not only fiscal performance, but personnel.

People who work in EDs are unique and challenging to manage; most do not like routine, enjoy bringing order out of chaos, are motivated, aggressive, and not content in a static environment. Keeping pace with an ever-changing field and with people who are easily bored is a challenging but rewarding job.

Today's ED manager must utilize strong organizational skills, effective interpersonal communication skills, and sound financial principles. The purpose of this chapter is not to prepare the emergency nurse to become an ED manager, but to provide an overview of managerial components to enhance communication between front line staff and ED management.

Organizational components of ED management, including goal setting, problem solving, and dealing with structure and change are provided in the first half of the chapter; management of people is discussed in the second half. More emphasis is placed on people than components because interpersonal issues are universal whereas organizational components vary significantly.

ORGANIZATIONAL COMPONENTS

An organization is a collection of people and processes that has an established system of performance. A collection of the most talented, motivated people in the world fails without a system for guiding their efforts. Without a system, confusion and chaos occur and overall output significantly decreases. For example, without a system for scheduling, most administrative time would be spent looking for people to work. Imagine a medical record without specific areas labeled for what should be recorded—time would be wasted trying to locate patient name, address, and orders. These same principles apply to less obvious areas, including goal setting and problem solving.

Organized systems for scheduling supply maintenance, staff distribution, and performance appraisal minimize confusion related to these and other essential processes. A systematic approach should also be used for identification and prioritization of departmental goals and performance problems.

Goals and Objectives

In emergency care, the only constant is change—usually rapid and often dramatic. Medical care changes, health care systems change, prehospital care changes—nothing seems to stabilize for more than a few days. Fighting daily "fires" can consume managerial hours and energy to the point that long-term goals are never met. Management by crisis does not allow personal or departmental growth. Conscious attention to identification of long-range goals and assessment of goal attainment is the most appropriate way to ensure consistent performance and growth for the manager and the department.

Goal-setting for the ED requires a cooperative effort among nurses, physicians, and hospital administration. Goals established independently may create multiple projects activated simultaneously, resulting in staff frustration, stress, and confusion. Without cooperation and consensus, team members may not understand or support objectives. Without front line support, projects may flounder, fail, and worsen an existing problem.

The first step in goal-setting is to define strategic goals for the department. Strategic goals represent the department's overall philosophy. Examples of overall strategic goals are "provide optimal emergency care"; "meet needs of all client groups"; and "provide opportunities for professional advancement."

An ED should have no more than five overall strategic goals. These philosophic goals represent the department's reason for existence and provide the basis for all other goal setting. Outlining these philosophies is therefore a very important part of the goal-setting process. Overall strategic goals are not revised annually.

Annual strategic goals, defined in writing, relate to one or more philosophic goals. For example, "ensure appropriate initial patient screening" is an annual goal and related directly to the overall goal of providing optimal emergency care. "Minimize patient processing time" is a goal that relates to meeting needs of the patient client group. Annual strategic goals represent *where you want to be* and therefore require that you first know where you are. A variety of tools are used to determine departmental status related to personnel, resources, volume, and service area.

Goal identification requires commitment, compromise, and common sense from those involved. Goals should be realistic and achievable. Tackling laboratory and radiology delays, medical record problems, new ED charts, facility redesign, and care of multiple trauma patients all in 1 year will result in frustration and discouragement at year's end. Two or three major goals should be set each year with a few minor goals set as needed.

Tactical objectives. Once annual goals have been identified, each goal should be broken down into tactical objectives. Writing objectives helps determine the cause of the deficiency and assists in resolution. "Ensure thorough documentation of all cardiac arrests" is an excellent goal, but the statement is insufficient basis for action. Telling staff to "improve your CPR documentation" will not be well received or prove productive. Tactical objectives for this goal may include:

- Establish criteria for CPR documentation
- Review 20 CPR charts and compare with criteria
- Assess cause of deficiency
- Implement staff education and charting format to correct deficiency
- Review results

A final step in the goal-setting process is formulation of the task outline, a listing of specific activities necessary to meet each objective. Each objective should have a task outline; however, outlines are not necessarily formal, typed, and submitted to a committee. Outlines can be jotted down and kept for reference so that as one step is completed, you can move rapidly to the next.

Goal setting is essential. No one can keep up with changes and new regulations and maintain systems already in progress unless an organized system for doing so exists.

Problem Identification and Resolution

Problem identification is more difficult than resolution. Once reasons for a deficiency are determined, correcting that deficiency, although sometimes tedious and time consuming, is usually easier than problem identification.

Many opportunities exist in ED management, problems abound and proliferate, and much effort is directed toward resolving them. Inadequately trained staff may be a barrier to appropriate patient triage; medicines in nonlockable cabinets may be a barrier to Joint Commission on Accreditation of Healthcare Organizations (JCAHO) approval; and personnel conflicts are barriers to teamwork. Each barrier represents an opportunity to use skill and creativity. Resolution requires not only problem identification but also differentiation of people problems from organizational, system, and process problems. Symptoms of the problem usually appear as difficulty with people, although the real problem may be the system.

Low morale is a symptom of disease, not the disease itself. High staff attrition rates are often symptoms of job dissatisfaction. Similarly, decrease in thorough charting with increased patient census may be a symptom of inadequate staffing. Problem resolution should focus on the problem not the symptom. Weekly requests for better charting will not produce results if there are simply not enough people to care for patients and thoroughly document that care at the same time. Working on symptoms alone does not produce long-term results and is a waste of valuable time.

Much is blamed on people when the system is at fault. Saying that a staff member does not care about doing proper chest compression is unfair if that person has never had basic life saving (BLS) or has not practiced for several years. Criticizing staff members for not reporting deficiencies when they have never seen results of their reporting is also unfair. Adequate documentation can be expected only if "adequate documentation" has been concretely outlined. Many complaints about inadequate performance can be traced to inadequate education, poor feedback, or poorly designed systems rather than laziness or apathy.

The cause of a significant decrease in overall output, efficiency, or effectiveness in a department is not likely to be that all staff members suddenly quit caring. Even isolated, person-specific deficiencies result from poor orientation or lack of positive feedback. When the manager has hired reasonably intelligent, well-intentioned people, probably 90% of all problems are system related.

A simple mechanism for differentiating symptom from disease and identifying people problems and system problems is to follow statements about problems with *because*.

- Morale is low *because* . . .
- Patients are leaving without a medical examination *because* . . .
- Theresa was rude *because* . . .
- Charting is inadequate *because* . . .

Use of *because* starts the thought process on the path to identifying the true problem. This technique should be taken to its conclusion. For instance, morale is low *because* there has not been enough feedback *because* the head nurse has not had time *because* there were too many simultaneous projects *because* of poor planning. Only when taken to the final stage can the real problem be determined. When looking for real problems, you only rarely arrive at *becauses* that end with laziness, apathy, or bad attitude. Even when you do, personal problems (family, school, money) usually have caused the behavior in a particular individual.

Once the problems have been identified, proceed to resolution decisions. Problems and solutions come in many sizes. Solutions range from 3-minute chats to 12-month projects, while some problems warrant "waiting it out."

When resolving problems, take care not to overtreat or undertreat the disease. The same type of decisions should be made as when caring for patients. A complete blood count, urinalysis, blood sugar, blood gases, electrolytes, radiographs, and lung scan on an emotionally upset patient with rapid respirations, numbness, and tingling relieved by paper bag breathing are costly and time-consuming overtreatment. Another example of overtreatment is a 12-person conference for an isolated abrupt exchange between staff members.

Conversely, a young patient with sudden onset severe headache and no prior history should not be sent home without neurologic examination. Similarly, a staff member going berserk during a cardiac arrest should not be written off as a "bad day."

Resolving deficiencies calls for common sense and good judgment. No one is always right in the decision-making process, so flexibility is essential. Treatment should fit the disease.

Administrative Structure

Finding the administrative structure that meets department needs is one of the greatest challenges faced by the manager. Administrative structure refers to assignment of responsibilities for people and functions—that entity on which organizational charts are based. A traditional administrative structure is presented in Figure 6-1.

Each staff category has defined area(s) of responsibility. No one structure works in every environment, so several attempts may be necessary to identify the best method of op-

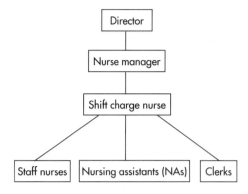

Figure **6-1**   Traditional administrative structure.

eration. Three consistent guidelines in developing an appropriate method for operating a department include identification of needs, creativity, and matching people with functions.

Defining needs in administrative structure is often instinctive, a "feeling" that certain activities are inefficient, not thorough, or inadequate. Feeling pressured for time indicates poor time organization, need for additional administrative help, or need to redistribute some duties.

One common error made when developing a management system is the tendency to see what is and not what could be. Tradition says that an official charge nurse is on each shift, that supervisors order supplies, and that only social workers do social service functions. Many managers are unable to clear out these tradition cobwebs and look at alternatives without preconceived ideas about the structure. After needs are identified, brainstorming and use of creative thinking about activities and categories can broaden available options.

Controversy exists over whether job responsibilities should be defined and someone sought to fulfill those responsibilities, or whether available resources should be used and people matched to responsibilities. In the real world a combination of both approaches is appropriate.

Matching people and functions is a challenge that can result in an odd distribution of duties. Everyone has areas of talent as well as areas of weakness. Compulsive superorganizers may not be outstanding in interpersonal relationships and vice versa. Some people are good teachers but cannot develop a budget. Matching combines the right people with the right job and balances talent in the department as a whole.

MANAGEMENT OF PEOPLE

The best systems developed are worthless without a manager with the ability to manage people. People run the system; the right people run it better. Placing the right people in a good system and managing them effectively produces an outstanding department.

People are complex. Much of what motivates them and causes them to respond so differently from each other is not well understood. Being responsible for a group of people, although frustrating, is also an incredible challenge and one of the most exciting parts of management. Information presented here is primarily a philosophy of management, although some "how-to" advice is included. The intent here is to convey concepts. People and leadership styles differ and each manager must develop his or her own specific techniques for dealing with other people.

Motivation

Inherent to people management is the necessity to motivate the individual. Intelligent individuals with significant potential for growth can be mediocre performers without motivation. Theories for staff motivation include hierarchy of needs, N Ach theory, expectancy theory, and motivation-hygiene theory.

Motivational theories

Hierarchy of needs. Maslow[2] identified five needs that serve as motivators (Figure 6-2). To understand the hierarchy, two basic assumptions must be accepted.

- A need emerges only when lower level needs have been met. An individual has little concern for self-actualization when having severe difficulty breathing.
- More than one need may operate simultaneously, but only one dominates.

Most managers are primarily concerned with the top two or three needs in the hierarchy. Physiologic and safety needs are generally adequately met in the work environment, so attention is directed toward higher motivational levels.

N Ach theory. McClelland[3] discusses what divides people in the world into two broad groups, "There is that minority which is challenged by opportunity and willing to work hard to achieve something and the majority which really does not care all that much." This minority, those with a high *n*eed for *ach*ievement (n Ach) are still a puzzle to psychologic researchers. According to McClelland, need for achievement is "a distinct human motive, distinguishable

from others."[3] People who score high in n Ach testing share several characteristics.

- Set moderately high, but achievable, goals for themselves.
- Respond only if they can influence outcome by doing work themselves.
- Show strong preferences for situations in which results of their effort are readily visible.
- Look for ways to "do things better."

No concrete answers can yet explain why certain people seem to have a higher level of n Ach than others. However, "evidence suggests it is not because they are born that way, but because of special training they get in the home from parents who set moderately high achievement goals, but who are warm, encouraging, and nonauthoritarian in helping their children reach these goals."[4] Can n Ach be increased in a given individual? McClelland's research suggests that it is possible to change an individual's thinking process and increase his or her need for achievement.

Expectancy theory. Developed by Vroom,[5] expectancy theory states that workers' motivation depends primarily on what they perceive as the result of a given behavior and the value they place on these results. For instance, if a staff nurse highly values promotion to charge nurse and believes that demonstrating commitment (e.g., schedule flexibility and educational participation) will produce desired promotion, she or he will probably be motivated to work extra shifts and attend lectures. A staff nurse who is content as a staff nurse and has no desire for promotion will probably have less motivation (or at least different motives) to put in additional time and energy. Vroom's theory therefore suggests that employees can be motivated by changing how they perceive *value* of the outcome of their behavior.

Motivation-hygiene theory. The motivation-hygiene theory developed by Herzberg[1] divides worker motivation into satisfiers (motivators) and dissatisfiers (hygiene or maintenance factors). When hygiene factors (dissatisfiers) are inadequate or absent, the result is worker dissatisfaction. Dissatisfiers are factors such as working conditions (lighting, space, and so on), salaries, relationships with management and co-workers, and company policies. If these factors or conditions are inadequate, the employee will be dissatisfied. Adequacy in all hygiene factors does *not*, however, produce motivated employees. Even if salary is adequate, co-worker and management relationships are good, working conditions acceptable, and company policies reasonable, the employee is not *necessarily* motivated to achieve or contribute.

Satisfiers (motivators) are such factors as achievement, responsibility, recognition, the work itself, and promotion. If these factors are available in the environment, employee satisfaction and motivation occur.

Motivation techniques. Managers do not study motivation theory solely to understand why people *do not* produce. Clearly the goal is to find motivation methods that encourage greater efficiency and productivity. Motivation is *not* a

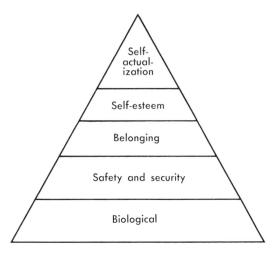

Figure **6-2** Maslow's hierarchy of needs. *(From Maslow A: Toward a psychology of being, New York, 1962, D Van Nostrand.)*

single interaction with another person, annual performance review, or once-a-week pat on the back, but should be an integral part of management style. When motivation is a natural outgrowth of what the manager thinks about people, techniques are easier to use.

Communication. We are naturally social creatures, so communication, verbal and nonverbal, is an integral part of our daily lives and of a motivational system. Communication is vital to motivation, and should include expectations, feedback, constructive criticism, recognition, and goals.

If you want complete vital signs on every patient but do not tell anyone, staff should not be criticized for failure to obtain these vital signs. Criteria used to make judgments about staff performance should be clearly defined and relayed to staff. The key here is for the manager to ensure expectations are clearly understood *without* creating a dictatorial atmosphere.

Any question or suggestion deserves a prompt response. When a staff member takes the time (and possibly has the good sense) to question a procedure or recommend improvement, a reply should be given as soon as possible. Even the worst suggestions warrant discussion and explanation of why they will not work.

Another area of feedback is constructive criticism. Staff should not be presented at their performance review with a list of errors that have not been previously discussed. Everyone makes mistakes, but timely discussion of these mistakes has the most positive result. Rules for constructive criticism that should never be broken are:

- *Never* criticize or reprimand an employee in the presence of others.
- *Always* ask for the person's version of the story. A logical explanation may exist for what you observed or heard from others.
- *Always* explain why the action was an error. People remember a correction if they understand the rationale behind it.

Recognition should be an integral part of motivational style. When was the last time you complimented someone on his or her handling of a difficult patient? When did you last express appreciation to a nurse, technician, or clerk who *always* does assigned duties? We all need recognition for accomplishments—large and small. *Take* time to notice and communicate. If someone makes a suggestion or unusual contribution, publicly recognize the effort.

The last communication practice in motivation, communication of goals, is often ignored. If you expect to receive support from staff, they must know the goal. Communicating goals includes *all* goals—from overall departmental goals for the year to the reason for instituting a new procedure. Again, people cooperate if the rationale is clear. If you are talking about departmental goals, explain mechanisms that will be used to accomplish the goal. For instance, if a goal for the year is to improve clerical efficiency, explain that you are planning to preprint the patient number on the charts and add an imprint maker, rather than make clerks work harder.

Staff involvement. The second component of a motivational system is staff involvement. To effectively involve staff members in growth and progress of the department, the manager should understand why and how.

Why should the staff be involved? The first reason is based on Herzberg's theory,[1] which states that satisfiers (motivators) are recognition, responsibility, and the work itself. Most of us are more enthusiastic about a project in which we have had direct input. Involving staff in goal setting and decision making also gives them some control over their work environment. Very few people respond positively to dictatorial leadership.

Secondly, staff should be involved because managers are not all-knowing. Unfortunately, no magic answers go with promotion. Experience, usually by trial and error, may have taught managers how *not* to do things, but they are not the only source of good ideas. Effective managers find good people and determine how best to utilize their talents.

How should the staff be involved? Every staff member is, at some level, "involved" in the progress of a department, either as a hindrance or help to progress. The adage "if you are not part of the solution, you are part of the problem" is true. Rarely is anyone a neutral force. Every time someone "complains," he or she is involved in identifying barriers to a goal. Although the barrier may be of a person's own making, it is still a barrier. Allowing individuals to be an asset to progress requires managerial skill and patience, but the benefits far outweigh the disadvantages.

Use of the word "allowing" is not accidental. Remember that managers do not "get" people involved, managers allow the individual to express a natural inclination, and establish mechanisms that encourage expression of that inclination.

What are the department's goals? Every member of the ED team should be able to list department goals—both ongoing, permanent goals and specific objectives for the year. One key to establishing successful mechanisms for staff involvement is ensuring that everyone knows the goals. When new staff members are oriented, they should be given a clear picture of overall philosophy of the department. When specific yearly, monthly, or weekly objectives are established, they should be shared with all members of the team.

Are the staff member's goals and departmental goals compatible? Everyone who seeks employment in your department probably has a reason for choosing that specific area. A critical care nurse may want to broaden his or her base of experience, a nursing student may want more clinical exposure, and a clerk may want exposure to health care to assist in future career decisions. Some staff may be looking for an exciting way to support their ski habit.

The manager's responsibility is to combine staff goals specific to emergency care with personal goals of *all* individuals and departmental goals in such a way that all can be fulfilled. This is no easy task, but is not as difficult as it may sound. Meeting these objectives simultaneously offers the manager another creative opportunity.

Methods established to promote involvement of staff members range from allowing staff to help establish annual objectives to allowing them to decide how to remove blood from the wall before the next trauma patient arrives. Opportunities for input and assistance are endless and vary from department to department, year to year, and individual to individual. The manager is responsible for creating methods best suited for the environment. Methods include assigning specific projects, establishing a mentor program for new employees, and soliciting ideas from staff.

Scheduling

Emergency care is stressful—mentally, physically, and emotionally. Scheduling operations for 24 hours a day, 365 days a year is not an easy task. When staff members are vacationing or ill, EDs do not have the luxury of working "short." Trying to fill every position every day tends to create rules and leads to decreased sensitivity to individual needs and differences. Dissatisfaction with work schedules can lead to decreased productivity, increased attrition, and low morale. Staffing schedules should be fair, consistent, and ensure patient safety while meeting individual needs and preferences. Indiscriminate use of power over the schedule can precipitate a critical morale level.

Create a staffing plan that meets ebb and flow of ED volume. When most patients arrive between 11 AM and 11 PM, scheduling the same number of staff around the clock is neither cost-effective or productive. Involve staff in determination of essential shifts. Consider various shift options including 6-, 8-, 10-, and 12-hour shifts. Post schedules early to allow staff to plan their personal time. Utilize written requests for days off or trade requests between staff to minimize variability and avoid claims of favoritism.

Self-scheduling has appeared as an option to increase staff control over their day-to-day schedules; however, ultimate control and responsibility still remain with the nurse manager. A 6-week schedule is posted for 2 weeks, during which full-time and part-time staff pencil in their desired schedule. After 2 weeks, per diem and on-call nurses may sign up to fill gaps in the schedule. After another week the nurse manager or designee reviews schedules to ensure that everyone is fulfilling their commitment for hours. Then the manager negotiates with staff to cover remaining gaps. Self-scheduling is not a perfect answer to scheduling dilemmas, but it is an option that increases staff nurse autonomy.

Performance Appraisal

Performance appraisal can be a motivating experience for both staff and reviewer when done in a positive, constructive manner. If not done appropriately, review can be a frightening, negative experience for staff and an energy drain for the reviewer. Performance appraisal is both formal and informal.

Formal performance appraisal is a structured method of looking at accomplishments and function. The most common mistake made in interpreting this definition is assuming the review process is a one-sided monologue. Good reviews are dialogues. Specific objectives are to establish rapport, discuss individual goals and how to achieve and provide feedback on performance, educate staff, and obtain feedback from employees related to the department and the management. These objectives should be included in each performance appraisal and documented for the personnel file. Most institutions use standardized assessment tools based on the job description to structure assessment and document performance.

Informal performance appraisal refers to casual assessment of performance. More specifically, informal reviews are discussions of single incidents or transient attitudes. Informal reviews take on many forms, including anecdotal records or casual queries such as "I heard there was a problem with the lab last night—what happened?" Informal reviews are conducted daily, even though we may not identify them as such. They are not restricted to discussing problems and negative behaviors. Informal reviews should be balanced with compliments and pats on the back. The process of informal review includes data collection, correction of misunderstandings, identification of desired future actions, and maintenance of daily contact with staff.

SUMMARY

A brief review of managerial concepts has been provided. Those interested in ED management are encouraged to expand knowledge of these and other essential skills through research and mentoring.

REFERENCES

1. Herzberg F: Dual-factor theory of job satisfaction, *Personnel Psychol,* Winter 1967.
2. Maslow AH: *Motivation and personality,* New York, 1954, Harper & Row.
3. McClelland D: That urge to achieve, *Think Magazine,* 1966.
4. Swansburg RC: *Introductory management and leadership for clinical nurses: a text-workbook,* Boston, 1993, Jones & Bartlett.
5. Vroom V: *Work and motivation,* New York, 1964, John Wiley & Sons.

look," observations should become specific, focusing on the immediate complaint and the specific system being evaluated first.

Auscultation. A stethoscope is used to identify sounds produced by various arteries, organs, and tissues. It does not amplify sounds but transmits them to the user's ear while reducing external noise interference. The diaphragm is useful when auscultating high-pitched sounds; the bell is employed to hear low-pitched sounds. But if too much pressure is applied to the bell against the skin, the bell acts like a diaphragm, and low-frequency sounds will not be appreciated.

Auscultated sounds are described in terms of pitch, intensity, duration, and quality. Noting presence or absence of sounds or deviation from normal sounds assists in the development of a diagnosis. Respiratory, cardiovascular, and gastrointestinal systems are routinely auscultated during examination. Findings for each are discussed in more detail later in this chapter under the Review of Systems.

Palpation. Hands become important tools when palpating skin temperature, skin texture, vibrations and pulsations, masses or lesions, muscle tenseness or rigidity, and deformities. Different parts of the hand are better equipped to feel different sensations. The dorsum of the hand is more sensitive to temperature changes, whereas the palm is more sensitive to vibratory sensations. Fingers are sensitive to touch, but sensation can be diminished by increasing pressure on fingertips, so light palpation is generally preferred to deep palpation. Pressure changes are used to palpate and distinguish one organ from another or to define the borders of organs. During examination of the abdomen, light palpation is generally followed by deep palpation in the process of identifying abdominal contents.

The preferred technique in light palpation is to use the fingertips of one hand to distinguish hard from soft, rough from smooth, and muscle tone. The preferred technique in deep palpation is to place the fingertips of one hand over and slightly forward of the fingertips of the other hand, which is placed over the area to be palpated. Both hands are used to press firmly and deeply over the area. Palpation with both hands can be employed to fix an organ in place with one hand while palpating its borders with the other, or by using one hand to entrap the organ between the fingertips.

Percussion. This is a technique for eliciting vibrations that can be heard and felt when a portion of the body is struck with the examiner's hand or fingers. The extent of the vibration varies depending on density, position, and size of the tissue underlying the area being percussed. Percussion is helpful in outlining borders of an organ, identifying pain and tenderness within an area of the body, identifying fluid within an organ or cavity, and evaluating lung fields for the presence of consolidation, fluid, or air.

Generally, sounds are described in terms of pitch, duration, intensity, and quality. Pitch is determined by the speed with which vibrations travel through the body, strike an organ, and bounce back to the examiner's fingers. When an organ is close to the skin surface, the pitch is *high* (not to be confused with *loud*) and is a result of the vibrations being returned rapidly to the examiner. Duration is the time a vibration lasts and is dictated by distance of the organ from the skin surface, and thus the amount of time available for the vibration to exist. A fairly solid tissue transmits a sound of short duration, whereas a hollow organ transmits a sound of reasonably long duration. Intensity of sound is assessed as loudness or softness of the sound heard when an area is percussed. A solid organ transmits a soft sound when percussed because the vibrations are traveling little if at all. The quality of the sound defines what type of organ is making the sound. For example, when the chest is percussed, a certain sound is heard if lungs are normal and the alveoli are inflated with air. This sound is described as *resonant* and has a different quality than would be heard if the chest was filled with bowel instead of normal aerated lung.

Bone produces a flat percussion note, so percussion is not usually carried out in areas where bone overlies cavities or organs. In addition, the deeper the organ, the more the sound is transmitted by the tissue lying above it, rather than the organ being evaluated. An organ that lies more than 5 cm below the surface is usually not detectable by percussion. Therefore trying to evaluate a kidney using the anterior approach to percussion is generally not helpful.

Finally, the patient's body must always be compared from side to side when eliciting percussion notes. Comparison makes it much easier to recognize normal sounds for each patient, and it helps distinguish changes in quality from organ to organ. If sounds are subtle, moving from side to side helps distinguish and differentiate what is being heard.

Olfaction. Olfaction can provide valuable patient information. Certain conditions are associated with specific odors, such as the smell of ketones in the breath of patients with diabetic ketoacidosis. Abnormal smells may also alert the nurse that the patient has been exposed to various agents (e.g., gasoline, alcohol, smoke, marijuana, cigarettes). Finally, the presence of some odors suggest that the patient has an infection or poor personal hygiene. Again, these findings must be considered in light of other assessment data.

Consultation

Invaluable information regarding the patient's status can be obtained from sources outside the ED. Obtaining previous medical records may provide not only past medical history, but also medications, previous assessment findings, abnormalities, and pertinent social information. An additional source of information is health care providers who have interacted with the patient in the past (e.g., private physician, home health nurses, health care workers in clinics, and hospital staff who have provided frequent or long-term care for a patient). Health care providers may offer valuable information not necessarily documented anywhere, but known from frequent interactions with the patient.

rates and in light of the clinical situation. Systolic pressure is a measurement of pump integrity; diastolic pressure is a measurement of vascular status. Normal pressures measured in the ED are not necessarily an indication that all is well. As previously mentioned, a healthy person may not exhibit signs of low circulating volume until all compensatory mechanisms have been exhausted. A change in position can cause a precipitous drop in pressure. Thus, anyone suspected of volume depletion should be evaluated for *postural vital sign* (orthostatic) changes. Box 12-3 discusses the procedure for orthostatic or postural vital signs.

If significant findings occur during a change to the sitting position, this test is considered positive for significant volume deficit. Fluid replacement should begin with volume expanders such as Ringer's lactate solution, normal saline solution, or other solutions appropriate for the situation. The source of volume depletion must be identified and controlled. If the sitting portion of the postural vital sign examination is positive, the standing portion may be deferred, since it will not yield additional information and may prove detrimental to the patient. If equivocal changes from lying to sitting exist or no changes occur at all, the patient should be moved to a standing position unless this change is contraindicated (e.g., in the case of a fractured leg). Positive findings are the same as those described for the sitting position.

Whenever evaluating blood pressure values, the findings are considered in relationship to the patient's history. If the patient is undergoing antihypertensive therapy, the values obtained during the ED visit may represent a significant deviation relative to the patient's "normal" pressure. Pulse pressure (the difference between systolic and diastolic pressures) represents the approximate stroke volume when all other variables are constant. Peripheral vascular resistance and elasticity of the vessel walls are critical determinants of the pulse pressure; therefore, approximating the stroke volume by measuring pulse pressure is more qualitative than accurate. However, the pulse pressure provides information about the status of the pump and the peripheral vessels, and indicates otherwise subtle hemodynamic changes.

Blood pressure can be obtained by auscultation, palpation, or with a Doppler depending on patient condition and the environment. Palpation does not provide information about the diastolic pressure (i.e., the peripheral vascular system), and the method used for assessment should be communicated so that others who obtain the pressure use the same method or correlate findings from another method. A single blood pressure recording yields little or no information. Serial pressures must be measured to monitor the hemodynamic status. Values are also affected by incorrect cuff size.

All vital signs must be taken and evaluated serially. The patient's condition is a continuum that can be assessed only through constant monitoring. Whenever therapy is instituted, all vital signs should be evaluated to assess the efficacy of treatment. Also, the vital signs should be repeated before a decision is made about disposition of the patient from the ED (discharged, admitted, or transferred to another facility).

Laboratory and other diagnostics. Laboratory and other diagnostic values described in Chapter 15 and elsewhere in this book are additional measurements obtained during patient assessment. They are interpreted in light of other parameters obtained during the assessment process.

Observation

Several techniques are involved in physical examination of any patient. The pattern of use varies with the body system being evaluated. With experience, the emergency nurse develops a routine for doing appropriate assessments in a timely manner.

Inspection. This is a key examination technique because observations obtained from visual inspection of the patient as a whole and of each system in particular help integrate what the patient says with what the physical appearance suggests. Inspection must always precede other techniques.

The emergency nurse first evaluates the patient's general appearance. Is the patient unkempt, malnourished, well groomed, or overweight? Does the patient appear to take good care of himself or herself? Or does he or she have poor hygiene? These observations help relate the general appearance to the illness. Checking the condition of the mucous membranes gives information about oxygenation and hydration. Observing body movement and posture provides information about pain, mental status, and mood, as well as clues to degree of debilitation. After this general "quick

Box **12-3**	**Orthostatic Vital Signs**		
Description	**Purpose**	**Indication**	**Significant findings**
BP and pulse supine, sitting, and/or standing with less than 1 minute between each value	Identify patients with potential volume deficits that have led to compensatory mechanisms such as severe vasoconstriction.	Patients with syncopal episode, dehydration, history of prolonged vomiting, diarrhea, sweating, diuretic therapy, gastrointestinal bleeding, burns, or obvious blood loss	Subjective feeling of dizziness or blurred vision. Decrease in blood pressure ≥20 mmHg and/or increase in pulse ≥20 beats per minute.

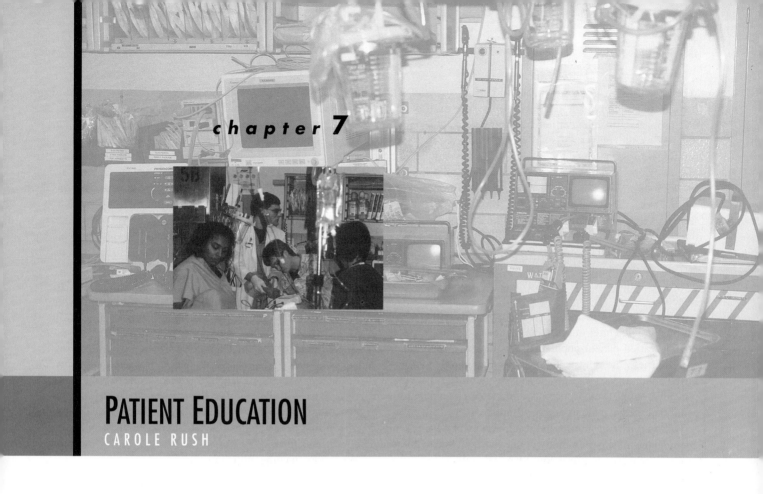

chapter 7

PATIENT EDUCATION
CAROLE RUSH

During the past several years, significant changes have affected the emergency nurse's responsibility for patient teaching. First, patient teaching is explicitly incorporated into the role and responsibilities of the professional emergency nurse as stated in the *Standards of Emergency Nursing Practice* and nurse practice acts of most states, and patient teaching is included in the nursing diagnosis index as "knowledge deficit." Second, documentation of patient teaching is mandated by both quality improvement and accreditation criteria. Third, the variety and sophistication of patient education materials have increased significantly. In the past, most patient education materials were "homemade" mimeographed copies of information chosen by interested nurses. Now, colorful, humorous, informative booklets and videotapes are published or produced by patient education departments and companies. Educational materials are also available from medical supply and pharmaceutical companies. In addition, some learning materials are published in languages other than English and in picture format for patients with limited reading abilities.

Although patient education has traditionally been an accepted component of emergency patient care, emphasis on the need for patient teaching has increased dramatically. Influential factors include fear of litigation, cost containment, and restriction of patient admissions. In many instances, patients formerly admitted from the emergency department (ED) are now treated and sent home. Promulgation of the Patient Bill of Rights by the American Hospital Association

in 1972 informed the public of the right of all hospital patients to be informed of procedures used in providing care, and self-care methods to be used after dismissal. The Patient Bill of Rights has been widely reprinted in the popular press and in some agencies is distributed to all admitted patients. Public awareness of the teaching responsibilities of health care professionals has increased significantly. In addition, the increased educational level of the general public and derogatory publicity regarding errors of omission and commission by health care providers have increased the number of malpractice suits. In an effort to contain rising health care costs, patient admissions have been restricted to those persons with illness or injury defined in specific diagnosis-related groups. Because of this economic situation, many patients formerly admitted are now discharged from the ED with specific instructions for home care and referral for follow-up care.

Compounding the fear of litigation and restricted admission is the public's focus on prevention of illness for both personal and financial reasons. Numerous national advertising campaigns focus on cholesterol control, prevention of heart and lung disease, and occupational and vehicular incidents. Many businesses and industries subscribe to health maintenance organizations that promote illness prevention and health maintenance.

All these efforts are aimed at containing escalating health care costs by decreasing use of hospital care. At the same time, the number of patients seen in EDs has increased.

Whether this increase is due to lack of personal physicians, limited office hours of nonemergency services, transportation problems, or financial reasons, many persons perceive the ED as the only consistently available access to the health care system. Even though numbers and acuity levels of emergency patients are increasing, staffing restrictions resulting from the nursing shortage have affected the ED as much as other hospital departments. Despite staffing shortages and increasing numbers of ED patients, effective patient teaching remains one of the top 10 priorities of local, state, and federal government. Patient education is perceived not only as a patient right but also as a means to contain health care costs and prevent expensive litigation.

Patient teaching in the ED is a special challenge. Constraints and potential impediments to teaching and learning include varied patient populations, multiplicity of illnesses and injuries, the physician, psychoemotionally compromised conditions of patients, various age groups of patients, typically tense ED environments, and increased anxiety levels of emergency patients and their families.

To minimize constraints and teach effectively, the emergency nurse must be familiar with the teaching and learning process, maintain current knowledge and skills regarding a large variety of health problems affecting all age groups, and be able to decrease the patient's anxiety level thus enhancing the learning opportunity. As with the use of any process involving knowledge and skill, familiarity with the sequential steps increases ease and effectiveness. Recall your first attempt at starting an intravenous infusion: initial attempts are awkward. However, repetition and familiarity with the equipment and process quickly improve skill and confidence.

Regardless of the constraints of time, number of patients, or nursing shortage, patient teaching is an integral component of professional emergency nursing care. Because patient teaching in the ED is necessarily "telescoped," that is, it focuses on immediate needs while the patient is provided referral for concomitant long-term care, familiarity with the process of patient teaching is essential.

THE TEACHING AND LEARNING PROCESS

One goal of patient education is to help patients and families cope more effectively with changes in health.[5] Patient education is a process similar to the nursing process. The steps are educational assessment, setting learning goals, planning teaching, implementation of the teaching plan, evaluation of learning, and documentation of teaching and learning.[9] Teaching and learning are two separate entities. Learning does not necessarily follow teaching. In the most general sense, teaching facilitates learning, whereas learning is evident through changes in behavior. Because time is limited in the emergency care setting, completing the patient education process is a challenge.

Educational Assessment

A comprehensive educational assessment of the patient includes assessing the individual, learning needs, learning styles, and readiness to learn. Assessing the individual focuses on special needs, support systems, health expectations, cultural considerations, economic considerations, and personal factors such as values, interests, and motivations. Assessing learning needs includes attention to the patient's current knowledge and personal goals as they affect the patient's health and ability to learn. Learning style is determined by personal preference, literacy level, and the patient's functional ability. The patient's readiness to learn can be assessed using the life stages identified in Erikson's stages of development, the needs level identified in Maslow's hierarchy of needs, the patient's motivation to learn, and any obvious lack of readiness to learn.

Comprehensive educational assessment is not always possible in the emergency care setting; however, interactive discussion with the patient and family throughout the emergency visit will shed light on their educational needs and expectations. The following questions facilitate identification of learning needs and can be adapted to almost any patient education situation.[5]

Why did you come to the hospital?
What did you think was happening?
What has the doctor told you?
What does it mean to you?
Do you know what caused your illness-injury?
How do you think this will change your life?
How has this illness-injury affected your family?
How can we help?

Learning Goals

Learning goals should be realistic, patient-centered, written, and flexible. Prioritize objectives based on what the patient "must know," "should know," and what it is "nice to know." The essentials or "must know" items should be taught first.

Planning Patient Teaching

Even when time is limited, it is possible to develop a teaching plan for patients and their families. Use identified learning needs from the educational assessment to determine what the patient should be taught. Focus on items the patient must know. Use moments throughout the entire visit when the patient's interest level is high and questions are asked. Summarize teaching when the patient is discharged. Remove distractions whenever possible. Make the patient comfortable; a patient in pain is not ready to learn.

In most EDs, discharge teaching occurs in the treatment area. However, some high-volume EDs have separate, centralized discharge areas where patients receive prescriptions, written instructions, and specific referrals for follow-up care. There are advantages and disadvantages for both sys-

---

Box 7-1 **Comparison of Discharge Teaching in Two Locations**

Patient care area	Separate centralized discharge area
Teaching done by primary nurse	Teaching done by nurse not familiar with patient, diagnosis, or care given
Nurse more likely to be familiar with what physician has already taught patient	Staff dedicated to discharge process ensure referrals are made
Overall length of stay may increase	
Overall ED patient flow slowed by patients occupying treatment space waiting for discharge teaching	Separate discharge area improves overall patient flow and may decrease length of stay

---

Table 7-1 **Teaching Media**

Materials	Examples of use
Objects and models	Model of spine to explain back pain
	Model of heart to explain angina
	Plastic food for diabetic diet teaching
Posters mounted in ED patient rooms or laminated for portable use	Back exercises
	Crutch walking
Videos	Show in waiting room to explain appropriate use of ED, describe injury prevention, etc.
Written discharge instructions with visual aids	How to take a child's temperature
	Treatment for vomiting and diarrhea
Toys	Stuffed bear with cast to teach children cast care

---

tems, which are summarized in Box 7-1. An ideal system for a high-volume ED may be a separate discharge room for each treatment area. The patient is moved to the discharge room to await instructions by the primary nurse. The treatment room is not occupied unnecessarily by a patient awaiting discharge instructions, and the patient can still receive discharge instructions from the primary nurse. A small waiting room provides space for the patient to wait for instructions while maintaining privacy.

Patient teaching in the ED is done by nurses and physicians involved in the patient's care. Patient teaching may also involve physiotherapists, respiratory therapists, and dieticians. In a low-volume ED, team teaching may occur. This type of collaborative teaching is less likely to occur in a high-volume ED. Regardless of how the organization provides patient education, all those involved must document the plan of care and teaching provided in the medical record.

Choosing the best method for patient teaching begins with the educational assessment. Discuss what usually works best with the patient and family. Demonstrate psychomotor skills such as crutch walking and dressing changes. Select teaching materials that fit the patient's learning needs, budget, and resources. Table 7-1 provides examples of various teaching media.

Teaching Material

Patient educational material may be developed by staff within the ED, a centralized educational department, or purchased as ready-to-use material from various resource companies including pharmaceutical companies, education groups, or specialty groups such as the American Heart Association, the American Trauma Society, and the American Au-

tomobile Association (AAA). Figure 7-1 is one example of a preprinted education sheet. Figure 7-2 shows the same sheet in Spanish. Computerized discharge instruction sheets are gaining popularity in many areas. There are advantages and disadvantages to each avenue for obtaining educational material.[11,12] Table 7-2 lists the pros and cons for each source.

When developing your own written material, write for a range of grade levels, for example, between the fourth and sixth grade levels.[3,4,5] Write for the level of the institution's population if this is known. Write in the active rather than the passive voice. A conversational style is effective so keep sentences short and express only one idea for each sentence. Use the second person "you" rather than the third person "the patient." Limit the number of words containing three or more syllables, that is, use "doctor" rather than "physician." Present the most important information first with adequate spacing to prevent eye strain. Keep the eye span to no more than 60 to 70 characters. (This sentence's eye span is 45 characters.) All–capital letter text is harder to read and strains the eyes.

Regardless of where educational material is obtained, material should be reviewed before use for applicability to the specific patient population served by the purchaser. Teaching material should be developed with consideration to accuracy, reading level, visuals, and referral information. Content should reflect current health care knowledge and practice and contain what the patient wants to know as well as what the patient needs to know. A question-and-answer format may be useful for patients to sift through and find the

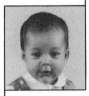

Diarrhea can be dangerous. It drains water and salts from your child. If these are not put back quickly, your child can get dehydrated and may need to be hospitalized. To protect your child follow these steps:

MANAGING DIARRHEA

1. As soon as diarrhea starts, give your child fluids. An oral electrolyte solution is the best fluid to give. This will put the water and salts back into your child's body that are lost with diarrhea.

- You can get these solutions at grocery and drug stores.
- If under 2 years old give ½ cup every hour using a small spoon. Call your doctor or public health clinic.
- If over 2 years old give ½ to 1 cup every hour.
- Keep giving the oral electrolyte solution until the diarrhea stops.
- If your child vomits, continue to give the oral electrolyte solution, using a teaspoon. Give one teaspoon every 2—3 minutes until vomiting stops. Then give regular amount.
- Do **not** give sugary drinks such as Gatorade,® cola drinks or apple juice. They can make your child's diarrhea worse.

2. Continue to feed your child as recommended by your doctor or public health clinic. Food will help your child stay healthy.

- If breast-fed continue to breast feed.
- If on formula continue to give formula.
- If on solid foods continue to give regular diet. Good foods to give include cooked meat, cooked cereal or bananas.

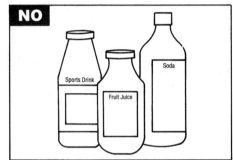

These have the WRONG amounts of water, salts and sugar.

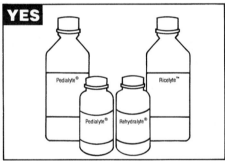

Oral electrolyte solutions have the RIGHT amounts of water, salts and sugar.

Your child may need medical help if the diarrhea is more serious than usual. You should call your doctor or public health clinic immediately if:

- the diarrhea lasts more than 24 hours,
- the diarrhea gets worse,
- there are any signs of dehydration:
  decreased urination
  sunken eyes
  no tears when child cries
  extreme thirst
  unusual drowsiness or fussiness

For more information or additional copies, phone (614) 624-7540.

Figure **7-1** Preprinted education sheet. (*Courtesy The National Oral Rehydration Therapy Project, Ross Products Division, Columbus, Ohio.*)

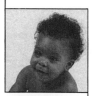

La diarrea puede ser peligrosa. Agota el contenido del agua y de las sales del cuerpo de su hijo. A menos que sean repuestas inmediatamente, su hijo corre el riesgo de deshidratarse y tal vez tenga que ser internado en el hospital. Para evitar esto, haga lo siguiente:

COMO CONTROLAR LA DIARREA

TAN PRONTO COMO empiece la diarrea, déle de tomar líquidos a su hijo. Lo mejor es darle un suero de tomar para la deshidratación (oral electrolyte solution). Esto repone el agua y las sales que ha perdido el cuerpo de su hijo por la diarrea.

- Puede conseguir esta solución en una farmacia o en una tienda de comestibles.
- Si su hijo es menor de 2 años, déle durante cada hora media taza de suero, utilizando una cucharita. Llame a su medico o a la clínica de salud pública.
- Si su hijo es mayor de 2 años, déle al menos la mitad de una taza o la taza entera, durante cada hora.
- Déle de tomar a su hijo el suero hasta que los síntomas de la diarrea desaparezcan.
- No importa si su hijo vomita, siga dándole de tomar el suero en cucharaditas. Déle una cucharadita cada 2 o 3 minutos hasta que deje de vomitar. Vuelva a darle la cantidad indicada según su edad.
- **No le** dé bebidas azucaradas como Gatorade,® refrescos, o jugo de fruta.

SIGA ALIMENTANDO a su hijo de acuerdo a las indicaciones de su médico o de la clínica de salud pública. Una buena alimentación mantiene a su hijo sano.

- Siga dandole pecho.
- Si le da fórmula infantil, siga dándosela.
- Si alimenta a su hijo con comidas sólidas, siga dándole la comida habitual. Entre las comidas indicadas están la carne cocida, los cereales cocidos, fideos o plátanos.

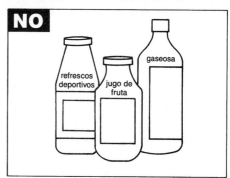

Estos contienen una cantidad
INADECUADA de sales y de azúcar.

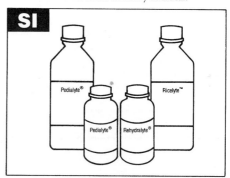

Los sueros de tomar para la deshidratación
(oral electrolyte solutions) contienen una cantidad
ADECUADA de sales y de azúcar.

SEÑAS DE PELIGRO DE LA DIARREA

Su hijo tal vez necesite atención médica si la diarrea es muy fuerte. Llame al médico o a la clínica de salud pública inmediatamente en caso de:
- diarrea que dura más de 24 horas,
- diarrea que empeora,
- síntomas de deshidratación:
  *orinar poco o menos frecuente
  ojos hundidos
  ojos sin lágrimas al llorar
  sed intensa
  demasiado sueño o inquietud*

Para obtener más información o copias adicionales, llama al (614) 624-7540.

*Figure **7-2*** Preprinted Spanish education sheet. (*Courtesy The National Oral Rehydration Therapy Project, Ross Products Division, Columbus, Ohio.*)

Table 7-2 Comparison of Sources for Educational Material

Source	Advantages	Disadvantages
ED staff committee	-Small group can accomplish tasks more quickly than large committee -Group is familiar with patient population and personnel available for teaching	-Group may be isolated from rest of hospital and existing materials due to lack of knowledge of that material -There may be inconsistency of information with material presented on the same subject by other departments -Increased cost to develop small amount of material for the department when compared to bulk order for the institution
Hospital education committee	-Eliminates duplication of efforts within the institution -Assures consistency of information within the institution -Promotes collaboration and contribution of a large number of health care professionals	-Large committee is tedious and takes longer to develop material -Increases production costs due to labor hours required to develop the material
Ready-made material	-Eliminates duplication of efforts and "reinventing the wheel" -May be more cost-effective than developing materials; some companies provide gratuitous products -Institution-wide use of materials helps standardize patient education	-Information may be too generic or basic -Information may conflict with some institutional policies and procedures
Computerized information	-Can be customized with patient name, diagnosis, medication regimen, discharge treatment, referrals, and physician involved -Personalized information may increase patient compliance with discharge instructions -Cost over time may be less than reordering printed supplies	-Initial cost of implementation may be prohibitive for some institutions -Requires multiple computers to ensure staff access and facilitate simultaneous processing of several patient instruction sheets -Staff must take time to enter the data for each patient -Most systems also require physician involvement with teaching process so the physician must take time to enter the data

topic of interest. Physician involvement in development and approval of teaching materials is recommended. It is also important to include referral information with discharge instructions. Provide resource information for business hours and evenings, weekends, and holidays.

Reading level. The average reading level for emergency care patients is between fourth and eighth grade levels.[6,7] Figure 7-3 is an example of instructions written at the fourth grade level.[8,9] Unfortunately many educational materials are printed for higher reading abilities. It is important to determine reading level for any printed materials used for patient education. Computer software programs that measure reading level are available. This feature is often part of a computerized grammar program. If this resource is not available, manual formulas can be used to calculate reading level. The SMOG formula predicts within 1.5 grade levels how difficult a passage is to read.

For discharge instructions that contain at least 30 sentences, identify 10 consecutive sentences each from the beginning, middle, and end of the selection. For these 30 sen-

Table 7-3 SMOG Table

Word count (Three-syllable words only)	Grade level
0-2	4
3-6	5
7-12	6
13-20	7
21-30	8
31-42	9
43-56	10
57-72	11
73-90	12
91-110	13
111-132	14
133-156	15
157-182	16
183-210	17
211-240	18

From Stewart KB: Written patient-education materials: are they on the level? *Nurs '96* 26(1):32k, 1996.

ABDOMINAL WARNINGS

What to do:

1. Stay home and rest for 24 hours or more if your doctor tells you.

2. Drink only clear liquids like apple juice, broth, or clear soda for the first 24 hours.

3. Take the medicines your doctor gives you. Ask your doctor before you take any medicines you have at home.

4. Keep your clinic appointment.

Watch for these Danger Signs:

1. Vomiting begins or gets worse.

2. Vomit blood or find blood in your stool.

3. Pain is not better in 24 hours.

4. Pain gets worse.

5. The pain is in the right lower abdomen.

6. Abdomen gets swollen.

7. Feel dizzy or faint.

8. Shortness of breath.

9. A temperature over 102 degrees (39 degrees C).

COME TO THE EMERGENCY ROOM IF YOU HAVE ANY OF THESE DANGER SIGNS.

Figure **7-3**   Instructions written at the fourth grade level. *(Courtesy Parkland Memorial Hospital, Dallas, Texas.)*

tences, count words containing three or more syllables, including repetitions. Count hyphenated words as one word. For numbers, count the syllables for each numeral. For example, the number 573 counts as seven syllables. Include proper nouns in your syllable count. Avoid using sentences that contain a colon in your count. If you do use one, count it as two sentences. When a word is abbreviated, count the number of syllables for the word when it is spelled out. Once you have the total number of words, use the SMOG table (Table 7-3) to determine grade level.

For discharge instructions that contain less than 30 sentences, count the number of sentences in the instructions. Use the conversion table (Table 7-4) to get the conversion number that corresponds to the sentences in the instructions. Count words with three or more syllables, then multiply the three-syllable word count by the conversion number to get an adjusted word count. Refer to Table 7-3 for the grade level of the material.

In addition to ensuring written words in patient education materials are effective, the author should pay attention to overall patient comprehension. One study evaluated patient comprehension of discharge instructions for a laceration, with and without visuals.[10] Researchers concluded the addition of illustrations improved patient understanding, especially among patients who are nonwhite, female, or have no more than high school education.[2]

Table **7-4** **SMOG Conversion Table**	
Number of sentences in selection	Conversion number
29	1.03
28	1.07
27	1.10
26	1.15
25	1.20
24	1.25
23	1.30
22	1.36
21	1.43
20	1.50
19	1.58
18	1.67
17	1.76
16	1.87
15	2.00
14	2.14
13	2.30
12	2.50
11	2.70
10	3.00

From Stewart KB: Written patient-education materials: are they on the level? *Nurs '96* 26(1):32k, 1996.

Visuals can be in the form of pictures, cartoons, anatomic diagrams, and photographs. As with the written word, simplicity is effective. Not all patient education materials are easily enhanced with illustrations. Figure 7-4 is an example of instructions with illustrations.

Implementing the Teaching Plan

Implementation of the patient teaching plan is the "meat" of the teaching and learning process; however, patient learning can only take place within the framework of a positive, helping relationship. This type of relationship relies on good communication skills and includes respect, trust, caring, acceptance, sincerity, and patient advocacy. Communication is a process by which information is given and received. Face-to-face communication includes both verbal and non-verbal messages.

Communication. Communication involves not only sending the message but also receiving and understanding the message. It can be verbal or nonverbal. It is the process through which the patient-caregiver relationship develops. The patient may base his or her perception on the level of the nurse's competence and what the patient sees as the level of communication and interpersonal skills the nurse has demonstrated. Usually the better the communication and the patient's perception of that communication, the more smoothly the therapeutic process goes.

The emergency nurse must be acutely aware of the following facts related to communication:

- Regardless of method, there is some form of communication in any relationship, even if it is nonverbal or does not involve physical contact.
- Communication can be formal or informal.
- All behaviors by the nurse, patient, and patient's family are forms of communication.
- It is impossible *not* to communicate.
- What you say may not necessarily be what the patient hears.

Verbal communication. Choose words carefully when communicating with patients or their significant others. Match spoken words with written information the patient will receive. Strategies for teaching patients throughout the life span and teaching patients with special needs will be discussed later in this chapter.

Listening is one way to hear the patient's concerns. Having the patient talk while you listen may relieve anxieties and facilitate information collection. Whenever possible, allow the patient to take the conversational lead. Listening is an active, physically visible process. Being able to listen is a learned skill, acquired through practice.

Nonverbal communication. Body position is important. The nurse should try to teach from a sitting position facing the patient to avoid being perceived as "talking down" to the patient. If the patient is lying down, raise the head of the bed to maintain eye contact. Patients can sense if staff is in a hurry. If time is limited, be honest with the patient about how much time is available to discuss his or her condition and aftercare. Allow time to listen. Many nonverbal messages such as eye contact, facial expressions, gestures, touch, and body position hold different meanings in different cultures. Cultural sensitivity will be discussed later in this chapter.

Although not often thought of as such, silence as an expressive, nonverbal response can be a useful tool in therapeutic communication. Remember, silence is the absence of words, but *not* the absence of activity. It may be a natural conclusion of verbally transmitted thoughts. Silence may be useful because it:

- Allows time to think
- May be helpful in finding solutions to problems and answers to questions
- Is a way to convey your feelings without words
- May promote acceptance or indicate anxiety in either you or the patient
- Can be used to pace, time, alienate, resist, or relax when employed carefully

Barriers to effective communication. Emergency care centers are usually busy, noisy places. Awareness of barriers to effective communication may help eliminate some of these distractions. Try to conduct teaching in a relatively quiet area. Lack of privacy can be an issue as many patient care areas are open. If a patient is in a private room, close the door. Personal attitudes and values about lifestyle, health behaviors, and learning can be projected to the patient, so avoid making judgments.

Teaching throughout the life span. An effective educator is able to individualize teaching strategies to accommodate the entire emergency patient population. Most emergency settings treat adult and pediatric clients. Pediatric facilities should be familiar with adult learning principles when teaching parents and other caregivers.

Children[13]

- Include the parent(s) or caregivers in teaching. They are most familiar with the child.
- Consider the child's stage of physical and cognitive development.
- Be truthful with children when explaining an illness, injury, or procedure. Do not tell a child a procedure does not hurt when it does.
- Allow children to express fears and ask questions.
- Don't explain a procedure too far in advance. This leaves time to imagine scary scenarios.
- Children need to know the reason for the hospital visit and to be reassured it is not because of bad behavior.

Adolescents (age 13 to 20 years)[1,13]

- Include parents with young adolescents, but use judgment with older teens. Parents should be informed of the patient's physical condition and specifics of treatment, but this can be accomplished with separate discussions.
- Any condition that will have an effect on physical appearance requires sensitivity. Body image is an important issue.

Crutch Walking

1. Remove the screw that holds the bottom peg and top of the crutch together.

2. Place the crutch under your arm.

3. Push the top of the crutch down on the bottom peg so that **3 fingers** fit between the top of the crutch and **under** your arm.

4. Put the screw back in the bottom peg and the top of the crutch to hold them together.

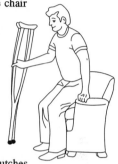

5. Remove the screw in the top of the crutch and the hand grip.

6. **Move the hand grip so your arm is bent just a little.**

7. Place the screw back into the top of the crutch and the hand grip to hold them together.

8. When walking with crutches, the top of the crutch must **not** touch your underarm.

9. Stand up straight.

10. Put the weight of your body on your hands and the hand grips.

11. **Stand on your good foot** and move both crutches in front of you.

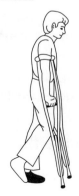

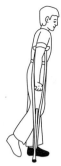

12. Resting your weight on your hands, **lift and swing your good foot** to where the crutches are.

13. **To sit down,** hold both crutches by the hand grip in one hand. Put your other hand on the chair and sit down.

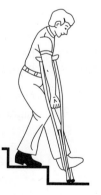

14. **To stand up,** hold both crutches by the hand grip in one hand. **Put your other hand on the chair** and stand up.

15. **To walk up stairs,** put your weight on the crutches and put your good foot on the step. Then put your weight on your good foot and lift the crutches up to the step that your good foot is on.

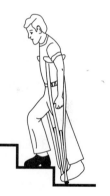

16. **To walk down stairs,** put your weight on your good foot and place the crutches on the step below you. Then put your weight on the crutches and step down with your good foot.

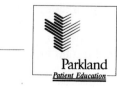

Parkland
Patient Education

IH-I-32

*Figure **7-4*** Instruction sheet with illustrations. *(Courtesy Parkland Patient Education, Parkland Memorial Hospital, Dallas, Texas.)*

- Use peer pressure in a positive way. Often teens come with peers to the ED. If appropriate, include peers in teaching as peer pressure may increase compliance.
  Young adults (age 20 to 40 years)[1]
- Give the patient a practical reason(s) for learning.
- Keep in mind that young adults often take good health for granted.

- If patient has young children, stress the need to recover and/or maintain health to allow care of children.
  Middle adults (age 40 to 60 years)[1]
- Patients are more aware of possible health problems than young adults.
- Use patients' life experiences as a foundation for new learning.

What to do for the Flu

The flu may cause one or more of the following:

- headache

- fever

- chills

- weakness

- lack of energy

- sore throat

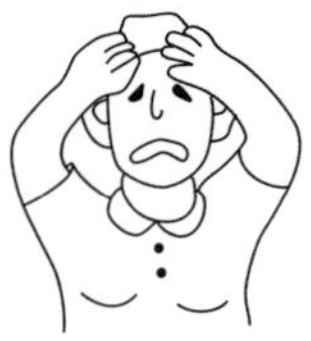

- body aches

- vomiting

- loss of appetite

- make you sick to your stomach

- cough

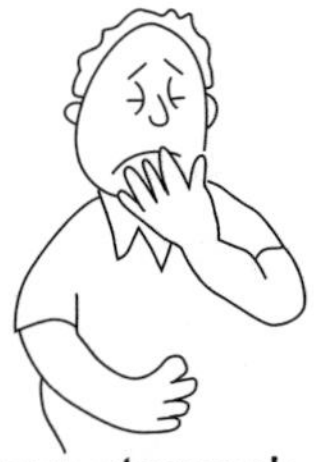

What to do when you have the flu:

1. Stay home and rest as much as possible.

2. Drink plenty of liquids. Lemon-lime sodas (like Sprite) and hot tea are good.

3. Eat small meals. Foods like chicken soup or broth, saltine crackers, plain toast, and gelatin are good.

4. Take your temperature every 4-6 hours

5. Take cool baths if you have a fever.

6. Antibiotics will not cure the flu. Take Acetaminophen (Tylenol) for fever, headaches or body aches. Usually you will take 2 tablets every 4 to 6 hours. Do not give Aspirin to children.

7. Come to the clinic if you are sick for over **1** week or if your fever goes higher than 102 degree Fahrenheit (38.8 degrees Centigrade).

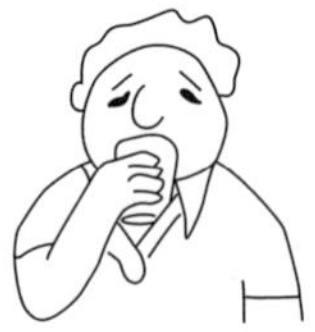

A

Decrease your chances of getting the flu:

1. Get a good night's sleep every night.
2. Eat 3 healthy meals each day.
3. Stay away from sick people.
4. Consider getting a flu vaccine before the next flu season.

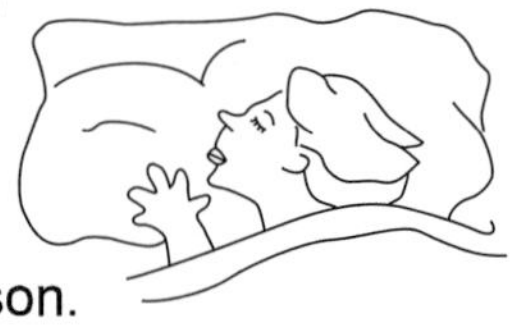

*Figure **7-5*** Standardized education sheet in (**A**) English, and (**B**) Spanish. *(Courtesy Parkland Patient Education, Parkland Memorial Hospital, Dallas, Texas.)*

Older adults (age 60 and over)[1]
- Motivate patients to learn by showing how acquisition of knowledge and skill will increase their quality of life.
- Use their past experiences to relate to current problems.

Teaching in special needs situations. Today's world is a complex blend of individuals with different physical, psychosocial, and cultural distinctions. Awareness of and sensitivity to these differences is essential for effective patient educa-tion in the ED. The Americans with Disabilities Act (ADA) of 1990 also has implications for patient education. ADA speaks to individuals with literacy problems, hearing impairment, and visual impairment. As world travel becomes more common, the emergency nurse must consider cultural differences as they relate to teaching and learning. Refer to Chapter 5 for further discussion of cultural aspects of health and illness.

Que hacer para la Gripe
(What to do for the Flu)

La gripe puede causar uno o más de los siguientes síntomas:

- dolor de cabeza
- fiebre
- escalofríos
- debilidad
- sentirse sin energía
- dolor de garganta

- dolor de cuerpo
- vómito
- pérdida de apetito
- sentirse enfermo del estómago
- tos

Que hacer cuando usted tiene la gripe:

1. Quédese en la casa y descanse lo más posible.

2. Tome muchos líquidos. Sodas de Lima-Limón (como Sprite) y también es bueno el té caliente.

3. Coma comidas pequeñas. Alimentos como caldo de pollo o consomé, galletas saladas, pan tostado (sin nada), y también es buena la gelatina.

4. Tomarse su temperatura cada 4 a 6 horas.

5. Si tiene fiebre tome baños pero que el agua esté a la temperatura del cuarto.

6. Antibióticos no curan la gripe. Tome **acetaminophen (acetaminofen) (Tylenol)** para la fiebre, dolores de cabeza o del cuerpo. Usualmente used tomará 2 tabletas cada 4 a 6 horas. No dé **(Aspirin) (Aspirina)** a los niños.

7. Venga a la clínica si usted está enfermo por más de 1 semana o si su fiebre sube a más de 102 grados Fahrenheit (38.8 grados Centígrados).

B

Reduzca sus probabilidades de que le dé la gripe:

1. Durmiendo bien todas las noches.
2. Comiendo alimentos saludables 3 veces cada día.
3. No se acerque a la gente que usted sabe que está enferma.
4. Considere vacunarse contra la gripe antes de la próxima estación de gripe.

*Figure **7-5,** cont'd   For legend see opposite page.*

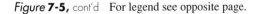

Literacy. Illiteracy is a major problem in today's society. Recent estimates place the level of functional illiteracy in the adult population at 13%. Functional illiteracy means the individual can recognize a majority of words, but understands only a small percentage of the words. Poor literacy skills are viewed in a negative light in Western culture. Do not assume money, educational level, or color dictate literacy level. Illiteracy does not correlate with intelligence; many self-made business people memorize sufficient information to succeed.[9]

Illiterate or low-literate patients have no clear identifying characteristics. A patient may be very polite, articulate, and willing to sign a document without understanding the written words. To determine the patient's reading ability, observe, listen, and ask questions. A non-threatening question to ask during assessment is "Do you like to read?" Usually people who read reasonably well like to read, whereas those who find reading difficult do not like to read. When given written materials, illiterate patients may give the excuse that their reading glasses are missing. Other patients may pass written materials to family or significant others to read.

When teaching patients who cannot read, use short, simple words, avoid medical jargon, and be consistent with chosen words. Teach essential information first, then repeat the information as necessary. Use analogies the patient can understand, with illustrations whenever possible. Have the patient restate, review, or demonstrate the information. Include available family and significant others to reinforce the teaching points.[9]

Hearing impairment. Many hearing-impaired patients may communicate that fact through gestures, written notes, or through family members. If alone, the patient may be constantly looking over his or her shoulder or appear uneasy. The patient may have a hearing aid, although these devices are not always visible in the external ear. Some hearing aids are designed to be concealed in the ear to avoid embarrassment. Patients' level of frustration may reflect how long they have been disabled and the effectiveness of their coping mechanisms.

When teaching patients who are hearing impaired, ask the patients if they can speech read, formerly called lip reading. If so, face the patient with adequate light on your face and speak slowly and deliberately. Gesturing can increase comprehension. Some patients and families may know sign language. A family member or significant other may be able to sign to the patient. Use a sign language interpreter when necessary. If the patient uses a hearing aid, make sure it is available; some patients may not wear the device all of the time. Reinforce verbal communication with written instructions and illustrations. Be patient; teaching will take more time than with patients who are not hearing impaired.[1]

Visual impairment. Visual impairment poses obstacles to communication for both the patient and the nurse. The patient may speak only when spoken to because of uncertainty of the presence and location of the other person(s). Communication can be compared to a telephone conversation. Legally blind persons often carry a white cane or stick. Some people use a seeing-eye dog to help guide their way. The visually impaired who still have some eyesight may use a magnifying glass to enlarge written words.

When teaching visually impaired patients, announce and identify yourself when you enter the patient's room or cubicle. Remember that verbal communication is more important than non-verbal messages. Maintain normal speech; talking louder will not make the message better understood. Avoid phrases such as "Do you see what I mean?" Explain all procedures. Touch is important to visually impaired persons; however, they do not need constant touch. For patients who still have some sight, consider enlarging written instructions and illustrations.[1]

Cultural diversity and foreign languages. Culture consists of values, social and family structure, religion, diet, customs, health beliefs, and expectations.[9] Sensitivity to cultural diversity is essential for the educator. Health care practices in conflict with the patient's values will probably not be followed. It is important to remain open-minded and nonjudgmental. Nurses can obtain information about cultures regularly encountered through their human resources department and library. Some institutions discuss basic cultural differences during orientation. If possible, incorporate all nonharmful components of the patient's desired cultural behaviors into the teaching plan. There is no need to speak more loudly, but speech should be slow and clear. Watch for facial expressions and other nonverbal cues that indicate confusion.

When teaching patients who speak a foreign language, try to learn a few words in those languages regularly encountered, and use reference books that translate English medical phrases into various other languages. Use professional interpreters if available; they should be familiar with medical terminology. Keep eye contact with the patient, use short units of speech, and wait for a response. Maintain rapport with the interpreter. Use family or friends to interpret as a last measure.[9] Figure 7-5,*A* shows an instruction sheet in English and Figure 7-5,*B* shows the same sheet in Spanish.

Evaluation of Learning

The next step in the teaching and learning process is evaluation. Since emergency care teaching sessions are often short, evaluation usually takes place upon discharge. The nurse evaluates whether the process is complete, needs reinforcement, or there are needs that must be referred to an outside agency.[13]

Ask the patient to repeat what has just been discussed, and ask the patient questions on the content discussed. Determine if the patient can perform a return demonstration of any skills taught. Other methods of evaluation may be used to evaluate learning. The patient may be telephoned after discharge to evaluate learning. Formal questionnaires on the comprehension of written tools may also be used. An informal review of written materials by a random se-

Columbus Hospital

2520 North Lakeview Avenue
Chicago, Illinois 60614

EMERGENCY DEPARTMENT AFTER CARE INSTRUCTIONS

PROVISIONAL DIAGNOSIS:

Follow-up In _____ Days At:

☐ PLEASE CALL FOR APPOINTMENT

Additional Instructions:

Please follow the instructions below as indicated for you:

☐ Abdominal Complaint
☐ Ankle Sprain
☐ Animal Bite
☐ Asthma
☐ Back Pain
☐ Burn Care
☐ Cast Care
☐ Chest Pain
☐ Cold - Adult/Child
☐ Constipation
☐ Crutch Walking/Crutches
☐ Culture
☐ Eye Injury
☐ Fever - Child
☐ Febrile Convulsion
☐ Frostbite
☐ General Medicine Physician Sheet
☐ Headache

☐ Head Injury - Adult/Child
☐ High Blood Pressure
☐ Itching
☐ Lice
☐ Neck Strain/Sprain
☐ Nosebleed
☐ Otitis Media (Earache)
☐ Pelvic Inflammatory Disease
☐ Seizure
☐ Shoulder Bursitis
☐ Strain, Sprain, Fracture
☐ Tetanus
☐ Tine Test
☐ Threatened Miscarriage
☐ Urinary Tract Infection
☐ Venereal Disease
☐ Vomiting/Diarrhea - Adult/Child
☐ Wound Care/Suture After Care

You were sutured. You have _____ sutures/staples
which must be removed in _____ days.

☐ You were prescribed sedatives or pain medications that may make you drowsy. Do not drink alcohol or operate machinery while you are taking these medications.

X-rays do not always show injury or disease. Fractures (breaks in the bones) are not always revealed on the initial x-rays, but may be revealed on subsequent x-rays. Your x-ray has been read on a preliminary basis. Final reading will be made by the radiologist in 24 hours. You will be notified of any additional findings.

The examination and treatment you have received in the Emergency Department has been given on an emergency basis only. (Should your condition worsen or any new symptoms develop, or should you not recover as expected, contact your Doctor or the Doctor you were given for follow-up care.) If you cannot contact the doctor, return to the Hospital Emergency Department.

_____
Signature of Patient or Responsible Person

_____
Signature of Witness   Date

Form

COLUMBUS HOSPITAL 2520 N. LAKEVIEW, CHICAGO, IL 60614

FOR _____ DATE _____

ADDRESS _____

℞

☐ May Substitute _____ M.D.

☐ May Not Substitute   DEA No. _____

☐ May Be Refilled   ☐ 1   ☐ 2   ☐ NR

PATIENT

COLUMBUS HOSPITAL 2520 N. LAKEVIEW, CHICAGO, IL 60614

FOR _____ DATE _____

ADDRESS _____

℞

☐ May Substitute _____ M.D.

☐ May Not Substitute   DEA No. _____

☐ May Be Refilled   ☐ 1   ☐ 2   ☐ NR

PATIENT

Figure **7-6** Standardized education documentation form. *(From Zimmerman PG: Emergency department aftercare instructions, J Emer Nurs 20(1):55, 1994.)*

lection of patients is helpful when you first introduce new materials.

Documentation

Documentation is the final component of the teaching and learning process, but it is no less important than the other steps. The Joint Commission on Accreditation of Healthcare Organizations' (JCAHO) manual contains a section on patient and family education. The manual specifically describes the institution's responsibility in this area. Many of the standards require careful documentation. It is recommended that all nurses involved with patient education be familiar with the current JCAHO standards. Basic information to include in documentation includes content taught, method(s) used, the patient's response, adjunct instructions provided, and referrals made. The date, time, and signatures of the patient and the educator should be included. If persons other than the patient were included in teaching, document their names and relationship to patient. All members of the health care team who participate in patient teaching are responsible for documentation. Institutional policies and procedures should be followed for all documentation.

Methods of documentation include written nurse's notes, standardized discharge forms, and computer-generated forms. Figure 7-6 is one example of a standardized documentation form. One copy of this form is given to the patient and another copy remains with the medical record. These forms can be translated into other languages. Computerized documentation can also produce a hard copy for the patient and one for the medical record.

SUMMARY

To ensure adherence to prescribed therapeutic, restorative, and preventive measures, the ED nurse is responsible for providing effective, individualized instruction regarding home care measures and the process involved in emergency care. This responsibility necessitates familiarity with sequential steps in the teaching and learning process. The process includes identifying learning needs, assessing the learning, establishing realistic goals, selecting and using appropriate teaching methods, allowing for learning time, evaluating the results, and documenting the instruction. Application of learning and communication principles is prerequisite to effective teaching. Because all emergency nurses must be familiar with the process involved in carrying out their professional role as nurse teacher, content regarding the patient teaching process is included in orientation and in-service educational programs. In addition, patient teaching is a criterion for quality improvement, clinical ladder, and performance evaluation.

Because knowledge of home care is a patient's right and also benefits the ED by reducing the number of call-backs and return visits, patient teaching can be considered an integral component of emergency patient care.

REFERENCES

1. Anderson C: *Patient teaching and communicating in an information age,* Albany, NY, 1990, Delmar.
2. Austin PE, Matlack R, Dunn KA et al: Discharge instructions: do illustrations help our patients understand them? *Ann Emerg Med* 25(3):317, 1995.
3. Boyd MD: A guide to writing effective patient education materials, *Nurs Manag* 18(7):56, 1987.
4. Chacon D, Kissoon N, Rich S: Education attainment level of caregivers versus readability level of written instructions in a pediatric emergency department, *Ped Emerg Care* 10(3):144, 1994.
5. Chatham MA, Knapp BL: *Patient education handbook,* Bowie, Mo, 1982, RJ Brady.
6. Fox MR, Baker C: *Understanding the illiteracy problem,* Alexandria, Va, 1989, Society for Human Resource Management.
7. Jolly BT, Scott JL, Feied CF et al: Functional illiteracy among emergency department patients: a preliminary study, *Ann Emerg Med* 22(3):573, 1993.
8. Pestonjee S: *Patient education booklet,* Dallas, Parkland Memorial Hospital.
9. Pestonjee S: The process of patient education, Dallas, Parkland Memorial Hospital.
10. Spandorfer JM, Karras DJ, Hughes LA et al: Comprehension of discharge instructions by patients in an urban emergency department, *Ann Emerg Med* 25(1):71, 1995.
11. Stewart KB: Written patient-education materials, *Nurs '96* 26(1):32j, 1996.
12. Vukmir RB, Kremen R, Ellis GL et al: Compliance with emergency department referral: the effect of computerized discharge instructions, *Ann Emerg Med* 22(5):819, 1993.
13. Winthrop E: *Mosby's patient teaching tips,* St Louis, 1995, Mosby.

SUGGESTED READING

Patient teaching

Canobbio M: *Mosby's handbook of patient teaching,* St Louis, 1996, Mosby.
Griffith H: *Instructions for patients,* ed 5, Orlando, Fla, 1994, WB Saunders.
McMahon E: *Teaching patients with acute conditions,* Springhouse, Pa, 1992, Springhouse.
Sodeman W: *Instructions for geriatric patients,* Orlando, Fla, 1995, WB Saunders.

Multiculturalism/languages

Bodiwala G, McCaskie H, Thompson M: *International translation guide for emergency medicine,* Oxford, Engl, 1993, Butterworth-Heinemann.
Kelland B, Jordan L: *CommuniMed: multilingual patient assessment manual,* ed 3, St Louis, 1994, Mosby.
Teed C, Raley H. & Barber J. (1983). *Conversational Spanish For the Medical and Health Professions.* New York: Harcourt Brace Jovanovich College Publishers.

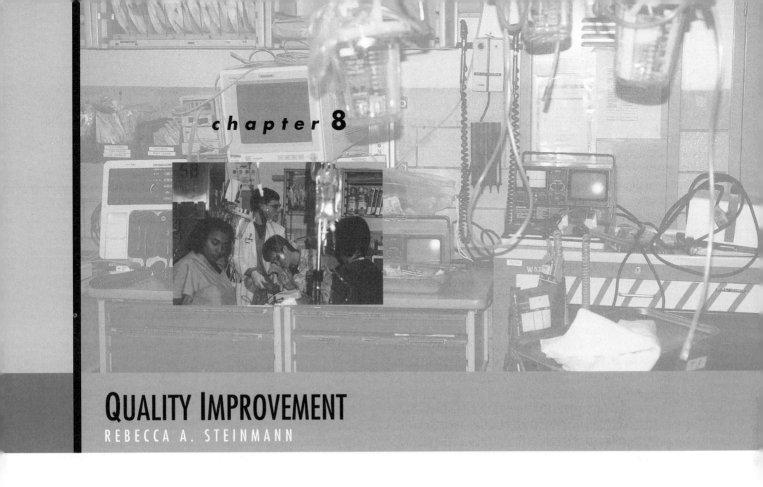

chapter 8

QUALITY IMPROVEMENT
REBECCA A. STEINMANN

Quality, cost, equity, and access are four basic concepts underlying the health care system. Quality is defined by *Webster's*[31] as "excellence, superiority; the degree of excellence a thing possesses." The multidimensional nature of health care makes quality difficult to define and assess. Consumers, health care organizations, providers, third-party payers, and regulatory agencies have expectations of how health care should perform and perceptions of what quality entails. Development of a comprehensive measurable definition of quality health care has been hampered by the diversity of definitions among and within these groups and the subjective perceptions of quality.

Assessment of quality in health care has traditionally been based on measuring the performance of organizations and providers against predetermined norms and standards of care. These standards tend to evaluate specific aspects of care, focusing on structure and process-oriented indicators of quality. Only recently has the health care community begun focusing on outcomes—the results of care—as measures of quality. Defining health care quality in terms of outcome portrays quality as a more universally defined and measurable entity. One outcome-based definition recommends assessing quality in health care through the efficacy of diagnostic/therapeutic procedures in accomplishing their goal, appropriateness of care based on cost and benefits of a particular course of action, and caring functions—interpersonal, supportive, and psychologic aspects of the patient-provider relationship.[6]

Today's hospital environment is characterized by rapid patient turnover; decreased length of stay; expanding ambulatory services; increased levels of severity, acuity, and nursing intensity; and older clients with multiple needs.[17] Health care providers are increasingly being judged, not just on individual knowledge and institutional capabilities for treating the ill and injured, but also on ability to actively improve quality of care while reducing use of resources. To be successful, health care organizations must be able to anticipate, understand, and proactively respond to multiple changes in the health care environment. Providers cannot be content with ensuring that patients are receiving good care based on established standards. Instead, providers are challenged to continuously evaluate the care delivered and seek opportunities to provide better care.

THE ROLE OF THE JOINT COMMISSION IN QUALITY ASSESSMENT

No entity has had a greater impact on quality assessment in health care organizations than the Joint Commission on Accreditation of Healthcare Organizations (JCAHO). Founded in 1951 as a voluntary accrediting agency, its mission has been to improve quality of care provided to the public. In the 1953 *Standards for Hospital Accreditation,* minimal standards for specific aspects of patient care were published, including standards for nursing services. In the 1970 *Accreditation Manual for Hospitals,* JCAHO began requiring organizational compliance with optimal standards of care.

JCAHO responded to concerns that organizations were auditing good care in quantity while avoiding problem patient care topics that needed review. JCAHO changed its emphasis in 1980, adopting quality assurance standards for hospitals that stressed the problem-focused (high-volume, high-risk) approach to quality assurance. In 1985, hospitals were required to demonstrate that quality of patient care was consistently optimal. Quality of patient care replaced the problem-focused approach to quality assurance with standards that specified systematic monitoring and evaluation of important aspects of patient care and services.

In 1986, JCAHO introduced "The Agenda for Change," a program reflecting their objective of basing accreditation decisions more directly on actual performance of health care organizations. This program included development and testing of clinical indicators of performance; review and revision of standards to refocus on aspects of care that affect quality and patient outcomes; and introduction of severity-adjusted measurements to the survey process. "The Agenda for Change" provides a model for quality assessment activities that emphasizes outcome management, incorporating Continuous Quality Improvement (CQI) methods and cross-organizational initiatives to evaluate and improve performance (Box 8-1).

The transition to CQI continued with revision of the Quality Assessment and Improvement Standards in 1992. Improvement standards promoted the change to more interdepartmental and interdisciplinary quality improvement activities; focused on process and system achievement not just individual performance; increased efforts to improve performance of the entire organization rather than focusing on outliers; and increased communication and collaboration. Organizational leadership was given responsibility for overseeing the quality improvement (QI) process, establishing QI responsibilities in the organization and setting strategic priorities for quality assessment and improvement.

In 1995, the Joint Commission[15] revised hospital standards, shifting to patient-centered and performance-focused standards organized around functions common to all health care organizations (Box 8-2). Each of these important functions is evaluated based on dimensions of performance—efficiency and appropriateness (described as "doing the right thing") and availability, timeliness, effectiveness, continuity, safety, efficiency, and respect and caring (dimensions of performance described as "doing the right thing well"). The survey process moved from traditional evaluation of specific departments and services to assessment of performance throughout the organization. Decreased emphasis was placed on activities conducted to pass the survey and more emphasis was placed on observation of actual performance and interviews with staff and patients.

Emergency nursing performance is evaluated within each of the patient-focused and organization functions delineated by JCAHO. Staff nurses are accountable for patient rights and organizational ethics, the assessment, care, and education of patients, and assimilating ED patients into the continuum of care. They are responsible for improving organizational function, managing the environment of care, managing human resources, managing information, and infection control. Nursing management of the ED is responsible for compliance with the leadership function. Each important function identified by JCAHO is further defined by standards delineated under that specific function. For example, standards listed under the management of information function specify that time and means of arrival must be documented for all ED patients and that the record include the patient's condition at discharge and instructions for follow-up care.

JCAHO plans to incorporate performance indicators into its accreditation process to further its emphasis on outcomes.

Box 8-1 Ten-Step Monitoring and Evaluation Process (JCAHO)

1. Assign responsibility for quality assessment activities
2. Delineate scope of care and service, i.e., identify key functions affecting quality of care
3. Identify important aspects of care and service, e.g., select-prioritize for ongoing monitoring
4. Identify indicators on measures of specific, objective events or occurrences
5. Establish thresholds for evaluation—a predetermined single event or level of performance that triggers intensive evaluation
6. Collect and organize data
7. Initiate evaluation
8. Take actions to improve care and services
9. Assess the effectiveness of actions and maintain the gain
10. Communicate results to affected individuals and groups

Box 8-2 Important Functions Evaluated by JCAHO

Patient-focused functions	Organization functions	Structures with functions
Patient rights and organizational ethics	Improving organization function	Governance
Assessment of patients	Leadership	Management
Care of patients	Management of the environment of care	Medical staff
Education	Management of human resources	Nursing
Continuum of care	Management of information	
	Surveillance, prevention, and control of infection	

Performance indicators are intended to further improve the ability of health care organizations to identify their areas of excellence and opportunities to improve patient care.

Quality Assurance

Quality assurance (QA) is a process established to ensure that patient care is consistent with established standards. Standards are statements of expected performance developed by authorities based on scientific knowledge. A standard may be structural, describing equipment, physical facilities, personnel, and resources of an organization; process-oriented, focusing on activities and interventions in the delivery of patient care; or outcome-oriented, defining measurable changes in the patient's health status as a result of care. Standards do not necessarily denote optimal level of achievement. They may simply denote an acceptable level of performance.

Traditionally, major components of a QA system included standards that described quality, a system for collecting information about the degree of achievement of standards, and a system for acting to bring performance into line with those standards. Operationally, each department or service was assigned the responsibility for overseeing monitoring and evaluation within the respective department. Each department or service delineated its separate scope of care and identified high-volume, high-risk, and problem-prone aspects of care. Each department or service identified indicators to correspond to these important aspects of care and established the level, pattern, or trend in data for each indicator that triggered intensive evaluation. A method of data collection was established and care was intensively examined only when the threshold for a given indicator was reached. Action was taken to improve care based on recommendations of those evaluating the care. Continued monitoring determined whether actions taken were effective. Results of QA activities were reported to the leadership within the department and to the organizational QA committee.

Quality assurance activities traditionally focused on retrospective chart audits. Critics argued that retrospective audits measured the quality of documentation, and questioned the relationship between quality of documentation and quality of care. Detractors further argued that QA focused on examining attainment of predetermined norms and standards of health care, without regard for consumer satisfaction and cost. Others charged that quality assurance is a misnomer since quality can never be assured or guaranteed.

One weakness inherent in departmentalized QA activities has been lack of action to improve care when problems crossed department or service boundaries. Health care can most effectively be improved by focusing on all key activities of the organization, coordinating efforts throughout the organization, using effective performance measures to collect reliable data, addressing processes with important direct or indirect effects on patient outcomes, and focusing primarily on opportunities to improve these processes.[16] All these principles are commonly associated with a continuous quality improvement approach to quality management.

Despite imperfections of the QA process, the degree to which processes of care adhere to acceptable standards continues to be an important measure in quality assessment. JCAHO standards continue to require ongoing monitoring and evaluation of specified high-risk situations, for example, patients receiving conscious sedation, patients restrained or secluded. Chart audits continue to serve as a mechanism to demonstrate compliance with these standards. Rather than limiting data collection to compliance with standards, the challenge is to incorporate data regarding various aspects of patient care delivery into audits that can indicate areas for improving the overall process (Figure 8-1).

Quality Improvement

Quality improvement (QI) is the organized creation of beneficial change.[18] Modern industry has revolutionized quality management by designing activities to determine customer needs as well as the products and processes required to meet those needs. Noting the success of Total Quality Management (TQM) and Continuous Quality Improvement (CQI) in transforming industry, health care organizations have embraced the quality orientation of Dr. W. Edwards Deming and other proponents of CQI. Deming's philosophy is detailed in his 14 points for transformation (Box 8-3).

The philosophic basis of CQI is grounded in a number of beliefs, such as:
- Improving quality by removing causes of problems in the system leads to increased productivity; 85% of problems

---

Box 8-3   Deming's 14 Points for Transformation of an Organization

1. Create constancy of purpose for improvement of product and service
2. Adopt the new philosophy
3. Cease dependence on inspection to achieve quality
4. End the practice of awarding business on the basis of price alone
5. Improve constantly and forever every process for planning, production, and service
6. Institute training on the job
7. Adopt and institute leadership
8. Drive out fear
9. Break down barriers between staff areas
10. Eliminate slogans, exhortations, and targets for the work force
11. Eliminate numerical quotas for the work force and numerical goals for management
12. Remove barriers that rob people of pride of workmanship; eliminate annual rating
13. Institute a vigorous program of education and self-improvement for everyone
14. Put everybody in the company to work to accomplish the transformation

SECLUSION/RESTRAINT AUDIT

Date of service: _____   Hospital ID # _____
Time into department: _____

Indicators:

1. Behavior necessitating seclusion/restraint documented in ED record.   Y   N

2. Physician order for seclusion/restraint recorded in ED record   Y   N

3. Time patient in seclusion/restraint documented   Y   N
      Time: _____

4. Seclusion/restraint flowsheet initiated   Y   N
      a. Observation of patient recorded q. 15 minutes   Y   N
      b. Toileting, nourishment, circulation checks recorded at least q. 2 hours   Y   N

5. Psychiatric consult ordered: Y   N
      Time consult called: _____
      Time consult arrived: _____   Time to consultation: _____

6. Chemical restraints ordered   Y   N
      <u>Medications administered</u>   <u>Time</u>

      _____   _____
      _____   _____
      _____   _____

7. Documentation of time seclusion/restraint discontinued   Y   N   NA
      Time: _____   Total time in seclusion/restraint: _____

8. Disposition recorded   Y   N
      Time: _____   Discharge   Admit   Transfer
      Total time in department: _____

Primary RN: _____   Attending Physician: _____

Comments:

Audit completed by: _____   Date: _____

Figure **8-1**   Seclusion/Restraint audit form.

can only be corrected by changing systems; less than 15% are under a worker's control.[29]
- The person doing the job is most knowledgeable about that job.
- People want to be involved and do their job well.
- Every person wants to feel like a valued contributor.
- More can be accomplished by working together to improve the system than by having individual contributors working around the system.
- A structured problem-solving process using graphic techniques produces better solutions than an unstructured process.
- Graphic problem-solving lets you know where you are, where the variations lie, the relative importance of the

problems to be solved, and whether changes have made the desired impact.

Quality improvement represents a paradigm shift in quality management strategies from quality assurance[3] (Table 8-1). The process of QI integrates the philosophies of customer focus, empowerment, leadership, and service, involving all employees in pleasing the customer and building quality into every system and process in the organization. It challenges providers to analyze the many processes through which care is provided to patients. Providers are challenged to redesign these processes to achieve greater efficiency in the delivery of health care services, reduce costs, and improve quality. Quality is defined as meeting the customers' needs, that is, doing the right thing right. An innovative ap-

Table **8-1**	**Comparing Quality Assurance and Quality Improvement**	
Characteristic	QA	QI
Definition of quality	No consensus on definition	Quality = customer satisfaction
Focus	Problem resolution; isolating outliers	Continuous improvement
Stimulus to act	Thresholds	Control limits (data range)
Leadership	Leadership rarely comes from top management and is delegated to a few	Leadership comes from the top and is delegated to all
Orientation	Detection orientation	Prevention orientation
Actions	Adversarial: emphasis on blaming when thresholds for compliance not met	Collegial: emphasis on finding root causes of failure to improve processes
Motivation	External requirements (JCAHO)	Self-motivation, professionalism
Scope	Segmented, department-oriented	Cross-functional, multidisciplinary
Cost	Rarely integrates determination of cost and quality	Quality cost measurement an integral part of evaluation process

proach defines quality by the formula, QP^4, where Quality is the sum total of People + Processes + Performance + Product (Q=P+P+P+P).[30]

Numerous process improvement models have been developed by health care organizations and quality consultants. One of the more commonly utilized models is the FOCUS PDCA model[4] of quality improvement based on Deming's work. FOCUS PDCA is an acronym for:

Find an opportunity for improvement.
Organize a team that knows the process.
Clarify current knowledge of the process.
Uncover root causes of process variation.
Start an improvement cycle based on theory.
Plan the process improvement.
Do the process improvement.
Check the results against the theory.
Act on the process and theory.

In practice, many organizations center quality improvement programs on the PDCA cycle itself (Figure 8-2). **P**lanning the process improvement involves defining measures of quality, measuring performance, analyzing the process, and identifying improvement actions. **D**oing the process improvement involves implementing improvement activities, usually as a pilot study. **C**hecking results of the improvement activities against the theory involves measuring benefits of the improvement activity. **A**cting on the process and theory involves adopting the change by standardizing the action or revising or abandoning the improvement activity. The PDCA cycle should sound familiar to nurses because it incorporates the four components of the nursing process—assessing, planning, implementing, and evaluating.

Emergency department staff have begun participating on QI teams addressing processes such as admissions, triage-registration, lab turnaround time, and x-ray turnaround time. A number of articles specific to QI activities in the ED have been published. The QI process has been used to redefine visiting policies,[19] develop projects to improve pediatric

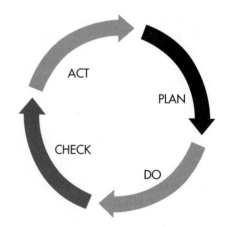

Figure **8-2** The PDCA cycle.

care,[21] decrease length of stay,[28] and improve outcomes of patients presenting with chest pain.[24] The multidimensional, cross-functional approach of QI activities is demonstrated in an article focusing on public health that advocates use of the ED for tetanus immunization to improve patient outcomes.[27] Box 8-4 presents a case study utilizing the QI process.

Tools for Quality Improvement

The core of quality improvement is the scientific process, a systematic model of problem solving. The QI approach advocates making decisions based on data rather than hunches, looking for root causes of problems rather than reacting to superficial symptoms, and seeking permanent solutions to problems rather than quick fixes.

An important QI concept is that of variance. Variance is defined as the degree of change, difference, discrepancy, or unreliability in a process. The source of variance in patient care processes can be found in one or more of five areas: materials, machines, management, manpower, and meth-

---

Box **8-4** **Case Study: Using the QI Process to Improve Time to Thrombolysis**

As part of a clinical research study, a community hospital began auditing the charts of all patients presenting with a diagnosis of acute myocardial infarction. Time from ED presentation to administration of thrombolytic agents consistently averaged over 90 minutes. These data were reported quarterly through QA committees over a period of 2 years. Independent attempts by the ED and the department of cardiology to reduce the time to thrombolysis proved largely unsuccessful. Administrators, recognizing an opportunity to improve patient care, developed a QI team composed of nurses, physicians, and management staff from the ED and the cardiac care unit (CCU), and staff from biometrics, pharmacy, and registration. The team was charged to develop a plan for decreasing time to thrombolysis to under 60 minutes.

A flow chart of the present situation was constructed by the team and compared to their "ideal" flow chart. A number of barriers to timely administration of thrombolytics were identified by the team. The average time to obtain an ECG was 25 minutes with a range of 0 minutes to 67 minutes. Emergency physicians could not order thrombolytics; they had to rely on contacting the patient's private physician and/or cardiologist on call. Patients waited until arriving in CCU to have thrombolytic therapy initiated. Therapy was frequently delayed waiting for the pharmacy to deliver the thrombolytic agents.

The team turned to benchmarking, obtaining data from top-performing institutions, to identify the processes enabling timely administration of thrombolytics. In these institutions, patients presenting with chest pain were immediately taken to a treatment room, ECGs were consistently obtained within 5 minutes of patient arrival, emergency physicians ordered thrombolytics based on preestablished protocols, emergency nursing staff initiated the thrombolytic agents, and thrombolytic agents were available in the ED reconstituted for use by the ED nursing staff.

The QI team adopted these best practices as the basis for decreasing time to thrombolysis at their own institution. To operationalize these processes all ED staff were instructed by the biometrics department in obtaining ECGs, with the expectation that the ED would obtain stat tracings, within 5 minutes of arrival, on all patients presenting with chest pain. This change in practice occurred immediately as ED personnel demonstrated competence in ECG performance. Emergency physicians were authorized by the medical board to order thrombolytic agents. An order sheet for thrombolytic therapy jointly developed by ED and CCU staff was approved by medical records. The ED nursing staff attended a mandatory 4-hour educational program to provide the knowledge base for administering thrombolytic agents with the expectation that these agents would be initiated in the ED. The ED was stocked with tPA and streptokinase and nursing staff was instructed on how to mix these agents to avoid delays from pharmacy.

Six months after the team was convened, the processes were in place to actually implement thrombolytic therapy in the ED. A 2-month pilot project was initiated during which the ED was assigned an on-site resource nurse from the CCU 24 hours/day to contact with any questions. During the 2-month pilot, time to thrombolysis decreased to 46.2 minutes. Minor modifications in various processes were made and ED thrombolysis continued. The average time to thrombolysis is currently 22.7 minutes.

---

ods.[5] The goal of QI processes is to reduce or control variance as much as possible to allow prediction of quality and outcome.

All quality assessment activities require available, accurate data. Quality monitoring has moved from a peer review system to a data-intensive system that emphasizes development of comprehensive data bases and statistical measures to define quality. The process of QI is dependent on data to assess the current status of a process and determine future goals for the process. A variety of tools complement the QI process.

Benchmarking is the continuous process of measuring performance against the best practices, those known as leaders in a particular field. Assessing present processes against those of the top performers identifies areas of improvement leading to superior performance. Numerous institutions are involved in providing data that are utilized in the benchmarking process.

A flow chart is a pictorial representation showing all the steps of a process. It can be useful in examining how various steps relate to each other. The flow chart is used to identify the actual process that a service follows. Comparing the actual flow chart to the ideal flow chart identifies opportunities for improving processes.

A check sheet is a simple form used to record how often certain events happen. This tool is useful in gathering data on the frequency of events.

A Pareto chart is a special form of vertical bar graph with the height of the bars reflecting the frequency or impact of problems. Based on the Pareto principle, which says that 80% of the trouble comes from 20% of the problems, this QI tool displays the relative importance of all the problems or conditions, allowing providers to focus improvement efforts on activities that can provide the greatest impact.

Cause-and-effect or fishbone diagrams represent the relationship between some effect and all the possible causes. The possible causes of a problem are detailed on the left-hand side of the diagram with the effect of the problem listed on the right-hand side. This tool is useful in identifying, exploring, and visually displaying the possible causes of a problem.

Run charts or time plots provide a visual representation of changes in a process over time, to see if the long-range average is changing. The ED may monitor patient census or waiting times using this tool.

Control charts are run charts or time plots with statistically determined upper and lower control limit lines drawn on either side of the average. This tool indicates how much variability in a process is due to random variation and how much is due to unique events or individual actions.

Cost of Quality Improvement

Quality improvement has an associated monetary value. A fundamental principle of CQI is reducing or controlling variance to decrease costs and allow prediction of outcomes. The QI activities are remedies that refine existing processes and strengthen controls. The cost of quality is the cost of doing things wrong. Organizations have the choice of investing in good quality or paying for poor quality.

The QI process is oriented towards prevention of poor quality. Deming theorized that there is a root cause for every failure, the cause is preventable, and that prevention is always cheaper than failure. Prevention costs are associated with proactive operational decisions and include nursing care delivery costs and equipment or supply costs incurred in an attempt to prevent an undesired patient outcome. Appraisal costs are associated with the time needed to collect, analyze, and review data with the staff, as well as determining and implementing corrective action. Failure costs are related to the cost of redoing work and damage control. In most health care organizations, failure costs account for 75% to 85% of total expenditures, preventative costs consume 10% of expenditures, and appraisal costs 15%.[2]

The goal of CQI is to reduce failure costs to zero—quality = zero defects. Decreasing failure costs improves productivity, increases patient and staff satisfaction, and reduces hospital liability. Health care organizations, providers, and third-party payers have focused on improved patient care with the expectation that consumers are willing to pay more for a higher level of service and will develop a greater degree of customer loyalty based on quality of care.

CUSTOMER SATISFACTION

The QI process defines quality as customer satisfaction. Related QI activities focus on customer service by emphasizing the best ways to meet customer needs. Rising interest on the part of consumers has produced more expectations of the health care system from clients. Expectations are influenced by the media, rising costs, diminishing resources, technologic complexity, ethical dilemmas, and previous exposure of self or friends to the system. The closer the expectations of care are to the care provided, the higher the perception of quality.

As early as 1966, Donabedian[10] proposed that consumer satisfaction is one method of assessing outcome and quality of care. Consumer dissatisfaction is not always an indicator of the quality of health care, but it does reflect a failure of the system to meet consumer expectations and/or needs. Meeting patients' needs can be described in terms of the quality of deliverables and service quality.[23] The quality of deliverables measures timely and accurate performance, features or additional perks associated with care, reliability,

durability, and serviceability. Characteristics of service quality include reliability, responsiveness, competence, access, courtesy, communication, credibility, and security.

Customers in the ED include patients, physicians, payers, and other hospital departments or employees. The ED staff contacts more customers than any other staff in other parts of the hospital. Approximately one third of hospital admissions come through the ED. The potential impact of emergency nursing on customer satisfaction is further advanced since nurses comprise the largest group of hospital providers in the ED. Satisfaction with nursing care has been found to be the most important factor in predicting overall patient satisfaction.[9]

Traditionally, patient satisfaction with emergency care has been measured through formal surveys, follow-up phone calls, and informally through patient letters and phone calls. An instrument to measure satisfaction with emergency nursing care based upon psychologic safety, discharge teaching, information giving, and technical competence has been piloted[7] and may provide practitioners with a tool for general use.

Many EDs have instituted a variety of programs aimed at improving patient satisfaction and therefore quality. Development of "fast track" areas has been a customer-driven effort to divert nonurgent patients from the mainstream ED and provide more timely service, often at a decreased cost. Many EDs have developed educational pamphlets describing emergency care. The pamphlets are given to patients at triage so that they know what to expect from their visit. Increasing numbers of organizations have developed customer service training classes for ED staff and have incorporated customer service education into general hospital orientation.

OUTCOMES

The aim of health care is to help the patient achieve the best health outcomes in the most satisfying and efficient manner. Outcomes are defined as the effects of care activities—measurable changes in the health status of persons, groups, or communities—that can be attributed to prior or concurrent care. Negative outcomes include mortality, morbidity, readmissions complaints, and cost. Positive outcomes include physical, mental, social, and psychologic wellbeing, improved functional status, and satisfaction. Customer definition of desired outcomes is critical since the perception of quality increases as expectations of care are met. Because outcomes represent the end result of care, major consumers in the health care economy are choosing outcome measures as the best means of assessing the quality of the health care they purchase.

A model for measuring health care excellence based on outcomes has been proposed. This model combines subjective-perceptual elements of quality with objective/clinical quality elements.[22] Subjective-perceptual elements of quality are based on opinions of health care consumers and include responsiveness of personnel, efficiency, caring and attention of nursing staff, and the caring and attentiveness of ancillary staff. Since these elements are subjective, the recommendation is they be measured in aggregate, looking for trends in performance. Objective-clinical elements of quality include deaths, infections, readmissions, drug reactions, unplanned surgeries, and complications.

Such models have served as the basis for development of institutional scorecards, a set of measures that provide a comprehensive view of key concepts of quality. In 1994, JCAHO began making individual institutional reports on 28 performance issues available for a fee. Other communities have seen health care organizations cooperatively engage in continuous performance review with publication of comparative scorecards in the local media. These initiatives facilitate the consumer's ability to make informed choices for quality care.

Managed care organizations have had a significant impact on the health care environment. These systems of care seek to influence selection and utilization of health services of an enrolled population and ensure that care is provided in a high-quality, cost-effective manner. Managed care demands demonstrated quality from its providers and demands measurement of value, a function of both quality and cost.[13]

Wide, unexplainable variation in outcomes of care, utilization of resources, and costs of care led major health care consumers to advocate increased funding for outcomes research. Efforts have been made by these groups to promote more rational medical decision-making and consistent practice by using practice guidelines to guide care. Pressure is increasing to standardize utilization of health care services through external review of the need for care.

A growing interest in managing quality by managing outcomes is evolving. The concept of outcomes management relies on use of standards and guidelines in selecting appropriate interventions, routine and systematic measurement of the functioning and well-being of patients, along with disease-specific clinical outcomes; pooling of clinical and outcome data on a massive scale, and dissemination of the results to each clinical decision-maker.[11] The Institute for Healthcare Improvement (IHI) asserts that sound science that could greatly improve costs and outcomes of current health care practices already exists. However, much of this science is unused.[25] The IHI's goal is to assist health care organizations to mobilize resources needed to make positive changes in outcomes by bridging the gap between what we know and what we do.

Outcomes have been difficult to measure in the ED where length of stay and patient/provider interaction is measured in minutes. Monitoring the patient's response to interventions and the patient's status at discharge or transfer are two important outcome measures in this environment. Many EDs are using follow-up calls to measure outcomes related to knowledge of discharge instructions, medications, and follow-up care (Figure 8-3).

CLINICAL COMPETENCE

Education is integral to maintaining skills and knowledge and directly affects the quality of care. Deming dedicated two of his fourteen points for organizational transformation to increasing the knowledge-base of the workforce—instituting training on the job and instituting a vigorous program of education and self-improvement for everyone. Clinical competence is an end result of education and training. Competent staff minimize variation in practice, a basic goal of CQI.

Clinical competence is enhanced by hiring staff members based on clearly defined job qualifications, orienting individuals appropriately, and maintaining knowledge and skills by incorporating new information and methods into practice. The Emergency Nurses Association (ENA) is an example of a competency-based orientation program designed to provide new staff with the basic knowledge and technical skills necessary to function in the ED.[12] Ongoing competency is demonstrated through participation in educational opportuni-

Date of Call: _____

Chart #	Patient's Name	Contacted	Child's Status
_____ _____		Y N	Better Worse Same
Understood D/C Instructions	Prescriptions Filled		Understood Rx
Y N	Y N NA		Y N
Plan for Follow-up care	Satisfied with Care		
Y N	Y N		
Comments:			

Initials: _____

Figure **8-3** Pediatric follow-up calls form.

ties and in-services as well as periodic evaluation of actual practice to demonstrate competency of technical skills.

The ED may require nursing staff to participate in annual or biannual proficiency testing of skills such as arterial blood gas sampling, defibrillation and cardioversion (Figure 8-4), hemodynamic monitoring, external pacing-temporary transvenous pacing, and chest tube set-ups. The EDs may also require Basic Life Support, Advanced Cardiac Life Support, Pediatric Advanced Life Support, and Trauma Nursing Core Course certifications-verifications to provide employees with a standard knowledge-base from which to practice emergency nursing.

JCAHO continues to require demonstration of specific competencies, for example, annual attendance of fire, safety, infection control, and blood-borne pathogen in-services.

A recent addition has been the requirement for direct-care providers to demonstrate age-specific competency, knowledge of physical development and physiologic norms, behaviors, psychosocial development, safety considerations, and general guidelines for care for all age groups to which they provide. Age-specific competency is a critical component of the emergency nurse's knowledge base. The majority of emergency nurses care for neonates, infants, toddlers, preschoolers, school-age, adolescent, adult, and geriatric patients. The accuracy of triage decision-making is dependent on knowledge of age-appropriate vital signs and patient behavior.

Clinical Care Paths

Standardizing patient care processes by using outcome-focused plans results in improved quality and decreased re-

Staff Member: _____   Date: _____

Signature of RN validating competency: _____

CRITICAL BEHAVIORS	Complies (Y/N)
1. Utilizes universal precautions.	
2. Identifies need for defibrillation e.g., V Fib/pulseless V Tach	
3. Identifies need for cardioversion e.g., PSVT	
4. Prepares patient placing defibrillator pads in appropriate positions.	
5. Turns on EKG recorder for continuous recording.	
6. Properly places paddles on the patient's chest wall.	
7. Charges defibrillator to proper energy requirement, 200 J.	
8. States "ALL CLEAR" and visually verifies that all personnel are clear of contact with bed, patient, and equipment.	
9. Depresses both buttons on paddles simultaneously until defibrillator fires.	
10. Assess for pulse and identifies rhythm.	
11. If first attempt unsuccessful, repeats steps 4-8 at 200-300 J.	
12. If second attempt unsuccessful, repeats steps 4-8 at 360 J.	
13. If third attempt unsuccessful, continues BLS and initiates ACLS.	
14. Documents procedure/response in patient record.	
15. Describes cardioversion-procedure & energy requirement.	
INTERNAL DEFIBRILLATION	Complies (Y/N)
1. Assembles equipment.	
2. Describes sterile procedure.	
3. Identifies energy requirements.	

Comments:

Figure **8-4** Competency checklist: defibrillation (external/internal) and cardioversion.

source utilization.[26] Clinical care paths, care maps, or pathways are interdisciplinary guides to the usual treatment pattern of patients with similar needs. Care paths are composed of predetermined care activities involved in the care of a patient from presentation through discharge, time frames in which activities are to be completed, and intermediate and expected outcomes of care. Similarities between care paths and case management programs abound. Case management, however, focuses on an entire episode of illness, including all settings in which the patient receives care. The uniform inclusion of outcome measures in these standardized plans affords providers and consumers a view of the patient's sequential progress and ultimate destination. Chapter 9 provides a more detailed discussion of case management and care maps.

Care paths will most likely be developed for the majority of inpatient conditions. The value of care paths lies in the agreement of the caregiving team on the critical steps in the care of a given group of patients. Monitoring variance and the success of interventions in accomplishing outcomes provides feedback during the process of delivering care, indicating the effectiveness of specific interventions or whether changes need to be made. By incorporating those interventions that are most successful in achieving desired outcomes, care paths offer providers a mechanism to constantly evaluate and improve care.

Many EDs have successfully instituted chest pain care paths and have collaborated to develop care paths incorporating both emergency and inpatient care for conditions such as asthma, pneumonia, congestive heart failure, GI bleeding, overdoses, CVA, head injuries, and sickle cell crisis. Care paths have been developed specifically for ED use in treating nonurgent conditions such as lacerations, sprains, and sexually transmitted diseases (STDs).

Care paths are improving quality. Nine of eleven studies measuring outcomes demonstrated improvement in quality by standardizing patient care processes.[14] A recent study described the effects of using an asthma care path in the ED. The average length of stay in the department decreased 50 minutes, regular admissions decreased by 27%, intensive care unit admissions decreased by 41%, return visits to the ED within 24 hours decreased by 66%, and patient care charges to payers decreased $395,000 for the year.[20]

NURSING ROLE IN QUALITY ASSESSMENT

Since the time of Florence Nightingale, nurses have been involved in the process of evaluating the quality of patient care. Florence Nightingale set standards for patient care and gathered data to support her observations. The first nursing audit was developed in 1957 at Theyer Hospital in Maine. In 1967, evaluation of care was defined as one of the four functions of the nursing process.[32]

However, it wasn't until the 1970s that nurses took an active role in development of standardized methods to determine the quality and effectiveness of nursing care. In 1973,

the American Nurses Association (ANA) published *Standards for Nursing Practice,* standards generic to all types of nursing. In 1983 the ENA (originally known as Emergency Department Nurses Association) published *Standards of Emergency Nursing Practice.* Professional standards identify nursing's role in the health care system and provide a framework for delivering patient care and evaluation of that care. Rather than defining a maximum or minimal level of performance, the ANA and ENA now define standards in terms of competency.

When JCAHO created QA standards in 1980, nursing responded by conducting audits specific to nursing care and establishing unit-based QA programs. Staff nurses were charged with identifying high-volume, high-risk situations, developing indicators to measure care, collecting data, and instituting remedial actions. The major thrust of nursing quality assessment focused on measuring processes and/or analyzing the degree of compliance with nursing care standards via randomized chart audits.

The CQI process, by focusing on active participation and communication, empowers all health care providers to examine their practice, identify areas for improvement, gather data, analyze it, and make recommendations for action. In a CQI environment, everyone has a responsibility for quality. Outcome measures have replaced compliance with standards as the focus of quality assessment measures. Nursing care outcomes, defined as measurable changes in the patient's state of health that are occasioned by nursing, include modification of signs and symptoms, knowledge, attitudes, satisfaction, skill level, and compliance. Documentation of what nurses do to affect patient outcomes must improve. Nursing should focus on clinical studies that demonstrate the cost-effectiveness of nursing and determine which treatment elements produce optimal outcomes for each type of patient. Ineffective interventions should then be replaced with more appropriate methods.

There is an urgent need for EDs to develop measurement tools, systems, and research to demonstrate the cost-effectiveness of quality nursing care in relation to positive patient outcomes. Aiken[1] concluded from studying outcomes literature that nurses influence who lives and dies in hospitals. Nurses must articulate their value in this health care environment.

SUMMARY

JCAHO has provided much of the leadership in health care quality assessment. Quality assurance programs focused on measuring the compliance of health care organizations and providers with established standards of care. Quality improvement programs focusing on measuring the performance of the many processes of care have been adopted as the quality management approach of the 1990s. The process of QI represents a change in paradigms. It emphasizes customer satisfaction and the role of education as a key to decreasing variance in processes. Care paths have been developed in increasing numbers to standardize patient care, improve quality, and decrease costs. Outcome measures have recently been adopted as the best assessment of health care quality.

Health care organizations are primarily in the business of patient care delivery. The majority of this care is provided by nurses. Nursing represents a major cost center to health care organizations. Accountability for the value of health services is shared not only by nurses but by all members of the health care team. High-quality care is dependent on the cooperative, collaborative efforts of multiple providers. In today's competitive health care environment, survival of the nursing profession may well rest in its ability to demonstrate the value of nursing care in promoting positive patient outcomes.

REFERENCES

1. Aiken LH: Charting the future of hospital nursing, *Image: J Nurs Sch* 22:72, 1990.
2. Beck KL, Larrabee JH: A simultaneous analysis of nursing care quality and cost, *J Nurs Care Qual* 9(4):63, 1995.
3. Bliersbach C: Quality improvement: one-third of the quality equation, *J Qual Assur* 13(5):58, 1991.
4. Burda D: Providers look to industry for quality models, *Mod Healthcare* 7(2):28, 1988.
5. Bush DL: Quality management through statistics, *J Qual Assur* 13(5):40, 1991.
6. Caper P: Defining quality in medical care, *Health Aff* 7(1):49, 1988.
7. Clark CA, Pokorny ME, Brown ST: Consumer satisfaction with nursing care in a rural community emergency department, *J Nurs Care Qual* 10(2):49, 1996.
8. Deming WE: *Out of the crisis,* Cambridge, 1986, Massachusetts Institute of Technology.
9. Doering ER: Factors influencing satisfaction with care, *Qual Rev Bull* 291, 1983.
10. Donabedian A: Evaluating the quality of medical care, *Millbank Q* 44:203, 1966.
11. Ellwood P: Outcomes management: a technology of patient experience, *N Engl J Med* 318(24):1549, 1988.
12. Emergency Nurses Association: *Orientation to emergency nursing: diversity in practice,* Park Ridge, Ill, 1993, The Association.
13. Fedora RD, Camp TL: The changing managed care market, *J Ambulatory Care Manag* 17(2):1, 1994.
14. Grimshaw JM: Effect of clinical guidelines on medical practice: a systematic review of rigorous evaluations, *Lancet* 342:1317, 1993.
15. The Joint Commission on Accreditation of Healthcare Organizations: *Accreditation manual for hospitals,* vol I, Oakbrook, Ill, 1996, The Joint Commission.
16. The Joint Commission on Accreditation of Healthcare Organizations, *Transitions: from QA to CQI, using CQI approaches to monitor, evaluate, and improve quality,* Oakbrook, Ill, 1991, The Joint Commission.
17. Jones KR: Maintaining quality in a changing environment, *Nurs Econ* 9(May/June):159, 1991.
18. Juran JM: *Juran on leadership for quality: an executive handbook,* New York, 1989, The Free Press.
19. Mason JD, Gunnels MD: Redefining emergency department visitor policies: a continuous quality improvement approach, *J Emerg Nurs* 20(6):562, 1994.
20. McFadden ER et al: Protocol therapy for acute asthma: therapeutic benefits and cost savings, *Am J Med* 99:651, 1995.
21. McGrath NE: Pediatric quality improvement in the emergency department, *J Emerg Nurs* 21(1):172, 1995.
22. Merry MD: What is quality care? a model for measuring health care excellence, *Qual Rev Bull* Sept: 298, 1987.
23. Nackel DG, Collier TA: Implementing a quality improvement program, *J Soc Health Syst* 1(1):1, 1989.
24. Oetker D, Cole C: Improving the outcome of emergency department patients with a chief complaint of chest pain, *J Nurs Care Qual* 10(2):58, 1996.
25. *Overview and status report:* Breakthrough series, Boston, 1995, Institute for Healthcare Improvement.
26. Peters DA: Outcomes: the framework for quality care, *J Nurs Care Qual* 10(1):61, 1995.
27. Provance L, Alvis D, Silfin E: Quality improvement and public health-tetanus immunization in the emergency department, *Am J Med Qual* 9:165, 1994.
28. Shea SS, Senteno J: Emergency department patient throughput: a continuous quality approach to length of stay, *J Emerg Nurs* 20(6):355, 1995.
29. Sholtes PE: *The team handbook: how to use teams to improve quality,* Madison, Wis, 1988, Joiner Associates.
30. Tackett SA: Quality assurance versus QP[4]: the missing link, *J Qual Assur* June/July: 8, 1989.
31. *Webster's New Collegiate Dictionary,* Springfield, Mass, 1981, Mirriam-Webster.
32. Yura H, Walsh MB: *The nursing process: assessing, planning, implementing, evaluating,* ed 5, Norwalk, Conn, 1988, Appleton & Lange.

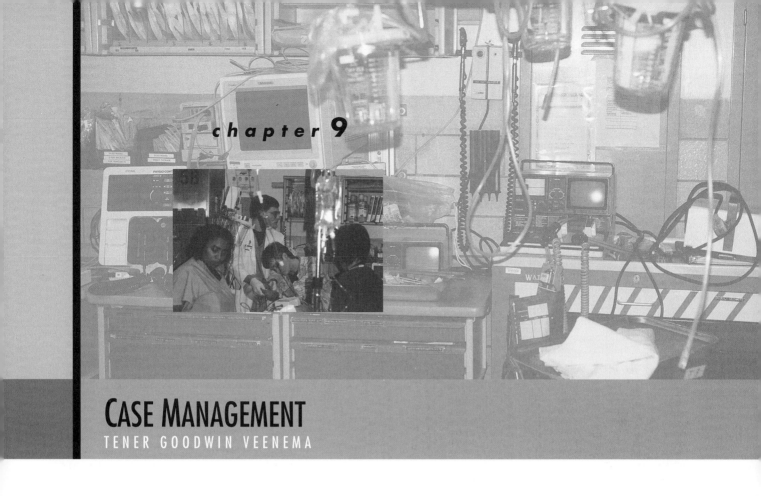

CASE MANAGEMENT

TENER GOODWIN VEENEMA

Widespread acceptance of the clinical guidelines and outcome measurement has driven emergency department (ED) medical directors and nurse managers to reconsider their present model of unit operation. Case management, a clinical system for strategic management of cost and quality patient outcomes, was originally implemented to address the needs of the acute inpatient population. The principles of case management can also be applied to EDs through work redesign to improve care delivery, enhance patient and provider satisfaction, and simultaneously control costs. Redesign focuses on reengineering care delivery systems through care maps, or clinical guidelines, enhanced collaboration and care coordination, and clearly defined time frames for care. Care management reflects the national shift from health care evaluation based on the process of care toward evaluation based on analysis of care outcomes.

Case management is not a new concept. It dates back to public health programs of the early 1900s. The concept became prominent during the 1960s and 1970s as social workers designed care systems for the mentally ill, the elderly, and disabled patients. The primary goal was to enhance access and coordinate health care services while decreasing fragmentation of care.[2] Nursing case management developed at New England Medical Center (NEMC) in Boston in direct response to economic pressures exerted on hospitals by implementation of the diagnosis-related groups (DRGs) prospective payment system. The NEMC model evolved from a 13-year history of primary nursing and an in-depth

investigation of nursing and physician practice patterns as they related to outcomes of care.[4] Specific goals of the NEMC model were increased nurse-physician collaboration in patient care, provider and patient satisfaction, and acceptable patient outcomes achieved within an effective time frame using resources appropriately.

A major force behind case management is the need to manage health care costs. Case management has also been strongly influenced by continuous quality improvement (CQI) and patient-centered care, which provide a framework for monitoring and managing clinical processes. Case management can decrease ED patient length of stay, avoid duplication of expensive health care resources, and identify system strengths and weaknesses. Emergency care is inherently challenging due to variability in volume and patient acuity. The emergency patient population is characterized by unpredictability and patients who present with complaints rather than clearly defined diagnoses. The problem for which the patient is seeking care is often unexpected and episodic. Acuity levels vary among patients presenting with similar complaints. High patient acuity with sudden, frequent changes in the patient's condition make compartmentalization of care into a series of predictable events difficult. Traditionally, patients present to the ED and receive care for their presenting complaint. With case management, administrators and providers utilize preestablished guidelines for patient care. A major paradigm shift is required to move providers from a reactive mode to a more proactive mode, creating a "gold standard" for delivery of emergency services.

Case management provides "a system of health assessment, planning, service procurement/delivery/coordination and monitoring to meet the multiple needs of clients."[1] With health care reform, capitation, and restrictive prospective payment systems, nursing must accomplish similar goals with fewer resources than ever before. Case management provides a framework for responding to changes in the health care industry by rethinking patient care needs and clinician roles. The focus of change is the provider and the focus of evaluation is the patient.

Reengineering patient care delivery systems using case management is based on the premise that quality is not an elusive goal for health care. Case management does require that ED medical directors, nurse managers, and administrators ask the following questions:

• What is required from each health care discipline to achieve realistic outcomes for patients with similar diagnoses or complaints?

• What is the best way to produce realistic outcomes?

• Who should be held accountable for outcomes?

• How can care be restructured so outcomes are consistently achieved?

• What cost-reduction strategies can be incorporated into clinical practice without sacrificing quality of care?

Answers to these questions are key components of the case management model—care maps, enhanced collaborative practice, care coordination, and time-framed clinical outcomes. The evaluation component of the model is variance analysis. Case management targets specific patient populations and operationalizes CQI programs where they matter most—at the patient care level. Used effectively, CQI provides a direct, powerful methodology to organize and coordinate services within a complex department, or a larger health care organization.

In many ways, the ED serves as a mirror for society at large. Societal issues such as increases in random and domestic violence, substance abuse, unemployment, homelessness, and the number of underinsured or uninsured patients have tremendous implications for how the ED functions. These crises of American society are reflected in the ED as increased ED visits for trauma, toxicology, premature birth, and infectious diseases such as hepatitis and AIDS. Visits for primary care have increased as the number of underinsured or uninsured has grown. As the number of Americans over the age of 65 increases, elderly patients with chronic health problems will have a significant impact on the ED. Advances in biomedical technology and pharmaceuticals have improved survival in the geriatric population, and in the neonatal population because of improved viability for preterm infants; long-term medical management of complex chronic conditions may lead to frequent ED visits. As the emphasis shifts from inpatient visits to ambulatory care, the role of the ED as gateway for the hospital will grow in scope and complexity. Fewer patients will be admitted to the hospital as bed access becomes more restricted by managed care providers. And, those admitted will have shorter inpatient stays due restrictions on coverage. If patients are discharged too early, increased recidivism will lead to additional ED visits. Providers will feel increased pressure to treat and release complex patient populations to avoid hospital admissions. Figure 9-1 illustrates these complex relationships.

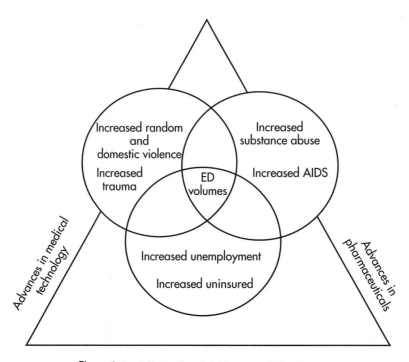

Figure **9-1** Effects of societal issues on ED volumes.

Lack of adequate health insurance has left many Americans without access to consistent primary care. EDs are now a leading provider of unscheduled primary and acute care, contributing to an already fragmented and overpriced health care system. As managed care permeates the health care market, fragmentation will no longer be tolerated. Provider discounts and capitation will limit reimbursement for ED visits and overall ED usage will be actively discouraged by managed care providers. To remain fiscally viable, the ED must analyze costs associated with providing emergency care and identify potential areas for cost reduction. The ED, a dynamic microsystem within a much larger, equally dynamic health care system, must position itself to grow and change in order to survive a highly competitive health care market. Collaborative efforts between hospital administration, physicians, and nurses using case management can meet the challenges of a capitated reimbursement system.

PLANNING

Design and development of an ED case management project requires identification of key participants early in project design, administrative commitment, provider support, and a realistic estimate of project development needs in time and resources. It is essential to develop a shared vision for the project and how it will look once implemented. Each project participant must realize there are various ways to implement this model. Each hospital must analyze the needs of its patient population and view these needs against its own priorities for cost containment and work redesign. This chapter provides a framework for applying key concepts of case management in the ED. Table 9-1 defines these key concepts.

COLLABORATION

One of the key components of case management is collaborative care. Collaboration is defined as "interactions between nurse and physician that enable the knowledge and skills of both professionals to synergistically influence the patient care being provided."[3] Critical attributes necessary for collaboration include shared planning and decision making, problem solving, responsibility, and cooperation. Case management strengthens interdisciplinary collaboration initially through team meetings outside the patient care areas. Health care providers are given the opportunity to discuss patient care issues in a forum that encourages constructive criticism and proactive decision making. Awareness grows regarding each provider's contributions and expectations as team members become clear about expectations for time lines, care activities, and resource utilization.

Conceptually, the ED is an ideal clinical location for case management because a collaborative practice model is already in place. Health care providers from a variety of disciplines provide patient care side by side, with ongoing communication about the patient's status. Physicians and nurses are already accustomed to an algorithmic approach to patient care by virtue of Advanced Cardiac Life Support (ACLS), Advanced Trauma Life Support (ATLS), and Pediatric Advanced Life Support (PALS) guidelines, which parallel time-framed standards of care for specific patient populations. This is the hallmark of the case management model.

The potential for creativity in developing collaborative practices in emergency care is limitless. Collaboration can be defined along patient service lines. For example, physicians and nurses could work as teams in their area of expertise. Partnerships might include a cardiovascular team, pulmonary team, or adolescent medicine team. Team partners could then participate in inpatient case management efforts to define standards of care, organize and oversee care of select patient populations, establish clinical outcomes, and identify system variances that are barriers to care. One potential outcome of this team concept includes continuity of

Table **9-1**	**Essential Case Management Concepts**
Concept	Definition
Case management	A patient care delivery system that focuses on achievement of outcomes within effective time frames with appropriate use of resources across the continuum of care. Crosses all service areas where the patient receives care, prehospital to postdischarge community health agencies. Incorporates diagnosis- or complaint-specific protocols including standard medical and nursing interventions. Defines accountability to ensure that cost and quality outcomes are achieved.
Managed care	A planned approach to care that delineates accountability for patient outcomes within specific time frames. May also refer to restricted reimbursement strategies by a prospective payment system. Key components include collaboration and appropriate resource utilization.
Care map/clinical pathway	Terms used interchangeably to describe a documentation tool that is part of the case management model. For their discussion in this chapter, *clinical pathway* is utilized. Other commonly used terms are anticipated recovery paths, care tracks, or critical care paths. The clinical pathway provides a time event picture of the patient's hospitalization.
Capitation	Restricted payment for health care. For example, a provider may negotiate reimbursement of $500 per vaginal delivery. If the institution provides the care for less, they keep the profit. If the care is more, the institution must absorb the expense.

patient care across service lines and after discharge. Teams could negotiate with home health agencies to create a comprehensive umbrella of care for certain patients.

Project Development

Administrative commitment to the case management project and resource availability are critical for successful implementation of case management. Administrative commitment refers to philosophic and financial support of the project, for example, personnel, secretarial support, computers, and external resources such as consultants, manuals, and videotapes. The ED medical director, nurse manager, program administrator, and members of the hospital executive committee must also be committed to the project. Administrative commitment can pave the way for project development and multidisciplinary approval of clinical pathways across service lines. When possible, commitment should be obtained in writing prior to start of the project.

Resource availability refers to personnel, time, and equipment required to implement the project. It is unlikely that hospital administration will create additional positions to facilitate development of the project since one of case management's primary goals is cost reduction. Existing staff usually incorporate project responsibilities into their present job responsibilities. Negotiations to ensure members of the project development team have time for essential tasks may be necessary. A coordinated effort not only ensures support, but also prevents duplication of effort by other committees within the institution. The management team should assess departmental readiness for change and educational needs related to the change. Preliminary data regarding patient volumes, acuity, length of stay, costs, resource utilization, and profit margins should also be collected.

After determination that case management is feasible and desirable, a steering committee must be created to begin formal work redesign. The steering committee may consist of ED management or other key individuals within the department who are interested and committed to the project. The importance of achieving a cross-section of professionals from within the department cannot be overemphasized. It is essential that all viewpoints are represented on the committee. The committee can expect to function 6 months to a year to get the project started. Figure 9-2 shows the relationship between the steering committee, nurse manager, project director, and other key players in the implementation process.

Project Director

Identification of one individual to organize and coordinate development of a case management system depends on the size of the project, resources available, and the time frame for project completion. Prior to embarking on case management, each ED should outline the project and assess what individuals are available to do the job. For a small project, one individual within the department may assume these additional responsibilities as part of his or her existing job. A small project might be one where the purpose is to design four to six clinical pathways and restructure the quality improvement program. This individual may be an experienced registered nurse with time and interest to devote to the project. With a larger project, such as development of 20 to 30 clinical pathways with concurrent variance tracking and implementation of a case management role, a full-time coordinator with specific skills is required. Ideally a solid clinical background coupled with exceptional verbal and written communication skills, some teaching experience, and research background are needed for the case manager role. In most instances, this position is held by an advanced practice nurse with a master's degree in nursing administration, business administration, or clinical nursing. In many large university settings, the project director is a physician whose interest lies in outcomes management. Extensive knowledge of clinical information systems, that is, data management, is an invaluable asset for a project director.

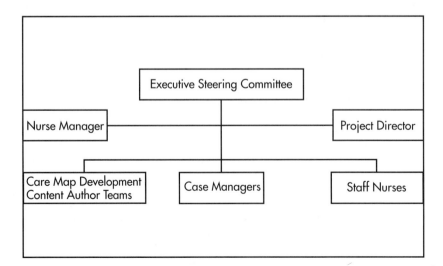

Figure **9-2** Case management organizational chart.

The project director must maintain close contact with the ED management team and the case management steering committee to ensure that all members of the team share the same vision for the project and that a unified approach is used as the project is unveiled. The project director must work well with the nurse manager, the medical director, and other members of the team to achieve consensus at project development meetings. Physicians, nurses, social workers, technicians, and administrators each bring their own agenda to the project. The project director must be able to negotiate and compromise to circumvent personal agendas and remain focused on the ultimate goal of improving patient care. The project director along with the steering committee must be empowered to make changes. Otherwise, clinical pathways may be written and positions restructured but real change will not occur.

Goals and the Vision Statement

Formulation of a clearly defined statement of the purpose for redesigning ED patient care delivery consistent with overall organization goals is imperative for the project's success. This responsibility belongs to the steering committee and should be completed before further work begins. Box 9-1 summarizes potential goals for case management in the ED. Measurement of goal attainment is determined by the individual ED.

In addition to articulation of goals for the case management project, a vision for overall design of the project should be developed. A clearly defined vision statement ensures all participants are working toward the same goal. Periodic review as the project evolves keeps everyone on track. The vision statement should be realistic for the specific situation, reflect goals the ED wishes to accomplish, and respond to the changing health care arena. Two examples of vision statements are:

- ALL patients will be placed on clinical pathways based on the presenting complaint identified at triage.
- SELECT patients will be placed in a case management plan that encompasses the entire episode of care.

Following completion of the statement of purpose, goals, and vision statement, a time line for the project should be completed prior to implementation. A realistic time line facilitates evaluation of progress, but is flexible enough to allow revision when necessary. The time line should be supported by all participants and contain specific time frames for each aspect of the project.

CLINICAL PATHWAYS

Clinical pathways bring the standard of care to the point of practice at the patient's bedside and function as a documentation tool that demonstrates standard of care and functional patient outcomes along a time line. A clinical pathway establishes a time-sequence relationship between standard of care and a specific patient type. Clinical responsibility for each professional discipline is described in clearly measurable outcomes. Box 9-2 identifies major components of a clinical pathway. Pathways serve many purposes in the ED, such as educational tools for resident house staff and new nursing staff. An ED staffed by multiple medical providers on a contractual basis, or traveling nursing agencies, may use pathways to convey the organization's standard of care. Finally, health care providers whose education and training are in a specialty other than emergency medicine find the pathway an invaluable reference tool.

Clinical pathways can be designed to incorporate regional and national standards of care. Pathways operationalize the organization's quality improvement program, making sure the right thing is done for the right patient, the first time and every time. Box 9-3 identifies ways clinical pathways can be used as a management tool.

Box 9-2 Clinical Pathway Components

Triage criteria
Prehospital care history
Assessment guidelines
High-risk indicators
Diagnostic studies
Treatments-medications
Patient activities
Consultations
Patient-family teaching
Discharge planning

Box 9-1 ED Case Management Goals

Increase the quality of patient care
Improve patient satisfaction
Decrease patient waiting times and ED length of stay
Increase multidisciplinary collaboration and improve provider satisfaction
Avoid duplication of expensive health care resources
Control spiraling health care costs
Ensure standard of care at the bedside
Identify system strengths and weaknesses

Box 9-3 Clinical Pathways as ED Management Tool

Provide unit-based quality improvement
Serve as educational tool for new staff
Facilitate research
Ensure continuity of care
Bring standard of care to point of practice

Clinical pathways for the ED can be created in a variety of formats. Most do not and should not look like inpatient care maps. Pathways are more than a new system for organizing and documenting care. When utilized effectively, pathways drive patient care and are an accurate reflection of care rendered. The standard columnar format of Day 1, Day 2, etc., used for inpatient pathways will not work. Attempting to structure patient care on an hourly basis does not always work. The ED clinical pathway views time in minutes and hours rather than days.

Successful ED clinical pathways are based on the premise that most emergency care is rendered within the first hour. Over 75% of the clinical pathway addresses assessments and interventions that take place within 60 minutes of the patient's arrival. A care map locked into a rigid chronologic time frame results in a document that is cumbersome, unbalanced, and rarely an accurate report of care rendered. A flexible time frame with reasonable ranges for care delivery or care map based on achievement of desired patient outcomes functions more effectively and accommodates the uniqueness of each patient. Clinical pathway construction in the ED requires development of several formats based on needs of the patient populations and types of services provided. One- or two-page formats can easily address needs of the nonacute patient with problems such as urinary tract infection-dysuria or dental pain. Figures 9-3 and 9-4 show two examples of this type of ED clinical pathway.

Needs of the more acutely ill patient can be met with an expanded format that incorporates repeated assessment and multiple interventions. Clinical pathways must also be designed to accommodate patient complications and comorbidities. The pathway may also be symptom based, or based on presenting complaint. Clinical pathways based on the patient's presenting complaint at triage allow the most flexibility in addressing clinical findings. The format of the care map should reflect the algorithmic approach inherent to emergency medicine and nursing, for example, current PALS guidelines could be included in a clinical pathway for major pediatric trauma. Pathways driven by DRGs are too narrow to function effectively in the ED. For example, a pathway designed to address DRG #198 Total Cholecystectomy has little value in the ED. A patient with abdominal pain may require a clinical pathway broad enough to accommodate a variety of possible diagnoses and patient responses. Figure 9-5 is an example of an expanded ED clinical pathway.

Clinical pathways interface with inpatient units, ambulatory clinics, private physicians, other health care facilities, and community agencies. Pathways may be generically designed to address the needs of a particular patient population or individualized to a specific patient. For example, an ED pathway for the asthma patient should interface with the pathway where the patient receives primary care. The patient's health history regarding treatment modalities and medications, baseline peak expiratory flow measurements, and criteria for seeking medical care can be captured on the pathway. In addition, subspecialty care can be included to reinforce the importance of consistent primary care, while communicating valuable information to ED personnel. Use of an interactive computer information system links the ED clinical pathway directly to the inpatient pathway for patients requiring admission. This facilitates communication across departmental lines, consistency of patient care, and prevents expensive and unnecessary duplication of diagnostic tests done in the ED.

Documentation

An important decision to make early in the design process is whether the clinical pathway will function as documentation tool or serve as a project management tool. Pathways that are an interdisciplinary documentation tool are more time consuming and challenging to write, however, ultimately function more effectively. Making pathways the sole documentation tool for the ED visit ensures compliance. Busy emergency care providers rarely use documents they do not write on. Pathways streamline documentation while increasing documentation accuracy. Patient care situations such as resuscitation, which previously required completion of many forms by medicine and nursing, can be reduced to one comprehensive pathway. Clinical pathways also blend easily into the hospital's clinical information system. Ideally, pathways online at a bedside terminal with an interactive software program allow ongoing individualization of the pathway as the patient progresses. Evaluation of outcome measurement can be calculated concurrently. Once implemented, annual review of the pathway by the development team ensures the content meets requisite practice standards and reflects current treatment modalities.

Designing clinical pathways in conjunction with the hospital's billing department ensures capture of appropriate charges and decreases revenue loss due to inadequate or insufficient documentation. Each pathway can be coded so that billing can be done directly from the care map, reducing lengthy chart reviews or additional paperwork.

Research

Clinical pathways are also excellent data collection tools for emergency care research. Historically, emergency medicine or nursing research required lengthy chart reviews or additional documentation on separate study forms. Clinical pathways facilitate departmental research by building specific data points directly into the pathway, allowing for more accurate collection of data and a larger sample size. Simultaneously, data provide a management tool for conveying current research findings for clinical application to patient care.

Piloting the Clinical Pathway

Before to piloting the pathway, all ED staff (nurses, physicians, patient care technicians, social workers) should be educated on the purpose of the pathway, overall project goals, and time frame for project implementation. Specifics regarding use of the pathway and plans for ongoing monitoring and revision should be discussed during this initial education. Regularly scheduled educational sessions help problem solving and keep staff updated. Each pathway should be piloted for a predetermined period to evaluate potential changes before the final draft is completed.

OUTCOME MEASUREMENT AND VARIANCE ANALYSIS

Clinical pathways allow accurate measurement of the quality of care through the identification of variations in outcomes. Traditional variance analysis categorizes ED variances into three main areas (Table 9-2). Ideally, variance data should be collected on all patients seen in the ED with analysis of variance replacing existing performance improvement activities; that is, chart audit, patient flow studies. It is important to collect meaningful data, that is, data regarding practice patterns, costs, length of stay, and resource utilization. Avoid the tendency to collect too much data. Aggregate variance analysis is done weekly or monthly as needed and can be reviewed at staff meetings or morbidity and mortality conferences. Variance analysis should not be part of the medical record.

Computerization is ideal for data collection and analysis. Manual data collection and variance analysis are cumbersome and time consuming, but should not prevent implementation of case management. Preplanning the process facilitates identification of variance sources and offers opportunities to improve systems, and ultimately, improve patient outcomes. Aggregate data can be analyzed to identify patterns and trends. For example, persistent delays in patient admissions may be tracked to their source, such as lack of transport personnel, housekeeping, communication problems. Variance analysis also offers opportunities for research to validate effectiveness of treatment and identify opportunities for improvements in patient care.

THE CASE MANAGER

It is important to remember the various ways to implement case management. The strength of any case management model lies in its ability to meet the needs of various patient care settings. Some case management models use clinical pathway and collaborative practice, whereas others go a step farther and designate a case manager. The case manager is a clinical expert with special interest and knowledge in care coordination. Traditionally, this role is best suited to an advanced practice nurse (clinical nurse specialist or nurse practitioner) who possesses the requisite leadership and communication skills. The role may also be successfully filled by an experienced staff nurse. Box 9-4 summarizes ED case manager responsibilities.

The ED case manager role will add significant project demands in time and money for recruitment, hiring, education, and orientation. This person can be a tremendous asset to the project director, steering committee, and physicians in developing and supporting the case management project while functioning as a care provider. The role does create opportunities for expanding professional practice for emergency nurses, and therefore deserves careful consideration.

Text continued on page 89.

Table **9-2**	**ED Variances**	
Source	Description	Example
System	Occurs when the system has not provided expected support.	Toxicology screen needed emergently is not completed because the laboratory is closed. CT not available 24 hours a day.
Provider	Clinician has not completed expected activity.	Hourly neuro checks are not documented on patient with closed head injury.
Patient	Patient does or experiences something unexpected that prolongs hospitalization.	Family refuses to take the patient home. Patient refuses a blood transfusion.

Box 9-4 ED Case Manager Responsibilities

Collaborate with physicians and other members of the health care team to develop patient-specific clinical pathways.

Serve as a direct care provider and collaborate with other nurses to ensure appropriate individualization of the clinical pathway.

Communicate with members of the health care team to solicit feedback regarding the plan of care for specific patient types and facilitate revision of the clinical pathway as needed.

Educate patients and their families regarding the case manager role through use of patient-friendly clinical pathways.

Monitor patient's clinical progress throughout the ED stay, admission to discharge.

Identify patient variance from the clinical pathway and collaborate with health care team members for variance resolution.

Identify additional patient populations appropriate for case management.

Compile aggregate variance data for specific patient types, communicate and analyze variances with members of the health care team, and develop strategies for variance reduction.

Incorporate findings of variance analysis into the ED quality improvement program.

Identify and implement strategies to reduce resource consumption.

Participate in case management–related research activities.

UNIVERSITY OF ROCHESTER
STRONG MEMORIAL HOSPITAL
SMH 689 MR
EMERGENCY DEPARTMENT CLINIC
OUTCOME BASED CARE MAP
FOR: DENTAL / ORAL AND MAXILLOFACIAL SURGERY

TRIAGE
Date: _____ Time of arrival: _____

Arrival: ☐ Emergency Medical Services ☐ Family member ☐ Self

Primary Dentist: _____ Location: _____

Patient sent in by Dentist: ☐ yes ☐ no ☐ other

Age _____ If under 18, page Eastman Dental Center Pediatric Resident after paging General Practice Dental Resident

VS T_____ P_____ R_____ BP_____ Hx of: ☐ Heart Murmur ☐ Prosthetic Heart Valve ☐ Prosthetic Joint Replacement

Weight (if < 18 years old) _____ ☐ Accompanied by Parent or Guardian

OUTCOME
Time Resident Paged _____

Time of arrival _____

CHIEF COMPLAINT
Toothache ☐ yes ☐ no

Location _____

Onset _____

Duration _____

Post Procedural Complication ☐ yes ☐ no

Date of procedure _____

Type of procedure _____

☐ Bleeding ☐ Persistent Pain ☐ Fever ☐ Swelling

Patient Triaged to Dental Clinic ☐ Yes ☐ No

Time: _____

Patient Taken to Dental Clinic by: _____

_____

If female, last menstrual period_____

TRAUMA
Have the teeth or jaws been traumatized? ☐ yes ☐ no

Time of occurrence_____

Type of trauma _____

Mechanism of trauma _____

Teeth brought to ED ☐ yes ☐ no

Facial lacerations ☐ yes ☐ no

Last tetanus_____

AVULSED TOOTH KEPT CLEAN, PLACED IN SALINE AND GIVEN TO DENTIST UPON HIS/HER ARRIVAL TO ED

☐ YES ☐ NO ☐ N/A

TETANUS GIVEN ☐ YES ☐ NO **TIME**_____

MANUFACTURER _____ **LOT #**_____

TRIAGE RN _____

HISTORY (to be completed by Provider)

History of Present Illness   Time _____

_____

_____

_____

Past Medical History
☐ Heart murmur ☐ CVA ☐ Rheumatic Fever ☐ Angina ☐ Hypertension
☐ Prosthetic heart valve ☐ Sickle cell anemia ☐ Hemophilia
☐ Other clotting factor syndromes ☐ Hx of prolonged bleeding
☐ Jaundice ☐ Hepatitis ☐ Other Liver Disease
☐ Hx of MI ☐ Pregnancy

☐ STD ☐ HIV ☐ AIDS ☐ TB ☐ Seizure Disorder
☐ Psychiatric Treatment ☐ Asthma ☐ Bronchitis
☐ Pneumonia ☐ Emphysema ☐ Cancer
☐ Radiation therapy ☐ Ulcers ☐ Other GI/GU
☐ Med Allergies ☐ Developmentally Disable ☐ Diabetes

Comments _____

_____

_____

Past Surgical History & Hospitalizations _____

_____

_____

Complications of Surgery or Adverse Drug Reactions _____

_____

Current Medications _____

_____

Rev. 4/94

Figure **9-3** Sample ED care map-short format. (*Courtesy University of Rochester, Strong Memorial Hospital, Rochester, New York.*)

Allergies:_____

_____

Type of Reaction:_____

_____

_____

[X] ED

ASSESSMENT 1

☐   Informed Consent Obtained
   ☐ Surgical   ☐ Sedation   ☐ Pediatric   ☐ Other

PHYSICAL EXAM

Extra Oral Exam: ☐ Swelling ☐ Large ☐ fluctuant ☐ airway compromised
                       ☐ Moderate   ☐ indurated   ☐ multiple spaces
                       ☐ Slight   ☐ extends past midline
            Location of swelling: _____
            Rate of Onset _____

      ☐ Erythema   Location:_____
      ☐ Sensitivity to Palpation   Site: _____
      ☐ Extraoral Lesion/Laceration   Location: _____
                         Approximate size: _____
           Comment: _____

Intra Oral Exam: ☐ Swelling   ☐ Large ☐ fluctuant   ☐ airway compromised
                       ☐ Moderate   ☐ indurated   ☐ uvula deviated
                       ☐ Slight ☐ tongue/floor of mouth elevated
            Location of swelling:_____

Traumatized Teeth: ☐ Fracture ☐ Tooth# _____ ☐ Class _____
                  ☐ Avulsion ☐ Tooth# _____
Toothache: Area/Tooth# _____
           Sensitive to: ☐ Hot   ☐ Cold   ☐ Percussion ☐ Palpation
Radiographic Survey _____
Assessment_____
☐ Oral Surgery Consult Called   ☐ Attending Consult Called
Diagnosis _____
Consent obtained ☐ Surgical procedure ☐ Sedation ☐ Pediatric ☐ other
Type Local Anesthetic_____
Amount _____ Type of Injection_____

Assessment:_____
_____
_____
_____
Plan: _____
_____
_____
_____

Treatment Rendered: Antibiotic Prophylaxis begun ☐ Yes   ☐ No
_____
_____
_____
_____
_____
_____

Dentist Signature: _____

DISPOSITION

☐ Admit to Floor_____
Report Called   ☐ Yes   Time _____
Transfer   Time _____
Admitting Attending _____
☐ OR ☐ OR Sheet Completed
Transfer   Time _____

Clothing and Valuables

☐ Family   ☐ Security   ☐ Cashier   ☐ Clothing Room

☐ Discharged Home:
Accompanied by:_____
Transportation: _____
Time:
Ambulatory: ☐ Yes   ☐ No
T_____   P_____   R _____   BP_____

OUTCOME

☐ Patient's pain controlled
☐ Patient discharge instruction sheet complete

Patient/Guardian demonstrates knowledge of:

   Discharge Medications   ☐ Yes ☐ No   ☐ N/A
   Activity Restrictions   ☐ Yes ☐ No   ☐ N/A
   Dietary Restrictions   ☐ Yes ☐ No   ☐ N/A
   Need for follow-up   ☐ Yes ☐ No   ☐ N/A

Follow-Up:

☐ Private Dentist   ☐ SMH Dental Clinic
☐ Eastman Dental Center   ☐ Other _____
Appointment Scheduled   ☐ Yes   ☐ No
Date _____   Time _____
Dentist Signature _____

Figure **9-3** cont'd   For legend see opposite page.

UNIVERSITY OF ROCHESTER
STRONG MEMORIAL HOSPITAL
SMH 71 MR
EMERGENCY DEPARTMENT
UTI/DYSURIA CLINICAL PATHWAY
Page 1 of 2

Date: _____

Time: _____

[X] ED

HISTORY

Estimated time for MD/NP and RN initial assessment 10-15 minutes.   Time _____

Onset of symptoms: _____   Dysuria: ☐ Yes ☐ No

Hematuria ☐ Yes ☐ No   Frequency: ☐ Yes ☐ No   Urgency: ☐ Yes ☐ No

Fever   ☐ Yes ☐ No   Degree of Fever: _____   Back/flank pain: ☐ Yes   ☐ No   Last sexual intercourse: _____

LMP: (female only) _____   Vaginal/penile discharge: ☐ Yes   ☐ No   Form of birth control _____

If patient is male with penile discharge, do NOT get U/A until after cultures obtained.

Pain with bowel movements (men only):   ☐Yes   ☐No

History of UTI in past: ☐ Yes   ☐ No   If yes, date last episode: _____

Number of UTI, within last year _____

History of urinary tract abnormality ☐ Yes   ☐ No   Recent Instrumentation: ☐ Foley   ☐ Cystoscopy   ☐ None

Other symptoms: _____

_____

_____

_____

Other Past Medical History: _____

Medications: _____

Allergies: _____

PHYSICAL EXAM

Triage Vital signs: HR: _____ BP: _____ T: _____ R: _____ Weight: _____ Signature: _____

General Appearance: ☐ Well   ☐ Mildly ill   ☐ Ill

State of hydration: ☐ Normal   ☐ Mildly dehydrated   ☐ Dehydrated

Abdomen: ☐ Non-tender   ☐ Tender (describe): _____

If female AND abdomen tender, or U/A negative, pelvic exam:

☐ Cervix Normal   ☐ Abnormal (describe): _____

☐ No discharge   ☐ Discharge (describe): _____

☐ Non-tender   ☐ Tender (describe): _____

If male OR abdominal tenderness, rectal exam: _____

CVA tenderness: ☐ Absent   ☐ Present (describe): _____

Other physical exam: _____

Figure **9-4**   Sample ED care map-short format. (*Courtesy University of Rochester, Strong Memorial Hospital, Rochester, New York.*)

UNIVERSITY OF ROCHESTER
STRONG MEMORIAL HOSPITAL
SMH 71 MR
EMERGENCY DEPARTMENT
UTI/DYSURIA CLINICAL PATHWAY
Page 2 of 2

Date: _____

Time: _____

$\boxed{X}$ ED

TESTS

Urine Dip: _____ Urine Micro: _____

☐ Urine Pregnancy _____

☐ Urine culture if: male with + U/A; diabetic, sickle cell, or other immunosuppressive state; renal system abnormalities; less than 2 weeks since last UTI; pregnant; or clinical symptoms of pyelonephritis.

☐ CBC not routinely indicated; obtain if patient appears clinically ill or suspicion high for other disease.

☐ Culture for GC/Chlamydia for vaginal/penile discharge or males < 40 years of age.

MD/NP ASSESSMENT AND PLAN

DIAGNOSIS: ☐ Cystitis   ☐ Vaginitis ☐ Cervicitis   ☐ Urethritis   ☐ Pyleonephritis   ☐ Other _____

_____

Treatment: Oflaxacillin contraindicated in children or pregnant women. If allergic to sulfonamides, consider oflaxacillin or cephalosporins.

Women: ☐ **Uncomplicated UTI** - Trimethoprim and Sulfamethoxazole DS bid x 3 days. Pyridium 200 mg tid x 2 days. Arrange follow up prn.

☐ **Complicated UTI** (fever > 38.5°C, flank pain, reasons for culture) - Trimethoprim and Sulfamethoxazole DS or Oflaxacillin 400 mg bid x 7 days and Pyridium x 2 days. Arrange follow up within 1-2 weeks

☐ **Cervicitis / Pelvic Inflammatory Disease** - Oflaxacillin 400 mg po x 1 or Ceftrioxone 250 mg IM AND Doxycycline 100 mg po bid x 14 days. Follow up within 1-2 weeks.

☐ **Vaginitis** - Metronidazole 500 mg bid x 7 days.

Men: ☐ **Penile Discharge** Ceftriazone 250 mg IM x 1 or Oflaxicillin 400 mg po x 1 AND Azithromycin 1 g po x 1 or Doxycycline 100 mg bid x 14 days, Arrange follow up in 5-7 days.

☐ Age > 40 or renal system abnormality-Trimethoprim and Sulfamethoxazole DS bid x 10 days or Oflaxacillin 400 mg bid x 10 days. Arrange follow up within 3-5 days.

☐ For age < 40 consider treatment as per penile discharge. If consistent with UTI, treat as per age>40.

Pyelonephritis (fever > 38.5°C AND flank pain, abdominal pain or nausea/vomiting)

☐ Give first dose antibiotics IV

☐ If appears ill, admit or observe for 6-8 hours and discharge if improved. Arrange follow up if discharge within 1-3 days.

☐ Admitted

Follow up: LMD _____   Time notified / appointment scheduled _____

MD/NP Signature _____   Date: _____

RN Signature _____   Date: _____

Figure **9-4** cont'd   For legend see opposite page.

UNIVERSITY OF ROCHESTER
STRONG MEMORIAL HOSPITAL
SMH35MR
Emergency Department
Asthma Clinical Pathway
Page 1 of 3

[X] ED

Drug allergies/reaction: ☐ No ☐ Yes

PMH	Medications	Significant Other
		☐ Present ☐ Notified
		☐ Yes ☐ No
		Clothing
		☐ with patient
		☐ with family
		☐ locked
		Valuables
		☐ with patient
		☐ with family
		☐ locked

Time: _____

HISTORY

INITIAL EVALUATION BY RN AND MD/NP SHOULD TAKE NO MORE THAN 10-15 MINUTES EACH

Duration of symptoms: _____

Circle any of the following symptoms that are currently present: wheezing   chest pain   fever

Cough   Shortness of breath   URI Symptoms   other: _____

Symptoms precipitated by:

URI   cold/heat exposure   smoke   dust/allergens   missed meds   other: _____

Current smoker? Y N   If no, does someone in home environment? Y N

Currently on steroids? Y N   If no, when was last dose? _____

When was last exacerbation? _____

When was last admission? _____

Has the patient ever been intubated/admitted to ICU? Y N   If yes, when? _____

Severity of symptoms at this time: _____

Treatment at home for this exacerbation: _____

EMS treatment for this exacerbation: _____

Other history: _____

_____

INITIAL PHYSICAL EXAM

Vitals: Temp_____   RR_____   BP_____   HR_____   Pulse ox_____

PEFR (best of 3 tries)_____   Predicted_____   Time_____   Initials_____

NOTIFY ATTENDING IMMEDIATELY FOR PEFR OF <25% PREDICTED! (See back of page 2)

Degree of respiratory distress: None   Mild   Moderate   Severe

Use of accessory muscles: None   Mild   Moderate   Severe

Cyanosis: None   Mild   Moderate   Severe

HEENT:

Cardiac:

Lungs: Wheezes: None   Mild   Moderate   Severe

Where?_____

Expiratory phase: Normal   Prolonged

Breath sounds: Normal   Decreased

Rales: Yes No   If yes, where?_____

Rhonchi: Yes No   If yes, where?_____

Mental Status:_____

Other physical exam _____

RN _____   MD/NP _____   Initials: _____

Figure **9-5** Sample ED care map-extended format. *(Courtesy University of Rochester, Strong Memorial Hospital, Rochester, New York.)*

UNIVERSITY OF ROCHESTER
STRONG MEMORIAL HOSPITAL
SMH35MR
Emergency Department
Treatment Sheet
Page 2 of 3
Drug allergies/reaction: ☐ **No** ☐ **Yes**

$\boxed{X}$ ED

<u>Lab Results</u>

```
_____
_____  Segs
_____  Bands
_____  Lymphocytes
_____  Monocytes
```

TREATMENT

☐   START O$_2$ 2-4 1 via NC for:☐ SaO$_2$ <94%   ☐ SaO$_2$ <90% and history of COPD ☐ all pregnant patients

☐   BEGIN   albuterol nebulization (2.5 mg) with O2 x 3 q20-30 min each (over 90 minutes total)
           After 3rd treatment, consult with medical provider for nebulization schedule (see assessment
            guidelines back of page 1)
           CHECK PEFR after each treatment

plt   PT_____
        PTT _____

☐   START steroids if patient requires >1 albuterol treatment (Relative contraindications: known varicella exposure within 3
            weeks, or active herpes)
      ADULT: Methylprednisolone 125 - 1000 mg IV **OR** ☐ Prednisone 60 -80 mg PO
      PEDIATRIC: Methylprednisolone 2 mg/kg IV **OR**   ☐ Prednisone 2 mg/kg PO
☐   For pts > 50 or with history of COPD add Ipratropium 0.5 mg to every Albuterol treatment

☐   CXR if high suspicion for pneumonia, foreign body, CHF; localized wheezing after therapy; first time wheezing.
      CBC if temperature >38.2°C
      ABG, Electrolytes, Theophylline level NOT ROUTINELY INDICATED

Total Bill	_____
AST	_____
ETOH	_____
Amylase	_____
Lipase	_____
CK-MB	_____
Other	_____

SECOND ASSESSMENT of patient should occur:
         ☐   For initial PEFR >40% predicted, after 3rd albuterol treatment
         ☐   For initial PEFR <40% predicted, after 1st albuterol treatment
           AND notify attending MD Time_____ RN/NP/MD_____

<u>REPEAT ASSESSMENT</u>   Time _____
Degree of respiratory distress: None   Mild   Moderate Severe
Use of accessory muscles: None   Mild   Moderate Severe
Cyanosis: None   Mild   Moderate   Severe
Lungs: Wheezes: None   Mild   Moderate   Severe   Where? _____
      Expiratory phase: Normal Prolonged
      Breath sounds: Normal Decreased
      Rales: Yes   No   If yes, where?_____
      Rhonchi: Yes   No   If yes, where?_____
Other physical exam:
      RN _____   MD/NP _____

ABG pH_____
      pCO$_2$_____
      PO$_2$_____
      SaO$_2$_____

U/A Dip_____
     Micro _____

_____

Urine Pregnancy_____
EKG _____
_____
_____
_____

<u>REPEAT ASSESSMENT</u>   Time _____
Degree of respiratory distress: None   Mild   Moderate Severe
Use of accessory muscles: None   Mild   Moderate Severe
Cyanosis: None   Mild   Moderate   Severe
Lungs: Wheezes: None   Mild   Moderate   Severe   Where?
      Expiratory phase: Normal Prolonged
      Breath sounds: Normal Decreased
      Rales: Yes   No   If yes, where? _____
      Rhonchi: Yes   No   If yes, where?_____
Other physical exam:

X-Rays _____
_____
_____
_____

      RN _____   MD/NP_____

PRIVATE MD/TIME NOTIFIED

Figure **9-5** cont'd   For legend see opposite page.

Continued

Sample Peak Expiratory Flow Rate Nomogram

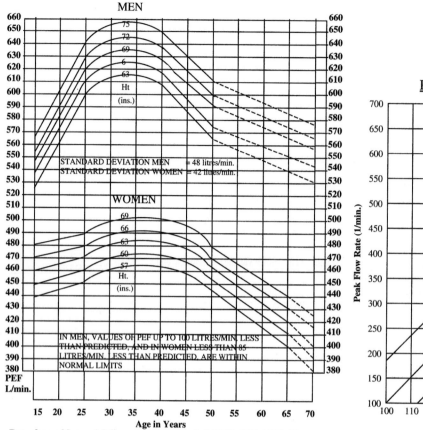

Data from: Nunn, AJ Gregg, I, *Brit. Med. J.* 1989; 298:1068-70

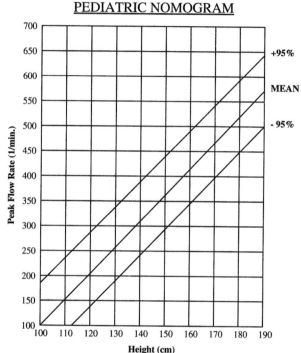

Data from: Godfrey S. et al., *Brit. J. Dis. Chest,* 1970; 64:15-24.

Table 1
Predicted Average Peak Expiratory Flow for Normal Males

(liters per minute)

Age	Height				
	60"	65"	70"	75"	80"
20	554	602	649	693	740
25	543	590	636	679	725
30	532	577	622	664	710
35	521	565	609	651	695
40	509	552	596	636	680
45	498	540	583	622	665
50	486	527	569	607	649
55	475	515	556	593	634
60	463	502	542	578	618
65	452	490	529	564	603
70	440	477	515	550	587

Data from: Leiner GC. et al: Expiratory peak flow rate Standard values for normal subjects. Use as a clinical test of venulatory function. *Am Rev Resp Dis* 88:644. 1963

Table 2
Predicted Average Peak Expiratory Flow for Normal Females

(liters per minute)

Age	Height				
	55"	60"	65"	70"	75"
20	390	423	460	496	529
25	385	418	454	490	523
30	380	413	448	483	516
35	375	408	442	476	509
40	370	402	436	470	502
45	365	397	430	464	495
50	360	391	424	457	488
55	355	386	418	451	482
60	350	380	412	445	475
65	345	375	406	439	468
70	340	369	400	432	461

Data from: Leiner GC. et al: Expiratory peak flow rate Standard values for normal subjects. Use as a clinical test of venulatory function. *Am Rev Resp Dis* 88:644. 1963

Table 3
Predicted Average Peak Expiratory Flow for Normal Children and Adolescents

(liters per minute)

Height (inches)	Males & Females	Height (inches)	Males & Females
43	147	56	320
44	160	57	334
45	173	58	347
46	187	59	360
47	200	60	373
48	214	61	387
49	227	62	400
50	240	63	413
51	254	64	427
52	267	65	440
53	280	66	454
54	293	67	454
55	307		

Data from Polger G. Promcdhat V: *Pulmonary function testing in children. Techniques and standards* Philadelphia W.B. Saunders. 1971

Note: These tables are averages and are based on tests with a large number of people. An individual's PEFR may vary widely. Further, many individuals' PEFR values are consistently higher or lower than the average values. It is recommended that PEFR objectives for therapy be based upon each individual's personal test which is established after a period of PEFR monitoring while the individual is under effective treatment.

Figure **9-5** cont'd   Sample ED care map-extended format. *(Courtesy University of Rochester, Strong Memorial Hospital, Rochester, New York.)*

UNIVERSITY OF ROCHESTER
STRONG MEMORIAL HOSPITAL
SMH35MR
Emergency Department
Vital Sign Record
Page 3 of 3

[X] ED

<u>RESPONSE TO THERAPY</u>   Time_____

☐   GOOD   ☐ Plan to discharge patient to home
☐   INCOMPLETE   ☐ Observe (planned duration)
☐ Admit
☐   POOR   Admit   ☐ Floor   ☐ ICU

ATTENDING NOTE   Time_____

Critical Care Time_____

MD _____

PROCEDURE NOTE Time_____

VITAL SIGN RECORD

Initials	Time	Temp	Pulse	RR	B/P	Pulse ox	PEFR	comments
					/			
					/			
					/			
					/			
					/			

INTAKE RECORD

Start time	Amount	Initials	IV gauge	End time	Amount

MEDICATION ADMINISTRATION RECORD

Albuterol nebulization dose: _____

#1 Time:	RN	#4 Time:	RN	#7 Time:	RN
#2 Time:	RN	#5 Time:	RN	#8 Time:	RN
#3 Time:	RN	#6 Time:	RN	#9 Time:	RN

Steroids Medication _____ dose: _____ Route: _____
Time: _____ RN _____

Other Medications _____ dose: _____ Route: _____
Time: _____ RN _____

<u>DISCHARGE PLAN COORDINATION</u>

<u>Patient/family teaching</u>
Assess patient's knowledge of asthma management and teach where needed.
Patient/family will demonstrate understanding of:
☐   proper use of medication
☐   precipitants of attack
☐   knowledge of symptom progression
☐   knowledge of ACTION PLAN for
increased severity of disease
☐   proper use of (if appropriate):
☐   inhaler and spacer device
☐   peak flow meter
patient discharged with peak flow meter ☐YES ☐NO ☐N/A

<u>Care coordination</u>
Ensuring appropriate and adequate outpatient plan
☐   Patient knows source of primary care and phone number
☐   Patient aware of need for follow-up visit within 5-10 days
☐   Assessment made for need for community health referral:
☐   Noncompliance with medical regimen
☐   lack of social support system
☐   poor coping skills
☐   frequent ED visits or admissions
☐   history of missed follow-up appointments
☐   If any indicator yes, make referral

RN _____

MD/NP_____

Figure **9-5** cont'd   For legend see opposite page.

Continued

Response to Treatment

1. <u>POOR RESPONSE</u>
   PEFR not improving
   OR
   PEFR < 40% of predicted
   OR
   persistent symptoms

   ADMIT/CONSIDER ICU
   1. Continuous to q 30 minute albuterol treatments
   2. Add ipratropium 0.5 mg to each treatment
   3. Consider parental therapy (epinephrine or terbutaline) magnesium, theophylline.
   4. Antibiotics only if indicated

2. <u>INCOMPLETE RESPONSE</u>
   PEFR > 40% or < 70% of predicted
   OR
   not doubled
   AND
   with mild to moderate symptoms

   OBSERVATION/ADMIT
   1. Continue hourly albuterol treatment
   2. Add ipratropium if appropriate

   3. Upon completion of 5 albuterol treatments if not good responder →Admit to Hospital
   4. Consider subcutaneous epinephrine, terbutaline, magnesium, or theophylline.
   5. Antibiotics only if indicated

3. <u>GOOD RESPONSE</u>
   Double initial PEFR
   AND
   PEFR > 70% of predicted
   OR
   patient without symptoms

   DISCHARGE
   1. Arrange for medical follow-up within 5-10 days/or while on steroids.
   2. Discharge Medications:
      Steroids:
      Adult: Prednisone 30-50mg po qd x 5 d (longer if appropriate)
      Pediatric: Prednisone 1mg/kg po qd x 5d (longer if appropriate)
   3. Antibiotics only if clearly indicated.
   4. Inhaled beta$_2$ - agonist prn.
   5. Consider inhaled steroids

<u>FUNCTIONAL PATIENT</u>
   Outcomes for Discharge:

   Patient able to speak in full sentences,
   Feels back to baseline

   RR at baseline,
   no FiO$_2$ requirements.
   O$_2$ Sat > 95% with mild or no
   wheezing

   Ambulatory in department without
   clinical deterioration.

Figure **9-5** cont'd   Sample ED care map-extended format. *(Courtesy University of Rochester, Strong Memorial Hospital, Rochester, New York.)*

TROUBLESHOOTING CASE MANAGEMENT

Implementation of any project that entails major restructuring of the work environment can lead to problems. Fortunately, solid planning and continuous vigilance over project development minimize many problems and circumvent others. This is particularly true for case management. Some problems associated with case management in the ED are presented below.

Inconsistent Use of the Clinical Pathway

Project managers often experience difficulty gaining widespread acceptance of the pathway concept. In addition to resistance to change, part of the problem may lie in the pathway development process. Each development team should be multidisciplinary, with each discipline involved in the patient's care represented. For example, the pathway development group for hip-femur fracture might include nursing, emergency medicine, orthopedics, radiology, and physical therapy. Representation from the inpatient orthopedic unit and the outpatient rehabilitation department may enhance communication across departmental lines and facilitate implementation of the pathway.

Select pathway authors for their clinical expertise and enthusiasm for the concept. Ensure content validity of each pathway through comprehensive review of the literature. Retrospective chart review can help identify organizational practice patterns for group review. Including key players in development ensures that everyone with an interest in the patient is involved, but keeps the group from becoming so large that consensus is impossible.

Loss of Momentum

The case management model is dependent on personnel, and may be subject to setbacks and delays with turnover of key personnel. Changes in either medical or nursing leadership can interfere with project progression. Recognize this weakness in the model and prepare in advance for leadership transfers in order to keep the project on course.

Data Collection

Before project implementation, identify what data are to be collected, what will be done with them, who will receive them, and how they will be protected. Several large case management projects have been interrupted for major revisions due to excessive collection of meaningless data. Collection of too much data overloads the system and confuses efforts to evaluate the program's effectiveness.

SUMMARY

Case management is designed to ensure continuity of care for patients across the continuum of the health care system. The ED case manager and project director should meet regularly with inpatient units and other critical areas to make sure ED clinical pathways interact easily with their respective inpatient clinical pathways. Ideally, case management should begin in the prehospital setting. Personnel should

network with EMS providers to design pathways for implementation in the field, for example, thrombolytics, trauma management. Appropriate EMS providers should participate in design of selected ED pathways.

Case management can address ED abuse by targeting patients who repeatedly bypass their primary care provider and go to the ED for routine complaints. Working with primary care providers to design pathways can ensure that ED care is consistent with the overall health care plan designed by the patient's primary provider. The ED case manager can review and encourage the patient to access the health care system appropriately. Patient-friendly pathways can be shared with the patient and family to allay their fears, establish patient/family health care goals, and to help them better understand their ED visit. This also creates the opportunity for patients to participate in decisions regarding their medical care.

Case management provides emergency personnel with a model for outcome-based care that facilitates achievement of clinical outcomes while conserving valuable resources. Case management cannot extinguish the chaos characteristic of many urban and community EDs; however, it can provide a sense of control for providers through its proactive design.

REFERENCES

1. Fuszard B et al: *Case management: a challenge for nurses,* Kansas City, 1988, American Nurses Association.
2. Ison A: Nursing case management: an innovative approach to care in the emergency department, *Topics Emerg Med* 13(3):335, 1991.
3. Veenema T: The ten most frequently asked questions about case management in the emergency department, *J Emerg Nurs* 20(4):289, 1994.
4. Zander K: Nursing case management: resolving the DRG paradox, *Nurs Clinics N Am* 23(3):503, 1988.

SUGGESTED READING

Baggs J, Schmitt MH: Collaboration between nurses and physicians, *Image: J Nurs Sch* 20:145, 1988.

Cronin C, Maklebust J: Case-managed care: capitalizing on the clinical nurse specialist, *Nurs Manag* 20(3):38, 1989.

Ethridge P, Lamb GS: Professional nursing case management improves quality, access, and costs, *Nurs Manag* 20(3):30, 1989.

Ethridge P et al: The professional nurse/case manager in changing organizational structures, *Series Nurs Admin* 2:146, 1989.

Lomas J, Anderson GM, Domnick Pierre K et al: Do practice guidelines guide practice? *N Engl J Med* 321(19):1306, 1989.

Lumsdon K, Hagland M: Mapping care, *Hosp Health Netw* 10, 1993.

Mayer G, Madden MJ, Lawrenz E: *Patient care delivery systems,* Rockville, Md, 1990, Aspen.

McCormac-Bueno M, Hwang RF: Understanding variances in hospital stay, *Nurs Manag* 24(11), 1993.

Nash DB: The state of the outcomes/guidelines movement, *Dec Imag Econ,* 1993.

Williamson A, Kives AA: Nurse-physician collaboration in emergency services, *Topics Emerg Med* 13(3):1, 1991.

Zander K: Managed care within acute care settings: design and implementation via nursing case management, *Health Care Super* 6(2):27, 1988.

Zander K: Nursing case management: strategic management of cost and quality outcomes, *J Nurs Admin* 18(5):23, 1988.

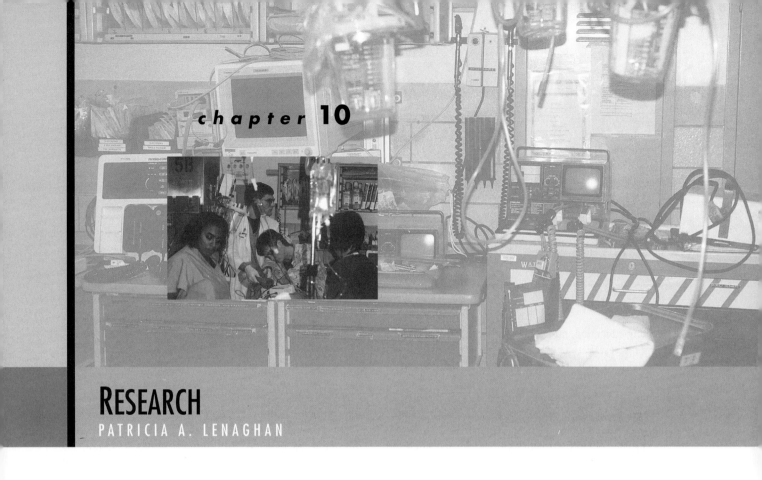

chapter 10

RESEARCH
PATRICIA A. LENAGHAN

The practice of nursing produces a never-ending stream of challenges to determine the best way to solve problems. Often nurses find solutions through logical reasoning, experience, trial and error, or even tradition. Although these methods are legitimate in some situations, the nurse must often search for the best way to solve problems. Research is any process designed to determine and confirm validity and accuracy.

In clinical settings, nurses rely on problem-solving ability acquired through experience. An experienced nurse may transfer knowledge gained from past experiences to other patients and situations. However, the knowledge may become outdated and stagnant in an ever-changing clinical environment. The traditional practice may have developed haphazardly from unsystematic methods; other methods may be more useful. Furthermore, this knowledge is often undocumented, so it is not accessible to others.

In clinical problem solving nurses use intelligence, experience, and formal systems of thought to arrive at a solution for the problem of a particular patient. The nursing process is based on this method. This method is not always formal, so we may not know if the solution was found in the best possible manner.

Research is the method used to determine truth as it best can be defined. It is not always possible to determine whether method A is better than method B, C, or D for solving problem X, but the nurse can determine that method A produces a more satisfied patient, less pain, and quicker re-

coveries. The goal of nursing research is to facilitate development of clinical nursing interventions that improve health outcomes and contribute to optimal delivery of health care. According to the American Nurses Association,[4] nursing research "develops knowledge about health and the promotion of health over a full life span, care of persons with health problems and disabilities and nursing actions to enhance the ability of individuals to respond effectively to actual or potential health problems."

The purpose of research is to provide new knowledge by finding valid answers to questions that have been raised or valid solutions to problems that have been identified. Unlike problem solving, research is related to care of patients in general, so the results benefit many. The final outcome of research occurs when these validated solutions to health care problems are implemented and there is improved health and/or more cost-effective care.

THE RESEARCH PROCESS

A researcher should proceed through a series of well-defined, logical steps to organize a study (Box 10-1). Other aspects of research from a nursing perspective include funding, protection of human subjects, informed consent, critiques, and how to apply research to nursing practice.

Problem Identification

Nursing research always begins with a question or a "researchable problem."[15] This problem may concern patient

---

care, nursing education, nursing administration, or any issue of nursing interest. Patient care or nursing practice problems generally address practice differences and what is ideal or desirable.

Deciding on a specific research question may be difficult for the beginning researcher. Nurses are particularly skilled at explaining things to other nurses and patients; however, envisioning how scientific inquiry can shed light on an old problem is more difficult. One of the best sources for researchable problems in nursing is personal experience. Many times an observation can be turned into a question such as:

- I wonder whether seeing the dying family member before death helps the family during their bereavement?
- I wonder whether using protocols for laboratory and radiographic examinations can expedite care in the emergency department?
- I wonder if drawing blood below or above IV sites has any bearing on the laboratory values?

Another source for problems to be researched is nursing literature. Most research studies make recommendations for future studies. Nursing practice is changed not by one study but by an accumulation of scientific results that indicates the best solution to a problem.[25] Start by reading literature in an area of interest to outline common themes and patterns you may wish to investigate.

Several nursing and federal organizations have published recommendations for research study. The Emergency Nurses Association, American Association of Critical Care Nurses, and American Nurses Association all have research priorities for clinical nursing.[1,4,17,27] The National Institutes of Health (NIH) also publish their priorities in the area of nursing research.

Literature Review

The purpose of the literature review is to explore work conducted in a particular area of interest, to help formulate or clarify the research problem. After critiquing previous research in a particular area, the researcher is more knowledgeable about what has been studied, more skilled in deciding how his or her study would best contribute to science, and more able to assess the feasibility of his or her study. Related research articles may be useful.

Librarians are excellent resources for the researcher conducting a literature review. They are familiar with the literature, literature retrieval, and library services. They are also familiar with the National Library of Medicine and community, state, and regional libraries that make up the Health Science Library Network.

The search for published articles about a specific problem usually begins with indexes to the literature or computerized data bases. The most commonly used indexes in nursing research are *International Nursing Index, Cumulative Index to Nursing and Allied Health Literature (CINAHL), Nursing Abstracts,* and *MedLine.* Abstract journals summarize articles that appeared in other journals. *Nursing Research* and *Psychological Abstract* both provide useful abstracts of nursing studies.

Computer searches provide the reviewer with complete bibliographic information, thereby saving time and energy. A computer search may be obtained by requesting one from a librarian or by conducting the search yourself. End-user systems are designed to allow reviewers to conduct their own computer searches in the library or at other locations.[33] The cost of a computer search depends on the type and extent of the search, as well as the data base used. Most libraries have specific request forms. The fees for computer searches are usually posted. Before requesting a computer search, the researcher should know the subject matter and how many years of research are included in the search. Many options are available. Literature in foreign languages can be searched or searches of literature in just English can be conducted. Nursing literature can be searched or a comprehensive search of all medical literature can be conducted.

When you receive the final search, you may see many or only a few pertinent articles. Review the articles most pertinent to the study. At the end of each article, there is a reference or bibliography. If current, these usually contain the best condensed citations you can find on that particular topic. Books are useful in that they contain references to other sources of information.

After you have selected articles that in some way contribute information to your research question, the next step is to critique and summarize them to see how they fit into the scope of your study. A good review reinforces the need for the study in light of what has already been done. What is accepted as truth from other studies is the groundwork on which new studies are based. A written literature review should include summaries of articles that differ from the proposed point of view. This indicates that the author conducted an exhaustive review of available knowledge.

A primary source of information is the description of an investigation written by the person who conducted it. A secondary source is a description of a study prepared by someone other than the original researcher. Both sources can be helpful, but written literature reviews should be based on primary sources whenever possible.[28] Nonresearch articles that contribute to ideas or theories about the problem may be included, but it is best to focus on primary research articles. LoBiondo-Wood and Haber[21] and Polit and Hungler[28] have provided guidelines for critiquing and writing literature reviews.

Theoretic Framework

One body organ does not function in isolation, nor does one bit of research. A theoretic framework is the abstract, logical structure of meaning that guides development of the study and enables the researcher to link the findings to a body of knowledge.[9] This framework consists of definition of concepts and propositions about the relationships of those concepts. This helps to organize rules or beliefs about what is observed, and provides a systematic way to organize information about a particular thing.

Examples of theories used in nursing are psychoanalytic theory, the theory of relativity, the theory of evolution, the theory of gravity, learning theory, systems theory, and the theory of homeostasis. Campbell[10] used the theoretic models of grief and learned helplessness to help explain women's responses to battering. The power of theories lies in the ability to explain the relationship of variables and the nature of this relationship. Theories also help stimulate research by giving direction. Questions and ideas formulated about what will occur in specific situations are called hypotheses. The hypotheses are tested in research to determine whether the information fits the theory.

The two components of a theory are the concepts and a statement of propositions. Concepts, the building blocks of a theory, are abstract characteristics, categories, or labels of things, persons, or events. Examples of nursing concepts are health, stress, adaptation, caring, and pain. Propositions are statements that define the relationships among concepts. A set of propositions may state that one concept is associated with another or is contingent upon another.

Conceptual frameworks represent a less formal, less well-developed system for organizing phenomena. These frameworks contain concepts that represent a common theme but lack the deductive system of propositions that give the relationship among concepts. Most research in nursing practice uses conceptual frameworks rather than theories.[28] These conceptual frameworks often lay the groundwork for more formal theories.

A conceptual model for nursing practice is a systematically constructed, scientifically based, and logically related set of concepts that identifies essential components of nursing practice. The model is a mental image of the realm of nursing and how it is put together and how it works. Fawcett[14] named four central concepts of the nursing discipline—person, environment, health, and nursing.

The past few decades produced several conceptual models of nursing practice—Peplau's developmental model for nursing practice, Newman's health care systems model, Orem's model of self-care, King's open system model, Johnson's behavioral systems model, Levine's conservation model, Rogers' model of the unitary person, and Roy's adaptation model. You may wish to use a nursing theory in your study or review relevant literature to determine how your research problem fits into what is already known.

Formulating Questions or Hypotheses

Before a problem can be researched, it must be narrowed, refined, and made feasible for study. The research interest can be stated as a question or a hypothesis. The research question should identify key variables under investigation. Often research questions begin with: "What causes. . .?" "Is there a relationship between. . .?" and "How effective is. . .?" For example, the research question might be "What effect does the presence of the parent in the child's room have on the child's experience of pain during fracture reduction?" The dependent variable is the child's pain experience and the independent variable is the presence of the parent in the room. The dependent variable is explained through its relationship with the independent variable. Both research variables must be specific. The goal is to determine whether a relationship exists between the two variables.

The independent variable is what is assumed to cause or thought to be associated with the dependent variable. Changes in the dependent variable are presumed to depend on the independent variable's effects. The dependent variable is what you want to explain or understand. Be specific about what you want to study in your research. If you try to measure too much, analyzing the data at the end of your project may be difficult. For example, it is known that many factors affect a child's perception of pain, but only one independent variable (parent's presence) is measured in the above study. The researcher can measure several variables if the study is well designed.

Often the dependent variable can have multiple causes. A study may be designed to examine several factors and their influence on a phenomenon. For example, you may want to know whether experience with triage or an educational program concerning triage influences ability to accurately perform triage. Both independent variables (education and experience) can influence triage performance ability (dependent variable).

Several dependent variables can be designated as measures of treatment effectiveness. Another question may be whether a comprehensive triage system has an influence on length of stay in the emergency department (ED), patient satisfaction, and patient outcome. Length of stay, patient satisfaction, and patient outcome are all dependent variables by which triage effectiveness is measured.

A hypothesis is a tentative prediction or explanation of the relationship between two or more variables. This prediction of expected outcomes is the basis of the research process. Hypotheses, which often stem from theories, are possible solutions or answers to research problems. The hypothesis is a prediction of the nature of the relationship between several variables. For example, one hypothesis might be that pediatric patients who are promised a reward at the end of a suturing procedure will cooperate and be more compliant than pediatric patients who are not promised a reward. In this example, the researcher is not only questioning whether a relationship between rewards and behavior exists but is also predicting outcomes from this relationship. The null hypothesis is often generated for statistical purposes, data analysis, and discussion.

Nursing Research Approaches and Designs

Experimental and quasiexperimental studies. Experimental studies differ from nonexperimental studies in that the researcher who conducts an experimental study actively participates in the research. He or she does not simply observe a phenomenon. To qualify as an experiment, the research design must possess manipulation, randomization, and control. Table 10-1 summarizes these characteristics.

Quasiexperimental design is similar to experimental design in that it also provides manipulation. However, quasiexperimental design lacks randomization or control. Randomization is usually lacking because the researcher cannot assign subjects to groups. When this occurs there is no guarantee that the experimental group and the control groups are similar. This design is called a *nonequivalent control group design.*

A *time-series design* is often used in nursing research when researchers are not able to randomize or have a control group. Because only one group is available for study, the phenomenon of interest is studied over a longer time and the experimental treatment is introduced during the course of the study.

Nonexperimental studies. When experimentation or quasiexperimentation is possible, these approaches are the best method for testing hypotheses. However, a number of research problems, especially those involving human subjects, do not lend themselves to experimentation. The independent variables, for example, diseases, widowhood, and injury, cannot be manipulated. Two broad classes of nonexperimental research, ex post facto or correlational research, and de-

scriptive research are utilized for these situations. The translation from Latin of *ex post facto* is "after the fact." This term indicates that research is conducted by use of variations of the independent variable in the natural course of events. Ex post facto studies are also known as explanatory studies, descriptive studies, causal-comparative studies, or comparative surveys. In conducting ex post facto research, the investigator does not have control of independent variables because they have already occurred. A retrospective study of ex post facto design looks at an existing phenomenon and tries to link it to others from the past. Epidemiologic studies are often ex post facto design. Many cancer research studies attempt to link past behaviors with current cancerous conditions. Prospective studies start with presumed natural causes and compare groups who have and do not have those independent variables. For example, a study of breast cancer may use two prospective groups, one with a family history of breast cancer and one without this history.

The purpose of descriptive research is to observe, describe, and investigate aspects of a phenomenon. For example, an investigator may wish to determine the percentage of ED patients who do not have a regular source of health care and why. Descriptive research studies include historical research, survey research, field research, case studies, evaluative research, and methodologic research.

Historical research provides an account of past events. The investigator systematically collects information relating to past occurrences and critiques the data. Generally, historical research is performed to test hypotheses or answer questions about causes, effects, or trends relating to past events that shed light on present behaviors or practices.[28] A researcher may wish to know the historical perspective of the nurse's role in prehospital care including air medical transport. This information could help identify trends and possibly predict future needs.

Survey research is designed to obtain information about distribution prevalence and interrelationships among variables. When this nonexperimental approach is used, intervention is not performed by the investigator but explained by the collection of data. A researcher may survey ED nurses to understand how retention may be affected by the increase in ED census, the occurrence of violence, and the

Table **10-1**	**Criteria for an Experimental Research Design**
Criteria	**Description**
Manipulation	The researcher must do something to at least some of the study participants.
Randomization	Subjects are randomly assigned to the experimental or control group. Each subject has an equal chance of being assigned to either group. Randomization assures the researcher that both groups are exactly alike and that the effect of the treatment or experiment is caused by the independent variable rather than individual differences.
Control	The research manipulates the independent variable by giving one group an experimental treatment. The control or comparison group does not receive the experimental treatment; this group receives normal treatment.

spread of infectious diseases. Surveys may be personal interviews, telephone interviews, or questionnaires. Political opinion polls are examples of survey research.

Field research is investigation of a certain situation in the natural setting. This qualitative research is aimed at describing and exploring the phenomenon to define behaviors, beliefs, and practices of individuals or groups in real situations. Anthropologists are probably the most widely recognized field researchers. Nurses conduct field studies in home environments and hospitals to determine what aspects of patients and their environment contribute to the well-being of patients.

Case study designs provide in-depth analysis of an individual, a small group, a family, a place, or an organization. Natural conditions are usually studied, and variables related to history, current characteristics, interactions, or problems are examined. Case studies usually focus on why the subject feels, thinks, or behaves in a particular way. Meier and Pugh[24] think that case studies are well suited to the study of clinical nursing problems, since case studies focus holistically on individuals. Case studies can be powerful because individuals or groups may describe a phenomenon not fully understood by science. For example, a case study of one patient's experience while in a coma, including smells, touch, and voices, can provide important information for families and health care providers to use to help patients recover from a coma.

Evaluative research is the use of scientific research methods and procedures to evaluate a program, treatment practice, or policy. This type of research uses analytic means to document the worth of an activity.[21] Experimental, nonexperimental, or quasiexperimental approaches can be used. Program goals or objectives should be the focus of the evaluation.

Methodologic research is controlled investigation of the ways of obtaining, organizing, and analyzing data.[28] This type of research addresses development, validation, and evaluation of research tools or techniques. For example, an investigator may want to develop or perfect a tool for measuring anxiety in the hospitalized cardiac patient. Measuring the level of anxiety in the patient is not the goal of this type of research; the goal is to determine the degree of accuracy with which the tool measures anxiety in all patients.

Data Collection

When you know what you want to study and whom you plan to use in your research, various techniques can be used to collect the needed information. The key to success in data collection is choosing or developing appropriate methods that will accurately describe the variables you wish to study. There are five types of data collection methods: physiologic and biophysical, observational, interviews and questionnaires, scale and psychologic measures, and records or available data.

Physiologic measurements fall into several major groups. Physical measurements are those used to measure character-

istics such as temperature, weight, height, cardiac output, muscle strength, and electrical activity of organs. Measurements of chemistry include hemoglobin levels, hematocrit percentages, blood sugar, and potassium levels. Microbiologic measurements provide counts and identification of bacteria. Radiographic studies, biopsies, computerized axial tomography, and magnetic resonance imaging are examples of anatomic or cytologic measurements. One advantage of physiologic measurements is objectivity because data are not influenced by the person performing the study. Physiologic measurements are relatively precise and sensitive.

Certain types of research problems are more amenable to direct observation methods where the researcher actually observes what he or she intends to study. For example, you may want to observe the response of parents to casting or suturing procedures performed on their children. The observation method is most useful for entities difficult to measure, such as interactions, nursing process, changes in behavior, or group processes.

Interviews and questionnaires allow subjects to report data for or about themselves. The purpose of questioning participants is to seek direct data such as age, religion, or marital status, or indirect data such as level of intelligence, anxiety, and pain. An instrument used or developed for interviews or questionnaires must measure the intended data. Newly developed instruments are often pilot tested. Pilot testing is performed on a small sample of people to evaluate effectiveness.

Instruments with scales are often used to make distinctions among subjects concerning the degree to which they possess a certain trait, attitude, or emotion. Scales are measuring instruments that permit comparisons in dimensions of interest.[28] For example, a researcher interested in knowing whether a nerve block or a local injection of anesthetic is more effective for relieving pain during fracture reduction would use a pain scale to measure pain.

Many scales and psychologic measures have been developed by researchers. To find the appropriate scale or instrument, review the literature related to what you are researching. Research texts discuss measurement methods at the end of most chapters on data collection methods.[28] Some texts provide nothing but instruments for measuring health and nursing care.[16,23]

Measurement and Sampling

Measurement and sampling depend on the population to be studied, the sample size used, and the data collection instrument's validity and reliability. The definition of population is not restricted to human subjects. A population can consist of records, blood samples, actions, words, organizations, numbers, or animals. Whatever the unit, a population is always made up of specific elements of interest.

A population can be defined to include thousands of individuals or narrowed to only a few hundred. The population is defined in a study by set criteria. For example, when studying emergency nurses, the researcher may choose nurses with 1, 5, or 10 years of experience. The researcher sets the criteria for inclusion in the study; the criteria define the population.

Because it is expensive and nearly impossible to include large populations, the researcher samples only a part of a large group. Samples represent a portion of the entire population to be studied. In Figure 10-1, all ED nurses represent the entire population; the sampling unit consists of ED nurses with 10 years of experience, and the sample is selected from those ED nurses with 10 years of experience.

The important factor in sampling is the researcher's ability to verify that the sample represents the entire population. This is known as representativeness. The researcher usually verifies representativeness by using probability and nonprobability sampling plans.

Probability sampling is the use of some form of random selection to choose the sample units. Every element in the population has a known, nonzero probability of being included in the sample. The goal of probability sampling is to ensure that the study population is represented.

The majority of human samples in most types of research, including nursing, are based on nonprobability.[28] There are three types of nonprobability sampling. *Accidental samples* are based on convenience, such as surveying the first 100 patients in the ED on a particular day. *Quota samples* are used when the researcher knows an element of the population and bases the sample on that element. For example, a researcher may know that 25% of ED nurses are men, so the

researcher makes sure that 25% of the sample consists of men. This increases the representativeness of the population. *Purposive sampling* occurs when the researcher handpicks cases to be included in the sample. Usually the researcher uses purposive sampling to ensure a wide variety of responses or because the choices are judged to be typical of the population. The extent to which you can generalize your results depends on the method by which you choose the samples. If you randomly pick the samples, results are more widely applicable.

No one simple equation is used to determine sample size; however, the largest possible sample should be used. Larger samples are more representative of the population. A procedure known as power analysis is often used by advanced researchers to estimate sample size.[13] Sample sizes should be determined according to population and the statistical procedures to be run on the data.

Instrument validity. Validity is the "degree to which an instrument measures what it is intended to measure."[28] Validity is content, constructs, or criterion-related. Although an instrument may appear to measure some aspect of a construct or element, the instrument must be evaluated to determine whether it really does provide such measurement.

Content validity is the degree to which an instrument measures the universe of content that it is said to represent or measure. Content validity is often determined by a panel of experts in the field to be evaluated. If you wanted to measure bereavement behaviors in the ED, you might ask social workers, members of the clergy, and emergency nurses to re-

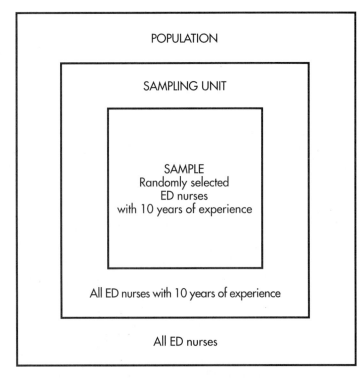

POPULATION

SAMPLING UNIT

SAMPLE
Randomly selected
ED nurses
with 10 years of experience

All ED nurses with 10 years of experience

All ED nurses

Figure **10-1**   Relationship of a study sample to the population.

view your instrument for measuring content related to grief.

Construct validity is the degree to which a tool measures the construct in the study. A *construct* is an abstraction developed for a scientific purpose. Construct validity is usually determined over time after data from research studies support the construct to a greater degree or question it further. For example, you may want to determine the sense of hope in trauma patients' families. The researcher's instrument must discriminate between families who possess hope and families who do not possess hope to ensure construct validity.

Criterion-related validity consists of predictive validity and concurrent validity. In each type, the subject's performance on one measure is used to infer the likely response on another measure.[5] *Predictive validity* is a measure used to predict future performance. For example, a nurse's score on a content knowledge test in emergency nursing predicts how well he or she will perform in practice. *Concurrent validity* is the degree to which an instrument can distinguish subjects who differ on a certain criterion measured at the same time.

Reliability. *Reliability* of an instrument refers to its ability to consistently and accurately measure a criterion. A test of reliability is whether the tool produces the same measurement when a measurement is repeated several times. The less an instrument varies in repeated measurements, the greater the reliability of the instrument. A thermometer that measures a temperature at 98.6° F one moment and 102° F the next is unreliable.

Data Analysis

After completing data collection, the researcher summarizes the data through a statistical procedure. The purpose of analysis is to answer the researcher's questions. The preliminary steps for data analysis include sorting, coding, or entering data into a computer. Researchers who use quantitative methods for data collection should plan for analysis before the research data are collected.

Statistical techniques give meaning to quantitative data. The techniques reduce, summarize, organize, evaluate, interpret, and communicate numeric data.[28]

Statistics are either descriptive or inferential. *Descriptive statistics* describe and summarize data. Examples are mode, median, mean, average, percentage, and frequency.

Inferential statistics are used to draw conclusions about a large population based on a sample from a study, to make judgments, and to generalize information. Inferential statistics are then used to test the hypotheses to determine whether they are correct. Two categories of inferential statistics are parametric and nonparametric.

Most statistical tests are *parametric tests,* which focus on population parameters, require measurements on at least one interval or ratio scale, and make assumptions about distribution of the variables.[28] *Nonparametric tests* are used when measured variables are nominal or ordinal. These tests do not make assumptions about distribution of variables.

Variability refers to the spread or dispersion of data, that is, range and standard deviation. *Range* is the spread between the highest and lowest scores. *Standard deviation* is the most commonly used variability test. The standard deviation is determined by first calculating deviation scores, or the degree to which a score deviated from the mean. Standard deviation indicates how far scores generally deviate from the mean.

Statistical tests. A *t*-test is a parametric test that determines whether a difference exists between the means of two groups.

Analysis of variance (ANOVA) is a parametric test used to determine the significance of differences between the means of two or more groups. The purpose is to then determine whether variability is due to the independent variable or other differences such as human or measurement error.

The *chi-square test* is a nonparametric test used when two sets of data can fall into various categories. A contingency table is used to test the significance of different proportions. The table is used to determine total frequencies for each category. The chi-square value is computed to determine actual observed frequency and to determine what would be expected if no relationship existed between the variables.

Correlation coefficients are used to describe a relationship between two measures. When two variables are totally unrelated, the correlation coefficient is 0. If two items are always positively related the correlation coefficient approaches 1.00. For example, temperature elevation usually correlates with white blood cell count elevation. A negative correlation occurs when one factor or variable increases while the other decreases. For example, increasing intracranial pressure has a negative correlation to level of consciousness. This correlation is called an inverse, or negative, relationship.

More sophisticated tests are being used in research because of the advancing skill of researchers and the rigorous attention to design of studies. Tests used to analyze three or more variables, termed multivariate statistical analyses, include multiple correlation, or multiple regression, analysis of covariance, and factor analysis.

Computer analysis. Computers are available at most universities and hospitals for statistical procedures. They are widely used to calculate and report results. A wide variety of software packages is available for performing necessary statistical procedures. Examples of prepackaged statistical programs are Statistical Analysis Systems, Statistical Package for the Social Sciences, and Biomedical Computer Programs.[11] A computer file must be made for data entry. The computer is then told how to read your data and what procedures to perform. Many research texts describe computer software programs, including cost, functions, and program sources.

Results, Conclusions, and Recommendations

Results are often reported in the form of tables and graphs. Data summarized in graphs and tables can be more easily interpreted and compared with research questions or hypotheses and theoretic framework. The visual image of data helps show the reader the results simply and clearly.

Interpretation of the findings is an extremely important aspect of conducting a study. Results are either positive, negative, serendipitous, or mixed.

Positive findings confirm what the researcher expected. Results are consistent with the logic and theoretic framework of the study. The null hypothesis is rejected when there is no relationship or difference between variables. The hypotheses are accepted.

Negative findings mean that nonsignificant results were discovered. The null hypothesis is accepted. The researcher must then evaluate alternative explanations for the negative results. Negative results can be attributed to sampling bias, measurement error, or design or measurement methods.

Serendipitous findings are those that were unexpected. These findings are usually not discussed in the problem statement because the factor or variable was not thought to be part of the conceptual or theoretic framework.

Mixed results contain some results that support the research questions and hypotheses and some that do not. Mixed results may lead the investigator to rethink the theory or to improve methods for study.

Conservative judgment should be used when considering the conclusions drawn from a study. Conclusions should be supported with facts, data, and results, not viewpoints or subjective judgments. Remember, correlation does not prove causation. Because two things are associated does not necessarily mean one causes the other. Alternative explanations for results should always be considered.

Recommendations stem from changes the researcher plans in sample, design, or analysis if the study is repeated. Recommendations may also be based on negative, mixed, or serendipitous findings. Other explanations for results should be discussed so progress can be made in future studies of the research problem. Implications of research such as how findings can be used to improve nursing or how to advance knowledge through additional research should be provided.

Communicating the Results

Once the research data are analyzed and conclusions are drawn, you have an obligation to yourself and to the profession to share this knowledge. The results have the potential to influence nursing care, and by reporting the results, nurses add to the available body of knowledge. Because the future of the profession depends on advancement of this knowledge, nurses must communicate with each other what has been discovered.

To communicate research results, you can write about them or give an oral presentation. Written reports are usually in the form of a thesis, a dissertation, or a journal article. Paper and poster presentations are opportunities to discuss your study with an audience.

Journal articles are the most useful means to reach a large group of professionals. Leading nursing journals that primarily publish nursing research articles include *Nursing Research, Research in Nursing and Health, Western Journal of Nursing Research, Applied Nursing Research, Clinical Nursing Research, Qualitative Health Research,* and *Advances in Nursing Science.* Clinical research is also published in other nursing and nonnursing journals. Specialty journals such as *Journal of Emergency Nursing* and *Heart and Lung* also publish research. The journal you select depends on the readership you want to reach.[34]

Swanson, McCloskey, and Bodensteiner[34] wrote a valuable report listing publishing opportunities for nurses. It includes facts about circulation, submission criteria, and acceptance rates for 92 U.S. journals that publish nursing and other health related research.

Because your manuscript must compete with those from other researchers, you may want to write a letter of inquiry (a query letter) to determine whether the editor is interested in your manuscript. A positive response increases the likelihood your article will be published. Send query letters to as many journals as you wish. However, do not submit your full manuscript to more than one journal. It is an unwritten ethical code between editors and authors that you may have your manuscript reviewed by only one journal at a time. This code prevents several journal editors from going through the time and work of reviewing an article, only to discover the article is being published in another journal. It is not ethical to submit exactly the same manuscript to two different journals, but you can report different information from your research in separate articles.

If your manuscript is not accepted for publication, you may submit it to another journal. Many researchers submit several times before they abandon hope of getting their results published. Many editors include "information for authors" at the beginning of their journals. Following these guidelines improves your chance of acceptance. You should ask colleagues, friends, and professional editors to read your manuscript for clarity and correctness.

Theses and dissertations are written mainly to fulfill requirements for a master's or doctoral degree. A thesis or dissertation has a limited audience and is the method least often used for dissemination of research results. These manuscripts are generally thorough and scholarly but too lengthy for most readers.

A paper presentation is an oral summary of your research results. It is usually read at scientific or professional meetings where members of the same field gather to share knowledge. Organizations require abstracts 6 to 9 months before the meeting date. Calls for abstracts are published in journals. The call usually lists requirements that your abstract must fulfil, such as length, format, deadline for submission, and any requirements regarding membership in that particular organization.

You will be allowed 15 to 30 minutes for your oral presentation of introduction, methodology, results, discussion, and time to answer questions. There will be a strict time limit. Practice your presentation so that you stay within the time frame. Include slides or other audiovisual aids in your professional presentation.

Sometimes professional organizations give researchers the option of a poster presentation. The organization will issue a call for abstracts or papers. A poster presentation combines a visual poster of your research and the opportunity to discuss your findings informally with interested persons.[29] Usually a poster session is set up at a specific site at the meeting to allow participants to walk among the researchers and their posters and ask questions. Following the guidelines for poster presentations will give your poster a professional appearance. Instructions regarding the size and number of poster boards are usually provided after the paper is accepted. You may wish to check with your hospital graphic arts department or biomedical department for help in preparing your poster.[20,22,31]

Writing an abstract. An abstract is a brief summary of the research study. It is located at the beginning of a journal article and of a bound copy of a thesis or dissertation. Some journals publish abstracts of articles that have appeared in other journals or that have been presented orally or as poster presentations at conferences.

Abstracts can be 250 to 1000 words long, depending on the space available. An abstract generally contains a statement about the research purpose of hypotheses, a description of the sample, a brief explanation of the data collection and analysis procedures, and a summary of important findings.

FUNDING

When seeking money to fund research, the researcher must follow formal guidelines. Most funding agencies release guidelines and standards for review to the public. When requesting grant funds, you should consider both the agency most appropriate for the project and the level of sophistication of the research.

The thousands of funding sources for research include federal, state, and local government agencies, private foundations, business and industry, university or hospital funds, private donors, and professional and scientific organizations. Public libraries and most university research departments have listings and current information regarding government and foundation sources. The source that is most helpful when looking for foundation money is the *Foundation Directory,* available at The Foundation Center, 888 Seventh Avenue, New York, NY 10106.

Many universities and hospitals have research funds for staff members. In many cases, these funds are more accessible and require less formal proposal preparation than other sources.

The American Nurses Foundation, Sigma Theta Tau, Emergency Nursing Foundation, and the American Association of Critical Care Nurses offer grants for nursing research. Grant applications are available from the executive offices of each institution.

The NIH has 12 freestanding institutes and the National Center for Nursing Research. Fundable research proposals

---

Box **10-2**　**NIH Research Priorities**
Low birth weight—mothers and infants
HIV infection—prevention and care
Long-term care for older adults
Symptom management
Information systems
Health promotion
Technology across the life span

---

submitted to the National Center for Nursing Research should be related to one of seven research priorities (Box 10-2).[7] The NIH is the primary source for nursing research funding.

Submitting a Proposal

The first step in submitting a proposal is to obtain specific guidelines from funding agencies. Agency deadlines, any restrictions, and investigator qualifications are all important components. Give consideration to any specific directions for preparation of your proposal. You may seek funding from more than one agency, but you must meet the specific requirements of each agency.

After writing a proposal, submit it to several of your peers for review. Select someone with knowledge of the content you are proposing to study. A second person who is not familiar with the content can review for style, clarity, and logical flow. Mistakes in grammar, spelling, and punctuation may cause reviewers to question your ability to perform scholarly research.

When a grant application is reviewed, one of the first things reviewers look for is the purpose of the study. The purpose must be stated clearly near the beginning of the proposal. The reviewers ask the following questions: Why is the study important? Who will benefit from the study? Is the study feasible? Are all ethical standards met? How well does this study contribute to what we already know?

Your grant proposal is evaluated by experienced researchers to first determine whether you followed the guidelines for submission. Read and follow the guidelines carefully. Deadlines are not usually flexible.

There are many more good research questions than there is money to fund them. If your proposal does not get funded, consider it a learning experience. The guidelines assisted you in clarifying your question and forced you to look closely at important components of your research. Consider the reviewer's comments as free expert advice, and use the advice to improve your proposal.

PROTECTION OF HUMAN SUBJECTS

The first federal guidelines requiring that grant applications for research involving human subjects be reviewed by an Institutional Review Board (IRB) were published in 1966 by the U.S. Public Health Service.[18] The purposes of these guidelines were to safeguard subjects' rights and welfare, ensure appropriate procedures for informed consent, and allow subjects to make independent decisions about risks and benefits. Any research activities supported by the Department of Health and Human Services were regulated by Congress in 1974.

In 1974, Congress established a National Commission for Protection of Human Subjects of Biomedical and Behavioral Research, which recommends legislative and regulatory action to govern agencies issuing research grants.

The National Research Act (PL 93-348) was passed on July 12, 1974. It regulated the ethics guidance programs for IRBs. This act requires that any institution applying for a grant or contract for any project involving a human subject in biomedical or behavioral research must show proof in the application that it has established an IRB. Agencies that receive no federal grants usually have a review mechanism similar to an IRB, sometimes referred to as a human rights committee or a research committee. Box 10-3 lists requirements that an IRB must guarantee before approving a research study.[12]

When risk to subjects is minimal, most IRBs have a process called *expedited review,* which usually shortens the review process.[12] A list of research categories eligible for expedited review is available from any IRB office. Keep in mind that IRBs usually have set meeting times during the year and that they may have many proposals to review. If you anticipate a starting date for your study, begin the IRB process early—several months in advance is *not* unrealistic. Every researcher should obtain the most up-to-date requirements for review from the institution's IRB office.

Studies usually exempt from the strict IRB requirements are those that use existing data, documents, records, or pathologic and diagnostic specimens, where these sources are available to the public or if the information is recorded so that the subjects cannot be identified.[12]

Box 10-3	Research Requirements by an Institutional Review Board

1. Risks to subjects are minimized.
2. Risks to subjects are reasonable in relation to anticipated benefits, if any, to the subjects and in relation to the importance of the knowledge that may be expected to result.
3. Selection of subjects is equitable.
4. Informed consent will be sought from each prospective subject or legally authorized representative.
5. Informed consent is appropriately documented.
6. The research plan makes provision for monitoring data collection to ensure subjects' safety (as needed).
7. When appropriate, provisions are made to protect subjects' privacy and confidentiality of data.
8. Additional safeguards are included if some or all subjects are likely to be vulnerable to coercion or undue influence.

Some institutions require progress reports. However, all institutions require final reports of the study, including the number of participants, study findings, and how these findings will be communicated. The IRB usually requests a copy of your publication or presentation to ensure that proper credit is given to the institution.

Informed Consent

The federal government has mandated the following elements of information when informed consent is obtained[12]:
1. A statement that the study involves research, explanation of purposes of the research, delineation of the expected duration of the subject's participation, description of the procedures to be followed, and identification of any procedures that are experimental.
2. A description of any reasonably foreseeable risks or discomforts to the subject.
3. A description of any benefits to the subject or to others that may reasonably be expected from the research.
4. A disclosure of appropriate alternative procedures or courses of treatment, if any, that may be advantageous to the subject.
5. A statement describing to what extent, if any, confidentiality of records identifying the subject will be maintained.
6. For research involving more than minimal risk, an explanation as to whether any medical treatments are available if injury occurs and if so, what they consist of or where further information may be obtained.
7. An explanation of whom to contact for answers to pertinent questions about the research and the subject's rights and whom to contact in the event of a research-related injury to the subject.
8. A statement that participation is voluntary, refusal to participate will not involve any penalty or loss of benefits to which the subject is otherwise entitled, and the subject may discontinue participation at any time without any penalty or loss of otherwise entitled benefits.

The language of the consent form must be understandable. The subject cannot be asked to waive rights or to release the researcher or institution from liability for negligence.[12]

The date, time, and signatures of the subject, researcher, and witness must be included on the form. The researcher should also include a phone number where he or she can be contacted about concerns.

Ethical considerations. In 1985, ANA issued its *Human Rights Guidelines for Nurses in Clinical and Other Research*[3] and its updated version of *Code for Nurses with Interpretive Statements.*[2] This code states that any proposed nursing research study should meet the following conditions:
• The study design is approved by an appropriate body.
• The individual has the right to freedom from intrinsic risks of injury.

- The individual has the right to privacy and dignity.
- All people have the right to choose to participate, to have full information, and to terminate participation without penalty.

CRITIQUES

A research critique is a critical appraisal of a research study performed systematically by someone with knowledge of both research and the content area. The goal is to determine how the new knowledge fits into what is already known. A decision concerning scientific merit is made so that readers can determine whether to incorporate the results into practice. A careful appraisal is made of the study's strengths and weaknesses. The information in a paper accepted for publication will not necessarily be adopted into practice. Usually several strong, similar research results are needed to change practice; therefore research is often replicated and refined. Each element of the research report is critiqued.

For adequate evaluation of research, expertise is required in the areas of study design, methods, sampling data analysis, and the content area under study. You may want to ask a nurse researcher in a local institution, school of nursing, or college for help in critiquing research. Beck[6] describes a 10-step process for critiquing all dimensions of a research report.

Phillips[26] devoted an entire text to critiquing and utilization of nursing research. Shelley[32] said that research critiques should provide answers to the following questions:

- What new knowledge, if any, has been generated?
- How does this new knowledge related to existing knowledge?
- What are the implications, if any, for practice?
- How might this research be extended or improved?

APPLICATION TO NURSING PRACTICE

The final step of the research process is to use the results to change nursing practice. Even if your findings have been disseminated in journals, at conferences, or in a paper, your useful data will not necessarily be put into practice. You must be the one to make research-based changes in practice. Often a group of research findings, called innovations, are used to change practice. Whether you are a researcher or a clinical nurse, you can identify these innovations and put them into practice.

Horsley[19] has described a seven-step process for producing research-based practice change. This process serves as an excellent resource for any nurse wanting to implement change. The steps of the process are:

1. Identify patient care problems systematically
2. Identify and assess research-based knowledge to solve identified care problems
3. Adapt and design the nursing practice innovation
4. Conduct a clinical trial and evaluate the innovation
5. Decide whether to adopt, alter, or reject the innovation

6. Develop the means to extend or diffuse the new practice beyond the trial unit
7. Develop mechanisms to maintain the innovation over time

Brett[8] studied organizational methods for integrating research into practice. She found that hospitals are having difficulty adopting innovations by nurses. Many organizations now support inclusion of research committees and nurse researchers on the organization's charts. Nursing research is often rewarded through clinical and career ladders. Joint appointments between academic and clinical settings promote research. Reading research-based literature and attending conferences that include research presentations contribute to the nurse's awareness of research findings and understanding of how this supports practice.

Brett[8] found conducting and publishing research did have a positive impact on adoption of findings into practice. Collaboration is one method for accomplishing research and changing practice. Rogers[30] states that collaboration allows joint discussion about problems, combines expertise, provides opportunities to develop and expand research skills, and provides an avenue for dissemination of findings into practice.

SUMMARY

Nursing research begins, for each nurse, with a "first" research project. Research is a set of logical steps that ensure meaningful and useful results. Start with a small project, and find resources that help you. Contact nurses in your hospital with advanced degrees who have done research. Faculty members of a nearby college or university may be looking for someone with clinical expertise with whom to collaborate on projects. Finally, look for research results when you are solving clinical problems. If you think there must be a better way to perform a particular aspect of nursing care, there probably is one. Review the literature to see if you can find an answer. If you cannot find one, you have the beginnings of a useful research study.

REFERENCES

1. American Association of Critical Care Nurses: Determining AACN's research priorities for the 90s, *Am J Crit Care* 2(2):110, 1993.
2. American Nurses Association: *Code for nurses with interpretive statements,* Kansas City, Mo, 1985, The Association.
3. American Nurses Association: Commission on Nursing Research: *Human rights guidelines for nurses in clinical and other research,* Washington, DC, 1985, The Association.
4. American Nurses Association: *Directions for nursing research toward the 21st century,* Washington, DC, 1996, The Association.
5. American Psychological Association: *Standards for educational and psychological tests,* Washington, DC, 1974, The Association.
6. Beck CT: The research critique: general criteria for evaluating a research report, *J Obstet Gynecol Neonatal News* 19(10):18, 1990.
7. Bloch D: Strategies for setting and implementing the National Center for Nursing Research Priorities, *Appl Nurs Res* 3(1):2, 1990.
8. Brett JL: Organizational integrative mechanisms and adoption of innovations by nurses, *Nurs Res* 38(2):105, 1989.

9. Burns N, Grove S: *The practice of nursing research, conduct, critique, and utilization,* ed 2, Philadelphia, 1993, WB Saunders.

10. Campbell J: A test of two explanatory models of women's responses to battering, *Nurs Res* 38(1):18, 1989.

11. Clochesy JM: Computer use and nursing research: statistical packages for microcomputers, *West J Nurs Res* 9(1):138, 1987.

12. Code of Federal Regulations: *Protection of human subjects,* Office of Protection from Research Risks, Reports: Sec 46.111, 46.101(b), 46.110, and 46.116(a), 1985, U.S. Department of Health and Human Services.

13. Cohen J: *Statistical power analyses for the behavioral sciences,* rev ed, New York, 1977, Academic Press.

14. Fawcett J: *Analyses and evaluation of conceptual models of nursing,* Philadelphia, 1984, FA Davis.

15. Fox DJ: *Fundamentals of research in nursing,* ed 4, East Norwalk, Conn, 1982, Appleton-Century-Crofts.

16. Frank-Stromborg M: *Instruments for clinical nursing research,* Norwalk, Conn, 1988, Appleton & Lange.

17. Funk M: Research priorities in critical care nursing, *Focus Crit Care* 16(2):135, 1989.

18. Gortner SR, Heath E, Sanders P: The institutional review board: a case study of no-risk decisions in health-related research, *Nurs Res* 30(1):21, 1981.

19. Horsley JA: *Using research to improve nursing practice: a guide,* New York, 1983, Grune & Stratton.

20. Lippman D, Ponton M: Designing a research poster with impact, *West J Nurs Res* 11(4):477, 1989.

21. LoBiondo-Wood G, Haber J: *Nursing research: methods, critical appraisal, and utilization,* ed 3, St Louis, 1994, Mosby.

22. McDaniel R, Bach C, Poole M: Poster update: getting their attention, *Nurs Res* 42:302, 1993.

23. McDowell J, Newll C: *Measuring health: a guide to rating scales and questionnaires,* New York, 1987, Oxford University Press.

24. Meier P, Pugh EJ: The case study: a viable approach to clinical research, *Res Nurs Health* 9:195, 1986.

25. Notter L, Hott J: *Essentials of nursing research,* ed 5, New York, 1994, Springer.

26. Phillips LR: *A clinician's guide to the critique and utilization of nursing research,* Norwalk, Conn, 1986, Appleton-Century-Crofts.

27. Piazza D, Lenaghan P, Bernardo L et al: 1992 ENA and ENF research initiatives, *J Emerg Nurs* 18(5):44A, 1992.

28. Polit DF, Hungler BP: *Nursing research: principles and methods,* ed 5, Philadelphia, 1995, JB Lippincott.

29. Rempusheski V: Resources necessary to prepare a poster for presentation, *Appl Nurs Res* 3:134, 1991.

30. Rogers B: Research and practice: collaborating for improved nursing care, *AAOHN* 36(10):432, 1988.

31. Ryan N: Developing and presenting a research poster, *Appl Nurs Res* 2(1):52, 1989.

32. Shelley SI: *Research methods in nursing health,* Boston, 1985, Little, Brown.

33. Smith LW: Microcomputer-based bibliographic searching, *Nurs Outlook* 37(2):125, 1988.

34. Swanson E, McCloskey J, Bodensteiner A: Publishing opportunities for nurses: a comparison of 92 U.S. journals, *Image* 23:33, 1991.

Unit III

Clinical Foundations of Emergency Nursing

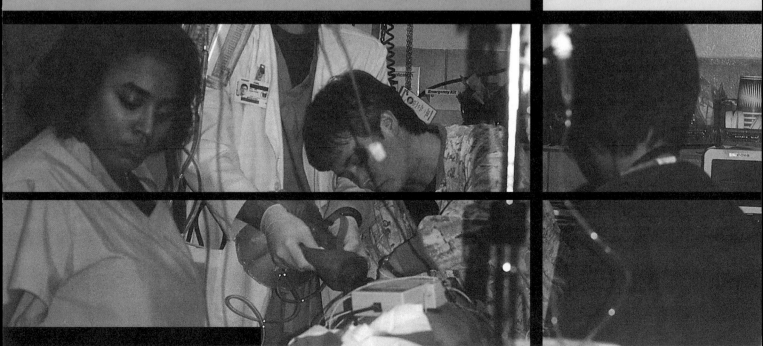

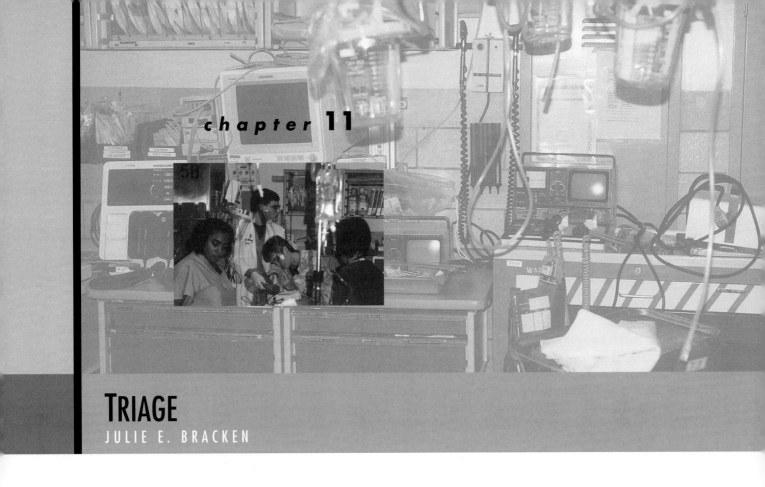

chapter **11**

TRIAGE

JULIE E. BRACKEN

Triage is a process used to determine severity of illness or injury for each patient who enters the emergency department (ED). Putting the patient in the right place at the right time to receive the right level of care facilitates allocation of appropriate resources to meet the patient's medical needs. Ingredients for an effective triage system are adequate space, supplies, a communication system, access to the treatment area, and an experienced professional supported by a multidisciplinary team.[10] In most EDs, a registered nurse fulfills this role. Joint Commission on Accreditation of Health Care Organizations (JCAHCO) standards identify the registered nurse as the appropriate person to perform triage.

The word *triage* is derived from the French verb *trier,* which means "to pick or to sort."[23] Triage dates back to the French military, who used the word to designate a "clearing hospital" for wounded soldiers. The U.S. military used *triage* to describe a sorting station where injured soldiers were distributed from the battlefield to distant support hospitals. After World War II, triage came to mean the process used to identify those most likely to return to the battle after medical intervention. This process allowed concentration of medical resources on soldiers who could fight again. During the Korean and Vietnam conflicts, triage was refined to accomplish the "greatest good for the greatest number of wounded or injured men."[26]

In the civilian arena, triage has two very different uses—disaster triage and daily triage.[4] Disaster triage is similar to military triage in that the goal is the greatest good for the greatest number of injured. Disasters include floods, hurricanes, earthquakes, bombs, collapsed buildings, fires, airline crashes, vehicular crashes, and tornadoes.[10] The primary difference between disaster triage and military triage relates to patient transport.[4,25] Table 11-1 compares priority categories used for military and disaster triage. During a disaster, transport for some victims is delayed to prevent overloading the receiving ED. Chapter 18 discusses disasters and emergency operations preparedness in greater detail.

Daily ED use of triage systems began in the early 1960s when demand for emergency services surpassed available resources. Space, equipment, and personnel could no longer handle the explosive increase in ED visits. From 1958 to the early 1960s, the nation's EDs reported 18 million visits.[23] This figure increased to more than 44 million by 1968 and to more than 99 million by 1990.[10] The greatest increase in patient numbers occurred in the nonurgent category. Reasons cited for increases include lack of available nonemergency services and lack of access to primary or urgent care providers.[10] The volume of patients with nonurgent problems increased as a growing number of underinsured or uninsured people used the ED for primary care.[20,27] The triage process evolved as an efficient way to separate patients requiring immediate medical attention from those who could wait.

TRIAGE SYSTEMS

The primary goal of an effective triage system is rapid identification of patients with urgent, life-threatening conditions.[11] Complementary goals include prioritizing care needs for all patients, regulating patient flow through the

ED, and determining the most appropriate area for treatment—the ED or an outside primary care area.[13]

Any triage system has primary and secondary functions. Primary functions include assessment and reassessment of the patient's chief complaint and related symptoms, taking a brief history, physical assessment, and measuring vital signs. Secondary functions include clerical tasks, directions, telephone advice, ambulance patient evaluation, ambulance dispatch, stocking of supplies, cleaning, equipment maintenance, crowd control, security, and information.[9,10] The extent to which a triage system encompasses all these functions depends on the daily census, available staff, presence of walk-in clinics or same-day clinics, type and availability of health care providers, availability of specialty treatment areas, and environmental, legal, and administrative constraints.[23,25]

ED triage systems vary widely. In 1982, Thompson and

Table **11-1** **Comparison of Military and Disaster Priority Categories**

Priority	Military	Disaster
1	**Immediate care** Shock, airway problems, chest injury, crush injury, amputation, open fracture	**Class I (emergent) Red** Critical; life-threatening—compromised airway, shock, hemorrhage
2	**Minimal care** Little or no treatment needed	**Class II (urgent) Yellow** Major illness or injury; requires treatment within 20 minutes to 2 hours—open fracture, chest wound
3	**Delayed care** Treatment may be postponed without loss of life; noncritical—simple fracture, nonbleeding laceration	**Class III (nonurgent) Green** Care may be delayed 2 hours or more; minor injuries; walking wounded—closed fracture, sprain, strain
4	**Expectant care** No treatment until immediate and delayed priority patients cared for; requires considerable time, effort, and supplies	**Class IV (expectant) Black** Dead or expected to die—massive head injury, extensive full-thickness burns

Modified from Thompson JD, Dains J: *Comprehensive triage: a manual for developing and implementing a nursing care system,* Reston, Va, 1982, Reston.

Table **11-2** **Comparison of Triage Systems**

Elements	Type I: traffic director	Type II: spot check	Type III: comprehensive
Assessment			
Staff	Nonprofessional	Registered nurse or physician	Registered nurse
Data	Chief complaint	Chief complaint: limited subjective and objective	Thorough assessment: complete, subjective and objective; education needs; primary health needs
Analysis			
Urgency category	2 categories: emergent; nonurgent	3 categories: emergent; urgent; delayed	4 categories: class I-IV
Nursing diagnoses	None	None	Present
Plan			
Alternatives	Treatment room; waiting room	Treatment room; waiting area; treat and discharge from triage;	Treatment room; waiting area with planned assessment
Diagnostic procedures	None	Inconsistent	Protocol driven
Documentation	Little; inconsistent	Variable	Systematic
Evaluation			
Reevaluation	None	None planned; at patient request	Planned; systematic
System	Difficult	Variable	Systematic

Modified from Thompson JD, Dains J: *Comprehensive triage: a manual for developing and implementing a nursing care system,* Reston, Va, 1982, Reston.

Dains identified the three most common triage systems—traffic director (Type I), spot checker (Type II), and comprehensive (Type III).[25] Differences between these systems are related to the depth of triage provided. Table 11-2 compares urgency categories, staffing patterns, documentation requirements, patient assessment and reassessment criteria, and use of diagnostic procedures found in these triage systems.

The comprehensive triage system may be provided as a single-tiered system, in which the nurse who first encounters the patient performs the interview, documents triage assessment, assigns triage acuity, and designates treatment areas. This system provides the most customer friendly triage process because the patient does not feel rushed and the nurse can establish rapport with the patient. The entire triage encounter is documented on a triage record or on the patient's medical record. Triage protocols and various interventions are initiated by the triage nurse. With this system, the triage area should be large enough to allow privacy for the interview without interfering with the triage nurse's ability to see patients as they come through the door. Large-volume EDs may require multiple triage nurses to maintain flow in this type of system.

A multitiered system is used in some large-volume EDs to expedite flow while providing rapid identification of patients with potential threats to life, limb, or vision. In this system, the first triage nurse sees each patient enter the ED, rapidly assesses the patient to determine chief complaint and identify immediate threats to life, vision, or limb. Acuity is determined from visual observations, a brief patient interview, and tactile examination of skin and quality of the pulse. The triage interview and vital signs are not obtained in the first tier. If the patient does not require immediate attention, a chart is completed before the patient is sent to the second tier of the system for the triage interview and taking of vital signs. Triage protocols are initiated at the second tier. With a multitiered system, the triage nurse is not occupied with comprehensive triage assessment, has constant visual access to everyone who enters the area, and can rapidly identify patients who require immediate attention.

Regardless of the process used, department structure should support the system. The triage area should be located by the front door, so that the first professional the patient encounters is the triage nurse. When a multitiered system is used, the first tier should provide immediate visual access to the front door without sacrificing security measures or exposing the triage nurse to unnecessary weather conditions. The process should flow from one step to the next without creating unnecessary walking for the patient or staff.

URGENCY CATEGORIES

Urgency categories are used in the triage process to rate patient acuity and to prioritize care. Rating systems vary with patient consensus and available resources. Most rating systems use predetermined criteria to classify patients into two or more categories. The most common system uses three classification levels: emergent, urgent, or nonurgent (Table 11-3).[10,11,13,19] The greater the number of urgency categories, the more discriminating an ED can be in meeting a patient's needs.[18] A comprehensive triage system uses four classifications. Table 11-4 summarizes these urgency categories by description, reassessment guidelines, and types of patients.

TRIAGE STAFFING

Historically, receptionists, ward clerks, nurse aides, emergency medical technicians, licensed practical nurses, registered nurses, physicians, and others performed triage. In 1985, Congress passed the Consolidated Omnibus Reconciliation Act (COBRA) that requires a medical screening for all ED patients before inquiries about finances, insurance, or

Table **11-3**	**Urgency Categories**
Category	Description
Emergent	Immediate care required; condition is threat to life, limb, or vision; "severe"
Urgent	Care required as soon as possible; condition presents danger if not treated; "acute" but not "severe"
Nonurgent	Routine care required; condition minor; care can be delayed

Table **11-4**	**Comprehensive Triage: Four Urgency Categories**			
Class	I	II	III	IV
Descriptor	Immediate; life-threatening	Stable; ASAP	Stable; no distress	Stable; no distress
Reassessment	Continuous	q15 min	q30 min	q60 min
Examples	Cardiac arrest, seizures, major trauma, respiratory distress, major burn	Open fracture, pain, minor burn, surgical abdomen, sickle cell, child, and fever	Closed fracture, laceration without bleeding, drug ingestion over 3 hr with no signs or symptoms	rash, constipation, impetigo, abrasion, nerves

Modified from Thompson JD, Dains J: *Comprehensive triage: a manual for developing and implementing a nursing care system*, Reston, Va, 1982, Reston.

ability to pay. COBRA, or the Emergency Medical Treatment and Active Labor Act (EMTALA), as it is now known, specifies that medical screening must be performed by a qualified individual.[7] The definition of a qualified individual is still an area of controversy, left open for interpretation. Use of a registered nurse as triage nurse to provide medical screening and prioritize patient care is widely recommended.[17] The Standards of Emergency Nursing Practice specify that a registered nurse should triage each patient.[6] Unfortunately, studies show that these nurses perform triage in only 59%-62% of all EDs.[2,22]

The triage nurse may be a dedicated position or may be done by all nurses working in the ED, rotating to triage for all or part of a specific shift. The most effective system is determined by the individual needs of each ED.

Triage Nurse Qualifications

The triage nurse decides the order in which patients receive medical attention.[13] A hallmark of an effective triage nurse is experience and skill in rapid assessment, and correct determination of patient urgency. The ability to recognize who is sick and who is not is a critical success factor for the triage nurse. In-depth knowledge and experience are essential.[10]

Triage areas are often chaotic and demanding. The triage nurse must determine priorities rapidly while under stress from incoming phone calls, multiple patient arrivals, visitors, and other events and people. To function effectively, triage nurses must have expert assessment skills, demonstrate competent interview and organizational skills, have an extensive knowledge base of diseases, and have the experience to look for subtle clues to patient acuity. Patients with an obvious critical condition do not present the greatest challenge to the triage nurse. The true test is recognition of subtle clues to a serious problem that can quickly deteriorate without immediate attention.[10,13]

The triage nurse is the first health professional the patient and family encounter in the ED; therefore, highly refined communication skills are essential. Triage nurses must be able to interpret assessment data while providing compassionate support to both patient and family. In-depth understanding of the human response to crisis helps the triage nurse maintain composure, which improves the public image for the ED and the hospital.[13]

The complexity of the triage role led to the recommendation from the Emergency Nurses Association that triage should be performed by a registered nurse with a minimum of 6 months emergency nursing experience.[5,6] Special training to provide the advanced skills and knowledge required in this role is also recommended. A survey by Purnell in 1993 revealed that only 43% of hospitals require special training (i.e., triage course, Advanced Cardiac Life Support, assessment, Certification in Emergency Nursing [CEN], extended orientation) for nurses working in the triage area. Only 9.5% require previous ED experience, with a range of 3 months to 3 years reported. Many hospitals acknowledge the desire to provide further education for triage nurses, but list multiple factors that prevent realization of this desire.[22]

Criteria regarding readiness for the triage role vary with each nurse and depend on the institution; sophistication of the triage system; the individual nurse's competence in assessment, clinical judgment, and decision making; and quality of the triage orientation process. Current legislation and legal implications affecting this role must be considered when designating new personnel. A risk management approach for the ED identifies strategies for preventing litigation.

Anecdotal information suggests that formal triage orientation and special training improve the triage nurse's effectiveness and comfort in the role. Written protocols to assist decision making as well as an internship or preceptorship allow the novice to grow with the assistance of an experienced triage nurse.

TRIAGE DOCUMENTATION

Documentation with the tiered triage system may use a triage record or a triage sticker. The triage record is often the first part of the ED nursing record (Figure 11-1). A triage sticker provides a method for documentation of essential initial triage information without the need for a separate triage sheet (Figure 11-2). The triage sticker is placed on the medical record to ensure continuity of documentation. Regardless of the system, triage documentation should provide a "snapshot" of the patient's chief complaint, appearance, and acuity. A focused assessment of the chief complaint is also necessary to prioritize care and identify appropriate treatment needs.

PATIENT ASSESSMENT

The goals of the triage process are to gather sufficient data to determine acuity, identify immediate needs, and establish a rapport with the patient and family. Use of the nursing process provides the necessary framework for a consistent approach for every patient.

Assessment

This is defined as a rapid systematic collection of data relevant to each patient.[6] Subjective data provide information disclosed by the patient or family; whereas objective data are observable, measurable information.[1] The triage nurse begins assessing the patient either with the first contact as the patient walks through the ED door, during a distraught call for help from a concerned person, or during a radio call from prehospital personnel. The triage nurse is expected to evaluate all patients entering the ED within 2 to 5 minutes of arrival.

In an ideal setting, the triage nurse begins with a self-introduction while assessing major threats to airway, breathing, or circulation (ABCs) (i.e., airway compromise, respiratory distress, excessive bleeding, and skin or mentation changes). The triage nurse provides immediate intervention for identified threats to ABCs and transports the patient to

EHS ⊕ Christ Hospital and Medical Center

Name _____
(Last, First, Middle Initial)

Age _____ Pt. Location _____

Sex _____

MR # _____

NURSING RECORD

Date _____ Time _____

| **Triage** | Chief Complaint | | | | | Allergies | | | |

| Vitals | | | | | | LMP | When Normal Abnormal | Tetanus | When |
| T | BP | P | R | WT. | | | | |

| Medications |

| Past Medical History |

| Accompanied by | Interventions | Acuity |

| Private Physician | Disposition ☐To Registration ☐Direct to ED ☐Other | **Triage Nurse** |

Figure **11-1** Triage record. *(Courtesy Christ Hospital and Medical Center, Oak Lawn, Ill.)*

Name _____ Age____ Date _____ Time _____

CC _____ Acuity **R Y G**

Potential Threats ☐None Apparent | **Visual**
☐Life   ☐Resp. Distress   ☐Altered LOC | ☐None Apparent   ☐Severe Pain
☐Vision ☐Chest Pain   ☐Suicidal | ☐Obvious Fracture   ☐Burn w/Blisters
☐Limb   ☐Overdose   ☐Violent | ☐Severe Bleeding

Appearance | **Color** | **Skin** | **Disposition**
☐Alert | ☐WNL | ☐WNL | ☐Registration   ☐Egleston
☐Cooperative | ☐Pale | ☐Cold | ☐Treatment Area   ☐Refusal of Care Signed
☐Ambulatory | ☐Flushed | ☐Hot | ☐Assessment
☐Wheelchair | ☐Cyanotic | ☐Diaphoretic | ☐ Other _____

RN Signature _____

Figure **11-2** Triage sticker. *(Courtesy Promina Kennestone Hospital, Marietta, Ga.)*

the appropriate treatment area. When no immediate threat is identified, the triage nurse proceeds with a brief interview. Eliciting the chief complaint, defined as the reason for seeking emergency care, is the first step.[10] This is a distinct challenge when the patient provides vague or global reasons for the visit. The triage nurse must focus the investigation on the history of the complaint and related symptoms and signs. The "PQRST" mnemonic is one example of a systematic approach to patient assessment (Table 11-5).

When sufficient information is obtained about the chief complaint and related symptoms, data are collected regarding medication usage, including prescribed and over-the-counter drugs and home remedy medications. The triage nurse then evaluates the patient's past medical history including hospitalizations. Immunization history is especially important in children[11]; however, a break in the skin or conjunctiva requires investigation of tetanus immunization status, regardless of age. Allergies to medication and environmental sources are then identified.

At an appropriate time during the interview other subjective data are acquired, including name of the primary health care provider. For female patients, the nurse obtains a menstrual history and obstetrical history, including gravida and parity. Screening for tuberculosis, child/elder abuse or neglect, and domestic violence victims is also performed.

Objective data is gathered during the interview. Vital signs (temperature, pulse, respiration, and blood pressure), body weight, and other physical data are acquired by inspection, palpation, percussion, and auscultation. Touching provides information on heart rate, skin temperature, and moisture. Smelling provides information on odors (i.e., ketones, alcohol, infections, and hygiene). Hearing provides information on cough quality, hoarseness, stridor, shortness of breath, tone of voice, logical thought, articulation patterns, and "what is not said." A wealth of information from nonverbal cues is obtained visually: facial grimaces, body movements, fear, obvious deformities, skin color, amount of

Table 11-5	PQRST Mnemonic
Component	Sample questions
P (provokes)	What provokes the symptom?
Q (quality)	What makes it better? What makes it worse? What does it feel like?
R (radiation)	Where is it? Where does it go? Is it in one or more spots?
S (severity)	If we gave it a number from 0-10, with 0 being none and 10 being the worst you can imagine, what is your rating?
T (time)	How long have you had the symptom? When did it start? When did it end? How long did it last? Does it come and go?

bleeding, cyanosis, use of personal space, appropriateness of clothing, and hygiene.[1,13]

Triage nurses must be highly skilled in asking the right questions and pursuing small details. Triage guidelines, protocols, decision trees, and algorithms aid in this process.[13] Computer programs exists to help structure the inquiry. Advanced interviewing skills support the communication process of giving and receiving information using verbal and nonverbal cues.

Questioning is a useful technique in the interviewing process. A mix of open (eliciting feelings and perceptions) and closed ("yes/no," factual) questions must be posed to obtain important data. Reflection, silence, displaying acceptance, showing recognition, verbalizing observations, sharing information, actively listening, and summarizing are all used in the monumental task of gathering data to make a good health care decision for each patient.[1] The nurse's style varies with each patient and situation.

Barriers to effective communication include language, vocabulary, cultural differences, patient developmental level, health status, anxiety, pain, and environmental issues, especially interview interruptions. The triage nurse has no control over interruptions during assessment[13]; however, every effort should be made to minimize interruptions. Gracious concern, a caring attitude, and willingness to listen help establish the necessary rapport with the patient and family.

DIAGNOSIS

Diagnosis is defined as analyzing information collected in the assessment phase to determine acuity needs. Assume that a more severe condition exists until proven otherwise to prevent undertriage.[6] Preliminary nursing diagnoses may be formulated and an initial data base established. Triage nurses must possess a span of knowledge to evaluate a vast variety of patient complaints.[13] Critical thinking at this step is mandatory to identify outcomes for each patient.

PLANNING

Planning is defined as determining a course of action for identified needs to meet the expected outcome.[6] The triage nurse differentiates urgency of problems and prioritizes care by assigning acuity level, designating an appropriate treatment area, communicating pertinent information to other team members, and identifying interventions to meet the expected outcome.[6]

IMPLEMENTATION

Implementation is defined as carrying out the plan of care.[6] The triage nurse initiates nursing interventions, performs diagnostic procedures and treatments defined in established protocols, communicates pertinent information to the patient and family, mobilizes necessary additional resources, and documents all activities in the patient's medical record. Examples of these activities include splinting, ice application, dressings, ordering radiology exams, administering fever or tetanus medications as per protocol, stocking emergency supplies and equipment, and ensuring isolation for immunocompromised or contagious patients (i.e., measles, chickenpox, tuberculosis).[11]

EVALUATION

Evaluation is defined as interpreting the patient's response to interventions. The triage nurse reassesses the patient based on acuity and within time frames established by the protocol; evaluates effectiveness of interventions; and revises the plan of care, expected outcomes, and acuity based on new or changing patient data.[6] Paying special attention to borderline patients can prevent catastrophic events.[19]

SPECIAL CONDITIONS
COBRA

In 1986 Congress passed COBRA, now called EMTALA, which applies to every hospital with an ED participating in the Medicare program. A medical screening examination to determine presence of an emergency medical condition or active labor is required for all persons who come to the ED. If qualified medical personnel determine an emergency medical condition or active labor to be present, the staff must stabilize the patient within the facility's capability. If a transfer to another facility is necessary, specific regulations govern the transfer.[7] (See Chapter 13.)

Many EDs use the triage encounter to provide the initial medical screening examination required by COBRA/EMTALA.[3,10,12,13,14] The triage process is then structured to screen the patient before any financial inquiries occur. To ensure that a "qualified" medical staff person is present, only an experienced, competent, and trained triage nurse should perform the examination.[3]

Managed Care

More and more consumers are choosing managed care plans for health care. Many of these plans require authorization before ED treatment; therefore, payment for the service is contingent on approval. This creates great concern for patients who are denied authorization; the triage nurse frequently advocates for the patient with the "gatekeeper" of the plan to determine where care can be provided in a safe manner.[3,10] The patient is always given the option to be evaluated in the ED, but must be informed of responsibility for payment. This creates special problems for the chronically ill elderly with limited economic and transportation resources, since the closest facility may not be affiliated with their plan.[8]

Referrals from Triage

A shortage of community resources and lack of awareness of access to available services are cited as reasons for nonurgent use of EDs. Referring patients to primary care settings, or "triaging out," provides delivery and continuity of care for the nonurgent complaints, reduces waiting times, and is cost effective.[10] Establishing links to primary care settings is a major component in developing a "triage out" program. Specially trained nurses guided by written protocols discuss and identify sources of alternative care. Patient agreement is required for this referral; then appointment information is provided. "Triage out" programs using feedback loops to evaluate patient satisfaction and safety report good results; this feedback is a necessary component to guarantee success.[12,14]

Telephone Triage

Telephone calls eliciting medical information and advice are problematic for EDs since evaluation of patients by phone is difficult if not impossible.[11] Most legal experts do not recommend giving advice and suggest the caller be directed to the ED. In situations such as cardiopulmonary resuscitation or childbirth, giving appropriate instructions until emergency medical personnel arrive may positively affect the outcome. Hospitals providing telephone information need standardized protocols and a mechanism for documentation so that every call can be logged, tape-recorded, or both.[11] Some EDs are providing special services to meet this consumer need for information. Trained nurses dedicated to telephone consultation using personal computers, specially designed software, telephone recording systems, and facsimile machines create an opportunity for EDs to strengthen their medical advice programs for the community.[15]

CONCLUSION

As the health care system evolves, responsibilities of the triage nurse change. The triage nurse is the initial contact for the patient and family in their emergency experience, and more importantly, this contact directly affects the final outcome for the patient. Although approaches vary, the common ingredient of a successful program rests with a qualified triage nurse.

REFERENCES

1. Bellack JP, Edlund BJ: *Nursing assessment and diagnosis,* ed 2, Boston, 1992, Jones & Bartlett.
2. Cadwell VS, Perkins P, Yates K: Use of registered nurse versus non-registered nurse triage in seventy-six California hospitals: an informal survey, *J Emerg Nurs* 29(6):21A, 1994.
3. Cordell B, et al: Managers ask and answer, *J Emerg Nurs* 19(6):533, 1993.
4. Emergency Nurses Association: *Emergency nursing core curriculum,* ed 4, Philadelphia, 1994, WB Saunders Co.
5. Emergency Nurses Association: Position statement: role of the emergency nurse in clinical practice settings, *J Emerg Nurs* 21(2):24A, 1995.
6. Emergency Nurses Association: *Standards of emergency nursing practice,* ed 3, St. Louis, 1995, Mosby.
7. Fiesta J: Emergency liability: Cobra's fangs, *Nurs Manage* 22(6):14, 1991.
8. Fulmer TT, Walker MK: *Critical care nursing of the elderly,* New York, 1992, Springer Publishing.
9. Geraci EB, Geraci TA: An observational study of the emergency triage nursing role in a managed care facility, *J Emerg Nurs* 20(3):189, 1994.
10. Handysides G: *Triage in emergency practice,* St. Louis, 1996, Mosby.
11. Kelley SJ: *Pediatric emergency nursing,* ed 2, Norwalk, CN, 1994, Appelton & Lange.
12. Kelly KA: Referring patients from triage out of the emergency department to primary care settings: one successful emergency department experience, *J Emerg Nurs* 20(6):458, 1994.
13. Kitt S: *Emergency nursing: a physiologic and clinical perspective,* Philadelphia, 1995, WB Saunders Co.
14. Kuensting LL: "Triaging out" children with minor illnesses from an emergency department by a triage nurse: where do they go?, *J Emerg Nurs* 21(2):102, 1995.
15. Martin C: Telephone consultation for a "managed care" population, *J Emerg Nurs* 21(2):155, 1995.
16. Merkley K, Nelson NC: Computerized charting by exception at triage, *J Emerg Nurs* 21(6):571, 1995.
17. Molitor L: *Emergency department triage handbook,* Gaithersburg, Md, 1992, Aspen.
18. Nelson MS: A triage-based emergency department patients classification system, *J Emerg Nurs* 20(6):511, 1994.
19. Nettina S, Gregonis S: Assigning priorities, *Nursing* 20(11):86, 1990.
20. Pane G, Farner M, Salness K: Health care access problems of medically indigent emergency department walk-in patients, *Ann Emerg Med* 20(7):59, 1994.
21. Pardee DA: Decreasing the wait for emergency department patients: an expanded triage nurse role, *J Emerg Nurs* 18(4):311, 1992.
22. Purnell L: A survey of qualifications, special training and levels of personnel working emergency department triage, *J Nurs Staff Devel* 9(5):223, 1993.
23. Rund DA, Rausch TS: *Triage,* St. Louis, 1981, Mosby.
24. Stock LM, et al: Patients who leave emergency departments without being seen by a physician: magnitude of the problem in Los Angeles county, *Ann Emerg Med,* 23(2):294, 1994.
25. Thompson J, Dains J: *Comprehensive triage: a manual for developing and implementing a nursing care system,* Reston, Va, 1982, Reston.
26. United States Department of Defense: *Emergency war surgery,* Washington, D.C., 1975, U.S. Government Printing Office.
27. Williams DG: Sorting out triage, *Nurs Times* 88(30):34, 1992.

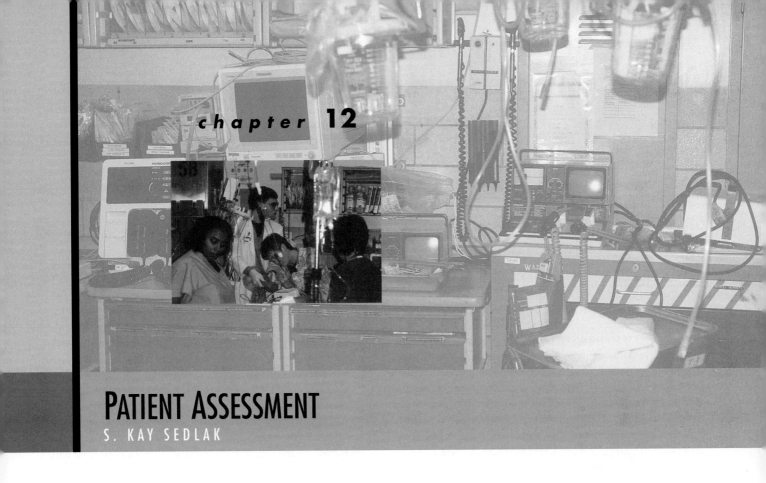

chapter 12

PATIENT ASSESSMENT

S. KAY SEDLAK

The basis of all care delivered to patients in the Emergency Department (ED) is an accurate and appropriate initial assessment. This is the first step of the nursing process. When sufficient data are gathered to identify specific patient problems, appropriate therapeutic interventions can then be initiated.

A rapid, primary assessment is indicated for all patients presenting to the ED, regardless of initial complaint, to ensure that potentially life-threatening conditions are identified and immediately addressed. The "ABC" mnemonic is used to direct this initial assessment. Table 12-1 describes this essential process. An experienced nurse automatically assesses the ABCs, promptly recognizes life-threatening conditions, and immediately initiates appropriate therapeutic actions.

All patients without life-threatening conditions receive a routine assessment based on facility protocol, identification of chief complaint, vital signs, medications taken, and presence of allergies. The triage nurse should correctly identify the patient's primary problem, as this determines priority for care and room placement. Certain complaints and findings support the need for a more focused assessment. A systematic approach ensures that important findings are not overlooked. This chapter addresses assessment in more detail according to specific body systems. Experience guides the nurse in identifying which systems to evaluate for the patient's complaint. Essential tools for the triage nurse include common sense, knowledge of anatomy and physiology, and ability to apply critical thinking to the situation. For example, the patient who comes to the ED with a laceration to the head may require medical management in addition to placement of sutures to repair the disruption in skin integrity. The inquisitive nurse may probe further to determine the cause of the laceration and any potential consequences (e.g., a Stokes-Adams attack with injury to brain tissue).

Ongoing assessment is indicated in certain patient conditions to identify a response to care rendered or to determine deterioration in a patient's status. No precise rules describe how often repeat assessment should be completed. Facility protocols may offer guidelines for specific situations, such as trauma score calculation for prehospital, on arrival, and 1 hour after presentation; repeat vital sign measurements every 15 minutes for patients receiving thrombolytic therapy; and follow-up pulse oximetry measurements every half hour following intravenous conscious sedation until the value returns to baseline. A high index of suspicion guides the experienced nurse in determining which follow-up measurements to obtain and appropriate intervals for doing so.

ASSESSMENT TOOLS

The ability to utilize a variety of assessment tools effectively is the hallmark of experience. Tools may be objective, subjective, verbal, or observed.

Subjective and Objective Data

During the assessment process, two types of information are obtained—subjective and objective. Subjective data are offered by the patient, family, or significant other. This infor-

Table 12-1   Assessment of the ABCs

Component	Description	Action
Airway	Represents patent airway	Identify and remove any partial or complete airway obstruction. Position airway to maintain patency. Insert oropharyngeal airway. Protect cervical spine.
Breathing	Determine presence and effectiveness of respiratory efforts. Identify other abnormalities in breathing (i.e., abnormal pattern, abnormal sounds, etc.).	Assist breathing with oxygen therapy, mouth-to-mouth ventilation, or bag-valve-mask ventilation. Intubate when necessary.
Circulation	Evaluate pulse presence and quality, character, and equality. Assess capillary refill, skin color and temperature, and the presence of diaphoresis.	Initiate chest compressions, medications, and/or intravenous fluid resuscitation as appropriate.

mation reflects their perception of the problem. While such information is quite valuable, it may also require clarification based on the patient's culture, feelings, and interpretation of the given situation. For example, a patient in denial about a particular health problem may not automatically offer critical information that facilitates identification of the condition. Subjective data are not readily visible to the nurse, but do assist in determining the direction of the focused survey.

Objective data are those that can be observed or measured. Methodologies used to collect objective data include inspection, auscultation, palpation, percussion, smell, and acquisition of laboratory reports and other diagnostic summaries. Objective information is considered factual. Certain objective findings indicate the need for more focused assessments. Gathering objective data offers the health care worker an opportunity to validate the patient's subjective information. Collectively, these data are the basis for identification of patient problems.

A variety of methodologies exist for collecting data, including interviewing the patient/significant other, obtaining measurements, performing skilled observations, and consulting with other resources. Ideally, all these assessment tools can and should be utilized; although often, particularly in the ED, this is not possible. For example, the patient may have an altered level of consciousness and be unable to give a history, or the patient's condition may not allow sufficient time for complete examination, or appropriate diagnostic tests may not be available at a given facility, particularly during nonbusiness hours. The skilled nurse adapts to such situations, relying even more on the ability to identify potential reasons for the patient's condition. Obtaining and interpreting available data become even more critical in such circumstances. The competent nurse anticipates potentially dangerous situations, then determines the extent and frequency of the assessment.

Patient Interactions

The general survey proceeds beyond the fundamental considerations of airway, breathing, and circulation to a more systematic observation of the patient. This includes observation of

- Affect and mood, including thought organization
- Quality of speech (normal, slurred, silent, unable to speak)
- General appearance (manner of dress, hygiene, color of skin, facial expression)
- Posture and motor activity (observe upright posture and motor activity while the patient walks, sits, undresses, and so on)
- Odors (breath, skin)
- Evaluation of degree of distress, based on preceding observations

The general survey can be conducted simultaneously with the primary survey. Combining the two may be difficult at first but becomes easier with practice. Often, the primary and general survey can be combined with the patient history interview. The determining factor for the interview is the patient's condition at the time. If immediate or unanticipated problems arise, the interview may be delayed and completed either during the physical examination or after the patient's condition has been stabilized.

History

The history interview for the ED patient focuses on the chief complaint. The questions, although open ended, should be directed by that complaint. The key to obtaining information about the chief complaint—the reason why the patient came—is to listen to what the patient says in trying to tell you what is wrong. What the patient tells you is by definition subjective and therefore demands objective assessment. The chief complaint should not be recorded as a diagnosis ("possible fractured left arm") but exactly as the patient describes the problem ("fell from step ladder, now pain and swelling in left arm"). Box 12-1 summarizes pertinent historical data.

If the patient initially comes to the triage area and is physically able to proceed through the triage process, the history can be completed there. If the patient enters the ED by am-

<table>
<tr><td>

Box 12-1   Pertinent Historical Data

History of present illness or injury
How and when injury or illness first occurred
Influencing factors
Symptom chronology and duration
Related symptoms
Location of pain or discomfort
What, if anything, the patient has done about the symptoms
Pertinent past medical history
Has this problem ever occurred before?
If so, was a medical diagnosis made? What was it?
Has the patient ever had surgery? For what reason? What was the result?
Is there any family medical history that may influence the patient's present complaint?
Does the patient have a private physician? (Obtain full name if possible)
Current medication (prescribed and unprescribed)
When was medication taken last?
Allergies
Age and weight
Tetanus immunization history if an injury is involved
Date of last menstrual period, if the patient is female

</td><td>

Box 12-2   PQRST Assessment

P   *(Provoking factors)*
Ask the patient what, if anything, provokes the pain or discomfort. Is there anything that makes it worse or relieves it? What was the patient doing when it began?
Q   *(Quality)*
Ask the patient to describe the pain in his or her own words. It is particularly important to avoid "feeding" descriptive terms to the patient; instead use open-ended questions to allow a personal description. (Can you tell me how your pain feels to you?)
R   *(Region or radiation)*
Ask the patient to point to the area of pain or discomfort, if possible. Ask if it travels anywhere, if there is pain any place else, if the pain moves from the region of onset.
A patient may not be able to isolate a single area of pain, particularly if the pain is visceral rather than cutaneous. In this case, ask if the patient can identify the general area for you. Do not touch the patient while he or she shows you where the discomfort is. This may obscure the answers and provide you with incorrect information.
S   *(Severity)*
Ask the patient to describe the severity of the pain using a scale of 0 to 10. On this scale, 0 is equivalent to no pain, and 10 is the most severe pain the patient has ever experienced. Ask if the pain affects normal activity, and if so, how it has affected activities of daily living. Watch while the patient moves or undresses, and assess the degree to which the pain compromises activities.
T   *(Time)*
The time of onset and constancy or duration of symptoms are assessed. Ask if the patient has had these symptoms before, what they were related to, and how they were treated.

</td></tr>
</table>

bulance or other vehicle and cannot be processed through the triage area, the nurse managing the patient in the treatment area generally has the responsibility to obtain the history and whatever information prehospital personnel may have regarding status or treatment before arrival. If the patient can respond to questions, any history obtained from others should be validated by the patient. Often, when anxiety from the transport diminishes, the patient remembers information he or she had not been able to recall previously.

Sometimes patients cannot describe their symptoms or reason for coming to the ED. When this occurs, attempts should be made to reach someone who can relate the history of the present complaint. If a patient is unresponsive and no one is available to provide the history, treating the patient becomes a more difficult and time-consuming process. However, treatment should not be delayed until a history is available.

The mnemonic "PQRST" (Box 12-2) has been used to great advantage in assessing complaints of pain or discomfort. It helps define the complaint by focusing on essential elements (i.e., provoking factors, quality, location, radiation, severity, and timing in terms of onset and duration).

Measurements

Vital signs

Vital signs are an important element of the assessment process and deserve much more than the casual attention they usually receive. These readings provide valuable infor-

mation, which when combined with the remainder of the physical examination findings, can greatly affect management of the patient. When signs and symptoms conflict with one another or with the vital signs, meticulous attention must be paid to all elements of the physical examination to determine the cause of the conflict. In the ED where a patient is usually new, determining if findings deviate from the patient's normal values is more difficult. Obtaining former medical records may assist in determining what is abnormal for a particular patient.

Vital signs are indicators of the patient's present condition. Serial values should be obtained if vital signs are to have any impact on identification of trends or developments in the clinical situation. Subsequent readings should be considered in light of the therapeutic interventions initiated. Also the body's compensatory mechanisms affect readings and vital signs must be viewed relative to other clinical findings. What may be considered normal blood pressure might be interpreted differently when considering that the value is only possible because of compensatory mechanisms (e.g., severe peripheral vasoconstriction).

Temperature. Temperature has been referred to as the "forgotten vital sign," particularly in critical patient situations. Practitioners often do not understand the significance of this measurement, and consequently neglect to obtain it. Temperature measurement is mandatory for all ED patients to identify hypothermia, hyperthermia, and other febrile conditions. Deviation from normal temperature may be the only clue of a significant medical problem. For most patients, an oral measurement is sufficient. The tip of the thermometer must be placed in the pocket of tissue at the base of the tongue against the sublingual artery. Temperature across the buccal cavity changes significantly with distance from this artery. Electronic thermometers, which may not read below 34.4° C, are commonly employed for this purpose. Pertinent assessment findings should alert the nurse to obtain the temperature by another methodology.

Rectal temperature may be obtained on pediatric patients and adults unable to cooperate with the oral route (e.g., a patient with altered level of consciousness). This approach does have limitations, such as temperature changes that lag behind core changes, the influence of blood temperature returning from the extremities, the insulating ability of fecal material, or the presence of hard stool limiting insertion of the thermometer to sufficient depth.

Some situations necessitate core temperature measurement. The gold standard for this value is pulmonary artery temperature. Several other approaches that correlate highly with this value but do not carry the same potential complications include urinary catheter thermistors, esophageal probes, and tympanic thermometers. With tympanic thermometers, placement is critical to ensure accurate readings.

Pulse. Increased dependence on electronic technology has decreased tactile assessment of the pulse. The electronically monitored pulse rate gives no indication of quality and other characteristics of the pulse. Equally important are rhythm disturbances that may not be identified unless these changes are seen on the cardiac monitor. Premature beats may be felt on palpation as missing beats or beats with less amplitude than preceding ones. Irregular rhythms, even subtle ones, can be felt as a chaotic rhythm.

In addition to describing the rate and rhythm of the pulse, the nurse should also describe the quality as bounding, normal, weak and thready, or absent. Other characteristic pulse qualities should be determined during cardiovascular assessment by actual palpation of peripheral pulses.

In context with other physical findings, the pulse is an important indicator of cardiac function. Changes in the pulse rate are often the first sign that compensatory mechanisms are being used to maintain homeostasis. In early volume depletion, a healthy person with an intact autonomic nervous system can retain normal pressures with only one subtle change—slight increase in pulse rate and amplitude. Any deviation from the normal range for the patient's age that cannot be related to psychologic or environmental factors should be considered an indication of an abnormal physiologic condition until proven otherwise.

Respirations. Assessing respirations as a part of the patient's vital signs identifies impairment of ventilatory function, attempts to isolate the cause, and provides timely intervention. When collecting vital signs, the nurse should not count the respiratory rate without completing a respiratory evaluation, in which other factors besides respiratory rate and rhythm are assessed.

Signs of respiratory effort include tracheal tugging, nasal flaring, use of accessory muscles, and retractions. Generally, a healthy person does not make any extra effort to breathe: airway noise is absent, the trachea is fixed midline, nasal cartilage is quiet, and sternocleidomastoid or intercostal muscles are not needed to help lift the chest cage. Suprasternal, intercostal, or substernal involvement in drawing on inspiration indicates an increase in the work of breathing.

An increase in anteroposterior diameter can generally be seen on casual observation and indicates chronic alveolar distension. Other changes in chest contour are funnel chest, pigeon chest, kyphosis, and kyphoscoliosis. These particular anatomic changes in contour may interfere with normal lung inflation and exacerbate respiratory conditions.

When a healthy person inspires, the chest expands symmetrically on both sides. When pulmonary or chest wall conditions exist, the chest may rise asymmetrically during ventilation. This asymmetry can be observed with the chest exposed and can also be palpated during inspiration.

The patient's tidal volume can be estimated by observing rise and fall of the chest during ventilation. The depth of ventilations is described as shallow, normal, or deep. A normal adult moves 300 to 500 cc of air at rest and as much as 2000 cc during exercise, with a corresponding increase in rate. A fast rate is not necessarily moving more volume, nor is a slow rate necessarily moving less volume.

Counting the respiratory rate is not measurement enough. All elements of respiration must be evaluated when assessing it as a vital sign. The days of rapidly calculating a 15-second rate are long over for the critical care nurse in an intensive care unit or ED.

Pulse oximetry. Oxygen saturation measurements have become a standard for patients with respiratory conditions or compromise. Knowledge of the patient's baseline value is helpful in determining severity of the present situation or response to therapy. The nurse should also be aware of the limitations of obtaining values with a finger or ear probe. Inaccurate readings occur with extreme peripheral vasoconstriction, hypothermia, and during administration of certain medications. Readings may also be affected by artificial nails and nail polish.

Blood pressure. Blood pressure varies with numerous factors, including patient condition, age, and gender; therefore it is not the most reliable indicator of physiologic changes except when considered with pulse and respiration

REVIEW OF SYSTEMS

The final step in the assessment process is a more detailed examination relative to the patient's chief complaint and clinical status. Health care workers find it helpful to develop a routine for this phase of the assessment process, whether it be head-to-toe evaluation or assessment according to systems. Using an organized approach to assessment ensures that key variables are not neglected. Table 12-2 highlights important variables to consider in a head-to-toe assessment. The following discussion describes assessment by the system approach. Assessment of systems is described in detail in applicable chapters.

Cardiovascular System

Physical assessment of patients with cardiac emergencies focuses on identifying their current cardiac status and the presence of potential complications. Symptoms suggestive of cardiac failure include neck vein distension (JVD), crackles, shortness of breath, and peripheral edema. Adequacy of coronary perfusion can be assessed by vital signs and the rate and quality of pulses.

Auscultation of heart sounds provides information about the integrity of heart valves, atrial and ventricular muscles, and the conduction system. Normally, each cardiac cycle produces two sounds, the first and second heart sounds. The *first heart sound (S_1)* is generally attributed to closure of the atrioventricular valves after ventricular filling. It signals onset of systole and is heard most loudly at the mitral and tricuspid auscultory areas (Figure 12-1). The pitch of the *second heart sound (S_2)* is slightly higher than that of the first. It represents closure of the aortic and pulmonic valves at the beginning of diastole and is best heard at the pulmonic and aortic auscultatory areas (see Figure 12-1). The *third heart sound (S_3)* and the *fourth heart sound (S_4)* are diastolic sounds not normally heard. An S_3 is also called a *ventricular gallop* and may occur in cardiac failure, increased preload, and abnormally slow rates. The term *atrial gallop* refers to an S_4 and indicates poor distensibility of the ventricles when the atria contract and force blood into them. When both an S_3 and an S_4 are heard, the sound is called a *summation gallop*.

Murmurs are produced by turbulent flow, increased flow, or regurgitant flow across valves. The severity of a murmur is described by the Levine Scale (Table 12-3). A *pericardial friction rub* has both a systolic and diastolic component related to cardiac movement. Pericardial friction rub increases in intensity during expiration and with the patient sitting forward. The sound is associated with inflammation of the pericardial sac and may herald pericardial tamponade.

The 12-lead electrocardiogram (ECG) assists in diagnosing cardiovascular disorders and provides information about rate, rhythm, previous or evolving infarctions, bundle branch blocks, electrical axis, atrial and ventricular enlargement, drug and electrolyte disorders, and pacemaker function. However, it represents only one moment in time. All patients

Table **12-2**	**Head-to-toe Patient Assessment**
Component	Potential abnormal findings
Head	Headache, dizziness, seizures, loss of consciousness, syncope, deformity
Eyes	Blurred vision, loss of vision, pain, discharge, conjunctival hemorrhages, jaundice, abnormal eye shape or size, abnormal pupil shape, size, or reactivity
Nose	Drainage, epistaxis, deformity, pain, obstruction
Ears	Discharge, earache, tinnitus, hearing problems, foreign body
Mouth	Bleeding gums, toothache, redness, enlarged tonsils, foul odor, hoarseness
Neck	Pain, enlarged thyroid, bruising, enlarged/tender lymph nodes, distended neck veins, deviated trachea
Chest	Wheezing, dyspnea, rales, use of accessory muscles, retractions, hypertension, angina, murmurs and/or thrills, abnormal heart tones, implanted devices (i.e., pacemaker, AICD, venous port)
Abdomen	Constipation, diarrhea, nausea, vomiting, indigestion, abdominal pain/tenderness, bleeding, ascites
Pelvis/perineum	Burning, frequency, hematuria, flank pain, decreased urination, dribbling, vaginal discharge, unilateral perineal swelling
Extremities	Pain, deformity, swelling, redness, abnormal range of motion
Skin	Rash, bruising, poor skin turgor, delayed wound healing, abnormal pigmentation

Table **12-3**	**Levine Scale for Heart Murmurs**
Grade	Description
I	Very faint, may not be heard in all positions
II	Quiet, but heard immediately when stethoscope is placed on the chest
III	Moderately loud. No thrill (i.e., tactile sensation associated with sound)
IV	Loud, usually associated with thrill
V	Very loud, may be heard without placing stethoscope completely on chest
VI	Extremely loud, may be heard without placing stethoscope on chest

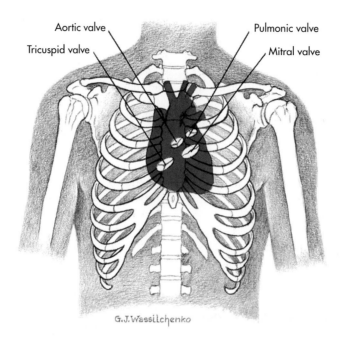

Figure **12-1**   Anatomic location of cardiac valves. *(From Canobbio MM:* Cardiovascular disorders: Mosby's clinical nursing series, *St. Louis, 1990, Mosby.)*

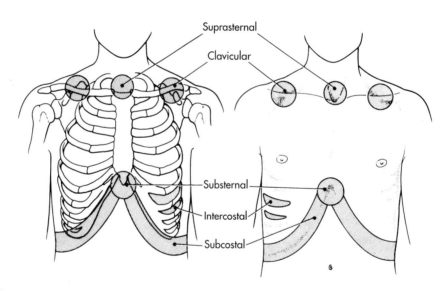

Figure **12-2**   Areas of respiratory retractions. *(From Scipien GM, et al:* Pediatric nursing care, *St. Louis, 1990, Mosby.)*

with a suspected cardiac problem should have continuous cardiac monitoring. Different leads may be selected based on what the nurse suspects. Lead II enhances identification of P waves; however, V_1 or MCL_1 are preferred in most situations. These leads are useful in distinguishing bundle branch blocks, differentiating between ventricular and aberrant conduction, and determining pacemaker wire location. During the evolution of a myocardial infarction, one may monitor the lead with the greatest ST segment elevation.

Respiratory System

Breath sounds can change drastically, depending on degree of pulmonary involvement and time span that pathologic condition has existed. Auscultation may reveal normal, decreased, absent, or abnormal sounds in various fields. Table 12-4 provides a summary of adventitious or abnormal breath sounds.

Use of accessory muscles to breathe is an abnormal finding that indicates increased work of breathing by location of the muscles involved (Figure 12-2).

Table **12-4** **Abnormal Breath Sounds**		
Abnormal		
Bronchial when heard over peripheral lung fields	High pitch; loud and long expirations	
Bronchovesicular sounds when heard over peripheral lung fields	Medium pitch with inspirations equal to expirations	
Adventitious	Crackles: discrete, noncontinuous sounds *Fine crackles* (rales): high-pitched, discrete, noncontinuous crackling sounds heard during the end of inspiration (indicates inflammation or congestion)	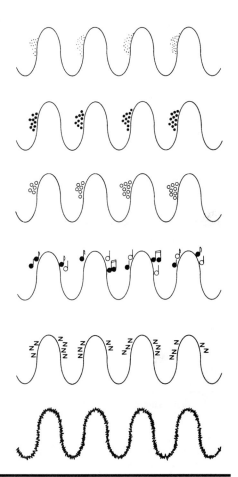
	Medium crackles (rales): lower, more moist sound heard during the midstage of inspiration; not cleared by a cough	
	Coarse crackles (rales): loud, bubbly noise heard during inspiration; not cleared by a cough	
	Wheezes: continuous musical sounds; if low pitched, may be called rhonchi *Sibilant wheeze:* musical noise sounding like a squeak; may be heard during inspiration or expiration; usually louder during expiration	
	Sonorous wheeze (rhonchi): loud, low, coarse sound like a snore heard at any point of inspiration or expiration; coughing may clear sound (usually means mucus accumulation in trachea or large bronchi)	
	Pleural friction rub: dry, rubbing, or grating sound, usually caused by the inflammation of pleural surfaces; heard during inspiration or expiration; loudest over lower lateral anterior surface	

Modified from Thompson JM et al: *Mosby's clinical nursing,* ed 4, St. Louis, 1997, Mosby.

Specific respiratory patterns offer clues to physiologic abnormalities. Deviant patterns are summarized in Table 12-5.

Neurologic System

The most important indicator of neurologic function is the patient's level of consciousness. Assessing consciousness in the order it may deteriorate is helpful. When cerebral hemispheres are intact, well oxygenated, and functioning normally, the patient responds with purpose to your normal speaking voice. The patient can answer questions readily and remains awake during the interview and examination. In short, the patient is fully conscious, and the nurse can proceed to evaluate the degree of orientation, beginning with the one thing the patient is least likely to forget—his or her name. The patient is asked where he or she is, what day or time it is, and what has happened. Allowing for possible patient confusion resulting from stress of the situation or even from the patient not having been told what hospital he or she was taken to, the patient's answers are assessed to evaluate orientation to person, place, time, and situation. These four areas of orientation are lost in a patient in a progressive order, beginning with disorientation to the situation, or amnesia for the situation. As a patient becomes less responsive, orientation decreases.

When the cerebral hemispheres become dysfunctional for any reason, level of consciousness and degree of orientation begin to deteriorate. Changes may be extremely subtle at first. Unless orientation is tested in the same way each time, subtle changes may be overlooked. Pupils, respiratory

Table 12-5 Respiratory Patterns

Name	Description	Etiology
Eupnea	Normal rate and rhythm	
Tachypnea	Increased respirations	Fever, pneumonia, respiratory alkalosis, aspirin poisoning
Bradypnea	Slow but regular respirations	Narcotics, tumor, alcohol
Cheyne-Stokes	Respirations gradually become faster and deeper, then slower alternating with periods of apnea	Increased intracranial pressure, cardiac and renal failure, drug overdose
Biot's	Faster and deeper respirations with abrupt pauses	Spinal meningitis, other central nervous system conditions
Kussmaul's	Faster and deeper respirations without pauses	Renal failure, metabolic acidosis, diabetic ketoacidosis
Apneustic	Prolonged, gasping inspiration, followed by short expiration	Dysfunction of respiratory center in pons
Central neurogenic hyperventilation	Sustained regular hyperpnea	Midbrain lesions
Ataxic	Completely irregular	Damage to respiratory center in medulla

Table 12-6 Glasgow Coma Scale

Activity	Points
Best motor response	
Obeys simple commands	6
Localizes noxious stimulus	5
Flexion withdrawal	4
Abnormal flexion	3
Abnormal extension	2
No motor response	1
Best verbal response	
Oriented	5
Confused	4
Verbalizes, inappropriate words	3
Vocalizes—moans/groans	2
No verbal response	1
Eye opening	
Spontaneously	4
To speech	3
To noxious stimulus	2
No eye opening	1

Box 12-4 Causes of Altered Level of Consciousness: AEIOU-TIPPS

A	Alcohol
E	Epilepsy/electrolytes
I	Insulin (hypoglycemia or hyperglycemia)
O	Opiates
U	Uremia
T	Trauma
I	Infection
P	Poison
P	Psychosis
S	Syncope

rate and patterns, and muscle reflexes and tone are assessed next. Glasgow coma scale (GCS) (see Tables 12-6 and 12-7) is used as a standardized objective measurement of neurologic function. It may be necessary to apply noxious or painful stimuli (e.g., press the nailbeds or squeeze the trapezius muscle) if the patient does not respond to verbal commands. When evaluating neurologic function, a GCS less than 8 suggests a comatose state. The patient's condition may impose certain limitations, such as with intoxica-tion, inability to move because of paralysis, inability to speak when intubated, or language barriers, that can render the total score invalid.

Box 12-4 offers a mnemonic for discerning potential causes for an altered level of consciousness.

Head, Ears, Eyes, Nose, and Throat

The head, face, and neck are inspected and palpated for any injuries or deformities, observing for any discharge from natural orifices. Oral mucosa is assessed for color, hydration, inflammation, and bleeding. The uvula should be smooth and pink; redness and swelling may indicate an allergic process. Asymmetry of facial expressions suggests abnormalities in the central nervous system.

The ears are inspected for any discharge, foreign bodies, deformities, lumps, or skin lesions. An otoscope is used to examine the tympanic membrane (TM). Pulling the auricle

Table 12-7 Pediatric Coma Scale

Eye opening

Score	>1 Year		<1 Year
4	Spontaneously		Spontaneously
3	To verbal command		To shout
2	No pain		To pain
1	No response		No response

Best motor response

Score	>1 Year		<1 Year
6	Obeys		Spontaneous
5	Localizes pain		Localizes pain
4	Flexion-withdrawal		Flexion-withdrawal
3	Flexion-abnormal (decorticate rigidity)		Flexion-abnormal (decorticate rigidity)
2	Extension (decerebrate rigidity)		Extension (decerebrate)
1	No response		No response

Best verbal response

Score	>5 years	2 to 5 years	0 to 23 months
5	Oriented and converses	Appropriate words/phrases	Smiles, coos appropriately
4	Disoriented and converses	Inappropriate words	Cries, consolable
3	Inappropriate words	Persistent crying and screaming	Persistent inappropriate crying and/or screaming
2	Incomprehensible sounds	Grunts	Grunts, agitated, restless
1	No response	No response	No response

TOTAL = 3 to 15

Modified from Goldberg SJ: *Prehospital pediatric life support*, St. Louis, 1989, Mosby. Reprinted with permission.

upward and back straightens the canal in an adult, in a child it is pulled downward and back. Using the largest speculum that comfortably fits in the patient's ear, the examiner inserts the tip slightly forward and downward into the canal. The TM normally appears shiny and pearl-gray or pale pink, whereas a reddened eardrum suggests inflammation, and blue discoloration suggests blood behind the TM. A tuning fork can be used to distinguish loss of hearing from an anatomical anomaly rather than a sensory abnormality.

A number of causes of eye problems exist: trauma, infection, systemic diseases, degenerative changes, and childhood or inherited disorders. Regardless of etiology, the standard assessment for eye problems includes visual acuity using a Snellen chart. Glasses are used for corrected vision when available. The smallest line the patient can read with each eye individually is noted and then together. Acuity is written as a fraction with the numerator indicating the distance from the chart (generally 20 feet) and the denominator describing the distance at which the line could be read by a person with normal vision. Therefore, 20/20 is a normal finding. Other determinations made for a person with an eye problem include the pres-

ence of pain/discomfort, any tearing or secretions, changes in appearance, and integrity of the extraocular muscles.

Gastrointestinal System

As with other systems, subjective data offered by the patient provide clues to assessment of the gastrointestinal system. Patients may give a history of nausea, vomiting, food intolerance, abnormal bowel habits, or changes in the character or amount of stool. Emesis or stool should be tested for blood and other laboratory diagnostics ordered by the physician.

The abdomen is first inspected for symmetry, distension, masses, pulsations, and scars. Listening to bowel sounds in all four quadrants is a key component of the abdominal exam. Hyperperistalsis is suggested by loud, frequent bowel sounds. In contrast, the absence of bowel sounds (after listening for 5 minutes) may indicate paralytic ileus. Palpation prior to auscultation may stimulate bowel sounds.

Palpation of the abdomen is always initiated away from the site of any pain. Sharp pain with rapid removal of your fingers is called rebound tenderness and may indicate peritoneal irritability. A rectal exam may be performed to determine rectal tone, the character of any stool, and the presence of blood.

Genitourinary System

Urinary disorders often can be identified by the patient's own subjective interpretation (e.g., changes in output, voiding pattern, or location of pain). Obtaining a urine sample for analysis can validate the nurse's suspicions. Urine should be examined grossly for color, clarity, and amount before being sent to the laboratory. Palpation of the kidneys may reveal pain such as costal vertebral tenderness or from masses.

Female patients, particularly those of reproductive age, warrant additional assessment for a broad spectrum of complaints. One should always consider the possibility of an unknown pregnancy and take a careful menstrual history, including the use of contraceptives. If the patient is pregnant fetal heart tones are assessed for presence, location, and rate. When a woman has a specific genital concern, a vaginal exam is indicated. Any discharge or bleeding should be noted and described by character and amount.

Males should be assessed for problems specific to their genitourinary anatomy, including the presence of a slow stream, inability to void, penile discharge, or warts.

Musculoskeletal System

Most problems with bones, joints, and muscles are associated with trauma. The skilled clinician, however, considers other possibilities including infectious, degenerative, nutritional, neurologic, and cardiac etiologies. Observation often provides critical data, such as deformity, redness, and swelling. Any effects of the patient's problem on activity and movement must be considered, and range of motion is compared against normal standards. Other concerns include impact on distal circulation and sensory changes. Figure 12-3 shows normal movement for various joints.

Integumentary System

The skin is the largest organ in the body and is located externally, so it is an excellent mirror of physiologic changes within the body. Assessment includes breaks in integrity, temperature, turgor, and the presence of rashes or perspiration. Various changes in pigmentation offer clues to patient problems (Table 12-8).

Endocrine System

The endocrine system impacts most, if not all, body systems. Complaints most commonly associated with endocrine disorders include fatigue and weakness, weight changes, polyuria and polydipsia, mental status changes, and sexual abnormalities. The focus survey should target the

Table 12-8 Color Changes in the Skin

Color	Cause	Location
Brown	Generic	Generalized
	Sunlight	Exposed areas
	Pregnancy	Localized (exposed areas, palmar creases)
	Addison's disease and some pituitary tumors	Localized (exposed areas, palmar creases) or generalized
Reddish	Polycythemia	Face, conjunctiva, mouth, hands, feet
	Excessive heat	Generalized
	Sunburn, thermal burn	Exposed areas
	Increased visibility of normal oxyhemoglobin caused by vasodilation from fever, blushing, alcohol, inflammation	Localized
	Decreased oxygen use in skin, as in cold exposure	
Yellow	Increased bilirubinemia caused by liver disease, red cell hemolysis	Exposed areas
		Sclera in initial stages, then generalized
Blue	Hypoxemia	Central (lips, tongue, nailbeds)
	Decreased flow to skin because of anxiety or cold	Localized, peripheral
		Central
	Abnormal hemoglobin from combination with methylene or sulfa drugs	
Pale or white	Obstructive, hemorrhagic, distributive, or cardiogenic shock	Generalized
	Renal failure	Generalized
	Fear or pain	Generalized and self-limiting

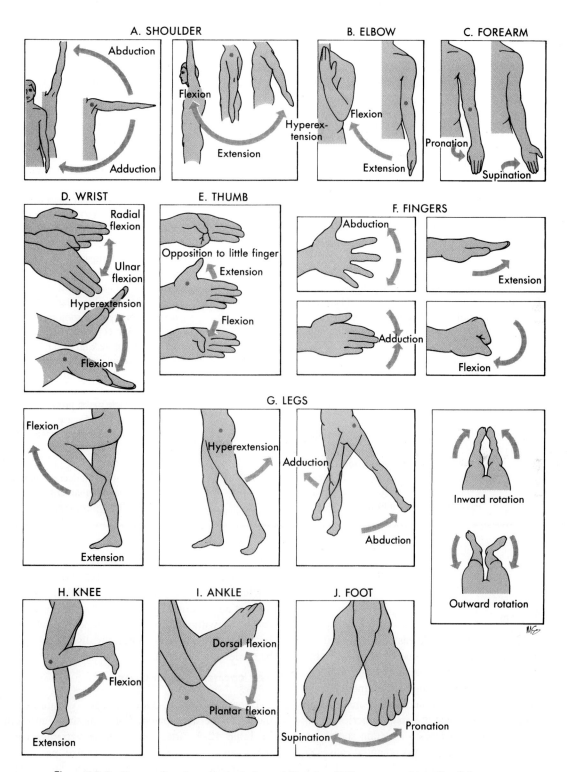

Figure **12-3** Range of motion, standards for mobility. **A** to **F,** Upper extremities. **G** to **J,** Lower extremities. *(From Beare P, Myers J:* Principles and practice of adult health nursing, *ed 2, St. Louis, 1993, Mosby.)*

Table **12-9**   **Age-Specific Assessment Considerations**

Assessment parameter	Pediatric	Geriatric
History	Consider mother's health during pregnancy; parent-child interactions; developmental level; childhood diseases; child unable to give pertinent data	May be influenced by patient's attitudes about aging; may respond slowly to questions; may be influenced by deterioration of the senses
Vital Signs	Faster heart and respiratory rates; BP approximately 70 and age × 2 mmHg; prone to hypothermia	Cardiac irregularities may be a normal variable; influenced by many medications; prone to hypothermia
Cardiovascular	Potential congenital heart problems; murmur and third heart sound may be normal variants	Cardiac output at rest decreases; development of coronary artery disease; heart less able to adapt to stress
Respiratory	Infants are obligate nose breathers; abdominal breathing until age 6 or 7; more susceptible to respiratory infections; airway smaller and more easily occluded	Increased anteroposterior chest diameter; decreased pulmonary function; decreased surface area for gas exchange
Neurologic	Must consider developmental stage; use pediatric coma scale	Degenerative changes; nerve transmission slows; may be impacted by changes in other systems
Head, Ears, Eyes, Nose, and Throat	20/20 visual acuity not obtained until age 7; anatomic differences in eustachian tube predispose to ear infection; hearing develops fully at age 5	Conjunctiva thinner and yellow; arcus senilis may appear, pupil smaller; lens loses transparency; prone to hearing loss
Gastrointestinal	Abdominal guarding more common in child with pain; air swallowed with crying causes abdominal distension	Digestion, GI tract motility, and anal sphincter tone decrease with age; prone to loss of appetite and constipation
Genitourinary	Ability to control urination between 2 and 3 years old; consider age of puberty	Renal function decreases after age 40; incomplete bladder emptying
Musculoskeletal	Bones flexible—greenstick fractures; subluxation common	Decreased muscle mass; prone to fractures; degenerative joint disease
Integumentary	Diaper rash; susceptible to contact dermatitis	Decreased mobility leads to stasis dermatitis and ulcers
Endocrine	Growth hormone abnormalities	Thyroid disorders
Hematopoietic	Anemias, leukemias, clotting disorders during childhood	Vitamin B_{12} absorption decreased; reduced hemoglobin and hematocrit
Immune	Passive immunity at birth	Decreased antibody response

specific presenting complaint. See Chapter 40 for additional discussion.

Hematologic System

Signs of bleeding diathesis include easy bruising and ecchymosis, spontaneous bleeding without an identifiable cause, bleeding from multiple sites, evidence of prior bleeding, petechiae, and anemia. Most signs are identified in a variety of other body systems. A detailed history may reveal concurrent diseases or conditions, previous surgeries or illness, medications, hereditary factors, or certain social behaviors (e.g., stress, alcohol, smoking) as potential causes of abnormal bleeding. Laboratory values are key to confirming the cause.

Immune System

Exposure to infectious materials can lead to many different outcomes. Key assessment data include a history of immunizations, prior disease history, and known exposures (including source and time frame). Fever is often an indicator that an infectious process is present; however, infection can occur without an elevated temperature. Because of the lymphatic system's role in fighting disease, lymph nodes can be tender and enlarged.

AGE-SPECIFIC ASSESSMENT

Depending on a patient's age, variations in assessment can be anticipated. Some of these are summarized in Table 12-9. Attention to these variables can enhance the assessment process and optimize patient outcomes. Refer to specific chapters on pediatric and geriatric emergencies.

SUMMARY

This chapter discusses essential elements of nursing assessment in the ED: purpose, tools, and components of the physical examination. Priority setting through knowledgable assessment and appropriate intervention contributes significantly to decreasing mortality and morbidity. This is particularly true for the early moments of the patient's visit, but it is also valid for the patient's entire stay in the ED.

Nursing assessment may be brief and confined to a narrow focus or may be a reasonably rapid and efficient evaluation of all systems affected by the current illness or injury. The extent of evaluation is the decision of the emergency nurse based on the patient's condition at that time, the chief complaint, and environmental factors. Regardless of the extent of this evaluation, a systematic approach to patient assessment is essential for the best patient care possible.

SUGGESTED READING

Cummins RO: *Advance cardiac life support,* Dallas, 1994, American Heart Association.

Jacobs BB, Baker P: *Trauma nursing core course,* ed 4, Chicago, 1995, Emergency Nurses Association.

Klein AR: *Emergency nursing core curriculum,* ed 4, Philadelphia, 1994, WB Saunders.

Potter DO: *Assessment: nurse's reference library,* Springhouse, Pa, 1982, Intermed Communications.

Sheehy SB: *Mosby's manual of emergency care,* ed 3, St. Louis, 1990, Mosby.

Smith S: *Sandra Smith's review for NCLEX-RN,* ed 7, Los Altos, Calif, 1992, National Nursing Review.

Tucker SM, et al.: *Patient care standards,* ed 5, St. Louis, 1992, Mosby.

Warner CG: *Emergency care: assessment and intervention,* ed 3, St. Louis, 1983, Mosby.

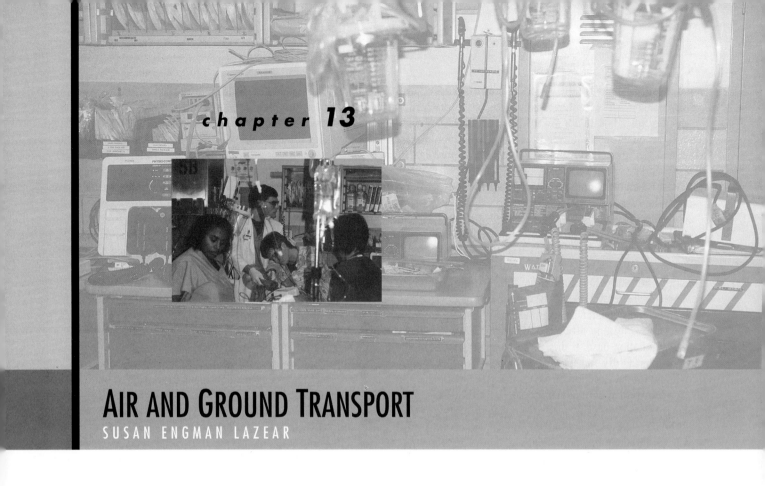

chapter *13*

AIR AND GROUND TRANSPORT

SUSAN ENGMAN LAZEAR

Transport of patients, whether by air or ground, is a unique aspect of emergency nursing. Emergency nurses may be involved in the actual transport, or with patient preparation and stabilization prior to transport. Regardless of the responsibility, the emergency nurse must be familiar with (1) how the practice of nursing and medicine differ in the transport environment, (2) how transport affects the patient, (3) equipment utilized in moving vehicles, (4) communication issues related to transport, and (5) relevant local, state, and federal regulations related to air and ground transport[2].

As transport systems have developed, so has transport nursing. Transport teams are staffed with a mix of personnel including nurses, physicians, paramedics, respiratory therapists, and emergency medical technicians (EMTs). Transport vehicles include modular and van-type ground ambulances, pressurized and nonpressurized aircraft, and helicopters. The focus of this chapter is air and ground transport of patients. Prehospital care issues are addressed as they relate to transport.

Transferring patients from one location to another is not a new concept. Throughout the ages, soldiers on the battlefield have been transported in all types of moving conveyances. Military needs provided the impetus for aeromedical evacuation operations. The first patients transported by air were flown in hot air balloons during the Prussian siege of Paris in 1870. During the 1960s and 1970s, Congress enacted numerous pieces of legislation addressing emergency medical care and transport. As recently as 1990, the Consolidated Omnibus Budget Reconciliation Act (COBRA) was revised to clarify guidelines for patient transfer. Emergency nurses are an integral part of the transport system—stabilizing patients prior to transport, providing care during transport, and ensuring patient safety throughout the transport process.

TYPES OF TRANSPORT

Patient transport occurs in two distinct environments: on the ground by ambulance or in the air by a rotor-wing vehicle (helicopter) or fixed-wing vehicle (airplane). Air and ground transport have both advantages and disadvantages; therefore, an informed decision to use air or ground transport must be made on the basis of many factors, such as out-of-hospital time, weather, terrain, work space, equipment, personnel, and proximity of a landing site.

Ground transport is most often accomplished utilizing a modular type vehicle that can easily accommodate two supine patients and a full crew. Access to the patient is excellent, and advanced life support (ALS) measures can be easily performed. These types of vehicles can also accommodate larger pieces of equipment such as infant isolettes, ventilators, and intraaortic balloon pumps. The level of care administered during transport varies with the level of training of transport personnel, from basic life support (BLS) to ALS. In choosing a transport vehicle, the referring physician must remember that, legally, the quality of care cannot diminish during the transport.

Ground transport is utilized in large urban areas requiring short transport times. Many rural areas have long ground transport times but do not always have the luxury of choosing between ground and air transport. Proliferation of air medical services into rural communities is making this choice a reality for many areas.

Adverse weather conditions influence the transport decision. When roads are impassable, air transport is usually the only alternative. Conversely, when the weather has grounded all air transport vehicles, ground transport is the only option. Another important transport consideration is transit time. For many critically ill or injured patients, the shorter the out-of-hospital time the better the patient's chance for survival. Finally, choice of a transport vehicle depends on the needs of the community. Some isolated rural areas have only one ground ambulance for a largely scattered population base. If this vehicle is taken out of service for an interfacility transport, the community is left without coverage for the duration of the transport.

Air transport should not be chosen indiscriminately. It has inherent dangers and is costly. Many third-party providers withhold reimbursement for flights considered nonemergent. Air medical transport should be considered an adjunct to, and not a replacement for, ground-based services. The advantage of fixed-wing transport is the ability to travel long distances at speeds greater than 250 mph. Care is provided in a pressurized cabin with sophisticated on-board medical equipment. Many fixed-wing aircraft can transport multiple patients. In some instances, family members are allowed to accompany the patient. All-weather navigational equipment allows for transfer during inclement weather. Fixed-wing transport requires suitable airfields to ensure safety of the crew and patient. Accessibility to such fields may be a problem in isolated areas.

Rotor-wing vehicles provide rapid point-to-point transport. Helicopters can reach most areas bypassing difficult terrain. Landing zones can be made at or near the patient to prevent lengthy ground transport time. Most helicopters operate within 150 miles of their base station to allow routine flights without refueling. One disadvantage of helicopters is that their use depends on certain minimum weather conditions, without which flights can be delayed or canceled. Helicopter cabin size and configuration can restrict access to the patient and limit in-flight interventions. Weight limitations restrict the number of passengers and the amount of equipment on board. When transferring by rotor-wing vehicles, comprehensive patient stabilization is required before departure.

TRANSPORT PROCESS
Transport Regulations

Local, state, and federal regulations impact patient transport in the air and on the ground. Emergency nurses facilitating a patient transfer need to be aware of these regulations and their choice of transport vehicle. Regulations also spec-

ify the emergency nurse's legal responsibilities before, during, and at completion of the transport.

Ground ambulance regulations are developed by each state, usually by the Department (Office) of Emergency Medical Services. Regulations must meet minimum standards outlined in federal regulations (i.e., equipment, personnel, licensure); however, state laws usually exceed these minimum standards, which vary significantly among states in many aspects. Ambulance capabilities range from BLS to advanced critical care capabilities. Personnel and equipment vary with services rendered. An emergency nurse preparing a patient for transport must assess the patient's needs during transport and then participate in choosing the most appropriate type of transportation for that patient.

Air transport is regulated by the Department of Transportation Federal Aviation Administration and must meet requirements of Part 135 operation. Regulations stipulate qualifications for the pilot-in-command and other flight crew members, maintenance requirements, and aviation management. States may require a transport service to meet the minimum requirements of an air ambulance to achieve ambulance licensure in their particular state. Voluntary accreditation, available through the Commission on Accreditation of Air Medical Services (CAAMS), is based on a program's compliance with patient care and safety standards.

Federal regulations for patient transport were stipulated in 1985 as part of COBRA and subsequently amended in 1990. COBRA states that all patients should have equal access to care and requires hospitals to ensure that proper care is provided. If a hospital cannot provide the care that the patient requires, it must transfer the patient to an appropriate facility. Specific COBRA mandates for an appropriate transfer are summarized in Box 13-1. The emergency nurse has the responsibility of ensuring adherence to these regulations.

Nurses participating in air transport must be cognizant of Federal Aviation Regulations (FARs) concerning in-flight safety and emergency procedures. The pilot in command of the aircraft is solely empowered with responsibility for safety of the transport, whereas transport personnel are charged with providing the patient with appropriate medical treatment.

Box 13-1   COBRA Mandates for Appropriate Transfers[1]

- The physician must certify in writing that benefits of transfer outweigh the risks.
- The transferring hospital treats the patient within its capacity to minimize patient risk.
- The receiving facility accepts the patient and provides appropriate medical treatment.
- Copies of all medical records, including treatment, certification, and consents, accompany the patient.
- Qualified personnel and appropriate transportation equipment are used for the transfer.

Prehospital Transport

In most parts of the country, prehospital transport can be initiated by citizens through the 911 emergency access number. Sophisticated prehospital emergency medical services programs provide patient transport to the nearest appropriate medical care facility. Emergency nurses may function as prehospital care providers, but their capacity to do so varies from state to state. Ground transport can also be initiated for interfacility transport of patients with medical needs that exceed the capabilities of the local hospital.

Helicopters are an integral part of prehospital transport; however, access to use is generally limited to medically trained personnel in the field. In 1992, the National Association of Emergency Medical Services Physicians (NAEMSP) developed guidelines for helicopter scene response that assist prehospital care providers in determining when a helicopter would be appropriate. However, every EMS community is unique, so these recommendations must be adapted to meet the needs of each patient population.

Interfacility Transfers

Every emergency nurse is occasionally involved with organizing and implementing an interfacility transfer. Effective organization includes assessment of the referring facility's capabilities, understanding the receiving facility's capabilities, and an in-depth knowledge of available EMS and transport systems. Implementation of the transport process is expedited if this knowledge is part of proactive referral strategy developed well in advance. Box 13-2 highlights components of an interfacility transfer.

Development of transfer strategies begins with objective assessment of the referring institution's personnel and facilities. Qualifications and availability of physicians and nurses to care for all patients who come to the ED must be examined. Facilities to be assessed include the intensive care unit; the operating room; and pediatric, obstetric, neonatal, and psychiatric units. The ability to perform advanced diagnostic testing and provide adequate blood and blood products must be analyzed. All these factors influence the level of care available to sick or injured patients.

Understanding the capabilities of the receiving institution is a part of the responsibility of the referring institution.

Box **13-2** **Components of an Interfacility Transfer**
• Physician-to-physician communication.
• Communication between the transferring facility personnel and the receiving facility personnel.
• Selection of appropriate transport vehicle and personnel.
• Consent for transfer signed by the patient or relative.
• Stabilization to limit effects of transport.
• Documentation before, during, and on completion of the transport.

Trauma patients are best cared for in centers designated by the American College of Surgeons Committee on Trauma as trauma hospitals. High-risk neonates benefit from care in a neonatal intensive care unit (NICU). Other areas of advanced specialized care include burn centers, limb reimplantation centers, pediatric centers, and high-risk obstetric centers.

The act of transferring a patient from one facility to another should be well documented and fall within legal guidelines identified by each institution. These guidelines must ensure that federal mandates (i.e., COBRA) have been met.

If a patient is unable to give consent due to their medical condition, and no family is located, a patient may be transferred under the implied consent law. COBRA assumes that the patient or the family would provide consent if able. A concentrated effort must be made to locate family members before this type of consent is invoked.

Stabilization

Field stabilization of the patient depends on the level of training of prehospital care providers. Care can range from basic stabilization to ALS instituted by highly trained paramedics, nurses, and/or physicians. Regardless of training, management of the airway, breathing, and circulation (ABCs) is paramount, and must be monitored throughout the transfer.

Preparation for interfacility transfer of an ill or injured patient depends on the specific illness, injury, age, and circumstance. Potential problems during transport must be identified before departure, and proper interventions must be undertaken at the referring hospital.

Airway and breathing

Airway patency during transport is of primary importance. Potential airway compromise must be anticipated before transport so that proper interventions can be accomplished under controlled circumstances rather than in the transport vehicle.

Endotracheal intubation should be considered in patients who might aspirate, have difficulty with chest expansion, or need ventilatory support (e.g., patients with altered level of consciousness, facial fractures, epiglottitis, or inhalation burns). Patients with chest wall injury, spinal cord injury, or neurologic dysfunction may require ventilatory assistance.

Chest tube placement for a possible pneumothorax or hemothorax should be done before transport. A closed drainage system or flutter valve should be in place to avoid recurrence of a pneumothorax.

Hemodynamic stabilization

To stabilize patients adequately before interfacility transfer, interventions to maintain an adequate pulse rate and blood pressure should be initiated. Interventions include control of bleeding, correction of hypovolemia, insertion of a foley catheter, and institution of cardiac monitoring.

Control of external bleeding sites with pressure or wound closure may be necessary. The use of splints for long-bone fractures and the pneumatic antishock garment (PASG) for pelvic injuries, if not contraindicated, provides stability and pressure to control bleeding. Applying the PASG before loading the patient and inflating the garment as needed are preferable to attempting to apply the garment in a moving vehicle. Air pressure in the PASG should be monitored carefully during the flight because of air volume increases occurring with altitude increases.

Proper intravenous (IV) access is needed to replace fluid loss. Large-bore IV cannulas (14-gauge or 16-gauge peripherally or 8.5-gauge subclavian) with blood or trauma tubing provide rapid fluid resuscitation routes. Having more than one IV route during transport obviates the need for restart in a moving vehicle. Use of plastic IV bags for fluid allows use of pressure bags if required. Blood prepared for transport and placed in a cooler may accompany the patient.

Patients requiring fluid management should have a bladder catheter (if not contraindicated) attached to a urometer to properly measure urinary output. In addition to measuring output, bladder drainage decreases patient discomfort during a long transport.

The cardiac status of the patient must be determined before transport. An electrocardiogram and rhythm strip should be obtained before departure to determine the need for any intervention before transport. Continuous monitoring should take place during transport.

Central nervous system stabilization

All attempts should be made to stabilize the patient's neurologic condition (i.e., maintain normal intracranial pressure, control seizure activity, and preserve the integrity of the spinal cord).

Maintenance of cerebral perfusion pressure in the head-injured patient includes measures to control increased intracranial pressure. Current therapeutics include hyperventilation, elevation of the patient's head if the spine is clear, and limited fluid administration. Hyperventilation is now under significant scrutiny by the medical community. Recent studies suggest that hyperventilation may actually worsen cerebral ischemia. As technological advancements improve methods that directly measure cerebral oxygenation, this and other therapeutic modalities may change. The receiving neurologist should be consulted to determine therapeutics, such as medications (i.e., mannitol, methylprednisolone, sedation, paralytics), patient position, and ventilation regimen.

Antiseizure medications should be used if a patient has seizure activity. Prophylactic medications to reduce the risk of seizure development during transport should be determined during the physician-to-physician consultation.

A patient with a suspected or documented spinal cord injury should be secured to a backboard to prevent movement of the spinal column. A rigid cervical collar should be used. Long transport times are not uncommon, and preventative measures should be undertaken to reduce the risk of pressure sore development. Administration of methylprednisolone for spinal cord injury should be initiated prior to transfer and continued throughout the transport according to established time dosage guidelines. Treatment should begin within 6 hours of the injury.

Musculoskeletal stabilization

Care of the patient with musculoskeletal injuries should include prevention of blood loss, fracture immobilization, wound care, and administration of medications such as pain medications or antibiotics.

Splints should permit assessment of distal pulses during transport. Air splints respond to pressure changes during air transport and should not be utilized in this environment. Pelvic fractures may be stabilized with a PASG and by placement of the patient on a backboard. Traction splints for femur fractures can be used in transport; however, length of the splint must be kept to a minimum so that the transport vehicle door can be closed properly. Free-swinging traction weights are avoided in transport due to the risk to medical crew members.

Patients transferred for limb replantation need special care. The amputated part should be preserved by wrapping in saline-moistened gauze and placing in a plastic bag. The plastic bag should be placed in a sealed container on ice inside a cooler. The part should not be allowed to freeze since this causes tissue destruction and prevents replantation.

Wound care prior to transport may be limited to control of bleeding, initial cleansing, and the application of a sterile dressing. Wounds to be sutured at the receiving facility must be kept moist with saline dressings to ensure tissue viability. Prophylactic antibiotics for open fractures may be ordered to reduce the risk of osteomyelitis.

Burn care includes calculation of the percentage of body surface area burned and fluid resuscitation (see Chapter 29). Fluid resuscitation must be continued throughout transport. The transport team must ensure that an adequate supply of fluid is available in the transport vehicle. Burns should be dressed with dry sterile dressings in accordance with local burn center protocols. Application of topical antibiotics is generally avoided. Constricting rings, necklaces, and clothing should be removed. If circulation impairment is present escharotomy should be performed prior to transport.

Emotional stabilization and psychosocial support

The patient who is about to be transferred has many physical and psychologic needs. Nurses can address these needs by recognizing the patient's many fears and questions.

Removing patients from home, family, and a familiar environment increases the stressors placed on them. They can exhibit fears of flying (if transported by air), fears of dying, and anger, which is often directed at the referring hospital for being unable to care for them. The need for the transport is often translated in a patient's mind to mean he or she is dying. Stressors increase the patient's anxiety causing increased heart rate and respiratory rate, diaphoresis, nausea, vomiting, and a general worsening of the patient's condition.

Personnel from the referring hospital and the transport crew should work together to alleviate the patient's fears by thoroughly explaining all procedures, noises, and reasons for the transport. A team member should interact with family members and include the family in all explanations. Transport personnel should work to instill confidence in the patient concerning the referring hospital. This confidence is important. If the patient survives, he or she will be returning to the home community and will be cared for by the referring hospital in the future.

The patient's family also has tremendous fears. If the patient is acutely ill or injured, this interaction may be the last they have with their loved one. The family may not understand the need for the transport. Time must be taken to explain the necessity for immediate transfer. The family may also have what is called the "Mecca syndrome," an inflated idea of what can be done for the patient at the receiving facility. The family may believe the receiving hospital will save the life of a patient, when in fact that may not happen.

A family member may want to accompany the patient. In helicopter transports, this possibility is usually out of the question because of space and weight limitations. However, depending on the type of ground ambulance or fixed-wing aircraft used, room may be available for a family member. Transport personnel should make the decision whether to allow the family member to come with the patient during a ground transport, but the final decision in air transport is the responsibility of the pilot in command. If the patient's condition deteriorates during flight, the family member has no place to go, and must watch all interventions. On the other hand, the family member's presence may alleviate some of the patient's anxiety, especially when the patient is a child. The decision should not be made until the time of the transport, since the patient's condition may change, and promises cannot always be kept.

To alleviate the family members' anxiety, they should be provided with as much information as possible about the receiving hospital. Maps, plans for patient admission, and a telephone contact gives them some direction after the patient departs. The family should be informed of the estimated length of transport and the expected time of arrival at the receiving hospital. This time should be calculated taking into consideration weather, unexpected delays, changes in time zone, and other factors. Overestimation of the time is always best—if the transport is completed sooner than anticipated, the family will feel relief. On the other hand, if the transport takes longer than expected, the family may fear the outcome of the transport itself.

One of the last things that should be done before departure is to allow the family time with the patient. The last remarks and the last kiss goodbye may be the most important few minutes of the transport.

Baseline diagnostic studies

Studies necessary for stabilization depend on severity and type of illness or injury. Each situation has different priorities. Baseline studies needed to make proper decisions regarding transfer should be performed while the transfer is being arranged. In severely injured patients, only tests that affect airway, breathing, and circulation should be performed.

The American College of Surgeons Committee on Trauma recommends performing the following studies, as time permits:

- Radiographs of the cervical spine, chest, pelvis, and any injured extremity
- Laboratory tests including hemoglobin content, hematocrit, arterial blood gases, urinalysis, toxic screens, blood alcohol content, and blood typing and crossmatching
- Electrocardiogram

Copies of all patient data and radiographs should be properly labeled and sent with the patient. Samples of peritoneal fluid, blood, and spinal fluid should accompany the patient when indicated. Laboratory data not completed at the time of transfer should be called in or sent by fax to the receiving center.

Documentation

Documentation of the transfer is essential. It confirms adherence to legal mandates, ensures compliance with established standards of care, and protects the caregiver in potential litigious situations. Documentation of prehospital care should include mechanism of injury, time of injury, time of EMS arrival, care provided in the field and during transport, and protocols or orders used during transfer. Documentation related to interfacility transfer includes the prehospital record, the ED record, and documentation of care during the transfer. Box 13-3 summarizes documentation requirements specific to interfacility transfer.

Care During Transport

Assessment and treatment to maintain patient stability during the transport is essential. Use of a pulse oximeter and cardiac monitor to monitor oxygenation, pulse rate, and rhythm are extremely beneficial. An ultrasound Doppler and stethoscope are useful when auscultation is difficult. The patient's level of consciousness should be monitored and recorded. Fluid intake and urinary output should also be documented.

Box 13-3   Documentation Requirements for an Interfacility Transfer

- Prehospital care record
- ED medical record
- Medical history
- Lab results
- Copies of x-rays
- Transfer record
- Protocols or orders used during transfer
- Signed transfer consent form
- Family information including contact person
- Contact information at referring hospital

The transport personnel should be prepared to implement interventions as needed to maintain patient stability. Protocols and physician's orders regarding specific interventions clarify expectations for the transporting team. Interventions that may be needed during transport include securing the airway, suctioning, administering fluids, performing emergency needle thoracotomy, applying the PASG, administering medications, and performing ALS measures. In unforeseen emergencies when sophisticated medical equipment and personnel are critical, diversion to a closer facility may be necessary. The location of these facilities must be known to prevent unnecessary delays.

All care during transport should be documented. A copy of the transport form should be inserted in the patient's chart at the receiving facility. Documentation should include patient assessment, interventions, and the patient's response to these interventions. Unusual events or effects of the transport on patient condition should also be noted.

Communication

Effective communication is the glue that holds the entire transport process together. Each component is essential and dependent on the others. When a call is placed to an emergency operations center, the dispatcher notifies appropriate units to respond. Radio communication is established, and pertinent information is transmitted. Depending upon case severity and local protocols, the mobile unit can be directly linked to the medical command center or the base station at the receiving hospital. Transmission of pertinent data is necessary so that the transport team can receive specific protocols for intervention.

During air transport by helicopter or airplane, the medical crew may be out of range of their base station. However, at no time is the aircraft out of touch with a ground station. The flight team intervenes according to standard protocols at the discretion of the flight team members. In the event of an emergency, the pilot in command can contact the ground station and ask to be patched through to medical control of the flight program.

Successful communication includes a complete loop in which all parties are notified and aware of the patient's status. This begins with the physician-to-physician contact that establishes the transport process. Communication is ongoing and should focus on essential information for the transporting and receiving personnel.

Communication techniques, radio codes, and communication technology are too extensive to be included here. The reader is referred to a number of excellent references if more in-depth information is desired. Regardless of technology used, every effort should be made to protect patient confidentiality during any communication. Use of patient names or other identifying factors is discouraged. A standard reporting format may be developed by the transport program to ensure quality assurance for each communication.

Medical Control

Organization of medical control varies from system to system. On-line medical control is direct communication between transport personnel and the physician (or physician-surrogate) via radio or telephone for the purpose of providing orders for patient care. Off-line medical control includes those administrative functions necessary to ensure quality of care. Each medical control officer is a physician who is directly responsible for care provided in transport. It is the medical control officer's responsibility to ensure proper training, orientation, and continuing education for those persons working under their control.

Transfer of Care

While the patient is in transit, the referring and receiving facilities share responsibility for care of the patient. Only after arrival at the receiving facility is the referring hospital's legal responsibility terminated. The time of arrival at the receiving hospital should be noted in the copy of the chart that remains at the referring facility.

GROUND TRANSPORT
Safety

All transport personnel must develop a positive attitude and a strict policy toward personal safety. Wearing seat belts or other restraining devices should be the first priority. Patient care may be limited during times of high risk to the medical care provider. Providers should consider the risks of potential hazards and take appropriate precautions. The Occupational Safety and Health Administration (OSHA) standards regulate minimal requirements for use of protective clothing. Ideal body protection is provided by approved helmets, safety goggles, reinforced boots, and gloves. Some states mandate specific equipment requirements. In some areas Voluntary Ambulance Specification Criteria (VASC) establish minimum equipment standards.

The risk of infectious disease is high in the prehospital care environment. Barrier protection should be used at all times. Bag-valve masks and pocket masks provide effective ventilation. The incidence of mycobacterium tuberculosis infection is increasing, and medical personnel need to reduce their risk of exposure. Prehospital care providers also have an obligation to reduce the risk of exposure to infectious diseases to other emergency care providers through careful handling of wounds and dressings as well as proper disposal of needles and other disposable equipment.

Patient safety is also a priority. Patients must be secured to the stretcher, and the stretcher should be secured to the transport vehicle. Stabilization measures should be undertaken to ensure patient safety throughout the transfer, including the use of a backboard, and restraining belts and tape.

Personnel

The level of care provided in ground transport depends on the level of the health care provider training. Jurisdiction over capabilities of these personnel is delegated to the state. However, federal legislation mandates certain minimum levels of care.

Basic EMTs provide BLS. Their basic level of training consists of 100 hours of classroom and field training with 10 hours of in-hospital observation. The EMT may receive additional training in administration of select drugs, use of advanced airway skills, and cardiac defibrillation. Persons with additional certification may be identified by the following titles: EMT-intermediate, EMT I to VI, cardiac rescue technician, EMT-advanced, EMT-defibrillator, EMT-cardiac, and others. These advanced trained EMTs can provide more advanced levels of care.

The EMT-paramedic must complete at least 212 hours of didactic training and 200 hours of hospital-based clinical rotations. Many training programs double this requirement. With successful completion of both written and practical examinations, the EMT can be state certified as a paramedic valid for 2 to 4 years. Paramedics are used extensively in urban emergency medical care systems, and their presence is becoming increasingly common in rural areas. Paramedics perform ALS measures and are considered the foundation of ALS care in the prehospital care environment.

Registered nurses are also found in ground transport programs. Training programs for nurses are essentially nonexistent, thus many nurses turn to paramedic training programs to achieve certification. In 1991, the Emergency Nurses Association developed the *National Standards Guidelines for Prehospital Nursing Curricula*. These guidelines intend to integrate the nurse's prior education and clinical experience with knowledge and skills needed by the prehospital nurse. Although the number of registered nurses working in the prehospital care environment remains low, it is increasing. These nurses continually push for recognition of their contribution to emergency care.

Equipment

Statutory law regulates equipment required in ground ambulances. The equipment listed in Box 13-4 is the minimum required for maintaining stability in the ill or injured patient during transport. Medical crew members must be familiar with operation of the equipment in the vehicle and any extra equipment brought to provide care for a particular patient. Crew members must also ensure that an adequate supply of disposable equipment is available to last throughout the transport, taking into consideration possible delays

that may extend the projected transport time. Oxygen must be available for the duration of the transfer. Table 13-1 shows duration of cylinder flow for two sizes of oxygen cylinders.

AIR TRANSPORT
Flight Physiology

Exposure to environmental factors occurs during air transport of patients. Problems encountered depend on changes in atmospheric conditions, vehicle designated configurations, motion of the aircraft, and the patient's condition. Some of these can be detrimental to the patient, but

---

Box 13-4   Equipment Needed for Transport

Airways
Nasal airway adjuncts
Oropharyngeal airway adjuncts
Endotracheal or nasotracheal tubes

Oxygen delivery system
Oxygen
Oxygen tubing
Oxygen cannulas
Oxygen masks
Bag-valve-mask device
Demand valve
Ventilator
Pulse oximeter

Suction equipment
Suction catheters
Catheter-tip syringe for gastric tube

IV equipment
IV fluids, pump, and tubing
EV restart equipment
Pressure infusion bag

PASG
Doppler device or sensitive stethoscope
Cardiac monitoring and resuscitation equipment
Cardiac monitor and defibrillator
Defibrillator pads
Recording paper

Emergency medications
Restraints

Table 13-1	**Duration of Cylinder Flow**						
Cylinder	2 L/min	4 L/min	6 L/min	8 L/min	10 L/min	12 L/min	15 L/min
E	5.1 hr	2.5 hr	1.7 hr	1.2 hr	1.0 hr	0.8 hr	0.6 hr
H	56 hr	28 hr	18.5 hr	14 hr	11 hr	9.2 hr	7.2 hr

with proper nursing care before and during transport, these harmful effects can be minimized or eliminated.

Atmospheric changes occur when the aircraft's altitude changes. Ascending into the atmosphere from sea level causes a decrease in atmospheric pressure, which in turn causes a decrease in the partial pressure of gases, decrease in temperature, and expansion of gases. The opposite occurs during descent. Four problems can develop in transport as a result of changes in atmospheric pressure: hypoxia, gas expansion, dehydration, and decreased temperature. Many of these effects are minimal unless the change in altitude is greater than 5000 feet.

Fixed-wing and rotary-wing vehicles are designed according to different principles. Most fixed-wing aircraft used in patient transport are pressurized, which allows for a comfortable cabin atmosphere when flying at high attitudes. Pressurization differentials allow for different cabin pressures at different atmospheres. Generally, the lower the altitude at which a plane is flying, the lower the cabin pressure that can be achieved. This ability to maintain a physiologically comfortable environment within the aircraft is a benefit when transporting patients who may be affected by atmospheric changes. Although pressurization allows for flights at high altitudes, even subtle changes in the environment may be harmful to a person whose condition is severely compromised.

If the pressurization system fails, pressurization within the cabin might be lost, causing a sudden change in atmospheric pressure. This rapid decompression causes the interior of the cabin to equalize with the pressures outside the cabin, resulting in sudden and often detrimental effects on the human body: a rapid loss of oxygen, sudden drop in temperature, and expansion of gas. A healthy person may be able to withstand these changes, but the condition of someone whose health is poor may deteriorate quickly. Those transporting patients should be aware of these effects and do everything possible before departure to minimize complications.

Rotary-wing vehicles are not pressurized, therefore these atmospheric changes are felt whenever the helicopter ascends and descends. Thus patients transported by helicopter may be at greater risk than those transported by fixed-wing aircraft.

Other problems that affect patient outcomes are influenced by the motion of the vehicle and constraints resulting from vehicle design.

Hypoxia

Many patients transported by air are hypoxic as a result of their condition. This hypoxic state is potentiated when changes in atmospheric pressure occur. As an aircraft ascends in altitude, the partial pressure of oxygen (PO_2) decreases, causing a decreased diffusion gradient for the oxygen molecule to cross the alveolar membrane. Table 13-2 shows the effects of altitude on PO_2.

Table **13-2**	Effects of Altitude on Partial Pressure of Ambient Oxygen	
Altitude (ft)	Atmospheric pressure (mm Hg)	Partial pressure of ambient oxygen (PO_2)
0	760	150
500	746	146
1000	733	144
1500	720	141
2000	707	138
2500	694	135
3000	681	133
3500	669	130
4000	656	128
4500	644	125
5000	632	123
5500	621	120
6000	609	118
6500	598	115
7000	586	113
8000	564	108
9000	543	104
10,000	523	100

Simple calculation of the diffusion gradient is accomplished by using the following formulas:

$$(\text{Atmospheric pressure} - \text{Water pressure}) \times (\text{percentage of oxygen}) = PO_2$$

and

$$\text{Alveolar } PO_2 - \text{Venous } PO_2 = \text{Diffusion gradient}$$

Room air is 21% oxygen. If the patient is receiving oxygen, the FiO_2 is used for the patient's oxygen therapy. Assuming that water pressure is equal to 47 mm Hg, the PO_2 at sea level is 150 mm Hg: $(760 - 74) \times (0.21) = 150$. At an altitude of 6000 ft the calculated PO_2 is 118 mm Hg: $(609 - 47) \times (.21) = 118$ mm Hg.

The decrease in PO_2 that occurs in the respiratory tree is approximately 45 mm Hg. Therefore, at the alveolar level, the PaO_2 at sea level is approximately 105 mm Hg and the PaO_2 at 6000 feet is about 73 mm Hg. The PO_2 of venous blood is approximately 40 mm Hg. Therefore the diffusion gradient at sea level is equal to 65 mm Hg $(105 - 40)$ and at 6000 feet is equal to 22 mm Hg. Patients with disease-induced hypoxia would be severely affected with this drop in diffusion gradient and are at increased risk of compromise during air medical transport. These patients include those with congestive heart failure, adult respiratory distress syndrome (ARDS), carbon monoxide poisoning, hypovolemic shock, inadequate amount of circulating hemoglobin, and stagnant hypoxia induced by low-flow states such as hypothermia. Altitude-induced reduction in PO_2 causes further deterioration in these patients if interventions are not performed to correct the problems related to hypoxia.

Signs and symptoms of hypoxia include changes in vital signs, tachycardia, pupillary constriction, confusion, disorientation, and lethargy. All of these signs may be caused by a number of other illnesses and injuries, making the diagnosis of hypoxia more difficult. Astute observation of the patient is necessary to detect and correct problems of hypoxia.

Transporting patients by pressurized fixed-wing aircraft can limit complications that develop as a result of this drop in the PO_2. Most aircraft used for air transport are able to maintain a sea level cabin pressure when flying below 7000 to 10,000 feet. At higher altitudes, the cabin can be pressurized. The maximum cabin pressure altitude is generally maintained well below 9000 feet. When cabin pressures are controlled, atmospheric changes that occur are limited, controlled, and within a tolerable range.

Before the patient is transported, stabilization measures can be taken to reduce the effects of atmospheric changes in oxygenation. Supplemental oxygen can be provided, and if the patient has previously required oxygen, the percentage of oxygen can be increased. This increase in oxygen delivery is performed as a prophylactic, temporary measure during the transport. When the patient arrives at the receiving institution, the oxygen can be decreased or terminated pending outcome of the arterial blood gas test.

Properly positioning the patient combats the effects of hypoxia. Ensuring proper chest excursion by loosening chest restraints on the stretcher allows the patient to breathe easier. In certain aircraft the head of the stretcher can be elevated to an angle of at least 30 degrees; however, in many rotary-wing transports this elevation is not possible because of limited head room.

The hypovolemic patient can receive transfusions to increase the hematocrit and oxygen-carrying capacity of the blood. Patients who are alert are generally anxious regarding their outcome, which causes an increased respiratory rate and a decrease in their oxygenation. Providing a calm environment and thoroughly explaining all procedures, noises, and so on can reduce the patient's feeling of helplessness. The case study in Box 13-5 demonstrates the effects of altitude changes on a patient.

Calculating the PO_2 of patients in various environments and situations tells only part of the story. The patient described in the case study, whose cardiac history is extensive, may also be anxious about leaving his loved ones behind and about the prognosis. While he may feel most comfortable in the sitting position, he must lie flat during the transport. Assessing the patient's vital signs and level of consciousness provides the best indicator of how he is tolerating the transport. All possible interventions to improve the patient's oxygenation status should be initiated. Continuous pulse oximetry should be used to adjust oxygen therapy.

Box 13-5 **Effects of Altitude Changes on a Patient**

A 58-year-old man requires transport from a small rural hospital to a university medical center for evaluation. He has a long history of cardiac disease and is currently receiving vasopressors for blood pressure support. The referring hospital is located at an altitude of 500 feet, whereas the medical center is at a 4000-foot elevation. During transport the helicopter must fly over a mountain range with peaks at altitudes more than 6000 feet.

At the referring hospital, the patient has a PO_2 of 150 mm Hg when breathing room air. When a nasal cannula was used, the PO_2 rose to 178 mm Hg, and the patient's pretransport blood gas levels during use of the nasal cannula were adequate. During transport, the helicopter must fly at an altitude of 6500 feet to ensure clearance of the mountains. During the time the patient is at this altitude his PO_2 will drop to 138 mm Hg if use of the nasal cannula is continued. To ensure that altitude-induced hypoxia does not develop, a nonrebreather mask can be applied. Use of this mask will raise the patient's PO_2 to approximately 400 mm Hg. At the medical center, at an altitude of 4000 feet, the patient's PO_2 when a nasal cannula is used is calculated at 152 mm Hg. This PO_2 may be inadequate for his current condition, necessitating the use of other oxygen delivery systems.

Gas expansion

According to Boyle's law, the volume of gas is inversely proportional to its pressure. As the transport vehicle ascends, atmospheric pressure decreases and gas expands. One hundred cubic centimeters (cc) of gas at sea level expands to 130 cc at an altitude of 6000 feet, 200 cc at 18,000 feet, and 400 cc at 34,000 feet. Gas expansion is a potential problem in all transports where the aircraft ascends, but is especially worrisome in an unpressurized fixed-wing aircraft flying above 12,000 feet.

Air is found in many places, including the pleural space when a pneumothorax is present, air splints, endotracheal tube cuffs, intravenous fluid bottles, and in the PASG. Table 13-3 lists various conditions and situations in which gas can expand, and nursing measures that can reduce the risk of complications.

If measures are taken during ascent to prevent gas expansion, such as removal of air from the PASG, an *opposite* measure must be taken during the aircraft's descent. For example, a patient with multiple trauma requires long-distance transport from a village in Alaska to a trauma center in Washington. The patient has been stabilized with use of the PASG before transport. As the aircraft departs from Alaska and ascends to a cruising altitude of 28,000 feet, the cabin pressure rises to approximately 8000 feet. Air volume in the PASG is now increased by at least one third. The PASG pants may now be too tight and compromise circulation to

Table 13-3   Effects of Gas Expansion on Patient Condition and Medical Equipment

	Complications	Therapeutic interventions
Patient condition		
Pneumothorax	Air expansion within pleural cavity, causing dyspnea	Insert flutter valve chest tube with water seal drainage
Bowel obstruction	Air expands, causing rupture	Insert nasogastric tube to suction; elevate head of bed
Plugged middle ear	Unable to equalize pressure	Valsalva maneuver in awake patient; ascend and descend slowly
Congested sinuses	Trapped air expands, causing pain	Vasoconstrictor sprays
Open skull fracture	Air in cranial cavity expands, causing herniation	Implement hyperventilation measures to reduce intracranial pressure
Colostomies, ileostomies	Air in bowel expands, causing increased motility	Insert rectal tube for decompression; change bag frequently
Gas gangrene	Air expands within tissues, leading to necrosis	Incision and drainage
Dental caries	Pain caused by air expansion	Administer local anesthetic
Equipment		
PASG, air splints	Air expands: pressure within garment or splints increases	Decrease volume at altitude
IV bottles	Air within bottle expands: fluid does not flow	Use plastic IV bags
Endotracheal tube cuffs	Air expands, causing tracheal necrosis	Decrease volume at altitude
Foley catheters	Air within drainage system expands: urine does not flow	Use a vent system Irrigate catheter
Oxygen flowmeters	Flow is increased under pressure	Monitor oxygen supply frequently
Volume ventilators	Volume of gas delivered increases	Measure tidal volume

the patient's lower extremities. By monitoring the patient's blood pressure, transport personnel can decrease air volume in the garment to ensure maximal benefit. During transport, the PASG should be monitored continually for changes in pressure to detect underinflation or overinflation. As the aircraft descends for landing at the receiving airfield, the PASG should be evaluated once again for effectiveness; usually air must be added.

Rotary-wing vehicles that fly low over flat terrain encounter few problems with gas expansion during transport. However, if transport requires traversing high-altitude areas, the aforementioned interventions are essential.

Dehydration

Another problem encountered during an increase in altitude is a drop in ambient humidity. Loss of humidification is enhanced in a pressurized fixed-wing aircraft, because system pressurization is achieved by recycling air and removing moisture from it. Patients who are dehydrated or diaphoretic are at increased risk for dehydration and possible fluid volume deficits. Supplemental intravenous fluids should be administered to prevent dehydration.

Other patients affected by dehydration include mouth-breathers and those who are intubated. These patients have lost the natural respiratory humidification mechanisms, so secretions become tenacious and difficult to mobilize. Pro-

viding humidified oxygen not only prevents drying of the respiratory tree but also counters effects of hypoxia.

Decreased temperature

As altitude increases, temperature decreases. For each 1000-foot gain in altitude, temperature drops 2° C until it reaches −55° C. During ascent, this temperature drop causes cooling of the aircraft. Although transport vehicles are heated, the fuselage becomes quite cold and radiates the cold into the interior of the cabin. The coldest area of the aircraft is against the outside walls. This cooling, although most significant during cold-weather months, is noticeable at all times of the year.

In addition to altitude-induced temperature changes, a number of environmental conditions affect air transport of patients. Of particular importance is a drop in environmental temperature. Interhospital transports require the patient be removed from the hospital, transported outside to the helipad or into an ambulance for transfer to the airfield, and subsequent transfer into the transport vehicle. The opposite occurs at the receiving end of the transfer. These multiple transfers expose the patient to changing environmental conditions, including cold weather. A patient requiring transport is less able to tolerate these stresses and can exhibit signs and symptoms of cold stress, including decreased level of consciousness, increased heart rate, and shivering. These symptoms increase the patient's oxygen demands. The previously hypoxic patient becomes increasingly hypoxic.

Awareness of an environmental drop in temperature allows adequate stabilization before the transport. Minimizing exposure to environmental conditions is of utmost importance. The interior temperature of the transport vehicle can be controlled in accordance with the patient's needs, not the needs of the transport crew. Maintaining an adequate supply of linen, and wrapping the patient in a rescue (Mylar) blanket is useful in cold environments. Caution should be used with Mylar blankets because they reflect back to the patient any radiated heat; if wrapped too tightly, the patient can become overheated. A cap can be put on the patient's head to reduce radiated heat losses.

When ambient air cools, changes in temperature cause gas molecules to contract. This change in gas molecules is similar to that which occurs with a decrease in altitude, with subsequent gas expansion within body cavities and equipment. This effect is most notable in the PASG and air splints. When the patient is transferred from a warm hospital interior to the cold outside, the volume of gas within the garment decreases, and the peripheral vasoconstriction effect on the venous system can decrease. As ambient temperature increases, the garment expands causing an increase in the patient's blood pressure. Change in gas volume must be compensated for during each change in environmental conditions.

Other problems that develop with cold environments include cooling IV solutions and crystallization of medications, most notably mannitol. A patient with cold stress resulting from changes in the environment requires warm IV fluids. Solutions stored in the aircraft or solutions exposed to the environment are quite cold and must be warmed before administration. If possible, solutions should be stored in the warmest spot in the cabin. If solutions remain cold, heat packs can be wrapped around the IV bag to warm the fluid. Some transport programs employ heating pads to keep the fluids warm. Drawbacks with such a system are the need for electricity to operate the pad and the risk of overheating the fluid, which may render the fluids useless. Mannitol should not be stored in an aircraft that is quite cold. Instead, it should be placed in the aircraft immediately prior to departure.

Acceleration and deceleration forces

Acceleration forces occur during takeoff and "climb-out." Blood pools in dependent areas, most commonly the lower extremities, causing fluid shifts that may not be tolerated by the severely compromised patient. Restoration of intravascular volume and proper positioning of the patient can minimize the effects of these forces.

Deceleration forces occur during slowing, stopping, or rapid descent. For the patient lying head forward in an aircraft, deceleration forces cause blood to pool in the head and upper body. Pooling produces what is known as "redout" as blood rushes to the head, causing an increase in blood within the ocular cavity. Deceleration forces are most harmful to a patient with increased intracranial pressure. The phenomenon may also adversely affect a patient with congestive heart failure.

The effects of acceleration and deceleration forces vary with the speed, angle, and duration of the forces. These forces are much more pronounced in a fixed-wing aircraft. In certain instances, the pilots can control these effects as long as safety measures and regulations are met. If a patient is known to be severely ill or injured, transport personnel should discuss this problem with their flight crew. A slow descent is often an option. If the airfield is long enough, a longer landing roll can decrease some deceleration forces that occur as the aircraft is slowed to a stop.

Positioning of the patient is crucial to counter these forces. In many aircraft, stretcher restraints are not interchangeable; therefore, the patient must be loaded head-first into the cabin. If the patient can tolerate a head-elevated position, the effects of these forces can be minimized, since fluid shifts would be centered at the core of the body rather than in the head.

Rotary-wing vehicles are also subject to acceleration and deceleration forces but to much less magnitude than fixed-wing aircraft. In addition to forward and rearward movement, helicopters are capable of lateral movements. Forces resulting from these movements are of little consequence. Because of the confined space of the helicopter, positioning the patient to counteract these forces is usually more difficult, if not impossible. Fortunately, pilot control is much greater in the helicopter.

Motion sickness

Changes in equilibrium caused by excessive motion can cause motion sickness. Nausea and vomiting may develop in the patient, the flight crew, and transport personnel. Prophylactic premedication is the best intervention available to limit these complications.

Other causes of motion sickness include hypoxia; excessive visual stimuli, such as the blinking lights on the aircraft control panel; stress, fear, unpleasant odors, heat, and poor diet. Gastric gas expansion occurring during ascent can worsen the problem. To prevent or limit these symptoms, transport personnel should provide adequate oxygenation, stare at a fixed visual reference, cool the cabin interior, attempt to limit stressors and fear, and have the patient lie in the supine position.

For crew members with motion sickness, premedication with transdermal scopolamine is the best treatment. However, these patches must be applied a few hours before departure. Since air medical transports are not usually scheduled, this preventive measure may not be possible. Often the crew members "recover" from their motion sickness when they focus their attention on the patient. However, they may experience residual symptoms after the flight.

Noise

Transport vehicles are inherently noisy. Engine noises create a constant loud hum that is not only distracting but also causes an increased level of stress. Reducing extraneous noise is often impossible, but limiting the sound input can be accomplished by the application of earplugs, cotton balls, or headphones. But when noise reduction devices are used for the patient, communication is also reduced. The patient who is not able to hear a conversation may become increasingly agitated, believing the crew is talking about him or her. Including the conscious patient in as much conversation as is appropriate is important. In a helicopter, which is extremely noisy, earpieces of the stethoscope can be inserted into the patient's ears. Then the crew can speak to the diaphragm for communication with the patient.

Noise also interferes with the ability to hear breath sounds, heart sounds, and blood pressure. Doppler devices are available to assist with detecting blood pressure but are of little use for hearing breath or heart sounds. Other assessment techniques are important to ascertain adequate ventilation, such as observing for bilateral chest wall movement, using pulse oximetry, and placing the stethoscope over the trachea to listen for air movement.

The flight crew may be familiar with noises of the aircraft, but the patient needs to be warned ahead of time. Many aircraft have audible warning signals to prevent accidents, but to the patient these alarms may signal that the aircraft is in danger of crashing. A preflight briefing should include the patient, and should be followed by continual reminders to alleviate these fears.

Long-term noise exposure is also a problem for the flight crew. Protective earplugs should be used to minimize the deleterious effects of noise over time. Periodic hearing tests are recommended to monitor changes in hearing.

Vibration

As a result of vehicle design, aircraft vibrate. The effects of vibration are much more noticeable in a helicopter, especially during takeoff and landing. This constant motion can cause equipment to loosen and become a danger during flight. The FAA regulations require that all equipment be secured during takeoff and landing. Equipment should be secured at all times in the event of unexpected turbulence.

The patient should be secured to the stretcher at all times. Before loading and unloading the patient from the aircraft, stretcher restraints should be checked for proper fit. During transport, straps may be loosened to allow the patient to move; however, restraints should never be fully released.

Continual vibration can also change equipment settings—constant jostling can cause knobs to slip, changing the functioning of the machinery. Ventilators are especially prone to this complication, so settings should be checked frequently during flight.

Immobilization

As a result of long transport times, prolonged immobilization of the patient can lead to pressure sores and venous stasis. Space limitations and inability to change the patient's position exacerbate these problems. The patient at greatest risk is one with a suspected spinal injury who is secured to a backboard.

Before departure, all splints, casts, and pressure areas should be padded. The patient secured to a backboard for a suspected cervical spinal injury can have a small towel or pad placed under the coccyx area to prevent pressure sores. In transport, proper positioning and assessment of range of motion should be performed within the space constraints. Assessing for areas of decreased perfusion should be part of the assessment of vital signs.

The length of the transport includes not only the time it takes to fly from the referring location to the receiving hospital, but also ground transport times, unexpected delays, and transfer times. For example, a patient injured in a motor vehicle crash at a remote site is secured to a backboard to protect the cervical spine. This patient is then transported by ground ambulance to the nearest hospital. After evaluation of injuries, the patient is found to require the facilities of a major trauma center. Radiographs of the cervical spine are inconclusive, so the patient must remain on the backboard during transport. Subsequently, the patient is taken by ground ambulance to the nearest airport, flown to the receiving airfield, and again transferred by ground ambulance to the trauma center. The total length of time that the patient is secured to the backboard exceeds 6 hours. The flight took only 1½ hours, but the patient was immobilized for five times that amount.

Consideration of injuries must take precedence during stabilization of the patient, but using padded splints, traction devices, and protecting bony prominences are a necessary follow-up, limiting preventable problems associated with immobilization.

Safety

Safety in air transport should be the primary concern of all persons involved. Most accidents occur in conjunction with helicopter transports; however, risk is also associated with fixed-wing transports. Issues of personal safety, patient safety, and infection control previously discussed for ground transport prevail also in air transport.

Fixed-wing transports

All equipment must be secured in accordance with FAA regulations. Meeting stringent requirements ensures that passengers and crew are not injured by flying objects during turbulence or if a crash occurs. Equipment not secured to the airframe itself should be kept in soft packs and placed on the floor during takeoff and landing. Emergency exits should *never* be blocked by equipment or extraneous items.

Ground personnel must be trained and briefed regarding aircraft safety. This briefing should include information on loading and unloading the patient. For instance, weight distribution is critical in aircraft, but ground personnel may not be aware of these requirements. Also, ground personnel should be trained to avoid hazardous areas, such as propellers and the exhaust cowling on a jet engine. No one should approach the aircraft until the pilot in command has given approval to do so.

The pilot in command is responsible for safety of the aircraft at all times and may determine whether to cancel a flight due to weather conditions. Most flight programs do not discuss severity of the patient's condition with the pilot until a decision has been made regarding weather. This relieves the pilot of undue stress when a life-or-death mission is being considered: the pilot should be able to make this decision without feelings of guilt or doubt affecting his or her judgment.

Everyone involved in the transport should be briefed prior to departure. Pilots should be informed of the patient's condition and specific needs related to takeoff and landing. For example, some patients are adversely affected by a short landing due to shifts in internal organs and fluids. Family members should be briefed on length of the flight, in-flight expectations, and the location and operations of emergency exits. Smoking is prohibited. Seat belts are required on landing and takeoff, although their use is preferred throughout the flight.

Fire extinguishers should be clearly marked, and all personnel should be trained in their use. Emergency procedures for rapid egress should be practiced on a regular basis.

Rotor-wing transports

Helicopter transports create a sense of drama. Many people assemble to watch a helicopter land and takeoff. Bystanders must be kept away from danger. A safe landing zone (LZ) should be established in a clearing that measures 60 feet by 200 feet, depending on the size of the helicopter. All wires, trees, and possible hazards should be marked *and* verbally described over the radio to the pilot. Smoke flares can be ignited to assist the pilot in locating the LZ. Flares are blown away from the helicopter during landing, which could ignite a fire. The patient, ground personnel, and bystanders should be at least 500 feet from the LZ and should turn their backs to the helicopter while it is landing. The rotor wash (wind created by the rotor blades) causes swirling dust, dirt, and gravel, which pose hazards to persons on the ground.

Ground personnel should wait to approach the helicopter until the pilot has given the signal that it is safe to do so. The helicopter should be approached from the downhill side, **never** the uphill side. Many accidents occur because persons approach the helicopter while the blades are still rotating. When blade rotation begins to slow, the blades drop, which may cause unexpected injury. A "hot" loading or unloading is one that is performed with rotor blades turning at idle power. This procedure should be used only in extreme circumstances and only by experienced personnel. Additional guidelines for helicopter safety are listed in Box 13-6. This information should be reviewed frequently and be readily available for review when a helicopter transport is expected.

Ensuring safe transport of the patient is the responsibility of all persons involved in the transport. All personnel, whether on the ground or in the air, should remain safety conscious at all times. Safety should be the number one priority.

Box 13-6   **Guidelines for Helicopter Safety**

Landing zone (LZ) size ranges from 60 to 200 sq ft, depending on size of the helicopter.

Select an LZ that is easily identifiable, as level as possible, and free of debris and overhead obstructions.

Mark one corner of the LZ with a smoke flare so the pilot can estimate wind speed and direction.

Flashing emergency lights are difficult to see in daylight. Landmarks such as intersections, waterways, distinctive buildings, or baseball or football fields are much easier to find from the air.

Turn off unnecessary lights and white lights such as strobe lights or headlights at night. These lights interfere with the pilot's night vision. *Never* direct a spotlight at an approaching helicopter.

Flags, cones, safety tapes, ambulance mattresses, poles used for intravenous infusion, other loose equipment, sticks, stones, and broken glass can be drawn into rotor blades or thrown during landing and liftoff.

Only persons such as fire fighters with proper personal protection, including safety goggles, should be permitted in the vicinity of the LZ.

Assign personnel to guard the area. Prohibit smoking and keep spectators at a safe distance.

Never approach the helicopter unless signaled to do so by the pilot or another air medical crew member. Keep low if the main rotor is still spinning.

Always approach the helicopter within the crew's line of sight and *never* from the rear or sloped side. If the aircraft is rear loading, approach cautiously with head down after being signaled by the pilot or crew.

Only flight crew members should lock, unlock, and otherwise handle aircraft doors.

Assist the flight crew only as requested. Never attempt to contact the pilot by radio during the helicopter's final approach unless an extreme emergency jeopardizes safety.

Personnel

Flight team configurations are many and varied. Emergency and critical care nurses are generally chosen to become flight nurses. They can work alone, as a member of a two-nurse team, or with a paramedic, an EMT, or an emergency physician. Respiratory therapists are also used, as a second member or third member of the team, when the patient is intubated and requires ventilatory support.

Flight nursing has developed into a subspecialty of emergency nursing. Flight nurses now go through rigorous training before joining a flight team. The National Flight Nurses Association (NFNA) has developed a flight nurse core curriculum to provide standardized training in such areas as flight physiology, stabilization, communications, and medicolegal issues. Initial training includes classroom and clinical experience. Preceptor programs are frequently used to allow the new flight nurse exposure to the transport environment. Recurrent training is also needed to maintain skills, update information regarding current therapies, and review current policies and procedures. Monthly "run" reviews provide quality improvement as well as sharing of learning experiences among staff members.

Nurses should be ACLS certified and trained in endotracheal intubation, chest tube insertion, and needle thoracotomy techniques. Depending on the capabilities of the program, additional education should include invasive line management, use of intraaortic balloon pumps, and pediatric neonatal ALS measures if children and neonates are transported. Development of the Flight Nurse Advanced Trauma Course (FNATC) demonstrates NFNA's commitment to improving educational opportunities available to flight nurses. Development of the certified flight nurse exam encourages flight nurses to achieve certification in flight nursing (CFRN). Flight nursing represents a unique opportunity for nurses to perform emergency care, critical care, and prehospital care during the same patient encounter.

Transport team members have a unique set of circumstances under which to work. Their interactions with the patient are short term and often rushed. The patients who are transported have an increased mortality because of the circumstances necessitating the transport. Following the patient's progress in the receiving hospital helps the crew alleviate their anxieties related to dealing with patients for the short term. Transport personnel must remember that they are often the only contact the family has with the receiving hospital. The crew can maintain contact with the family, explaining interventions and other procedures. Maintaining contact and follow-up with the referring personnel also provides the transport crew with opportunities to communicate about the patients and helps instill a sense of commitment and pride in their jobs.

Equipment

Equipment used in air transport must be based on the level and type of medical care the patient requires during the transport. Because of space and weight limitations, not all equipment can be carried in the transport vehicle. Before departure, a decision must be made concerning what equipment and how much should be taken. A limited amount of backup supplies should be on hand in the event of unexpected delays.

All medical equipment must be easily secured during take off, flight, and landing. Equipment requiring alternating current (AC) should have a backup battery source, or an alternative, hand-operative device should be available. All equipment should be protected from electromechanical interference. Equipment with diaphragms such as oxygen analyzers may not function in the pressurized cabin of a fixed-wing aircraft. All equipment should be tested inflight before it is used on a patient.

Required vehicle equipment and medical equipment is listed in Box 13-7. Specialized equipment is now available for transport vehicles, but before such equipment is pur-

---

Box 13-7　Equipment for Air Medical Transport

Vehicle equipment

Communication system
Adequate lighting with ability to isolate pilots from lights
Electrical outlets (110 v AC)
Locking hooks for IV bags and bottles
Fire extinguisher
Survival gear appropriate to environment over which transport occurs
Sharps disposal container
Trash receptacle

Medical equipment

Oxygen tanks with flow meters
Air cylinders if ventilator is to be used
Portable and permanent suction devices with regulators
Cardiac monitor with defibrillator
Radio-shielded Doppler device
Stretcher with approved securing mechanisms
Blood pressure cuffs
Emesis basin
Urinal and bedpan
Additional items
　Infusion pumps
　Backboards
　PASG
　Cervical collars
　Heimlich valves
　Water seal drainage sets
　Cervical spine immobilizer

Universal precautions equipment

Goggles
Gloves
Gowns
Masks

Patient-specific equipment

---

chased, an in-flight test should be performed. Some types of equipment have specialized accessories that render the equipment difficult to use and costly. For example, some IV infusion pumps require specialized infusion tubing that must be changed before the transport. Time spent repriming tubing can delay the transfer.

Expendable items should be placed in soft packs whenever possible. Product packing materials may be removed to eliminate extraneous bulk. Space-efficient equipment packs include burn, neonatal, IV, trauma, and medication packs. Pediatric equipment may be kept in a separate pack to reduce the quantity of equipment taken on all transports.

Arranging equipment so that it is prepared for use is recommended. Intravenous solutions should be in plastic bags, with tubing secured to the bag with a rubber band. Nasogastric tubes should be banded together with connectors. This organization, completed before the transport, can expedite

Table 13-4	Effects of Altitude on Flow Rates		
Flowmeter (L/min)	Flow rate at altitude (calculated)		
	2000 ft	5000 ft	8000 ft
2	2.1	2.4	2.6
4	4.2	4.7	5.3
6	6.3	7.1	7.9
8	8.4	9.4	10.6
10	10.5	11.8	13.2
12	12.6	14.1	15.8

interventions and limit the need to open many compartments to find one or two items.

Equipment of any type should be lightweight and compact. Aluminum cylinders of oxygen, which weigh one third the weight of steel tanks, are available. Pocket-type Doppler devices can be removed from the aircraft and taken with transport personnel.

Adequate equipment should be available to care for the patient during the entire transport and during any unexpected delays. To calculate the amount of equipment necessary, estimate the length of the transport, including transfer times, then multiply that figure by one half. To estimate the amount of oxygen remaining in a standard "E" cylinder, the following formula is used:

$$\text{PSI} \times 0.3 \text{ L/min} = \text{hr in cylinder}$$

Altitude and pressure changes can cause changes in flow rates. Table 13-4 shows the effects of altitude on flow rates.

Medications are commonly carried in hard plastic cases to prevent breakage. The types and amounts of medications carried depend on the types of patients transported and medical protocols of the transport program. Narcotics should be in locked carrying cases that can be secured and should be counted at each shift change.

In-Flight Responsibilities

During transport, vital signs should be obtained at least every 15 min. Depending on the patient's condition, vital signs may be taken more frequently. Changes in patient condition usually occur during ascent and descent when pressure changes occur in the aircraft. The patient's response to transport should be monitored during these times.

An advantage of air transport is that transport personnel are never farther than a few feet from their patient. This closeness allows astute observation of the patient and the ability to pick up subtle changes in condition. However, noise, distractions, and space limitations within the transport vehicle can distort certain cues. The crew must pay careful attention and monitor the patient closely for problems that

may develop as a result of changes in atmosphere or the transport itself.

Patients with respiratory distress

Warm, humidified oxygen should be administered to all patients. The percentage of oxygen should be increased for those receiving oxygen therapy before the transport. Gas expansion within the pleural cavity can cause the size of a previously undetected pneumothorax to increase, which may result in respiratory compromise. A flutter valve should be placed to reduce pressure within the chest cavity (Table 13-3). If the patient had a chest tube placed before transport, the tube should never be clamped during flight. A one-way (Heimlich) valve can be placed between the chest tube and the drainage set to prevent air from reaccumulating in the chest cavity with accidental disruption of the system.

Pulmonary secretions become more tenacious with dehydration and decreased ambient humidity. Instillation of sterile saline before suctioning enhances removal of secretions. Hyperventilation can accompany cold stress or it can be caused by excessive noise and vibration. Measures should be taken to warm the patient and allay the patient's fears and anxieties.

Immobilizing the patient on the stretcher interferes with chest expansion and can lead to underventilation and subsequent atelectasis. Elevating the patient's head improves oxygenation and gas exchange and helps limit pulmonary congestion that occurs as a result of acceleration and deceleration forces.

Mechanical volume ventilators used in the transport environment must be constantly monitored for delivery of adequate tidal volumes, since gas expansion can affect the volume of gas delivered. Oxygen flow rates of at least 15 L/min are required to operate ventilators. This can rapidly decrease oxygen supply. Should the ventilator fail, the patient must be ventilated with a resuscitation bag.

Patients with cardiovascular conditions

Hypoxia presents the greatest risk for the cardiac patient during transport. It can lead to increased myocardial irritability and ventricular ectopy. Providing supplemental oxygen and positioning the patient for optimal gas exchanges is imperative. Interventions to decrease oxygen demand include keeping the patient warm, allaying fears, and preventing motion sickness.

Placing a nasogastric tube can prevent decreased venous return caused by gastric distension. However, placement must be performed with caution since vagal stimulation and bradycardia can develop. The decision to employ a nasogastric tube should be made on a patient-by-patient basis.

Acceleration forces cause pooling of blood in the lower extremities with subsequent poor cardiac return. The opposite effect develops as a result of deceleration forces, where cardiac congestion and transient fluid overload develop. The patient in congestive heart failure is severely affected by these factors. Pretransport diuresis can help prevent these problems.

Specialized equipment associated with cardiac patients needs special attention. Patients with pacemakers should be monitored for pacemaker malfunction that can occur as a result of radio and navigational equipment signals. Intraaortic balloon pumps are now available for use during transport. Only trained personnel should use these devices, since the risk of balloon dislodgment and equipment malfunction is increased in the transport environment. During transport, close monitoring of pressures within the balloon is imperative to detect changes that may result from gas expansion.

Patients with multiple traumatic injuries

Hypoxia and gas expansion can rapidly cause deterioration of the pulmonary and cardiovascular systems. Pulmonary embolus should be considered a possibility when increasing dyspnea develops. Thoracic injuries should be identified and stabilized before transporting the patient.

The effect of gas expansion on the PASG, air splints, and endotracheal tube cuffs has been discussed previously. Free air in the peritoneal cavity resulting from bowel injury or peritoneal lavage should be aspirated if possible.

Adequate resuscitation of the trauma patient usually includes fluid and blood support. Measures must be taken to ensure that blood products are properly stored. In the event that their use is unwarranted, they can be returned to the blood bank for future use.

Patients with head injuries

Patients with an isolated injury or a head injury in conjunction with other injuries, are at significant risk from air transport. Increased intracranial pressure decreases the level of arterial oxygen saturation, which may result in hypoxia caused by changes in the partial pressure of oxygen. This hypoxia can cause seizure activity, so seizure precautions should be used at all times.

Noise, vibration, vomiting, and an increased metabolic rate associated with cold stress all increase intracranial pressure. In-flight measures, including hyperventilation, should be used to reduce these untoward effects and prevent unnecessary rises in intracranial pressure. Induction of paralysis can also help control intracranial pressure; however, posturing and other clinical indicators of patient status are forfeited. The patient should be positioned to minimize effects of gravitational forces.

Burn victims

Burns of the face, head, and neck may cause massive swelling, reducing the airway. Prophylactic intubation before transport prevents the need for intubation in the poorly lit, cramped interior of the aircraft. Supplemental oxygen should be administered to all patients with suspected smoke inhalation; it combats the effects of hypoxia. Providing cool humidified oxygen to the patient with suspected oropharyngeal burns helps reduce swelling.

Loss of the skin causes massive fluid shifts and loss of temperature-regulation. Evaporative heat loss increases in the burned area, and the burn victim becomes increasingly dehydrated and cold. All wounds should be covered with absorbent dressings to control heat loss and limit contamination of the wounds. Dressings should not be moistened with saline solution or other fluids, because this procedure enhances hypothermia. Using a Mylar blanket to cover the patient helps limit heat loss.

Patients with burns require large amounts of fluids and dressings; therefore adequate supplies must be available throughout the transport of a burn victim. Escharotomies may become necessary when fluid shifts occur during take-off and descent.

Maintaining sterility of the transport environment is impossible. Meticulous care to prevent contamination should be taken at all times. Wearing masks and gowns over transport clothing helps limit transfer of bacteria. Topical antibiotics may be applied before the transport; however, this procedure delays evaluation of the burn wound when the patient arrives at the receiving hospital, since the antibiotic first must be removed.

Patients with high-risk obstetric conditions

Hypoxia and fluid shifts increase uterine irritability and can lead to premature labor. Hypoxia of short duration has little effect on the fetus, but prolonged maternal hypoxia can lead to fetal distress and subsequent fetal demise. Supplemental oxygen should be provided to the patient throughout transport.

Pressure from a distended stomach increases uterine irritability and increases pressure on the diaphragm causing dyspnea. Nasogastric tube placement may be uncomfortable for the pregnant woman. The tube decompresses the stomach and decreases the risk of aspiration from delayed gastric emptying.

Pregnancy increases blood volume by approximately 45%-50%. This increased volume must be replaced if the woman is hypovolemic. Pregnant women can lose a significant portion of their circulating blood volume before hypovolemia is evident. Fluid shifts accompanying acceleration and deceleration forces can cause decreased uterine blood flow. Proper positioning is essential for the pregnant patient.

The pregnant patient should be placed in the left lateral decubitus position during transport. Safely securing the patient to the stretcher in this position is often difficult. The patient may have to be secured in the supine position during loading and unloading. The woman should be returned to the left lateral decubitus position as soon as the aircraft reaches cruising altitude or with signs of fetal distress.

Preeclampsia and eclampsia cause an increase in nausea and vomiting associated with motion. These patients are also sensitive to extraneous stimulation; noise and vibration may increase blood pressure. Dim lighting and earplugs for the patient help prevent overstimulation.

All personnel who transport high-risk obstetric patients must be familiar with the techniques of childbirth and neonatal resuscitation. Equipment for delivery and resuscitation must be readily available. If delivery is imminent, the transport should reroute to the nearest hospital to avoid in-flight delivery regardless of the final destination. Keeping a newly delivered infant warm, dry, and oxygenated is the priority for newborn care.

Pediatric patients

The problems associated with transport of children are the same as those for adults. However, interventions must take into account the unique anatomic and physiologic features of children. Since equipment of the appropriate size varies with age and weight of the child, a large assortment of choices must be available.

Pediatric patients have smaller vital capacities than adults and are more prone to the effects of hypoxia. Children may not be able to tolerate or cooperate with application of an oxygen mask. In these cases, the oxygen mask can be placed in front of the child's face and oxygen can be blown at the child. A family member accompanying the child can assist with administration of oxygen by holding the mask and encouraging the child to cooperate.

Because the gastric cavity of a child is small, the child has a greater tendency to develop complications from gastric gas expansion. Many nasogastric tubes for children do not have a sump port and should not be used, since absence of the sump port makes emptying the stomach more difficult.

The greater ratio of surface area to body mass in children makes them more susceptible to evaporative heat losses. The proportionally larger surface area of the head and neck also enhance radiated heat loss, which puts the child at great risk for hypothermia. A stocking cap and extra linen help keep the child warm.

Securing children to a standard stretcher is difficult because stretcher restraints are not easily moved to accommodate a smaller size. Extra straps may be necessary to keep the child secured. One method of transporting a child less than 5 years of age is to place the child in a car seat and secure the car seat to the stretcher restraints. Using and providing familiar items such as car seats, toys, and security blankets help alleviate the child's fear of the unknown.

If the child's condition is stable, including a family member in the transport may be advantageous. The family member can comfort the child, help explain procedures, and provide diversionary activities as warranted, to keep the child occupied.

Other in-flight responsibilities include documentation of all interventions, vital signs, and changes in the patient's condition. Changes in environmental conditions such as with takeoff and landing should also be documented, since changes in the patient's condition may be secondary to the effects of transport rather than to changes in the disease process or condition itself. Throughout the transport, safety must be the number one consideration.

CONCLUSION

Air and ground patient transport has improved outcomes for many. Proper stabilization procedures should anticipate potential problems that may be encountered during transport. Employing specialized equipment and personnel trained in transporting patients ensures that the patient is transported in a highly sophisticated environment.

The future may bring consolidation of transport programs. To ensure viability, air transport programs must work together, consolidate and provide a consortium approach to transport. Incorporating ground transport with air transport will improve appropriate utilization of these services.

Newer therapies are being instituted in the prehospital care environment (e.g., thrombolytic therapy). As computerization and information sharing grows, medical control officers can make informed decisions while the patient is still in transport. As these decisions are made, therapies can be instituted immediately rather than waiting for the patient's arrival in the ED. This increased responsibility requires that transport personnel are continually updated in current methodologies. Many studies have confirmed the benefits of early therapy; and transport personnel may assume more responsibility in the future.

Sophistication of air and ground transport is limited by the size and weight of most medical equipment. As miniaturization continues and transport equipment becomes lightweight and truly transportable, transporting patients will develop into an even more specialized aspect of emergency nursing.

This chapter is dedicated to the memory of Marna Bloom Fleetwood, RN, and Amy Riebe, RN, MN, who lost their lives on September 11, 1995 while performing a job they loved and excelled in—transporting patients.

REFERENCES

1. Commission on Accreditation of Ambulance Services: *Standards for the accreditation of ambulance services,* Dallas, 1991, The Commission.
2. McCloskey K, Orr R: *Pediatric transport medicine,* St. Louis, 1995, Mosby.

SUGGESTED READING

American Academy of Pediatrics, Task Force on Interhospital Transports: *Guidelines of air and ground transport of neonatal and pediatric patients,* Elk Grove Village, Ill, 1993, The Academy.

Association of Air Medical Services: Position paper on the appropriate use of emergency air medical services, *J Air Med Trans* 9:29-33, 1990.

Guidelines Committee of the American College of Critical Care Medicine, Society of Critical Care Medicine and American Association of Critical Care Nurse Transfer Guidelines Task Force: Guidelines for the transfer of critically ill patients, *Crit Care Med* 21(6):931-937, 1993.

Lee G: *Flight nursing: principles and practice,* St. Louis, 1991, Mosby.

National Association of Emergency Medical Services Physicians: Air medical dispatch: guidelines for trauma scene response, *Prehospital and Disaster Medicine* 7(1):75, 1992.

National Flight Nurses Association: *Standards of flight nursing practice,* ed 2, St. Louis, 1994, Mosby.

Youngberg BJ: Medical-legal considerations involved in the transport of critically ill patients, *Crit Care Clin* 8(3):501-514, 1992.

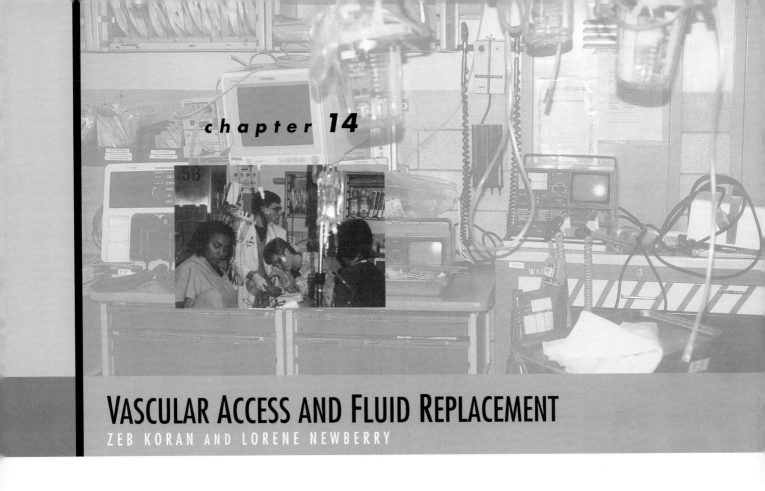

chapter **14**

VASCULAR ACCESS AND FLUID REPLACEMENT

ZEB KORAN AND LORENE NEWBERRY

Circulatory assessment and related interventions are a cornerstone of emergency interventions for emergency patients, regardless of the complaint or symptoms. Patients in the emergency department (ED) often require temporary vascular access for medications, fluid and electrolyte replacement, or transfusion of blood or blood products. Routine vascular access involves insertion of catheters into peripheral veins of hands and arms. Site selection depends on urgency of the situation and the condition of the patient's veins. Central veins may be used for invasive hemodynamic monitoring or when peripheral access is not possible. Needle insertion into bone marrow is also used for emergency fluid replacement. Patients also may have catheters or ports for long-term vascular access.

Fluid replacement is used for patients with subtle and overt volume losses. Solution, rate, and amount is determined by patient condition, underlying pathology, and current fluid imbalance. Maintenance fluids are used for patients with no oral intake, whereas aggressive fluid replacement is indicated for patients with significant volume depletion. Patients with hematologic disorders, cancer, or frank blood loss may also require blood or blood products replacement. Vascular access options and various aspects of fluid replacement are described in the following sections.

ANATOMY AND PHYSIOLOGY

Low-pressure vessels located throughout the body receive blood from capillary beds and return it to the heart. Small venules flow into increasingly larger veins, which eventually flow into the inferior and superior venae cavae. Vessel diameter varies among patients and with location on the body. Surface vessels in hands and arms are primary access points; however, vessels in the neck, legs, feet, and head may also be used. Figure 14-1 shows the location of major vessels of the body. Valves located along veins prevent backflow (Figure 14-2); therefore, intravenous catheters must be inserted in the same direction as venous flow. Elderly patients lose collagen in vessel walls, which causes significant thinning over time. Vessels may also sclerose and become torturous with aging.

Veins in the upper extremities include digital veins on the dorsal aspect of fingers, metacarpal veins on the dorsum of the hand, cephalic veins, basilic veins, and median veins (Figure 14-3). Figure 14-4 illustrates veins of the hand and fingers. Cephalic veins are located at the radial aspect of the dorsal venous network with the accessory cephalic vein originating from the union of dorsal veins. The basilic vein, which originates from the union of dorsal veins on the ulnar aspect of the arm, can be seen when the elbow is flexed. The union of veins from the palmar aspect of the hand creates the median antebrachial vein. The antecubital fossa, a depression in the anterior elbow, contains the median cephalic vein or median basilic vein.

The dorsal venous network on the foot and saphenous vein on the ankle flow into the larger femoral vein (Figure 14-5). These vessels are rarely used for routine vascular ac-

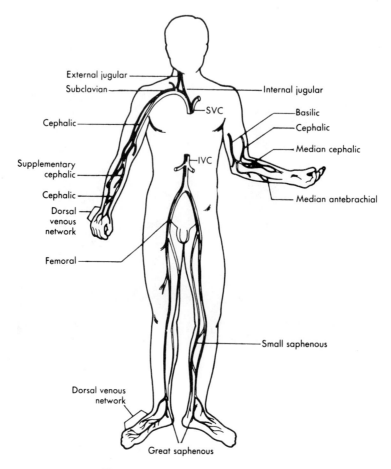

Figure **14-1**　Major veins of the body.

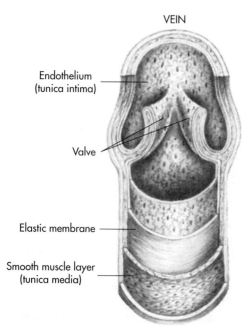

Figure **14-2**　Vein cross section. *(Modified from Thompson JM, et al:* Mosby's clinical nursing, *ed 3, St. Louis, 1993, Mosby.)*

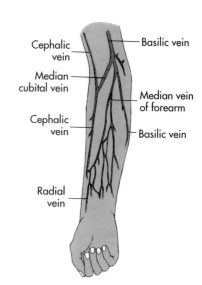

Figure **14-3**　Veins in the upper arm. *(Modified from Potter PA, Perry AG:* Fundamentals of nursing: concepts, process, and practice, *ed 4, St. Louis, 1997, Mosby.)*

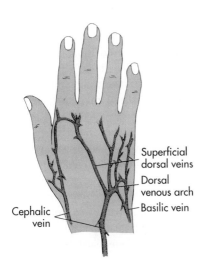

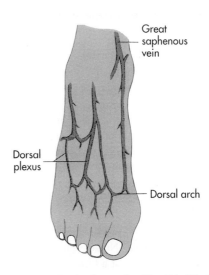

Figure 14-4 Veins in the hand. *(Modified from Potter PA, Perry AG: Fundamentals of nursing: concepts, process, and practice, ed 4, St. Louis, 1997, Mosby.)*

Figure 14-5 Veins in the foot and ankle. *(Modified from Potter PA, Perry AG: Fundamentals of nursing: concepts, process, and practice, ed 4, St. Louis, 1997, Mosby.)*

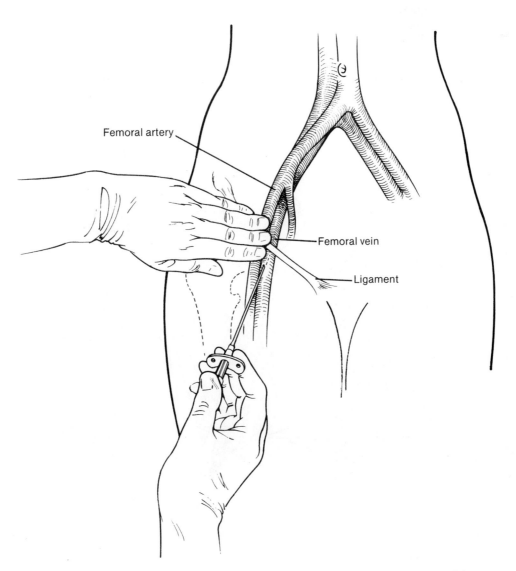

Figure 14-6 Femoral vein. *(Modified from Meeker MH, Rothrock JC: Alexander's care of the patient in surgery, ed 10, St. Louis, 1995, Mosby.)*

cess due to associated complications. The femoral vein located medial to the femoral artery is used for access to the central circulation in some patients (Figure 14-6).

Peripheral veins of the neck flow into the subclavian vein and can be used for vascular access (Figure 14-7). The external jugular vein is visible in most patients on the lateral aspect of the neck. The internal jugular vein is located beneath and medial to the external jugular. Subclavian veins are used for access to the central circulation.

VASCULAR ACCESS

Insertion of peripheral intravenous catheters is a routine skill for emergency nurses. Nurses may also insert central catheters; however, this is not a basic skill for the majority of emergency nurses. Catheters are usually inserted into peripheral veins of the hand, arm, or neck. Veins in the foot and leg are rarely used due to increased incidence of embolism and phlebitis. Nurses also use and maintain established vascular access points.

Vascular access is obtained using aseptic technique. Initial insertion attempts should begin with distal veins and progress up the extremity. Proximal veins are not routinely used unless patients need immediate fluid replacement, such as in trauma patients or patients in hypovolemic shock.

Proximal veins are also used for patients receiving drugs with an extremely short half-life (e.g., adenosine). Scalp veins have no valves, so fluid can be infused in either direction and are easily visualized, making them an ideal alternative in infants.

Insertion of intravenous catheters is not without risk to the patient and the emergency nurse. Potential complications for the patient include infection and hematoma (Box 14-1). The emergency nurse risks exposure to potentially infectious blood through needle stick or direct contact. Extreme care should be taken to minimize risks through use of universal precautions and appropriate disposal of needles. Intravenous catheters with safety features such as self-capping needles

Box **14-1**   **Complications of Intravenous Catheters**
Hematoma at insertion site
Fluid infiltration
Phlebitis
Embolism of blood, air, or catheter fragments
Infection
Cellulitis

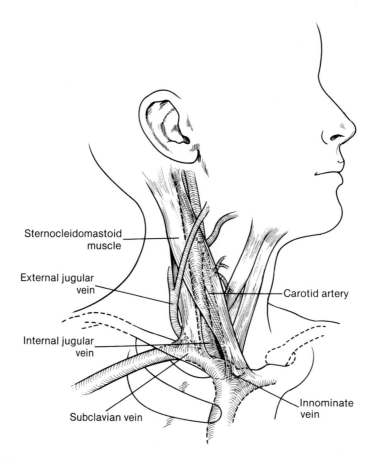

Figure **14-7**   Veins in the neck. (*Modified from Meeker MH, Rothrock JC:* Alexander's care of the patient in surgery, *ed 10, St. Louis, 1995, Mosby.*)

and retracting needles are available; but are not used routinely in most facilities.

Catheter Selection

The size and type of catheter are determined by urgency of need and patient size, age, and vasculature. Blood should flow easily around the catheter after insertion. Larger diameter catheters are used for administration of significant volumes, colloid solutions, or blood/blood products, whereas smaller diameter catheters are used for routine vascular access. All intravenous catheters now use a catheter-over-needle design. Intravenous needles without catheters are available, but should not be used. Catheters used for peripheral access include a butterfly or winged catheter (Figure 14-8) and straight catheter-over-needle (Figure 14-9). Winged catheters are inserted easily and can be stabilized with minimal effort; however, these catheters are not ideal for rapid fluid replacement. Catheters-over-needles are ideal for aggressive fluid replacement, but can present problems with stabilization, particularly in distal veins of the hand. Dual lumen peripheral catheters must be flushed before insertion to activate a hydrolytic lubricant on the outside of the catheter.

Insertion

Aseptic technique is essential to protect the patient from infection during intravenous catheter insertion. Gloves should be worn for site preparation and catheter insertion. The selected insertion site should have adequate circulation and be free of infection. Peripheral veins in hands and arms are the first choice for intravenous access. Other sites include veins of the lower extremities, or the external jugular, internal jugular, and femoral veins. Lower extremities are not routinely used due to potential complications such as phlebitis and embolism.

The external jugular vein is accessible in most patients, but requires turning the neck for access. Lowering the patient's head distends the vein and decreases risk of air embolism during insertion. Use of the external jugular vein is not recommended for patients with suspected neck injury. Use of the internal jugular vein is also contraindicated in these patients. Internal jugular access is not used during cardiac arrest since cardiac compressions must be stopped for insertion. Other problems associated with use of the internal jugular vein include hematoma development, which compromises respiratory effort. The femoral vein is an excellent choice in cardiac arrest since cardiac compressions can continue. Figure 14-10 shows cannulization of the femoral vein. Femoral access also provides an opportunity for hemodynamic pressure monitoring. Complications associated with femoral vein access include hematoma and infection.

Once a site is selected, a tourniquet is placed proximally to distend vessels for easy insertion (Figure 14-11, *A*). Because veins may be more prominent in elderly patients, a tourniquet may not be required. Tourniquets may actually rupture vessels due to increased pressure in fragile veins. Gently tapping or rubbing vessels below the tourniquet increases vessel size by dilation. When vessels are not easily visualized or palpated, applying warm towels over the vein for 5 minutes causes vasodilation and can facilitate catheter insertion (Figure 14-11, *B*).

Skin preparation begins with initial cleansing using alcohol to remove fat and other residue. Povidone-iodine (betadine) solution is the bactericidal agent of choice unless the patient has an allergy. The solution is applied directly over the insertion site in a circular pattern moving slowly outward (Figure 14-12). The ideal bactericidal effect requires that the solution remain on the skin for 30 seconds. The surface is then wiped with sterile gauze.

Anesthesia is not routinely used for catheter insertion unless time permits, and a large bore needle must be used. After site preparation, Lidocaine 1% may be injected at the insertion site for immediate anesthetic effect. *Emla* cream applied topically over the insertion site for approximately 15 to 20 minutes is an alternative to injection if time is not an issue.

Once the site is prepared, the catheter is inserted by stabilizing the vein to prevent movement during puncture. With needle bevel up, skin is punctured using the smallest angle possible between skin and needle (Figure 14-13). Veins may be entered on the top or side. The catheter is advanced slowly until blood flashes into the catheter, then the catheter is advanced over the needle into the vein. The tourniquet is then removed, and intravenous tubing is connected. One-way valves are recommended to prevent bleeding from the

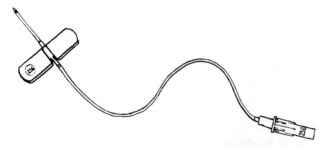

Figure **14-8** Butterfly or winged infusion set.

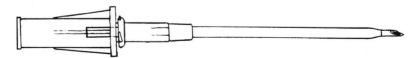

Figure **14-9** Catheter-over-needle.

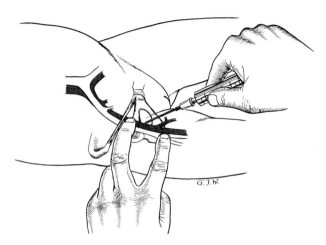

Figure **14-10**   Femoral venous catheterization technique. *(From Daily EK, Schroeder JS: Techniques in bedside hemodynamic monitoring, ed 5, St. Louis, 1994, Mosby. Modified from Chameides L: Textbook of pediatric advanced life support, Dallas, 1994, Copyright American Heart Association.)*

A

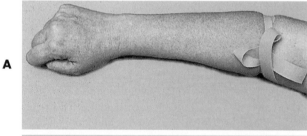

B

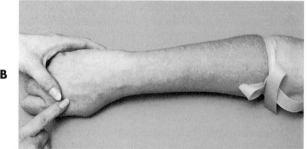

Figure **14-11**   **A,** Placement of tourniquet. **B,** Technique for increasing vessel size by dilation. *(From Potter PA, Perry AG: Fundamentals of nursing: concepts, process, and practice, ed 4, St. Louis, 1997, Mosby.)*

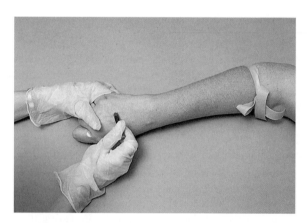

Figure **14-12**   Application of solution over insertion site. *(From Potter PA, Perry AG: Fundamentals of nursing: concepts, process, and practice, ed 4, St. Louis, 1997, Mosby.)*

catheter during subsequent tubing changes. If fluid therapy is not required, catheters may be capped with a one-way valve and sterile cover. The catheter and tubing should be secured with tape according to hospital policy; however, tape should never be applied directly over the insertion site. Clear, occlusive dressings such as *Opsite, Tegaderm,* or *Bio-*

clusive should be applied over the insertion site. Sites should be labeled with the date, time, catheter size, and initials of the person inserting the catheter.

Central Venous Access

The subclavian, external jugular, and cephalic veins are used for short- and long-term vascular access. Short-term central venous access is indicated when peripheral access cannot be obtained or when the patient's condition requires hemodynamic monitoring. Long-term vascular access is indicated for prolonged intravenous therapy, total parenteral nutrition, extended antibiotic therapy or therapy with caustic drugs such as vancomycin, and in patients with debilitating

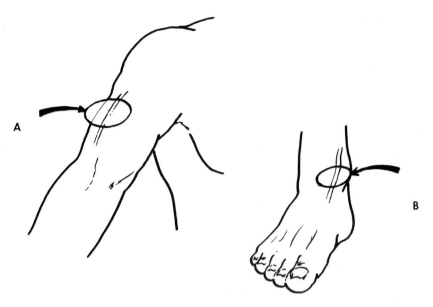

Figure **14-20** Common sites for venous cutdown. **A,** Cephalic vein. **B,** Saphenous vein.

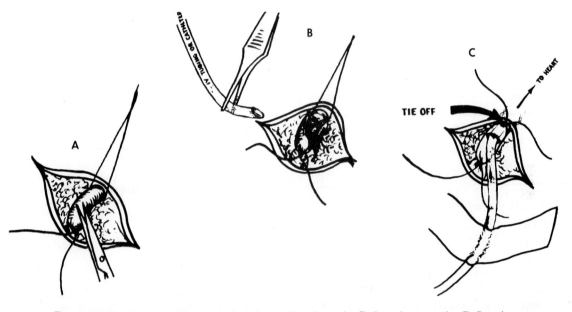

Figure **14-21** Venous cutdown. **A,** Isolating and cutting vein. **B,** Inserting cannula. **C,** Suturing cannula in place.

skin and respiratory tract account for more than 1500 ml/day of fluid loss. Calculation of basal fluid needs is based on patient size calculated as body surface area. Box 14-3 gives formulas for maintenance fluids and for volume replacement. Isotonic, hypotonic, and hypertonic fluids may be used as maintenance fluids. Isotonic fluids provide greater intravascular volume because more fluid remains in the vascular space. Hypotonic fluids shift fluid into intracellular spaces and are more useful for preventing cellular dehydration. Hypertonic fluids move fluid from cells to the extravascular space and may be used to promote diuresis. Table 14-3 gives examples and describes use of these maintenance fluids.

Crystalloid and colloid solutions are used for volume replacement. These fluids may be isotonic, hypotonic, or hypertonic. Crystalloid solutions increase intravascular volume through actual volume administered, whereas colloids pull fluid into the vascular space through osmosis. Synthetic and natural colloid solutions are available. Examples of crystalloid and colloid solutions and actions for each are presented in Table 14-4.

Blood and Blood Products

These naturally occurring colloid solutions are used to replace blood losses and replenish clotting factors. Blood loss

---

Box 14-3   Formulas For Fluid Administration

Basal fluid maintenance

1500 ml/m^2 BSA/24 hr = ml/24 hr (calculate as ml/hr)

General guidelines: Up to 10 kg = 100 ml/kg/24 hr

11-20 kg = 50 ml/kg/24 hr plus 100 ml/kg for first 10 kg

>20 kg = 20-25 ml/kg/24 hr plus 50 ml/kg for each kg 11 through 20 plus 100 ml/kg for first 10 kg

Volume replacement with crystalloids

Administer 3 ml for each ml lost. Fluid challenges/options are:

IV bolus 20 ml/kg D5% RL in children

IV bolus of 200-300 ml RL in adult surgical patients

IV bolus of 200-300 ml NS in adult medical patients

Volume replacement with colloids

Administer 1 ml for each ml lost

Volume replacement for measured losses

Gastric Losses: Replace 1 ml for each ml lost q 4 hr. Use D$_5$ ½NS plus 30 mEq K/L

Intestinal Losses: Replace 1 ml for each ml lost q 4 hr. Use D5%LR.

Basal urine output

Up to 30 kg = 40 ml/kg/24 hr (2 ml/kg/hr)

>30 kg = 1200 ml/24 hr (17-18 ml/kg/hr)

Modified from Kidd PS, Sturt P: *Mosby's emergency nursing reference,* St. Louis, 1996, Mosby.

NS = normal saline

RL = Ringer's lactated solution

Table 14-3   Maintenance IV Fluids

Solution type	Examples	Uses
Isotonic	0.9% Normal saline (NS)	Expands intravascular volume. Used for dehydration (e.g., diabetic ketoacidosis, hyperosmolar non-ketotic coma) and packed red blood cell administration.
	Ringer's lactated solution	Expands intravascular volume. Used for maintenance fluid when patient is NPO.
Hypotonic	NS 0.45% NS 0.2% Dextrose 5% and water (D$_5$W)	Shifts water into intracellular spaces. Useful in preventing dehydration and assessing renal status. D$_5$W may be used in adult patients for mixing IV medications. Used for maintenance fluid when patient is at risk for free water loss.
Hypertonic	Dextrose 5% in NS Dextrose 10% in NS Dextrose 10% in water Dextrose 5% in 0.45 NS Dextrose 20% in water	Shifts fluid from intracellular to extracellular space. Used in water intoxication states created by too much hypotonic fluid administration. Used for maintenance fluid to promote diuresis.

Modified from Kidd PS, Sturt P: *Mosby's emergency nursing reference,* St. Louis, 1996, Mosby.

---

depletes the body of blood cells and clotting factors, so whole blood replacement is ideal in frank blood loss. However, whole blood is expensive, not readily available, and has greater risk for transmission of infectious diseases. Packed red cells (PRBC) are used more often for blood replacement. Other blood products used for component replacement include platelets, fresh frozen plasma, and albumin. Table 14-5 summarizes administration of these and other blood products in adults; Table 14-6 summarizes administration of these products in children. Blood products are always administered using normal saline. Dextrose solutions cause cellular edema as fluid shifts into the intracellular space.

Before blood administration, a blood sample should be obtained for type and crossmatch. Two specimens should be obtained if large volume replacement is anticipated. Ideally, complete type and crossmatch should be done on all blood before administration; however, this procedure can take 40 minutes or more. Type-specific blood or blood that is not completely crossmatched may be given in patients with critical blood loss. Type 0 blood may be given for patients with

extreme blood loss who cannot wait for type specific blood. Table 14-7 summarizes type and crossmatch procedures.

Blood administration is not without risk. Blood processing procedures have reduced the risk for transmission of infectious diseases; however, transfusion reactions can occur because of transfusion of incompatible blood, patient allergy, or depletion of clotting factors (Table 14-8). Unrecognized transfusion reactions represent a significant threat to the patient's life. Before transfusion, blood and patient identification should be checked carefully. During the transfusion, the patient should be carefully monitored for signs of reaction including fever, chills, urticaria, and breathing difficulty.

Table **14-4** **Fluid Resuscitation Summary***		
Crystalloids	Description/indication	Action(s)
0.9% Normal saline†	Isotonic	• May produce fluid overload • 25% of volume administered remains in vascular space
0.45% Normal saline	Hypotonic, moves fluid from vascular space to interstitial and intracellular spaces	• Decreases blood viscosity • May promote hypovolemia • May promote cerebral edema
5% Dextrose	Hypotonic	• 7.5 ml/100 ml infused remains in vascular space • Inadequate for fluid resuscitation
Ringer's solution	Isotonic	• Does not provide free water or calories • Expands intravascular volume and replaces extracellular fluid losses
Ringer's lactated solution†	Isotonic, contains multiple electrolytes and lactate	• May produce fluid overload • May promote lactic acidosis in prolonged hypoperfusion with decreased liver function • Lactate metabolizes to acetate, may produce metabolic alkalosis when large volumes are transfused
Hypertonic saline (7.5%)	Hypertonic, pulls fluid from interstitial and intracellular spaces into vascular space	• Requires smaller amount to restore blood volume • Increases cerebral oxygen drive while decreasing ICP • May promote hypernatremia • May promote intracellular dehydration • May promote osmotic diuresis • Controversial
Synthetic colloids	Description	Action(s)
Dextran‡	(Comes in 40, 70, and 75 molecular weight)	• Associated with anaphylaxis • Reduces Factor VIII, platelets, and fibrinogen function, so increases bleeding time • May interfere with blood type and cross match, glucose, and erythrocyte sedimentation levels • Risk of fluid overload
Hetastarch‡		• May increase serum amylase levels • Associated with coagulopathy • Risk of fluid overload

Modified from Kidd PS, Sturt P: *Mosby's emergency nursing reference*, St. Louis, 1996, Mosby.
*Dosages are not listed because of variability in patient response and need.
†Fluid overload using these agents may occur because of large amount required for volume lost (3:1 ratio).
‡Fluid overload using these agents may occur in cases of preexisting pulmonary and/or heart disease.

Continued

Table **14-4**	**Fluid Resuscitation Summary*-cont'd**	
Natural colloids	Description	Action(s)
Fresh frozen plasma	Contains all clotting factors	• Potential to transmit blood-borne infection • Can cause hypersensitivity reaction • Blood volume expander
Plasma protein fraction (Plasmanate)	Does not contain clotting factors	• May cause hypersensitivity reaction • May cause hypotension with rapid infusion • Blood volume expander
Albumin‡	5% iso-oncotic 25% hyperoncotic "salt poor"	• Preferred as volume expander when risk from producing interstitial edema is great (e.g., pulmonary and heart disease) • Hypocalcemia
Whole blood	Can be administered without normal saline; reduces donor exposure	• Hyperkalemia, hypothermia, and hypocalcemia • May require greater amount than packed RBCs to increase oxygen-carrying capacity of blood • Rarely used, not cost-effective
Packed RBCs	Administer with normal saline	• Deficient in 2, 3-diphosphoglycerate and may increase oxygen affinity to hemoglobin and decrease oxygen delivery to tissue • Hypothermia, hyperkalemia, and hypocalcemia
Experimental agents	Description	Action(s)
Liposome encapsulated hemoglobin hypertonic saline (7.5%)	NOT APPROVED BY FDA	• Improves skeletal muscle oxygen tension • Expands vascular volume quickly • Improves tissue oxygenation
Hypertonic saline (7.5%) with Dextran 70	Combined crystalloid and colloid therapy	• Promotes rapid expansion of blood volume and promotes retention of volume in vascular space • Controversial

Modified from Kidd PS, Sturt P: *Mosby's emergency nursing reference,* St. Louis, 1996, Mosby.
*Dosages are not listed because of variability in patient response and need.
†Fluid overload using these agents may occur because of large amount required for volume lost (3:1 ratio).
‡Fluid overload using these agents may occur in cases of preexisting pulmonary and/or heart disease.

Table 14-5	Blood Component Administration in Adults					
Blood component	Uses	Blood type	Infusion rate	Filter	Volume	Comments
Whole blood	Acute or chronic anemia, aplastic anemia, bone marrow failure, congestive heart failure, chronic renal failure, hepatic coma	*Must* be ABO compatible	2-4 hr Max: 4 hr	Required	500 ml	Rapid infusion if need is urgent. Clotting factors deteriorate after 24 hr.
Packed red blood cells	Acute massive blood loss, hypovolemic shock	*Must* be ABO compatible	2-4 hr Max: 4 hr	Required	250 ml	Hgb rises 1 g/dl; Hct rises 3% after 1 U.
Leukocyte-poor red blood cells	Thrombocytopenia, platelet function abnormality	Need *not* be ABO compatible	2 hr	Required	Variable	
Fresh frozen plasma	Hypovolemia combined with hemorrhage caused by deficiencies	*Must* be ABO compatible	1-2 hr, rapidly if bleeding	Use component filter	250 ml	Notify blood bank— takes 20 min to thaw; use in 6 hr of thawing. Do not use microaggregate filter.
Platelets	Hemophilia, von Willebrand's disease, hypofibrinogenemia, factor XIII deficiency	Need *not* be ABO compatible	Rapidly as patient tolerates	Use component filter	35-50 ml U	Usually 6-10 U are ordered. Request that blood bank pool all units. Do not use microaggregate filter.
Albumin	Shock caused by burns; maintains blood volume in patients with hypovolemia; hypoproteinemia	Need *not* be ABO compatible	1-2 ml/min in normovolemic patients	Special tubing	Varies	Comes in 5% and 25%; can increase intravascular volume quickly; infuse cautiously.
Cryoprecipitate	Repeated febrile reaction; reaction from leukocyte antibodies and patients who are candidates for organ transplants	*Must* be ABO compatible	30 min	Use component filter	10 ml/unit	Usually 6-10 U ordered; request that blood bank pool units. Unstable to heat and storage.
Granulocytes			2-4 hr	Use component filter	300-400 ml	VS q 15 min during infusion. Granulocytes have a short life span. Transfuse as soon after collection as possible.

Table 14-6 Blood Component Administration in Children

Blood component	Usual dose	Infusion rate	Comments
Whole blood	20 ml/kg initially	As rapidly as necessary to restore volume and stabilize the child	Administration is usually reserved for massive hemorrhage.
Packed RBCs	10 ml/kg, not to exceed 15 ml/kg	5 ml/kg/hr or 2 ml/kg/hr if congestive heart failure develops	1 ml/kg will increase Hct approximately 1%. Infuse within 4 hr. If necessary, divide the unit into smaller volumes for infusion.
Platelets	1 unit for every 7-10 kg	Each unit over 5-10 min via syringe or pump	The usual dose will increase platelet count by 50,000/mm^3.
Fresh frozen plasma	Hemorrhage: 15-30 ml/kg Clotting deficiency: 10-15 ml/kg	Hemorrhage: rapidly to stabilize the child Clotting deficiency: over 2-3 hr	Monitor for fluid overload.
Granulocytes	Dependent on WBC counts and clinical condition, 10 ml/kg/day initially	Slowly over 2-4 hr because of fever and chills, side effects commonly associated with infusion	Granulocytes have a short life span. Transfuse as soon after collection as possible.
Albumin 5%	1 g/kg or 20 ml/kg	1-2 ml/min or 60-120 ml/hr	Monitor for fluid overload. Type and crossmatch are not required.
Albumin 25%	1 g/kg or 4 ml/kg	0.2-0.4 ml/min or 12-24 ml/hr	Monitor for fluid overload. Type and crossmatch are not required.

Modified from Kidd PS, Sturt P: *Mosby's emergency nursing reference,* St. Louis, 1996, Mosby.

Table 14-7 Type and Crossmatch Procedures

Procedures	Tests	Time required (minutes)
Complete type and crossmatch	ABO-Rh typing Full crossmatch Antibody screening*	30-45
Incomplete type and crossmatch†	ABO-Rh typing Saline-immediate-spin crossmatch	5-10
Type†	ABO-Rh typing‡	5-10
Type and screen	ABO-Rh typing Antibody screening*§ (Saline-immediate-spin crossmatch when ordered for transfusion)	30-45

Modified from Rosen P et al.: *Emergency medicine: concepts and clinical practice,* ed 3, St. Louis, 1992, Mosby.
*Additional time is required if antibodies are found.
†Physician requesting the incomplete type and crossmatch must take full responsibility for adverse effects.
‡Most blood banks will not release type-specific blood without saline-immediate-spin crossmatch.
§After release, screening is completed for less common antibodies.

Table **14-8**	**Transfusion Reactions**			
Reaction	**Cause**	**Prevention**	**Assessment**	**Intervention**
Hemolytic	Blood incompatibility	Type and crossmatch; infuse first 50 ml slowly	Fever, chills, dyspnea, tachypnea, lumbar pain, fever, oliguria, hematuria, tightness in chest; collect blood and urine samples	Discontinue immediately; fatality may occur after 100 ml infused Start NS or RL* Consider diuretics; monitor BUN, serum creatinine
Allergic	Antibody reaction to allergens	Screen donors for allergy; administer antihistamines before transfusion	Hypersensitivity, chills, hives, wheezing, vertigo, angioneurotic edema, allergic itching Anaphylaxis, dyspnea, bronchospasm, hypotension, decreased responsiveness, generalized edema	Stop infusion; give antihistamine, steroids, and antipyretics Stop infusion; administer epinephrine, start NS or RL* Anticipate intubation
Pyrogenic	Infusing chilled blood	Screen donors; use aseptic technique in administration	Fever, chills, nausea, lumbar pain	Stop infusion
Hypothermic	Infusing chilled blood	Give at room temperature; use warming coils for rapid infusion	Chills	Slow infusion; cover client
Circulatory overload	Infusion of large amounts of blood, especially to clients with cardiac disease or extremes of age	Infuse slowly; check drip rate frequently	Rales, cough, dyspnea, cyanosis, pulmonary edema, increased CVP	Stop infusion; treat pulmonary edema
Air embolism	Entry of air into vein	Use proper infusion technique; avoid giving under pressure; check connections to tubings; avoid Y-tubes; use filter; use plastic containers	Chest pain, dyspnea, hypotension, venous distension	Stop infusion; position on left side; give oxygen; embolectomy may be performed
Hypocalcemic	Precipitate from acid citrate dextrose Calcium dilution with massive transfusions	Use blood immediately	Numbness, tingling in extremities May contribute to development of diffuse intravascular coagulation	Stop infusion; give calcium as ordered
Hyperkalemic	Hemolysis of red blood cells releases potassium	Use blood immediately	Nausea, vomiting, muscle weakness, bradycardia	Stop infusion

Modified from Barber J, Stokes L, Billings D: *Adult and child care: a client approach to nursing,* ed 2, St. Louis, 1977, Mosby.
*NS = normal saline
 RL = Ringer's lactated solution

SUMMARY

Intravenous lines provide a route for administration of medications, fluids, blood, and blood products. Venous access and fluid replacement can save the patient's life or create significant threats to health if vigilance is not used with catheter insertion and fluid administration. Consistent use of universal precautions, sharps disposal, and aseptic technique protect the patient and the emergency nurse. Assessment and reassessment during fluid replacement can identify symptoms related to fluid overload, and anaphylaxis and other side effects.

REFERENCES

1. Bernardo LM, Bove M: *Pediatric emergency nursing procedures,* Boston, 1993, Jones and Bartlett.
2. Kitt S, et al., editors: *Emergency nursing: a physiologic and clinical perspective,* ed 2, Philadelphia, 1995, WB Saunders Co.
3. Lewis SM, Collier IC, Heitkemper MM: *Medical-surgical nursing: assessment and management of clinical problems,* ed 4, St. Louis, 1996, Mosby.
4. Proehl JA: *Adult emergency nursing procedures,* Boston, 1993, Jones and Bartlett.

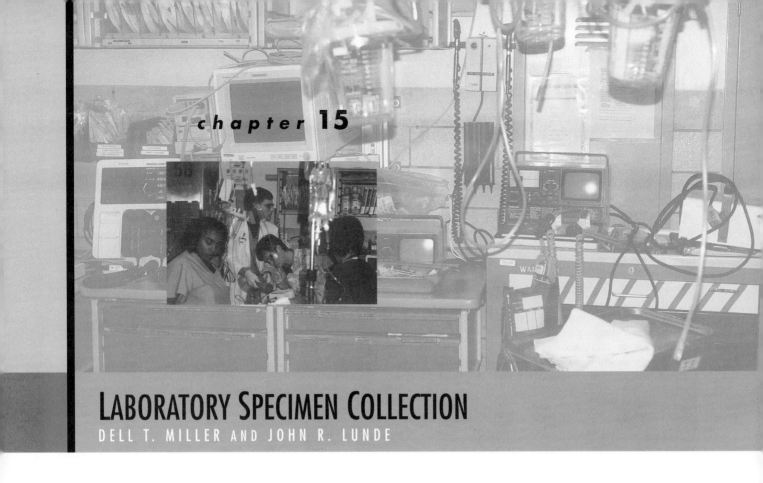

chapter **15**

LABORATORY SPECIMEN COLLECTION

DELL T. MILLER AND JOHN R. LUNDE

The act of obtaining blood specimens has been practiced since antiquity. Specimens are used to diagnose and monitor the disease process to determine patient treatment. Appropriate diagnosis and treatment of acute disorders in the emergency department (ED) depend on accurate collection and interpretation of laboratory data. A viable specimen is the key to the entire practice of laboratory medicine and vital to the practice of emergency care. Emergency personnel are often called on to obtain specimens for laboratory analysis. The process is not complicated, but does require attention to detail and accuracy.

BLOOD COLLECTION

Blood for analysis may be collected from the venous, arterial, or capillary system. In general, the majority of blood specimens are venous samples. Collection of blood from the arterial system has a higher risk for complications; therefore, collection of arterial samples is usually limited to arterial blood gas (ABG) analysis. Capillary specimens are collected primarily from infants and children. Regardless of collection site or specimen type, the specimen must be collected using aseptic technique to minimize the risks of infection to the patient and to avoid contaminating specimens. Personnel collecting the specimen should always use universal precautions and review laboratory orders before specimen collection to ensure that the proper tube is used for each test. Box 15-1 identifies general rules of safety for specimen collection.

Collection Systems

Venous or arterial blood may be collected from a primary venipuncture or may be withdrawn from existing access points such as venous access ports, central venous catheters, or arterial catheters.

Evacuated blood collection system

The evacuated blood collection system (EBCS) is the most widely used and recognized collection system available. EBCS allows collection of multiple specimens with a single venipuncture (Figure 15-1). The key element in the system is an evacuated specimen tube. Vacuum in the tube pulls blood into the tube after the blood vessel has been cannulated. Tubes have color-coded stoppers to indicate additives present. Table 15-1 lists tubes by color, the additives present in the tube, and what the additive does. As with intravenous (IV) and intramuscular needles, these needles are color-coded for length and diameter.

Nonevacuated collection system

The nonevacuated collection system is not used as frequently as the EBCS, but is a valuable collection system in certain circumstances. This system uses manual pressure rather than a vacuum to withdraw blood, and is recommended when the vacuum in the EBCS causes the vein to collapse preventing blood collection, such as in the very young or the very old. One example of this system is a butterfly attached to a syringe.

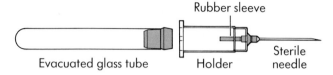

Figure **15-1** Evacuated blood collection system.

Box 15-1	**General Guidelines for Specimen Collection**

Use universal precautions.

Use aseptic technique.

Review laboratory orders before collection to confirm tests and tubes required for each test.

Identify the patient before specimen collection. Confirm medical record identification number.

Tell the patient what you are going to do.

Position the patient for safety and specimen collection.

Label all specimens with patient name and identification number.

Do not collect the specimen from a site proximal to an intravenous catheter.

Venous Collection

The venous system is the primary source for blood specimens used for laboratory testing. Only a few of the many veins in the human body are actually accessible for venipuncture or IV cannulation, so care must be exercised to guard limited resources for future specimen collection and IV therapy. Most venous specimens are obtained from primary puncture in the antecubital area. Figure 15-2 highlights veins in this area. The vein is selected after visual inspection; however, this should never be the sole method for selection. Palpating for location, size, fullness, and softness of the vein wall is also performed. Figure 15-3 illustrates the technique for venipuncture and specimen collection. The tourniquet is never left on for more than 2 minutes because hemoconcentration can affect test results. The tourniquet is released and reapplied before preparing the puncture site.

With the exception of coagulation tubes, which must be filled completely, most tubes contain an adequate volume of blood when they are at least half full. A general rule of thumb is that the tube should contain one part additive to nine parts blood. Tubes that do not contain an adequate amount of blood proportionate to the additive can lead to erroneous results. Also, tubes should be filled in a specific order to prevent specimen contamination from additives in the tubes: tests are collected for blood cultures first, then red top tubes, blue top coagulation tubes, and finally purple top hematology tubes. The patient's condition is always a determinant of which tests are most important; therefore the priority of collection should reflect this.

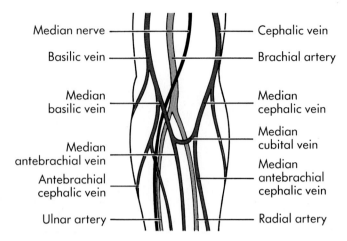

Figure **15-2** Superficial arteries and nerves in antecubital fossa.

Table 15-1	**Commonly Used Evacuated Specimen Tubes**	
Stopper color	Additive	Action; notes
Red	None	—
Red/black	Inert silicon gel	Acts as a separator between red blood cells and serum after centrifuging
Purple	Ethylenediamine tetraacetic acid (EDTA)	Chelates calcium from the blood, thus preventing clotting; the potassium salt of EDTA is usually used
Blue	Sodium citrate	Same action as for EDTA; the anticoagulant of choice for coagulation studies
Black	Sodium citrate	Same action as for EDTA; used for red blood cell sedimentation studies
Gray	Potassium oxalate	Same action as for EDTA; is also a glycolytic inhibitor for glucose determinations
Green	Heparin	Prevents clotting by deactivating thrombin and thromboplastin; both sodium and lithium salts are used

---

Failure to obtain blood may be caused by several problems. The needle may go through the vein and must be withdrawn slowly watching for blood in the tube. The needle may not puncture the vein, and venipuncture must be attempted at another site; however, multiple sticks are not to be attempted. If the specimen cannot be obtained after two attempts, someone else should stick the patient. Tubes can lose vacuum be-

A   **B**   **C**

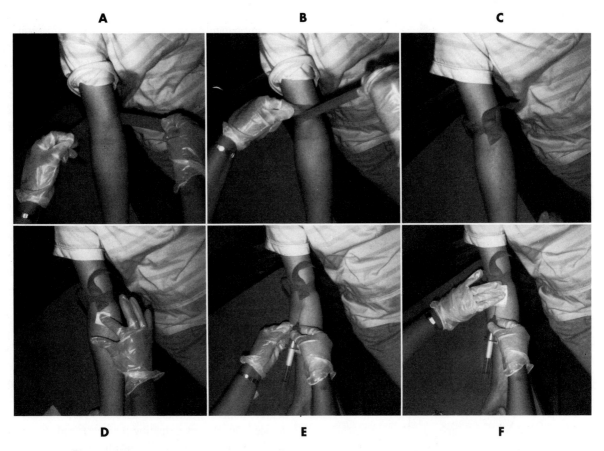

D   **E**   **F**

Figure **15-3**   Venipuncture procedure. **A,** Wrap tourniquet around arm. **B,** Pull one end taut while holding other in place. **C,** Loop opposite end under taut end to form slip knot. **D,** Cleanse puncture site with 70% isopropyl alcohol, followed by providone iodine, using circular motion. **E,** Insert EBCS needle into skin at 20- to 30-degree angle to arm with needle bevel up. **F,** As needle is removed, place pressure on site.

cause of age or a puncture that opens the tube to outside air. When this occurs, another tube must be inserted. If the vein is small and fragile, the vacuum may cause the vein to collapse. In this situation, a needle and syringe are the best alternative. Alternative sites for specimen collection, such as the femoral vein, should be considered. Blood may also be collected when an IV catheter is inserted. A catheter can be used to withdraw the blood, or a Luer lock adapter can be used to fill the tubes directly from the IV.

Capillary Collection

Capillary specimens are obtained from infants, children, and adults where multiple blood samples must be taken over a period of time (e.g., glucose testing in diabetic patients). The basic capillary collection system uses a lancet to puncture the skin and a container to collect the specimen. The containers are similar to blood tubes for venous samples in that they contain various additives; however, the requisite volume is smaller.

In children younger than 1 year of age, the heel or great toe is preferred.[6] Figure 15-4 illustrates preferred sites in the foot. The ring finger of the nondominant hand is preferred for capillary sticks on children and adults (Figure 15-5). Lancets are used that minimize depth of penetration. A penetration greater than 2.4 mm has been associated with development of osteomyelitis and sepsis. The area is warmed for 3 to 5 minutes with a heel warmer or cloth soaked in warm water to increase circulation and facilitate specimen collection. Povidone iodine affects results, falsely elevating potassium, phosphorus, uric acid, and bilirubin levels and should be avoided. The first drop of blood is discarded because it contains fluids from the tissues rather than the capillaries. Moderate pressure is adequate since excessive pressure can cause hemolysis, bruise the heel, and contaminate the specimen with tissue fluids. Collection from the finger is the same procedure as collection from the heel or toe. The lancet should puncture the pulp of the finger.

For blood sugar analysis, the finger is held over the analysis strip and the blood is dropped onto the strip. This provides the best sample for the test. If a platelet count is ordered, this test is drawn first. Platelets clump, so the count is often lower in capillary specimens.

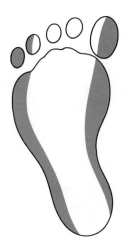

Figure **15-4**   Shaded areas represent areas on infant's foot that are used for obtaining blood specimen.

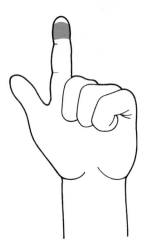

Figure **15-5**   Shaded area represents area commonly used for obtaining blood specimen from fingertip.

Venous Access Devices

In addition to primary venipuncture, venous samples may also be collected from intermittent infusion catheters, indwelling central venous catheters, and implanted central venous access devices.[3] General rules of asepsis and the use of universal precautions also apply to collection from these access points.

Intermittent infusion catheters

If a patient has an intermittent infusion catheter, blood may be collected from this site provided that collection does not endanger the integrity of the catheter. The process is the same as that for blood collection from a primary venipuncture with a few exceptions. If the catheter has an access port that must be punctured by a needle, the port must be carefully cleaned before use. After the port is punctured, 3 to 5 ml of blood is withdrawn and discarded before the venous specimen is collected.[4] Blood cultures are never drawn from an indwelling catheter because of the risks for contamination.

Central venous access devices

Many patients have long-term indwelling central venous catheters. The catheter tip is located in the superior vena cava or other large vessel. Access ports may be located subcutaneously or externally. Catheters located in the central circulation are at greater risk for systemic complications if contamination occurs. In addition to gloves and aseptic technique, masks are recommended to prevent droplet contamination.

External devices

Hickmann and Groshong catheters are long-term devices with external ports (Figure 15-6). The ports for these catheters are usually located at the 4th or 5th intercostal space. When blood is collected from these devices, 3 to 5 ml of blood is withdrawn and discarded before the sample is obtained. Once the specimen is obtained, the catheter should be flushed with saline. A dilute heparin solution can be used to flush the Hickman catheter; however, heparin should not be used with the Groshong catheter.

Internal devices

The Port-a-Cath Mediport and Bard Implanted Port are examples of an internal central venous access device, which is surgically implanted in subcutaneous tissue with the tip in the superior vena cava. The device has a self-sealing diaphragm that is ideal for multiple sticks (Figure 15-7). A 90-degree, noncoring needle is used to access the device. The device is located by palpating the chest, and stabilized with the thumb and forefinger. The needle is inserted into the center of the device at a 90-degree angle until it touches the bottom of the device. The device is then flushed with 5 ml of saline to ensure patency, and 5 ml of blood is withdrawn and discarded.

Arterial Systems

Arterial blood is usually obtained for ABG analysis. Blood may be collected from the radial, brachial, and femoral arteries. The radial artery is the preferred site for arterial puncture (Figure 15-8) because there is collateral circulation to the hand via the ulnar artery, the vessel is easily accessible for palpation and stabilization, and the surrounding tissue is relatively insensitive. The brachial artery (Figure 15-8) is the second choice for arterial collection; disadvantages include the lack of collateral circulation, vessel instability, and close proximity to the brachial nerve. The femoral artery (Figure 15-8) is used when no other site is available. Special precautions must be taken when collecting blood from this site because of the increased risk for hematoma formation and other complications.

Before the radial artery is punctured, an Allen's test is usually performed to ensure collateral circulation to the hand.[5] Box 15-2 and Figure 15-9 describe this test. If the test is positive, collateral circulation to the hand is present and the specimen can be collected.[1] Hyperextending the wrist moves the artery closer to the surface and aids stabilization and puncture. The needle is inserted at a 45-degree angle to

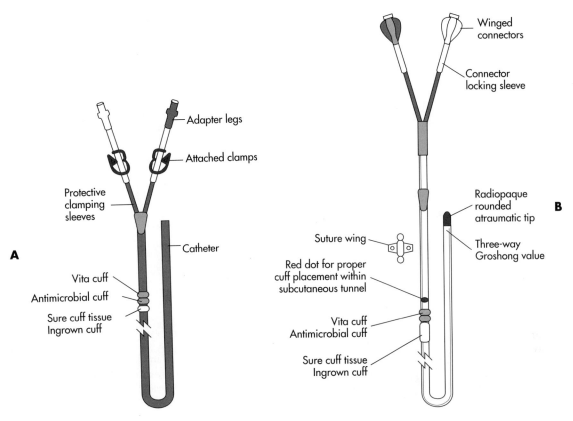

Figure **15-6** External central venous access devices. **A**, Hickman Dual-Lumen Catheter. **B**, Groshong Dual-Lumen Catheter. *(From Kidd PS, Sturt P:* Mosby's emergency nursing reference, *St. Louis, 1996, Mosby.)*

Box **15-2**   **Procedure for Allen's Test**

Flex arm with hand above level of the elbow.

Have patient clench fist. This forces blood from the hand.

Place pressure on both arteries simultaneously, then ask patient to open the hand. The hand should appear blanched.

Remove pressure from the ulnar artery. The blanched area flushes within seconds if collateral circulation is adequate.

If the area flushes quickly, this is recorded as a positive Allen's test. The test is negative if the blanched area does not flush quickly.

A negative Allen's test means collateral circulation is inadequate to support circulation to the hand; therefore, an alternative site should be selected.

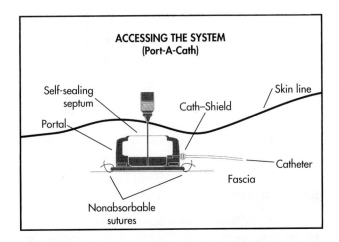

Figure **15-7** Implanted access device. *(Modified from Kandt KA:* An implantable venous access device for children, *MCN 16:88–91, March/April 1991.)*

the skin. This minimizes the actual opening into the arterial wall and promotes closure once the needle is removed. Brachial punctures may be performed at a 45- to 60-degree angle, whereas the femoral vein is punctured at a 90-degree angle. Figure 15-9 shows needle placement for radial artery puncture. Once the specimen is collected, pressure should be applied to the puncture site for at least 5 minutes, or for 10 minutes if the femoral artery is punctured or if the patient

is on anticoagulants. The specimen is placed on ice if analysis is delayed. Most venous blood tests can be collected from an arterial stick.

Arterial specimens may also be drawn from an existing arterial line. Similarly, a discard sample of 3 to 5 ml is collected before collection of the actual specimen. Care should

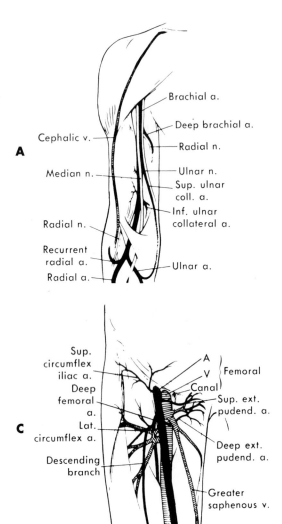

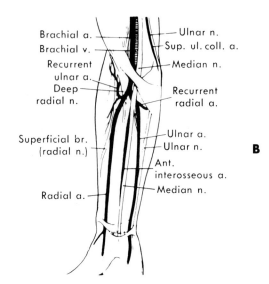

Figure **15-8** **A,** Brachial artery, continuation of axillary artery. **B,** Radial artery extends from neck of radius to median side of styloid process. **C,** Femoral artery branches from abdominal aorta and branches to superficial epigastric, superficial circumflex iliac, external pudendal, deep femoral, and descending geniculate arteries. *(Modified from Budassi SA: J Emerg Nurs 3(2):24, 1977.)*

be taken to prevent introduction of air into the system during the process. In some institutions, the discard sample is returned to the patient after the actual specimen is collected; however, this is more common with neonates and infants.

URINE SPECIMENS

Urine testing is one of the world's oldest laboratory tests. Ancient Greeks used a "taste" test to determine the presence of sugar in the urine. Urine tests are used to assess renal function, diagnose disease, and confirm pregnancy. Urine normally contains numerous metabolic end products and water. Obtaining a good urine specimen is just as important as obtaining a good blood specimen.

The basic urine specimen is a clean-catch, midstream specimen. Catheterization or a percutaneous bladder tap may also be used. A specimen collection bag is used for infants, and is placed on the infant before venipuncture. Catheterization is often recommended for female patients to

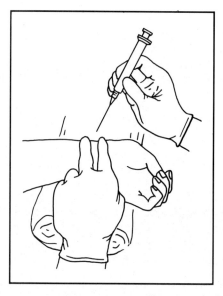

Figure **15-9** Puncture of radial artery.

minimize contamination from the vagina. A small female catheter, available in size 5 or 8 Fr, is recommended to minimize discomfort. When catheterization is necessary in infants, a size 5 or 8 Fr catheter is recommended. If sexual assault is suspected, the genitalia should not be cleaned before specimen collection. The specimen should be placed in a dry, sterile container and analyzed within 1 hour of collection. Specimens more than 2 hours old should not be submitted for analysis. Accelerated chemical changes, decomposition of cellular contents, and growth of bacteria can alter test results. When toxicologic screening is required, 30 to 50 ml of urine is necessary. Special regulations apply to collection of specimens in the case of a criminal action or an on-the-job injury.

BODY FLUID SPECIMENS

In addition to blood and urine, laboratory analysis is done on pleural fluid, synovial fluid, amniotic fluid, peritoneal fluid, gastric fluid, and cerebrospinal fluid. If a cell count is required on body fluid, it should be placed in a tube containing EDTA or heparin to prevent clotting. Fluid for chemistry analysis is put in a red top tube. Synovial fluid for crystal analysis should be placed in tubes containing heparin. If the fluid is to be cultured, it is usually left in the collection syringe. The syringe should be capped to ensure an anaerobic environment. Emesis and gastric fluids are used primarily for toxicologic analysis. Complete information about suspected substances should be provided along with the specimen. Amniotic fluid must be protected from light as soon as the sample is obtained and during transport to the laboratory. This prevents light breakdown of bilirubin in the specimen.

Cerebrospinal fluid may be submitted in three to five tubes containing 0.5 to 1 ml of fluid each. Tubes are filled in order with Tube 1 filled first. Various facilities and physicians prefer to submit particular tubes for specific tests. In general, Tube 1 is used for chemistry analysis, Tube 2 for cell and differential counts, and Tube 3 or 4 for microbiology (i.e., culture, gram stain). Tube 5 is held for any special testing that may be required. When obtaining a sample is difficult, microbiology testing is usually given priority over other tests. Cerebrospinal fluid should be transported promptly to the laboratory for processing.

SPUTUM SPECIMENS

Sputum may be collected for culture, gram stain, and other tests. It should be obtained before giving antimicrobial therapy. Many institutions have a high-fail rate for sputum collection, collecting saliva and oral secretions more often than sputum. The delays in definitive therapy as a result create a significant financial burden, because cultures must be repeated. Also, broader spectrum antibiotics are ordered when the organism is not identified, which leads to longer therapy while the test is repeated. Box 15-3 describes the procedure for sputum collection.[5]

Box **15-3** **Sputum Collection**

Explain the procedure and the purpose of sputum collection to the patient.
Remind the patient that sputum must be coughed up from the lungs and that saliva is not the specimen required.
Provide sterile container.
Ask patient to rinse mouth before collection to decrease specimen contamination.
A total of 5 ml sputum is required.
Instruct the patient to take several deep breaths and cough to expectorate the specimen.
Aerosolized warm saline solution may be given if the patient is unable to produce a specimen.

STOOL SPECIMENS

Stool specimens may be collected for cell counts, presence of ova and parasites, and cultures. A fresh, warm stool is preferred for a culture. A small amount of stool is collected from a bedpan and placed in a dry, sterile container. Care is taken not to contaminate the sample with urine. Therapy should be withheld until specimens are obtained. Specimens for parasitology should be submitted as soon as possible. Unpreserved specimens must be examined for trophozoites within 1 hour. A specimen can be preserved for later examination by dividing it into three portions: one unpreserved, one mixed with polyvinyl alcohol (PVA), and the third mixed with 10% formalin. Stool samples are usually obtained for three consecutive days.

MICROBIOLOGY SPECIMENS

Microbiology specimens are referred to as aerobic or anaerobic specimens. Aerobic specimens are obtained when the organism to be identified can be grown in the presence of oxygen (e.g., *Streptococcus* and *Staphylococcus*). Anaerobic specimens are obtained when the organism to be identified grows without oxygen. Examples include the *Clostridia* species that causes gangrene or botulism.

Specimens are placed on a designated transport medium after collection. Various swabs with transport media are available commercially for aerobic and anaerobic cultures. Specimens, particularly anaerobic specimens, should be transported to the laboratory as soon as possible after collection. When rapid monoclonal antibody testing for *Streptococcus* is available, two throat swabs should be submitted: one swab for a confirmatory culture, and one for rapid testing.

GUIDE TO SELECTED LABORATORY RESULTS

Evaluation of laboratory results is based on comparison of the patient's results to a range of normal values for a given test. A range is usually plus or minus two standard deviations from the mean result for a representative, healthy population. Most health care facilities publish ranges of normal values for the area and population they serve. Normal ranges discussed in this text are generally accepted values for the identified test. Values for a specific institution may vary.

Arterial Blood Gases

Results reported for ABGS are a combination of measured values and calculated values. The pH, PCO_2, and PO_2 values are measured, whereas the HCO_3, O_2 saturation, and base excess values are calculated. Normal values are identified in Table 15-2.[5] Normal PO_2 values vary with elevation above sea level.

Actual interpretation of ABG results is a two-step process. The acid-base status is determined first, then the patient's oxygen status is determined. Acute and chronic acid-base disturbances include metabolic and respiratory acidosis and metabolic and respiratory alkalosis. Table 15-3 highlights ABG results associated with these acid-base disturbances. Common causes of acid-base disturbances are identified in Table 15-4.

Electrolytes

Body fluid is composed primarily of water and dissolved substances called electrolytes, which carry a negative or positive charge. An anion carries a negative charge, whereas a cation carries a positive charge. Electrolytes are measured in millequivalents per liter (mEq/L) with a balance of cations and anions in the body. Normal ranges for intravascular electrolytes are listed in Table 15-5. The amount of each electrolyte within the cells varies. Table 15-6 lists causes for major electrolyte imbalances. (Refer to Chapter 40 for more discussion on electrolytes.)

Complete Blood Cell Count

The complete blood cell count (CBC) is used to determine the patient's hematologic status. Historically, a CBC has been reported in two parts: the cell count and the differential count. The cell count was done by machine, and the differential count was done manually. Electronic particle counters have made this process almost obsolete, providing an automated cell count and differential count; however, if the automated differential count reported is abnormal, a manual count is then done.

Table 15-2	Normal Arterial Blood Gas Values
Component	Normal range
pH	7.35 to 7.45
PCO_2	35 to 45 mmHg
PO_2	80 mmHg
HCO_3	22 to 28 mEq/L

Table 15-3	Assessment of Arterial Blood Gas Values		
Condition	pH	PCO_2	HCO_3
Acute metabolic acidosis	<7.30	<30	Depressed
Chronic metabolic acidosis	Normal	Depressed	Depressed
Acute respiratory acidosis	<7.30	>50	Normal
Chronic respiratory acidosis	Normal	>50	Elevated
Acute metabolic alkalosis	>7.50	Elevated	Elevated
Chronic metabolic alkalosis	Normal	>50	Elevated
Acute respiratory alkalosis	>7.50	<30	Normal
Chronic respiratory alkalosis	Normal	<30	Depressed

Table 15-4	Common Causes of Acid-base Disturbances
Acid-base disturbance	Causes
Metabolic acidosis	Renal failure, diabetic ketoacidosis, starvation, lactic acidosis, hepatic collapse, ingestion of methanol, ASA, or other acids
Metabolic alkalosis	Extended IV therapy, diuretics, diarrhea, gastric suction or vomiting, steroid therapy, excessive use of $NaHCO_3$
Respiratory acidosis	COPD, respiratory arrest, primary alveolar hyperventilation, pulmonary edema
Respiratory alkalosis	CNS trauma, CNS infection, carbon monoxide poisoning, anemia, anxiety, psychosis, pain, hyperventilation, hypoxia

Table 15-5	Normal Ranges of Electrolyte Values	
Electrolyte	Serum	Urine
Sodium (Na)	136 to 142 mEq/L	80 to 180 mEq/24 hr
Potassium (K)	3.8 to 5.0 mEq/L	40 to 80 mEq/24 hr
Chloride (Cl)	93 to 105 mEq/L	110 to 250 mEq/24 hr
Carbon dioxide (CO_2)	24 to 30 mM/L	—
Magnesium (Mg)	1.8 to 3.0 mg/100 ml	6.0 to 8.5 mEq/24 hr
Calcium (Ca)	8.5 to 10.5 mg/100 ml	100 to 250 mg/24 hr

The cell count of the CBC provides normal values for leukocytes, erythrocytes, hemoglobin and hematocrit (Table 15-7). Normal CBC values vary with the age and sex of the patient. The differential count provides information on red cell morphology and the percentage distribution of leukocytes. See Chapter 44 for discussion of these cell types. The differential is also helpful in evaluation of malaria and other parasites as well as in identification of abnormal cells.[2]

Table 15-6 Causes of Electrolyte Imbalance

Imbalance	Causes
Hyponatremia	Excess sweating, excess intake of water, diuretics, adrenal insufficiency, renal failure
Hypernatremia	Diarrhea, decreased water intake, salt water ingestion, impaired renal function, febrile illness, inability to swallow, burns, diabetes insipidus
Hypokalemia	Diarrhea, vomiting, diuretics, burns, heat stress, ulcerative colitis, potassium-free IV fluids, metabolic acidosis, steroids
Hyperkalemia	Acute/chronic renal failure, burns, crush injuries, metabolic acidosis, potassium-sparing diuretics

Urinalysis

Urine is composed of 95% water and 5% solutes. Solutes normally found in urine include nitrogenous wastes such as creatinine, uric acid, and urea. Urine also contains electrolytes and pigments derived from bile. A urinalysis tests for the presence of abnormal constituents such as protein, glucose, white blood cells, red blood cells, and ketones. Protein in the urine may indicate glomerulonephritis. Glucosuria may be caused by insulin deficiency, stress, or renal disease. White blood cells indicate infection, whereas red blood cells are seen with inflammation, trauma, kidney stones, or posturethral catheterization. Incomplete oxidation of fat leads to ketones in the urine, often seen with diabetes or starvation.

The most commonly used form of urine testing is a reagent tablet or a dipstick. Each strip contains pads that show reactions to specific components of the urine, such as protein, bilirubin, ketones, glucose. Urinary pH, specific gravity, color, and appearance are also included in the urinalysis.

CONCLUSION

Analysis of various laboratory tests is the foundation for many diagnostic and therapeutic challenges. Without the benefit of sound specimen collection, diagnosis and treatment for many patients is needlessly delayed. This can place the patient's life in danger, increase potential complications, and add to overall cost of health care. A certificate of waiver for ED laboratory testing covers urine dipstick, urine preg-

Table 15-7 Components of Complete Blood Cell Count

Component	Normal values	Comments
White blood cell count	$5\text{-}10,000/\text{mm}^3$	
Red blood cell count	Male $4.6\text{-}6.2\ \text{ml/mm}^3$ Female $4.2\text{-}5.4\ \text{ml/mm}^3$	
Hemoglobin level	Male $14\text{-}18\ \text{g}/100\ \text{ml}$ Female $12\text{-}16\ \text{g}/100\ \text{ml}$	A conjugated protein responsible for oxygen and CO_2 transport in the blood
Hematocrit	Male $40\%\text{-}54\%$ Female $37\%\text{-}47\%$	Percentage (volume) of red blood cells in a volume of blood, generally equal to the hemoglobin level $\times\ 3 \pm 2$
Mean corpuscular volume (MCV)	$82\text{-}92\ \mu\text{m}^3$	Average volume of red blood cells in a sample
Mean corpuscular hemoglobin (MCH) content	$27\text{-}37\ \mu\text{g}$	Average hemoglobin content of red blood cells in a sample
Mean corpuscular hemoglobin concentration (MCHC)	$32\%\text{-}36\%$	Average hemoglobin content in 100 ml of blood
Platelets	$150,000\text{-}400,000/\mu\text{L}$	Platelets aid in hemostasis and maintenance of vascular integrity

nancy, glucose, and stool hematocrit. However, positive results must be confirmed by laboratory analysis.

REFERENCES

1. Emergency Nurses Association: *Emergency nursing core curriculum,* ed 4, Philadelphia, 1994, WB Saunders.
2. Ignatavicius DD, Workman ML, Mishler MA: *Medical-surgical nursing: a nursing process approach,* ed 2, Philadelphia, 1995, WB Saunders.
3. Kitt S et al: *Emergency nursing—a physiologic and clinical perspective,* Philadelphia, 1995, WB Saunders.
4. Smith R: A nurse's guide to implanted ports, *RN* pp. 48-52, April 1993.
5. Thompson JM et al: *Mosby's clinical nursing,* ed 3, St. Louis, 1993, Mosby.
6. Wong DL: *Whaley & Wong's essentials of pediatric nursing,* ed 5, St. Louis, 1997, Mosby.

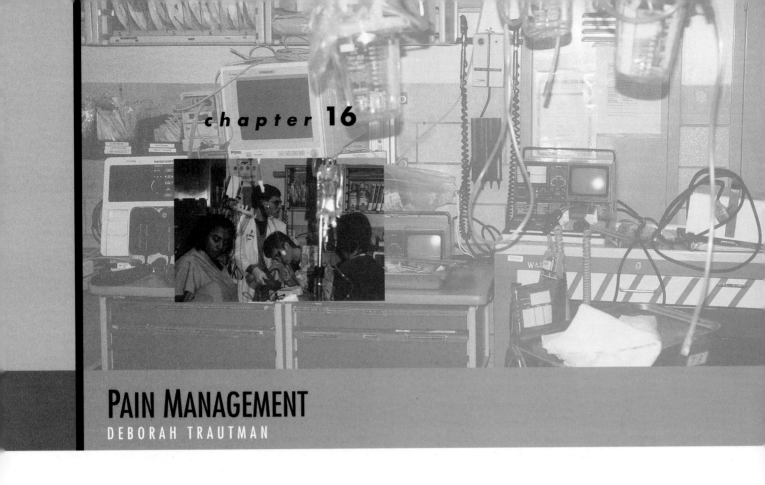

chapter 16

Pain Management

DEBORAH TRAUTMAN

In the practice of emergency nursing, patients are encountered who need assistance in the relief of acute pain. Pain is the most frequent complaint that motivates people to seek emergency medical care. Emergency nurses are challenged to manage acute pain of patients with unique needs in an often chaotic environment. The relief of acute pain and suffering should be a primary goal in treating an acutely painful injury or illness. Unfortunately, emergency nurses and physicians often fail to address pain management adequately. Traditionally, prompt management of pain in the emergency department (ED) has been neglected. Relief of pain is not universally accepted as essential in emergency care.

Effective pain management may be neglected for several reasons; however, three prominent reasons usually emerge: (1) emergency nurses and physicians often believe that treating pain early may delay or complicate the workup or examination of the patient; (2) they may not believe or understand the patient's complaint of pain; and (3) they may be reluctant to use narcotics because of fear of addiction or uncontrollable life-threatening side effects such as respiratory depression. Consequently, inadequate pain management occurs often in the ED; therefore, education about ED pain management is essential. Emergency nurses have an obligation to advocate effective pain relief for their patients. This advocacy can be facilitated by increasing one's knowledge of pain, emphasizing a more prominent role in helping patients and physicians manage acute pain, and monitoring treatment plans to ensure safe and effective pain management for ED patients.

DEFINITION OF PAIN

Attempts at defining pain vary widely; however, the definition most commonly accepted in nursing is "whatever the experiencing person says it is, existing whenever he or she says it does, including both verbal and nonverbal behavior."[9] Pain is subdivided into two types: acute and chronic. McCaffery[10] defines acute pain as "an episode lasting from a second to less than six months." Chronic pain is usually defined as pain that lasts for 6 months or longer. Additionally, acute pain is usually a symptom of an identifiable disease, persisting only as long as the disease itself and responding to adequate pain management. Chronic pain may be associated with chronic tissue disease, may not have an identifiable cause, may last longer than the normal healing period for an acute injury or disease, and may not respond to standard analgesic interventions. Chronic pain management is beyond the scope of emergency care. This chapter focuses exclusively on management of acute pain.

To understand acute pain management, the nurse must recognize that acute pain has two components: the actual physical stimulus and the patient's cognitive and emotional interpretation of that stimuli. Although removal or treatment of the actual physical stimulus is the most reliable and therapeutic approach to pain control, nursing interventions and the nurse's role in particular can greatly influence the patient's interpretation of pain. A patient's interpretation of pain is influenced by a variety of factors such as culture, religious beliefs, coping styles, and trust and fear about the ED visit.

A calm, empathetic nurse can do much to minimize a patient's fears and facilitate early pain management. In a study of 148 patients, Copp[4] found that patients frequently shared ideas on how nurses and physicians could help them with their pain. Box 16-1 summarizes these ideas. These are important points for the nurse to incorporate into the role of assisting with pain management. Traditionally, many nurses considered their role in pain management to be simply administering physicians' orders. This is an antiquated belief that minimizes the nurse's contribution to patient care. The emergency nurse's role is vital to facilitating early relief of pain and suffering. The nurse should assure the patient that the health care team believes that the patient is in pain and will treat the pain soon and effectively.

PATHOPHYSIOLOGY

Pain is a multidimensional phenomena consisting of psychologic and physiologic components.[8] Physical, neurologic, and biochemical properties comprise the physiologic aspect of pain. Somatic sensation is initiated by a variety of somatic receptors.[17] Pain, one type of somatic sensation, is associated with specific receptors known as nociceptors. Stimulation of nociceptors results in the sensation of pain. Mechanical, thermal, or chemical irritation can depolarize nociceptors and initiate action potentials in the afferent nerve fibers, which conduct impulses toward the brain or spinal cord; efferent nerve fibers carry impulses away from the brain or spinal cord.

Three primary theories of pain perception exist. The specificity theory proposed by Muller proposes that specific receptors exist for pain. Wolland and Seridan developed the pattern theory, which states that multiple receptors form specific patterns of pain sensation. The gate theory developed by Melzak and Wall suggests that sensory input from peripheral fibers is transmitted to the dorsal horn of the spinal cord where it is modulated and then transmitted to the brain for perception.[15] A recent theory postulates that the classic pain pathway is dual. "The sensation of pain that is experienced arrives in the central nervous system by means of two pathways: (1) a sensory discriminate system that encodes the capacity to analyze the nature (e.g., burning or pricking), location, intensity, and duration of nociceptive stimulation,

and (2) an affective, motivational component that gives rise to the unpleasant character of painful sensation."[5] Inhibitory and augmentive controls exist. Prevention and treatment are guided by knowledge of the pathophysiology.

PATIENT ASSESSMENT

Management of acute pain begins with the initial nursing assessment. A concise, comprehensive assessment is essential. Not all patients adequately verbalize key components of their pain due to language barriers, fever, and other factors. Assessment indices include both subjective and objective measures. Because of the broad scope of nursing literature on patient assessment, the following discussion is limited to a brief summarization of nursing assessment of pain. For more detailed assessment techniques, see McCaffery and Beebe.[11]

An initial focused assessment should be conducted to collect data about the patient's pain. Carpenito[3] defines focused assessment as "the acquisition of selected or specific data as determined by the nurse and the client or family or by the condition of the client." Assessment of pain includes location, quality, intensity, onset, duration, and aggravating or alleviating factors.

Techniques such as facilitation (saying "mmm-hmm" or "go on"), reflection, repeating key phrases the patient said in a question format, and clarification of ambiguous statements facilitate collection of data pertinent to the chief complaint.[1] Prompting the patient by asking leading questions should be avoided. Adequate assessment of a patient's pain is hampered when the nurse makes inferences about the patient's pain.[10]

Objective data include, but are not limited to, physical description of the patient, any facial expressions, and measurement of pulse rate, blood pressure, and respiratory rate. After the initial assessment, the emergency nurse must ensure ongoing assessment and evaluation of the patient's pain. This ongoing assessment facilitates evaluation of treatment.

Assessment of pain in the pediatric patient is often difficult because of the child's inability to communicate. The child is observed for change in facial expression and body position. Numbers expressing severity of pain can be used for older children.

MANAGING PAIN

Managing pain is a multifaceted, multidimensional process. Physical, social, cultural, and psychologic needs, beliefs, and experiences all influence the process. The nurse's role in management of pain cannot be overstated. Essential nursing actions related to pain management are described in Box 16-2. Incorporating these components into the nursing role facilitates an effective nursing approach to and the probability of successful pain management. The nurse should avoid letting personal attitudes, beliefs, or values influence perceptions of the patient's pain or selection of pain control interventions.

Box 16-2 Essential Nursing Actions for Pain Control

- Establish an effective, supportive relationship with the patient.
- Believe, collaborate with, and respect the patient's response to pain and its management.
- Educate the patient about the occurrence, onset, and duration of pain; methods of pain relief; and preventive measures.
- Inform the patient what he or she is likely to experience while in the ED to minimize fear of the unknown.
- Maintain current knowledge and competencies.
- Monitor the patient's response and effectiveness of treatment.
- Communicate frequently and effectively with the patient and physician regarding the treatment plan and its effectiveness.
- Ensure patient safety at all times. Monitoring the patient facilitates assessment of treatment effectiveness and minimizes potential adverse occurrences.
- Maintain a calm, empathetic manner.
- Research the multidimensional nature of pain, its assessment, and subsequent management. Use this research in practice.

Box 16-3 Pain Control Interventions

- Medication
- Physical comfort
- Verbal reassurance
- Massage
- Distraction
- Relaxation techniques
- Breathing techniques
- Imagery

Box 16-4 Essential Aspects of Pain Control

No one universally superior method of pain management exists.

The goal of pain management is to prevent pain whenever possible. Pain relief is more effective if initiated soon after onset of pain.

The underlying cause of pain is an important consideration in selecting analgesia.[14]

A calm, quiet patient does not preclude the presence of pain.

A patient's refusal to accept pain medication may be related to fear of addiction, sedation, loss of control, or method of administration.

A patient's request for specific pain medication does not automatically mean he or she is a drug seeker.[14]

A patient's tolerance for pain is not directly proportional to the amount of analgesia required to relieve pain.

All pain is real. Pain is what a patient says it is.

Burke and Jerrett[2] found that tradition, intuition, and stereotypes influence interventions selected for pain management. Researchers studied student nurses' perceptions of the best interventions for people of various ages who were in acute pain. Age was identified as a factor that influenced both the number and type of interventions selected. In this study, student nurses selected more interventions for adolescents and adults, and fewer interventions for infants, toddlers, children, and the elderly. Of 8 possible intervention types (see Box 16-3), a mean of 3.3 types was selected for infants, 5.0 for adults, and 4.5 for the elderly. Additional research is indicated; however, nurses should be careful not to let personal belief negatively influence practice.

Pain management interventions include invasive techniques such as medication and noninvasive techniques such as imagery. When selecting a technique for a specific patient, the nurse should remember that each patient is unique and no one universally superior pain control method exists for all patients. Patients should be evaluated individually and interventions tailored to each patient and his or her situation. Box 16-4 identifies essential aspects of pain control. General principles of invasive and noninvasive pain management are discussed at top right.

Narcotics

Narcotic analgesics or opiates provide effective relief of acute pain. Narcotics can be classified as narcotic agonists, narcotic agonist-antagonists, and narcotic antagonists. Narcotic classification is summarized in Box 16-5.

Morphine is the prototypical opioid agonist with which all other opioids are compared.[12] Morphine and other narcotic analgesics directly affect the central nervous system, causing analgesia, changes in mood and emotion, respiratory depression, bronchoconstriction, miosis (pupil constriction), nausea, vomiting, and decreased gastric motility. Cardiovascular effects of narcotics are variable and require close monitoring of vital signs. Although morphine does not dramatically alter heart rate and blood pressure when administered in the right dosage, higher dosages can decrease heart rate and blood pressure. The efficacy of narcotic agonist-antagonist analgesics depends on proper dosage, rates of administration, and frequency of use (Table 16-1). Use of narcotic agonist-antagonist analgesics in patients addicted to narcotics can precipitate withdrawal and seizures.

Health professionals' fears of inducing addiction result in ineffective pain management. Physical dependence on narcotic agents may occur; however, repeated doses over a period of time are required to develop dependency. Questions and concerns arise when ED nurses are faced with administering narcotics to a known substance abuser. A substance abuse patient or narcotic addict has a right to effective pain management. Nurses should discuss the treatment plan with the patient and physician, the goal being to deliver humane care to a person with pain who happens to be a narcotic addict by relieving the pain and keeping the person out of

Table 16-1 Narcotic Agonist-Antagonist Analgesics

Drug	Average oral dose (mg)	Average parenteral dose (mg)	Duration (hr)	Comments	Precaution
Pentazocine (*Talwin*)	50 to 100	30 to 60	2 to 3	Suppositories available	Increase stroke work; high incidence of psychotomimetic effects
Nalbuphine (*Nubain*)	40	10 to 15	3 to 4	Minimal if any hemodynamic effects; ceiling on respiratory depression; low-abuse potential	Can precipitate withdrawal if dependence on narcotic agonist
Butorphanol (*Stadol*)	Not available	1 to 4	2½ to 3½		Cardiovascular effects similar to pentazocine; can precipitate withdrawal
Buprenorphine (*Buprenex*)		0.3 to 0.6	5 to 6	Partial agonist can be given sublingually; long analgesic action	Not completely antagonized by naloxone

withdrawal.[11] A substance abuse patient needs larger than usual doses. In the ED environment, the primary goal remains relief of acute pain, not drug rehabilitation.

Narcotics often cause nausea and vomiting; therefore, antiemetics such as promethazine are given in conjunction with these drugs.

Nurses should also be aware of mistakes that commonly occur with administration of narcotic analgesics, including the wrong dose, route, frequency of administration, and choice of drug.

Wrong dose

The most important factor in achieving adequate analgesia with a given narcotic is titrating the dose to achieve the desired degree of analgesia. A wide interpatient variability exists for effective analgesia concentration. The approach of treating all patients with 75 mg of meperidine (Demerol) or 10 mg of morphine is ineffective in many patients. Doses should be individualized for each patient.

Wrong route

The most commonly used route for parenteral administration of narcotics is an intramuscular injection (IM). This route has several disadvantages and should not be the primary route of choice. Intravenous (IV) and subcutaneous routes are preferred. Disadvantages of IM injections include
- Painful administration
- Delayed onset of action
- Inability to predict effect
- Inability to titrate dose easily
- Diurnal variation in level achieved
- Disease state may affect level achieved
- Level depends on muscle used

Wrong frequency of administration

An error that commonly occurs is failure to repeat narcotic administration frequently enough. Patient-controlled analgesia is an analgesia administration system designed to enable maintenance of optimal serum analgesic levels throughout a therapeutic course.[6] This system provides the patient with the ability to administer small IV doses without excessive sedation. Although patient-controlled analgesia is not widely used in the ED setting, its advantages suggest that it would be beneficial for some ED patients.

Wrong drug

In general, most narcotics can effectively produce the desired degree of analgesia if the proper dose is given. The exceptions to this rule are oral codeine and propoxyphene (*Darvon*). Codeine at any dose is not very potent, and propoxyphene has little justification for use; many studies have shown that propoxyphene is no more effective than placebo, or only marginally so.[13] Morphine, meperidine, fentanyl, and midazolam (*Versed*) are considered effective for use in the ED.

Nitrous Oxide

Nitrous oxide, a sedative analgesic agent, is a mixture of 50% nitrous oxide and 50% oxygen. Nitrous oxide is self-administered through a demand valve. Its benefits include rapid onset, safety, ease of administration, short duration, effectiveness, and cost.[15] A potential side effect may be cardiovascular depression when it is used concomitantly with narcotics. Research indicates that a 50:50 combination provides a safe, low-risk treatment modality without major side effects.

Contraindications include impairment of consciousness, inebriation, inability to understand instructions, dyspnea, cyanosis, presence or suggestion of pneumothorax, decompression sickness or air embolism, severe chronic lung disease, and abdominal pain with distension or suggestion of obstruction.

A primary nursing responsibility in nitrous oxide administration is patient education. The ED nurse should instruct patients to breathe normally. Deep or rapid breathing produces hyperventilation, which causes light-headedness and minimizes effective inhalation. The gas should be self-administered.

Box 16-5 Narcotic Classification

Agonists

Naturally occurring alkaloids and semisynthetic opiates
    Natural
        Morphine
        Codeine (methylmorphine)
    Semisynthetic
        Oxymorphone *(Numorphan)*
        Hydromorphone *(Dilaudid)*
        Hydrocodone *(Vicodin, Hycodan)*
        Heroin (diacetylmorphine)
        Oxycodone *(Percodan, Tylox)*
Meperidine and related phenylpiperidines (synthetic)
    Meperidine *(Demerol)*
    Alphaprodine *(Nisentil)*
    Diphenoxylate (in *Lomotil)*
    Fentanyl *(Sublimaze)*
    Alfentanil
    Sufentanil *(Sufenta)*
Methadone and related drugs
    Methadone *(Dolophine)*
    Propoxyphene *(Darvon)*
Morphine derivatives
    Levorphanol *(Levo-Dromoran)*
    Dextromethorphan

Agonist-antagonists

Nalorphine type
    Pentazocine *(Talwin)*
    Nalbuphine *(Nubain)*
    Butorphanol *(Stadol)*
Morphinelike drugs
    Buprenorphine *(Buprenex)*
    Meptazinol
    Profadol
    Propiram

Antagonists

Allyl-substituted compounds
    Nalorphine *(Nalline)*
    Naloxone *(Narcan)*
    Naltrexone *(Trexan)*
    Nalmefene

Box 16-6 Commonly Prescribed Nonnarcotic Analgesics

Acetaminophen *(Tylenol)*
Acetylsalicylic acid (aspirin)
Nonacetylated salicylates *(Dolobid, Trilisate)*
Acetic acids (indomethacin, sulindac, tolmetin)
Propionic acids (ibuprofen *[Motrin, Advil, Nuprin, Medipren]*,
    fenoprofen *[Nalfon], Ansaid*, naproxen *[Naprosyn]*)
Oxicams *(Feldene)*
Ketorolac tromethamine *(Toradol)*

---

nervous system, nonnarcotics affect the peripheral nervous system. Nonnarcotic agents act by inhibiting prostaglandin synthesis, which minimizes pain, edema, and inflammation.[12] Nonsteroidal antiinflammatory drugs (NSAIDs) are indicated for mild to moderate pain, and are frequently prescribed for musculoskeletal injuries, headaches, arthritis, dysmenorrhea, pleuritis, pharyngitis, ureteral colic, and other common painful conditions.[15] Major side effects from NSAIDs include gastrointestinal hemorrhage, renal failure, platelet dysfunction, and anaphylaxis; acute hypersensitivity may also occur. Concomitant use with a narcotic analgesic agent augments pain relief.

Ketorolac *(Toradol),* an NSAID available for short-term management of pain, is a potent injectable analgesic, antiinflammatory, antipyretic agent, which inhibits prostaglandin synthesis. Use is not recommended for obstetric preoperative medication or analgesia. Contraindications include demonstrated hypersensitivity to ketorolac, angioedemå, bronchospasm with aspirin or NSAIDs, and complete or partial syndrome of nasal polyps. The recommended initial dosage is 30 or 60 mg every 6 hours IV or IM as needed. Lower dosages are recommended for patients who weigh less than 50 kg or patients older than 65 years of age. Side effects are minimal but may include drowsiness, dyspepsia, gastrointestinal pain, nausea, diarrhea, edema, headache, and diaphoresis. Routine use with other NSAIDs is not recommended; however, ketorolac can be used concomitantly with morphine and meperidine without adverse effects.[16]

Local Anesthesia

Local anesthetics are often used for minor surgical procedures performed in the ED. Onset of rapid nerve block occurs within minutes and reverses within minutes or hours. Lidocaine, bupivacaine, procaine, and topical tetracaine *(Pontocaine)* are frequently used agents. A comparison of these agents is presented in Table 16-2. Mixing lidocaine with sodium bicarbonate decreases pain associated with the lidocaine injection.

Numerous local anesthetic mixtures are used as topical anesthetics for children who require sutures. Three mixtures are described in Table 16-3. A sterile cotton ball is soaked with the medication and applied to the laceration for a mini-

Family or friends must be instructed not to assist the patient. The risk of overdose is minimal if the gas is self-administered: when the patient becomes drowsy, the mask or mouthpiece simply falls away. The patient should be placed on a pulse oximeter to be continuously monitored for oxygen saturation during the procedure. In addition to patient education, the ED nurse should ensure that equipment is maintained. Daily inspection with a cleaning schedule is optimal.

Nonnarcotic Analgesics

Nonnarcotic analgesics (see Box 16-6) are widely used in emergency medicine. Unlike opiates that affect the central

Table 16-2	Local Anesthetic Agents*		
Agent	Uses	Dose and rates	Contraindications
Lidocaine	Peripheral nerve block: caudal, epidural, spinal; surgical anesthesia	Dependent on route; 0.5%, 1%, 1.5%, 2% with or without epinephrine; 4% without epinephrine; topical 5%; viscous	Hypersensitivity; children less than 12 years of age, elderly; liver disease
Bupivacaine	Peripheral nerve block: epidural and caudal	Dependent on route; 0.25%, 0.5%, 0.75% with or without epinephrine	Hypersensitivity; children less than 12 years of age, elderly; liver disease
Procaine	Peripheral nerve block: spinal, epidural; perineum, lower extremity infiltration	Dependent on route; 1%, 2%, 10%	Hypersensitivity; children less than 12 years of age, elderly; liver disease
Tetracaine, topical (*Pontocaine*)	Pruritus, sunburn, toothache, sore throat, oral pain, rectal pain, control of gagging	Apply to affected area; 1 oz for adults; ¼ oz for children; 2% solution aromatic spray; liquid; ointment; gel	Hypersensitivity; infants less than 1 year of age, application to large areas

*Modified from Skidmore-Roth L: *Mosby's 1991 nursing drug reference*, St. Louis, 1991, Mosby.

Table 16-3	Topical Anesthetic Mixtures	
	Ingredients	Comments
LET	Lidocaine, epinephrine, and tetracaine	Inexpensive. Is not a controlled substance.
TAC	Tetracaine, adrenaline, and cocaine	Cocaine is a controlled substance, so the solution must be locked in the narcotic cabinet and counted. This solution is expensive because of the cost of the cocaine.
ZAP	Xylocaine, adrenaline, and *Pontocaine*	Inexpensive. Is not a controlled substance.

mum of 20 minutes. Approximately 50% of patients do not require further anesthesia for sutures.

Other options for local anesthesia include mixing long-acting anesthetics such as *Marcaine* and *Sensorcaine* with shorter acting anesthetics such as lidocaine. This mixture causes rapid anesthesia while providing longer pain control. A BIER block is used for closure of extensive extremity lacerations. A tourniquet is applied to the affected extremity, and lidocaine without preservatives is injected intravenously.

The patient's blood pressure, pulse rate, and respiration rate should be monitored during treatment with injectable agents because systemic toxicity may occur if the dose is too high. Lidocaine and bupivacaine with epinephrine should not be used on the digits, penis, ears, or nose because of vasoconstrictive effects. In explaining the procedure, the ED nurse informs the patient that pain will be blocked but touch and pressure will remain intact. Pain management is facili-

tated if the patient is assisted into a comfortable position before initiation of the procedure and when distraction techniques are used. Research has shown that music provides an effective distraction during the procedure.[14] The numbing effects of local anesthetics provide a safe mechanism for pain control in the ED.

Noninvasive Pain Relief Methods

Cutaneous stimulation, distraction, hypnosis, imagery, and relaxation are psychologic approaches to pain management. These approaches are briefly discussed.

Cutaneous stimulation

This method applies to cutaneous techniques that stimulate the skin for the purpose of pain relief, such as massage, vibration, superficial heat and cold, ice application and massage, methanol application to the skin, and transcutaneous electrical nerve stimulation. Effects of cutaneous stimulation are variable; nursing skill and preparation are required before this method is used as a pain management intervention. Emergency nurses should receive an initial orientation and continuing education for these techniques.

Distraction

Distraction facilitates pain management by assisting the patient in focusing on a stimulus other than the pain. Usually distraction minimizes, but does not entirely alleviate, pain. For distraction to be effective, the object of that distraction must be of interest to the patient. Research indicates that music has beneficial pain relief qualities. In September 1989, a study was conducted to determine whether music significantly reduces the anxiety and pain associated with laceration repair in the ED.[14] Adult patients 18 years of age and older, who were not under the influence of analgesics or alcohol or other mood-altering substances, were included. Patients were randomly assigned to one of two groups. A control group received standard laceration repair with lidocaine only. A music group received standard laceration repair with lidocaine and music. Patients in the music group were permitted to select from a variety of audio cassette tapes and to listen to their choice of music through a headset. Measured psychologic variables included Spielberger State-Trait Anxiety Inventory, a visual analog pain-rating scale, and a brief questionnaire. Pain (P) scores were significantly lower ($p < 0.001$) in the music group (mean of 2.04) when compared with the control group (mean of 5.92). The authors concluded that music can be a safe, effective, inexpensive, noninvasive adjunct to pain management in the ED.

Hypnosis, imagery, and relaxation

Hypnosis is rarely used in emergency nursing, because few nurses have the knowledge or skills necessary to induce a trancelike state. However, the nurse functioning in the capacity of patient advocate can assist the patient in pursuing this method of pain management by referring the patient to available community resources for continued pain management. Self-hypnosis for pain management is becoming more widely accepted among health care professionals. Nurses interested in courses on hypnosis can obtain information by contacting the American Society of Clinical Hypnosis, 2250 East Devon Ave., Suite 326, Des Plaines, IL 60018.

Using one's imagination to control pain is a form of distraction that produces relaxation. This technique does not imply that the pain sensation is imaginary. McCaffery and Beebe[11] identified four types of imagery: (1) subtle or conversational, (2) simple, brief symptom substitution, (3) standardized imagery techniques, and (4) systematically individualized imagery techniques. In all four types, the imagination is used to develop images that promote pleasant sensations and diminish pain perception. For example, a patient may have decreased pain when imagining lying on the beach listening to the sound of waves washing over sand. Assisting in creating this imaginary setting, the nurse can assist with pain management. Effectiveness of imaging depends on familiarity of the image and its pleasantness for the patient.

Relaxation techniques promote a state free from anxiety. When the patient is relaxed, skeletal muscle tension is minimal. Deep breathing is one way to promote relaxation. The nurse can instruct the patient to inhale deeply through the nose and exhale slowly through the mouth. Repeating this sequence several times while concentrating on muscle relaxation is an effective approach for pain management in the ED. It is simple to use and can be taught quickly and easily to most patients.[7]

CONCLUSION

Pain is an all too often occurrence in any health care arena, but it is even more so in the ED. Pain management in emergency nursing is challenging but also rewarding. As Dunwoody suggests "few things we do for patients are more fundamental to the quality of life than relieving pain."[6]

REFERENCES

1. Bates B: *A guide to physical examination,* ed 3, Philadelphia, 1983, JB Lippincott.
2. Burke SO, Jerrett M: Pain management across age groups, *West J Nurs Res* 11:164, 1989.
3. Carpenito LJ: *Nursing diagnosis: application to practice,* Philadelphia, 1983, JB Lippincott.
4. Copp LA: The spectrum of suffering, *Am J Nurs* 90(8):35, 1990.
5. Cross, S: Pathophysiology of Pain, *Mayo Clinic Proc,* 69, 375-383, 1994.
6. Dunwoody CJ: Patient controlled analgesia: rationale, attributes, and essential factors, *Orthop Nurs* 6(5):31, 1987.
7. Fincke MK, Lanros NE: *Emergency nursing: a comprehensive review,* Rockville, Md., 1986, Aspen Publications.
8. International Association for the Study of Pain Subcommittee on taxonomy. Pain terms: A list with definition and usage. *Pain,* 6, 249-252, 1979.
9. McCaffery M: *Cognition, bodily pain and man-environment interactions,* Los Angeles, 1968, University of California.
10. McCaffery M: *Nursing management of the patient with pain,* ed 2, Philadelphia, 1979, JB Lippincott.
11. McCaffery M, Beebe A: *Pain: clinical manual for nursing practice,* St. Louis, 1989, Mosby.
12. McGuire L: Administering analgesics: which drugs are right for your patient, *Nursing* 20(4):34, 1990.
13. Miller RR et al: Propoxyphene hydrochloride: a critical review, *JAMA* 23:996, 1979.
14. Paris PM et al: Use of music to reduce anxiety and pain associated with laceration repair, *Ann Emerg Med* 20(4), 1991.
15. Paris PM, Stewart RD: *Pain management in emergency medicine,* Norwalk, Conn., 1988, Appleton & Lange.
16. *Product information:* Toradol, Palo Alto, Calif, 1990, Syntex Laboratories.
17. Vander AJ, Sherman JH, & Luciano DS: *Human physiology: the mechanism of body function,* New York, 1994, McGraw-Hill.

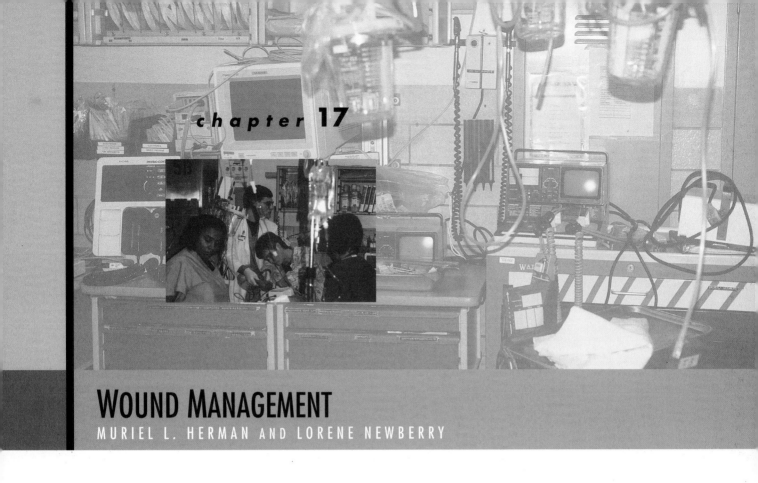

WOUND MANAGEMENT

MURIEL L. HERMAN AND LORENE NEWBERRY

chapter **17**

Emergency nurses encounter many patients with soft tissue injuries that can greatly alter a person's appearance. Unless life-threatening bleeding or neurovascular compromise are present, patients with surface trauma are not a triage priority. Wound management in the emergency department (ED) includes careful assessment, cleansing, wound closure, and discharge care. Basic principles of wound care are promotion of optimal healing, prevention of infection, and reduction of scar formation.

ANATOMY AND PHYSIOLOGY

Skin is the largest organ of the body and is composed of the epidermis, dermis, and subcutaneous tissue (Figure 17-1). The *epidermis,* or outer layer, generates cells that promote wound healing. Thickness of the epidermis varies with location; epidermal thickness is significantly greater in the soles of the feet and palms of the hand than in the eyelids. Thickening of epidermal layers, or calluses, may be caused by poorly fitted shoes, repetitive actions such as plucking guitar strings, or manual labor such as raking the yard. The *dermis* is a tough connective layer that forms the thickest layer of the skin and contains the lymphatic vessels, blood vessels, and nerves. Collagen found in the dermis provides tensile strength, and elastin allows skin to resist deformation. Sensory receptors for pain, touch, pressure, heat, and cold are found in the dermis, whereas hair follicles and sweat glands are found between the epidermis and dermis. The *subcutaneous layer* stores fat below the dermis and pro-

vides insulation against heat loss. Heat conduction in fat is one third that of other tissues. Fat also provides protection against injury and acts as an energy storage site.

Skin regulates body temperature through sweating and evaporation. Insensible fluid loss through skin and lungs accounts for 450 to 600 ml/day or 12 to 16 calories/hr of heat loss.[5] Skin also provides innate immunity because of macrophages, mast cells, and Langerhans cells in the skin that respond to antigens and pathogens,[5] and because of the presence of normal skin flora (i.e., coagulase-positive and coagulase-negative staphylocci, streptocci, and diptheroids).

WOUND HEALING

Healing occurs in three cumulative phases or layers (inflammatory, fibroplasia, and collagen maturation) with each layer creating the pathway for the next layer to occur (Figure 17-2). After injury occurs, blood flows into the wound and coagulates forming a clot. Beneath the clot, a network of fibrinogen strands form to unite wound edges. Scab formation begins within 2 hours to minimize fluid loss and prevent bacterial invasion.

Once scab formation begins, inflammatory processes start, and the wound becomes painful and edematous. Vasodilation in injured tissues leads to protein leakage and antibody release, which create a medium for white blood cells (WBCs) that arrive at the site 6 hours after the injury. White blood cells attack bacteria through phagocytosis using neutrophils to surround and engulf bacteria providing a short-

183

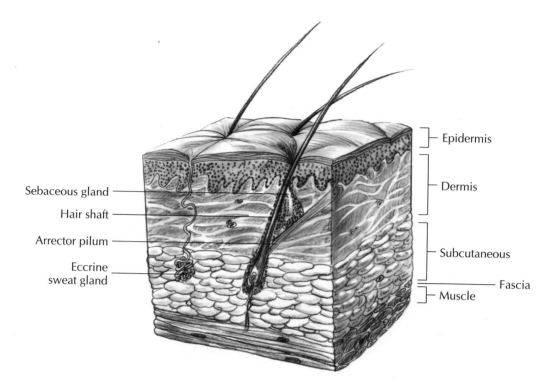

Figure **17-1** Epidermis, dermis, and subcutaneous tissue. *(From Davis P et al.:* Surgery: a problem solving approach, *ed 2, St. Louis, 1995, Mosby.)*

term defense against infection, whereas monocytes provide a long-term defense against infection.

Within 24 hours of injury, fibroblasts generate new epidermis. Fibroblast activity peaks in approximately 6 days during which time lymphatic vessels, blood vessels, and supporting tissues are repaired. New capillary beds form and mesh with damaged tissue providing oxygen and proteins for tissue growth. During fibroblast activity, collagen is produced for dermal scar tissue. Scar tissue is initially translucent, grayish-red, bleeds easily, and can be damaged with minimal force. Tensile wound strength is weakest 3 days after injury.

Collagen fibers initially develop randomly; however, within 2 weeks, fibers reorganize into thick fibers along stress lines and increase in strength over weeks or months. The amount of scarring is determined by heredity, stress, and movement of the affected area. Healing, with increasing collagen density and nerve regeneration, may actually take years. It is significantly affected by conditions such as obesity, infection, diabetes mellitus, and malnutrition. Effects of these and other factors on wound healing are described in Table 17-1.

WOUND EVALUATION

Initial assessment of wounds follows assessment and stabilization of airway, breathing, and circulation (ABC). Mechanisms of injury can provide clues to the severity of in-

jury. Wounds caused by small objects may be superficial, whereas crush injuries caused by a large dog's bite can cause significant deep tissue damage. Appearance of the wound provides clues to the difficulty of wound closure. Jagged edges require more skill to close and may not heal as well. The time since injury is critical, since delayed care increases the risk for complications such as infection. Special closure techniques are required for wounds that are more than 12 hours old.

Patient age, physical condition, current health status, and occupation also affect wound healing. Medical conditions such as diabetes mellitus or the use of medications such as corticosteroids delay wound healing. Aspirin and nonsteroidal antiinflammatory drugs affect coagulation and healing. Patient occupation influences long-term wound management and patient compliance with wound care. From an occupational point of view, lacerations on the fingers are more difficult for pianists than for public speakers. An allergy history and immunization status should also be evaluated during initial assessment.

The patient should be assessed for associated injuries such as fractures, dislocations, or neurovascular compromise, and possible fractures or dislocations should be splinted. Tendon or bone injuries, the presence of a foreign body, and peripheral nerve damage should also be considered. A wound culture should be obtained before irrigation for wound contamination. The wound can be cleaned with

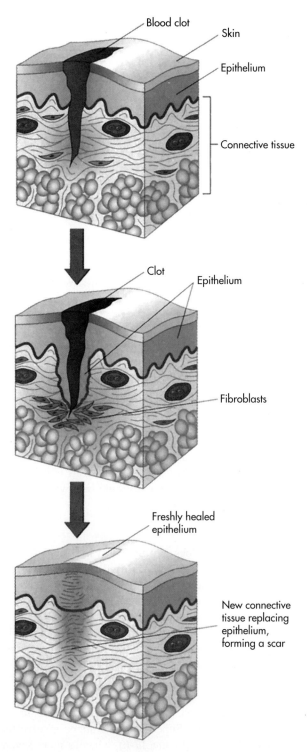

Figure **17-2** Healing of a minor wound. *(From Thibodeau GA, Patton KT: Anthony's text of anatomy and physiology, ed 15, St. Louis, 1996, Mosby.)*

isotonic saline or other acceptable solutions (Table 17-2); however, hydrogen peroxide should not be used because it causes absorption of oxygen in the wound and cell destruction, and gives no protection against anaerobes. Soaps with strong cleaning agents or those containing alcohol may cause further tissue damage. Wounds with heavy contamination should be irrigated for 5 minutes or more with local anesthesia injected or applied topically before vigorous scrubbing. Puncture wounds are soaked for 10 to 15 minutes; however, soaking of other wounds should be avoided. The area surrounding lacerations is usually shaved because hair is a source of contamination; however, eyebrows should never be shaved because the hair may never grow back. Eyebrows also function as landmarks for wound alignment and closure.[8]

Devitalized tissue is debrided before wound closure. Wounds may be closed by primary intention, secondary intention, or tertiary intention. The type of closure depends on the age of the wound, presence of infection, and amount of contamination present. Figure 17-3 illustrates types of wound closure. *Primary intention* with sutures, staples, or steri-strips within 12 hours of the injury is the ideal method of closure since this technique has the least scarring. Table 17-3 describes wound healing with primary intention closure. Following wound closure, the wound is covered with a thin layer of antibiotic ointment followed by a nonadherent dressing. Types of wound dressings are described in Table 17-4. *Secondary intention* is used for wounds with devitalized tissue, severe contamination, or infection. Wound edges are not closed initially so that the wound granulates form tissue from the inside out. *Tertiary intention,* or delayed wound closure, occurs days after injury.

SPECIFIC WOUNDS

Wounds are categorized into six basic types: abrasions, abscesses, avulsions, lacerations, puncture wounds, and bites. Their severity varies with the cause of injury and amount of tissue damaged; however, patient age, health status, medications, and preexisting conditions affect overall wound severity and healing. Occupation is also a factor in wound care. Wounds may be a minor inconvenience that do not alter lifestyle or impact work requirements. More severe wounds may cause significant discomfort and affect self-care and work. In some cases, lifestyle is permanently altered.

Abrasions

Abrasions occur when skin is rubbed or scraped against a hard surface. Friction removes the epithelial layer and can also remove part of the epidermis, which leaves deeper layers of skin exposed. Examples of abrasions are floor burns, carpet burns, or brush burns (Figure 17-4). Abrasions have the same physiologic effect as a second degree burn, so a significant risk of infection exists because of the loss of skin

Table **17-1**   **Factors Delaying Wound Healing**

Factor	Effects on wound healing
■ Nutritional deficiencies:	
Vitamin C	Delays formation of collagen fibers and capillary development
Protein	Decreases supply of amino acids for tissue repair
Zinc	Impairs epithelialization
■ Inadequate blood supply	Decreases supply of nutrients to injured area, decreases removal of exudative debris, inhibits inflammatory response
■ Corticosteroid drugs	Impair phagocytosis by WBCs,* inhibit fibroblast proliferation and function, depress formation of granulation tissue, inhibit wound contraction
■ Infection	Increases inflammatory response and tissue destruction
■ Mechanical friction on wound	Destroys granulation tissue, prevents apposition of wound edges
■ Advanced age	Slows collagen synthesis by fibroblasts, impairs circulation, requires longer time for epithelialization of skin, alters phagocytic and immune responses
■ Obesity	Decreases blood supply in fatty tissue
■ Diabetes mellitus	Decreases collagen synthesis, retards early capillary growth, impairs phagocytosis (result of hyperglycemia)
■ Poor general health	Causes generalized absence of factors necessary to promote wound healing
■ Anemia	Supplies less oxygen at tissue level

*WBCs = white blood cells

From Lewis SM, Collier IC, Heitkemper MM: *Medical-surgical nursing: assessment and management of clinical problems,* ed 4, St. Louis, 1996, Mosby.

and its protective properties. Fluid loss also occurs because of loss of surface area.

Foreign bodies left in the skin stain the epidermis and cause permanent scars or a "tattoo." Cleansing is critical in management of abrasions to prevent tattooing. Local anesthesia by topical application or infiltration should be used for abrasions with heavy contamination. Topical antibiotic ointment and nonadherent dressings are used; however, abrasions may occasionally be left open to air. Dressings should be changed daily until eschar forms. Clothing or sunblock should be used for 6 months to prevent discoloration by the sun of fragile new tissue.

Abscess

Localized collection of pus beneath the skin causes an abscess. Pus may eventually erupt; however, wound management does not include waiting for this to occur. The wound is cleaned, infiltrated with local anesthesia, and drained. An elliptical area of tissue may be removed to facilitate drainage, then the wound is packed loosely with iodoform or similar material and covered with loose dressing. Antibiotics are indicated when the patient has a fever.

Avulsion

Avulsion is full-thickness skin loss where approximation of wound edges is not possible. A degloving injury is a severe avulsion injury where skin is peeled away from hand, foot, or the greater portion of an extremity. Figure 17-5 shows a degloving injury of the ring finger. Tendons and

muscles may also be injured with this type of avulsion. Management includes local anesthesia by injection or topical application followed by irrigation and debridement of devitalized tissue. A split-thickness skin graft is necessary with large avulsions. The wound should be covered with a bulky dressing to protect exposed tissue.

Contusions

Blunt trauma that does not alter skin integrity causes a contusion or bruise. Swelling, pain, and discoloration occur as a result of extravasation of blood into damaged tissues. Following assessment of neurovascular status, therapeutic interventions include cold packs and analgesia as necessary. Large wounds or those located in an extremity should be carefully observed for cellulitis or the development of compartment syndrome.

Lacerations

Lacerations are open cuts caused by shearing forces through dermal layers. Superficial lacerations involve the epidermis and dermis (Figure 17-6), whereas more severe injuries involve deeper layers including subcutaneous tissue and muscle (Figure 17-7). Initial interventions focus on controlling bleeding and assessing neurovascular function distal to the injury. Anesthesia should be used to facilitate the removal of foreign bodies and the excision of necrotic or devitalized tissue. Exploration is indicated when possible damage to underlying structures is possible. Wound closure involves the approximation of edges followed by closure

Table **17-2** **Antiseptic Solutions**

Agents	Antimicrobial activity	Mechanics of action	Tissue toxicity	Indications and contraindications
Povidone-iodine solution (iodine complexes) (*Betadine*)	Available as 10% solution with polyvinyl-pyrolidine (povidone) containing 1% free iodine with broad rapid-onset antimicrobial activity	Potent germicide in low concentrations	Decreases PMN migration and life span at concentration >1% May cause systemic toxicity at higher concentrations; questionable toxicity at 1% concentration	Probably safe and effective wound cleanser at 1% concentration 10% solution is effective to prepare skin about the wound
Povidone-iodine surgical scrub	Same as the solution	Same	Toxic to open wounds	Best as a hand cleanser; never use in open wounds
Nonionic detergents *Pluronic F-68* *Shur Clens*	Ethyleneoxide is 80% of its molecular weight Has no antimicrobial activity	Wound cleanser	No toxicity to open wounds, eyes, or intravenous solutions	Appears to be an effective, safe wound cleanser
Hydrogen peroxide	3% solution in water has brief germicidal activity	Oxidizing agent that denatures protein	Toxic to open wounds	Should not be used on wounds after the initial cleaning; may be used to clean intact skin
Hexachlorophene (*pHiso Hex*) (polychlorinated bis-phenol)	Bacteriostatic (2% to 5%) Greater activity against gram-positive organisms	Interruption of bacterial electron transport and disruption of membrane-bound enzymes	Little skin toxicity; the scrub form is damaging to open wounds	Never use scrub solution in open wounds Very good preoperative hand preparation
Alcohols	Low-potency antimicrobial most effective as 70% ethyl and 70% isopropyl alcohol solution	Denatures protein	Kills irreversibly and functions as a fixative	No role in routine care
Phenols	Bacteriostatic >0.2% Bactericidal >1% Fungicidal 1.3%	Denatures protein	Extensive tissue necrosis and systemic toxicity	Never use >2% aqueous phenol or >4% phenol plus glycerol

Modified from Rosen P et al.: *Emergency medicine*, ed 3, St. Louis, 1993, Mosby.

with a tape closure, staples, or sutures. Deeper wounds are closed in layers. Once the wound is closed, a thin layer of antibiotic ointment is applied followed by a nonadherent dressing.

Puncture Wounds

Puncture wounds are caused by tissue penetration with a sharp object such as knife blade or injection from high-pressure nail guns or paint guns, which can exert pressures of up to 2000 psi.[9] Injection injuries cause more severe damage to underlying tissues than indicated by the appearance of the surface wound. Infection is reported in 10% to 15% of puncture wounds. A greater risk for infection exists in wounds that are more than 6 hours old; large and deep; contaminated with foreign matter and debris; from the outdoors; from penetration through footwear; and in patients with underlying disease such as diabetes mellitus or immunosuppression.[9] Risk for wound contamination increases with high-pressure injuries. Management includes necrotic tissue removal followed by drain placement and sterile

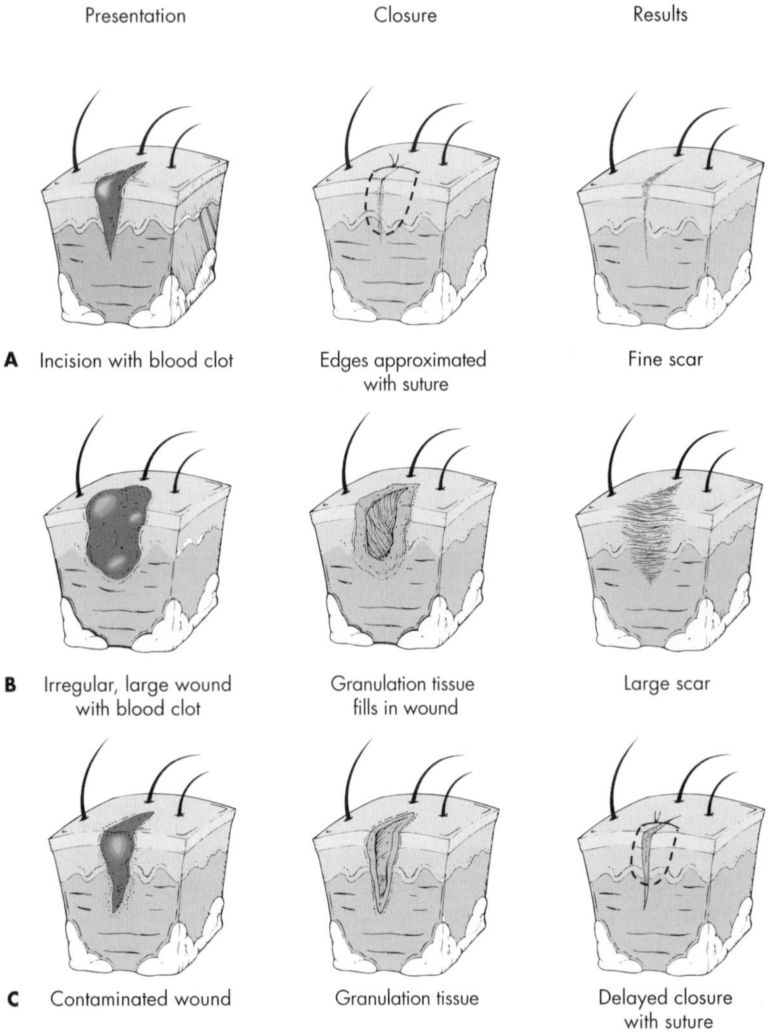

Presentation   Closure   Results

A Incision with blood clot   Edges approximated with suture   Fine scar

Figure **17-3** Types of wound healing. **A,** Primary intention. **B,** Secondary intention. **C,** Tertiary intention. *(Modified from Lewis SM, Collier IC, Heitkemper MM: Medical-surgical nursing: assessment and management of clinical problems, ed 4, St. Louis, 1996, Mosby.)*

B Irregular, large wound with blood clot   Granulation tissue fills in wound   Large scar

C Contaminated wound   Granulation tissue   Delayed closure with suture

Table **17-3**	**Phases in Wound Healing**
Phase	Activity
■ Initial (3 to 5 days)	Approximation of incision edges; migration of epithelial cells; clot serving as meshwork for starting capillary growth
■ Granulation (5 days to 4 weeks)	Migration of fibroblasts; secretion of collagen; abundance of capillary buds; fragility of wound
■ Scar contracture (7 days to several months)	Remodeling of collagen; strengthening of scar

Modified from Lewis SM, Collier IC, Heitkemper MM: *Medical-surgical nursing: assessment and management of clinical problems,* ed 4, St. Louis, 1996, Mosby.

dressing application. Impaled objects should be stabilized until safe removal is possible. A foreign body can be removed if the object is small, and its removal does not cause further damage. Some objects may be left in place or removed surgically.

Bites

Bites may be caused by animals or humans and involve contusions, avulsions, lacerations, and puncture wounds. Teeth can crush or tear tissue causing extensive damage. An estimated 1 to 2 million Americans are bitten by animals each year, with dog bites accounting for 80% to 90% of these injuries and cat bites reported in 5% to 18%.[9] Exotic animals such as primates, felines, alligators, and camels also cause bite injuries. Regardless of the source, bite wounds are considered contaminated. Infection, abscess, cellulitis, septicemia, osteomyelitis, tenosynovitis, rabies, tetanus, and loss of body parts are potential complications of bite wounds.

Human bites result from fighting or sexual activity, or can be self-inflicted. Infection is the greatest risk with human

Table 17-4	**Types of Wound Dressings**	
Type	Description	Examples
Gauze	Provides absorption of exudate; supports debridement if applied and kept moist; can be used to maintain moist wound surface and as filler dressings in sinus tracts	
Nonadherent dressings	Woven or nonwoven dressings may be impregnated with saline, petrolatum, or antimicrobials; minimal absorbency	Telfa Exu-Dry Vaseline gauze Xeroform
Transparent adhesive	Semipermeable membrane permits gaseous exchange between wound bed and environment; minimally absorbent so fluid environment created in presence of exudate. Bacteria do not penetrate membrane.	Opsite Biocclusive Tegaderm Acu-Derm Polyskin Blisterfilm
Hydrocolloid	Occlusive dressing does not allow O_2 to diffuse from atmosphere to wound bed. Occlusion does not interfere with wound healing; not used in infected wounds; supports debridement and prevents secondary infections; available in powder, wafer, and paste form	DuoDerm Restore Intact Intrasite Tegasorb Ultec
Foam	Nonadherent wafers with absorptive capacity; have limited permeability and are not totally occlusive; supports debridement in exudative wounds	Allevyn Lyofoam Synthaderm Epilock
Absorption dressing	Large volumes of exudate can be absorbed; supports debridement; maintains moist wound surface; placed into wounds and can obliterate dead space; made up of dextranomer beads, copolymer starches, and calcium alginate	Bard Absorption Hydragan Sorbsan Kaltostat Duoderm Paste Debrisan Sorbsan
Hydrogel	Debridement because of moisturizing effects; maintains moist wound surface; provides limited absorption of exudate; available as sheet dressings and granules	Vigilon Elasto Gel Intrasite Gel Geliperm

Modified from Lewis SM, Collier IC, Heitkemper MM: *Medical-surgical nursing: assessment and management of clinical problems,* ed 4, St. Louis, 1996, Mosby.

bites since human saliva contains 10 bacteria/ml of saliva including *Staphylococcus aureus,* streptococci, *Proteus, Escherichia coli, Pseudomonas,* and Klebsielleae. More than 3% of these organisms are penicillin-resistant *S. aureus.* Hepatitis B virus may also be transmitted through human saliva; however, risk for HIV infection appears to be low.[9] Management of human bite wounds includes neurovascular assessment, wound exploration, copious irrigation, debridement of devitalized tissue, and application of a bulky dressing. The wound is initially left open. Prophylactic antibiotics should be given within 3 hours of arrival at the ED.

Animal bites carry a risk of infection, tetanus, and rabies. Infection occurs in 5% to 15% of dog bite wounds and in a significant number of cat bite wounds. An increased risk for infection exists in persons over 50 years old, and in those with hand wounds, deep puncture wounds, and delayed treatment of more than 24 hours. Up to 33 organisms have been identified in dog saliva.[1] Cat saliva contains *Pasteurella multocida,* an extremely virulent organism that can lead to septic arthritis and bacteremia. Dog bites are more likely to be associated with crush injuries because of compressive forces of the canine jaw of up to 400 psi in some breeds. Fifty-seven percent to 86 percent of all cats bites are puncture wounds caused by the cat's long, slender fangs.[9] Most dog bites occur on the extremities, head, and neck, with fewer bites on the trunk. Children are more likely to have wounds on the head and neck. Most cat bites are found on the arm, forearm, and hand. Treatment for cat and dog bites is essentially the same: cleaning, debridement, and wound closure for small wounds. Prophylactic antibiotics are recommended for high-risk patients, whereas rabies and tetanus prophylaxis should be considered for all patients.

ANESTHESIA

Closure may be done with tape closure, sutures, or staples. *Local anesthesia* is required for sutures and staples, and lidocaine is preferred for local and regional anesthesia because of its greater potency, decreased irritation, and long-lasting anesthetic effect. Lidocaine with epinephrine is used for lacerations in highly vascular areas. One disadvantage of lidocaine is its greater toxicity in larger doses. Other anesthetic agents are procaine, mepivacaine *(Carbocaine),* bupivacaine *(Marcaine* or *Sensorcaine),* and tetracaine *(Pontocaine).* Agents may be used to infiltrate the wound area or may be applied topically. Table 17-5 highlights anesthetic agents used for local infiltration and nerve blocks. Mixing sodium bicarbonate 8.4% (Neut) with lidocaine decreases the pain associated with infiltration.[8] A warm lidocaine solu-

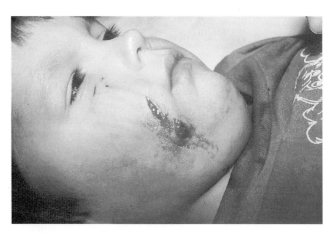

Figure **17-6** Superficial laceration. *(Courtesy Thomas Lintner, MD.)*

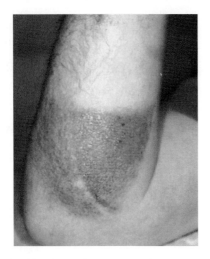

Figure **17-4** Abrasion. *(From National Association of Emergency Medical Technicians in Cooperation with the Committee on Trauma of the American College of Surgeons, Pre-Hospital Trauma Life Support, ed 3, 1994.)*

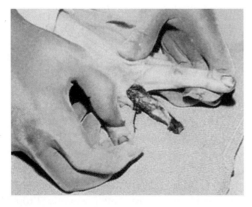

Figure **17-5** *Degloving injury of finger. (From Grossman JA:* Atlas of minor injuries, *St. Louis, 1993, Gower Medical Publishing.)*

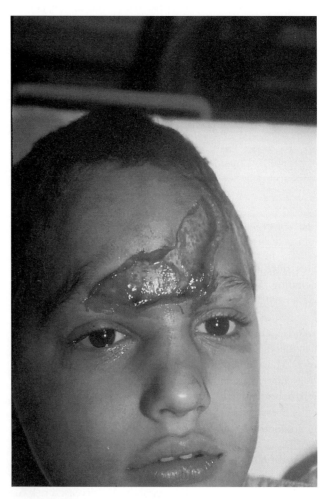

Figure **17-7** Deep laceration. *(Courtesy Thomas Lintner, MD.)*

Table 17-5   Local Anesthetic Agents

Agent	Dose route (maximum recommended doses)	Special considerations
Lidocaine: with epinephrine*	7 mg/kg sc	Use as local anesthetic before wound closure.
Lidocaine: without epinephrine	4 mg/kg sc	Administer to wound edges only.
Procaine: with epinephrine*	14 mg/kg sc	Use as local anesthetic before wound closure.
Procaine: without epinephrine	8 mg/kg sc	Administer to wound edges only.
Bupivacaine: with epinephrine*	4 mg/kg sc	Use as local anesthetic before wound closure.
Bupivacaine: without epinephrine	1 mg/kg sc	Administer to wound edges only.

*Do not use agents with epinephrine in areas with decreased blood flow (e.g., digits).
Modified from Kidd PS, Sturt P: *Mosby's emergency nursing reference*, St. Louis, 1996, Mosby.

Table 17-6   Topical Anesthetics

Drug	Concentration (%)	Duration (min)	Maximum adult dose (mg)
Cocaine	4	30	200
Lidocaine (Xylocaine)	2-4	15	200
Tetracaine (Pontocaine)	0.5	45	50

From Rosen P, et al.: *Emergency medicine*, ed 2, vol 1, St. Louis, 1988, Mosby.

tion also causes less pain and can be warmed by running the vial under warm tap water.

Topical anesthetics are ideal for the management of minor lacerations in children. Available solutions include TAC (tetracaine, Adrenalin, and cocaine) and XAP (xylocaine, Adrenalin, and pontacaine), which is also called LET (lidocaine, epinephrine, and tetracaine). Cocaine solutions should be used cautiously because of potentially deleterious side effects such as CNS stimulation and vasomotor collapse. These solutions obviate the need for needle infiltration but do require a minimum of 20 minutes for adequate anesthesia. Infiltration is required when the desired anesthetic effect is not achieved. A cotton ball is saturated with anesthetic solution and applied directly to the laceration. A clear dressing such as tegaderm applied directly over the cotton ball holds the cotton ball in place and prevents absorption of the solution when tape is used. A white ring around the wound is caused by the vasoconstrictive effects of epinephrine. Anesthetic effect varies slightly with each solution because of duration of the individual agents (Table 17-6). Solutions containing cocaine are controlled substances and significantly more expensive. Viscous lidocaine may be applied to abrasions before cleaning but is not used as an anesthetic for wound closure.

Regional anesthesia, or Bier block, may be selected when a greater anesthetic effect is desired. A tourniquet is placed proximal to the wound, and the anesthetic agent is injected distal to the injury. After wound repair, the tourniquet is re-

leased, and the anesthetic agent is slowly absorbed. A *local nerve block,* or digital block, for anesthesia is accomplished by injecting the anesthetic agent along the nerve to abolish afferent and efferent impulse conduction. The anesthetic agent is aspirated before each injection to prevent parenteral lidocaine injection.

One alternative to local and regional anesthesia is nitrous oxide. The patient inhales a 50% mixture of nitrous oxide and oxygen during short, painful procedures such as debridement. Self-administration limits the amount of nitrous oxide used while providing the appropriate level of anesthesia.

WOUND CLOSURE

Primary wound closure uses a tape closure (steri-strips), sutures, or staples. Table 17-7 describes advantages and disadvantages for each. The technique chosen depends on wound size, depth, and location. *Tape closure* is used for superficial linear wounds under minimal tension or as an adjunct after suture removal in patients with thin, frail skin such as the elderly or steroid-dependent patients (Figure 17-8). Tape closure is also more easily accomplished in obese patients since adipose tissue tends to evert wound edges.[8] Tincture of benzoin is applied to skin before tape application to ensure adherence. A tape closure may also be used after deeper layers are closed with sutures. Dressings may or may not be applied over the tape closure. An anesthetic is not necessary, and a lower risk of infection is associated with tape closure. Tape strips remain in place until they fall off.

Sutures approximate and attach wound edges, which decrease infection, promote wound healing, and minimize scar formation. A local anesthetic applied by infiltration or topically is required for suturing. Different stitches are used to close various wounds depending on the depth, location, and tension of the wound. Figure 17-9 shows various stitches and their uses. Sutures may be absorbable or nonabsorbable, which means they are composed of natural or synthetic material, respectively. Essential qualities of suture material are security, strength, reaction, workability, and infectious potential. Table 17-8 describes these qualities for various su-

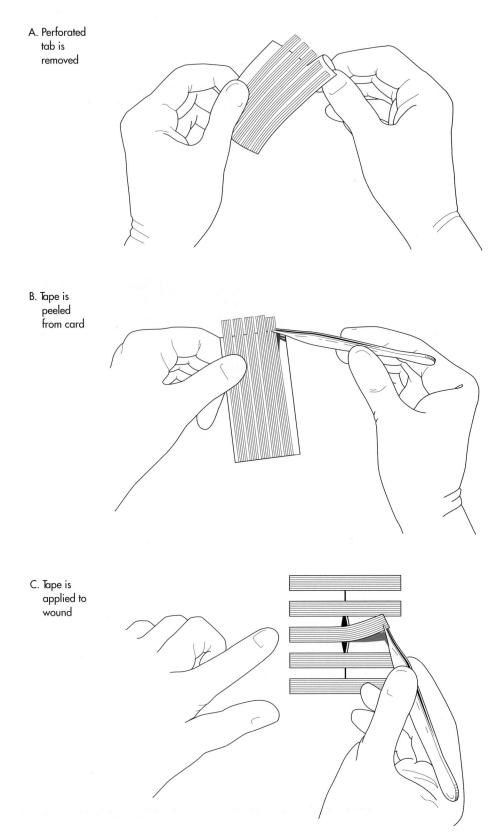

A. Perforated tab is removed

B. Tape is peeled from card

C. Tape is applied to wound

Figure **17-8** Tape closure **(A–D).** *(From Meeker MH, Rothrock JC:* Alexander's care of the patient in surgery, *ed 10, St. Louis, 1995, Mosby. Courtesy 3M)*

D. Additional
tape placed
parallel to
wound to limit
shear stress
on skin

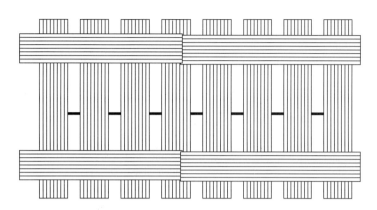

Figure **17-8,** cont'd   Tape closure (**A–D**). *(From Meeker MH, Rothrock JC:* Alexander's care of the patient in surgery, *ed 10, St. Louis, 1995, Mosby. Courtesy 3M)*

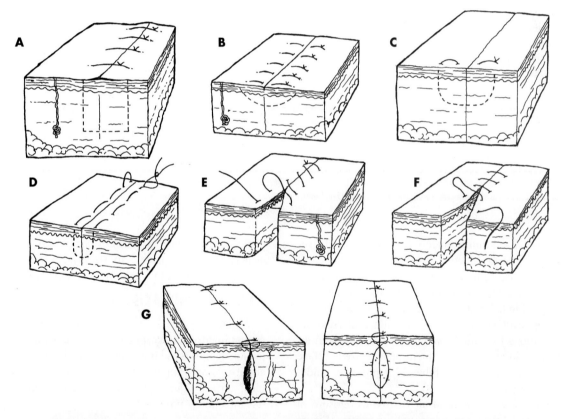

Figure **17-9** Stitches for suturing. **A,** Simple interrupted sutures: pairing skin edges together evenly; edges are slightly elevated but flatten with healing. **B,** Vertical mattress suture: assures eversion on healing. **C,** Horizontal mattress suture: closely approximates skin edges and has slight amount of eversion, especially in areas under tension. **D,** Half-buried horizontal mattress sutures: good with flaps, V-shaped wounds, and parallel lacerations. **E,** Subcuticular suture (continuous intradermal suture): good for wounds where sutures should be left in place for longer periods, as in wounds under a great deal of tension. **F,** Continuous suture: good when suture marks will not show, as in scalp. **G,** Buried sutures: reduce dead space and reduce surface tension in wound.

Table **17-7**	**Wound Closure Methods**	
Method/use	Advantages	Disadvantages
Steri-strips		
May be used for partial-thickness lacerations or small superficial lacerations without signs of adjacent tension	Eliminate need for anesthetic Decrease tissue trauma Decrease risk for infection	Potential for wound edge inversion Less strength than sutures
Approximate wound edges, applying steri-strips uniformly; use benzoin or mastisol on adjacent skin to secure adhesiveness of steri-strips.	—	—
Sutures		
May be used for simple and more involved lacerations; closure of deep wounds done in layers; suture selection is matter of individual choice.	Definite closure of wound edges. Patient able to shower; dressing not always needed after 24 hrs	Local anesthetic used Follow-up appointment needed for suture removal
Absorbable suture used for deeper layers; examples are plain or chromic catgut and the synthetics, *Dexon* and *Vicryl*.	—	—
Nonabsorbable suture used for skin closure and must be removed	—	—
Examples are silk or synthetics (nylon, polyprophylene).		
NOTE: Synthetics have decreased wicking action that decreases scarring potential.		
Staples		
May be used for linear lacerations to scalp, trunk, and extremities*	Rapid method of closure; produces less inflammation	Provides less precise approximation; should not be used when magnetic resonance imaging of affected part may be conducted

*From Markovchick V: Suture materials and mechanical after care, *Emerg Med Clin North Am* 10:673-689, 1992.
Modified from Kidd PS, Sturt P: *Mosby's emergency nursing reference,* St. Louis, 1996, Mosby.

ture materials.[9] Ideal suture material is strong, easily secured, and resistant to infection, and causes minimal local reaction. Sutures cause minimal discomfort after insertion; however, they act as a foreign body and can cause local inflammation. A thin layer of antibiotic ointment is applied after suture application followed by a nonadherent dressing. Recommendations for suture removal vary with wound location. Wounds in areas of movement or increased surface tension should remain longer. Table 17-9 provides guidelines for suture removal.

Staples are a fast, economical alternative for closure of linear lacerations of the scalp, trunk, and extremities (Figure 17-10). Wounds closed with staples have a lower incidence of infection and tissue reactivity, but do not provide the same quality of closure as sutures. Scars are more pronounced; therefore, staples are only recommended for areas where a scar is not apparent (i.e., scalp).[9] Staples should not be used in areas of the scalp that have permanent hair loss because of poor aesthetic results. Local anesthesia may not be used when only one or two staples are required since pain from the infiltration of anesthetic agents is greater than the

pain associated with insertion of one or two staples. Staples usually remain in place 7 to 10 days. A special staple remover (Figure 17-11) is required for removal.

WOUND PROPHYLAXIS

Wounds are at risk for local and systemic infection from contaminants, surface organisms, tetanus, and rabies. Protection against these infectious agents begins with cleansing and irrigation. Prophylactic antibiotics are not indicated for most surface injuries unless severe contamination or obvious infection is present.

Tetanus Prophylaxis

Tetanus is a systemic infection caused by *Clostridium tetani,* a gram-positive, spore-forming, anaerobic bacillus. Once activated, the bacillus is extremely resistant to almost anything, including sterilization. The incubation period for tetanus is 2 days to 2 weeks or more. *Clostridium tetani* spores are present in soil, garden moss, and anywhere animal and human excrement are found. Spores may contaminate wounds, but remain dormant in tissue for years. Once *C.*

Table 17-8 Suture Materials for Wound Closure

Type	Description	Security	Strength	Reaction	Workability	Infection	Comment
Nonabsorbables							
Silk		++++	+	++++	++++	++	Nice around mouth, nose, or nipples, but too reactive and weak to be used universally
Mersilene	Braided synthetic	++++	++	+++	++++		Good tensile strength; some prefer for fascia repairs
Nylon	Monofilament	++	+++	++	++	+++	Good strength; decreased infection rate; but knots tend to slip, especially the first throw
Prolene Polypropylene	Monofilament	+	++++	+	+	++++	Good resistance to infection; often difficult to work with; requires an extra throw
Ethibond	Braided coated polyester	+++	++++	++½	+++	+++	Costly
Stainless steel wire	Monofilament	++++	++++	+	+	+	Hard to use; painful to patient; some prefer for tendons
Absorbables							
Gut (plain)	From sheep intima	+	++	+++		+	Loses strength rapidly and quickly absorbed; rarely used today
Chromic (gut)	Plain gut treated with chromic salts	++	++	+++		+	Similar to plain gut; often used to close intraoral lacerations
Dexon	Braided copolymer of glycolic acid	++++	++++	+		++++	Braiding may cause it to "hang up" when tying knots
Vicryl	Braided polymer of lactide and glycolide	+++	++++	+		+++	Low reactivity with good strength; therefore, nice for subcutaneous healing; good in mucous membranes
Polydioxanone	Monofilament	++++	++++	+	Excellent	Unavailable	First available monofilament synthetic absorbable sutures; appears to be excellent

From Swanson NA, Tromovitch TA: *Int J Dermatol* 21:373 1982.

tetani enters the circulatory system, bacilli attach to cells in the central nervous system causing depression of the respiratory center in the medulla. Symptoms may be mild or severe and include local joint stiffness and mild trismus or inability to open the jaw. Severe tetanus is characterized by severe trismus, back pain, penile pain, tachycardia, hypertension, dysrhythmias, hyperpyrexia, opisthotonos, and seizures.

Prevention of tetanus includes immunization and scrupulous wound care, particularly for tetanus-prone wounds (Box 17-1). Tetanus immunization is part of the childhood immunization regimen and continues with regular tetanus immunizations in adults. Tetanus toxoid provides active immunization whereas tetanus immune globulin provides passive immunization. Persons who are inadequately immunized against tetanus should receive active or passive protection depending on the type of wound and their individual immunization status. Table 17-10 reviews recommendations for tetanus prophylaxis for clean and tetanus-prone wounds.

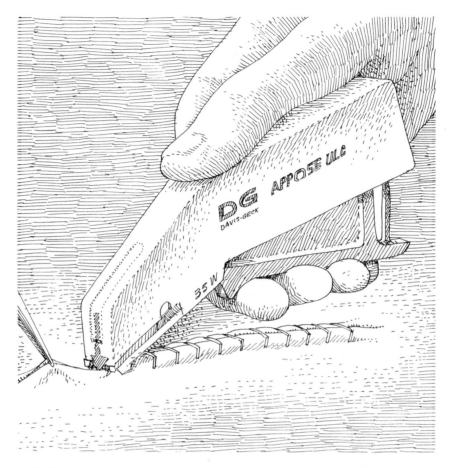

Figure **17-10** Application of skin staples. Staples are centered over incision line, using locating arrow or guideline, and placed approximately one quarter inch apart. *(From Meeker MH, Rothrock JC:* Alexander's care of the patient in surgery, *ed 10, St. Louis, 1995, Mosby. Courtesy Sherwood, Davis, and Geck, Danbury, Conn.)*

Table **17-9**	**Guidelines for Suture Removal**
Location	Removal date
Eyelids	3-5 days
Eyebrows	4-5 days
Ear	4-6 days
Lip	3-5 days
Face	3-5 days
Scalp	7-10 days
Trunk	7-10 days
Hands and feet	7-10 days
Arms and legs	10-14 days
Over joints	14 days

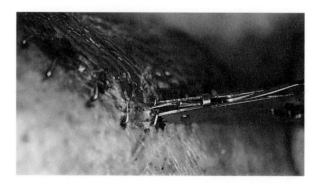

Figure **17-11** Staple remover. *(From Potter PA, Perry AG:* Fundamentals of nursing: concepts, process, and practice, *ed 4, St. Louis, 1997, Mosby.)*

Table 17-10   Tetanus Prophylaxis

Type of wound	Patient not immunized or partially immunized	Patient completely immunized: time since last booster dose	
		5 to 10 yr	10 yr+
Clean minor	Begin or complete immunization per schedule: toxoid 0.5 ml	None	Tetanus toxoid 0.5 ml
Tetanus-prone	Human tetanus immune globulin, 250-500 U; toxoid, 0.5 ml, complete immunization per schedule; antibiotic therapy as indicated	Tetanus toxoid 0.5 ml; antibiotic therapy if indicated	Tetanus toxoid 0.5 ml; tetanus immune globulin, 250-500 U; antibiotic therapy if indicated

From Trunkey DD, Lewis FR: *Current therapy of trauma*, ed 3, St. Louis, 1991, Mosby.

Box 17-1   Tetanus-Prone Wounds

Greater than 6 hr old
Stellate or avulsed
Caused by missile, crushing mechanism, heat, or cold
Obvious signs of infection
Devitalized tissue
Contaminants such as dirt, feces, soil, saliva

Box 17-3   Rabies Immunization

Passive immunity	**Active immunity**
Rabies immune globulin (RIG) 20 IU/kg	Human diploid cell vaccine (HDCV)
Half dose IM and half dose injected locally into wound	1 ml IM days 0,3,7,14,28 1 ml IM only days 0 and 3 if preexposure immunization

---

Box 17-2   Sources of Rabies Exposure

Domestic*	Wild
Cats	Raccoons
Dogs	Skunks
Cattle	Bats
Horses	Foxes
Goats	
Sheep	
Llamas	
Swine	

*Listed in order of frequency

Box 17-4

NURSING DIAGNOSES FOR SURFACE TRAUMA

Fluid volume deficit
Pain
Altered tissue perfusion
High risk for infection
Impaired skin integrity

Rabies Prophylaxis

Rabies exposure can occur with bites from wild and domestic animals. Rabies should be considered if an attack was not provoked, involved a domestic animal not immunized against rabies, or involved a wild animal. Rabies is a neurotoxic virus found in saliva of some mammals. Incubation period is 4 to 8 weeks. After inoculation, the rabies virus travels by peripheral nerves to the central nervous system causing encephalomyelitis, which is almost always fatal. Sources of rabies in wild and domestic animals are listed in Box 17-2. Carnivorous wild animals are always considered rabid, so immediate rabies prophylaxis should be administered. Domestic animals that show sign of rabies are destroyed, and a laboratory analysis is performed; those that appear healthy are observed for 10 days with prophylaxis required if the animal exhibits signs of rabies. Prophylaxis is always given when the animal cannot be found. Rodents such as rats, chipmunks, hamsters, gerbils, and squirrels rarely carry rabies; however, local authorities should be consulted for confirmation.

Rabies immunization includes the administration of rabies immune globulin (RIG) and human diploid cell vaccine (HDCV). Rabies immune globulin provides passive immunization, and HDCV provides active immunization. Box 17-3 summarizes rabies immunization.

CONCLUSION

Skin is the first barrier between the body and the rest of the world. Loss of skin integrity affects the ability to resist infection, retain fluids, and regulate body temperature. Changes caused by surface trauma such as scarring or tattooing affect body image and can cause significant anxiety for the patient. The emergency nurse can reduce potential complications related to these wounds through assessment, scrupulous wound care, and thorough discharge teaching. Priority nursing diagnoses for patients with surface trauma are listed Box 17-4.

REFERENCES

1. Dire DJ: Emergency management of dog and cat bite wounds, *Emerg Med Clin North Am* 10:719-736, 1992.
2. Emergency Nurses Association: *Emergency nurses core curriculum,* ed 4, Philadelphia, 1994, WB Saunders.
3. Emergency Nurses Association: *Trauma nurse core course provider manual,* Park Ridge, Ill, 1995, The Association.
4. Feliciano DV, Moore EE, Mattox KL: *Trauma,* ed 3, Stamford, Conn, 1996, Appleton & Lange.
5. Guyton AC, Hall JE: *Textbook of medical physiology,* ed 9, Philadelphia, 1996, WB Saunders.
6. Kidd PS, Sturt P: *Mosby's emergency nursing reference,* St. Louis, 1996, Mosby.
7. Kitt S, et al.: *Emergency nursing: A physiologic and clinical perspective,* ed 2, Philadelphia, 1995, WB Saunders.
8. Strange GR, et al.: *Pediatric emergency medicine: A comprehensive study guide,* New York, 1996, McGraw-Hill.
9. Tintinalli JE, Ruiz E, Krome RL: *Emergency medicine: A comprehensive study guide,* ed 4, New York, 1996, McGraw-Hill.

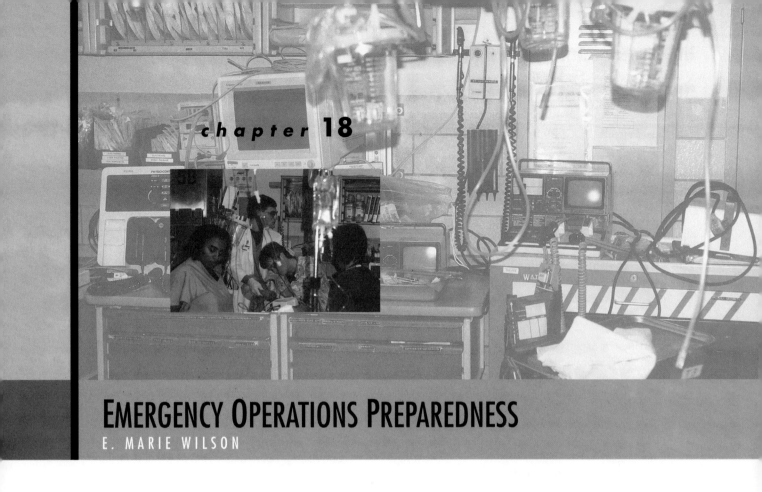

chapter **18**

EMERGENCY OPERATIONS PREPAREDNESS

E. MARIE WILSON

An emergency is a serious situation or occurrence that happens unexpectedly and demands immediate action.[1] A disaster—an occurrence causing widespread destruction and distress, or a catastrophe with fatal or ruinous results—generally implies great destruction, hardship, or loss of life.[1] A mass casualty incident (MCI) occurs when the number or needs of patients exceeds available resources.[8]

The term disaster is somewhat imprecise as a description of a specific event; therefore, the term "emergency operations" has replaced "disaster" in the vocabulary of those responsible for hospital planning. Emergency operations planning (EOP) is a framework for managing a wide variety of sudden or unexpected events. Effectively managing the emergency may prevent evolution into a full-blown disaster.

The emergency department (ED) is the primary focus for emergency planning; however, each department in the facility should be integrated into the plan. Coordination of the hospital plan with public safety services is critical. These services then collaborate with county, regional, state, and national agencies. Specific principles that govern EOP in the prehospital setting also apply to EOP in the hospital. Understanding and application of these principles facilitate emergency planning (Box 18-1). This chapter describes general EOP concepts, discusses hospital-wide and department planning, and integrates these concepts with the community at large.

GENERAL PLANNING CONCEPTS

An EOP committee should be authorized at the highest level of an organization with the chairperson appointed by, and accountable to, the president or chief operating officer. Authority delegated to the chairperson of the planning committee is commensurate with the desired quality of the plan and planning process. The plan is a strategic statement that provides overall direction and philosophy for emergency operations. Persons with authority to make tactical decisions should be clearly identified, so that staff have a framework for making decisions.

PLANNING PROCESS

The chairperson of the planning committee draws together people and organizational components who play a role in emergency operations. The chairperson should be a leader who can hold planners accountable for their assigned tasks and for gaining consensus from the staff of departments they represent. A strong plan is built as a consensus document with contributions from front-line staff.

During initial planning efforts, the chairperson should obtain authority to proceed. Responsibility for hospital emergency operations planning is ideally held by someone at the level of vice-president or above. Without direct involvement at the highest administrative levels, consensus across departmental lines may be difficult to obtain.

Box **18-1**	**Disaster Management Principles**

Prevent occurrence
Minimize casualties
Prevent further casualties
Rescue the injured
Provide first aid
Evacuate the injured
Provide definitive care
Facilitate reconstruction and recovery

From Sanford JP: Civilian disasters and disaster planning. In Burkle SM Jr, Sanner PH, Wolcott BW, editors: *Disaster medicine*, New York, 1984, Medical Examination Publishing. By permission of Appleton & Lange.

Plans written by experts as advice to supervisors during an emergency do not provide essential operational details or give consideration to organizational authority. Planning should be done by staff with the authority to execute the plan during an emergency operation. An emergency nurse is not qualified to direct how the medical ICU or pharmacy meets their obligations in an emergency. Conversely, a floor supervisor is not prepared to assist an emergency nurse with triage.

An operating procedure should be established for the planning committee with a core group of department heads and administrators. Each department should develop individual operating procedures (OPs) that are reviewed by the core planning group to prevent overlap of authority and ensure that OPs provide a seamless plan of action. When overlap does occur or an identified need for additional resources exists, department representatives can then negotiate a strategy to coordinate functions.

Participants should be empowered to make decisions during emergency operations. Employees are most efficient when doing tasks with which they are familiar. Expansion or elaboration of routine activities is best done by staff familiar with daily operations; therefore, front line staff should be enlisted to help formulate department OPs. Department heads may want to assign the department plan to a writing group of department staff. Participants should be authorized to find and solve problems. A triage nurse who assesses patients every day is the best person to triage incoming patients during an emergency operation.

Many hospitals review emergency operations plans before accreditation inspections; however, effective, efficient planning requires frequent evaluation with revision as needed. Employees involved in planning should be encouraged to note everyday events that provide useful information for plan revision. Any change in daily procedures or the environment should warrant review of the existing plan.

Plan evaluators should test their plan through drills; however, overemphasis on the drill can focus too much on failure (i.e., who makes the first or worst mistakes), whereas emphasis more on the plan concentrates on success (i.e.,

does the plan work as written, have people been trained to implement the plan?). Priority time should be applied to thinking through and documenting the plan. Drills should be viewed as exercises or lessons designed to teach skills and should focus on teaching staff how to carry out assigned duties under stressful situations rather than on finding faults and deficiencies. Teachers or preceptors should coach and teach as the exercises progress. The goal of a drill is to strengthen the problem-finding and problem-solving abilities of staff rather than only show whether they can carry out a predetermined list of tasks.

Evaluation should also focus on planning and training rather than on individuals. Staff members generally do a job to the best of their ability; therefore, mistakes made during the exercise are probably due to the plan being flawed or staff not being trained to execute the plan. Critique of the drill should address whether elements of the plan worked as designed and then consider whether the plan should be changed to reflect staff actions or more education should be provided. Problems identified during a drill may occasionally lie with the scenario rather than the plan. Unrealistic scenarios, or victims who are not convincing, can affect the staff's ability to role-play, which is an integral part of the exercise.

Emergency operations planning should be incorporated into the hospital's continuous quality improvement (CQI) program. Too often, exercises are evaluated without follow-up, and changes recommended in the critique are not made. Lack of follow-up can lead to a repeat of identified problems. Continuous quality improvement serves as a technique to constantly improve performance through process evaluation and follow-up. See Chapter 8 for a discussion of CQI principles.

HOSPITAL PLAN

Hospital plans should be flexible to respond to a variety of events with differing levels of intensity. An EOP plan based on a core emergency response can be expanded to meet the demands of any situation. One structure for central authority and control is easier to remember than 12 or 15 different situational structures. A single emergency operations plan for many different situations is more effective than numerous individual plans. Separate plans usually contain more areas of similarity than differences; however, this redundancy does not increase efficiency during emergency operations. Plans written by experts to provide technical advice may not follow a logical sequence of events, and may use bureaucratic prose that is difficult to remember when emergency strikes. During stressful emergency situations, staff should not have to read a plan. Efficiency increases when staff can remember one basic plan that requires only incremental changes for the situation at hand.

A hospital emergency operations plan should delegate authority to solve problems, rather than list every imaginable problem together with a proposed solution. Persons who work in an area are usually the best ones to solve problems in that area. They confront the problems better than anyone can by forecasting problems and identifying solutions. Solutions are time-, place-, and situation-specific; what works now may not work 10 minutes from now. Therefore, the authority and ability to solve problems as they arise must be the central focus of an emergency operations plan. Table 18-1 identifies key elements of the hospital emergency operations plan.

The structure of hospital leadership may change during an emergency operation. Administrators who have made a special study of emergency operations are often assigned lead roles. Such assignments should contain full authority from the president or CEO to make all decisions. In an emergency response, authority held centrally at the Hospital Emergency Operations Center (HEOC) allows the hospital to function as a unit rather than a series of independent departments. The HEOC should delegate autonomy to departments to make decisions within departmental boundaries. When the required response crosses department lines, the HEOC makes essential decisions and communicates those decisions to each department. For example, the need for additional staff in the ED to move patients is communicated to the HEOC, which may then pull staff from nursing units. When no longer needed, staff then return to their respective units.

The HEOC can be viewed as the hub of an operational wheel with spokes for different types of emergencies including MCIs, fire, telephone outage, power outage, oxygen system out, bomb, hazardous material (HAZMAT) in the community or hospital, flooding, hospital evacuation, and hostage situations (Figure 18-1). Each spoke represents an appendix to the emergency operations plan, which identifies plan adjustments that can be made to accommodate each situation.

In the hub-and-spoke-design operational plan, authority to move resources within a department is retained within each department, whereas authority for moving resources between departments is held at the HEOC. Distribution of authority in this manner ensures the most efficient use of resources. For example, if each department calls housekeeping directly, no priority can be set, so housekeeping becomes overwhelmed with requests, and no department gets sufficient help. Total hospital planning for HEOC responsibilities is a complex, collaborative effort. All departments, in addition to their own planning, should contribute to the EOP plan to ensure a coordinated response to community and facility emergencies.

Departmental Response

Many emergency situations do not require a full response by the hospital; therefore the plan should contain provisions for gradual escalation of response as details of an incident become known. Provisions should consider travel time for staff, and child care for those who must respond. The hospital may want to make arrangements for child care as part of the plan for full response. Specialized departments such as admissions, public relations, security, social services, dietary, and purchasing should collaborate extensively with clinical departments, preparing appendices to the plan to meet all types of response needs.

Public relations. Media experts should manage representatives from news agencies who descend on the hospital at the first hint of unusual activity. Reporters should be channeled away from patient receiving and care areas. Public relations staff should collaborate with admissions to obtain casualty lists, and with clinical specialists to provide background and interviews on injuries. The more reporters' needs are met, the less they need to wander around the facility in search of patients, witnesses, or stories. Patient confidentiality is an issue during news coverage; however, the public nature of the event itself means special handling is required.

Table **18-1**   **Key Elements of the Hospital Emergency Operations Plan**

Element	Description/rationale
Table of contents	Essential for quick reference
Authorization letter	Signed and dated by CEO; gives authority to the plan
Purpose and scope	Sequential outline of procedures, duties, responsibilities for departments during all phases of the incident
Definition of terms	Clarifies staff understanding of all aspects of operations
Chain of command	Clearly identifies leadership roles during the incident
Activation process	How plan is put into action; includes mobilization and staging of supplies and personnel; identifies notification steps for key personnel
Patient management plan	Describes triage procedure; patient flow; destination for critical, urgent, and noncritical patients; command posts; visitor and family areas; media plan
Communication plan	Addresses global communication (i.e., from the institution to outside agencies, within the institution, and within various departments); addresses communication alternatives if phone outage occurs
Special incidents	Defines actions for bomb threats, hazardous material spills, radiation incidents, and fires. May include management of military personnel, pediatric patients, and patients with burn injuries

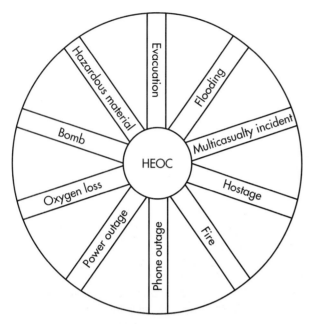

Figure **18-1** Operational wheel for emergency operations.

Security. Access to the grounds and building should be controlled so that everyone is directed appropriately. Wandering around is inappropriate for visitors, patients, or staff. Security-sensitive areas include the ED entrance, which is likely to see heavy activity; side doors to the building and loading areas that can provide easy access for unauthorized persons; and dead-end driveways, which may be used for disruptive activities.

Communication. A facility's internal system of communication is integral to the success of the hospital's response. Fail-safe mechanisms in this area are important to ensure communications if technology-dependent systems fail. Equally as important as the technology of communication is defining who needs to talk to whom about what. Defining the flow of necessary information during planning minimizes stress on the communications system, ensures that the HEOC has essential information to coordinate interdepartmental resources and responses, and provides various departments with information necessary to respond to specific problems.

Social services. Crisis intervention has a critical role in the ultimate recovery of patients, families, and the community. Chaplains, counseling teams, bereavement specialists, and others function in a variety of settings during the emergency response. Arriving families and friends should be met and escorted to a designated area until news is available, and they can make plans based on knowledge instead of fear. Accommodations to meet diverse needs should be included in planning, specifically addressing infants, children, elderly, and the disabled.

Many communities now have critical incident stress debriefing (CISD) teams to provide peer counseling for rescue workers including hospital personnel. Effects of working in the high-stress climate of an emergency operation can be minimized or delayed until some time after the event ends.[8,11] Some workers need immediate help while others may take weeks or months to recognize need for counseling to cope with their reactions. Planners should ensure that community resources are available quickly and at low cost for every worker.

Dietary. Workers in high-stress situations need food for energy; however, they can seldom take time away to eat or drink properly. High-energy foods that can be eaten with a minimum of utensils and fuss should be transported to front-line staff. Families, reporters, and others who are now guests of the hospital also require eating facilities, preferably in areas where these people are concentrated, so that travel to another location is not required.

Admissions. Many persons arriving at the ED are not identified, and some patients may not be identified for several hours or days. A mechanism of identification should be available at the triage area using a hospital identification number or other numeric system. Some hospitals prepare charts and have a numbered bracelet, requisition slips, order sheets, nurses' notes, and other materials readily available. Admissions staff may keep a master list of identification numbers for all patients as well as patient disposition and location. As the incident progresses, identifications can be matched with this list to compile a roster of all patients received. Patients arriving from the scene may have triage tags (usually on the ankle), which denote severity of injuries and other pertinent information such as treatment before arrival. Tags should be placed on the in-patient chart to facilitate cross identification of numbers.

Logistics. While distribution of supplies from storerooms is relatively easy, replenishing those supplies from outside sources is more difficult. Planners must locate alternative vendors who can reliably deliver supplies on short notice in difficult conditions. What role the hospital will play in providing supplies for on-scene operations should be determined in advance. If the hospital is responsible for replenishing supplies for on-scene operations, planners should identify ways to collect and transport supplies.

A new concept in emergency operations logistics refers to accounting for all materials with potential reimbursement from outside sources for supplies used. In such cases, staffing costs may also be included, so purchasing and human resources should work closely to ensure that all costs of an emergency operation are documented.

EMERGENCY DEPARTMENT PLANNING

Creating ED OPs follows much the same model as the hospital emergency operations plan. The same planning process can be used by substituting departmental staff for hospital administrators. Since an effective plan reflects the thinking of those who use it, persons who collaborate to produce their department's response plan usually remember best what is contained in the plan. Staff who have to think through the plan before writing it as a formal document usually find it easy to remember content and pertinent actions.

As with the hospital plan, a core plan should be the primary focus of ED planning efforts followed by the development of appendices to address particular situations likely to impact the ED. The hub-and-spoke concept is just as valid here as in the hospital plan. A plan should be created that closely resembles daily operations of the department. Disruption of normal flow can be detrimental. For instance, instead of moving the ambulance receiving area if it gets too crowded, a better solution would be finding a way to move vehicles out of the way more quickly. Likewise, triage and making room assignments can be delegated to someone with essential experience. Using a physician or supervisor unfamiliar with these functions creates a problem, not a solution.

The department plan should be written using the premise that employees will continue in their usual roles or assume specific responsibilities. Pooling staff in the cafeteria or other locations is not as effective as leaving employees to work in their units doing usual tasks until needed for special assignment. Employees pooled in a central location may feel useless and unneeded. Employees who arrive in response to a call for help and go to their assigned department can help staff who are already on duty to get ahead in routine tasks, so that if any staff are reassigned, impact on the unit is not as great. A master sign-in sheet is helpful when large numbers of ED staff are called in. When calls come from family about an ED employee, the secretary can check the log-in sheet for staff presence in the ED. Since staff cannot respond to every phone call during an emergency operation, this is a simple method for providing information to the person on the phone. A binder with alphabetical tabs facilitates staff log-in and makes it easy for secretaries to obtain information.

Each employee should know his or her position in the organization, specific assignment, whom to report to, and whom to supervise. While most employees function well in their daily tasks, emergency operations add stress, so supervisors should observe staff performance carefully during emergency operations to ensure compliance with the emergency operations plan. Staff supervision during emergency operations should be clearly defined and linear in nature. Shared supervision is confusing in the best of times, and much worse during emergency operations. If a supervisor is reassigned, assigned staff should be reassigned to another supervisor or to a new role under the same supervisor. This maintains supervisory functions and minimizes staff confusion.

Communication is essential for the success of the response. It increases staff performance and alleviates stress that comes from not knowing what is going on in the community or at the scene. Use of portable phones or hand-held radios facilitates communication between triage and treatment areas. This type of communication is critical in an ED with a large floor plan. Informing staff of essential information related to the incident is also critical, particularly during a response of long duration. Departmental functions should also be communicated to the HEOC, so that coordination among departments can be maintained.

All employees should know their responsibilities when the emergency operations plan is invoked. In most cases, this is enhancement of daily activities. Staff preparation is also critical. The situation is worsened if staff have not called their family to explain why they will not be coming home. Box 18-2 lists common sense steps for staff preparation. Employees should remain in their assigned areas to ensure coverage and prevent overloading in critical areas by those who are sightseers, interfering with operations and draining resources needed for the emergency operation.

Successful hospital emergency operations rest on the principles of control and coordination, different strategies for different emergencies, and department plans or standard OPs drawn for emergency operations. The main plan and appendices defining departmental responsibilities should be published for general distribution. Standard OPs are the nuts and bolts of how a department functions to discharge its responsibilities. Procedures should remain within the department with one copy in the HEOC.

COMMUNITY PLANNING

Hospitals are in a unique leadership position to foster and support EOP for communities. Hospitals are an integral part of the community plan in some areas, but in other areas community plans have been done by public safety agencies without hospital participation in the planning process. If no plan exists for surrounding communities, the hospital should take the lead in getting the process started.

The table of contents of a community EOP plan are similar to that of a hospital plan. Fire, police, emergency medical services, and other organizations have appendices to support the incident command system, which establishes

---

Box **18-2**	**Common Sense Steps in Staff Preparation for Emergency Operations**

Contact family to prevent multiple calls of inquiry.
Use the bathroom—breaks may not be possible for a long time.
Check rooms for necessary supplies.
Prepare appropriate medical record documents such as nurses' notes and ED chart.
Obtain a stethoscope, pen, and scissors.

Data from Promina Kennestone Hospital Emergency Center: *Emergency center disaster plan,* Marietta, Ga, 1990, Promina.

the command post (similar to the HEOC) to coordinate operations.

Command information from the scene should go to one central place within the hospital. A communication link between the command post in the field and the HEOC should be established early in the incident. Community and hospital plans should contain information on establishing this linkage and should assign responsibility for who should establish this linkage. The community may also have an Emergency Operations Center, but these centers rarely involve hospitals. A liaison may be needed to coordinate activities between the HEOC and the community's operations center, especially if the situation directly impacts the hospital's daily operations. The hospital should continue to play its defined role in the community emergency operations plan as long as normal operations are possible.

Hospitals have the ability to communicate with EMS personnel at the scene to get information on numbers, types, and other characteristics of the injured. At most incidents with casualties, protocols define who will communicate with the hospital. This is usually the same person with the authority to manage on-the-scene treatment and receive orders from hospitals receiving patients. Hospitals can position themselves to control patient flow and volumes. Unless weather or safety restrictions are present, the hospital can request a 15- to 20-minute delay in patient delivery to allow the hospital to accommodate volume. Critical patients may be diverted in certain situations while patients with minor injuries can remain at the scene until the hospital can more easily accommodate them.

Understanding field operations is important because the hospital may become the field if an emergency incident occurs in the facility. When this occurs, hospital administrators are no longer in charge of the emergency scene. In many states, law places authority and responsibility for all scene operations with the chief fire officer until he declares the incident under control. As the Incident Commander, the senior fire official delegates authority to various specialist groups, such as extrication, fire suppression, and medical teams. Hospital planners should be sure they understand how the Incident Commander in their town will handle an event at their facility.

For almost all incidents, the local community is able to care for the injured and manage the impact of the incident with local or regional resources. Occasionally, assistance from outside agencies must be obtained, so resources from county, regional, state, and national agencies with specialized services should be at the disposal of communities with special needs. To make use of these resources, planners should identify contact points and response times to the locality within the plan. The Federal Emergency Management Agency through the National Disaster Medical System has medical assistance teams that can be sent to major catastrophes to provide patient care. System objectives are de-

---

Box 18-3 **National Disaster Medical System Objectives**

Provide medical assistance to a disaster area in the form of medical assistance teams, supplies, and equipment.

Evacuate patients who cannot be cared for on the scene to designated locations elsewhere in the nation.

Provide hospitalization in a nationwide network of hospitals that have agreed to accept patients in the event of a national emergency.

From Department of Defense: The national disaster medical system concept. In *Disaster medical assistance team organization guide*, Washington, DC, 1985, U.S. Government Printing Office.

---

scribed in Box 18-3. Teams are activated at the request of the governor of the state with a response of at least 48 hours after activation. Planners should contact the state Office of Emergency Management and other agencies to determine what help may be available. In most cases, operations in communities must rely on local resources for the first 12 hours of an emergency.

OTHER CONSIDERATIONS
Regulatory Oversight and Accreditation

Some states require hospitals to have a disaster or emergency operations plan as a condition of their license to operate. California, for instance, requires that hospitals have an incident command system established to manage emergency operations. Some states loosely require the hospital to have a disaster plan but do not identify specific criteria for the plan, while others have no regulatory requirement. Planners should be sure that their hospital meets or exceeds requirements in their state.

Accrediting agencies require emergency operations planning and drilling, although standards usually are not rigorous. Voluntary agencies, such as the Joint Commission on the Accreditation of Healthcare Organizations, have definitive criteria for judging hospital plans and exercises, which can be used as an impetus to improve planning. The American College of Surgeons, in the process for verification of trauma facilities, has specific requirements for EOP. Hospitals may not plan for or practice emergency operations unless it is required for licensure or accreditation.

Education. As with any new procedure, employees should receive education about the emergency operations plan. Each time the plan is revised (ideally once a year), each department should brief employees on each shift. Relatively minor revisions can be done at a regular staff meeting, whereas major changes are better presented in a special meeting. An interactive workshop using scenarios with audience participation to devise solutions to problems presented is an ideal way to educate staff on major changes in the plan.

New-employee orientation should include thorough coverage of the emergency operations plan and department operating procedures. Review of the plan 3 months later provides an opportunity for questions about emergency procedures. By then, employees have more knowledge of how their department operates routinely and can discuss the plan more realistically.

Exercising the plan. Exercises, or drills, are the clinical component of EOP and education. During an exercise, participants have an opportunity to practice skills and decision-making capabilities developed during the planning process and in special classes. The most common forms of exercises are tabletop, functional, and full-scale exercises.

Tabletop exercises provide a relatively low-stress way for participants to review roles during play with others. This exercise is well suited to HEOC operations where scripted scenarios provide stimulation for interdepartmental collaboration to solve presented problems. Exercises are usually run by a facilitator experienced in emergency operations and who understands the facility's plan. The facilitator prepares the scenario, presents the incident, and guides players through individual thought processes used in making correct decisions. Coaching and teaching are key components that enable players to formulate solutions that are easy to remember. Exercises also identify flaws in the plan that may require adjustment. Multiple tabletop exercises may be held during planning to test various proposals before they are included in the plan.

Functional exercises test interrelated components of the plan and are especially useful for activities that cross department lines, such as admission procedures, security, or media relations. Various problems, such as prioritization of injured patients, supply access, and visitor control, can be posed in rapid sequence with time intervals similar to those seen in a real event.

A full-scale exercise is usually held in cooperation with public safety agencies. Such exercises test all areas of the plan as well as education and response of hospital staff and other participating personnel. Planning for the exercise usually takes several months and involves setting goals, creating a scenario, formulating extent of play, soliciting volunteer patients, and recruiting faculty/evaluators. Unfortunately, some planners spend more time planning the exercise than they do exercising the plan. Goals for all participants should be well defined and measurable. The scenario should provide a fair test for identified goals and should result in a document that describes expectations of how far each area will go in response to the scenario. Volunteer patients should be prepared mentally and physically for the part they will play to ensure that the scenario provides realism and evokes proper responses. Faculty/evaluators should be persons with experience in emergency operations as well as in teaching or coaching, so that players can learn as they implement plans and procedures.

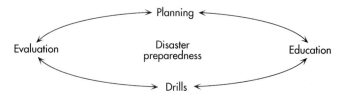

Figure 18-2 Dynamic process of emergency operations preparedness.

Evaluation. Everyone who participates in an exercise should be given an opportunity to comment on lessons learned, usually during a critique held immediately after the exercise. The exercise facilitator and faculty/evaluation sector leaders should present brief oral remarks with a formal written report compiled by the facilitator from written reports of each sector leader. The written report forms the basis for departmental meetings and administrative activities that revise the plan as necessary. Focused, detailed sessions may be necessary for individual departments, but the immediate critique gives an opportunity for positive reinforcement, acknowledgment of participant contributions, and a strategic view of further activities. Evaluation reports of deficiencies should focus on shortcomings of the plan, education, or scenario, assuming that each participant acts to the best of his or her ability during an exercise. When actions fall short, failure is probably the result of the plan not identifying the best responses, the player not being educated in responses called for by the plan, or the scenario being unrealistic and failing to evoke desired responses. Actual events should be critiqued and evaluated similarly to exercises. With actual events, the critique does not take place immediately after the event is finished; however, the less time that passes from event completion to critique, the more effective the critique.

As part of the hospital's CQI process, results of the exercise or event evaluation and subsequent critique sessions should be returned to the EOP committee. The committee should then consider each comment and recommendation to develop changes in the plan, departmental appendices, or content of educational sessions.

CONCLUSION

Preparing for emergency operations is a continuous cycle of planning, education, exercising, and evaluation (Figure 18-2). Periodically, literature should be reviewed for advances in technology of emergency responses and innovative response patterns. A growing interest exists in this aspect of medical and nursing care, so the body of knowledge is rapidly expanding. A notebook or file folder devoted to articles about EOP and responses can enhance planning and execution during the next emergency operation. As Christopher Robin said, "Planning is something you do, so when you do it, it's not all messed up."

REFERENCES

1. *American Heritage Electronic Dictionary,* 1992, Houghton Mifflin.
2. Coleman R: Loma Prieta: Emergency planning revisited, *IEMS News,* April 15, 1990.
3. Delehanty RA: The emergency nurse and disaster medical assistance teams, *J Emerg Nurs* 22(3):184-189, 1996.
4. Department of Defense: The national disaster medical system concept. In *Disaster medical assistance team organization guide,* Washington, DC, 1985, US Government Printing Office.
5. Early E: Darnall Army Community Hospital's response to the Killeen massacre, *J Emerg Nurs* 18(4):316-318, 1992.
6. Hindman D: Planning a disaster drill: checklists for success, *J Emerg Nurs* 16(4):298-299, 1990.
7. Joint Commission on Accreditation of Healthcare Organizations: Hospital emergency preparedness. In *1996 Accreditation Manual for Hospitals,* Chicago, 1996, The Committee.
8. Kitt S, et al: *Emergency nursing: A physiologic and clinical perspective,* ed 2, Philadelphia, 1995, WB Saunders.
9. Lippman H: When the disaster drill is for real, *RN* 54-58, September 1992.
10. Luce ZR: A practical hospital emergency plan, *Contingency J* 47:20-21, May/June 1991.
11. Miller DM: Care for the caregivers, *RN* 58-60, September, 1992.
12. Promina Kennestone Hospital Emergency Center: *Emergency center disaster plan,* Marietta, Ga, 1990, Promina.
13. Sanford JP: Civilian disasters and disaster planning. In Burkle SM Jr, Sanner PH, Wolcott BW, editors: *Disaster medicine,* New York, 1984, Medical Examination Publishing.

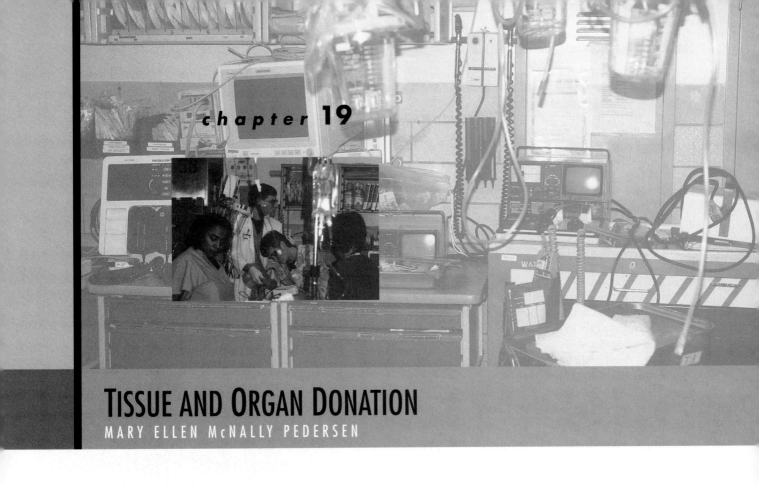

chapter **19**

TISSUE AND ORGAN DONATION

MARY ELLEN McNALLY PEDERSEN

A critical issue faced by emergency nurses is tissue and organ donation. In the past, the emergency nurse was peripherally involved with donation of organs and tissues. As technology and availability of professionals to recover tissue and organs increase, donation has become more commonplace in the emergency department (ED). Emergency nurses and other health care professionals must be prepared to offer the family or next of kin of a patient who dies the opportunity for donation.

OVERVIEW

Each time a patient dies in the ED, the patient should be considered a potential organ or tissue donor. Box 19-1 summarizes organs and tissues that can be donated. Almost any person who dies can become a tissue donor, excluding anyone with a systemic infectious disease. The most common potential donor is a tissue donor, yet this opportunity is frequently overlooked by health care professionals. Many needed tissues are lost because no one remembers to offer the family the option of tissue donation. More importantly, the family of the person who has just died may not be given the opportunity to carry out the wishes of the patient to donate tissues and organs. The potential donor may have expressed this desire by signing a donor card, completing an advanced directive or living will, or previously discussing these preferences with his or her next of kin. Organ donor wishes are included on the backs of driver's licenses in some states. At a time when family stress is greatest, the wish to

donate is not considered the first priority and is frequently forgotten. Health care professionals should help provide this opportunity. Countless people are waiting for a new cornea, bone, or other tissue (Table 19-1). Their lives may not hang in the balance, as when one is waiting for a heart, liver, lung, or heart and lung transplantation, but quality of life can be greatly enhanced by tissue transplantation. Transplantation surpasses conventional means of treatment.

As common as tissue donation, organ donation is also available when a person suffers a severe brain injury or a prolonged anoxic event. Such situations result in eventual death of brain tissue, rendering the patient dead and supported only by mechanical means. Potential donors are typically victims of traumatic injuries secondary to a motor vehicle crash, a gunshot wound to the head, a ruptured cerebral aneurysm, arteriovenous malformation, severe stroke, or a severe anoxic event resulting from prolonged cardiac arrest.

A person declared dead by brain-death criteria who is a potential organ donor is also considered a tissue donor. A patient in asystole, however, is a potential tissue donor only, because visceral organ donation requires an intact circulatory system. A donor on a ventilator may require vasopressors to maintain blood pressure, urine output, fluids and electrolytes, and alterations of ventilatory settings to maintain adequate ventilation and perfusion. Before a patient is considered for potential organ donation, he or she must meet criteria for brain death or be in the process of evaluation for

Box **19-1**   **Transplantable Organs and Tissues**

Organs	Tissues
Kidneys	Cornea
Heart	Bones
Lungs	Pancreatic islet cells
Pancreas	Bone marrow
Intestines	
Liver	

Table **19-1** **Number in U.S. Awaiting Transplants**	
Number in U.S.	Transplant needed
32,725	Kidney
6629	Liver
294	Pancreas
44	Pancreas islet cell
1366	Kidney-pancreas
3600	Heart
219	Heart-lung
2083	Lung
77	Intestine
47,037	

UNOS National Patient Waiting List Weekly Update of July 10, 1996. Used with permission from Lifelink of Georgia.

these criteria. Ultimately, the patient must be declared dead by brain-death criteria for actual donation to take place.

All too often the family of the patient declared dead according to brain-death criteria are not offered the option of organ and tissue donation. For example, a 1985 Gallup poll described a situation in which 20,000 potential donors were identified and only 3000 became actual organ donors.[11] More recent data support this same phenomenon. Reports from the United Network of Organ Sharing (UNOS) suggest that between 1990 and 1994 approximately 10,000 to 14,000 potential internal organ donors existed. The actual number of donors during the same time period ranged from 4500 and 4900.[17] The most commonly cited reason for this lack is the health care professional feeling uncomfortable in dealing with death and broaching the subject of donation,[4,18] and wanting to avoid greater suffering for the family. The result of this hesitation, however, is that the supply of organs and tissues does not meet the demand. As of March 1996, approximately 40,000 people were waiting for a solid organ transplant (UNOS Communication). By the late 1980s, this widening gap between potential organ donors and recipients stimulated development and enactment of amendments to the Uniform Anatomical Gift Act on a state-by-state basis. These creative adjustments redefined the potential donor in an effort to expand availability of greatly needed organs for transplant. Many states mandated that the health care professional or hospital designee offer each family at the time of the patient's death the option of tissue and organ donation as deemed medically appropriate. Sensitivity to the family's cultural, religious, and emotional situation must be considered. More often than not, the family appreciates that the option is offered because something positive can result from the death of a loved one.[3] The family may not wish to hear more about donation and may decline to donate, but at least they are given the opportunity to make that decision and should be supported in their decision, whatever it might be.

Redefinition of the potential cadaver donor population includes expansion of age limits, and consideration of patients on a case-by-case basis who have a history of high blood pressure, diabetes, and evidence of minor cardiac and respiratory difficulties. Transplant programs have begun to incorporate the option of a living, nonrelated kidney donation into their programs for those needing a kidney transplant. Kidney transplants are now done between husband and wife or between a person and significant other where a reasonable tissue match exists. Work is also being done with a nonheart-beating kidney donor, with differing levels of success. Segmental liver and lung transplants are being carried out in different areas of the country offering new hope to those who wait.

HISTORICAL PERSPECTIVE

Throughout time, humanity has been intrigued with the idea of finding a way to maintain and extend life to its fullest. Current technologies permit replacement of a diseased organ with one that is healthy, using transplantation techniques to restore life and health.

Tissue transplantation is described in the historical literature as early as 1682, when Meekren made an attempt to replace a portion of a soldier's cranium with the skull bone of a dog.[6] Historical literature describes pancreatic transplantation and details transplantation of a sheep's pancreas into a human by Williams in 1893. This took place before a description and isolation of islet cells in the pancreas had been made. Corneal graft surgery was undertaken by Wolf in 1800,[17] and in 1881 skin grafting was tried as a temporary means of treating a severe burn.[8] Further work in skin grafting was carried out by Sir Peter Medawar, who used skin grafts treated with cold refrigeration in the 1940s.[17] Medawar was also awarded the Nobel Prize for his work in immune response and the rejection phenomenon,[9] which to a great extent has been the basis for further study in transplantation. Advances in the last 15 years in immunosuppressive therapies have greatly enhanced the potential for many transplantation procedures previously hampered by tissue rejection complications.

Work in whole-organ transplantation began somewhat later than tissue transplantation. In 1902, Ullman attempted the transplantation of kidneys in a goat model. His work and the research of others was spurred on by an ever increasing number of people suffering from end-stage renal disease.[17]

Many attempts at dialyzing patients who have renal failure were made as early as the 1860s by Grahm using his wooden hoop dialyzer.[16] However in the 1940s Kolft designed the dialysis machine on which current dialysis is based.[15] Merrill and his colleagues at the Peter Bent Brigham Hospital in Boston implemented dialysis therapy in 1954.[8] This work was based on Kolft's work as the method of choice for treating patients in end-stage renal failure.

Simultaneously, research in renal transplantation occurred because great numbers of people required dialysis. Dialysis remains a lengthy, expensive, and limited modality for patients with renal failure. The first kidney transplantations were performed at the Peter Bent Brigham Hospital in 1954 between living, identical twins by Murray (Nobel Prize winner, 1990) and Harrison.[17] These autografts were successful. Further work with living, related (sibling, parent) donors and cadaveric donors continued with moderate success.

As kidney and tissue transplantation became an effective treatment modality, the possibilities of other whole-organ transplantation became a reality. The first liver transplantation was performed in 1963 in Denver, Colorado by Thomas Starz.[13] The first lung transplantation was performed by Hardy at the University of Mississippi in 1963,[13] and the first kidney and pancreas transplantation was by Lillehei at the University of Minnesota in 1967.

Most significant of all events in the arena of transplantation was the first heart transplantation in 1967 by Christiaan Barnard in Cape Town, South Africa.[13] The first heart and lung transplantation was performed by Shumway in 1981 at Stanford University.[13] Each of these extrarenal transplantations was somewhat limited in restoring life for the person receiving the new organ; however, each transplantation was the beginning of a new technologic era. This activity and further innovative research resulted in several new areas of concern. Of greatest consequence was prevention of rejection, infection, and other issues related to allograft survival. Research efforts continue to probe and perfect different modalities of transplantation, and many research groups are delving into the efficacy of xenographs, genetic manipulation of specific animal models, and the use of mechanical bridges until a much needed organ or health care alternative becomes available.

Issues such as determination of death by brain-death criteria, the health care professional's comfort level when offering donation to families, and the ongoing need for public education about donation to prepare families before the time of crisis are diligently being addressed by the medical and transplantation communities.

LEGISLATIVE OVERVIEW

Transplantation was a thriving technology in the late 1960s. Survival rates improved, and legislators began taking notice of this unique medical practice. Two key documents were developed in 1968, one legislative and the other professional, relating to effective medical practice. These were known respectively as the Uniform Anatomical Gift Act and the Harvard Criteria for Determination of Brain Death.

The Uniform Anatomical Gift Act of 1968 was adopted as law in all 50 states. Organ and tissue donation became accepted legal and medical practice. This law allows a person to decide to become an organ or tissue donor. A person may carry a donor card, or a sticker may be affixed to a driver's license signifying intent to donate in the event of death. It helps if the family is aware of the potential donor's wishes. The donor card serves as a tool of communication to ED staff, emergency medical personnel, and the family. For practical purposes, consent from the next of kin is sought in all cases of donation. The critical point staff must communicate in teaching the family, patient, or community groups about donation is that each person should make his or her own decision about donation and then share that decision with the family. A person filling out the donor card must be 18 years of age or older and must have two witnesses, preferably known to the card carrier, who sign the card on behalf of the donor.

In the donation process, the next of kin has the integral role of giving final permission for donation. The order of priority for next of kin is (1) spouse, (2) adult child, (3) parent, (4) sibling, and (5) guardian. (The order of priority varies slightly from state to state.) The next of kin acting for the deceased must be 18 years of age or older. In most situations of traumatic death, many family members are involved in the care and decision making for the patient. Decision making on behalf of the patient is difficult at best. When the issue of donation is discussed, many families become confused about the wishes of their loved ones, particularly if no discussion has taken place regarding donation. Often dissension exists among family members that can be painful and distressing. However, the best decision is one with which all family members are comfortable. The next of kin with highest priority has the final decision-making power. Whether the patient ever expressed the desire either to donate or not to donate, the family should be encouraged to honor the deceased's wishes.

The Uniform Anatomical Gift Act not only provides a person with the opportunity to donate organs and tissues but also protects that person if he or she chose not to donate.

Throughout the years the Uniform Anatomical Gift Act has been amended to assist in meeting the growing need for transplantation organs and tissues. The amendment of greatest note was development of the "required request" or "required referral" clause. The concept of required request was the direct result of a Congressional investigation in the early 1980s surrounding the difficulties a private citizen might have obtaining an organ for transplant because of a shortage of organs and lack of third-party funding for organ transplant. Albert Gore, as senator from Tennessee, spearheaded an inquiry by a committee of experts to determine the shortcomings and inequities of the organ transplant process. This led to enactment of the Organ Transplantation Act (PL 98-507), which mandated formation of the Organ Transplantation Task Force to critically review the medical, ethical, economic, and legal issues surrounding donation and transplantation. The report of the Organ Transplantation Task Force, published in 1986,[6] outlines conclusions and recommendations for the donation and transplantation community. Key conclusions which affect the emergency nurse and other health care professionals are: (1) families were not approached consistently concerning the option to donate tissues and organs for transplantation and (2) health care providers were hesitant to approach families with the option of donation. Recommendations included (1) encouraging states to enact some form of required request legislation, mandating that hospitals implement and develop organ and tissue donation policies; (2) encouraging states to enact the Uniform Determination of Death Act; and (3) encouraging and supporting increased professional and public education.[9]

Aside from the development of the task force, the Organ Transplantation Act required the Department of Health and Human Services (DHHS) to establish a single national network for the distribution and management of organs and tissues for transplantation. The Organ Procurement and Transplantation Network was created and is administered by the secretary of the DHHS. A private, nonprofit agency, the United Network of Organ Sharing (UNOS), serves as a network and accomplishes the objectives of the secretary. UNOS is located in Richmond, Virginia and serves as a clearinghouse for organs and tissues recovered for transplantation.

Subsequent to the task force recommendations, required request legislation evolved in 44 states in the form of amendments to state anatomical gift acts. The rationale behind the legislation is summed up nicely by ethicist Arthur Caplin, PhD:

> In enacting required request legislation, our society has indicated its collective desire that people routinely be given the option of organ and tissue donation as a last act of respect for the dead and their families and as an expression of concern for those who will die unless more organs and tissues are made available.[4]

The goal of the required request law is to ultimately increase the number of organs and tissues available for transplantation and more importantly, provide the grieving family with the option of tissue and organ donation for a family member. Each state law has its own idiosyncrasies with slightly different requirements, but essentially all ascribe to these goals. In response to state legislation throughout the United States, Congress incorporated into the federal Consolidated Omnibus Budget Reconciliation Act (COBRA) of 1986 (PL 99-506) a requirement that hospitals receiving Medicare funding develop a policy to achieve the following[14]: (1) families of potential donors are made aware of the option of organ or tissue donation and their option to decline to donate, (2) discretion and sensitivity are encouraged with respect to the circumstances, views, and beliefs of such families, and (3) an organ procurement agency designated by the secretary of DHHS is required to be notified of potential donors.

Ten UNOS regions have been designated in the United States by DHHS (Figure 19-1). Within each region, a single designated Organ Procurement Organization (OPO) theoretically serves to advise hospital administration, nurses, and medical professionals concerning issues related to tissue and organ donation and provide respective hospitals with services necessary for recovery and placement of organs and tissues. In many regions, a number of isolated OPOs merged to share the responsibility of the organ and tissue donation process and to eliminate competition for organs. When an emergency nurse identifies a potential tissue and/or organ donor the local organ procurement agency should be contacted as soon as possible.

THE DONATION PROCESS

When a patient dies in the ED, he or she should be considered for donation of some tissue or organ. Three key pieces of information that must be documented in the medical record for the donation to take place are:

1. Determination and declaration of death
2. Medical examiner's approval (as required by state law)
3. Consent from the next of kin

Determination of Death

A patient must be declared dead for the donation process to begin. The Uniform Determination of Death Act plays an integral role in identifying which criteria must be met to determine death. Death in a person is defined as either of the following criteria[7]:

I. A person with irreversible cessation of circulatory and respiratory function is dead.
   A. Cessation is recognized by an appropriate clinical examination.
   B. Irreversibility is recognized by persistent cessation of functions during an appropriate period of observation, trial of therapy, or both.
II. A person with irreversible cessation of all functions of the entire brain, including the brainstem, is dead.
   A. Cessation is recognized when evaluation discloses two findings:
      1. Cerebral functions are absent.
      2. Brainstem functions (pupillary reflex, corneal reflex, gag reflex) are absent.
   B. Irreversibility is recognized when evaluation discloses three findings:
      1. Cause of coma is established and is sufficient to account for loss of brain functions.
      2. Possibility of recovery of brain functions is excluded.
      3. Cessation of all brain functions persists for an appropriate period of observation, trial of therapy, or both.

These commonly accepted criteria have been adopted as the standard of practice. Traditionally, death was believed to occur when a person's heart stopped beating. As technology evolved, a patient could be maintained on mechanical support devices, so determination of death by brain-death criteria became a recognized practice, and has been described by

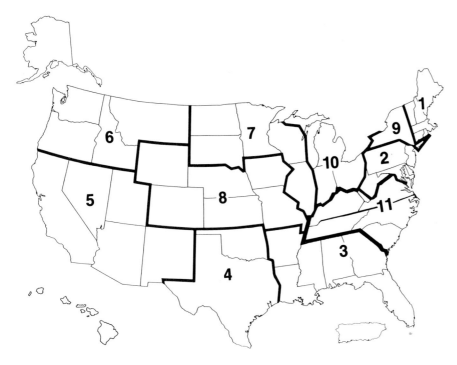

Figure **19-1** UNOS regional map.

many neuroscience professional groups, most notably the Harvard Group, in the *Harvard Criteria for Determination of Brain Death*.[7] The process of determining death by brain-death criteria when appropriate has become more specific as a result of (1) a restating and updating of the criteria by the President's Commission for the Study of Ethical Problems in Medicine and Biomedical and Behavioral Research, (2) an evolution of the definition of brain death, and (3) increased levels of comfort and experience with application of the criteria on the part of neuroscience physicians and hospital personnel.

After death has been determined, it must be documented in the patient's medical record, including the time of death. Then the patient is evaluated as a potential tissue and organ donor. Criteria used to determine whether a patient is a suitable candidate for donation change frequently. Emergency nurses and other health care professionals should contact their respective organ procurement agency to determine suitability for donation before speaking to the family.

Medical criteria that may prevent donation of organs and some tissues from a patient include the presence of a documented septicemia, communicable disease such as hepatitis, or the possibility that the patient is at high risk for human immunodeficiency virus. All other persons can be considered potential candidates for donation of tissues or organs. Frequently an error is made in determining that a patient diagnosed with metastatic cancer is ineligible for tissue donation. Almost any person with most forms of cancer, including cancers that have metastasized, is eligible to donate corneas for transplantation and/or research. Again, the key is to contact the regional procurement agency to determine suitability for donation before discussing donation with the family.

Emergency nurses referring potential donors to the regional procurement agency must employ referral policies approved within their respective institutions. If no policy exists, contacting the local procurement agency can be of benefit; the agency can help design a program to suit the hospital's needs and comply with state law.

When a nurse calls the local procurement agency, guidelines shown in Figure 19-2 for required information are recommended. A typical referral pattern for tissue or organ donation is outlined in Figure 19-3.

Medical Examiner's Approval

The medical examiner must be notified when a donation takes place under certain circumstances, including:
1. Homicide
2. Suicide
3. Accidental death
4. Death within 24 hours of admission
5. Patient is admitted in comalike state and dies
6. Death of a person 18 years of age or less
(Medical examiner regulations vary slightly from state to state.)

Each state has specific criteria. Before these criteria are included in a donation policy, the hospital should contact the state medical examiner for more information. For example, the medical examiner's office in Rhode Island requires notification of death and request for approval of donation *without* exception, for all persons who are potential tissue or organ donors. Documentation of this notification is essential for donation to take place. Notation of communication with the medical examiner should be included in the patient's medical record.

WORSHEET

(Does not need to be saved)

ORGAN AND TISSUE DONOR REFERRAL GUIDELINE

(800) _____ - _____

24 HOUR HOTLINE

Name of Patient _____ MR# _____

Age _____ Date of Birth _____ Admission Date _____

Time of Death _____ Cause of Death _____

Past Medical History _____

_____

- ☐ Ocular History/including Surgeries _____
- ☐ Anticoagulation Therapy   Yes / No
        What type? (Heparin, Coumadin, ASA, TPA, Steptokinase, etc. _____.)

- ☐ History of Positive Blood Culture   Date _____

        Name of Antibiotic given _____ Date _____

- ☐ Cancer Patient, had   ☐ Chemotherapy   ☐ Radiation therapy
        If so, date and type of last therapy given

        Date _____   Type _____

- ☐ Social History _____

- ☐ Family Status-Next of Kin _____

- ☐ Attending Physician _____

- ☐ Medical Examiner Case   Yes / No,   Called: ☐ Approve donation
  24 hour phone: (800) _____ - _____   ☐ Disapprove donation

Comments: _____

_____

_____

_____

Figure **19-2** Organ and tissue donor referral guideline.

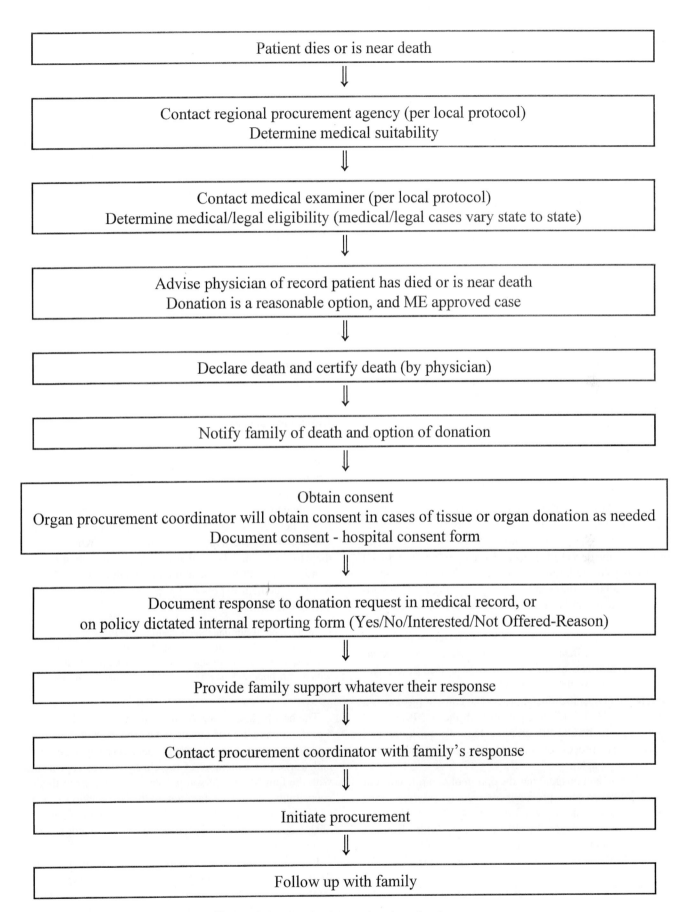

Figure **19-3** Organ and tissue donation referral pattern.

Hospital Requirements

Required-request mandates resulted in the development of organ and tissue donation hospital policy requirements that focus on offering donation to families at the time of death of a family member. Implementation of this law dictates documentation of all aspects of the request for donation including a sound practical policy supported by administration, development of user friendly documentation tools, and education of all staff involved in the process about how to offer tissue and organ donation. The education process must address staff around the clock in all areas of practice.

Three essential forms in the documentation process are necessary when a tissue or organ donation takes place. First is the consent form; it must be completed when a family indicates the desire to donate organs. The second is the hospital's internal reporting form that documents the request for donation and the next of kin response to the request. This document must be completed for every person that dies in the hospital regardless of the family decision to donate. This document is frequently required for compliance with some state laws and is helpful with federal law compliance. Lastly, a state reporting form may be required in some states. It summarizes the hospital's annual tissue and organ donation activity.

The internal reporting form can be an extremely helpful tool when attempting to educate staff and determine an area of need within an institution. In states where hospitals are required to complete such documentation, many institutions have developed a two-page duplicate copy form. One copy is for the medical record and one is for the hospital record keeping department. The form documents patient age, location where death occurred, the offer of donation, the reason for not offering donation, family response, next of kin relationship to the deceased, consent for organs and tissues, and what was recovered. Information can be placed in a database so that potential donors and tissues stemming from the donation process can be tracked over the course of the year. Figure 19-4 is an example of this form.

Documentation of the next of kin's consent must be included in the medical record. Usually permission for donation of tissues and organs is written on a specific consent form provided by the local OPO or a state-mandated form with hospital-specific amendments. The consent process is a delicate one and requires a person with the sensitivity and knowledge to handle the grieving family's questions and concerns. The process of consent is discussed in more detail later in this chapter.

Each state and hospital has the option of creating consent forms; however, most procurement agencies provide forms and prefer use of the consent form they developed. This document is modified periodically to comply with changing laws. If consent forms are not available in the ED, the local procurement agency or UNOS provides them promptly. (Figure 19-5).

The last form of documentation required is dictated by state law. Many states require an annual report on donation data. Data must be tabulated and submitted to the state department of health or other state regulatory body for review, licensure, and certification of the institution. This also provides the hospital with much needed feedback concerning how best to provide donation education within the hospital community. Data can also be reported annually for verification of Medicare and Medicaid funding, as required by federal regulations pertaining to COBRA of 1986 and 1990. (This verification has not yet been mandated.)

A policy or program to manage tissue and organ donation must be developed in each institution, and can be only as strong as those who manage and are committed to it. Whether this program is managed by a donation liaison staff member who works with the procurement agency's donation coordinator, by a donation committee, or by a dedicated emergency nurse, with significant commitment the program will evolve successfully. Documentation during the program's first year is the best measure of the program's strengths, and permits ongoing assessment and correction of shortcomings. Successes can and should be shared with other institutions as a contribution to the overall tissue and organ donation process. Failures should be shared when successful solutions have been implemented.

Obtaining Consent

Offering the family or next of kin the option of donation is one of the more difficult yet potentially rewarding responsibilities that emergency nurses assume in their professional careers. Providing a family with the option of donation may give them a measure of comfort and consolation. The comfort is not necessarily experienced at the time of the death, but later when the death has been realized. Knowing that their loved one has been able to help another often helps a family cope with the loss and continue their lives. The following statement expresses the positive effect of donation during one family's grief.[15]

At the time of our daughter's death it was difficult to think and make choices. Now, it [donation] has helped our grieving to know that in spite of our tragedy and loss several other people are blessed with health, hope and the promise of life. Rob and Jan Rivera, Denver, Colorado

The best person to approach the family about donation is a professional who has developed a rapport with the family, such as the primary nurse, the primary care physician, a social worker, or a member of the clergy who has spent time with the family. The person designated to carry out this responsibility should be familiar with the donation process and comfortable with feelings about death and the donation of tissues and organs. Much thought and knowledge are required to assume this responsibility.

Emergency nurses are in an ideal position to offer the family the option of donation. They have been working with the family and patient throughout the admission and have in most situations developed the greatest rapport with the family.

GEORGIA EYE BANK, INC.
LIFELINK OF GEORGIA

CONSENT FOR DONATION OF ANATOMICAL GIFT

I, the _____ of _____ do hereby give consent to Georgia Eye Bank, Inc. and/or
    (Relationship)   (Name of Donor)

LifeLink of Georgia or any person authorized by said organizations to recover from the body of the deceased patient the following anatomical gift(s) for the purpose of transplantation, therapy, medical research and/or education. I further consent to the release of medical records for the purpose of determining and documenting the suitability for donation; to examination(s) needed to ensure medical acceptability of the donation, and to the drawing of blood and/or tissue samples needed for laboratory testing. These tests include but are not limited to: blood typing, hepatitis, syphilis, cytomegalovirus, and human immuno deficiency virus.

I further acknowledge that I have read this document or that I have had it read to me in its entirety and that I fully understand it.

Please indicate by checking appropriate box
Y=Consent Granted; N=Consent Refused; N/A=Not Medically Suitable;

	Y	N	N/A		Y	N	N/A
1. WHOLE EYES	—	—	—	**TISSUES**			
				8. Heart Valves	—	—	—
ORGANS				9. Bone: Lower Extremities	—	—	—
2. Kidneys	—	—	—	10. Bone: Upper Extremities	—	—	—
3. Heart	—	—	—	Humerus/Ulna/Radius			
4. Liver	—	—	—	11. Bone: Ribs	—	—	—
5. Pancreas	—	—	—	12. Mandible	—	—	—
6. Lungs	—	—	—	13. Skin	—	—	—
7. Other	—	—	—	14. Dura	—	—	—
				15. Other	—	—	—

INCLUDE FOR ORGAN AND/OR TISSUE DONATION ONLY

I hereby consent to the removal of adjacent tendons, ligaments, muscle, fascia and blood vessels, as well as the spleen and lymph nodes, for tissue typing and testing. I understand and consent that in all cases when bone tissue is donated a complete autopsy will be performed.

_____
Next of Kin Signature

Funeral Arrangements: Open Viewing/Primary Cremation
                                    No Viewing

_____
Print Name

Funeral Home:_____

_____
Street

_____
Signature of Witness

_____
City/State/Zip

_____
Print Name

_____
Area Code/Telephone

_____
Signature of 2nd Witness

_____
Signature of Person Presenting the Option of Donation

_____
Print Name

_____
Print Name/Title

_____
Date/Time

_____
Hospital or Agency

7/93   HDRL-002

WHITE - CHART,   YELLOW - LLGA   PINK - GAEB

Figure **19-4**   Consent form for donation of anatomical gift. (*Used with permission from LifeLink of Georgia and Georgia Eye Bank, Inc., 1997.*)

LIFELINK CADAVER DONOR INFORMATION SHEET   UNOS # _____

LL # _____ BONE # _____ HV # _____ OTH. # _____ REF # _____

REFERRAL DATE __ / ___ / __ TIME _____ LOCAL ____ IMPORT ____ OPO _____

LIFELINK PROGRAM: (Circle One)   LLFL   LLGA   LLPR   LLSW   Ph./Fax: _____

LOCAL VASCULAR AND TISSUE REFERRALS   (Circle One) **VASC. / TIS.**

Donor Name _____

Age _____ Sex _____ Race _____ Eth. _____

DOB __ / ____ / ___ Hgt _____ Wgt _____

U.S. Born: Yes / No   If no:

Yrs. in U.S.: _____ yrs. Citizen: Yes / No

Admit Date _____ Time _____ ABO _____

Hospital/ME/FH _____

Referring Institution _____

Referring Person _____

Phone _____ Unit_____

Med. Rec. # _____

Pronounced ___ / ____ / ___ Time _____

Attending M.D.: _____

Consulting M.D.: _____

Cause of Death Code: _____

Mechanism of Death Code: _____

Circumstances of Death Code: _____

M.E. Case? Yes / No Autopsy? Yes / No

M.E. Name: _____

County: _____

M.E. Phone: _____

M.E. Comments: _____

M.E Permis.? Yes / No M.E. # _____

Phys. Performing Autopsy: _____

Location of Autopsy: _____

Funeral Home: _____

F.H Phone: _____

F.H. Contact: _____

F.H. Follow-up Name: _____

          Date: _____ Time: _____

Refrigerated: Yes / No Time:_____

Eye Tissue Referred: Yes / No

Eye Bank Coord.: _____

Past Medical/Social History: _____

_____

Clinical Course: _____

_____

_____

_____

Cardiac / Respiratory Arrest: Y / N Amt. of Time: _____

CONSENT INFORMATION

Med. Suit.: Vas- Yes / No_____ Bone- Yes / No_____ Skin- Yes / No_____ Other- Yes / No_____

Family Initially Approached By: _____ Code: _____

Person Requesting Consent: _____ Code: _____

Name of NOK Approached: _____ Code: _____

Family Refusal Reason: _____ Code: _____

Consent For: (If No, Code) Ki_____ H_____ Li_____ Lu_____ Pa_____ Int_____

          B_____ HV_____ Du_____ Sk_____ Eyes_____ Corneas_____ Research_____

IMPORT REFERRALS ONLY

Referring Coord. _____ Ph: _____ Clamp Date: _____ Clamp Time: _____

Potential Recipient Name:_____ Org.:___Accept: Yes / No If no, Code: _____

Potential Recipient Name:_____ Org.:___Accept: Yes / No If no, Code: _____

Potential Recipient Name:_____ Org.:___Accept: Yes / No If no, Code: _____

_____   _____   _____   _____

Primary Coordinator Signature   Date   Second Coord. Signature (if applicable)   Date

LLDIS1.10/1/94

Figure **19-5** Documentation for hospital management of organ/tissue donation. *(Used with permission from LifeLink of Georgia, 1997.)*

VITAL SIGNS

Date				
Avg.B/P				
Low B/P				
Duration				
HR				
Temp				
CVP				
PCWP				
Card.Out.				
SVR				
UOP/HR				
Low UOP				

Pressor History

HEART & LUNG DATA

EKG	
CXR	
ECHO	
CATH	
BRONCH	

LUNG MEASUREMENTS

Xiphoid	_____ cm
Nipple Line	_____ cm
Base	_____ cm
Rt. AP	_____ cm
Lt. AP	_____ cm

CHEMISTRIES/BLOOD WORK

Date			
Time			
NA +			
K +			
CL-			
CO2			
GLUC			
BUN			
Creat			
CA++			
Mg++			
PO4- -			
CPK			
CPK/MB			
SGOT/AST			
SGPT/ALT			
TOTAL BIL			
DIRECT BIL			
LDH			
GGTP			
ALK PHOS			
AMYLASE			
LIPASE			
WBC			
Hgb			
Hct			
PLT			
PT			
PTT			

MEDICATIONS/FLUIDS

Date	Type	Dose	Duration

BLOOD GASES

Date			
Time			
PH			
PC02			
P02			
02SAT			
HC03			
BE			
F102			
TV			
IMV			
PEEP			

SEROLOGY

	PRE	POST	CONF.
Date			
Tech			
Anti-HIV I			
Anti-HIV II			
Anti-HTLV I			
Anti-HTLV II			
RPR-VDRL			
Anti-CMV			
HBsAg			
Anti-HBC			
Anti-HCV			
IGM			
HBsAb			

P = Positive   N = Negative   U = Unknown
C = Can't Disclose   ND = Not Done   I = Indeter.

CULTURES

CULTURE	DATE	RESULTS
Blood		
Urine		
Sputum		

Figure **19-5** cont'd   For legend see opposite page.

However, the nurse should discuss with the attending physician the potential for donation. If the physician is not comfortable with offering the option of donation to the family, the emergency nurse will then be in a position to provide the family with the opportunity. Each institution may have an established protocol for offering donation to a family, and this protocol should be given consideration before proceeding.

Many institutions have a program in which certain staff members are educated in the art of obtaining consent and are available to offer donation to the family. These staff members are often referred to as *requestors* or *initiators* of consent for donation. The emergency nurse caring for the patient who has just died may not be familiar with the process of obtaining consent. The requestor can be a great resource and can assist with the process. The nurse can also talk to the local OPO for support in this matter; a coordinator from the agency can obtain consent from the family in person or over the telephone. An ED education program can be requested concerning methods of obtaining consent and initiating the donation process.

Before the family is made aware of their option, they must be told the patient has died. The family must be comfortable with the knowledge that everything possible was done to prevent death and that all available treatments were carried out to maintain the life of their family member. The family's sense of devastation is extreme; members are grieving and unlikely to believe that death has occurred. Discussion of anything immediately following the discussion of death may be impossible. The family needs a period of time to grieve and to grasp what has happened before they are asked to make another critical decision.[12]

Waiting until the family gives a verbal or nonverbal cue that they are ready to discuss what is to happen next is essential. In the case of potential brain death, when tissues and organs may be donated, the situation usually involves a sudden, unexpected event, and the person who dies may be young and previously healthy. This patient is usually transferred to an intensive care setting, where a series of tests is administered to establish that criteria for brain death have been met. When death is declared by these criteria, the family can be given a bit more time to adjust to the fact that death has occurred. Understanding death in this instance is difficult for most families: their loved one is breathing, warm, and looks alive. The family must accept that ventilatory support of the patient who is brain dead is strictly mechanical and has nothing to do with life and survival. If the support systems are removed, the patient's heart would stop beating and all signs of life would disappear. Helping the family understand that death has occurred is difficult. Information must be provided for the family by the primary physician in terms they can understand and must be educationally reinforced by the primary nurse and other available health care professionals.

When the patient in the ED is declared dead by the more conventional criterion of cardiac asystole, death is physically more obvious to the family. Grasping the reality of the event is poignant. Death as a result of cardiac arrest is recognized as a tangible end point. Family members have less time to consider possible options or treatments and less time to adjust to their loss.

Emotions can be labile. Adjusting to the idea of death is always difficult. The family will be in shock, engulfed by many different emotions and feeling. They may have had little to do with this particular family member recently, or they may feel responsible for the death. Families often ask themselves what could have been done to prevent death or how this death might have been made easier. Before the option of donation is broached, family members need time to gain control of their thoughts and adjust if possible to the reality that a family member has died and is not going to return home. Their lives will never be the same, and as difficult as it may seem, they must continue to live without this loved one.

The first step in the initiation process of donation, identifying the next of kin, can be straightforward or complex, depending on the family situation. (Reviewing the order of priority of the next of kin outlined earlier in the chapter would be prudent.) One must also differentiate between the next of kin and the family spokesperson. For example, the wife of a 70-year-old man in cardiac arrest may not come to the hospital when her husband is admitted and dies. However, in the absence of a son or daughter, a close family friend accompanies the patient and relays information to the next of kin by telephone. It is not appropriate in this case to offer the family friend the option of donation. One must initiate the process of donation by talking with the wife on the telephone and, if appropriate, obtain consent over the telephone. The nurse must keep in mind when obtaining consent over the telephone, that two witnesses must sign the consent form indicating that the next of kin has given permission to donate tissues and organs by telephone.

If family members choose to come to the ED to see the patient who has just died, they will need time to say goodbye and to make plans and various arrangements. The family must be provided with a private room or location that is comfortable, quiet, and gives them an opportunity to share their feelings of loss and grief with each other or experience that grief alone. Realizing that the family member is dead is the greatest hurdle the family must overcome. Viewing the body of the person who has just died is a critical step in this process.

An assessment of what the family knows or what they have been told is of great importance in offering the option of donation. If they are not yet able to accept that death has occurred, it is not time to talk about donation. The family must hear the words *death* and *dead* when references are made to the status of their family member. A common error in health care is to refer to the death euphemistically. For example, the nurse may say that the patient "has just expired" or "passed on" or "will no longer be with us," or that "there is no hope" or "it is over." Saying the word *dead* when talking to the family is straightforward and prevents misinterpretation. Because of shock and denial, the family may not comprehend the impact of the message that there is "no hope for their loved one." This understanding is critical in the case of the family of a patient considered dead by brain-death criteria.

The family essentially "becomes the patient" after death of their loved one. It is important to determine how the family members are working together as a unit. Who is the "strong right arm" of the family? Who is asking the questions? Who is the spokesperson or next of kin? What was the family's relationship to the deceased? How does the family make decisions? General observations of the family's behavior are essential when initiating the process of donation in a way that is comfortable both for the family and for the nurse.

Other goals when assessing the family should include assessment of the family's cultural and religious background and its impact on how they will handle the concept of donation. A decision not to offer donation because of religious and cultural biases based on assumptions about the family's last name and background has no place in the process. The choice belongs to the family.

When a family says no to donation, that response is perfectly reasonable. Donation is not an option for every family or every person. Whatever the decision about donation, it is the right one for that family or person and should be accepted. The nurse's role is to give the family the choice of donation along with the right information about donation, and to support the family's decision.

Family Education

The family needs information about donation so they can decide what is right for them and if it is what the family member would have wished. Detailed, understandable information is essential. The family must never be coerced into a decision about donation and its benefits.

The family needs to know that if they grant permission for donation, it will be carried out promptly. A slight chance exists of changes in physical appearance related to the incisions required for different donations. The family should know that this will cause no disfigurement that would prevent an open casket or alter funeral arrangements. For example, even after donation of bone, the body can be prepared for an open casket funeral.

The family also needs to know that they will be required to participate in an extensive medical and social history review before donation is possible. This history is carried out in response to FDA regulations effective July 1, 1995, permitting distribution of tissues and organs for transplant. A typical multitissue donation case study is given in Box 19-2.

Tissue and organ retrieval occurs after permission is given by the family, and recovery teams can be arranged to recover the tissue. Recovery teams may be in the same facility, or they may be 500 miles away, so transportation

---

Box 19-2   Case Study: Multitissue Donor

A 54-year-old man is admitted to the ED in cardiac arrest at 2:30 am. He is in asystole and is declared dead at 3:15 am. His wife gives permission to donate organs and tissues. "Anything he can donate is fine . . . he always wanted to be an organ donor." The medical examiner approves the donation for corneas, bone, skin, and heart for valves.

---

arrangements may be complex. When eyes, corneas, heart for valves, and skin are the only tissues to be recovered, the entire donation could take place in the morgue, since an operating room would not be required. However, if bone was included in the donation, an operating suite and sterile aseptic technique are essential for most bone procurement teams across the country.

Procurement of internal organs takes place in an operating suite. The multitissue, multiorgan procurement procedure is usually completed in 4 to 5 hours. Delays in the procurement process should be reported to the family promptly. The regional procurement agency provides technical staff to recover the eyes, valves, and skin. If the family made special funeral arrangements, they should inform the emergency nurse or coordinator of those plans.

A donation coordinator from the local OPO is available for support in the case of any donation. In most donations of internal organs, the coordinator attends the patient and family at the hospital, obtains consent from the family, explains the process of donation to the family, and coordinates the entire donation from start to finish. In the case of tissue donation only, the coordinator is less likely to be at the hospital but is available for consultation and ensures that necessary support is available. The coordinator works with the emergency nurse, other contact staff at the hospital, and the respective procurement teams.

THE PROCUREMENT PROCESS

Tissue and organ donors are managed differently. The tissue donor has been declared dead, with no heartbeat. The potential organ donor has been declared brain dead, but the heart is still beating. Management of the tissue or organ donor is discussed in the following sections. These patients must be managed carefully to ensure viable tissues and/or organs for transplant.

Tissue Procurement: Eyes, Corneas, Bone, Heart for Valves, and Skin

Tissue procurement is less complex than internal organ procurement. The coordinator from the procurement agency arranges for arrival of recovery teams and works with nursing staff in the operating suite of the hospital to set up surgery time and conditions convenient for all parties involved.

Maximum time allowed for recovery of tissue after asystole is approximately 10 hours for bone, 6 to 10 hours for heart valves, and 24 hours for corneas and skin. These time limits vary, depending on the procurement agency and availability of refrigeration. The preferred time of recovery is that time closest to asystole.

The process of recovering bones is usually carried out using sterile technique. Usually all four limbs, including both femurs, proximal tibia, fibula, and proximal humerus, are prepared for recovery. Occasionally a mandible, hemipelvis, every other rib, tissues from the limbs such as tensor fasciae latae, Achilles tendon with a block of calcaneus, and others are recovered.[6] The surgical procedure lasts approximately 1½ to 4 hours, depending on the experience of the team and the number of tissues to be recovered. A single incision is made along each limb so that the respective bones can be extracted. A prosthetic device made of polyvinyl chloride telescopic tubing or in some cases wooden dowels are used to replace bones as a means of reconstruction. Aside from the single incision made along the outer aspect of the limb, no disfigurement associated with the procurement process should be apparent. After procurement of the bone, it is stored in a freezer at −70° F, is freeze-dried, or processed into chips for later use. The uses of bone are extensive, ranging from replacement of bone invaded by a tumor to replacing bone in neurosurgical cases when bone has been removed.

The bone recovery process is difficult to observe and participate in, particularly if staff in the operating room are not accustomed to this type of procedure. If this is the case, before the procurement is performed, an educational in-service program should be provided for the staff by the regional procurement agency. The donation coordinator who oversees development of hospital's program in conjunction with the hospital's liaison should organize an educational program of this type to facilitate the education and enhance the comfort level of operating room staff who will eventually be involved in this process.

After death, the eye donor should be maintained in a refrigerated room if available. The head should be elevated at 20 degrees, and the eyes should be taped closed with paper tape. Cool compresses can be placed over the eyes to prevent swelling and ease the procurement process. Recovery of eyes is a clean procedure using sterile technique. It requires 20 to 30 minutes. Two methods of recovery are commonly used: recovery of the entire globe of the eye, or a corneal punch procedure. The eye tissue is packed in preservative solution, and the container is placed on ice and dispatched to the respective eye recovery center for processing. Corneas are generally transplanted within 24 to 48 hours for the treatment of keratoconus and other diseases of the cornea. If the globe of the eye has been recovered, the orbit is filled with ample cotton and a cap similar in contour to the eye to eliminate any disfigurement resulting from the absence of the globe. The technical staff recovering the eyes must be skilled in these procedures and in many states must be certified in the techniques of recovery.

For recovery of heart for valves, the entire heart is removed from the donor. The aortic and pulmonary valves are dissected from the heart and are eventually used as replacement valves. Aortic root replacement, repair of tetralogy of Fallot, and pulmonary atresia can also be performed using valve parts. The chest is opened from the xiphoid process to the sternal notch. The ribs and sternum are retracted, and the heart is mobilized. Cardiectomy of the heart includes dissection along the great vessels extending distally from the heart as far as possible. The heart is then removed from the chest, placed in sterile Ringer's lactated solution, packed in a sterile container, double-bagged sterilely, and packed on ice for shipping to a processing center. The valves are dissected from the heart, their integrity examined, and the entire heart examined for pathologic conditions. Serologic examinations are performed, and after a brief period of quarantine, usually 40 days, the valves are released for homograft transplant according to size and need. The donor has a single incision on the chest that does not prevent an open casket if the family so wishes.

If the process of skin recovery is available in the region, this procedure can also take place in the morgue. A clean room and sterile technique are required. By use of a dermatome, skin is recovered from the buttocks, thighs, back, and abdomen. A split-thickness graft, removed from the top surface of the body, is barely visible unless the donor has a dark tan or is of high pigment. Once the skin is recovered it is treated with antibiotics, prepared surgically for grafting, and stored at −70° F. The recovered skin is used for temporary grafts in the care of severely burned patients to provide protection from infection, fluid shifts, and other complications of burns.

Solid-Organ Procurement: Heart, Lungs, Liver, Pancreas, and Kidney

Recovery of solid organs for transplant may be complex and requires cooperation of team members representing many different disciplines. Before the process can begin, the family or next of kin must give their consent for the specific organs and tissues to be donated. The time of death, as determined by brain-death criteria, must be documented in the record, and the medical examiner's approval (when required) must be in place before proceeding.

Many hours of hemodynamic maintenance of the donor may be necessary before the actual procedure takes place. The donation coordinator works with the family to address their concerns and with the intensive care unit staff to manage the donor until the time of the procurement. Hemodynamic parameters of donor management have been worked out over time and if met, facilitate procurement of the healthy organs for transplant. The hemodynamic parameters of donor management are summarized in Box 19-3. The goals are the same in the pediatric patient but adjusted for weight and size of the potential donor. The potential donor may not necessarily exhibit these parameters, but the patient must be considered for donation.

Box **19-3**	**Hemodynamic Parameters for the Organ Donor**

Systolic BP $\geq$ 100 mmHg
PaO$_2$ 100 mmHg
SaO$_2$ $\geq$ 95%
CVP 5-15 mmHg
Urine output 100-500 ml/hr
Hematocrit $\geq$ 25%
Temperature > 95 to < 102° F

Once the patient is declared dead by brain-death criteria, management for preservation of organs for transplantation can begin. The donor's blood pressure is extremely labile, and diabetes insipidus can develop due to herniation, which results in an imbalance of fluids and electrolytes. Management of the donor includes balancing of fluid and electrolytes, use of pressors such as dopamine and dobutamine, and treatment of developing diabetes insipidus. Antidiuretic hormone replacement using a pitressin supplement via an intravenous drip, intranasally, or by injection is frequently instituted. Management of the pulmonary status of the donor should ensure that blood gas levels reflect extremely well-oxygenated organs. Hematocrit is monitored closely to prevent lowered oxygen transport, which may result from excessive bleeding caused by related trauma. All laboratory values must be reviewed, including fluid status, and evaluated for overhydration or underhydration. Numerous laboratory studies, including electrolyte, BUN, creatinine, hematologic studies, liver function tests, cardiac enzyme assessment, an electrocardiogram, an echocardiogram, TEE, cardiology consultation, arterial blood gas tests, pulmonary consult, and evaluation of radiographs of the chest, are carried out to determine the health of the organs to be recovered.

After the patient has been accepted as a donor and all organs to be recovered have been assigned to a receiving patient, recovery teams convene at a stated time convenient to all parties. The host hospital has final determination of operating time; however, most donations of organs occur during the late hours of the night. The hospital is asked to provide operating room staff and anesthesia support.

The donor is transported to the operating room fully supported by mechanical means and is hemodynamically maintained in the operating room according to the goals outlined previously. The donor is maintained throughout the organ dissection and mobilization of the respective tissue until organs and tissues are freed for immediate removal and preservation. After the last aspects of the dissection have been completed, the aorta is clamped, and cardioplegia takes place. Quick cooling and in situ flushing of the organs is then accomplished. After flushing of the organs has been completed, they are removed from the donor, examined individually in a sterile back basin, flushed again if required, and packed in a sterile container for transport and immediate

transplant (in the case of heart, heart and lung, and single lung) For kidneys, approximately 24 hours may elapse before transplantation takes place. For the pancreas and liver, this number ranges from 6 to 20 hours, the preferred time being approximately 15 hours. This flexibility of preservation time in the case of the kidneys, liver, and pancreas is largely the result of the development of the preservation fluid "U.W." by Dr. Folkert O. Belzer of the University of Wisconsin during the late 1980s. This preservation fluid greatly enhanced the procurement process, allowing time for transportation of organs and prospective tissue typing of the donor with the recipient. Prospective tissue typing is primarily carried out between kidney donor and recipient and in some cases between heart, heart and lung, and single-lung donor and recipient.

FINANCIAL CONSIDERATIONS

The process of donation of tissues and organs is an expensive one. The family of the donor should never be issued a hospital bill that accrued during the hospital stay until the organ procurement agency has had an opportunity to review the charges and take care of all charges related to the donation process. Families must be made aware of this, if at all possible, when they speak with the coordinator. If the family members receive a bill, they are encouraged to contact the organ procurement agency, which ensures proper payment of the bill.

In the United States, payment for organ transplant is usually made by third-party payors. In 1972, the End-Stage Renal Disease Act was enacted, allowing patients with end-stage renal disease coverage by Medicare for treatment of dialysis and kidney transplantation. All persons were given the opportunity for treatment essential to life. For liver and heart transplantation, most third-party payors cover the cost of the transplantation surgery and postoperative care. However, in many states, third-party reimbursement is not available in the case of heart and lung, pancreas, and lung transplantation, since these transplants are still considered experimental. A great deal of controversy exists regarding the expense of transplantation, with emphasis on the number of people helped, cost, and life expectancy after the graft and the transplantation. Table 19-2 presents the cost range for solid-organ transplantations.

Costs vary from center to center but serve as a guideline for actual costs. Many states cannot justify the cost of transplantation in these times of cost containment when so few people benefit. Oregon, for example, reallocated Medicaid monies previously designated for transplantation, except in the case of kidneys and corneas, to other areas of the governmental budget that were felt to better serve a greater number of people such as pregnant mothers, and infants and mothers at high risk.[16] How the money is spent and who pays for these highly specialized, technologically advanced procedures are questions considered daily. The ethics of choosing one cause over another is grappled with continually.

Table **19-2**	**Estimated Charges for Organ Transplantation (1993 Dollars)**	
Organ	Estimated first-year charge	Estimated annual follow-up charge
Heart	$209,100	$15,000
Liver	302,900	21,900
Kidney	87,700	10,400
Pancreas	65,000	1,600
Heart-lung	246,000	18,400
Lung	243,600	18,400
Cornea	8,000	0
Bone marrow	167,200	27,600

Modified from: *Financing Transplantation: what every patient needs to know,* United Network of Organ Sharing, 1993.

ETHICAL ISSUES

Numerous ethical issues relate to donation and transplantation of organs and tissues. Those that affect the daily practice of the emergency nurse include the nurse's role in offering the family the option of donation, the comfort level of the emergency nurse in this area of nursing care, and how best to deal with examination of one's feelings regarding this option. Occasionally the emergency nurse is also faced with a death determined by brain-death criteria, maintaining the patient declared dead so that others may benefit, and dealing with a family's grief and confusion. These and other questions, including determining who will receive the organ and who will pay for the transplant, issues related to sale of organs and tissues, required request and presumed consent, and how far the art of transplantation should be expanded to extend life, are routinely reviewed on a global level and addressed in numerous forums. The answers are always complex and are an ongoing concern.

The key to effective nursing care is to individually assess one's personal and professional feelings, examine the literature on the respective issues, and make a decision consistent with personal beliefs. If a nurse is uncomfortable with donation and with offering the family the option of donation, the nurse should separate from that aspect of practice and pass the responsibility on to a peer more comfortable with the process. Thus families, potential donors, and potential recipients are better served.

CONCLUSION

Many issues surrounding the role and responsibility of the emergency nurse relate to tissue and organ donors. The emergency nurse has the responsibility to provide the family with the option of tissue and organ donation when a patient dies in the ED. The *Emergency Nurses Association Position Statement of 1987* clearly indicates this responsibility.

The Emergency Nurses Association believes emergency nurses should be knowledgeable in identification of potential donors and life support of donor patients, and in accessing resource personnel from state and/or local transplant teams. It is within the role of the emergency nurse, and is not mandated by federal law, to initiate discussions regarding organ donation and to facilitate, coordinate, and intervene with families as appropriate.

For too long, the concept of donation has been associated solely with trauma victims: patients maintained and declared dead by brain-death criteria in the intensive care setting. Almost any person who dies can be a donor of some tissue or organ for transplantation. This is an integral part of the emergency nursing care for patients and families in crisis.

REFERENCES

1. American Council on Transplantation: *From here to transplant,* Alexandria, Va., 1987, The Council.
2. American Hospital Association, American Medical Association, and United Network for Organ Sharing: *Required request legislation: a guide for hospitals on organ and tissue donation,* Chicago, 1988, American Hospital Association, American Medical Association, and United Network for Organ Sharing.
3. Batten HL, Prottas JM: Kind strangers: the families or organ donors, *Health Affairs,* p. 38, Summer 1987.
4. Caplin AL: Professional arrogance and public misunderstanding, *Hastings Cent Rep,* p. 37, April 1988.
5. Childress JF: Obtaining the gift of life: ethical issues in the procurement of organs for transplantation. In Hodges LW, editor: *Social responsibility: business, journalism, law, medicine,* Lexington, Va., Washington and Lee University, 21:65-85, 1995.
6. DeBoer H: The history of bone grafts, *Clin Orthop* 226:292, 1988.
7. *Defining death: medical, legal, and ethical issues in the determination of death,* President's Commission for the Study of Ethical Problems in Medicine and Biomedical Research, Washington, DC, 1981.
8. Dekker ML: Bone and soft tissue procurement, *Orthop Nurse* 8(2):33, 1989.
9. Department of Health and Human Services: *Organ transplantation: issues and recommendations,* Report of the Task Force on Organ Transplantation, Washington, DC, 1986, US Department of Health and Human Services.
10. Emergency Nurses Association: *Role of the emergency nurse in organ procurement: ENA position statement,* Chicago, 1987, The Association.
11. Gallup Poll 1985: *The US public's attitudes toward organ transplant/organ donation,* 1985, The Gallup Organization.
12. Garrison RN, et al.: There is an answer to the organ shortage, *Surg, Gynecol, and Obstet* vol 173, November 1991.
13. Grenvik A: Ethical dilemmas in organ donation and transplantation, *Crit Care Med* vol 1012, 1988.
14. Laudicina SS: *Medicaid coverage and payment policies for organ transplants: findings of a national survey,* George Washington University, 1988, US Department of Health and Human Services.
15. National Kidney Foundation: *For those who give and grieve: a booklet for donor families,* Washington DC, 1990, The Foundation.
16. Newberry MA: *Textbook of hemodialysis for patient care personnel,* Springfield, Ill, 1989, Charles C. Thomas.
17. Tilney NL: Renal transplantation between identical twins: a review, *World J Surg* 10(3):381, 1986.
18. United Network for Organ Sharing: *Organ and tissue donation: a reference guide for clergy,* 1995, UNOS.

unit IV

MAJOR TRAUMA EMERGENCIES

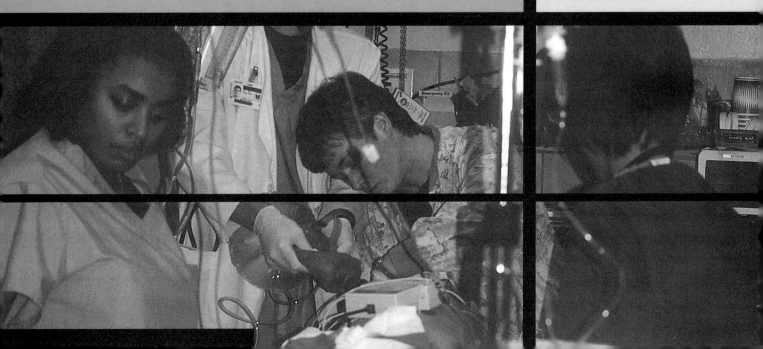

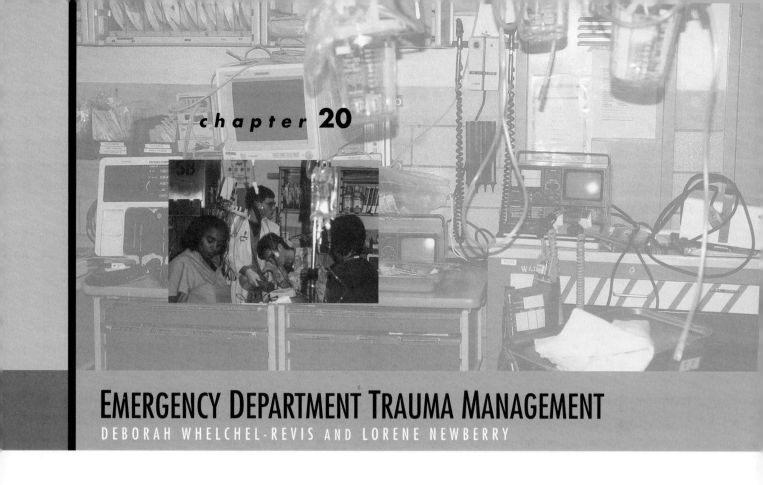

chapter 20

EMERGENCY DEPARTMENT TRAUMA MANAGEMENT

DEBORAH WHELCHEL-REVIS AND LORENE NEWBERRY

Trauma is the leading cause of death in the United States for people in the first four decades of life.[4] Incidence is not limited to densely populated areas but occurs in all geographic regions of the country. Trauma care is ideally provided in institutions that specialize in trauma; however, trauma centers are not as widely distributed as the patients who require care. Most trauma patients are assessed, stabilized, admitted, or transferred by emergency departments (ED) in nontrauma centers. Emergency nurses in these facilities are challenged by trauma situations similar to those seen in designated trauma centers. While trauma centers have treatment areas, staff, and physicians dedicated to assessment, stabilization, and long-term care of injured patients, most EDs must provide trauma care while facing a myriad of other problems (e.g., heart attacks, asthma, and abdominal pain). The volume of trauma patients may not be as great as in trauma centers, but the intensity faced by the emergency nurse and requisite knowledge are similar. This chapter describes departmental and staff preparation, ED trauma management, and transfer criteria for the emergency nurse in a nontrauma center ED.

PREPARATION

Trauma patients may arrive by ambulance, police car, private automobile, or helicopter. Team members should be ready with minimal notice; advance notification does not always occur. An assignment board with member names and responsibilities enhances communication. Members should assume their responsibilities as soon as notification is received. Trauma literature strongly supports a systematic approach to assessment as a means to prioritize care and save time. Krantz writes "satisfactory outcomes for injured patients are strongly influenced by the initial care delivered particularly in the so called 'golden hour'. Approximately 60% of all hospital deaths from trauma occur during this crucial period and inadequate assessment and resuscitation may contribute to the preventable death of 35% reported in some series."

Successful trauma care depends on preparation of the ED and staff. Given unlimited funds all EDs can create an ideal trauma resuscitation area; however, this is not realistic for most facilities. Each ED has architectural strengths and weaknesses that require creative solutions for maximum use of space and efficiency of personnel. Consideration should also be given to community needs related to trauma, ED volume, institutional resources, and number of treatment bays in the ED. Figure 20-1 is an example of a single-patient resuscitation area that can accommodate two patients during emergency operations. Components considered in the creation of a trauma resuscitation area include size, equipment, and radiographic capabilities (Table 20-1). Equipment should be available to assess and treat immediate life-threatening problems such as tension pneumothorax, airway compromise, and blood loss (Box 20-1).

Location of the room is also important. Given the luxury of placing the room anywhere, the best choice is unique

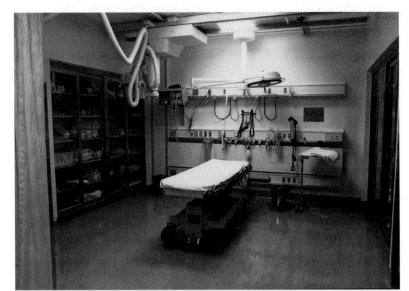

Figure **20-1** ED trauma resuscitation bay. Note overhead x-ray and surgery light. *(Courtesy Promina Kennestone Hospital, Marietta, Ga.)*

Table **20-1** **Components for Ideal ED Trauma Resuscitation Area**

Component	Description/comments
Treatment space	• Allow sufficient space for exam stretcher, trauma team, supplies, and traffic around the bed. • Walls should be leaded for stationary x-ray unit. • Locate supplies logically around room (e.g., airway supplies at head of bed, splinting supplies near foot of bed).
Overhead radiograph capabilities	• Ceiling tracks facilitate use and eliminate need for portable machine. • Tracks may interfere with ceiling-mounted IV holders. • May not be able to provide adequate oblique films in some situations. • Adjacent dark room provides best turnaround time for films.
Procedure tables	• Maintain large procedure tables for trays (e.g., thoracotomy, venisection, peritoneal lavage). • Create storage space under counters when tables are not used.
Surgical lights	• Choose a model that provides adequate lighting for gross surgical procedures (i.e., ED thoracotomy). • Two mid-sized lights might be preferable to one large OR light. • Positioning can be a challenge with radiograph tracks.
Wall suction	• One suction unit for each bed for gastric, nasotracheal, and two pleural drainage systems.
Scrub sink	• Foot controls and plaster trap increase effectiveness.
Radiograph view box and hot light	• Ability to view three films simultaneously is desirable. • Build in hot light to decrease counter clutter.
Hemodynamic monitoring	• Hardwire units for each bed to monitor cardiac rhythm, NIBP, pulse oximetry as a minimum. • ICP, arterial pressure, and PA pressure monitoring should be available.

for each institution, depending on the location of the ambulance door, operating room, CT scanner, radiology, intensive care unit, and helipad. An adjacent ambulance ramp decreases transit time from door to room, but may not be ideal if most patients arrive by helicopter. Crowd control is also an issue with room placement. If the room is near the waiting area or staff entrance to the department, the room is more likely to attract unnecessary observers. Flow should be analyzed to determine existing traffic patterns in the department.

After creation of the trauma resuscitation area, trauma team composition should be determined. A team approach has proven most efficient in combating time until treatment—the worst enemy faced by an injured patient. Team composition varies with available human resources, but a multidisciplinary team with medical, nursing, and other specialties represented is ideal (Table 20-2). Team members may originate in the ED or come from other areas of the institution, such as the intensive care unit or postanesthesia care unit. Notification methods for team members include overhead paging and beepers. Team members may be assigned to procedures, such as establishing IV access, or to a specific anatomic area, such as head, left arm, etc. Responsibilities should be clearly defined in writing and reviewed regularly with all members.

<table>
<tr><td colspan="2">*Box* **20-1**   **Essential Supplies, Instruments, and Trays**</td></tr>
<tr><td colspan="2">
Intubation supplies with blades, handles, and tubes easily accessible
Chest tube insertion trays with chest drainage bottles
Thoracotomy tray including rib spreaders, vascular clamps, long-handled instruments, pledgets, and cardiac sutures
Autotransfusion supplies
Blood and fluid warmer
Venous access supplies for peripheral and central access with range of sizes
Diagnostic peritoneal lavage tray
Defibrillator with pediatric and internal paddles
Transport monitor with ECG, NIBP, pulse oximetry, and end tidal CO_2
Dressings, suture supplies, splinting material, restraints
Rapid sequence induction medications
Ventilator
Tracheostomy and cricothyrotomy supplies
</td></tr>
</table>

Documentation of the trauma resuscitation is an essential aspect of trauma care to protect the patient, institution, and staff providing care. Forms should allow rapid, comprehensive description of care with minimal effort. Many institutions utilize trauma flowsheets rather than a narrative script. Figure 20-2 shows a flowsheet used by a busy, designated trauma center in a large metropolitan area. Flowsheets should include areas for documentation of vital signs, identified injuries, treatment provided, staff providing care, and patient disposition. Injuries may be marked on anatomic sketches or identified by location on the body.

Trauma care is so intense that problems can arise despite prior preparation, usually from confusion or irritation over large or small issues. Which physician is in charge? Where are the lead aprons? Where are physician order sheets? Prevention of all conflicts may not be possible; however, with thought for basic issues these can be minimized. Box 20-2 provides practical tips for ED management that may help eliminate or reduce some irritants. These tips are somewhat generic, so each institution should analyze previous trauma resuscitations to identify common themes that lead to conflict in their area. Have there been repeated complaints related to inadequate supplies, missed x-rays because no one was in charge, or physician concern over staff education?

Table **20-2**	**Multidisciplinary Trauma Team**
Discipline	**Role**
Emergency Nursing	Assesses patient and provides ongoing care
	Documents and coordinates care
	Administers medication
Emergency Medicine	Provides initial assessment in many institutions
	Determines notification priority for other specialties (e.g., surgery, neurosurgery, orthopedics)
	Intubates and provides initial airway management
	Maintains awareness of need to complete essential tests such as cervical spine films
Surgery	Acts as team leader in trauma centers
	Focuses on surgical management of trauma
Pulmonary Services	Provided by anesthesiology in some institutions
	Intubates, manages airway and ventilations
	Collects lab specimens and obtain ECG in some situations
Radiology Services	Complete of essential radiographs and special procedures
	Provides final interpretation on-site or through use of teleradiography
Laboratory	Collects specimen and analyzes sample
	Utilizes hematocrit and ABG machine placed in the ED, resuscitation area, or central lab
Social Services	Contacts family, minister, and others
	Provides immediate support to family during resuscitation
	Obtains vital information and documents valuables
	Provided by designated patient representative in some institutions
Ancillary Staff	Includes nursing assistants, patient care technicians, and other nonlicensed personnel
	Removes clothing, transports patient, and performs procedures such as ECG, splint application, dressing wounds, and urethral catheterization

Grady Health System®
80 Butler Street
Atlanta, GA 30335

Allergies

Date:____________________

Arrival Time:____________________

ED Notification Time:__________ DOB__________ Age:__________ Mechanism of injury:__________

Time Trauma Team Called:__________ Sex:__________

Stat ☐ Resp ☐ LMP:__________ Approximate time of injury:__________

Transported by:__________Service LOC duration:_____ Last Tetanus__________

☐ground ☐ air Safety belt: ☐ yes ☐ no ☐ unkown Helmet ☐ yes ☐ no ☐ unknown

Prior Medical Hx:__________ Current Meds__________

Emerg. Med. Attending

____

Emerg.Med. Resident

____

	Surgery Attending	Surgery Resident	ORTHO	NSQ.
Called				
Responded				
Arrival				

Morehouse ☐ Emory ☐

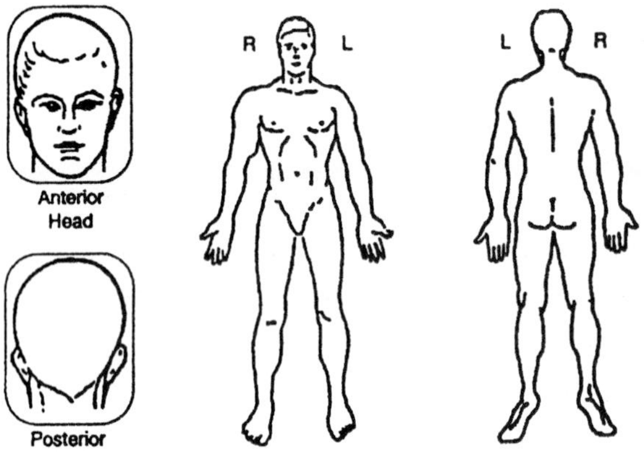

Anterior Head
Posterior Head
R
L
L
R

A. Abrasion
B. Burn
C. Contusion
D. Deformity
E. Ecchymosis
F. Fracture
G. GSW
H. Edema
I. Avulsion
J. Tenderness
K. Scar
L. Laceration
M. Amputation
N. Stab
☐ IV's on arrival

Airway ☐ clear ☐ obstructed
C-spine: ☐ immobilized ☐ cleared
Breathing: ☐ normal ☐ labored
☐ shallow ☐ assisted ☐ intubated
☐ absent ☐ trach deviation
Circulation: ☐ carotid rhythm__________
Skin: ☐ cool ☐ warm ☐ dry ☐ wet
☐ pale ☐ flushed ☐ cyanotic ☐ mottled
Chest: ☐ decreased ☐ R ☐ L
☐ absent ☐ R ☐ L
☐ asymmetrical ☐ symmetrical
Extremities: (Circle if NOT present)
Upper: Moves sensation - pulses ☐ R
: Moves - sensation - pulses ☐ L
Lower: Moves sensation - pulses ☐ R
Moves sensation - pulses ☐ L

Time	BP	Pulse	Resp	Temp	0_2 Sat	GCS	NURSES NOTES

Page 1 of 2 WHITE - Medical Records YELLOW - Trauma Center PINK - Emergency Dept. 12/96

Figure **20-2** ED trauma flow sheet. *(Courtesy Grady Health System, Atlanta, Ga.)*

TIME PROCEDURE

_____ Rigid C-Collar _____ Headrolls/tape _____ Spineboard
_____ 0₂: Device _____ % _____ Device _____ % _____
OGT _____
_____ Trauma Labs:
  - ☐ Chem 19 ☐ UDS
  - ☐ Amylase ☐ UA
  - ☐ PT - PIT ☐ ABG
  - ☐ CBC ☐ T & CM
  - ☐ Beta HCG
_____ CT
_____ US + ☐ - ☐
_____ Radiology
_____ Peritoneal Lavage:
  In _____ cc Out _____ cc
  Blood: Positive Negative
_____ Foley # _____ OGT _____
  Blood: With dip stick _____ Positive _____ Negative
_____ Chest Tube: Right _____ Fr. Left _____ Fr.
_____ Autotransfusion: _____ cc
_____ Rectal Tone: Normal Absent
_____ Stool Guaiac: Positive Negative
_____ Prostate _____

INTAKE AND OUTPUT					
CRYSTALLOIDS			PTA _____ cc Total		
Time	IV#	Solution	Amount	Site	Total Infused
TOTAL CRYSTALLOIDS ABSORBED					

BLOOD COMPONENTS (include autotransfusion)					
Time	Unit#	Solution	Amount	Site	Total Absorbed
TOTAL BLOOD PRODUCTS ABSORBED					

GLASGOW COMA SCALE - ADULT

1. Eye Opening:
Spontaneous	4
To Voice	3
To Pain	2
None	1

2. Verbal Response:
Oriented	5
Confused	4
Inappropriate Words	3
Incomprehensible Words	2

3. Motor Responses:
None	1
Obeys Commands	6
Purposeful Movement (Pain)	5
Withdraw (Pain)	4
Flexion (Pain)	3
Extension (Pain)	2
None	1

TOTAL _____

GLASGOW COMA SCALE - PEDIATRIC

1. Eye Opening:
Spontaneous	4
To Speech	3
To Pain	2
None	1

2. Best Verbal:
oriented/smiles,cries	5
confused	4
inapprop./inapp. cry	3
incomprehensible/grunts	2
no response	1

3. Best Motor:
Spontaneous	6
Localizes Pain	5
Withdraws to pain	4
Decorticate (Flexion)	3
Decerebrate (Extension)	2
None	1

REFERENCE TOTAL _____

MEDICATIONS ALLERGIES _____

Time	Med	Dos	Route	Initial
	Tetanus/0.5cc		IM	

MD Signature:

Admission: OR ☐ ICU ☐

DISPOSITION SUMMARY:

Time family notified: _____ Time out of ED: _____
By whom: _____
Clerk Disposition of: Clothing _____ valuables _____ #

Admitted to:
- ☐ Surgery ☐ Ortho
- ☐ Neuro Surg. ☐ Home
- ☐ Morgue ☐ Other _____

Nurse Signature: _____ Nurse II: _____

M ONITOR

WHITE - Medical Records   YELLOW - Trauma Center   PINK - Emergency Dept.

Figure **20-2,** cont'd   For legend see opposite page.

Box **20-2**　**Practical Tips for ED Trauma Management**

Personnel/trauma team

Determine team composition then post daily assignments. Assign tasks such as IV access, vital signs, application of ECG electrodes.

Decide which physician is in charge.

Designate a primary nurse who owns the patient and is responsible for coordination of care.

Designate a recorder for the initial resuscitation and identify a documentation area.

Don personal protective equipment (gown, goggles, gloves) and lead aprons before patient arrives.

Establish protocols for patient assessment, trauma labs, trauma surgeon notification, and trauma surgeon back up.

Provide interpreter services.

Develop a trauma flow sheet.

Room/supplies

Keep sufficient lead aprons hanging in room.

Stock large sharps containers.

Organize supplies by system or process (e.g., abdominal, thoracic, hemodynamic).

Place IV access supplies on both sides of the room.

Use large trash and linen containers in the room.

Place essential forms and phone numbers at the documentation area.

Install at least one dictation line and two phones in the area.

Put intubation supplies at the head of the bed.

Stock prenumbered trauma charts and forms at the documentation area.

Create a separate pediatric resuscitation area or cart stocked with pediatric supplies.

Table **20-3**　**Life-Threatening Airway Problems**

Problem	Signs and symptoms	Interventions
Airway obstruction (complete or partial)	• Dyspnea, labored respirations • Decreased or no air movement • Cyanosis • Presence of foreign body in airway • Trauma to face or neck	Airway opening maneuvers 　• Jaw thrust 　• Chin lift 　• Suction Airway adjuncts 　• Nasal airway 　• Oral airway 　• Endotracheal tube Surgical airway 　• Cricothyrotomy 　• Tracheostomy
Inhalation injury	• History of enclosed space fire, unconsciousness, or exposure to heavy smoke • Dyspnea • Wheezing, rhonchi, crackles • Hoarseness • Singed facial or nasal hairs • Carbonaceous sputum • Burns to face or neck	• Provide high-flow oxygen (100%) via nonrebreather mask or bag-valve device • Prepare for endotracheal intubation as soon as possible

From Kidd PS, Sturt P: *Mosby's emergency nursing reference,* St. Louis, 1996, Mosby.

INITIAL RESUSCITATION

Trauma care begins with primary assessment—an organized approach for the evaluation of airway, breathing, circulation, and neurologic function. An organized approach includes a rapid, initial survey that focuses on identification of injuries that pose an immediate threat to the patient's life (e.g., airway obstruction, tension pneumothorax, and hemorrhage). Emergencies related to the airway include airway obstruction secondary to edema (Table 20-3). The emergency nurse should prepare for endotracheal inhalation, tracheostomy, or cricothyrotomy. Emergencies identified during a primary assessment of breathing include tension pneumothorax, sucking chest wound, and flail chest (Table 20-4). Needle decompression of tension pneumothorax should not be delayed until completion of chest radiograph. Hypovolemia and external hemorrhage may be identified during an assessment of circulation (Table 20-5). Direct pressure should be applied to control external hemorrhage while large-bore intravenous catheters should be inserted

for fluid resuscitation using crystalloid solutions (Ringer's lactate or 0.9% NaCl). Defibrillation pads can be used to cover sucking chest wounds, and tape can be used initially to stabilize a flail segment. Blood is not routinely administered; however, the emergency nurse should anticipate this need in patients with gunshot wound to the chest and abdominal, or other wounds with significant blood loss.

Secondary assessment is a more complete evaluation including vital signs, a history, a head-to-toe examination, and an inspection of the back (Box 20-3). Potentially life-threatening injuries identified by secondary assessment include hypothermia, pelvic fractures, and spinal cord injury. Certain injuries suggest the presence of concomitant injuries that should alert the emergency nurse to the need for careful assessment and ongoing monitoring (Table 20-6).[6] Obvious fractures should be immobilized and open wounds covered with sterile saline gauze.

Diagnostic studies including laboratory analysis and radiographic examination are obtained following assessment

Table 20-4 Life-Threatening Breathing Problems

Problem	Signs and symptoms	Interventions
Tension pneumothorax	• Dyspnea, labored respirations • Decreased or absent breath sounds on affected side • Unilateral chest rise and fall • Tracheal deviation away from affected side • Cyanosis • Jugular venous distension • Tachycardia and hypotension • History of chest trauma or mechanical ventilation	• Provide high-flow oxygen (100%) via nonrebreather mask or bag-valve device. • Perform rapid chest decompression by needle thoracostomy on affected side. • Place chest tube on affected side.
Pneumothorax	• Dyspnea, labored respirations • Decreased or absent breath sounds on affected side • May have unilateral chest rise and fall • May have visible wound to chest or back • History of chest trauma	• Provide high-flow oxygen (100%) via nonrebreather mask or bag-valve device. • Place chest tube on affected side. • Place occlusive dressing over any open chest wound and secure on three sides with tape.
Hemothorax	• Dyspnea, labored respirations • Decreased or absent breath sounds on affected side • May have unilateral chest rise and fall • Tachycardia and hypotension • May have visible wound to chest or back • History of chest trauma (usually penetrating)	• Provide high-flow oxygen (100%) via nonrebreather mask or bag-valve device. • Place chest tube on affected side. • Consider autotransfusion.
Sucking chest wound	• Dyspnea, labored respirations • Visible, sucking wound to chest or back • Decreased or absent breath sounds on affected side	• Provide high-flow oxygen (100%) via nonrebreather mask or bag-valve device. • Cover wound with occlusive dressing and secure on three sides with tape. • Watch for signs of tension pneumothorax and remove dressing during exhalation if they are noted.
Flail chest	• Dyspnea, labored respirations • Paradoxical chest wall movement • Chest pain • Tachycardia	• Provide high-flow oxygen (100%) via nonrebreather mask or bag-valve device. • Prepare for intubation and mechanical ventilation.
Full-thickness circumferential burn of thorax	• Dyspnea, labored respirations • Shallow respirations • Obvious circumferential burns to thorax	• Provide high-flow oxygen (100%) via nonrebreather mask or bag-valve device. • Prepare for immediate escharotomy.

Modified from Kidd PS, Sturt P: *Mosby's emergency nursing reference*, St. Louis, 1996, Mosby.

Table 20-5 Life-Threatening Circulation Problems

Problem	Signs and symptoms	Interventions
External hemorrhage	• Obvious bleeding site	• Direct pressure • Elevation
Shock	• Tachycardia • Weak, thready pulses • Cool, pale, clammy skin • Tachypnea • Altered mental status • Delayed capillary refill • Oliguria or anuria	• Provide high-flow oxygen (100%) via nonrebreather mask or bag-valve device • Place two large-bore IV lines with warm isotonic crystalloid solution infusing (Ringer's lactate solution or 0.9% NaCl) • Administer fluid bolus (2 L in adults or 20ml/kg in children) • Prepare to administer blood

Modified from Kidd PS, Sturt P: *Mosby's emergency nursing reference*, St. Louis, 1996, Mosby.

Box **20-3**	**Secondary Assessment**

E = Expose patient

F = Fahrenheit—Keep patient warm

- Blankets
- Warming lights

G = Get vital signs

- In addition to obtaining a complete set of vital signs, consider:
  - Cardiac monitor and pulse oximeter (SpO_2)
  - Urinary catheter if not contraindicated
  - Gastric tube
  - Laboratory studies

H = History/head-to-toe examination

History	• Mechanism, injuries, vital signs, and treatment (MIVT)
	• Patient-generated information
	• Past medical history
Head and face	• Inspect for wounds, ecchymosis, deformities, drainage from nose and ears, and pupils.
	• Palpate for tenderness, note bony crepitus, deformities.
Neck	• Remove the anterior portion of the cervical collar to inspect and palpate the neck. Another team member must hold patient's head while collar is being removed and replaced.
	• Inspect for wounds, ecchymosis, deformities, and distended neck veins.
	• Palpate for tenderness, note bony crepitus, deformities, subcutaneous emphysema, and tracheal position.
Chest	• Inspect for breathing rate and depth, wounds, deformities, ecchymosis, use of accessory muscles, paradoxical movement.
	• Auscultate breath and heart sounds.
	• Palpate for tenderness; note bony crepitus, subcutaneous emphysema, and deformities.
Abdomen and flanks	• Inspect for wounds, distension, ecchymosis, and scars.
	• Auscultate bowel sounds.
	• Palpate all four quadrants for tenderness, rigidity, guarding, masses, and femoral pulses.
Pelvis and perineum	• Inspect for wounds, deformities, ecchymosis, priapism, blood at the urinary meatus or in the perineal area.
	• Palpate the pelvis and anal sphincter tone.
Extremities	• Inspect for ecchymosis, movement, wounds, and deformities.
	• Palpate for pulses, skin temperature, sensation, tenderness, deformities, and note bony crepitus.

I = Inspect posterior surface

Posterior surfaces	• Maintain cervical spine stabilization and support injured extremities while the patient is logrolled.
	• Inspect posterior surfaces for wounds, deformities, and ecchymosis.
	• Palpate posterior surfaces for tenderness and deformities.
	• Palpate anal sphincter tone (if not performed previously).

Modified from Emergency Nurses Association: *Trauma nursing core curriculum*, ed 4, Park Ridge, Ill, 1995, The Association.

Table **20-6**	**Sentinel Injuries and Associated Findings**
Injury	**Associated injuries**
First rib fracture	Heart and great vessel injury (i.e., subclavian vein and artery), head and neck injury
Scapula fracture	Brachial plexus injury, pulmonary contusion, great vessel injury, CNS injury
Sternal fracture	Myocardial contusion, great vessel injury, pulmonary contusion
Lower rib fractures	
Left	Spleen lacerations
Right	Liver lacerations

and treatment of life-threatening injuries. Blood work varies with each institution but should include as a minimum a complete blood count (CBC), and type and crossmatch. Table 20-7 identifies common laboratory tests obtained in trauma patients and provides clinical implications for each. Radiographic examinations vary with institutions and patient assessment. Specific studies and related clinical implications are provided in Table 20-8. Special procedures such as angiography, diagnostic peritoneal lavage, and ultrasound are indicated for some patients (Table 20-9). When the patient must be taken from the ED to the radiology department, a transport monitor, oxygen, and documentation forms should be taken with the patient.

Trauma patients should be carefully monitored throughout resuscitation for changes in condition and development

Table 20-7   Common Laboratory Tests

Laboratory test	Clinical implications
Complete blood count (CBC)	• Hematocrit and hemoglobin may be normal or above normal despite acute hemorrhage. Normal values do not exclude hemorrhagic shock.
Electrolytes	• Baseline data • Rule out electrolyte imbalance
Protime (PT) Prothrombin time (PTT)	• Baseline data • Rule out coagulopathies
Amylase	• Baseline data • Elevated value may indicate possible intraabdominal injury.
Lipase	• Baseline data • Elevated value may indicate possible intraabdominal injury.
Lactate	• Baseline data • Elevated level correlates with acute hemorrhage, shock, and increased anaerobic metabolism.
Arterial blood gas (ABG)	• Assess ventilatory and respiratory status. • Acidosis, especially in the presence of normal or decreased $PaCO_2$ level correlates with shock. • Base deficit of -6 or greater correlates with acute hemorrhage and shock. • Decreased PaO_2 and SAO_2 and an elevated $PaCO_2$ may indicate an airway or breathing emergency.
Liver function tests (LFTs)	• Baseline data • Elevated values may indicate liver damage.
Type and crossmatch	• Prepare for administration of blood and blood products.
Urinalysis	• Dip for blood.

Modified from Kidd PS, Sturt P: *Mosby's emergency nursing reference,* St. Louis, 1996, Mosby.

Table 20-8   Common Radiographic Examinations

Radiographic examination	Indication	Clinical implications
Chest x-ray	Chest trauma or pain Shortness of breath	• Anteroposterior examination with patient in supine position if immobilized. • Should be taken immediately upon arrival if possible. • Do not delay treatment of a suspected tension pneumothorax for a chest x-ray.
Pelvis x-ray	Blunt trauma Pelvic pain or instability Blood at urethral meatus	• Anteroposterior examination with patient in supine position. • Should be taken early in the resuscitation.
Cervical spine x-ray	Blunt trauma Trauma above nipple line Neck tenderness Neurologic deficit	• Cross-table lateral film usually obtained early in resuscitation. • Immobilization should be maintained until spine is radiographically and clinically cleared.
Thoracic and lumbar spine x-ray	Blunt trauma Back pain or trauma Neurologic deficit	• Patient should be logrolled until spine is cleared radiographically and clinically.
Extremity x-rays	Extremity trauma, deformity, or pain	• Suspected fractures should be immobilized before radiographs.
Heat CT*	Head trauma Loss of consciousness Focal neurologic findings Altered level of consciousness	• Transfer to a definitive care facility should not be delayed to obtain a head CT.
Abdominal CT	Abdominal trauma or pain Altered level of consciousness Unreliable clinical examination	• Transfer to a definitive care facility should not be delayed to obtain an abdominal CT.

*CT = Computerized tomography
From Kidd PS, Sturt P: *Mosby's emergency nursing reference,* St. Louis, 1996, Mosby.

Table 20-9   Common Special Procedures

Procedure	Indication	Clinical implications
Angiography	Suspected vessel injury Cerebral blood flow study	• Be prepared to assess and intervene in the event of an anaphylactic reaction. • Insertion site must be watched closely for bleeding after procedure.
Ultrasound	Abdominal trauma Unable to perform diagnostic peritoneal lavage or abdominal CT	
Diagnostic peritoneal lavage	Abdominal trauma or pain, especially in a hemodynamically unstable patient	• Gastric and bladder decompression must be done before performing a diagnostic peritoneal lavage. • This procedure does not evaluate the retroperitoneal space.
Transesophageal echocardiogram	Widened mediastinum Significant chest trauma	• Patient is usually rolled on side for procedure. • Patient may be sedated during procedure.

From Kidd PS, Sturt P: *Mosby's emergency nursing reference*, St. Louis, 1996, Mosby.

Table 20-10   Criteria for Early Transfer of Trauma Patient

System/location	Injury
Central nervous system	Penetrating injury or open fracture with or without cerebrospinal fluid leak Depressed skull fracture Glasgow Coma Scale (GCS) <14 or GCS deterioration Lateralizing signs Spinal cord injury or major vertebral injury
Thoracic	Major chest wall injury Widened mediastinum or other suggestions of great vessel injury Cardiac injury Patients requiring prolonged ventilation
Pelvis	Unstable pelvic ring fracture Unstable pelvic fracture with shock or continued hemorrhage Open pelvic injury Acetabular fractures
Major extremity injuries	Fracture/dislocation with loss of distal pulses Open long-bone fractures Ischemic extremity
Multiple injuries	Head injury with face, chest, abdominal, or pelvic injury Burns with associated injury Multiple long-bone fractures Injury to two or more body regions
Comorbid factors	Age <55 years Pediatric patient Cardiac or respiratory disease Insulin-dependent diabetic Morbid obesity Pregnancy Immunosuppression

of life-threatening problems. Patients may go to surgery after minimal ED management, remain in the ED for extensive diagnostic tests, or be transferred for specialty care. Patients transferred usually include those with burn injuries, pediatric trauma, and spinal fracture. Transfer to a trauma center should be considered for patients with multiple injuries, cardiac injury, and comorbid factors. Table 20-10 reviews criteria for early transfer to a trauma center.[1]

CONCLUSION

The importance of ED trauma management cannot be overstated. All EDs provide trauma care, with emergency nurses holding a pivotal role. Staff and departmental preparation minimize confusion and decrease time required for definitive care. A systematic approach to assessment and intervention improves patient outcomes through early recognition of potentially life-threatening injuries and intervention for identified problems.

REFERENCES

1. American College of Surgeons: *Resource document for optional care of trauma patients,* Chicago, 1993, ACS.
2. Childs SA: Musculoskeletal trauma: implications for critical care nursing practice, *Crit Care Nurs Clin North Am* 6:483-490, 1994.
3. Day R: Major trauma outcomes in the elderly, *Med J Austral* 160:675-678, 1994.
4. Feliciano D, et al.: *Trauma,* ed 3, Stamford, Conn, 1996, Appleton & Lange, pp 123-141.
5. Gallo K: Emergency department assessment of the adult trauma patient, *J Trauma Nurs* 1:451-461, 1994.
6. Kidd PS, Sturt P: *Mosby's emergency nursing reference,* St. Louis, 1996, Mosby.
7. Myers MB: Standing orders for trauma care, *J Emerg Nurs* 20:111-117, 1994.
8. Rotz NP: Application of the case management model to a trauma patient, *Clin Nurse Spec* 8:180-186, 1994.
9. Schmidth J: Management of multiple trauma, *Emerg Clin North Am* 11:29-47, 1993.
10. Shoemaker WC: Resuscitation from severe hemorrhage, *Crit Care Med* 24:12-23, 1996.
11. Weigelt JA: Resuscitation and initial management, *Crit Care Clin* 9:657-668, 1993.

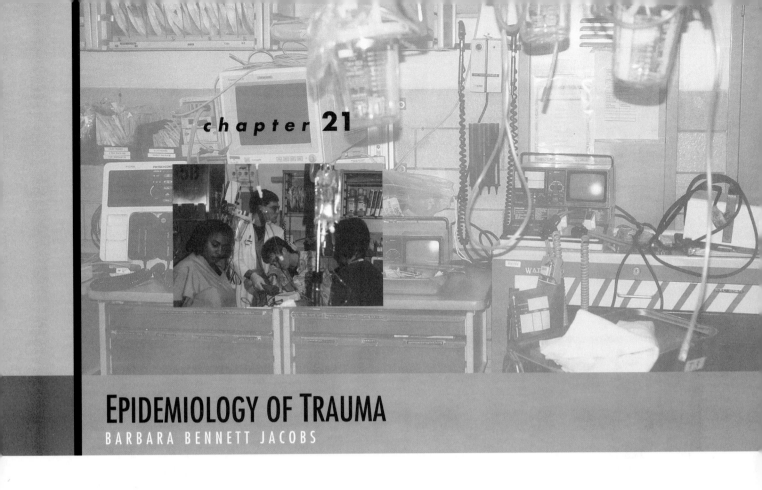

chapter 21

EPIDEMIOLOGY OF TRAUMA

BARBARA BENNETT JACOBS

Epidemiology is the study of "distribution and determinants of disease frequency in man."[14] To view trauma or injury from an epidemiologic perspective implies that the view consists of data elements such as age, gender, race/ethnicity, and geographic characteristics. These elements can form a frequency and distribution pattern that lends itself to further research and identification of causal factors. Frequency and distribution of injuries in the United States is the basis for planning and constructing injury prevention and control strategies.

Injury comes from the Greek word meaning "wound." The term "accident" is less frequently used by injury scientists and preventionists since the term connotes unexpectedness, random occurrence, and to some extent, inability to be prevented. Loimer, Driur, and Guarrnieri examined usage of the word "accident" from early writings. Philosophers such as Aristotle and Maimonides used "accident" to describe essential qualities of humans such as one's shape.[13] Therefore, use of the word "accident" in biblical, religious, legal, and statistical circles stems from a connotation of random and unexpected reality. Many publications from the U.S. Government continue to use the word accident; however, the words "injury" or "trauma" are preferable to describe the magnitude of this public health dilemma. Nurses who care for victims of trauma clearly recognize the need for prevention and control strategies to curb trauma mortality and morbidity. Perception of such trauma as preventable rather than as an act of random unexpectedness is essential for success

of preventive strategies. Throughout this chapter, the terms "trauma" and "injury" are interchangeable while the term "accident" is used only when the term is used by a reporting agency.

MORTALITY IN THE UNITED STATES

Mortality statistics, derived from death certificate data, are published annually by the National Center for Health Statistics. Deaths that occur 2 years before the publication date are analyzed. Eight years of data are used to give some perspective on trauma deaths over time. In 1986, 2,105,361 deaths occurred in the United States compared to 2,286,000 in 1994.[18,26] Table 21-1 summarizes deaths and death rates for 1986–1994.[18,26]

The National Center for Health Statistics counts injury deaths by the International Classification of Disease (ICD) "E" codes or the cause of death (i.e., motor vehicle crash, suicide, homicide). ICD codes also include accidents and their adverse effects (E800-949), suicide (E950-959), homicide and legal intervention (E960-978), and "all other external causes." When categories are combined to identify rate of injury death in the United States, trauma is the fourth leading cause of death for all groups and ages combined in 1994.[26] However, some controversy exists concerning the accuracy of this aggregate data.

Table 21-2 depicts causes of injury-related death from 1986–1994.[18,26] Table 21-3 presents death rates for leading causes of death in the United States for these same years. In

Table **21-1**	U.S. Deaths and Death Rates, 1986–1994	
Year	Number of deaths	Death rate/100,000 population
1986	2,105,361	873.2
1987	2,170,000	872.4
1988	2,171,000	882.0
1989	2,150,466	866.3
1990	2,148,463	863.8
1991	2,169,518	860.0
1992	2,175,613	852.9
1993	2,268,553	880.0
1994	2,286,000	876.9

Table **21-2**	U.S. Injury Deaths, 1986–1994 (Death rate/100,000 population)		
Year	Accidents and adverse effects	Suicide/homicide, legal intervention, and all other causes	Total of all injuries
1986	95,277	55,755	151,032
1987	94,840	54,380	149,220
1988	97,500	55,280	152,780
1989	95,028	55,841	150,869
1990	91,983	58,228	150,211
1991	89,347	59,840	149,187
1992	86,777	58,878	145,655
1993	90,523 (35.1)	60,538 (23.5)	151,061
1994	90,140 (34.6)	59,380 (22.7)	149,520

Table **21-3**	Death Rates for Leading Causes of Death in the United States, 1986–1994 (Death rate per/100,000 population)				
Year	All causes	Heart disease	Malignant neoplasm	Cerebrovascular disease	All injuries
1986	873.2	317.5	194.7	62.1	62.6
1987	872.4	312.4	195.9	61.6	61.6
1988	882.0	311.3	199.3	61.2	62.1
1989	866.3	295.6	199.9	58.6	60.8
1990	863.8	289.5	203.2	57.9	60.4
1991	860.3	285.9	204.1	56.9	59.1
1992	852.9	282.5	204.1	56.4	57.0
1993	880.0	288.4	205.6	58.2	58.6
1994	876.9	281.6	206.0	59.2	57.3

Table **21-4**	Injury Deaths and Death Rates for U.S. Males and Females, 1993 (Death rate/100,000 population)		
Injury category	Male deaths (death rates)	Female deaths (death rates)	Total deaths (death rates)
Accidents and adverse effects	60,117 (47.8)	30,406 (23.0)	90,523 (35.1)
Suicide	25,007 (19.9)	6095 (4.6)	31,102 (12.1)
Homicide/legal intervention	20,290 (16.1)	5719 (4.3)	26,009 (10.1)
All other injury causes	2521 (2.0)	906 (0.7)	3427 (1.3)
Total	**107,935** (**85.8**)	**43,126** (**32.6**)	**151,061** (**58.6**)

1994, 149,520 deaths from all injuries (accidents and their adverse effects, suicides, homicides/legal intervention, and other external causes) had a combined death rate of 57.3. In 1993 and 1994, injuries ranked as the fourth leading cause of death.[25,26] Death rates for injuries were comparable to cerebrovascular diseases. For the 9 years reviewed, injuries ranked as the third leading cause of death for the first 7 years. However, in 1993 and 1994 cerebrovascular disease ranked third because of an increase in the death rate for these diseases.

Between 1992 and 1993, a 3.2% increase in crude death rate from accidents and their adverse effects occurred with the most significant increase in the 25 to 34 age group. However, the highest death rate from accidents continues to be for those over the age of 85. In 1993, 8994 trauma deaths occurred in the 85 year-and-over category with a death rate of 263.3. In comparison, in the 25 to 34 age group, 14,022 deaths occurred with a corresponding death rate of 33.5. The greatest number of deaths occur in younger age groups; however, likelihood of dying from injury is almost eight times greater in the older age group.

Gender and age variances in injury deaths are related to the type of injury. Accidents and their adverse effects exclude suicides and homicides and account for more deaths among males than females. In 1994, 58,790 male deaths and 31,350 female deaths occurred with death rates of 46.3 and 23.5 respectively.[26] Table 21-4 compares injury deaths and death rates for males and females for the year 1993. Complete data in these categories are not yet available for 1994. Injury deaths and death rates by age for 1994 are summarized in Table 21-5.[26] The leading causes of death by age group are ranked in Table 21-6.

Leading causes of death vary by age as seen in Table 21-6. Accidents and their adverse effects are the leading cause of death for persons aged 1 to 24 years. When homicide and suicide deaths are added to deaths from accidents and their

Table **21-5** **Injury Deaths and Death Rates in the U.S. According to Age, 1994 (Death rate/100,000 population/age group)**

Age (years)	Death rate (accidents)	Number (accidents)	Death rate for suicides	Number of suicides	Death rate homicide/ legal intervention	Homicide/legal intervention*
<1	35.3	980	—	—	8.0	*
1-14	11.7	6270	0.7	390	1.7	920
15-24	39.0	14,000	14.0	5350	21.6	7770
25-34	30.7	12,690	16.0	6610	15.4	*
35-44	30.7	12,790	15.4	6430	10.6	*
45-54	27.3	8140	13.2	3940	5.9	*
55-64	32.4	6800	14.5	3050	4.5	*
65-74	41.2	7700	16.2	3040	3.3	*
75-84	1029	11,240	24.0	2620	3.4	*
>85	267.7	9430	27.0	950	4.8	*
Unknown	—	110	—	40	—	*
Total	**34.6**	**90,140**	**12.4**	**32,410**	**9.1**	**23,730**

*All numbers not available until 1994 Final Mortality Report is released.

Table **21-6** **Leading Causes of Death in the United States Ranked by Age Groups, 1994**

Cause of death	1-4 years	5-14 years	15-24 years	25-44 years	45-64 years	65+
Accidents and adverse effects	1	1	1	2	4	
Heart disease	5	5	5	4	2	1
Cerebrovascular disease					3	3
Congenital anomalies	2					
Malignant neoplasm	3	2	4	3	1	2
Homicide	4	3	2			
Suicide		4	3	5		
Chronic obstructive pulmonary disease					5	4
Pneumonia and influenza						5
Human immunodeficiency virus				1		

adverse effects in the 25 to 44 age group, injuries become the leading cause of death for persons 1 to 44 years.

Injury deaths and death rates also vary by race. As calculated by the National Center for Health Statistics and using its terms for explanation, whites have a higher death rate from suicide (13.1) compared to blacks (7.0). Blacks have a higher death rate from accidents and their adverse effects (39.5) compared to whites (35.0). Homicide/legal intervention death rate for blacks is 40.2 compared to 5.7 for whites. Blacks have a higher overall injury death rate for all categories of injuries combined of 89.0 compared to an overall death rate for whites of 55.0[26] (Table 21-7). Seventy-eight percent of all injury deaths occur in the white population, 19% in the black population, and 2.8% in all other races. However, the overall injury death rate is 1.6 times greater in the black population than the white population.

FIREARM DEATHS

Provisional data from the National Center of Health Statistics are available regarding deaths from injuries caused by firearms in 1994.[26] Of 39,730 deaths from firearms, 20,540 (52%) were suicides and 17,190 (43%) were due to homicide/legal intervention (Table 21-8). Suicide using a firearm (87%) is overwhelmingly a problem with males and is more prevalent when the victim is male and white (79%). Homicide/legal intervention using a firearm is more prevalent among males (84%); 44% of the victims are black, 38% are white. From an epidemiologic perspective, this data should be viewed with an appreciation for the population ratio, which is quite different for blacks and whites in the United States. The death rate from all firearm injuries for the white population is 13.0 compared to 32.3 for the black population. One of the most striking differences in these groups is that the death rate among white males who use a

Table **21-7**	**Injury Deaths and Death Rates in the United States by Race, 1993 (Death rate/100,000 population)**		
Injury category	Number of deaths (death rates, whites)	Number of deaths (death rates, blacks)	Number of deaths for other races
Accidents and their adverse effects	75,218 (35.0)	12,707 (39.5)	2598
Suicide	28,035 (13.1)	2259 (7.0)	808
Homicide/legal intervention	12,286 (5.7)	12,937 (40.2)	786
All other external causes	2581 (1.2)	751 (2.3)	95
Total	**118,120** **(55.0)**	**28,654** **(89.0)**	**4287**

Table **21-8**	**U.S. Deaths from Firearms, 1994 (Death rate/100,000 population)**				
Age groups	Accidents by firearm missiles	Suicides by firearms	Homicide/ legal intervention by firearms	Deaths by firearms, undetermined purpose	Total
<1	—	—	—	—	**—**
1-14	230	180	410	70	**890**
15-24	600	3760	6740	150	**11,250**
25-34	310	3850	4900	40	**9100**
35-44	200	3560	3020	40	**6820**
45-54	130	2460	1150	30	**3770**
55-64	50	1940	540	10	**2540**
65-74	60	2240	250	—	**2550**
75-84	20	1930	100	40	**2090**
85+	—	610	10	10	**630**
Age un- known	—	10	50	—	**60**
Total	**1600**	**20,540**	**17,170**	**390**	**39,700**

firearm to commit suicide is 15.3 compared to 8.5 for black males. The death rate for black males who die from a firearm in the homicide/legal intervention category is 48.9 compared to 6.2 for white males.

From a probability sample of 91 U.S. hospitals, researchers from the National Center for Injury Prevention and Control, estimate for a 2-year period (1992–1994), 34,485 unintentional, nonfatal firearm injuries occurred.[33] Injuries occurred primarily to males (87%) with 61% of all injured between 15 to 34 years of age. Seventy percent of the sample sustained firearm injuries that were self-inflicted with 38% requiring hospitalization. Hargarten et al. studied firearm fatalities in the city of Milwaukee, Wisconsin and found of the 705 firearm fatalities, 74% were homicides, 25% were suicides, 0.3% were unintentional firearm deaths, and the remaining could not be classified. The Raven MP-25 handgun was the weapon identified in 32% of the homicides and 77% of suicides. Overall, handguns were used for 85% of the fatalities.[10]

Hutson et al. studied the relationship of gangs to homicides in Los Angeles County, California for a 16-year period (1979–1994).[11] Of 27,302 homicides committed over this extensive period, almost 27% were gang related. Researchers found a statistically significant difference ($p <$ .001) between the percent of homicides related to gangs in 1979 (18.1%) and that in 1994 (43%). "Street gangs" were "responsible" for over one third of all homicides in the Los Angeles County area. More than 25% of the gang-related homicides, from an area that accounts for 66% of the county, were "drive-by" shootings with 64% of the victims "documented members of violent street gangs."

General Estimates of Nonfatal Injuries

The incidence and rate of injury that occur but do not cause death are more difficult to determine. However, a few

Table **21-9**	**U.S. States with Accidents and Their Adverse Effects, 1993 Death rate >2500 persons**
State	Number of accidents and adverse effects (rate/100,000 population)
California	10,684 (34.2)
Florida	7,120 (51.9)
New York	6,144 (33.8)
Texas	6,009 (33.3)
Pennsylvania	5,212 (43.3)
Ohio	4,771 (43.1)
Illinois	4,325 (37.0)
Michigan	3,459 (36.6)
North Carolina	2,833 (40.7)

available statistics reflect the wide magnitude of the injury-occurrence problem. Each year, 1 out of 4 U.S. citizens sustains an injury.[1] Ten percent of patient visits to physicians' offices are related to injuries.[32] For every single injury death, an additional 19 persons are hospitalized for nonfatal injuries and 354 receive some form of medical care.[1]

Geographic Differences

Table 21-9 shows the actual number of accidents per 100,000 population.[26] Death rates vary with population number, so states with the highest death rates are Mississippi (59.5), California (56.4), and New Mexico (51.4).

Geographic differences occur with regard to death rate with suicide, homicide, and motor vehicle crashes. The highest homicide rate is in the District of Columbia, the highest suicide rate is in Nevada, and the highest death rate from motor vehicle crashes is in Mississippi (Table 21-10). The states with the highest suicide rates are all mountain states.[26]

MOTOR VEHICLE CRASHES

The Fatal Accident Reporting System (FARS) and General Estimates System (GES) are compiled annually by the National Highway Traffic Safety Administration (NHTSA) in a report called *Traffic Safety Facts*. Changes over time reflect interesting issues associated with motor vehicle crashes. In 1966, the fatality rate per 100 million miles traveled in the United States was 5.5; in 1994 the rate declined to 1.7.[34] Between 1966 and 1994, the fatality rate per 100,000 population declined from 26.02 to 15.62; however, the actual number of fatalities did decrease significantly. In 1966, 50,894 fatalities occurred compared to 40,676 in 1994 (Table 21-11). Additional facts related to 1994 crashes are summarized in Box 21-1. Table 21-12 summarizes the types of vehicles involved in fatal and nonfatal crashes for this same year.

RELATIONSHIP OF VIOLENCE TO INJURIES

Assaultive violence has been defined as "both nonfatal and fatal interpersonal violence where physical force or other means is used by one person with the intent of causing harm, injury, or death to another."[30] Definitions become clouded when legal and nonlegal terms are interchanged. Violence has numerous mechanisms of injury and numerous vehicles and vectors of transfer from the environment to the human victim. The issue however is one of "intent" to cause harm. All kinds of abuse (i.e., sexual, verbal, and physical) can be viewed as violent acts. Beatings, assaults, attempted murders, and homicides also fit the definition of violence.

The Crime Victim Research and Treatment Center of the Medical University of South Carolina reported in the *Rape*

in America study that 618,000 women over the age of 18 were raped in a one-year period in the United States.[4] Researchers also concluded 12.1 million women in the United States have been victims of at least one forcible rape. Child abuse incidence is primarily an estimate. Schafran reported "at least 20% of American women and 5-10% of American men experienced some form of abuse as children."[31,6] The Centers for Disease Control and Prevention estimate that approximately 2000 child fatalities per year in the United States are caused by neglect or abuse.[5]

Grisson, Schwarz, Miles, and Holmes reported on causes of injury to women during 1987–1990 as part of the Philadelphia Injury Prevention Program.[7] Surveillance from 11 participating emergency departments found 11,654 injured women 15 years of age and older during the 4-year study period. Of these victims, 804 were hospitalized (7%) and 86 died. Falls were the most frequent mechanism of injury associated with admission; however, over time, violence became the leading cause of injury with a 55% increase over the study period. Overall rate for violence-induced injuries in 1990 in this study was 33.2 per 1000 women compared to 29.5 for falls and 15.8 for motor vehicle events.

Table **21-11**	U.S. Traffic Deaths, Fatality Rates (per 100,000 Population), and Fatality Rates (per 100 Million Miles Traveled), Selected Years 1966–1994		
Year	Number of deaths	Fatality rate/ 100,000 pop.	Fatality rate/ 100 million miles traveled
1966	50,894	26.02	5.5
1970	52,627	25.80	4.7
1974	45,196	21.18	3.5
1979	51,093	22.75	3.3
1984	44,257	18.72	2.6
1989	45,582	18.36	2.2
1994	40,676	15.62	1.7

Table **21-10**	U.S. States with Highest Rates for Motor Vehicle Crashes, Suicides, and Homicides, 1993 (Death rate/100,000 population)	
Motor vehicle death rates	Homicide death rates	Suicide death rates
Mississippi (32.9)	Dist. of Columbia (72.4)	Nevada (23.4)
Alabama (26.5)	Louisiana (21.3)	Wyoming (22.4)
New Mexico (25.3)	Mississippi (18.6)	Arizona (18.4)
Arkansas (24.6)	Alabama (13.9)	Montana (18.4)
Tennessee (23.5)	California (13.8)	Idaho (17.2)

Table **21-12**	Types of Vehicles Involved in U.S. Fatal and Nonfatal Crashes, 1994		
Type of vehicle	Number in fatal crashes (percent)	Number in nonfatal crashes	Total involved in all crashes
Passenger car	30,149 (54.9)	2.742 million	2.772 million
Light truck	16,289 (29.7)	893,000	909,289
Large truck	4615 (8.4)	95,000	99,615
Motorcycle	2325 (4.2)	53,000	55,325
Bus	258 (0.5)	14,000	14,258
Other	480 (0.9)	5000	5480

Box 21-1   Factors Related to 1994 Motor Vehicle Collisions

- 40,676 traffic-related deaths with an estimated 3.215 million injuries
- 34,293 occupants and 6383 pedestrians, pedalcyclists, and other nonmotorists killed
- 23,695 (58%) drivers, 10,502 (26%) passengers, 6383 (15.7%) nonmotorists (i.e., pedestrians, pedalcyclists)
- 2304 motorcycle occupants killed and another 56,000 injured
- 53,174 drivers involved in fatal crashes, 39,739 males and 13,430 females; 44.66 males and 15.6 females per 100,000 licensed drivers/gender
- 28.1% drivers in 21-24 age group and 14.1% in 16-20 year-olds involved in fatal crashes had blood alcohol ≥0.10
- 41% of fatalities involved alcohol; lowest percentage from 1982–1994 and represents 3.5% decrease from 1993
- Occupant fatality rates were highest in 16-20 age group (30.67), 21-24 (26.26), and those over 74 (20.79).
- 36,223 fatal crashes; more occur Saturday 6 p.m. to 3 a.m.; 56.9% on rural roadways, 42.5% urban roadways; 67% on nondivided roads, 29% on divided roads
- Vehicles involved in more fatal crashes were passenger cars.
- 40% fatal crashes were collisions with another motor vehicle, 28.4% collisions with a fixed object, 19.7% collisions with object not fixed (pedestrian, parked car), 9.7% rollovers
- 55% fatal motorcycle crashes were collisions with another vehicle while moving
- 91 fatalities involved emergency response vehicles—26 ambulances, 9 fire trucks, and 56 police cars
- 21 fatalities and 15,000 injuries involved buses
- 21,903 fatalities related to cars; 19,616 victims (90%) in front seat with 14,610 in left front; 2019 in back seat with 934 on right and 744 on left
- Fatalities in cars only 35.6% using restraints, 55.4% unrestrained
- 53% motorcycle fatalities wearing helmets, 43% were not
- Arkansas, Delaware, and Texas have highest percentage of alcohol-related fatal crashes in United States whereas South Carolina, Ohio, and Utah have the lowest
- Wyoming, New Mexico, and Mississippi have highest fatality rate per 100,000 population, whereas Rhode Island, Connecticut, New Jersey, and New York have the lowest.
- All 50 states, Puerto Rico, and the District of Columbia have safety belt laws and child restraint laws with varied degrees of applicability.

Abuse among pregnant women is not uncommon. In a study of 691 black, Hispanic, and white women who sought prenatal care, 17% of the sample had been abused at least once.[17] Of 236 Hispanic women, 62% were married, compared to 7% of the 267 black women, and 40% of the 188 white women. Overall, 95% were below the poverty level. Sixty percent reported two or more incidents of abuse. Sixty-four percent of the black women abused were abused by a boyfriend (58%) or husband/exhusband (6%), whereas 91% of the Hispanic women were abused by their husbands/exhusbands (50%) or boyfriend (41%), and 77% of the white women were abused by their boyfriend (44%) or husband/ex-husband (33%).

Murder-suicide events are another manifestation of violence in the United States. Although the actual incidence is difficult to determine, researchers from Cornell University published data related to review of previously published studies on this issue.[16] Relevant demographic determinants derived from studies are summarized in Box 21-2.

Researchers also studied filicide-suicide, when a parent murders a child then takes his or her own life. A father is more likely to commit suicide after killing a child than a mother, with depression a significant characteristic in murderous mothers. The term "family annihilator"[3] describes

---

Box 21-2   Demographic Determinants of Violence

Majority of murder-suicides related to "amorous jealousy"
Typical victim is married, "recently estranged," or "involved in a love relationship"
Mean age of "offender" is 39.6 years
93%-97% of "offenders" are male
50%-86% of "offenders" are white
Over 85% of "victims" are female
Most common means of murder-suicide is firearms

---

the "senior male of a household" who experiences "cumulative financial, marital, or other social stresses on the family" and feels he can relieve the family stress by annihilating them. Extrafamilial murder-suicide, unfortunately, may claim more adult victims than those involved in the murderer's realm of discontent. Such a person is often distressed over employment or financial issues and seeks out those perceived as the source of such distress (i.e., fellow employees, supervisors, teachers, etc.). In this type of murder-suicide, the weapon is usually a firearm. The murderer may also kill bystanders or anyone who interferes in the pursuit of intended victims.

The violence and injury issue is often difficult to analyze, making strategic planning for prevention even more difficult. Rosenberg suggests two approaches to the violence issue.[30] One is a biologic approach, which views violence from characteristics such as age, gender, and previous psychiatric illnesses. The sociologic approach puts cultural, structural, interactionist, and economic issues in view. A combination of identifiable risk factors and sociologic factors is the most likely scenario. From a cultural perspective, learned behavior specific to a cultural group may exist. From a structural perspective, violence may be a result of social forces, such as poverty. From an interactionist perspective, violence results from human interactive processes; and from an economic perspective, violence is a choice when faced with violent or nonviolent solutions to conflict resolution.

WEATHER-RELATED DEATHS

Although risk of death from natural occurrences such as lightning, hurricanes, or other weather events may be viewed as the most uncontrollable risk, disaster preparedness is an effective prevention strategy. The Centers for Disease Control and Prevention reported on two hurricanes that struck the United States in 1995, Hurricane Opal in April and Hurricane Marilyn in September.[3] Hurricane Marilyn affected Puerto Rico and the U.S. Virgin Islands of St. Thomas, St. John, and St. Croix. The hurricane was so severe (category 2) that 80% of all residential housing in St. Thomas was damaged or destroyed. Ten deaths were reported from this storm: one secondary to electrocution while preparing a TV antenna and nine related to the impact of the storm. Of these nine, seven were due to drowning and considered boat related with one due to head trauma while on a boat. The last death was a 107-year-old woman who died of "natural causes" while in a shelter. Hurricane Opal was a category 3 storm that struck Florida, Alabama, Georgia, and North Carolina. The storm claimed 27 lives, with one death before the storm, 13 during impact, and 13 after impact. Three of the deaths, although storm related, were not "accidental": one was due to chronic obstructive pulmonary disease, two due to myocardial infarctions. The remaining deaths resulted from falling trees, electricity failure (one from carbon monoxide from a gas generator, three from house fires caused by candles burning), motor vehicle-related incidents, and one electrocution from a downed wire.

BURNS

Burn death data are not as retrievable as deaths from injuries from motor vehicles crashes, suicides, and homicides. Of 54,400 to 100,000 persons hospitalized each year from burns, approximately 6000 die.[2] The most frequent cause of death from fire in a dwelling is inhalation injury from toxic products of combustion. Most deaths are caused by exposure to hydrogen cyanide, carbon monoxide, products of decomposition, and products of combustion that yield nitrogen oxides, acid gases, aldehydes, and alcohols. Scald burns are more frequent in the younger age group (5 and under) and the elderly over age 65. However scald burns are not usually lethal. Clothing ignition deaths occur mostly in the elderly; 75% of such deaths are those over age of 65. Of approximately 80 deaths per year from lightning, the largest incidence is in those age 10 to 19 years with the death rate seven times greater in males. Southern states have the highest death rates from burns with the highest incidence in the winter followed by spring, fall, and summer respectively.

INJURY PREVENTION AND CONTROL

Injury prevention and control strategies generally fit into three categories: education and persuasion, legal regulation of behavior, and engineering or technologic advancements to provide "automatic protection" to people. Leon Robertson, a leading injury research scientist from Yale University, recently reported in *The American Journal of Public Health* that vehicle-related deaths from 1975 through 1991 decreased as a result of "minimum safety standards, crashwor-

Table **21-13** **Haddon's Strategies for Injury Prevention**[8]	
Strategy	Application to firearm injuries
Prevent creation of the hazard	Do not manufacture firearms
Reduce amount of the hazard	Pass gun control laws
Prevent release of an existing hazard	Manufacture weapons with safety locks
Modify rate or spatial distribution of the hazard	Reduce power and velocity of projected missiles
Separate hazard in time and space from that which is to be protected	Keep firearms in area inaccessible to children
Separate hazard by material barrier from that which is to be protected	Store firearms in locked cases, boxes, or other secure places
Modify relevant basic qualities of the hazard	Manufacture real firearms that look less like toys
Make what is to be protected more resistant to damage from the hazard	Have populations at risk wear protective devices (e.g., police should wear bullet-proof vests)
Counter damage already done by the hazard	Implement 911 ambulance access
Stabilize, repair, and rehabilitate the object of the damage	Transport gunshot victims to trauma centers

thiness improvements, seat belt use laws, and reduced alcohol use."[28] As evidenced by Dr. Robertson's analysis, all three injury-prevention strategies contributed in some degree to reduction in vehicle-related fatalities.

Although reports related to use of motorcycle helmets indicate reduced fatalities, three states (Colorado, Indiana, and Iowa) do not have legal requirements for helmet use, and 22 states require helmet use only for certain riders (e.g. 18 or 21). Twenty-five states plus the District of Columbia and Puerto Rico require helmet use for all motorcycle riders.[34] Age is frequently the variable that identifies legal requirement for helmet use despite the fact that head injury or death of an 18-year-old is no less devastating than death or injury of a 17-year-old. Krause et al. reported on the effects of the motorcycle helmet use law that went into effect in California in 1992.[12] During the pre-law year (1991), 523 fatalities occurred with a motorcycle fatality rate of 70.1/100,000 registered motorcycles compared to 51.5/100,000 in 1992. Data show a 37.5% decrease in fatalities (from 523 in 1991 to 327 in 1992) and 25.5% reduction in fatality rate.[12] Rowland et al. reported on the outcome and hospitalization costs of motorcyclists hospitalized.[29] Researchers found of 2090 motorcycle crashes in Washington state, 409 (20%) riders were hospitalized and 59 (2.8%) were killed. Unhelmeted riders were more critically injured than helmeted riders, had three times greater incidence of head injury, a greater likelihood of being readmitted, stayed in the hospital longer, and incurred a mean hospital cost ($16,460 compared to $12,689, respectively).

Recognizing the importance of prevention to curb the injury epidemic, Ricardo Martinez, Administrator of the NHTSA, summarized his "perspective" of injury prevention[15]: "Injury is disease process that results from energy transmission to a human host in a permissive environment. Common forms of energy release that cause injury are mechanical, electrical, thermal, and chemical. Injury prevention takes a scientific approach that identifies high-risk persons and problem injuries, develops and implements effective countermeasures, and evaluates the results. Injury prevention countermeasures can be directed at human and behavioral factors, vectors of energy (i.e., motor vehicles, firearms, or heaters), and environmental factors (i.e., lightning, roadways, or home). These countermeasures can be implemented through the "four Es" of injury prevention: education and information efforts, enforcement and regulation, engineering and technology, and economic incentives." Many of the principles Martinez postulated are found in the works of William Haddon, Jr., MD, the first director of NHTSA. Table 21-13 summarizes Haddon's 10 strategies for injury prevention and control.[8] Table 21-14 lists three sources of information related to injury prevention.

Haddon is also credited with designing a matrix that combines three phases of the injury event with three contributing factors to the event[9] (Table 21-15). Although originally designed for highway safety to develop injury strategies, the nine cells of the matrix identify areas where prevention programs can focus efforts to reduce falls in the elderly who live in nursing homes and other situations.

CONCLUSION

In the 14th century, "accident" meant "to happen by chance; a misfortune; an event that happens without foresight or expectation." This meaning is associated with the French word *accidence,* which may be a corruption of the Latin verb *accidere,* meaning "to fall down" or "to fall to."[13] Fortunately, today's consumers and health care providers see trauma as a preventable event rather than as an accident.

Table **21-14** **Information Sources for Injury Prevention**

Source	Location/phone number
National Center for Injury Prevention and Control	Atlanta, Georgia (404) 448-4365
National Highway Traffic Safety Administration	Washington, DC (202) 336-4198
National Center for Health Statistics	Hyattsville, Maryland (301) 436-8500

Table **21-15** **The Haddon Injury Matrix**

Phases	Human factors	Vehicle/vector factors	Environmental factors
Pre-event	Reduce use of sedatives	Correct defects in safety equipment	Use of safety bars, handrails, side rails on beds
Event	Consider reduction in severity of preexisting medical conditions	Cover exposed skin areas with protective barriers to reduce severity of injury	Reduction of clutter in the patient's environment
Post-event	Consider if patient is on anticoagulants and effects on subsequent bleeding from injury	Have patients avoid areas where they become trapped after a fall	Comprehensive emergency response systems

Efforts across the country have reduced morbidity and death caused by injury. However, a review of data in this chapter emphasizes the fact that much work needs to be done. The emergency nurse is challenged to become active in local, state, and national trauma prevention programs. Only through efforts by health care providers, consumers, legislators, and injury prevention scientists will trauma become a disease with no victims.

REFERENCES

1. Adams PF, Benson V: Current estimates from national health interview survey, *Vital Health Stat,* 184, 1992.
2. Baker SP, et al.: *The injury fact book,* ed 2, New York, 1991, Oxford University Press.
3. Centers for Disease Control: Deaths associated with hurricanes Marilyn and Opal; United States September-October, 1995, *MMWR,* 45:32-38, 1996.
4. Crime Victim Research and Treatment Center: *Rape in America,* 1992, Medical University of South Carolina.
5. Durfee MJ, Gellert GA, Tilton-Durfee D: Origins and clinical relevance of child death review teams, *JAMA* 267(23):3172-3175, 1992.
6. Finkelhor D: Current information on the scope and nature of child sexual abuse, *The future of children,* Summer/Fall 31, 1994.
7. Grisso JA, et al.: Injuries among inner city minority women: a population-based longitudinal study, *Am J Public Health,* 86(1):67-72, 1996.
8. Haddon W: Advances in the epidemiology of injuries as a basis for public policy, *Public Health Rep* 95:411-421, 1980.
9. Haddon W: A logical framework for categorizing highway safety phenomena and activity, *J Trauma* 12:197, 1972.
10. Hargarten SW, et al.: Characteristics of firearms involved in fatalities, *JAMA* 275(1):42-45, 1996.
11. Hutson HR, et al.: The epidemic of gang-related homicides in Los Angeles county from 1979–1994, *JAMA* 274(13):1031-1036, 1995.
12. Kraus JF, et al.: The effect of the 1992 California motorcycle helmet use law on motorcycle crash fatalities and injuries, *JAMA* 274(19):1506-1511, 1994.
13. Loimer H, Driur M, Guarnieri M: Accidents and acts of God: a history of the terms, *JAMA* 86(1):101-107, 1996.
14. Mahon B, Pugh T: *Epidemiology principles and practice,* Boston, p. 1, 1970, Little Brown and Co.
15. Martinez R: Injury prevention a new perspective, *JAMA* 272(19):1541-1542, 1994.
16. Marzck PM, Tardiff K, Hirsch CS: The epidemiology of murder-suicide, *JAMA* 267(23):3179-3182, 1992.
17. McFarland J, et al.: Assessing for abuse during pregnancy, *JAMA* 267(23):3176-3177, 1992.
18. National Center for Health Statistics, U.S. Department of Health and Human Services, Public Health Service, *Monthly vital statistics report: Advance report of final mortality, 1986,* 39(6), 1988.
19. National Center for Health Statistics, U.S. Department of Health and Human Services, Public Health Service, *Monthly vital statistics report: Advance report of final mortality, 1987,* 38(5), 1989.
20. National Center for Health Statistics, U.S. Department of Health and Human Services, Public Health Service, *Monthly vital statistics report: Advance report of final mortality, 1988,* 39(7), 1990.
21. National Center for Health Statistics, U.S. Department of Health and Human Services, Public Health Service, *Monthly vital statistics report: Advance report of final mortality, 1989,* 40(8), 1992.
22. National Center for Health Statistics, U.S. Department of Health and Human Services, Public Health Service, *Monthly vital statistics report: Advance report of final mortality, 1990,* 41(7), 1993.
23. National Center for Health Statistics, U.S. Department of Health and Human Services, Public Health Service, *Monthly vital statistics report: Advance report of final mortality, 1991,* 42(2), 1993.
24. National Center for Health Statistics, U.S. Department of Health and Human Services, Public Health Service, *Monthly vital statistics report: Advance report of final mortality, 1992,* 43(1), 1993.
25. National Center for Health Statistics, U.S. Department of Health and Human Services, Public Health Service, *Monthly vital statistics report: Advance report of final mortality, 1993,* 44(7), 1996.
26. National Center for Health Statistics, U.S. Department of Health and Human Services, Public Health Service, *Annual summary of births, marriages, divorces, and deaths: United States, 1994,* 43(13), October 23, 1995.
27. National Committee for Injury Prevention and Control, Injury prevention meeting the challenge, *Amer J Prev Med,* 5(3):2, 1989.
28. Robertson L: Reducing death on the road: the effects of minimum safety standards, publicized crash tests, seat belts, and alcohol, *American Journal of Public Health,* 86(1):31-33, 1996.
29. Rowland J, et al.: Motorcycle helmet use and injury outcome and hospitalization costs from crashes in Washington State, *Amer J Public Health,* 86(1):41-45, 1996.
30. Rosenberg ML, Mercy JA: Assaultive violence. In Rosenberg ML, Fenley M editors: *Violence in America,* p. 14, New York, 1991, Oxford University Press.
31. Schafran LH: Topics for our times: rape is a major public health issue, *Amer J Public Health,* 86(1):15-17, 1996.
32. Schappert SM: National ambulatory medical care survey: 1992, summary, *Vital and health statistics,* Hyattsville, Md, 1994, National Center for Health Statistics.
33. Sinaver N, Annest JL, Mercy JA: Unintentional, nonfatal firearm-related injuries, *JAMA,* 275(22):1740-1743, 1996.
34. United States Department of Transportation, National Highway Traffic Safety Administration, *Traffic safety facts, 1993,* Washington, DC, DOT HS 808 292, August, 1995.

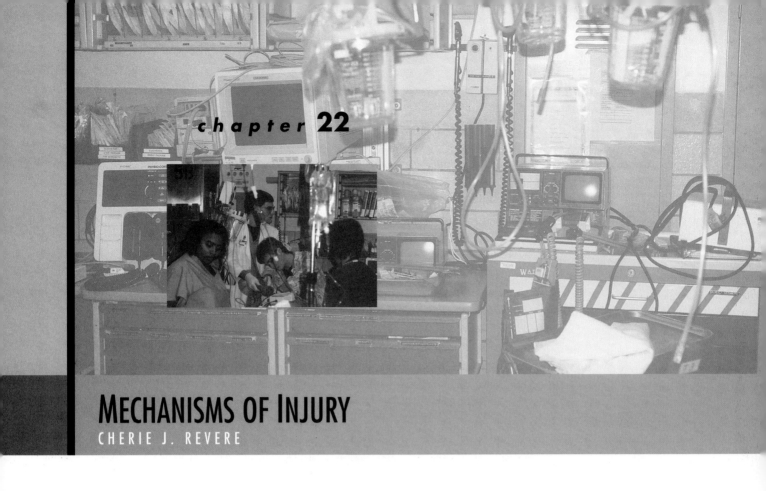

chapter 22

MECHANISMS OF INJURY

CHERIE J. REVERE

Trauma is the most frequent cause of death for children and adults under 45 years. The high social, personal, and economic costs associated with traumatic injuries makes trauma a major public health problem in the United States. Trauma is also the main cause for loss of work years because the younger population is affected more often. An estimated 4 million productive work years are lost each year. One of three Americans are injured annually, 340,000 permanently disabled, and more than 160,000 die. Injuries are the number one reason patients seek treatment or see physicians. Treatment of injuries accounts for 25% of hospital, clinic, and emergency department (ED) visits.

Trauma is now recognized as a disease process with mechanisms of injury a part of the etiology. Strong assessment skills are essential for health care providers because treatment of trauma patients is contingent on locating all injuries. Unfortunately, even with strong assessment skills, some injuries go undetected if the "index of suspicion" is not sufficient. Providing trauma care without understanding or recognizing the mechanism that produces injuries is not optimal trauma care. Understanding mechanisms of injury and using a high index of suspicion enable the care giver to predict and locate occult injuries more quickly and save time initiating essential treatment. Injury should be considered present until definitively ruled out in a hospital setting.

Injury is defined as physical harm or damage to a person. When an uncontrolled or acute source of energy makes contact with the body and the body cannot tolerate exposure to that acute energy, injury results. Energy originates from several sources, kinetic (motion or mechanical), chemical, electrical, thermal, or radiation. Absence of heat and oxygen causes injuries such as frostbite, drowning, or suffocation. Kinetic energy is defined as energy that results from motion. A basic component in producing injury is the absorption of kinetic energy. Box 22-1 defines essential concepts for understanding mechanisms of injury.

Severity depends on the wounding agent. Velocity and missile mass affect severity of gunshot wounds, whereas deceleration injuries depend on the rate of deceleration, victim body mass, and area of energy dissipation. Burn severity is determined by duration of contact and temperature.

Personal and environmental factors that affect injuries include sex, age, underlying disease processes, and nutrition. Risk factors amenable to prevention measures are sex, age, alcohol, race, income, geographic region, and temporal variation.

Males are 2.5 times more likely to be injured or involved in an accident than females because of their participation in more hazardous activities and greater risk taking. The high rate of injury in persons between 15 and 24 years may be caused by experimentation with drugs and alcohol in combination with poor judgment. Elderly persons ($\geq$75 years) have the highest death rate from injuries that may be associated with existing medical conditions.

Alcohol is a major factor in all types of trauma, including motor vehicle crashes (MVCs), family violence, suicides,

Box 22-1	**Essential Concepts for Mechanisms of Injury**
Acceleration:	Change in rate of velocity/speed of a moving object.
Acceleration/deceleration:	Increase in velocity/speed of object followed by decrease in velocity/speed.
Axial loading:	Injury occurs when force is applied upward and downward with no posterior or lateral bending of the neck.
Cavitation:	Creation of temporary cavity as tissues are stretched and compressed.
Compression:	Squeezing inward pressure.
Compressive strength:	Ability to resist squeezing forces or inward pressure.
Deceleration:	Decrease in velocity/speed of a moving object.
Distraction:	Separation of spinal column with resulting cord transection, seen in legal hangings.
Elasticity:	Ability to resume original shape and size after being stretched.
Force:	Physical factor that changes motion of body at rest or already in motion.
High velocity:	Missiles that compress and accelerate tissue away from the bullet, causing a cavity around the bullet and the entire tract.
Inertial resistance:	Ability of body to resist movement.
Injury:	Physical harm or damage to a person.
Kinematics:	Process of looking at an accident and determining what injuries might result.
Kinetic energy:	Energy that results from motion.
Low velocity:	Missiles that localize injury to a small radius from center of the tract with little disruptive effect.
Muzzle blast:	Cloud of hot gas and burning powder at the muzzle of a gun.
Shearing:	Two oppositely directed parallel forces.
Stress:	Internal resistance to deformation, or internal force generated from application load.
Tensile strength:	Amount of tension tissue can withstand, and ability to resist stretching forces.
Tumbling:	Forward rotation around the center, somersault action of the missile can create massive injury.
Yaw:	Deviation of bullet nose in longitudinal axis from straight line of flight.

homicides, and altercations. Alcohol increases severity of injury and causes or contributes to injury-producing events. Injury and death rates vary with race and income. For blacks and whites, the higher the income, the lower the death rate. MVCs decrease in a depressed economy, while homicide and suicides increase. The highest homicide rate occurs in the black population, the highest suicide rate is seen in whites and Native Americans, and the lowest death rates occur in Asian Americans.

Injury rates are also characterized by physical environment or geographic area. Homicides and suicides occur more in urban areas, whereas unintentional injuries or accidents are more numerous in rural areas. Injury and death rates are greater on weekends and peak on Saturday. More injuries are seen in July, probably due to summer activities.

Along with the wounding force, recognition of the subsequent tissue response is important to evaluating injuries. When tissue limits are surpassed, injury occurs that results in physiologic and/or anatomic damage. A central nervous system (CNS) injury is a physiologic injury that may cause permanent damage despite healing. Skeletal fractures are anatomic damage that can heal without permanent disability. Understanding mechanisms of injury affects outcome because common injury patterns can be predicted and identified.

KINEMATICS

Kinematics is the process of looking at an accident and determining what injuries are likely to occur given the forces and motion involved. Physics is the foundation on which kinematics is based. Understanding essential laws of physics is the first step toward understanding kinematics.

Newton's first law of motion states that a body at rest remains at rest and a body in motion remains in motion unless acted on by an outside force. Stationary objects set in motion by energy forces can be seen as pedestrians struck by a vehicle, blast victims, and persons with gunshot wounds. Moving objects interrupted or acted on to stop their motion are the same as persons falling from a height, or vehicles hitting a tree or braking to a sudden stop.

The second essential law of physics, the Law of Conservation of Energy, states that energy is neither created nor destroyed but changes form. As a car decelerates slowly, the energy of motion (acceleration) is converted to friction heat in braking (thermal energy).

Trauma may be penetrating or blunt. Penetrating trauma causes a break in the skin that communicates to the outside. The injury pattern associated with penetrating trauma is related to the energy created and dissipated by the wounding agent and the surrounding area. Damage is contingent on velocity of the wounding agent and underlying structures that are damaged. With blunt trauma, where trauma is without communication to the outside, injuries are less obvious, so the extent of injury is difficult to diagnose.

Patient Assessment

Initially, trauma patients may not appear seriously injured due to strong compensatory mechanisms that maintain adequate vital signs. All members of a trauma team must anticipate injuries by recognizing potential patterns of injury related to the energy and force of the accident. Assessment, resuscitation, and stabilization efforts based on patterns and mechanisms recognized in each patient enable health care providers to recognize hidden or internal injuries and avoid potentially harmful diagnostic interventions.

Health care providers should match injuries to reported mechanisms. Patients, family, and friends may have reasons to fabricate, falsify, or deny the actual event. Therefore, injuries identified in the examination must match the reported mechanism. Eliciting a careful history of the injury during initial assessment of a trauma patient is vital. Accurate information, especially about mechanisms surrounding injuries, can reduce morbidity and mortality in many circumstances.

When assessing a trauma patient, the emergency nurse should note mechanisms associated with major force or energy transfer (e.g., pedestrian hit by vehicle traveling at speed $\geq$20 mph; falls $\geq$20 feet; MVC with major vehicular damage; speed change $\geq$20 mph; vehicle rollover; ejected occupant; or death of occupant).

Some injuries are significant because of potential complications, such as two or more long bone fractures; flail chest; penetrating trauma to the head, neck, chest, abdomen, or groin; and any combination of these patterns with burns $\geq$15% of head, face, or airway. Patients with significant injuries require close monitoring for complications or changes in hemodynamic stability.

Certain questions provide valuable information regarding the mechanism of injury and are helpful in assessing potential injuries. What type of vehicle was the patient driving (large or small)? What was the estimated speed at the time of crash? Were seat belts or restraint devices used? Were the devices applied appropriately? Were airbags installed and did they deploy? Where was the patient in the vehicle (driver, front or rear seat passenger)? If ejected, how far was the patient thrown or found from the vehicle? How much damage was done to the vehicle? Where was the majority of damage? Occupants have injuries at the same site as the vehicle damage. The emergency nurse should ask about steering wheel deformity for all drivers. If the patient fell, what was the approximate height of the fall? Were any objects struck during the fall? What was the surface where the patient landed? In what position was the patient found after the fall?

With penetrating injury, the wounding agent (i.e., knife, gun, arrow, ice pick) must be ascertained. What was the size and length of the agent? With guns, what was the caliber and distance from weapon to patient? Patients with penetrating trauma must be assessed for other types of trauma, such as falls or assaults. Patients may be exposed to more than one type of energy.

A detailed history is not always possible and is often impractical. Valuable information can be obtained from family members, emergency medical service personnel, police, fire fighters, bystanders, or eyewitnesses; however, these resources are often overlooked in a hectic ED. Management of life-threatening injuries has priority over obtaining a detailed history; however, every effort should be made to obtain as much historical data as possible.

Once resuscitation is accomplished, rapid examination or assessment should be performed. Patients with penetrating trauma are easier to assess than those with blunt trauma because injuries are usually focused in one area. Surface trauma may or may not be present with blunt injuries; therefore, assessment tends to be more difficult. During a secondary survey, missed injuries can be found by systematically examining the patient who is completely undressed. Maintaining a high index of suspicion for probable injuries for certain mechanisms and performing a detailed physical assessment minimize risks of missed injuries.

SPECIFIC CONCEPTS
Blunt Injury

Blunt trauma is an injury with no opening in the skin or communication to the outside environment. Definitive diagnosis of blunt trauma is difficult, and the extent of injuries is less obvious than penetrating ones; however, these injuries may be more life-threatening. Depending on the tissue injured and properties associated with this tissue, certain diagnostic studies are more helpful than others. Air-filled organs, such as lungs and bowel, are subject to explosion injuries. Crush injuries to solid organs (liver and spleen) may present with minimal external signs of injury, but blunt trauma energy is transmitted in all directions, so organs or tissues burst or break if pressure is not released.

Automobiles are responsible for at least half of blunt injuries. Blunt abdominal trauma accounts for 1% of all trauma admissions, but is associated with a 20%-30% mortality rate due to chest and head injuries.

MVCs, falls, contact sports, and assaults are examples of common blunt forces. Direct impact, when a wounding agent and body surface make contact, causes the greatest injury. Injuries result from energy released upon impact with the body. Various body tissues respond differently; tissue may move and displace with impact, or rupture from the force.

Common forces in blunt trauma are acceleration/deceleration, shearing, and compression. Acceleration/deceleration injuries occur with increased velocity/speed of a moving object followed by a sudden decrease. Shearing injuries occur when two oppositely directed parallel forces are applied to tissue. Compression injuries occur with a squeezing inward pressure applied to tissues. An example of these forces is seen with blunt injury to the thoracic aorta. Rapid deceleration causes the aorta to bend and stretch. Shearing damage occurs when vessel elasticity is exceeded by stretching forces. Shearing damage causes the aorta to dissect, rupture, tear, or form an aneurysm.

Before collision, the occupant and vehicle are moving at the same speed. At the time of collision, the vehicle and the occupant decelerate to a speed of zero, but at different speeds. Deceleration forces are transferred to the body in three points of collision (Figure 22-1). The first collision occurs when the automobile strikes another object. As the vehicle stops, the unrestrained driver or occupant continues to move forward. The second collision occurs when the driver or occupant impacts the steering wheel, windshield, or other structures in the car. The body stops; however, internal organs continue to move until they impact another organ, cavity wall or structure, or they are restrained suddenly by vasculature, muscles, ligaments, or fascia—the third collision point. Different damage occurs with each collision; therefore each point must be considered separately to avoid missed injuries.

One way to estimate injuries in an MVC is to look at the vehicle. Since this is not possible in the ED, the emergency nurse should ask prehospital providers about vehicular damage. Some EMS providers take instant snapshots allowing hospital personnel to see vehicular damage first hand. The picture showing mechanisms of injury can then become a permanent part of the medical record.

Frontal impact. This type of impact occurs when the vehicle front impacts another object. The first collision results in damage to the front end. The more severe the damage, and the faster the car was traveling, the greater the probability for severely injured victims because of the high level of energy involved.

Multiple injuries are produced when an unrestrained body comes to a sudden stop. Interior structures, such as the windshield, steering wheel, dashboard, or instrument panel, injure the occupants when contact is made. Once the vehicle stops occupants in the front seat continue to move down and under, or up and over, the dashboard.

Down and under. The first path an occupant may travel after frontal impact is down and under. With this path, the occupant continues forward movement downward and into the steering column or dashboard. The knees impact the dashboard; however, most energy is absorbed by the upper legs. This mechanism causes midshaft femur fractures, patella dislocations, and posterior dislocations/fractures of acetabulum or femoral head. This classic knee-femur-hip injury is caused by transfer of energy from the knee through the femur into the hip (Figure 22-2). When one of these injuries is identified, the patient should be carefully evaluated for other injuries.

Up and over. Continued forward motion from frontal collision carries the body up and over, so the chest, abdomen, or both impact the steering wheel. Head injuries, such as contusions and scalp lacerations, skull fractures, facial fractures, cerebral hemorrhage and/or cerebral contusions can occur when the head or face impact the steering wheel or dashboard.

The brain does not stretch easily, so as one part of the brain moves in one direction, the rest follows. The skull stops suddenly after impacting the steering wheel, windshield, or another stationary object, but the brain continues to move forward and impacts the inside of the skull. This area of the brain is compressed and may sustain ecchymosis, edema, or contusion. The other side of the brain continues to move forward and may be disrupted and shear away from tissue and vascular attachments (Figure 22-3). This impact can cause two separate injuries, shear injury and compression injury, to the same organ.

When the head impacts, injury to the cervical spine can also occur. A spider web effect of the broken windshield

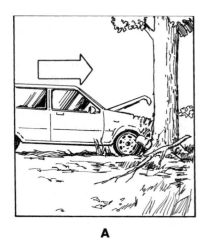
A

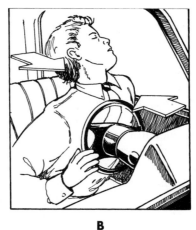
B

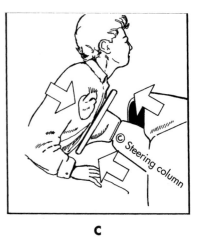
C

Figure **22-1**   The three collisions of an MVC. **A,** Auto hits tree. **B,** Body hits steering wheel, causing broken ribs. **C,** Body hits steering wheel, causing myocardial contusion.

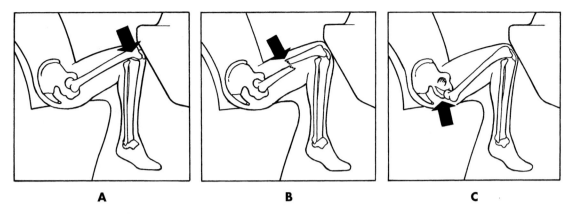

Figure **22-2** Down and under pathway. **A,** Dislocation of the knee. **B,** Fracture of the femur. **C,** Dislocation from the acetabulum.

suggests that a possibility exists for cervical spine injury. If prehospital providers report a spider web effect, care givers must maintain a high index of suspicion for occult spinal injury.

Chest injuries occur as the thorax is compressed against the steering wheel. Injuries include fractured ribs and sternum, anterior flail chest, myocardial contusion, and pulmonary contusion. The abdomen can also impact the steering wheel causing compression injuries. Ruptured hollow organs such as the stomach and bladder spill contents, whereas fractured or ruptured solid organs such as the liver and spleen are associated with significant blood loss. Organs in the abdominal cavity are attached to the abdominal wall by the mesentery, ligaments, and vasculature. As organs continue forward motion, attachments are torn or lacerated. Thoracic vertebral injuries occur as energy travels up or down the thoracic spine; however, these injuries are less common because the thoracic vertebrae are so well protected.

The steering wheel is often referred to as a modern day battering ram, the most lethal weapon in the vehicle. When steering wheel deformity is reported, the index of suspicion for neck, face, thoracic, or abdominal injuries should increase. Injuries caused by impact with the steering wheel may be readily visible, or represent only the tip of the "injury" iceberg. Lacerations of the chin and mouth; contusion and ecchymosis of the neck; traumatic tattooing of the chest and abdomen; and bruising of the chest and abdomen may be obvious or subtle. Internal occult injuries may be secondary to compression forces, shearing forces, and the displacement of kinetic energy. Figure 22-4 illustrates injuries commonly seen with steering wheel impact.

Certain organs are more susceptible to shear injuries because of ligamentous attachments (e.g., liver, spleen, bowel, kidneys, and aortic arch). Lungs, diaphragm, heart, and bladder are commonly injured by compression forces. Respiratory distress in trauma patients may be caused by injuries such as pneumothorax, flail chest, and pulmonary

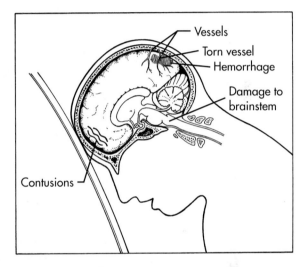

Figure **22-3** Brain injury.

contusion. A diaphragmatic hernia and ruptured diaphragm also cause respiratory distress in a trauma patient and are characterized by bowel sounds in the chest. If a trauma patient has a contused chest wall, myocardial contusion should be considered.

In frontal and lateral impacts, a mechanism sometimes called the "paper bag effect" leads to pneumothorax. The driver or occupant sees the accident about to happen, inhales deeply, and holds the breath. The glottis closes and seals the lungs. As the chest impacts, the lungs burst like paper bags (Figure 22-5).

Frontal impacts are also characterized by extremity injuries. Fractures of the lower extremities, ankles, and feet occur when the occupant extends the feet, or are secondary to vehicle intrusion into the passenger compartment. An unrestrained back-seat passenger doubles the risk for injury to front-seat occupants during frontal impact.

Rear impact. Rear-impact collision occurs when a stationary object or a slower moving object is struck from behind.

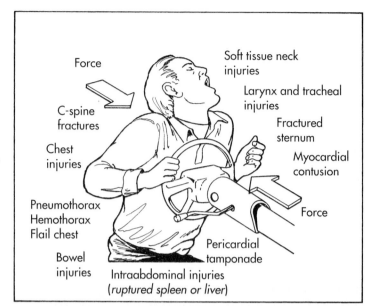

Figure **22-4** Steering wheel injuries.

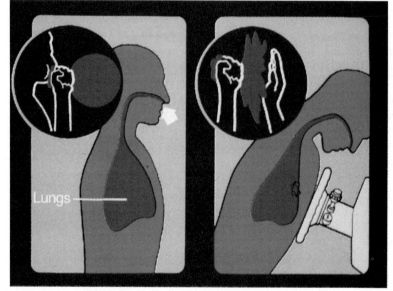

Figure **22-5** Compression of lung against closed glottis by impact on anterior or lateral chest wall produces effect like that of compressing a paper bag when opening is closed tightly by hands. Paper bag ruptures and so does lung. *(From National Association of Emergency Medical Technicians in Cooperation with the Committee on Trauma of the American College of Surgeons, Pre-Hospital Trauma Life Support, ed 3, 1994.)*

Initial impact accelerates the slower moving or stationary object and may force the vehicle into a frontal collision. When the vehicle suddenly accelerates, hyperextension of the neck may occur, especially when head rests are not properly positioned. Strained and torn neck ligaments also occur. Figure 22-6 demonstrates how these injuries occur. If the vehicle strikes another object or is slowed by the driver applying the brake, rapid forward deceleration occurs. The crash then involves two points of impact, rear and frontal, which increases the chance for occupant injuries. Injuries common to each mechanism must be assessed.

Side impact. When a vehicle is struck on either side, most injuries are dependent on vehicle deformity as the vehicle remains in place or moves away from the point of impact. If

the vehicle remains in place, energy is transferred or changed to vehicle damage rather than the energy of motion. Trauma to the occupants can be more severe because of intrusion into the interior compartment.

With side-impact or lateral collisions, occupants generally receive most injuries on the same side of their body as the vehicle impact. A second collision may occur between occupants if another passenger is in the vehicle. The head and shoulder of one occupant may impact the other occupant's head and shoulder. When a patient has an injury on the side opposite the impact, care givers should assess both occupants for associated injuries.

Figure 22-7 illustrates injuries from a side-impact collision. Flail chest, pulmonary contusion, and rib fractures are

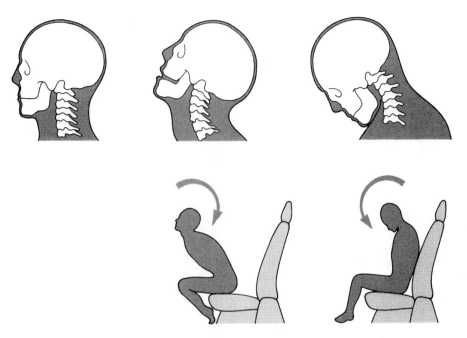

Figure **22-6** Rear-impact collision results in hyperextension of neck. *(From Neff JA, Kidd PS: Trauma nursing: the art and science, St. Louis, 1993, Mosby.)*

possible chest injuries. Numerous musculoskeletal injuries can occur. Energy from the impact can pin the occupant's arm against the car causing injury to the chest wall and clavicle, or force the femoral head through the pelvis causing a pelvic or acetabulum fracture. Strain on the lateral neck can cause spinal fractures or ligament tears. Side impacts can cause spine fractures associated with a neurologic deficit more often than rear collisions. Other injuries include a ruptured liver when impact is on the passenger side, and a ruptured spleen when impact is on the driver's side.

Rotational impact. When the corner of one vehicle strikes another stationary vehicle, a vehicle traveling in the opposite direction, or a slower vehicle a rotational impact occurs (Figure 22-8). The part that is hit on the second car stops forward motion, while the rest of the vehicle rotates around until all energy is transformed. As the car is hit the occupant's forward motion continues until it impacts with the side of the car as the vehicle begins rotating. Injuries that occur in rotational impacts are a combination of those seen in frontal and lateral impacts.

Vehicle rollover. Rollover is when a car flips, regardless of whether the motion is end-over-end, or side-over-side. In rollovers, injuries are sometimes difficult to predict. Occupants frequently have injuries in the same body areas where damage occurs to the vehicle. Just as the vehicle impacts at different angles, several times, so does the occupant's body and internal organs.

Ejection. This refers to when an occupant is thrown from the vehicle. Occupants who are ejected sustain injuries at the point of impact and when energy is transferred to the entire body. Spinal fractures occur at a higher rate in ejected per-

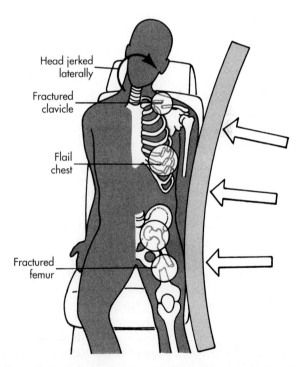

Head jerked laterally

Fractured clavicle

Flail chest

Fractured femur

Figure **22-7** Potential injury sites in lateral-impact collision. Injury is still possible in lateral crash with airbag inflation; however, injuries are usually fewer with airbag inflation than without. *(From Neff JA, Kidd PS: Trauma nursing: the art and science, St. Louis, 1993, Mosby.)*

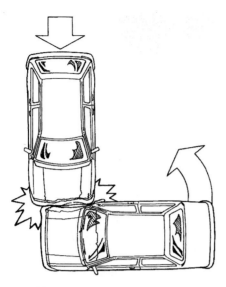

Figure **22-8** Rotational impact.

Spinal

Cervical vertebral fractures from flexion forces
Neck sprains 2° to hyperextension
Lumbar vertebral fractures 2° to flexion-distraction forces

Thoracic

Soft tissue injuries of the chest wall associated with belt placement
Sternal fractures with or without myocardial contusion
Rib fractures ≤3 if restrained; ≥4 if unrestrained
Trauma to breast in females

Abdominal

Soft tissue injuries (contusions, abrasions, ecchymosis)
"Seat belt" friction burns or abrasion where seat belt rests
Injuries to small bowel 2° to crushing and deceleration
Ruptured aorta 2° to longitudinal stretching of the vessel
Injuries to the liver, pancreas, gallbladder, and duodenum 2° to crushing forces

sons. Increased mortality is associated with ejection, and those at greatest risk are unrestrained occupants.

Restraints. Restraint systems are designed to prevent injuries and decrease the severity of injuries by allowing occupants to decelerate at the same rate as the vehicle rather than being thrown against interior structures or being ejected from the vehicle. Injuries can be reduced with the use of restraints. Occupants who are ejected have a much greater chance of dying than occupants who remain in the vehicle. Restraints also keep occupants from striking each other within the compartment; therefore, restraints worn properly reduce fatalities and the severity of injuries. The most effective restraint system is the three-point restraint, which is a shoulder harness and lap belt. Three-point restraints decrease severity of the "second" collision, reducing facial, head, abdominal injuries, and long-bone fractures.

Injuries caused by a shoulder-lap belt fastened loosely or worn above the anterior iliac crease include compression to abdominal organs such as pancreas, liver, spleen; possible rupture of the diaphragm with herniation of abdominal organs; and lumbar spine anterior compression fractures. Diaphragmatic rupture occurs from increased intraabdominal pressure from the misplaced lap belt. Lap belts worn alone allow injuries to the face, head, neck, and chest, while shoulder belts worn without a lap belt can cause neck injuries—even decapitation.

Properly used restraints transfer energy from the impact to the restraint system instead of to the occupant. Injuries received when seat belts are used properly are generally non-life-threatening, or the chance of sustaining a life-threatening injury is greatly reduced. Box 22-2 describes injuries that occur even with proper seat belt usage.

Airbags. Newer cars are now equipped with at least a driver-side airbag. Some vehicles also have passenger-side airbags. Airbags are designed to protect front seat occupants in frontal deceleration collisions. Airbags inflate from the center of the steering column and/or the dashboard at impact (Figure 22-9), cushion the head and chest, and then rapidly deflate. Injuries reported from airbag deployment include facial trauma, such as tattooing, ecchymosis, and corneal abrasions. Episodes of minor trauma from airbags are becoming more commonplace as these life-saving devices are installed in more cars. Temporary hearing loss has also been reported. Abrasions and ecchymosis from airbag deployment are seen on forearms. Infants and children placed in the front seat have been seriously injured or killed by inflating airbags. Injury may also be caused by inflation of side airbags.

Because MVCs account for over half the injuries associated with blunt trauma, preventive measures are an ongoing concern. Research has shown that the number of MVCs can be reduced by changes in highway design, enforcement of speed limits, and improvements in vehicle design. Box 22-3 shows how changes in highway design can reduce the number of MVCs that occur.

Enforcing the speed limit also reduces injuries from MVCs, since speed is a determining factor in the severity of injuries. The greater the speed/velocity, the more energy dissipated, and the more severe the injury. Injury is also affected by the size and design of vehicles. Small cars are associated with more injuries and deaths than larger cars. Making all cars larger is not the only answer, since a great number of deaths from MVCs occur in single-car crashes involving large and small vehicles. Changes in interior design can decrease injuries seen in occupants. If auto racing designs were incorporated into all privately owned vehicles, likelihood of escaping a collision without injury would increase dramatically.

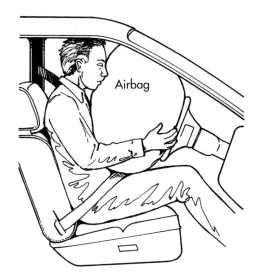

Figure **22-9**   Inflated airbag.

Pedestrians. When a pedestrian is struck by a vehicle, certain injuries can be predicted. Children and adults have different injuries because of their size differences and orientation to the vehicle.

Very small children are rarely thrown clear of the vehicle due to their low center of gravity, size, and weight. A child may be knocked down and under the vehicle then run over. Multisystem trauma should be suspected in any child hit by a car. A combination of injuries referred to as Waddell's triad often occurs when a child is struck by a car (Figure 22-10). Waddell's triad is characterized by injuries to the chest, head, and femurs. Frontal impacts usually occur because children tend to freeze and face the approaching vehicle. The femur and/or chest of the child impacts the bumper or hood depending on the child's size. The child is then thrown backwards (rarely clear) impacting the upper back or head with the ground or pavement, where contralateral skull injuries occur.

Adults struck by a vehicle sustain significant injuries to the abdomen and chest in combination with head and musculoskeletal injuries. Adults try to protect themselves by turning sideways, so impact is lateral. Upper and lower leg impact with the bumper and hood of car cause bowing of both legs, with fractures above and below the joint of impact. This may also cause ligament damage to the opposite knee from associated strain. Figure 22-11 shows points of impact when an adult is struck by a vehicle.

Another common injury in an adult pedestrian is a fractured pelvis. As the victim folds over, the upper femur and pelvis strike the front of the hood. The top of the hood is then struck by the abdomen and chest. The victim then travels off the hood and onto the pavement or into the windshield. The victim may be able to protect the face and head with the arms during this forward motion. If the victim is thrown any distance, he or she can be run over by a second

Separate opposing streams of traffic.
Eliminate intersections, overpasses, and underpasses.
Create wider shoulders and remove obstacles from roadside.
Install breakaway barriers.
Use road surface materials that decrease skidding.

vehicle. Tire mark impressions may be found on the clothing or skin of victims who are run over.

Motorcycle crashes. Injuries occurring from motorcycle crashes depend on the amount and type of kinetic energy and the part of the body impacted. Head, neck, and extremity injuries occur more frequently with motorcycle crashes due to lack of a protective encasement. Clues to the amount of force sustained during a collision include length of skid marks, deformity of the motorcycle, and stationary objects impacted. The condition of a driver of a motorcycle is often similar to an occupant ejected from a vehicle. Three types of motorcycle impacts with predictable injuries are head-on impact, angular impact, and ejection.

Head-on impact. During a head-on impact, the motorcycle impacts an object that stops the bike's forward motion. The bike flips forward so the rider impacts or travels over the handlebars. As the rider impacts the handlebars, abdominal and chest injuries and shearing fractures of the tibia can occur. Bilateral femur fractures occur if the rider's feet remain on foot pegs at the time of impact. A helmet may protect the rider's head, but does not protect the neck. If the rider impacts the head and neck, injuries may still occur. The chance of a head injury increases 300% when a helmet is not used.

Angular impact. When a cycle is hit at an angle and collapses on the rider, the angular impact injures the side that is crushed between the rider and ground or the object impacted. Injuries tend to occur in lower extremities such as open fractures of the tibia/fibula, crushed legs, ankle dislocation, and soft tissue injuries.

Ejection. When a rider is thrown off the motorcycle, injuries occur to whatever body part is hit. Energy from the impact is absorbed by the rest of the body. Ejection from a motorcycle has a high potential for severe injuries.

Laying the bike down. Laying the bike down is a maneuver used by professional riders to separate themselves from the bike when they see an impending collision. This maneuver slows the rider as the bike is turned sideways, and the rider drags the inner leg. The most common injuries seen with laying the bike down are minor fractures, abrasions, and crush injuries to lower legs.

Bicycle crashes. Several mechanisms for bicycle collisions exist; the most common are collisions with a motor vehicle or pedestrian, and falling off the cycle. Approximately 90%

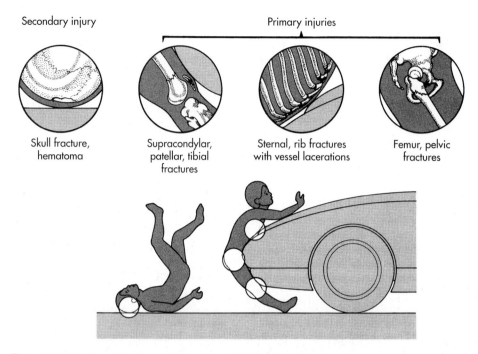

Secondary injury | Primary injuries

Skull fracture, hematoma

Supracondylar, patellar, tibial fractures

Sternal, rib fractures with vessel lacerations

Femur, pelvic fractures

Figure **22-10**   Potential primary injury sites of child pedestrian. *(Modified from Neff JA, Kidd PS:* Trauma nursing: the art and science, *St. Louis, 1993, Mosby.)*

of all deaths related to bicycles are the result of a collision with a motor vehicle. A rider usually loses control and falls off due to hazardous ground surfaces, performing stunts, speeding, or generalized lack of skill.

Bicycle crashes have certain common patterns of injuries. The spokes of a bicycle wheel can fracture the feet if feet are caught in the wheel. These injuries are generally seen in second riders and may cause the person to be thrown and sustain other injuries. Properly installed wheel guards decrease spoke-related injuries.

When a rider is thrown over the handlebars, as a bike impacts an object and tips forward, the rider without a helmet may suffer injuries similar to someone ejected from a car (i.e., head, neck, and chest injuries). If the rider impacts the middle bar or seat, straddle injuries such as vaginal tears, scrotal injuries, and perineal contusions occur.

Bicycle-mounted child seats are another cause of injuries with bicycle use. The child may fall from the seat, the seat can detach from the bicycle, the bike can tip over, or the child's extremity may be caught in wheel spokes. Head and facial injuries are common and often severe. Child seats mounted on bicycles do not provide protection to the child's head and face, and the child is not developmentally ready for self-protection; therefore, helmets should be worn by all children in bicycle-mounted seats.

Injuries can occur to bicycle riders from rearview mirrors that extend from trucks or vans. Significant head, neck, and facial injuries as well as severe deep lacerations to the head and neck can occur and are often fatal.

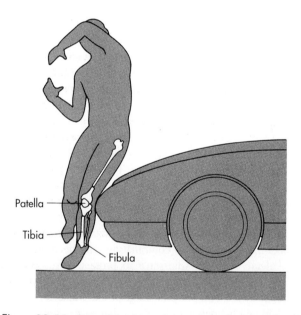

Patella

Tibia

Fibula

Figure **22-11**   Potential primary injury sites of adult pedestrian. *(From Neff JA, Kidd PS:* Trauma nursing: the art and science, *St. Louis, 1993, Mosby.)*

All-terrain vehicles. All-terrain vehicles have two basic designs: three-wheeled or four-wheeled vehicles. Four-wheeled vehicles offer easier handling and more stability than three-wheeled vehicles, which are prone to rollover when turned sharply due to a higher center of gravity. Some states have enacted laws defining the minimum operator age and requiring helmets for all riders.

The three most common mechanisms of injury associated with all-terrain vehicles are rollover, a rider falling off, and the vehicle impacting a stationary object causing forward deceleration of the rider. Injuries depend on which part of the rider's anatomy impacts and the mechanism involved. Head, spine, and chest injuries involving the ribs, sternum, and clavicles have been reported.

Falls. Vertical deceleration is the mechanism associated with falls. Severity of injuries with persons who fall or jump depends on the height of the fall. Falls are severe when the distance is three times greater than victim height. Different patterns of injuries are seen with different types of falls. Small children tend to land on the head since it is the biggest part of their body. Certain injuries occur when a person lands feet first (i.e., bilateral calcaneus fractures, compression fractures of the vertebrae [usually thoracolumbar], and bilateral Colles fractures). This trio of injuries is called the "Don Juan Syndrome." Energy initially causes bilateral calcaneus fractures, then displaces upward, and causes other injuries including femur fractures, hip dislocations/fractures, vertebral compression fractures, and basilar skull fractures. Wrist fractures occur from acute flexion as the person falls forward onto the outstretched arms. Deceleration forces of this nature can also cause secondary renal injuries.

If a person lands on other areas of the body, injuries occur at those impact points and as energy is distributed to the rest of the body. If the impact is on the wrist, energy is transferred upward through the elbow and shoulder, whereas impact on the knee transfers energy upward to the hip. Another point of impact may be the head, as seen in diving injuries. With this impact, injuries occur because weight and force of the torso, pelvis, and legs bear down on the head and cervical spine. This type of injury is known as a compression injury or an axial loading injury. Vertebral bodies are compressed and wedged producing vertebral fragments that can pierce the cord.

Sports-related injuries. Injuries associated with sports are generally caused by compressive forces or sudden deceleration. Other injuries can be caused by twisting, hyperflexion, or hyperextension. Factors that affect injury include lack of protective equipment, lack of conditioning, and inadequate training of the participant. Mechanisms associated with recreational sports and sportslike activities are similar to those involved in MVCs, motorcycle collisions, and bicycle crashes. Potential mechanisms associated with individual sports are numerous; however, general principles are the same as with falls and MVCs.

- What energy/forces impact the victim?
- What parts of the body are affected by the energy/force?
- What are the obvious injuries?
- What injuries are associated with the involved energy/force?

Table **22-1**	**Sports-Related Injuries**
Sport	Potential injuries
Boxing	Cumulative brain damage, ocular injuries, lacerations, nasal fractures
Gymnastics	Spinal cord injuries, extremity fractures, sprains, strains
Football	Spinal cord injuries, head injuries, knee strains, fractures, lacerations
Skiing	Head injuries, lower extremity fractures, exposure to elements
Ice hockey	Facial fractures, soft tissue injuries, lacerations
Running	Lower extremity injuries, strains, sprains
Baseball	Head injuries, ocular injuries, fractures, lacerations, sprains, strains
Basketball	Lower extremity sprains, strains, fractures, lacerations, contusions
Horseback riding	Head injuries, bite wounds, crush wounds

Damaged equipment, such as broken snow skis or helmets, can help establish impact. Table 22-1 describes injuries associated with various sports.

Penetrating Trauma

Injuries caused by foreign objects set in motion that penetrate the body are called penetrating trauma. Energy created by the foreign object is dissipated into the surrounding tissues or areas. Evaluation and assessment of penetrating trauma depend on the wounding agent, how energy is dissipated, distance from victim to weapon, and characteristics of the tissues struck. Examples of penetrating trauma include gunshot wounds, stab wounds, and impalements. The tissue penetrated and underlying structures damaged determine the severity of the injury. Victims of penetrating trauma may also suffer blunt injuries, for instance, secondary to falling down a flight of stairs after being shot.

A variety of objects can produce penetrating injuries, including those thrown from a lawn mower or industrial machinery. However, in today's society the majority of penetrating injuries are caused by knives and guns.

Stab wounds. These wounds are considered low-velocity injuries, and therefore low energy. Minimal secondary trauma occurs. Damage is the result of the sharp cutting edge of the wounding agent. For patients with penetrating trauma, the projected path of the weapon can be identified by knowing the position of the attacker and the victim, weapon used, and gender of the attacker. Women tend to stab downward whereas men tend to stab upward. Determination of gender is not considered absolute, because intentional injuries do not always fit a specific pattern.

Damage from a stab wound depends on the location of the penetrating object. Tissue damage is generally isolated to the area of penetration; however penetrating injuries with a single wound can penetrate several body cavities causing lethal injuries. For example, the weapon can enter the tho-

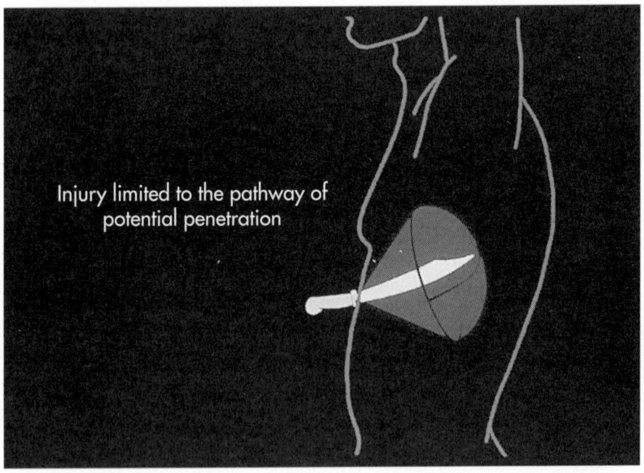

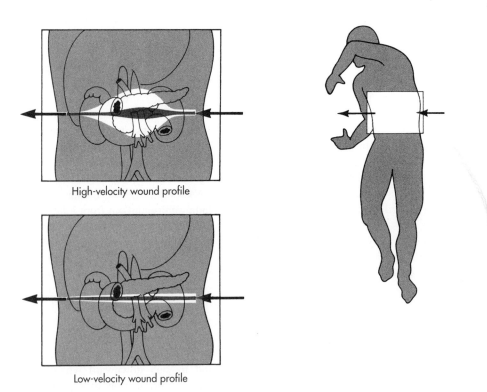

Figure 22-12 Movement of knife blade inside victim produces damage, limited to path of penetration. *(Modified from National Association of Emergency Medical Technicians in cooperation with the Committee on Trauma of the American College of Surgeons, Pre-Hospital Trauma Life Support, ed 3, 1994.)*

racic and abdominal cavity with just one penetration. Chest wounds at the level of the nipple or below can also involve the abdominal cavity and underlying organs.

More than one wound may exist, and small entrance wounds can hide extensive internal damage caused by weapon movement. Internal damage is directly proportional to length of the wounding object (Figure 22-12) and to the density of tissue affected.

Impalements. These are low-velocity injuries that occur as a result of falls or MVCs, or secondary to a flying or falling object. Impaled objects should be stabilized and removed only when the patient is in a controlled environment where surgical support is available.

Gunshot wounds. Most penetration wounds by firearms are from handguns, shotguns, and rifles. Missile velocity determines tissue deformation and extent of cavitation. Velocity is generally described as low velocity or high velocity. Low-velocity missiles travel at 1000 to 3000 ft/sec and have little disruptive effect on tissues. Injuries are localized at the center of the tract with a small radius of distribution. The temporary cavity is 2 to 3 times the diameter of the missile. Low-velocity missiles push tissues aside along the path.

High-velocity missiles travel over 3000 ft/sec and cause more serious injuries due to high cavitation and energy transfer. High-velocity missiles create a cavity around the bullet and the bullet tract by compressing and displacing tissue. As kinetic energy is transferred from the bullet to the

High-velocity wound profile

Low-velocity wound profile

Figure 22-13 Potential injury path of high- and low-velocity bullets. *(From Neff JA, Kidd PS: Trauma nursing: the art and science, St. Louis, 1993, Mosby.)*

tissue, the cavity enlarges. A tract temporarily displaces tissue laterally and forward as the missile moves forward. Behind or following the missile, negative pressure contaminates the wound by pulling in foreign material. These cavities can be 30 to 40 times the diameter of the bullet. Wounds often require debridement because of extensive tissue disruption. Figure 22-13 shows the cavitational differences with low-velocity and high-velocity bullets.

Entrance and exit wounds with high-velocity missiles differ with types of tissues and body areas hit. Exit wounds may be larger when the missile travels through smaller structures such as an extremity because all energy has not dissipated by the time the bullet exits; cavitation and missile movement is still occurring. Exit wounds tend to be small in dense tissue because cavitation is complete and most energy is dissipated. If the bullet fragments while traveling through the tissues no exit wound is found. Figure 22-14 compares entrance and exit wounds.

Bullet yaw and tumbling are the most important factors in tissue destruction, next to velocity. Bullets become unstable in flight as velocity increases. Yawing refers to deflection or deviation of the nose of the bullet from a straight path. Tumbling refers to the continuous forward rotation around the center of the bullet causing the bullet to somersault, creating massive tissue destruction. Figure 22-15 demonstrates these movements. Yawing and tumbling increase with impact producing more damage as temporary and permanent cavity size increases.

Deformation of the bullet is another important factor when assessing gunshot wounds. Energy production increases when missiles change shape on impact. Types of bullets that produce greater kinetic energy include soft-nosed, flat-nosed, and hollow point bullets that mushroom on impact.

Another feature of gunshot wounds is the muzzle blast seen with close-range wounds or when the gun is pressed against the skin. Immediately on firing, a cloud of burning powder and hot gas is released from the muzzle. If a muzzle blast is evident, tattooing from burning particles, abrasions, and burn marks at the entrance wound is seen (Figure 22-14).

Blast Injuries

Blasts are not as common in the United States as in other countries. However, the potential for hazardous explosions at chemical plants, oil refineries, shipyards, and other industrial settings does exist. Explosions can occur anywhere because of the large amount of volatile materials carried by rail or truck. Blasts occur when explosives are detonated and changed to gases. As the gas expands, an equal volume of air is displaced and travels after the blast wave. Disruption of tissue, evisceration, and traumatic amputation can occur from this mass movement of air. When the explosive casing ruptures, the casing fragments become high-velocity projectiles.

Due to the greater density of water, the blast wave travels more rapidly and farther in water than air. Consequently injuries associated with underwater blasts are usually more severe. Closed-area explosions cause more damage than open-area ones due to potential inhalation of smoke and toxic gases.

Blast injuries can occur in three phases or impact points. Figure 22-16 diagrams how the injuries occur from an explosive blast. As explosives change to an expanding mass of heated gas, primary injuries occur due to concussive effects of the pressure wave. Concussion injuries are frequently overlooked because they are not obvious and may occur without external signs of trauma. However, these injuries are usually the most severe. Injuries associated with this mechanism include CNS injuries, rupture of gas-containing organs, and tearing of membranes and small vessels. The as-

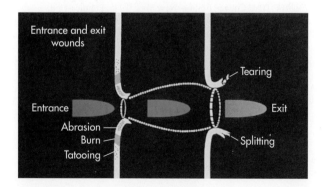

Figure **22-14** A spinning missile produces a 1-2 mm abraded edge along wound if it enters straight. If it enters at angle, abraded side is on bottom of missile, with more skin contact, and covers a much wider area. Difference in entrance and exit wounds is also depicted. Exit wounds are generally longer and more explosive. *(Modified from McSwain N et al.: The basic EMT: comprehensive prehospital patient care, St. Louis, 1996, Mosby.)*

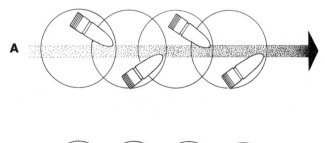
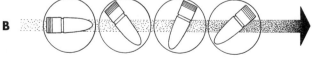

Figure **22-15** Effect of bullet movement on wounding potential. **A,** Yawing. **B,** Tumbling.

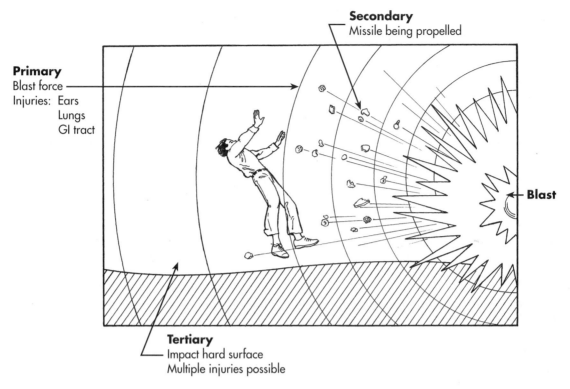

Figure **22-16**   Effects of an explosive blast.

sociated heat wave can also cause burns on areas of the body facing the explosion.

Fragments such as glass, rocks, or metal debris become high-velocity projectiles causing secondary injuries. Examples of injuries include impalements, fractures, traumatic amputations, burns, and soft tissue injuries such as contusions, abrasions, and lacerations.

The third point of impact occurs when the victim is thrown through the air and becomes a missile. Tertiary injuries associated with this mechanism are similar to those seen when persons are ejected from vehicles or fall from heights, and generally occur at the point of impact.

CONCLUSION

Treatment of trauma patients depends on locating all injuries and rapidly intervening to correct those that are life-threatening. Consideration of mechanisms of injury is essential to identify patients with possible underlying injuries that require further evaluation and treatment.

SUGGESTED READING

Halpern J: Mechanisms and patterns of trauma, *J Emerg Nurs,* 15(5):380-388, 1989.

Kidd P: Assessment of the trauma patient. In Neff J, Kidd P, editors: *Trauma nursing: the art and science,* St. Louis, 1993, Mosby.

McSwain N et al., editors: *Prehospital trauma life support,* Akron, 1990, Emergency Training.

McSwain N, Paturas J, Wertz E, editors: *Pre-hospital trauma life support,* St. Louis, 1994, Mosby.

Neufeldt V, Editor in Chief: *Webster's new world dictionary of American English.* Third College Edition, New York, 1986, Prentice-Hall.

Rea R, editor: *Trauma nursing core course,* Chicago, 1986, Award Printing.

Sheehy S, Marven J, Jimmerson C: *Manual of clinical trauma care: the first hour,* St. Louis, 1989, Mosby.

Vansie M: Mechanisms of injury. In Bayley E, Turke S, editors: *A comprehensive curriculum for trauma nursing,* Boston, 1992, Jones & Bartlett.

Weigelt JA, Klein JD: Mechanism of injury. In Cardona V, et al., editors: *Trauma nursing: from resuscitation through rehabilitation,* ed 2, Philadelphia, 1988, WB Saunders.

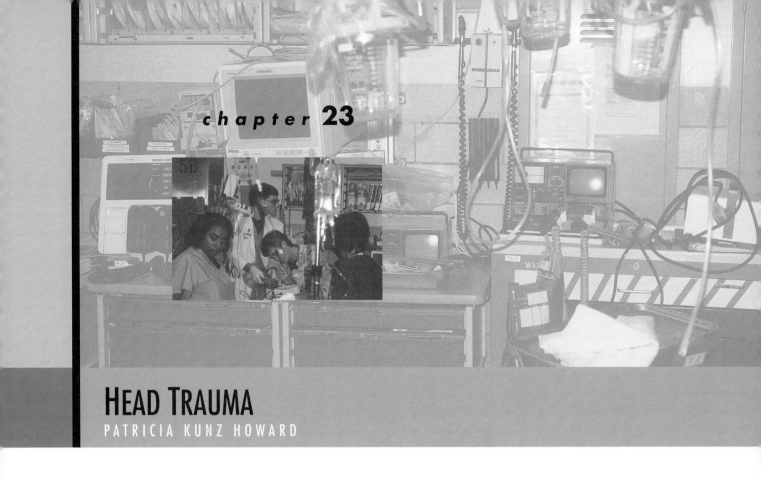

chapter **23**

HEAD TRAUMA

PATRICIA KUNZ HOWARD

Half of all annual trauma deaths in the United States can be attributed to head injuries. More than 100,000 people sustain head injuries that cause permanent disabilities.[10] The cost of traumatic brain injuries to our society is devastating from a financial and psychosocial impact. Annual expenditures for care of victims with traumatic brain injury exceed $5 billion. Injuries permanently change the lives of the victim and the family.

Traumatic brain injuries (TBI) occur most frequently as a result of motor vehicle crashes. Changes in momentum cause stress and deformation of brain tissues including neuronal, axonal, and vascular structures.[2] A small percentage of patients with severe TBI have concomitant fracture of the cervical spine. Alcohol is a recognized contributing factor in the incidence of TBI. Alcohol places the victim at greater risk for injury and makes assessment of the head-injured victim more complex. Other causes of TBI include falls, recreational injuries, and penetrating trauma (i.e., gunshot and stab wounds). This chapter discusses assessment and patient management of various head injuries. A brief review of anatomy and physiology is included.

ANATOMY AND PHYSIOLOGY

The hair, scalp, skull, meninges, and cerebrospinal fluid (CSF) protect the brain from injury (Figure 23-1). The scalp consists of five layers of tissue: skin, subcutaneous tissue, galea aponeurotic, ligaments, and periosteum. The skull is composed of the frontal, parietal, temporal and occipital bones. Figure 23-2 illustrates the relationship between components of the nervous system. Cranial bones join with the facial bones to form the cranial vault, a rigid cavity that can hold 1400 to 1500 ml. Other bony structures of import are depressions at the base of the skull called the anterior, middle, and posterior fossae. The frontal lobe is located in the anterior fossae; parietal, temporal, and occipital lobes in the middle fossae; and brain stem and cerebellum in the posterior fossae.

Three layers of meninges surround the brain and provide additional protection. The outermost meninge is the dura mater (meaning tough mother), which consists of two layers of tough fibrous tissue. The inner layer of the dura mater forms the falx cerebri and tentorium cerebelli. Potential spaces located above (epidural) the dura mater and below (subdural) the dura mater are at risk for hematoma formation because the middle meningeal artery lies in the epidural space, and veins are located within the subdural space. The middle meningeal layer is the arachnoid mater (spiderlike), a fine, elastic layer. Below the arachnoid mater, the subarachnoid space contains arachnoid villi, fingerlike projections that form channels for CSF absorption. Adhering to the surface of the brain is the pia mater (meaning tender mother).

The cerebrum consists of two hemispheres separated by a longitudinal fissure. Each lobe of the cerebrum is responsible for specific functions. The frontal lobe coordinates voluntary motor movements and controls judgment, affect, and

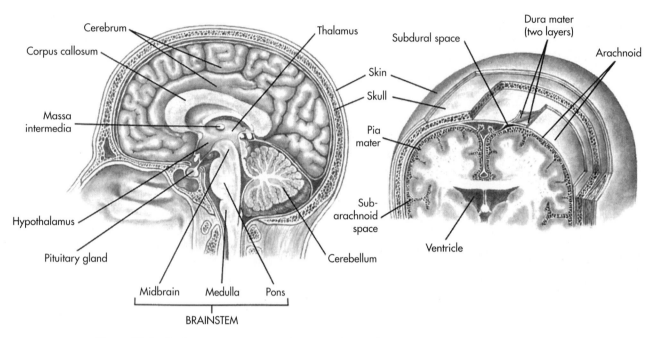

Figure **23-1**   Brain structures. *(From Thompson JM, et al.: Mosby's clinical nursing, ed 4, St. Louis, 1997, Mosby.)*

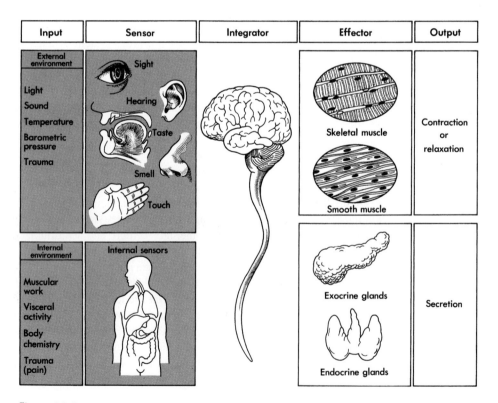

Figure **23-2**   Components of the nervous system. *(From Mosby's medical, nursing, and allied health dictionary, ed 4, St. Louis, 1994, Mosby.)*

personality. Hearing, behavior, emotions, and dominant-hemisphere speech are controlled by the temporal lobe. Sensory interpretation occurs in the parietal lobe, whereas the occipital lobe is responsible for vision.

The cerebellum is located in the posterior fossae adjacent to the brain stem and is separated from the cerebrum by the tentorium cerebelli. Primary functions of the cerebellum are integration of motor function, maintenance of equilibrium, and maintenance of muscle tone.

The brain stem consists of the midbrain, pons, and medulla. While each structure has important pathway functions, the medulla contains the cardiac, respiratory, and vasomotor centers. The reticular activating system (RAS), also located in the brain stem, is responsible for arousal, the lowest level of consciousness, which is interpreted as awakeness. Cranial nerves originate in the brain stem. Table 23-1 describes the function of each cranial nerve.

PATIENT ASSESSMENT

After ensuring adequate control of airway, breathing, and circulation, the nurse should perform a complete, concise neurologic assessment. A subtle change in level of consciousness is the earliest indication of deterioration in the head-injured patient. Assessment of the level of consciousness should be directed toward acquiring the highest level response with the least stimulus. The Glasgow Coma Scale (GCS) (see Box 23-1) is measured as a component of neurologic assessment.[13] Completing the GCS allows assignment of numerical values to clinical findings and assists in recognition of trends in neurologic changes. Interpretation of the GCS must be correlated with other clinical assessment findings. Presence of other physiologic conditions such as hypotension, hypothermia, alcohol, or substance abuse may artificially lower the total GCS score. Patients with a total GCS ≤ 8 have sustained a severe head injury in the absence of associated physiologic parameters previously identified.

Normal pupillary response to direct light examination is constriction. A consensual reaction (constriction of the opposite pupil) should occur with direct light examination. Unilateral pupil dilatation may indicate early compression of the third cranial nerve. Anisocoria or unequal pupils are a normal finding in 20%-25% of the population, so assessment of reactivity in the dilated pupil is critical. Bilateral fixed and dilated pupils are indicative of impending transtentorial herniation. Figure 23-3 illustrates pupil reactions at different levels of consciousness.

Abnormal motor responses include inequality in movement from side to side and posturing. Decorticate posturing

---

Box **23-1**	**Glasgow Coma Scale**

Eye opening

Spontaneously 4
To verbal command 3
To pain 2
No response 1

Best motor response

Obeys commands 6
Localizes pain 5
Withdraws from pain 4
Abnormal flexion 3
Abnormal extension 2
No response 1

Best verbal response

Oriented 5
Confused 4
Inappropriate words 3
Incomprehensible sounds 2
No response 1

Total 3-15

Table **23-1**	**Cranial Nerves and Their Functions**	
Cranial nerves	**Function**	**Physiologic effects**
I. Olfactory	Sensory	Smell
II. Optic	Sensory	Vision
III. Oculomotor	Motor	Extraocular movement of eyes; raises eyelid; constricts pupils
IV. Trochlear	Motor	Allows eye to move down and inward
V. Trigeminal	Motor and sensory	Facial sensation, mastication and corneal reflex
VI. Abducens	Motor	Allows eye to move outward
VII. Facial	Motor and sensory	Movement of facial muscles; closes eyes, secretes saliva and tears
VIII. Acoustic	Sensory	Hearing and equilibrium
IX. Glossopharyngeal	Motor and sensory	Gag reflex, swallowing and phonation
X. Vagus	Motor and sensory	Voluntary muscles for swallowing, involuntary to visceral muscles (heart, lungs)
XI. Spinal Accessory	Motor	Turn head, shrug shoulders
XII. Hypoglossal	Motor	Tongue movement for swallowing

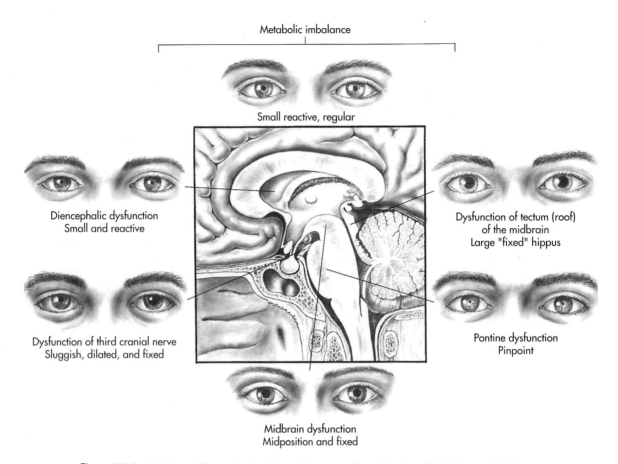

Metabolic imbalance

Small reactive, regular

Diencephalic dysfunction
Small and reactive

Dysfunction of tectum (roof)
of the midbrain
Large "fixed" hippus

Dysfunction of third cranial nerve
Sluggish, dilated, and fixed

Pontine dysfunction
Pinpoint

Midbrain dysfunction
Midposition and fixed

Figure **23-3**   Pupils at different levels of consciousness. *(From Huether SE, McCance KL:* Understanding pathophysiology, *St. Louis, 1996, Mosby.)*

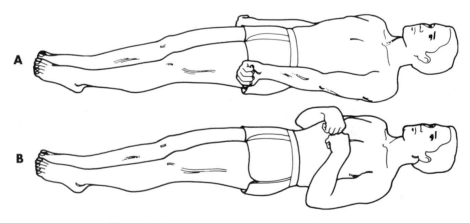

Figure **23-4**   **A,** Decerebrate posturing and **B,** decorticate.

is rigid flexion with arms flexed toward the core and lower extremities extended. This type of posturing is associated with lesions above the midbrain. Rigid extension of the arms with wrist flexion and rigid extension of lower extremities is decerebrate posturing. This type of posturing is associated with an insult to the brain stem. Figure 23-4 illustrates decerebrate and decorticate posturing. Lateralization occurs when patients with TBI present with unilateral decorticate

and decerebrate posturing. Posturing may be spontaneous or elicited by verbal or painful stimuli.

Additional Assessment Parameters

Integrity of the brain stem is evaluated by the oculocephalic (Doll's eye) reflex and the oculovestibular reflex with the ice water caloric test. A Doll's eye examination is performed to evaluate brain stem integrity only after the cer-

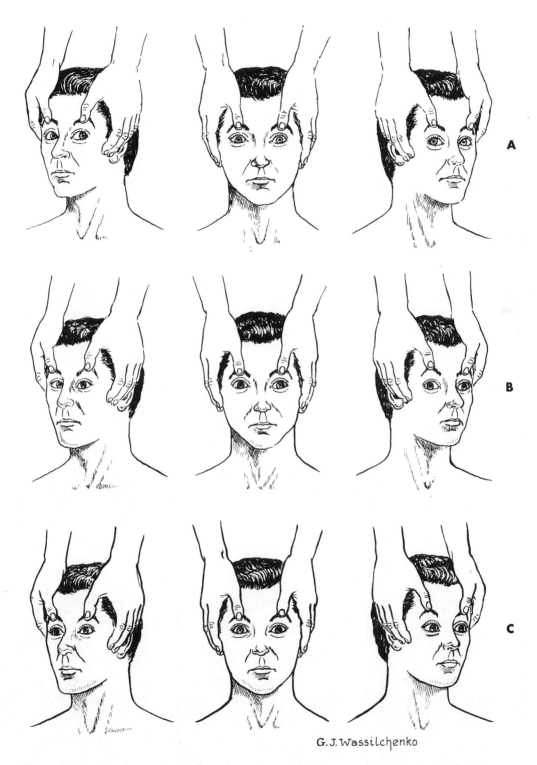

Figure **23-5** Test for oculocephalic reflex response (doll's eyes phenomenon). **A,** Normal response—eyes turn together to side opposite from turn of head. **B,** Abnormal response—eyes do not turn in conjugate manner. **C,** Absent response—eyes do not turn as head position changes. *(From Rudy EB:* Advanced neurological and neurosurgical nursing, *St. Louis, 1984, Mosby.)*

vical spine has been cleared. To perform the Doll's eye examination, briskly rotate the head to the right or left. If the brain stem is intact, eyes deviate away from the direction the head is rotated (normal exam). Loss of brain stem integrity is presumed when eyes remain midline with rotation of the head or do not move with rotation. Figure 23-5 illustrates these three responses.

Oculovestibular response is evaluated by injection of ice water in the ear of an unresponsive patient. Normal response is conjugate deviation of eyes. No movement, dysconjugate movement, or asymmetrical movement indicates interruption in the functional connection between the medulla and midbrain. Figure 23-6 illustrates evaluation of this reflex. Severe dizziness and vomiting occur with this test in a conscious patient, so the ice water test is contraindicated in semiconscious or conscious patients. Another contraindication is tympanic membrane rupture.

PATIENT MANAGEMENT

Initial stabilization of the head-injured patient is directed toward restoration of circulating volume, maintenance of blood pressure, oxygenation, and ventilation. The first priority of care for the head-injured patient is rapid resuscitation. Current recommendations for treatment of severe head injury specify that treatment for increased intracranial pressure should be initiated only in presence of signs of transtentorial herniation (i.e., unilateral or bilateral pupillary dilation, asymmetric pupillary reactivity, motor posturing, or continued neurologic deterioration after physiologic stability has been restored).[3] Figure 23-7 illustrates the mechanism that causes herniation. Due to the frequency of concomitant cervical spine trauma, cervical spine immobilization should be maintained until adequate radiographic exams have ruled out cervical spine trauma. Prevention of

secondary injuries begins with recognition of factors that correlate with further brain injury, such as hypoxia, hypercapnia, hypotension, and cerebral ischemia secondary to increased intracranial pressure. Hypoxia during the immediate postinjury period, reported in more than one third of all head-injured patients, substantially increases morbidity and mortality associated with head injury.[1] The presence of a secure airway, adequate ventilatory rate, and volume resuscitation decrease the incidence of hypoxia, hypercapnia, and hypotension. Diagnostic evaluation for head injury is initiated after stabilization of the ABCs. Tests performed are often determined by available resources; however, most EDs have access to radiographs and CT scan. Table 23-2 discusses the diagnostic tests with regard to purpose and advantages.

After initial stabilization, the emergency nurse should consider other interventions that promote return of optimal neurologic function. General guidelines for the care of the head-injured patient include ensuring a patent airway, ventilatory support as indicated, hemodynamic stability (SBP > 90 mm Hg), ongoing neurologic assessment, administration of pharmacologic agents as needed (i.e., neuromuscular blocking agents, anticonvulsants), and other interventions based on patient condition. An integral component of caring for head-injured patients is inclusion of the family or significant other in the plan of care. Head injuries can be overwhelming for the family; psychosocial support and education regarding the injury cannot be overemphasized.

Intracranial Pressure (ICP)

In the adult patient, the skull is a closed box containing the brain, CSF, and blood. For intracranial pressure (ICP) to remain within normal limits (0 to 15 mm Hg) an increase in blood, CSF, or brain mass must be accompanied by a recip-

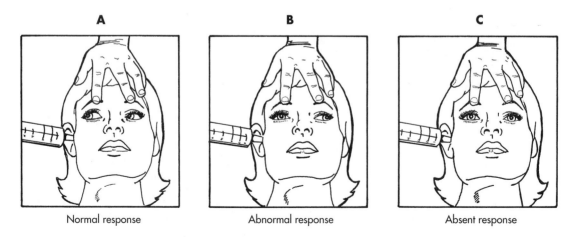

| Normal response | Abnormal response | Absent response |

Figure **23-6** Test for oculovestibular reflex (ice water caloric test). **A,** Normal response—conjugate eye movements. **B,** Abnormal response—dysconjugate or asymmetric eye movements. **C,** Absent response—no eye movements. *(From Huether SE, McCance KL:* Understanding pathophysiology, *St. Louis, 1996, Mosby.)*

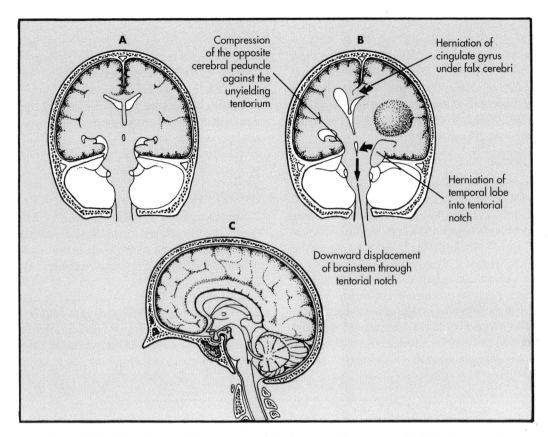

Figure **23-7**   Herniation. **A,** Normal relationship of intracranial structures. **B,** Shift of intracranial structures. **C,** Downward herniation of the cerebellar tonsils into the foramen magnum. *(From Huether SE, McCance KL:* Understanding pathophysiology, *St. Louis, 1996, Mosby.)*

Table **23-2**	**Diagnostic Evaluation for Head Injury**	
Diagnostic exam	Purpose	Comments
Cervical spine radiographs	Visualization of all 7 cervical vertebrae to rule out injury	Tomograms or CT scan of the cervical spine may be necessary to completely rule out injury
Skull radiographs	Evaluate for skull fractures	Bone windows from CT scan may give more definitive evidence of basilar skull fractures
CT scan	Detect intracranial injuries—bleeds, hematomas, cerebral edema	Patients may require sedation to obtain adequate CT

rocal decrease of the other components. An ICP greater than 20 mm Hg represents intracranial hypertension. Failure to reduce ICP may cause ischemia and necrosis of brain tissue. Cerebral blood flow is maintained through autoregulation as cerebral blood vessels dilate and constrict to preserve adequate blood flow to the brain. Cerebral perfusion pressure (CPP) is calculated by subtracting ICP from mean arterial pressure (MAP). To ensure adequate cerebral blood flow, CPP must be greater than 60 mm Hg. Recent recommendations for care of severe head injuries advocate maintaining a CPP greater than 70 mm Hg to prevent primary

cerebral ischemia and the resultant secondary injury that may occur.[1]

Recommended indications for management of intracranial hypertension include an abnormal admission CT scan with a GCS of 3 to 8; and a normal CT scan with two of the following: age greater than 40 years, abnormal posturing, or systolic blood pressure less than 90 mm Hg. Intracranial pressure monitoring aids in detection of intracranial mass lesions, limits unnecessary use of adjunctive therapies to control ICP, maintains normal ICP by draining CSF, helps determine prognosis, and may improve outcome.[1] The ultimate goal of

ICP monitoring is to optimize cerebral perfusion while preventing secondary brain injury. Studies have shown that ventricular catheters with an external strain gauge are the most accurate means of monitoring intracranial pressure. Intraparenchymal catheters with a fiber optic tip may drift and are not as accurate. Many facilities use a fiber optic monitor and an external strain gauge device simultaneously to ensure accurate ICP monitoring (Figure 23-8).

Hyperventilation

Recent studies have shown that chronic prophylactic hyperventilation should be avoided during the first 5 days following severe TBI. Cerebral blood flow studies illustrate substantial reduction in cerebral blood flow within the first few hours of injury where absolute blood flow values are consistent with ischemia.[1,3] Hyperventilation reduces cerebral blood flow without consistently decreasing ICP. In addition, autoregulation may be interrupted and further compromise blood flow to the injured area. Hyperventilation should be instituted when other means do not control ICP and should be employed to minimize adverse effects. When hyperventilation is used, maintain $pCO_2 \geq 25$ mmHg.

Mannitol

Mannitol is an osmotic diuretic that reduces ICP by changing the osmotic gradient, which causes fluid to leave cerebral extracellular tissues and move to intravascular beds. Movement of fluid reduces total brain mass, therefore decreasing intracranial pressure. Mannitol should be administered at doses of 0.25 to 1 gm/Kg when signs of transtentorial herniation are present or progressive neurologic deterioration is evident. The patient's overall volume status should be assessed before administration of mannitol.

Neuroprotective Agents

Neuroprotective agents to protect the brain from secondary injury are being used investigationally across the United States. Pharmacologic adjuncts are believed to affect three key mediators of reperfusion injury: oxygen-free radicals, lipid peroxidation, and excitatory amino acids. For each of these mediators, neuroprotective agents are being utilized to counteract secondary injury effects. (See Chapter 37 for additional discussion of neuroprotective agents.)

Oxygen radical scavengers synthesize with oxygen radicals to produce a less harmful substance. Reduction in circu-

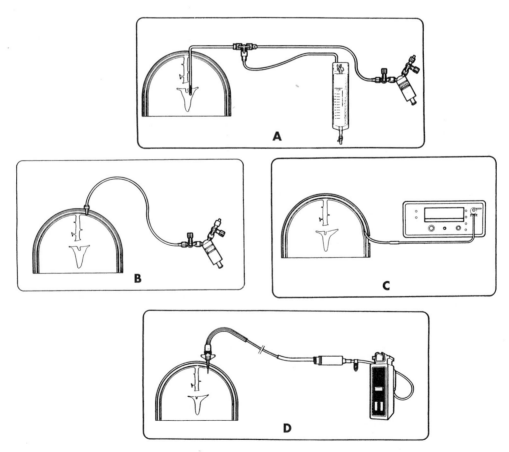

Figure **23-8** **A,** Ventricular pressure monitoring system. **B,** Subarachnoid pressure monitoring system. **C,** Epidural pressure monitoring system. **D,** Intraparenchymal pressure monitoring system. *(From Thelan LA et al: Critical care nursing: diagnosis and management, ed 2, St. Louis, 1994, Mosby. Courtesy Camino Laboratories, San Diego, Calif.)*

lating oxygen radicals gives better control of ICP, subsequently lessening cerebral ischemia.

Lipid peroxidation is inhibited by lazaroids, synthetic nonglucocorticoid steroids that suppress cellular membrane breakdown. Lazaroids assist in stabilization of cell membranes, impede neuronal deterioration, and deter secondary brain injury.

Excitatory amino acids (EAAs) are liberated during an ischemic event. Presence of EAAs produces a hypermetabolic state that extends the injury by overwhelming neurons. N-methyl-D-aspartate (NMDA) antagonists restrict the effects of EAAs at an injury site. This action reduces metabolic activity and protects tissues from ischemia.

Additional Treatment Modalities

The fluid of choice for TBI patients is 0.9% NaCl or Ringer's lactate solution. Dextrose solutions should be avoided due to increased cerebral edema. Barbiturate therapy may be considered for patients with refractory intracranial hypertension. Hemodynamic stability should be confirmed before induction of a barbiturate coma. Early seizure activity should be treated with appropriate anticonvulsants. Prophylactic use of anticonvulsants is not recommended for prevention of late post-injury seizure activity. Paralytics in conjunction with sedation may help control ICP. Currently no evidence exists to support routine use of glucocorticoids in head injury. Follow-up of patients who received steroids following a head injury reveal no difference in outcomes. If cervical spine in-

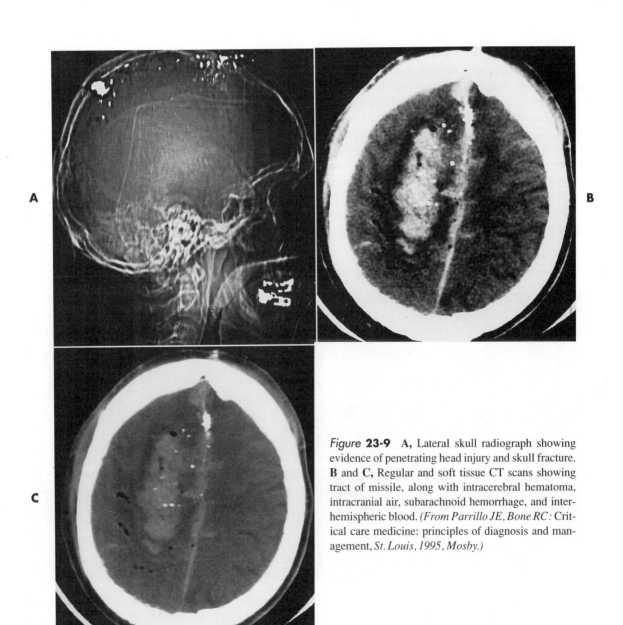

Figure **23-9** **A,** Lateral skull radiograph showing evidence of penetrating head injury and skull fracture. **B** and **C,** Regular and soft tissue CT scans showing tract of missile, along with intracerebral hematoma, intracranial air, subarachnoid hemorrhage, and interhemispheric blood. *(From Parrillo JE, Bone RC:* Critical care medicine: principles of diagnosis and management, *St. Louis, 1995, Mosby.)*

jury has been ruled out and the patient is hemodynamically stable, elevating the head of the bed can help decrease ICP.

SPECIFIC HEAD INJURIES

Head injuries may be grouped into focal injuries or diffuse injuries. Focal injuries have an identifiable area of involvement whereas diffuse injuries involve the entire brain. Examples of focal injuries include skull fractures and hematomas. Diffuse injuries include concussion and diffuse axonal injury. Penetrating injuries to the head cause significant focal injuries along the path of the bullet (Figure 23-9).

Focal Head Injuries

Scalp lacerations. The scalp protects the brain from injury by acting as a cushion to reduce the energy transmission to underlying structures. Excessive force applied to the scalp often causes a laceration; because the scalp has an extensive vascular supply with poor vasoconstrictive properties, lacerations bleed profusely. Bleeding is controlled with direct pressure to the affected area followed by wound repair as indicated, and tetanus prophylaxis.

Skull fractures. Skull fractures occur when energy applied to the skull causes a bony deformation. Clinical presentation of skull fractures is directly correlated to type of fracture, area involved, and damage to underlying structures. A linear skull fracture is nondisplaced and usually associated with a minimal neurologic deficit (Figure 23-10). Supportive care is usually all that is required for optimal neurologic recovery.

When energy displaces the outer table of bone below the inner table of the adjoining skull, a depressed skull fracture occurs (Figure 23-11). Surgical elevation is required when depressed bone fragments become lodged in brain tissue. Open depressed skull fractures are surgically elevated and repaired as soon as possible because of an increased risk of infection.

A basilar skull fracture develops when enough force is exerted on the base of the skull to cause a deformity. The base of the skull includes any bony area where the skull ends, and is not limited to the posterior aspect of the skull. A basilar skull fracture may be visualized on a radiograph; however, this is not always true. Approximately 25% of basilar skull fractures are not seen on radiograph; therefore, diagnosis is usually made on the basis of clinical findings. Basilar skull fractures that overlay the middle meningeal artery may cause a subgaleal hematoma. Disruption of the middle meningeal artery is the cause of more than 75% of epidural hematomas. A basilar skull fracture may also cause intracerebral bleeding.

Neurologic changes that occur with a basilar skull fracture range from mild changes in mentation to combativeness and severe agitation. Combative behavior is often considered a hallmark of a basilar skull fracture. Clinical manifestations of basilar skull fracture include periorbital ecchymoses (raccoon eyes) from intraorbital bleeding, Battle's sign (ecchymosis over the mastoid process) 12 to 24 hours after the initial injury, hemotympanum (blood behind the tympanic membrane caused by a fracture of the temporal bone), and CSF leak from the nose or ear caused by a tem-

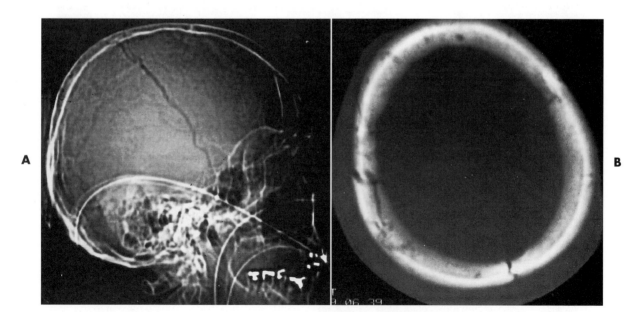

Figure **23-10** **A,** Lateral CT topogram showing extensive linear skull fracture. **B,** Bone windows of CT scan of same patient showing fracture. *(From Parrillo JE, Bone RC:* Critical care medicine: principles of diagnosis and management, *St. Louis, 1995, Mosby.)*

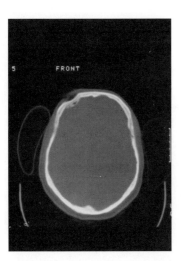

Figure 23-11 CT scan of depressed skull fracture right frontal region.

poral bone fracture. If the tympanic membrane is intact, fluid drains through the eustachian tube and appears as CSF rhinorrhea. However, absence of visible CSF does not eliminate the possibility that the patient may have a basilar skull fracture. If a CSF leak is possible, test the fluid on filter paper. Formation of two distinct rings is called the "halo" or "ring" sign and indicates presence of CSF. Clear fluid should be tested for glucose, a normal finding in CSF.

Diagnostic interventions include skull radiographs and a CT scan in some patients. Additional interventions focus on protecting the patient from injury, preventing infection, and using nasal drip pads as needed for rhinorrhea. Nasal packing is not recommended. Frequent neurologic assessment with ongoing reassessment is essential for early identification of deterioration in neurologic function.

Contusion. Cerebral contusion is a bruise on the surface of the brain that occurs from movement of the brain within the cranial vault (Figure 23-12). When an acceleration-deceleration injury occurs, two contusions may result, one at the initial site of impact (coup) and one on the opposite side of the impact (contra-coup). The clinical presentation varies with size and location of the contusion. Commonly occurring symptoms include altered level of consciousness, nausea, vomiting, visual difficulty, weakness, and speech difficulty. Interventions focus on preservation of neurologic function, control of pain, and adequate hydration.

Epidural hematoma. Epidural hematoma is bleeding between the skull and dura mater (Figure 23-13) resulting from a direct blow to the head. A skull fracture and injury to the middle meningeal artery may also be present. A torn middle meningeal artery with arterial bleeding leads to a rapidly forming hematoma, with an associated morbidity and mortality of more than 50%. Approximately half of the patients with an epidural hematoma have no evidence of skull frac-

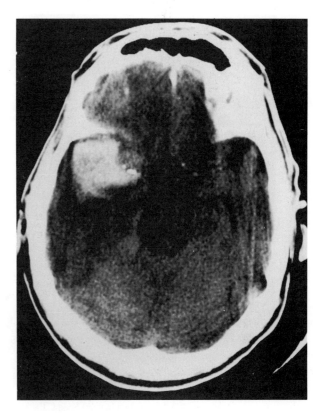

Figure 23-12 CT: contusion. *(Courtesy of Laurence Cromwell, MD, Department of Radiology, Dartmouth-Hitchcock Medical Center.)*

ture. Signs and symptoms include a brief period of unconsciousness followed by a lucid period, followed by another loss of consciousness. This brief lucid period is considered a hallmark of an epidural hematoma; however, it does not occur in all patients. If alert, the patient with an epidural hematoma complains of severe headache and may exhibit hemiparesis and a dilated pupil on the side of injury.

Subdural hematoma. Subdural hematomas occur more frequently than other intracranial injuries and have the highest morbidity and mortality of all hematomas. Bleeding into the subdural space between the dura mater and arachnoid leads to a subdural hematoma (Figure 23-14). A subdural hematoma may be acute, subacute, or chronic. When acute, the hematoma usually results from dissipation of energy that ruptures bridging veins in the subdural space. Clinical features are loss of consciousness; hemiparesis; and fixed, dilated pupils. Surgical intervention within 4 hours of injury has the best potential for neurologic recovery.

Subacute subdural hematomas develop 48 hours to 2 weeks after injury. The clinical presentation is a progressive decline in level of consciousness as the hematoma slowly expands. The brain compensates due to slow blood collection over time, so decline in neurologic function occurs

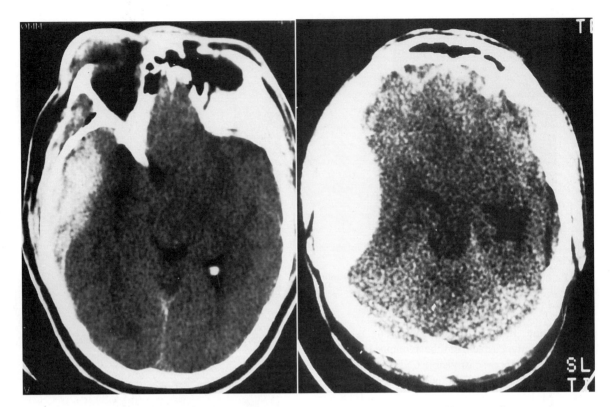

Figure **23-13** Nonenhanced head CT scan displaying right ventricular epidural hematoma in young male, resulting from motor vehicle collision. *(From Parrillo JE, Bone RC:* Critical care medicine: principles of diagnosis and management, *St. Louis, 1995, Mosby.)*

gradually. After the subdural is drained, the patient improves quickly with little or no lasting neurologic deficit.

Chronic subdural hematomas, seen frequently in the elderly, progress slowly. Blood collects over 2 weeks to months; by the time a person is examined, the causative mechanism may have been forgotten. Chronic subdural hematomas are tolerated by the elderly due to brain atrophy associated with aging. As the brain decreases in size, the space within the cranial vault increases. A hematoma collects over time without obvious changes in neurologic status until its size is sufficient to produce a mass effect. Treatment of a chronic subdural consists of burr holes and a subdural drain. Patients become more alert after the subdural is drained.

Other focal injuries. Intraventricular hemorrhage (Figure 23-15) and intracerebral clots (Figure 23-16) are types of focal injuries. Management depends on the size of the clot and source of bleeding. Surgical evacuation is usually necessary in concert with medical management of increased intracranial pressure.

Diffuse Brain Injuries

Concussion. A concussion can occur as a result of a direct blow to the head, or from an acceleration or deceleration injury where the brain collides with the inside of the skull. Brief interruption of the reticular activating system may occur causing transient amnesia. Amnesia usually requires no

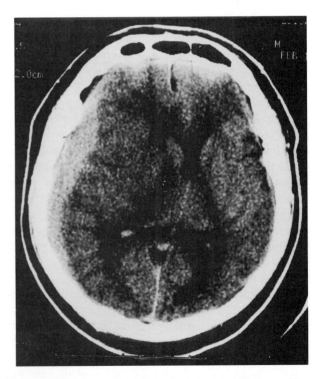

Figure **23-14** CT: Acute subdural hematoma. *(Courtesy of Laurence Cromwell, MD, Department of Radiology, Dartmouth-Hitchcock Medical Center.)*

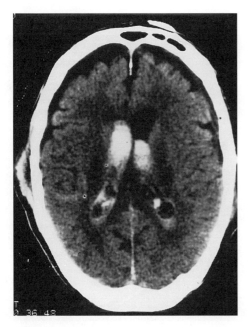

Figure **23-15** CT scan of head showing intraventricular hemorrhage secondary to motor vehicle collision. *(From Parrillo JE, Bone RC:* Critical care medicine: principles of diagnosis and management, *St. Louis, 1995, Mosby.)*

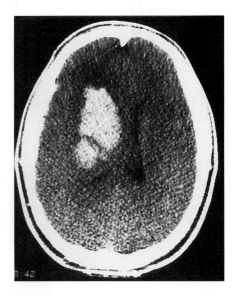

Figure **23-16** Nonenhanced head CT scan showing large right hemispheric clot in 26-year-old male patient who sustained closed head injury from a motor vehicle collision. Note mass effect on right lateral ventricle. *(From Parrillo JE, Bone RC:* Critical care medicine: principles of diagnosis and management, *St. Louis, 1995, Mosby.)*

therapeutic intervention other than observation for development of potential complications. A classic concussion is characterized as loss of consciousness followed by transient neurologic changes such as nausea, vomiting, temporary amnesia, headache, and a possible brief loss of vision.

Care for a concussion patient includes observation, especially with prolonged loss of consciousness (greater than 2 to 3 minutes). With protracted nausea and vomiting, hospital admission may be considered to avoid dehydration. Nonnarcotic analgesia may be administered for headache. Narcotics affect the level of consciousness and interfere with ongoing patient assessment. Patients with a concussion may be discharged with a responsible adult who will observe the patient overnight for possible complications, such as confusion, difficulty walking, an altered level of consciousness, projectile vomiting, and unequal pupils. Discharge teaching includes instructions on how to assess neurologic status in the home and when to contact the primary care provider.

Headache, memory loss, and difficulty with activities of daily living are characteristic of postconcussion syndrome, which can occur up to 1 year after the patient's initial injury. Interventions include supportive treatment and recognition that this is a true physiologic consequence of what was perceived as a minor head injury.

Diffuse axonal injury. The phrase "diffuse axonal injury" (DAI) illustrates the major pathophysiologic events associated with the most severe form of TBI. This injury is almost always the result of blunt trauma that causes shearing and disruption of neuronal structures. Prognosis for diffuse ax-

Box **23-2**

NURSING DIAGNOSIS FOR HEAD INJURY

Airway clearance, ineffective
Pain
Tissue perfusion, altered cerebral
Aspiration, risk
Gas exchange, impaired
Injury, risk
Mobility, impaired physical

onal injuries depends on the degree of injury (mild, moderate, or severe) and the amount of damage from any secondary injury.

Mild DAI is characterized by a loss of consciousness for 6 to 24 hours. Initially, the patient may exhibit decerebrate or decorticate posturing but improves rapidly within 24 hours. Return to baseline neurologic status may occur over days, and periods of amnesia may be present.

Moderate DAI is a coma lasting longer than 24 hours, possibly extending over a period of days. Brainstem dysfunction (decorticate/decerebrate posturing) is evident almost immediately and may continue until the patient begins to wake up. Patients with moderate diffuse axonal injury usually recover but rarely return to full pre-injury neurologic function.

A   **B**

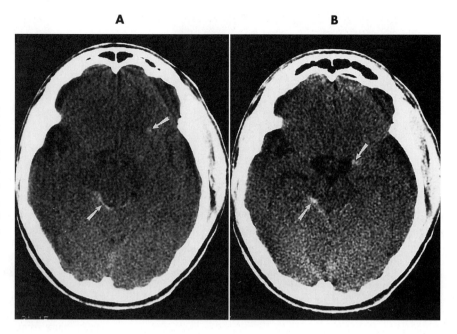

Figure **23-17**   A and **B,** CT scans of head in a patient with coma secondary to motor vehicle collision. Scans show punctate hemorrhage in left frontal lobe and midbrain and subarachnoid hemorrhage in perimesencephalic cisterns. This picture is suggestive of diffuse axonal injury. *(From Parrillo JE, Bone RC:* Critical care medicine: principles of diagnosis and management, *St. Louis, 1995, Mosby.)*

Severe DAI is characterized by brainstem impairment that does not resolve. Victims of severe DAI remain comatose for days to weeks. Autonomic dysfunction may also be present. Overall prognosis for severe diffuse axonal injury is extremely poor. Early CT scans may be unremarkable; however, serial exams reveal areas of edema and microvascular hemorrhage (Figure 23-17). Treatment for all degrees of DAI includes general supportive care, prevention of further brain injury, and support for the family.

CONCLUSION

Head injuries are a major cause of traumatic deaths in the United States and cause significant long-term disability. Recognition and prevention of secondary injuries related to ischemia, increased ICP, and hypoxia are essential components of care for these patients. Box 23-2 summarizes nursing diagnoses for these patients.

REFERENCES

1. American Association of Neurological Surgeons Joint Section on Neurotrauma and Critical Care: *Guidelines for the management of severe head injury,* Park Ridge, Ill, 1995, The Association.
2. Bandak F: On the mechanics of impact neurotrauma: a review and critical synthesis, *J Neurotrauma* 12(4):635-649, 1995.
3. Fortune J, et al.: Effect of hyperventilation, mannitol, and ventriculostomy drainage on cerebral blood flow after head injury, *J Trauma* 39(6):1091-1099.
4. Gennarelli T: Cerebral concussion and diffuse brain injuries. In Cooper P: *Head injury,* Williams and Wilkins, 1987, Baltimore.
5. Hickey JV: *Neurological and neurosurgical nursing,* ed 4 Philadelphia, 1996, JB Lippincott.
6. Hilton G: Experimental neuroprotective agents: nursing challenge, *Dimens Crit Care,* 14(4):181-188.
7. Lucatorto M, Taylor J: In Neff J and Kidd P, editors, *Trauma nursing: The art and science,* St. Louis, 1993, Mosby.
8. Marshall S, et al.: *Neuroscience critical care pathophysiology and patient management,* Philadelphia, 1990, WB Saunders.
9. Mitchell P: Central nervous system I: closed head injuries. In Cardona V, et al., editors: *Trauma nursing from resuscitation through rehabilitation,* ed 2 Philadelphia, 1994, WB Saunders.
10. National Safety Council: *Accident facts, 1995 edition,* Itasca, Ill, 1995, The Council.
11. Sosin D, Sniezek J, Waxweiler R: Trends in death associated with traumatic brain injury, 1979 through 1992, *JAMA* 273(22):1778-1780.
12. Teasdale G, Jennett B: Assessment of coma and impaired consciousness: a practical scale, *Lancet* 2(81), 1974.
13. Walleck C, Mooney K: In Barker E, editor: *Neuroscience nursing,* St. Louis, 1994, Mosby.

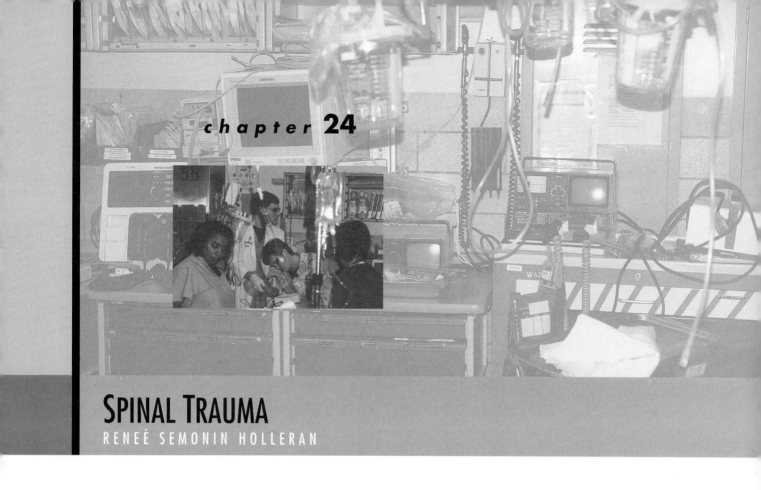

chapter **24**

SPINAL TRAUMA

RENEÉ SEMONIN HOLLERAN

Trauma to the spinal column and the spinal cord can result in devastating and life-threatening injuries. Each year, approximately 10,000 acute spinal cord injuries occur in the United States. The majority of those injured are males under the age of 30. The estimated cost for care ranges from $225,000 to $400,000 with an overall cost to society of 4 billion dollars per year.[2,8,9,19]

The spinal cord may be injured in a number of ways. The most common mechanisms of injury remain motor vehicle crashes, accounting for as many as 49% of acute spinal cord injuries.[18] Motor vehicle crashes cause spinal cord injuries by rollovers, occupant ejection, and collisions with pedestrians. Other mechanisms include falls, direct blows to the head or neck, penetrating wounds from guns or knives, and sports injuries. Over the past decade, in-line skating, snow boarding, and bicycling have become more frequent sources of spinal cord injuries in addition to diving and football.[11]

In the past, many who suffered acute spinal cord injuries died from respiratory complications such as aspiration and pneumonia. Today, establishment of spinal-cord–injury care systems have decreased complications from acute spinal cord injuries and improved survival of those injured.[9]

Care of the patient with spine trauma begins in the prehospital environment with rapid identification of injury or the potential for injury based on the mechanism of injury followed by appropriate patient immobilization. Five percent of patients with major trauma have an unstable cervical spine injury and two thirds of these persons have neurologic deficits.[4] Once in the emergency department (ED), the patient should be fully evaluated to rule out concomitant life-threatening injuries such as tension pneumothorax or intraabdominal bleeding.

Emergency care of the patient with spine trauma requires an organized multidisciplinary approach. Patient survival and quality of life from the acute injury depend on the emergency care a patient receives. This chapter discusses anatomy and physiology of spine trauma; mechanisms of injury; patient assessment and initial interventions; specific injuries; and current research related to management of acute spine injury.

ANATOMY AND PHYSIOLOGY
Anatomy

The spinal cord regulates body movement and function through transmission of nerve impulses. It is an integral part of the central nervous system, extending from the superior border of C-1 to the superior border of L-2. It tapers in the lower thoracic area and terminates in a cone-shaped structure known as the conus medullaris. The cauda equina contains the spinal nerve roots that exit below the conus medullaris.[8,19] The spinal cord travels through a canal within the vertebrae, covered by three layers of meninges: the pia, the arachnoid, and dura.

The human body has 7 cervical, 12 thoracic, 5 lumbar, and 1 sacral vertebrae (Figure 24-1). The vertebral column provides support for the head and trunk and protection for the spinal cord. A vertebral body is composed of the body, a

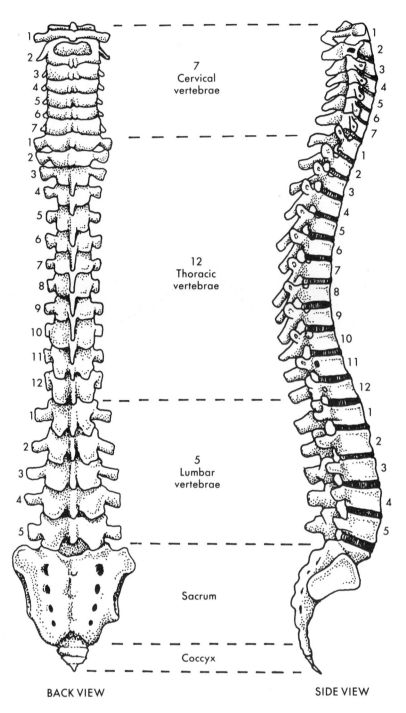

Figure **24-1**   Vertebral column.

7
Cervical
vertebrae

12
Thoracic
vertebrae

5
Lumbar
vertebrae

Sacrum

Coccyx

BACK VIEW   SIDE VIEW

vertebral arch, and a vertebral foramen. The arch of the vertebra is composed of two pedicles, two laminae, four facets, two transverse processes, and the spinous process, which can be palpated.[8]

The cervical vertebrae are the most mobile part of the spine, so this area is the most frequent site of injury. The rib cage keeps the vertebrae from T1 to T10 stable and relatively immobile. The second most common site of injury is the thoracolumbar junction at T11 to L2. This is a transition area between the rigid thoracolumbar region and the more mobile lumbar region.[4]

Ligaments connect the vertebral bodies and provide support and stability to the vertebral column. They also keep the spinal column from excessive flexion and extension. Between the vertebral bodies are discs that act as shock absorbers and articulating surfaces for the adjacent vertebral bodies.[8,19]

Physiology

The primary function of the spinal cord is to regulate function and movement of the body by transmitting nerve impulses between the brain and the body. The spinal cord is an extremely delicate collection of nervous tissue. A cross-

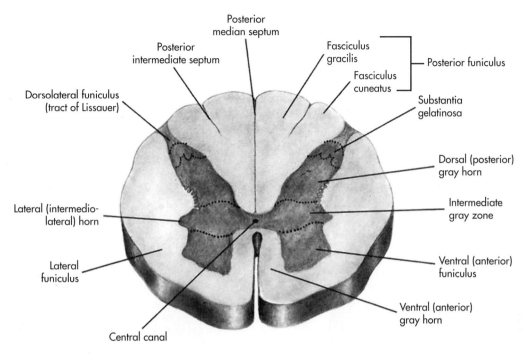

Figure **24-2** Cross section of spinal cord illustrating subdivisions of white and gray matter. *(From Rudy EB:* Advanced neurological and neurosurgical nursing, *St. Louis, 1984, Mosby.)*

sectional view of the spinal cord (Figure 24-2) reveals an H-shaped core composed of gray matter. The gray matter is divided into posterior, horizontal, and anterior columns and nine laminae. The posterior gray matter mediates sensory impulses for processes, such as proprioception, pressure sense, vibratory sense, and movement. The horizontal gray matter contains interconnecting neurons that form the first part of a two-neuron pathway for the sympathetic nervous system. The central canal pierces the horizontal gray matter. The anterior part of the gray matter contains the motor cell bodies that form the final common pathway for all impulses going to skeletal muscles. The motor cell axons pass out of the spinal cord by way of the ventral root and end at the muscles' motor end plates.[19]

The white matter of the spinal cord is formed by axons of the cells within the gray matter; axons of sensory cells in the dorsal ganglia; and descending tracts from the brain, brain stem, and cerebellum. These fibers are organized into tracts in the white matter and run parallel to the spinal cord's vertical axis. The tracts ascend to and descend from the brain and to other parts of the spinal cord. The spinal cord is composed of multiple tracts. Table 24-1 lists some of these tracts and describes their functions.[9,19]

Spinal nerves. The spinal cord has 31 pairs of spinal nerves that provide pathways for involuntary responses to specific stimuli. They innervate voluntary striated muscle. Each of these nerves has a posterior root that transmits sensory impulses and an anterior root that transmits motor impulses. The nerves are paired and correspond to specific spinal cord segments. The nerves are listed as follows: 8 cervical

Table **24-1** **Examples of Spinal Tracts and Their Functions**	
Spinal tract	**Function**
Dorsal columns (ascending)	Conscious muscle sense, touch, vibration
Lateral spinothalamic tract (ascending)	Pain and temperature
Ventral spinothalamic tract (ascending)	Light touch
Ventral pyramidal tract (descending)	Voluntary control of skeletal muscle
Extrapyramidal tract (descending)	Automatic control of skeletal muscle
Dorsal spinocerebellar tract (ascending)	Unconscious muscle sense
Lateral pyramidal tract (descending)	Voluntary control of skeletal muscle

Data from Jaworski M, Wirtz K: Spinal trauma. In Kitt S, et al., editors: *Emergency nursing*, Philadelphia, 1995, WB Saunders and Walleck C: Central nervous system II: spinal cord injury. In Cardona V, et al., editors: *Trauma nursing*, ed 2, Philadelphia, 1994, WB Saunders.

nerves, 12 thoracic nerves, 5 lumbar nerves, 5 sacral nerves, and 1 coccygeal nerve. The dorsal root of these nerves supplies a distinct region of the body surface known as a *dermatome* (Figure 24-3). Assessment of the 28 dermatomes provides information about injury to sensory areas of the spinal cord.

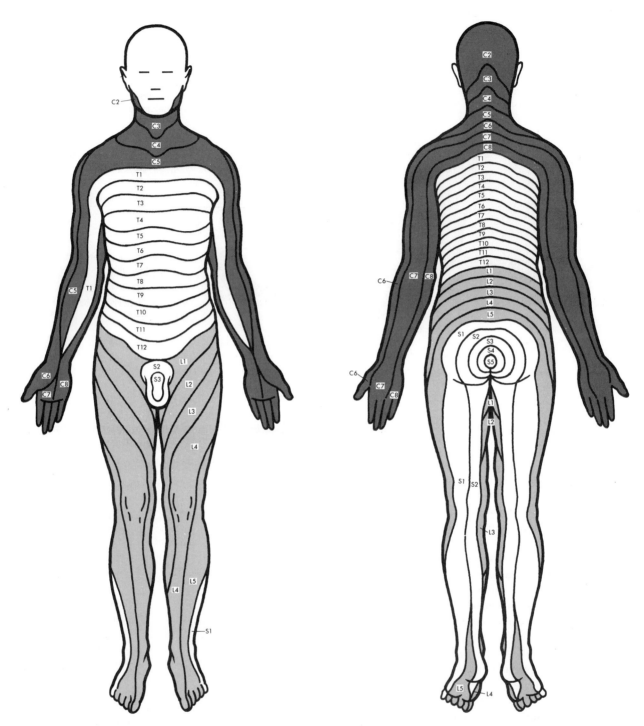

Figure **24-3** Sensory dermatomes. *(From Rosen P et al.: Emergency medicine, ed 3, vol 1, St. Louis, 1992, Mosby.)*

A group of muscles innervated by a single spinal segment, known as *myotomes,* contain the distribution of spinal cord motor activity. As with the dermatome, these fibers correspond to a specific segment of the spinal cord. The innervated muscles and patient's response are summarized in Table 24-2.[9,19]

Vascular supply. The vascular supply for the spinal cord comes from the vertebral artery and a series of spinal rami ar-

teries that enter the intervertebral foramina at various levels.[9] The anterior spinal artery supplies blood to two thirds of the spinal cord. The remaining one third of the spinal cord's blood supply is carried by the two posterior arteries, which originate from the vertebral artery. Unlike other structures in the body, spinal cord arteries cannot develop adequate collateral blood supply when they are blocked or injured.[9,19]

Table **24-2**	Spinal Nerve Muscle Innervation and Patient Response	
Nerve level	Muscles innervated	Patient response
C-4	Diaphragm	Ventilation
C-5	Deltoid	Shrug shoulders
	Biceps	Flex elbows
	Brachioradialis	
C-6	Wrist extensor	Extend wrist
	Extensor carpi radialis longus	
C-7	Triceps	Extend elbow
	Extensor digitorum communis	Extend fingers
	Flexor carpi radialis	
C-8	Flexor digitorum profundus	Flex fingers
T-1	Hand intrinsic muscles	Spread fingers
T-2 to L-1	Intercostals	Vital capacity
	Abdominal	Abdominal reflexes
L-2	Iliopsoas	Hip flexion
L-3	Quadriceps	Knee extension
L-4	Tibialis anterior	Ankle dorsiflexion
L-5	Extension hallucis longus	Ankle eversion
S-1	Gastrocnemius	Ankle plantar flexion
		Big toe extension
S-2 to S-5	Perineal sphincter	Sphincter control

Table **24-3**	Categories of Movement That May Result in Spinal Cord Injury	
Category	Mechanism of injury	
Hyperextension	The head is forced back, and the vertebrae of the cervical region are placed in an overextended position.	
Hyperflexion	The head is forced forward, and the cervical vertebrae are placed in an overflexion position.	
Axial loading	A severe blow to the top of the head causes a blunt downward force on the vertebrae and the spinal column.	
Compression	Forces from above and below compress the vertebrae.	
Lateral bend	The head and neck are bent to one side, beyond the normal range of motion.	
Overrotation and distraction	The head turns to one side, and the cervical vertebrae are forced beyond normal limits.	

PATIENT ASSESSMENT

Primary and secondary assessment of an injured patient is performed by the emergency nurse with initiation of critical interventions as appropriate. Since all patients with multisystem injuries or significant mechanisms of injury may have a spinal injury, each patient should be completely immobilized. Spinal immobilization involves manual immobilization of the patient's head until a hard cervical collar, lateral head support such as sand bag or rolled sheets, and backboard have been applied (Figure 24-4). The entire spine should be immobilized with a backboard and straps across the chest, abdomen, and knees. Once the patient's critical needs have been met, the emergency nurse may then perform a more focused assessment related to spinal injury.

The initial assessment of the patient with spine trauma begins with obtaining a history including the mechanisms of injury, and results of inspection, palpation, and percussion focused on the spine and spinal cord.

Mechanisms of Injury

Mechanisms of spine injury may come from blunt and/or penetrating forces. The vertebrae, spinal cord, and nerve roots may be injured as a result of fractures, dislocations, or subluxation. The cord may also be injured through direct

penetration by a bullet, knife, or other sharp object. Six basic types of movement can injure the spinal cord. These are illustrated in Figure 24-5, and summarized in Table 24-3.

When obtaining information from the patient with a suspected spine injury, the emergency nurse should ask the patient about neck pain, changes in sensation or movement since the accident, and loss of consciousness. If the patient is unconscious, prehospital history may be the only source of information about the patient immediately after the accident. The emergency nurse should acquire as much history as possible from the prehospital care providers.

History

Spinal cord injury should be suspected with any of the following: a history of significant trauma and altered mental status from intoxication; a history of seizure activity since the accident; any complaint of neck pain or altered sensation in their upper extremities; a complaint of neck tenderness; a history of loss of consciousness; an injury above the clavicle; a fall greater than three times the patient's height; a fall that results in a fracture of the heels; an unrestrained (no seat belt) person with facial injury; significant injuries in a motor vehicle crash that result in chest and intraabdominal injuries; and a motorcycle crash.[13] The patient may complain of a feeling of "electric shock" or "hot water" running down the back. A history of incontinence before arrival in the ED may be reported. Priapism may be noted in male patients.

Inspection

The emergency nurse should observe the patient for obvious signs of spinal injury including abnormality in the vertebral column, cervical edema, and entrance or exit wounds in

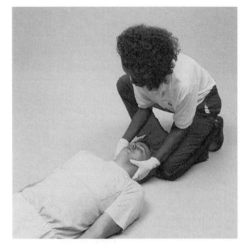

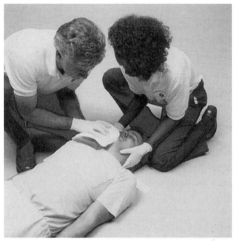

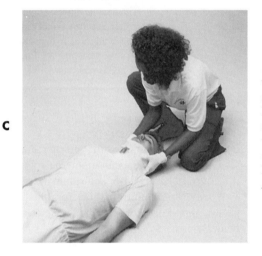

Figure **24-4**   Spinal immobilization. **A,** Manual in-line immobilization is applied and this position is maintained throughout the procedure. **B,** A collar is positioned and secured with Velcro straps. **C,** Support is maintained for the patient with spread fingers until the patient is secured to a short or long spine board. *(From Sanders M:* Mosby's paramedic textbook, *St. Louis, 1994, Mosby.)*

the neck, chest, or abdomen. The patient's ventilatory pattern and effort can indicate a cord injury. Injuries to the spinal cord above C-6 interfere with ventilation. Use of abdominal muscles rather than the diaphragm to breathe suggests injury to the cord at level C-3 to C-5.

The emergency nurse should observe the patient's ability to move and to perceive pain during procedures such as intravenous insertion or arterial punctures. The patient may be holding his or her head forward, which suggests a level C1 to C2 injury, or may have his or her arms folded across the chest indicating a level C5 to C6 injury. Priapism indicates a cervical spine injury because it occurs with a loss of sympathetic nervous system control and parasympathetic stimulation.[8,9]

The emergency nurse should observe the patient for a cerebral spinal fluid (CSF) leak from the nose or ears. Confirm the presence of CSF with a halo test or dextro stick. The patient must be carefully checked for ecchymosis, tracheal deviation, or hematoma in the posterior pharyngeal area, which may indicate spinal injury, particularly in penetrating neck trauma.

Palpation

The patient's spinal column should be palpated for pain, tenderness, and deformity. If the cervical collar is removed for this procedure, manual immobilization must be maintained. Skin temperature can be assessed by palpation. A patient with a spinal cord injury becomes poikilothermic, because of loss of sympathetic tone, assuming the temperature of the surroundings. Injury above the T-4 level usually disrupts the sympathetic nervous system causing vasodilation below the level of the injury. If the patient is diaphoretic, the diaphoresis is present above, rather than below, the level of the injury.

Strength and equality of movement of all four extremities should be evaluated. Table 24-2 summarizes specific responses and their relationship to spinal motor nerve innervation. A quick motor evaluation should include flexion and extension of the arms, flexion and extension of the legs, flexion of the foot, extension of the toes, and sphincter tone.[8]

Sensory status may be assessed by evaluation of dermatomes (Figure 24-3). A brief assessment includes using a safety pin or cotton swab so that the patient can distinguish

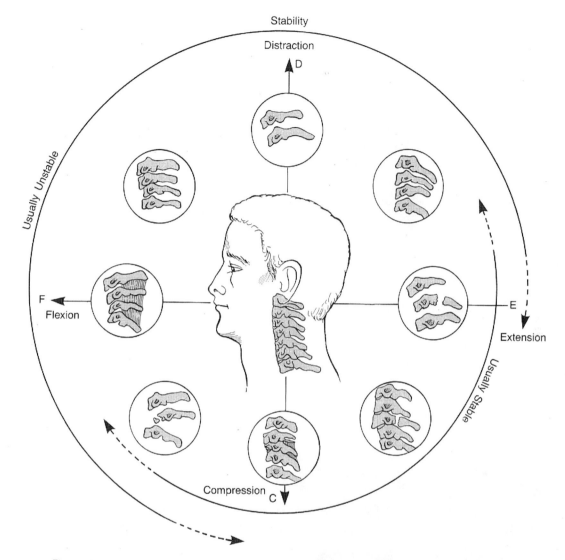

Figure **24-5** Mechanisms of injury to the spine. The mechanism of cervical injury (flexion versus extension) determines the type of cervical spine fracture or dislocation. *(From Moore EE, et al: Early care of the injured patient, ed 4, 1990, American College of Surgeons.)*

between sharp and dull. Test the top of the shoulder, at the nipple line, the umbilicus, and the great toe on each side.[8]

Percussion

The emergency nurse can assist with or perform an assessment of the patient's reflexes. These are summarized in Table 24-4.

Radiographic Evaluation

Radiographic evaluation of the injured patient is performed to assess alignment, identify fractures or ligamentous injuries, and to identify spinal cord compression by bone or soft tissues.[4] Anteroposterior (Figure 24-6) and lateral (Figure 24-7) x-ray views of the spine show all seven cervical vertebrae and the C7-T1 junction. When a satisfactory cross table is obtained, the C-spine series should be

Table **24-4** Reflexes Tested in Spinal Trauma	
Reflex	Spinal cord level
Biceps	C5-6
Brachionadialis	C5-6
Triceps	C7-8
Superficial abdominal (above umbilicus)	T7-T10
Superficial abdominal (below umbilicus)	T11-L1
Cremasteric	T12-L1
Knee jerk	L3-L4
Ankle jerk	S1
Anal wink	S2-S4
Bulbocavernosus	S3-S4
Plantar response	Brain-cord continuity

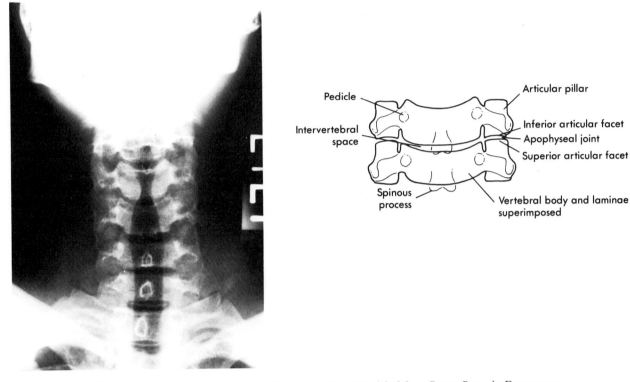

Figure **24-6** Anteroposterior view of cervical spine. *(Modified from Rosen P et al.:* Emergency medicine, *ed 3, vol 1, St. Louis, 1992, Mosby.)*

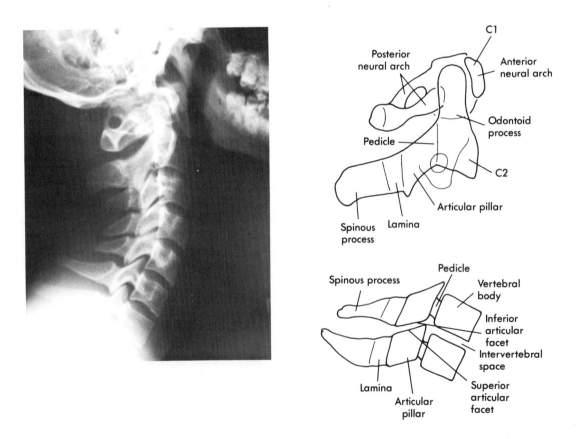

Figure **24-7** Lateral view of cervical spine. *(Modified from Rosen P et al.:* Emergency medicine, *ed 3, vol 1, St. Louis, 1992, Mosby.)*

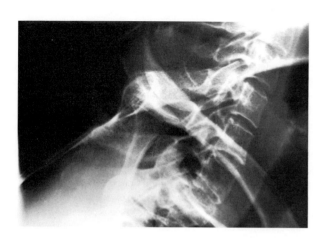

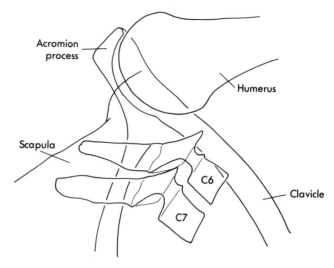

Figure **24-8**   Swimmer's view of cervical spine. *(Modified from Rosen P et al.:* Emergency medicine, *ed 3, vol 1, St. Louis, 1992, Mosby.)*

completed. A swimmer's view (Figure 24-8) is performed when all the cervical vertebrae cannot be visualized, and an open-mouth series is used to evaluate integrity of the odontoid body, C-1 and C-2 vertebrae.[9] Any patient with a history of a fall or significant chest and abdominal trauma should have films of the thoracic and lumbosacral spine.

Computerized tomography (CT) facilitates evaluation of soft tissue damage, the patency of the neural canal, and compression of the spinal cord. A CT scan is indicated for patients with subluxation, fractures, neurologic deficits with no apparent abnormalities, severe pain without obvious injury, and when C-7/T-1 junction cannot be visualized.[4,9]

Magnetic resonance imaging (MRI) has emerged as an excellent diagnostic tool for spinal cord injury. An MRI does not show bone well, so it should be used in conjunction with a CT scan. In a study done by Schroder and colleagues[14] the CT scan revealed all acute bony injuries, but did not consistently identify longitudinal ligament lesions, intramedullary hemorrhages, and vertebral disc herniations. The MRI on the other hand identified all medullary and paravertebral soft tissue changes, dislocations, and spondylophytes narrowing the spinal channel.[14] Schroder et al. thought that when the patient's condition allowed, an MRI should be performed before a CT. An unstable patient should not be taken for an MRI. The MRI is of particular importance in a pediatric patient who has suffered a spinal cord injury without radiographic abnormality (SCIWORA).[4,11]

STABILIZATION

Initial stabilization of a patient with trauma to the spine begins with recognition and treatment of life-threatening injuries such as airway and vascular compromise. The airway is evaluated while maintaining C-spine control. Therapeutic interventions are directed at ensuring an adequate airway, maintaining ventilations, and preventing further injury.

Airway Management

The patient with cervical spine trauma is at risk for hypoxia, respiratory arrest, and aspiration. The emergency care team also needs to initiate interventions to minimize postinjury edema. The airway may be at risk from a spinal cord injury that compromises the muscles of respiration or from localized edema that can cause airway obstruction, particularly in penetrating neck trauma. Advanced airway management such as endotracheal intubation should be considered early. Cricothyrotomy may be necessary if the patient has extensive facial trauma or anatomic landmarks cannot be located due to injury. Any airway maneuvers require that the cervical spine remains adequately immobilized. Nasal intubation is preferred for patients with spinal cord injury who do not have facial or cranial injury. Intubation via the nasal route can be accomplished with minimal manipulation of the spine.

Cervical Spine Immobilization

The emergency nurse must ensure that the patient is correctly immobilized. Box 24-1 summarizes this procedure. The equipment required to immobilize the cervical spine includes a rigid cervical collar, a lateral head immobilizer, and a backboard.

A rigid cervical collar is applied to decrease head and neck movement. When applying a cervical collar, the emergency nurse should follow directions for size selection and application. Someone should always provide in-line immobilization during this process. Rigid cervical collars should not obstruct the patient's mouth or airway or interfere with ventilations, and should be applied after the patient's head has been placed in a neutral in-line position.[13]

Box **24-1**   **Cervical Spine Immobilization Procedure**

1. Assess airway; ensure patency using the jaw thrust or chin lift maneuver; do not hyperextend the neck; if endotracheal intubation is necessary and not possible without hyperextension, consider nasotracheal or digital intubation or cricothyrotomy to ensure the airway.
2. Evaluate the cervical spine by observation; palpate each spinous process, note deformity, crepitus, pain, and instability. Talk to the patient; inform the patient of each step of the process to alleviate anxiety and movement and to elicit cooperation.
3. Apply gentle in-line manual immobilization by placing hands on either side of the head and stabilizing the neck in a neutral vertical position. Once immobilization has been applied, it must be maintained until a comparable or better alternative has been implemented or until the possibility of cervical spine injury has been ruled out by radiographic findings or computed tomography scan.
4. Have other members of the team assist by gently placing a spine board under the patient while one care giver continues to maintain immobilization. Synchronize the log roll maneuver with absolute cervical spine protection.
5. Secure the patient to the long board. Undress the patient completely if possible, and pad bony prominences liberally. Remove any sharp or bulky objects. Place chest, hip, and leg straps across the patient and snugly attach straps to handles or cutouts in the board. Secure the straps diagonally from the chest to the hips. Pad behind the head and neck to support the cervical spine, always maintaining a neutral position. Secure the patient's head to the spine board using adhesive tape that is 2 inches wide. Tape across the eyebrows, and secure the ends of the tape to the spine board. Exercise extreme caution to ensure that straps and tape do not interfere with respirations or emesis. A lateral head immobilization device may be used instead of tape.
6. When satisfied that the cervical spine is absolutely immobile, release manual immobilization.
7. Be prepared to logroll the patient, using the backboard, if emesis occurs. Be sure to have adequate suction equipment on hand.
8. If a short spine board or another short device is used, it should be used in conjunction with a long board or scoop stretcher. Short boards should only be used to facilitate extrication.
9. If the patient is wearing a helmet, leave it in place, as long as the airway is not compromised and immobilization can be accomplished. See Box 24-2 for helmet removal procedure.

Modified from Sheehy SB, Marvin JA, Jimmerson CL: *Manual of clinical trauma care: the first hour,* St. Louis, 1989, Mosby.

Helmet Removal Procedure

A variety of helmets are available for those who participate in sports where head protection is recommended (e.g., motorcycling, bicycling, kayaking, ice hockey, football, and automobile racing). Careful removal of this protective device is imperative for protection of the cervical spine.
1. Never attempt to remove the helmet by yourself—two people are needed to remove it. An adequate airway usually can be achieved with the helmet in place, especially when the potential exists for complicating an injury during a difficult helmet removal.
2. One person applies in-line immobilization by placing hands on each side of the helmet with fingers on the patient's mandible, pulling carefully. Remember to cut or remove the chin strap.
3. A second person concurrently receives the weight of the patient's head by placing the fingers of both hands on the occipital region and the thumbs at the angles of the mandible. The second person is now in control of the head and neck.
4. The first person then removes the helmet by pulling laterally and carefully sliding it off. If the helmet has full face protection, the eye covering must be removed first. If it cannot be removed, tilt the helmet, *not the head,* back to pass the face protector over the patient's nose. Then pull the helmet laterally.

Modified from Sheehy SB, Marvin JA, Jimmerson CL: *Manual of clinical trauma care: the first hour,* ed 2, St. Louis, 1994, Mosby.

Placing the patient on a backboard does not completely immobilize the spine. The head must be stabilized laterally. This can be accomplished with a commercial head immobilizer composed of a back, side pillows and straps, towel rolls and tape, or by taping the patient's head to the backboard. Tape or straps should never obstruct the patient's airway. The patient should be secured to the backboard at the chest, abdomen, and knees.

If the patient has a helmet in place, it should be removed. Box 24-2 and Figure 24-9 illustrate this procedure. ED personnel should practice this procedure for safe and efficient performance.[13]

Circulation Management

Fluctuations in the patient's blood pressure may be directly related to spinal shock. Injury to the spine may cause loss of sympathetic vasomotor tone that causes hypotension and bradycardia. With disruption of the sympathetic nervous system in spinal trauma, a drop in blood pressure from vasodilation does not cause a compensatory increase in the

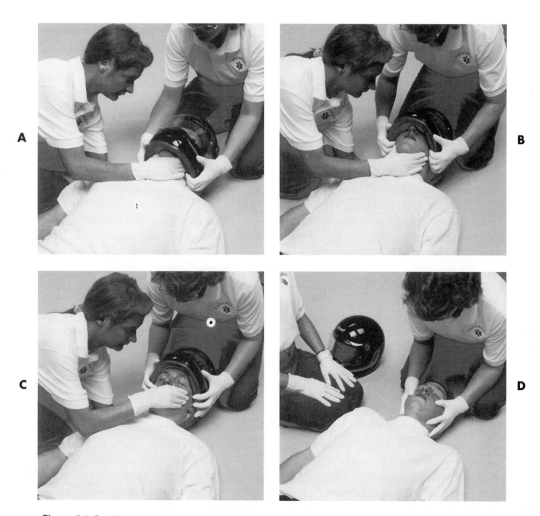

Figure **24-9**   Helmet removal. **A,** The helmet and the head are immobilized in an in-line position. The patient's mandible is grasped by placing the thumb at the angle of the mandible on one side and two fingers at the angle on the other side. The other hand is placed under the neck at the base of the skull, producing in-line immobilization of the patient's head. **B,** The sides of the helmet are carefully spread away from the patient's head and ears. **C,** The helmet is then rotated to clear the nose and removed from the patient's head in a straight line. **D,** After removal of the helmet, in-line immobilization is applied as well as a rigid cervical collar. *(From Sanders M:* Mosby's paramedic textbook, *St. Louis, 1994, Mosby.)*

heart rate. When hypotension occurs, injuries such as a tension pneumothorax or intraabdominal bleeding, which also causes hypotension, should be ruled out.

In the patient who has a spinal cord injury, hypotension may be the result of spinal shock or secondary to hypovolemia for other injuries. If the cause of the patient's hypotension is not clear, intravenous crystalloid solutions should be started to correct hypovolemia.[4] A pulmonary artery catheter should be inserted as soon as possible to monitor fluid resuscitation and prevent complications from excessive fluid administration. Blood loss should be corrected before vasoactive medications are used.

Pharmacological Management

If the patient arrives in the ED within 8 hours of injury, high-dose methylprednisolone should be administered. In 1990, Bracken and colleagues[3] demonstrated neurologic improvement in patients with spinal cord injury who received methylprednisolone within 8 hours of injury. The patient receives an initial bolus of methylprednisolone of 30 mg/kg over 15 minutes followed 45 minutes later by a continuous infusion of 5.4 mg/kg for 23 hours. Administration of methylprednisolone is the current standard of care for spinal cord injury; however, recent research has begun to question its effectiveness.[6] George and colleagues[6] found that patients who received high-dose methylprednisolone were at greater risk for pneumonia, decubitus ulcer formation, and urinary tract infections. Early administraton within 8 hours of injury did not improve the functional status of the patient as assessed by mobility and the Functional Independence Measures (FIM).[6] Further research is needed to determine whether high-dose methylprednisolone is effective or may actually place the patient at risk for post-injury complications.

Additional Interventions

The patient with an acute spinal cord injury needs a foley catheter to decrease bladder distention and to monitor urinary output during resuscitation. A nasogastric or orogastric tube should be inserted to protect the patient from aspiration. A histamine blocker should be given to prevent the development of gastric ulcers.[4]

The emergency nurse needs to remember that the patient with a spinal cord injury has lost the ability to control body temperature. The patient should be kept warm and protected from unnecessary exposure. Warm blankets or a commercial warmer such as a Bear Hugger should be used to keep the patient warm and prevent cold stress, particularly if the patient receives a large amount of intravenous fluids. Fluids should be warmed before administration.

Cervical Tongs and Halo Skeletal Fixation

Unstable cervical fractures may initially be stabilized in the ED with application of cervical tongs, which provide consistent traction and minimize cord compression. Two types currently used are Gardner-Wells tongs (Figure 24-10) and Crutchfield tongs (Figure 24-11).

In some EDs, halo fixation devices are applied, which provide the most rigid immobilization of all cervical orthotic devices and have been used since 1959.[2] A halo device may be used for stabilization of Jefferson (C1) fractures; type III odontoid fractures; type II hangman's fractures (C-2); single-column cervical spine injuries; and management of cervical fractures in patients with ankylosing spondylitis. Halo traction devices are contraindicated when the patient has an unstable skull fracture or traumatized skin where the pins are inserted.

When cervical stabilization is applied in the ED, the emergency nurse may assist with this procedure. The procedure should be explained to the patient, and, if the patient's condition permits, sedation should be administered to decrease anxiety and ensure patient comfort. Box 24-3 summarizes the procedure for the application of a halo device.[2]

Complications related to application of a halo skeletal fixation device include pin loosening, which causes loosening of the crown; infection at the pin site; development of pressure sores; loss of cervical reduction; pin-site swelling; difficulty swallowing; and puncture of the dura.[2] Emergency nurses should be familiar with these complications because patients often come to the ED after discharge with some of these conditions.

PSYCHOSOCIAL CARE

Injury to the spine elicits a tremendous amount of anxiety and fear from both the patient and the family. The major concern of many patients and families is whether the patient will be able to move, walk, or "be the same" again. Unfortunately, this cannot be answered fully in the ED. The emergency nurse's concern should be based upon honesty. All questions should be answered, and all procedures should be explained. The family should be allowed to see the patient as soon as possible and remain there. Care of these patients can be quite challenging. Being truthful from the beginning and focusing care on prevention of further injury are important emergency nursing interventions.

SPINAL CORD INJURIES

Injuries to the spinal cord are the result of primary and secondary injuries. The primary injury is a direct injury from blunt or penetrating forces. Secondary injury is a consequence of vascular changes; the release of catecholamines, endorphins, and enkephalins; lipid peroxidation; lysosomal

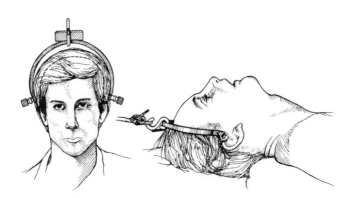

Figure **24-10**   Gardner-Wells tongs. (*From Stauffer ES: In Evarts CM, editor:* Surgery of the musculoskeletal system, *New York, 1983, Churchill Livingstone.*)

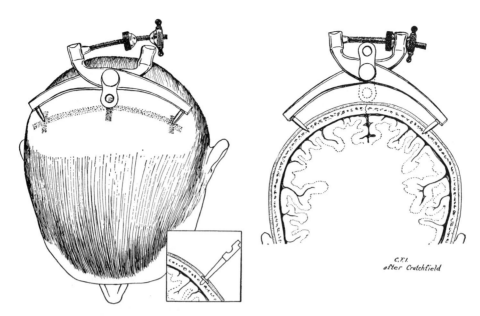

Figure **24-11**   Crutchfield tongs for skeletal traction in fractures or fracture-dislocations of cervical spine. Inset: Special drill constructed with flange that allows it to penetrate outer table only. *(From Crenshaw AH, editor:* Campbell's operative orthopedics, *ed 7, vol 4, St. Louis, 1987, Mosby.)*

Procedure for Application of Halo Traction

1. Determine the ring's crown size by holding it over the crown of the patient's head.
2. Measure the patient's chest circumference to determine the size of the vest.
3. Identify sites for pin insertion on the patient's head. Evaluate for trauma to these areas.
4. Shave pin site areas and cleanse the skin with antiseptic solution.
5. Assist the physician in anesthetizing the pin site area. This is usually done with injection of 1% lidocaine.
6. Administer sedation if the patient's condition permits it.
7. Assist the physician in insertion of the pins.
8. Ensure that the appropriate weight has been added to the traction. Weight may vary from 5-10 lb. depending on stability of the injury or the presence of a dislocation, which must be reduced.
9. Tape tools to the halo vest for emergency use.
10. Obtain cervical spine films after application of the halo device.

From Botte MJ, et al: Halo skeletal fixation: techniques of application and prevention of complications, *Clin Orthop* 239:12-18. 1989.

enzymes; and adenosine triphosphate.[7,10,11] Acute spinal cord injury causes physiologic derangement of the gray and white matter, which decreases oxygen tension, and disrupts vasomotor tone and autoregulation. Injuries to the spinal cord may be complete or incomplete. Injuries of the vertebral column may occur with or without associated spinal cord injury. Figure 24-12 describes specific injuries of the vertebral column.

Complications related to spinal cord injury are related to location of the injury. An injury to the cervical spine puts the patient at risk for pulmonary and ventilatory problems; and injury between T-1 and T-4 causes loss of sympathetic tone. A low-thoracic spine injury causes loss of abdominal muscle functions, decreased respiratory reserves, and gastric distension. Injury to the lumbosacral area of the spinal cord may cause loss of temperature regulation and bowel and bladder function, and the development of decubitus ulcers, and may put the patient at risk for developing deep venous thrombosis and pulmonary emboli.[7]

Spinal Shock

When a complete injury occurs, motor and sensory functions cease below the level of injury. Pain, touch, temperature, and inhalation are evaluated as part of a sensory evaluation. Spinal shock is generally seen with injuries above the T-6 level. Disruption of the sympathetic nervous system causes flaccid paralysis, loss of sphincter tone, bradycardia, and hypotension. Other signs of spinal shock include cool dry skin and bounding peripheral pulses.

If the patient's injury indicates the potential for spinal shock, the emergency team should quickly rule out other potential causes of shock. Blood loss from thoracic and abdominal injuries may be the cause of the patient's shock state, particularly if the patient's spinal cord injury is not the only injury. Management of spinal shock is discussed in the initial management section of this chapter.

Cervical

Jefferson (C-1)	Hangman (C-2)	Odontoid (C-2)

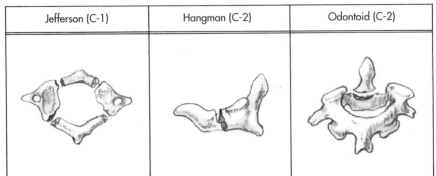

Facet dislocation	Body compression	Burst	Other

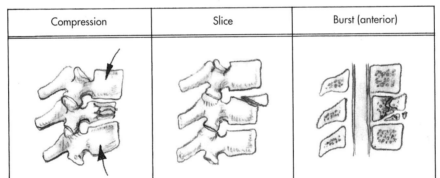

Thoracic/Lumbar

Compression	Slice	Burst (anterior)

Burst (posterior)	Chance	Dislocation	Other

Figure **24-12** Common vertebral column fractures. *(Modified from* Orthopaedic knowledge update—I, *Chicago, 1984, American Academy of Orthopaedic Surgeons.)*

Incomplete Spinal Cord Injury

The most common type of incomplete cord injury is a complete cord lesion with lumbar-root sparing.[15] Other types of incomplete spinal cord lesions are central cord syndrome, anterior cord syndrome, posterior cord syndrome, Brown-Séquard syndrome, and nerve root injuries. Confirmation of an incomplete lesion is based on evaluation of sensory and motor functions as defined by the American Spinal Injury Association.

Central cord syndrome. Central cord syndrome (Figure 24-13) is caused most frequently by hyperextension and is seen most often in elderly patients after a fall. This syndrome causes loss of function in the upper extremities; lower extremity function is not affected. Bowel and bladder function are maintained.

Anterior cord syndrome. Anterior cord syndrome (Figure 24-14) usually results from occlusion of the anterior spinal artery, a herniated nucleus pulposus (rupture disk), or transection of the anterior portion of the cord. The patient has hyperesthesia, hypoalgesia, and incomplete or complete paralysis. The patient is able to feel vibrations and has proprioception because the posterior column is preserved.

Brown-Séquard syndrome. Hemisection of the cord in the anteroposterior plane is known as Brown-Séquard syndrome (Figure 24-15). The most common cause is a penetrating injury such as a gunshot wound or a missile fragment penetration. Brown-Séquard syndrome is characterized by ipsilateral (same side) paresis or hemiplegia and contralateral (opposite side) decreased sensation to pain and changes in temperature. A person can feel one side of the body but not the other, and can move that side but not the other.

Nerve root injuries. Injuries to nerve roots often occur as a result of spinal cord trauma. Common symptoms include hypoalgesia, pain, or referred pain.

Penetrating Injuries

Penetrating injuries to the spinal cord are usually the result of gunshot wounds and stab wounds. The emergency nurse should look for entrance and exit wounds. Presence of cerebral spinal fluid indicates spinal cord perforation. If the missile passes through the abdominal viscera into the spinal cord, the patient is at great risk of central nervous system infection.

If the patient is brought to the ED with the wounding object in place, the emergency nurse should leave the object in place and stabilize it. Bullets and wounding objects are evidence and should be handled carefully.

Swelling from soft tissue injury that may occur with penetrating injury can put the patient in danger of airway obstruction. Soft tissue injury to abdominal and thoracic structures can also produce life-threatening complications in the patient with a penetrating neurologic injury. Many of these patients go to the operating room for resuscitation and stabilization.

Spinal Cord Injury Without Radiographic Abnormality

Spinal cord injury is relatively uncommon in young children because anatomical differences allow for more laxity in the child's neck ligaments. However, more common in the pediatric population than in adults, is a phenomenon called SCIWORA (spinal cord injury without radiographic abnormality). This injury usually occurs at the cervical or thoracic levels of the cord. The child has spinal cord injury with neu-

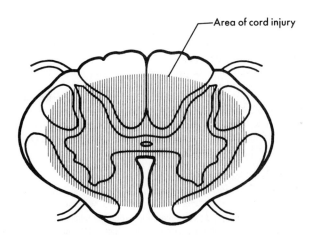

Figure **24-13** Central cord syndrome. *(Modified from Rosen P et al.: Emergency medicine, ed 3, vol 1, St. Louis, 1992, Mosby.)*

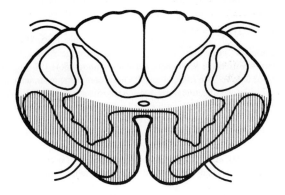

Figure **24-14** Anterior cord syndrome. *(Modified from Rosen P et al.: Emergency medicine, ed 3, vol 1, St. Louis, 1992, Mosby.)*

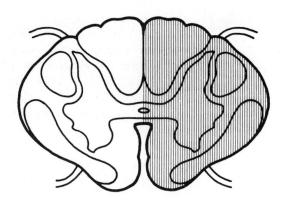

Figure **24-15** Brown-Séquard syndrome. *(Modified from Rosen P et al.: Emergency medicine, ed 3, vol 1, St. Louis, 1992, Mosby.)*

rologic deficits; however, no evidence of bony injury exists. As previously discussed, an MRI has been found invaluable in diagnosing this injury.[11]

Autonomic Dysreflexia

Autonomic dysreflexia is a complication of spinal cord injury above the T-6 level. This life-threatening emergency is seen in patients after spinal shock has resolved. Multiple stimuli below the level of injury can trigger this response. Stimuli include a full bladder, full rectum, or decubitus ulcer. When triggered, the sympathetic nervous system overreacts below the level of the lesion due to a lack of control from higher nerve centers.

Signs and symptoms of autonomic dysreflexia include sudden severe headache, hypertension, sweating, cardiac dysrhythmia (tachycardia or bradycardia), flushing above the level of the injury, and coolness below the level of the injury. The patient may also complain of nasal stuffiness and appear quite anxious.

Treatment of autonomic dysreflexia begins with identifying the cause of the sympathetic response. Assessing for a full bladder or constipation, the nurse can begin to rapidly relieve the problem. Medications that may be administered are ganglionic blockers such as apresoline, or Hypertsat, procardia, and atropine sulfate. All of these drugs must be given cautiously with close monitoring of the patient's blood pressure to prevent a precipitous drop.

Once the emergency is over, the emergency nurse should work with the patient and family to develop interventions to prevent another occurrence.[19]

CONCLUSION

Spinal trauma is not as common as other types of injury, but its consequences are devastating. It affects approximately 200,000 people each year and is extremely expensive.[5,17] Patients are generally young and require extensive physical and psychosocial care. Emergency care of these patients involves resuscitation and rehabilitation to decrease and prevent further injury to the spinal cord. Box 24-4 identifies pertinent nursing diagnoses for the patient with spinal cord injury.

Current research focuses on treating the effects of any secondary injuries that occur with spinal cord damage. Drugs presently being evaluated include B-glycosides, growth factors, Ginkgo biloba, and thyroid releasing hormone (TRH).[1,10,16] Other experimental research is looking at cord transplantation and early surgical decompression.[1,12] The most successful way to lessen spinal trauma is prevention. Use of seat belts, helmets, and other safety devices are some methods used to prevent spinal injury. Teaching children, adolescents, and adults the consequences of risky behavior such as snow boarding may eventually help decrease the uncommon but lamentable consequences of this injury.

REFERENCES

1. Bernstein JJ, Goldberg WJ: Experimental spinal cord transplantation as a mechanism of spinal cord regeneration, *Paraplegia* 33(5):250-253, 1995.
2. Botte MJ, et al.: Halo skeletal fixation: Techniques of application and prevention of complications, *Clin Orthop* 239:12-18, 1989.
3. Bracken MB, Shepard MJ, Collins WF: A randomized, controlled trial of methylprednisolone or naloxone in the treatment of acute spinal cord injury: Results of the Second National Acute Spinal Cord Injury Study, *New Engl J Med* 322:1405-1411, 1990.
4. Chiles BW, Cooper PR: Acute spinal injury, *New Engl J Med* 334(8):514-520, 1996.
5. Devivo MJ, Ivie CS: Life expectancy of ventilator-dependent persons with spinal cord injuries, *Chest* 108(1):226-232, 1995.
6. George E, et al.: Failure of methylprednisolone to improve the outcome of spinal cord injuries, *Am Surg* 61:659-664, 1995.
7. Hickey R, Sloan T, Albino M: Acute spinal cord trauma. In Shoemaker WC, et al., editors: *Textbook of critical care,* pp 1457-1465, Philadelphia, 1995, WB Saunders.
8. Jacobs B, Baker P: *Trauma nursing core course,* Park Ridge, Ill, 1995, Emergency Nurses Association.
9. Jaworski M, Wirtz K: Spinal trauma. In Kitt S, et al., editors: *Emergency nursing* pp 357-376, Philadelphia, 1995, WB Saunders.
10. Koc RK, et al.: Lipid perioxidation in experimental spinal cord injury: Comparison of treatment with Ginkgo biloba, TRH, and methylprednisolone, *Res Exp Med* 195(2):117-123, 1995.
11. Medina FA: Neck and spinal cord trauma. In Barkin R, editor: *Pediatric emergency medicine,* pp 230-260, St. Louis, 1992, Mosby.
12. Pettijean ME, et al.: Thoracic spinal trauma and associated injuries: should early spinal decompression be considered? *J Trauma* 39(2):368-372, 1995.
13. Sanders MJ: *Mosby's paramedic textbook,* St. Louis, 1995, Mosby.
14. Schroder RJ, et al.: Comparison of the diagnostic value of CT and MRI in injuries of the cervical vertebrae, *Aktuelle Radiologie* 5(4):197-202, 1995.
15. Spivak JM, Vaccaro AR, Colter JM: Thoracolumbar spine trauma: evaluation and classification, *J Am Acad Orthop Surg* 3(6):345-352, 1995.
16. Spivak JM, Vaccaro AR, Colter JM: Thoracolumbar spine trauma: principles of management, *J Am Acad Orthop Surg* 3(6):353-360, 1995.
17. Spoltore TA, O'Brien AM: Rehabilitation of the spinal cord injured patient, *Orthop Nurs* 14(3):7-14, 1995.
18. Thurman DJ, et al.: Risk factors and mechanisms of occurrence in motor vehicle-related spinal cord injuries, Utah, *Accid Anal Prev* 27(3):411-5, 1995.
19. Walleck C: Central nervous system II, Spinal cord injury. In Cardona V, et al., editors: *Trauma nursing,* ed 2 pp 435-465, Philadelphia, 1994, WB Saunders.

Box **24-4**

NURSING DIAGNOSES FOR SPINAL CORD INJURY

Ineffective airway clearance
Impaired gas exchange
Ineffective breathing pattern
Risk for aspiration
High risk for injury, secondary to injury of spinal cord
Ineffective thermoregulation
Fluid and volume deficit
High risk for impaired skin integrity
Impaired verbal communication
Ineffective individual coping
Anticipatory grieving

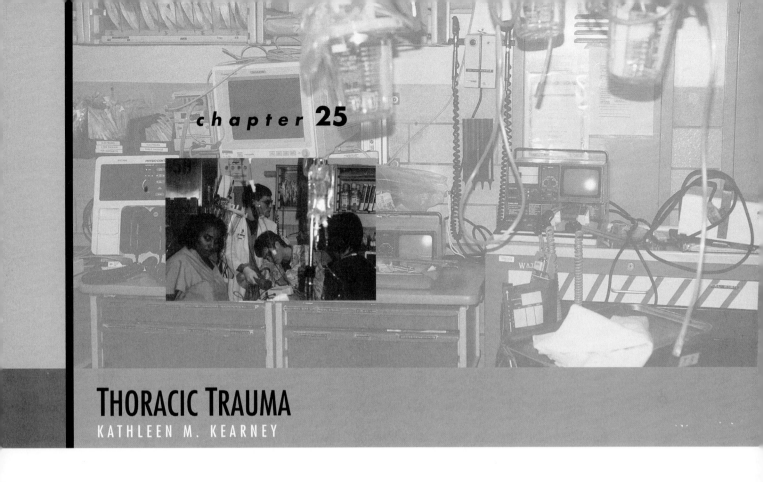

chapter 25

THORACIC TRAUMA

KATHLEEN M. KEARNEY

Thoracic trauma, whether blunt or penetrating, affects structures and organs within the thoracic cavity, an area that extends from the top of the sternum to the diaphragm. Thoracic trauma accounts for 20% to 25% of trauma deaths and is a contributing factor in an additional 25%.[14]

Thoracic injury and treatment has been described for centuries; however, not until the end of World War II did a chest tube connected to underwater seal drainage become standard treatment for many thoracic injuries.[43] Endotracheal intubation, anesthesia, and chest roentgenography, developed in the nineteenth and early twentieth centuries, as well as advances in the past 50 years such as improved ventilatory assistance, antibiotics, blood gas analysis, and specialized nursing care have increased survival in patients with thoracic injuries.[43] Despite the ability to diagnose and treat many previously fatal thoracic injuries, thoracic trauma remains the second leading cause of death in trauma victims preceded only by injuries to the brain and spinal cord.

Thoracic trauma may be caused by blunt or penetrating mechanisms. Blunt injuries are caused by motor vehicle crashes, falls, crush events, and assaults. Gunshot wounds and stab wounds account for most penetrating injuries, although impalement injuries are also implicated. Burns caused by thermal energy, electricity, or radiation may also damage the thorax.

Approximately 70% of thoracic injuries are due to blunt trauma sustained in motor vehicle crashes.[6] With blunt trauma, energy is transferred to the thorax and underlying structures through forces that are unidirectional, compressive, indirect, acceleration/deceleration or explosive. Extent of injury depends on the magnitude, direction, and duration of applied energy and the anatomic area to which energy is being directed.[29]

Penetrating trauma causes injury in different ways. Stab wounds are low velocity, so injury is localized to the weapon's path. Characteristics of the weapon used (i.e., length, width, sharpness) and what the assailant does once the weapon impacts the victim (i.e, twists or pulls the knife out) determine severity of injury. With impaling injuries, speed and how the victim impacts the object, such as landing on a fencepost while trying to jump over versus falling 20 feet onto the fencepost, determine severity. Gunshot wounds create temporary and permanent cavities along the path of the bullet. Permanent cavities are due to direct damage from the bullet, whereas, temporary cavities occur because tissue stretches radially as the bullet passes through the body. Tissue damage caused by a gunshot wound depends on the type of gun and type of bullet. Bullets with hollow or soft points cause more damage because they expand or fragment on impact and increase the size of the permanent cavity. High-velocity weapons cause more extensive damage because tissue is stretched more along the bullet path causing a larger temporary cavity. The full extent of an anatomic injury may be difficult to ascertain because of bullet ricochet off internal structures. Bullets may also damage bone, causing fragments that act as missiles and worsen injuries.

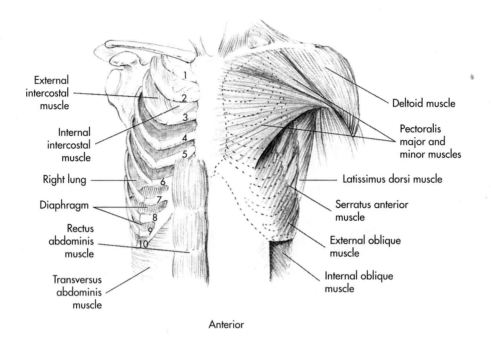

External
intercostal
muscle

Internal
intercostal
muscle

Right lung

Diaphragm

Rectus
abdominis
muscle

Transversus
abdominis
muscle

Deltoid muscle

Pectoralis
major and
minor muscles

Latissimus dorsi muscle

Serratus anterior
muscle

External oblique
muscle

Internal oblique
muscle

Anterior

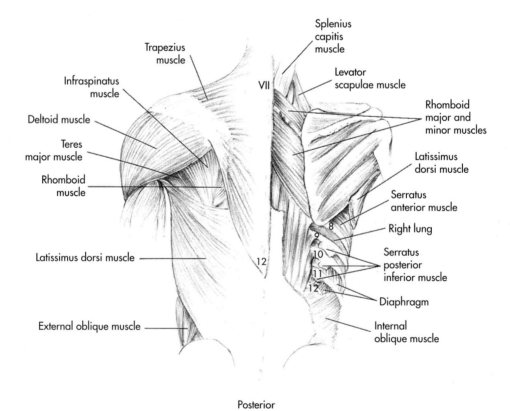

Trapezius
muscle

Infraspinatus
muscle

Deltoid muscle

Teres
major muscle

Rhomboid
muscle

Latissimus dorsi muscle

External oblique muscle

Splenius
capitis
muscle

Levator
scapulae muscle

Rhomboid
major and
minor muscles

Latissimus
dorsi muscle

Serratus
anterior muscle

Right lung

Serratus
posterior
inferior muscle

Diaphragm

Internal
oblique muscle

Posterior

Figure **25-1** Bony structure of the chest wall and the anterior and posterior musculature. *(From Davis JH, et al.:* Clinical surgery, *St. Louis, 1987, Mosby.)*

Thoracic trauma requires systematic assessment for potentially lethal injuries followed by rapid intervention. This chapter discusses assessment and treatment of various thoracic injuries. A brief discussion of anatomy and physiology is provided to enhance understanding of essential information.

ANATOMY AND PHYSIOLOGY

The thoracic cavity skeleton includes the sternum, ribs, costal cartilages, and thoracic vertebrae (Figure 25-1). Fairly mobile, the thorax expands easily to facilitate respiratory efforts. Ribs attach posteriorly to thoracic vertebrae and anteriorly to the sternum. Seven upper ribs are joined directly to costal cartilages, whereas ribs 8 to 10 interface indirectly with the sternum through fusion of costal cartilage. Ribs 11 and 12 do not interface with the sternum. The diaphragm forms the inferior border of the thorax while the superior border is continuous with structures of the neck.

Internal thoracic structures are composed of organs and structures of the pulmonary, cardiovascular, and the gastrointestinal systems (Figure 25-2). Pulmonary structures are located in the pleural space, whereas cardiovascular and gastrointestinal structures are located in the mediastinum, a cavity between the two pleural spaces.

Pulmonary System

Lungs are cone-shaped organs above the diaphragm that extend approximately 1.5 inches above the clavicles. Each lung is located in a cavity lined with a serous membrane called the pleura. The *visceral pleura* covers the lungs themselves; *parietal pleura* covers the rib cage, diaphragm, and pericardium. A potential space between these layers is the pleural cavity. Pleural cells secrete *pleural fluid,* which separates the lungs but allows membranes to remain in contact and move without creating friction.

Normal breathing occurs through the processes of ventilation (Figure 25-3), which moves air in and out of the lungs, and respiration, which exchanges gases across alveolar capillary membranes. During inspiration, phrenic nerve stimulation causes the diaphragm to contract and pull downward. As the diaphragm pulls downward, external intercostals pull the chest wall out, which enlarges the thoracic cavity. As lung capacity increases, intrathoracic pressure becomes negative (i.e., lower than atmospheric pressure). This negative intrathoracic pressure draws air into the lungs. During expiration, this process is reversed as the diaphragm relaxes and moves up. Intercostal muscles compress the chest so that the lungs recoil passively. Intrathoracic pressure becomes more positive as lung capacity diminishes. Increasing positive intrathoracic pressure forces air out of the lungs.[2,32]

Cardiovascular System

The heart is located in the mediastinum, positioned with the right ventricle anteriorly beneath the sternum. The pericardium, a three-layered sac that surrounds and protects the heart, is a fibrous envelope separated from the heart by the pericardial space, a potential space between the parietal pericardium and the visceral pericardium, or *epicardium.* The heart's middle layer is the *endocardium,* and the inner muscular layer is the *myocardium.* The pericardium contains pericardial fluid (5 to 30 ml), which prevents friction during

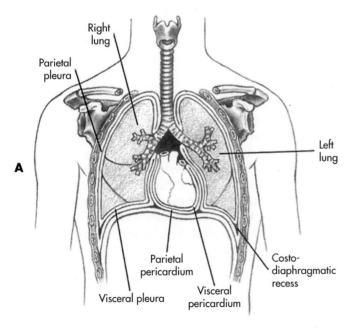
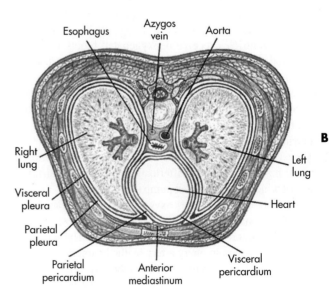

Figure **25-2** Chest cavity and related structures. **A,** Anterior view. **B,** Cross section. *(From Thompson JM, et al.: Mosby's clinical nursing, ed 4, St. Louis, 1997, Mosby.)*

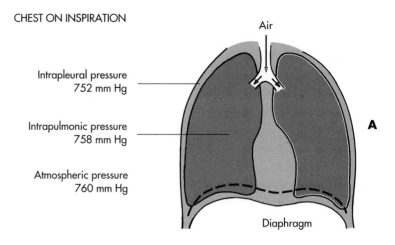

CHEST ON INSPIRATION

Air

Intrapleural pressure
752 mm Hg

Intrapulmonic pressure
758 mm Hg

Atmospheric pressure
760 mm Hg

Diaphragm

A

Figure **25-3** **A,** Contraction of diaphragm increases vertical dimensions of lungs. **B,** Relaxation of diaphragm decreases vertical dimensions of lungs. *(From Wade JF: Comprehensive respiratory care, ed 3, St. Louis, 1982, Mosby.)*

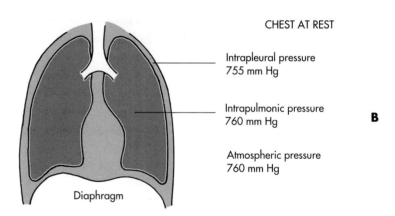

CHEST AT REST

Intrapleural pressure
755 mm Hg

Intrapulmonic pressure
760 mm Hg

Atmospheric pressure
760 mm Hg

Diaphragm

B

contraction. The outer parietal pericardium is the fibrous pericardium, which attaches to the sternum, great vessels, and diaphragm to hold the heart in place.

Four muscular chambers, called atria and ventricles, contract rhythmically as they fill and empty with blood. The right atria and ventricles receive deoxygenated blood and pump the blood to the lungs for oxygenation. Oxygenated blood then enters the left side of the heart, which sends blood to the systemic circulation. The left heart is a high-pressure system, the right heart a low-pressure system. Valves separate chambers to prevent regurgitation of blood back into the atria and ventricles. Cardiac function and output depend on contractility, heart rate, preload (volume achieved during diastolic filling of the ventricles), and afterload (the force, or resistance, against which the heart must pump to eject blood).

The thoracic aorta carries oxygenated blood to various tissues. Three anatomical parts of the aorta are recognized: ascending aorta, aortic arch, and descending aorta. The aortic arch is attached to the pulmonary artery by the ligamentum arteriosum. Near the ligamentum, a portion of the aorta branches off to form the left subclavian artery. At this point of the aorta, just distal to the ligamentum, the aorta is relatively immobile and is at increased risk for disruption. Over 85% of aortic injuries caused by acceleration/deceleration forces occur here.[19]

Also in the mediastinum is the trachea posterior to the heart, the esophagus posterior to the trachea, the phrenic nerve, and the diaphragm. Other thoracic cavity structures include the thymus gland in the anterior mediastinum behind the sternum, the esophagus, and subclavian and common carotid arteries.

PATIENT ASSESSMENT

The patient with an obvious or suspected thoracic injury must be promptly assessed since these injuries can produce death within minutes. Rapid assessment of airway, breathing, and circulation (ABC) followed by rapid, essential interventions is paramount. Control of the cervical spine occurs simultaneously with assessment of the patient's airway. Breathing rate, depth, and effort are assessed after airway patency is ensured. If an open chest wound is present, a three-sided occlusive dressing should be applied. Vaseline gauze, defibrillator pads, or gauze taped on three sides are all effective. After the dressing is applied, the patient must be monitored for development of tension pneumothorax. Supplemental oxygen should be administered with a nonrebreather mask at 100% or bag-valve mask as appropriate. Circulation is assessed by palpating pulse rate and character. Obvious bleeding is controlled with direct pressure and fluid resuscitation.

Box **25-1** **Initial Assessment of Thoracic Trauma**

Airway with C-spine control, *Breathing, Circulation*
Bilateral breath sounds
Respiratory stridor
Tracheal deviation
Sucking chest wounds
Subcutaneous emphysema
Distended neck veins
Paradoxical chest wall movement
Upper abdominal injury
Shortness of breath
Cyanosis
Skin color and temperature
Wound size and location
Intercostal and accessory muscle use
Heart sounds
Vital signs

Box **25-2** **Additional Assessment of Thoracic Trauma**

Assess pain
Obtain patient history
Identify mechanism of injury
Determine time of the injury
Determine what the patient remembers about the event

Box **25-3** **Therapeutic Interventions for Thoracic Trauma**

Maintain patent airway
Promote adequate ventilation
Provide high-flow oxygen
Cover open chest wound
Assist with chest tube insertion or needle decompression
Monitor bleeding from chest
Initiate two large-bore intravenous lines
Facilitate essential radiographs—cervical spine, chest, and pelvis
Monitor cardiac rhythm continuously
Monitor blood pressure, respiratory rate and effort, pulse oximetry, and level of consciousness every hour or more often if indicated by patient condition.
Document urine output and patient response to therapeutic interventions

---

Two large-bore intravenous lines should be started using lactated Ringer's or other appropriate crystalloid solution. Box 25-1 highlights an initial assessment of a patient with thoracic trauma; Box 25-2 presents additional assessment data that should be obtained during the secondary assessment. Therapeutic interventions are listed in Box 25-3.

SPECIFIC THORACIC INJURIES

Thoracic injuries include injuries of the chest wall, pulmonary system, cardiovascular system, and esophagus. Acuity is determined by the effect of the injury on ventilation and circulation. Figure 25-4 compares normal ventilatory movement seen in the presence of a sucking chest wound with that seen in flail chest.

Chest Wall Injuries

Rib fractures. The exact incidence of rib fractures is unknown, but experts estimate a regional trauma center can expect 10% of all trauma admissions to have rib fractures.[46] The most common mechanism of injury associated with rib fractures is a motor vehicle crash.

Rib fractures may occur in a single rib or multiple ribs. Fractures occur most often in the fourth through tenth ribs and are not themselves considered life-threatening. Rib fractures result from a direct or indirect blunt force or crush injuries. The patient often has tenderness and shallow respirations to avoid moving the chest wall. Subcutaneous emphysema or crepitus may also be present. Radiographs assist with diagnosis; but are only 70% accurate for rib fractures.[46] Fractures that separate the sternum from costal cartilage are not evident on a radiograph.

Treatment for most rib fractures is analgesia and good pulmonary toilet. Pain management is essential because even one or two rib fractures can result in disability from pain.[29] Oral or intravenous analgesia are used for many patients; however, intercostal nerve blocks may be appropriate for some patients.

Good pulmonary toilet, such as coughing and deep breathing, are used to prevent complications including pneumonia or atelectasis. Incentive spirometry may also be used. Patients with multiple rib fractures are usually admitted for observation. Those with severe injuries (8 or more fractured ribs, massive flail injury) may require internal fixation with plates and screws.[20] First and second ribs are well protected by the clavicle, so a significant blunt force is required to fracture these ribs. Great vessel injuries should be considered when the first or second rib is fractured. Other injuries associated with upper rib fractures are injuries to the clavicles, scapulae, trachea, and lungs. Lower rib fractures (9 through 12) are associated with injuries to the spleen, liver, or other abdominal contents, depending on location of the fracture(s).

Rib fractures in an elderly patient are a particular risk for complications because of diminished vital capacity that occurs with aging. Impaired ventilation worsens in all patients during the first few days after injury secondary to increasing chest wall edema and decreasing compliance. In an elderly patient with a rib injury and diminished capacity, serial assessment is essential to prevent complications. Patients with decreased pulmonary function from asthma or COPD also require careful assessment since vital capacity in this population is also decreased.

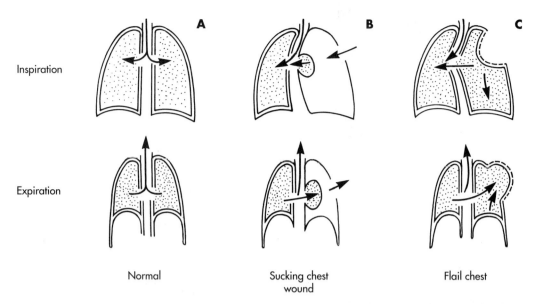

Figure **25-4** Comparison of ventilatory movement in normal and injured chest. *(From Johnson J, Kirby CK:* Surgery of the chest, *ed 4, Chicago, 1970, Year Book Medical.)*

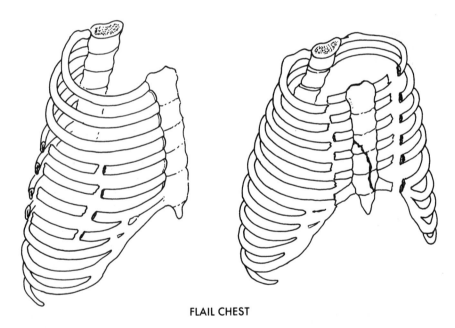

FLAIL CHEST

Figure **25-5** Fracture of several adjacent ribs in two places with lateral flail or central flail segments. *(From Rosen, et al.:* Emergency medicine, *ed 3, vol 1, St. Louis, 1992, Mosby.)*

Children have thin chest walls, and their bony thorax is more pliable. Consequently, energy is easily transmitted to underlying thoracic structures without fracturing ribs. When rib fractures do occur in children, concurrent thoracic and abdominal injuries may be severe.[18]

Flail chest. A flail chest is defined as fractures in two or more adjacent ribs in two or more places, or bilateral detachment of the sternum from the costal cartilage (Figure 25-5). Flail chest is usually associated with a massive crush injury or a high-speed motor vehicle crash. This injury creates a free-floating, unstable segment that moves in opposition to normal chest wall movement (Figure 25-6). The flail segment moves in when the patient inspires and out with exhalation. A flail chest causes hypoventilation of both lungs followed by atelectasis and eventually hypoxia. The injury is usually associated with an underlying pulmonary contusion that worsens the injury due to loss of compliance, increased airway resistance, and decreased gas diffusion.[27]

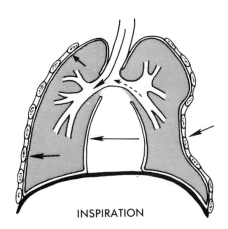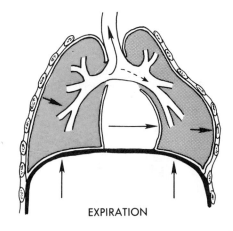

INSPIRATION   EXPIRATION

Figure **25-6** Chest wall movement with flail chest. On inspiration, flail section sinks in as chest expands, impairing ability to produce negative intrapleural pressure to draw in air. Mediastinum shifts to uninjured side. On expiration, flail segment bulges outward, impairing ability to exhale. Mediastinum shifts to injured side. Air may shift uselessly from side to side in severe flail chest (broken lines). *(From Rosen et al:* Emergency medicine, *ed 3, vol 1, St. Louis, 1992, Mosby.)*

Diagnosis of flail chest is usually made by direct observation. The affected area moves paradoxically from the rest of the chest. However, muscular splinting of the chest immediately after injury may mask a flail chest until hours later when muscles become fatigued and paradoxic movement becomes obvious.[1,6,27] With flail chest, the thorax moves in an uncoordinated manner, so air movement is extremely poor. Palpation of the chest wall indicates abnormal motion and crepitus. The patient complains of pain and difficulty breathing. Radiographs may not be helpful since costochondral separation may not appear. Arterial blood gas values reflecting respiratory failure ($O_2 < 60$ mm Hg and $CO_2 > 45$ mm Hg on room air) aid in diagnosis.[1,33]

Treatment consists of ensuring adequate oxygenation, administering fluids carefully, and providing pain relief with intercostal nerve blocks. Fluids are limited due to associated pulmonary contusion and potential development of adult respiratory distress syndrome (ARDS). Intubation and mechanical ventilation is not required for all patients, but patients should be monitored carefully for any change in respiratory status that indicates a need for more aggressive management (i.e., changes in respiratory rate, arterial oxygen tension, and work of breathing).[1] Patients who require mechanical ventilation are usually managed with continuous positive end expiratory pressure. Continuous positive airway pressure may be used for some patients.

Sternal fracture. Sternal fractures occur when tremendous force is applied to the chest, as with a steering wheel impact. The most common site of fracture is the junction of the manubrium and body of the sternum.[6] In addition to pain, a sternal fracture has significant potential for underlying cardiac injury including myocardial contusion and pericardial tamponade.

The patient may experience dyspnea and localized pain with movement, and may hypoventilate to avoid chest wall movement. Chest wall ecchymosis, sternal deformity, or crepitus may also occur. Treatment includes pain relief, a baseline electrocardiogram (ECG), and serial patient examinations. If the fracture is displaced, operative reduction may be required.[20] If cardiac symptoms are present, an echocardiogram may be obtained to check for cardiac tamponade. Otherwise, patients are treated symptomatically.

Pulmonary Injuries

Laryngeal injury. Fracture of the larynx is a rare, life-threatening injury.[19,20,28] Common mechanisms of injury include striking the anterior neck on the steering wheel or dashboard, karate blows, or "clothesline" injuries when a snowmobiler or motorcycle rider hits a clothesline, wire, or tree limb with direct anterior neck impact.[28] The patient presents with hoarseness, subcutaneous emphysema, and crepitus. Injury is suggested with a history of blunt trauma to the neck; however, initial diagnosis may be difficult if initial presentation is subtle, such as local tenderness or crepitus. A lateral soft tissue radiograph of the neck or a CT scan may be necessary to confirm diagnosis. Intubation is indicated for the patient with severe respiratory distress or complete obstruction. In cases where intubation is hampered by the injury itself, tracheostomy is recommended.[1,45] Cricothyrotomy is usually performed in the ED, with tracheostomy reserved for operative management.

Penetrating trauma to the larynx is readily apparent and requires immediate surgical intervention. Associated injuries to the carotid artery or jugular vein may occur. Penetrating missile injuries have been associated with extensive tissue destruction related to the blast effect.[1] Injury to the cervical spine must also be considered in any patient with an injury to the neck.

Tracheal injury. Trauma to the trachea may be blunt or penetrating; mechanisms of injury are often the same as for laryngeal injuries. Blunt injuries can be subtle or acute. Noisy breathing may be the only indication of partial obstruction, whereas absent breathing suggests complete obstruction. If the patient has an altered level of consciousness, diagnosis is more difficult. Diagnostic evaluation includes bronchoscopy, a CT scan, and laryngoscopy. Treatment includes operative interventions for severe blunt or penetrating injuries. Less acute injuries may be managed with intubation or tracheostomy.

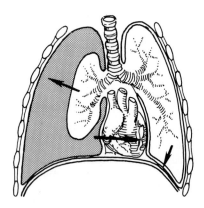

Figure **25-7** Closed pneumothorax. Simple pneumothorax is present in right lung with air in pleural cavity and collapse of right lung. *(From Rosen et al: Emergency medicine, ed 3, vol 1, St. Louis, 1992, Mosby.)*

Bronchial injury. Major bronchial injuries are unusual and often overlooked.[1,28] Blunt trauma to the chest that causes bronchial injury has a high mortality because of a delayed or missed diagnosis of the injury.[28] Stab wounds or gunshot wounds of the bronchus are often identified during an operation performed for other reasons. Many patients die at the scene of the accident.[1] Most injuries occur within 1 inch of the carina. Signs and symptoms include hemoptysis, subcutaneous emphysema, mediastinal crunch (Hamman's sign), or tension pneumothorax with mediastinal shift. With bronchial disruption into both pleural spaces, bilateral tension pneumothoraces have occurred. The patient may present with dyspnea, tachycardia, and diminished or absent breath sounds. Persistent emphysema or air leak following chest tube insertion should increase the index of suspicion for this injury; bronchoscopy confirms the diagnosis. Treatment may be limited to airway support until inflammation and edema resolve; however, surgical intervention is required for patients with a significant tear.

Pneumothorax. Pneumothorax refers to accumulation of air in the pleural space resulting in a partial or complete collapse of the lung as intrapleural pressure is lost (Figure 25-7). Pneumothorax may be due to blunt or penetrating injuries. The laceration of lung tissue, often associated with

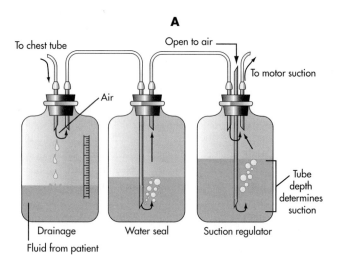

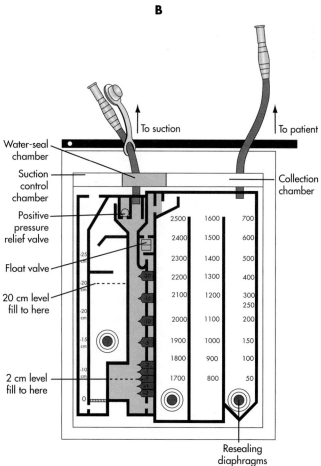

Figure **25-8** Chest tubes and chest tube drainage systems. **A,** Three-bottle water-seal suction. Bottle I is drainage bottle. Vertical piece of tape should be applied to outer surface of drainage bottle. Time and fluid level should be marked hourly on tape. Bottle II is water-seal bottle. Bottle III is suction control bottle. Length of glass tube below water surface determines amount of suction. **B,** Pleurevac disposable chest suction system. *(From Lewis SM, Collier IC, Heitkemper MM: Medical-surgical nursing: assessment and management of clinical problems, ed 4, St. Louis, 1996, Mosby.)*

rib fractures and subsequent air leak, is the most common cause of pneumothorax with blunt trauma.

A patient with a pneumothorax complains of chest pain and shortness of breath. Auscultation of the lung on the injured side shows decreased or absent breath sounds; percussion demonstrates hyperresonance. Normal breath sounds can occur as a result of resonance within the thoracic cavity. Tachycardia and tachypnea are usually present. If air accumulates in the mediastinum, a crunching sound called *Hamman's crunch* occurs. With each contraction the heart beats against air trapped between the heart and chest wall. Radiographs aid diagnosis of pneumothorax.

Pneumothorax is treated with chest tube placement in the fourth or fifth intercostal space, along the anterior axillary line.[1] The chest tube is connected to an underwater drainage system with suction attached to facilitate lung reexpansion. Box 25-4 identifies essential components for chest drainage systems and discusses general nursing implications. Figure 25-8 illustrates a typical chest drainage system. A radiograph following tube placement is done to confirm tube placement and lung reexpansion. The patient is positioned upright after tube placement to prevent pressure forming from abdominal organs against the diaphragm. High-flow oxygen is continued.

Open pneumothorax. Open pneumothorax, or "sucking chest wound," occurs when an opening in the chest is more than two thirds the diameter of the trachea. Air preferentially moves into the chest through the chest wall rather than through the trachea. The injury is usually a result of penetrating trauma to the chest wall; however, blunt trauma may also cause an open chest wound. An open chest wound causes loss of intrathoracic pressure (Figure 25-9). As the patient breathes, air is drawn into the chest but cannot escape. Pressure increases, and a tension pneumothorax may develop. The patient has chest pain, shortness of breath, and may be hypotensive. Breath sounds may be decreased or absent on the affected side, and a "sucking" sound may be heard with each breath. Bubbles often occur around the wound as air escapes through the blood. Immediate treatment consists of placing a sterile, nonporous, three-sided occlusive dressing over the injury. Taping three sides allows air to escape but prevents air from entering the wound. After placement of this dressing, the patient should be carefully monitored for tension pneumothorax. If a tension pneumothorax develops, the taped dressing must be removed immediately, with chest tube insertion to follow. Definitive treatment of the open chest wound is operative closure.

Tension pneumothorax. Tension pneumothorax is a life-threatening condition that occurs when accumulation of air in one pleural space forces thoracic contents to the opposite side of the chest (Figure 25-10). Initial lung injury allows air into the pleural space with inspiration; however, air cannot

---

Box **25-4** **Chest Drainage Systems—Components and Management**

Fluid collection chamber

Fluid drains from the patient through a long tube to a collection chamber, marked for assessment of drainage.

Water seal chamber

Allows air to pass out via bubbles through the bottom of the chamber. Often calibrated for measuring intrathoracic pressure, may have float valve to protect patient from high negativity.

Suction control chamber

Improves drainage and helps overcome the air leak. Keep suction control at 10 to 20 cm H_2O. Works by adding or removing water from the chamber with a regulator that adjusts to negative pressure changes, suction source or patient variations, and through a restrictive orifice mechanism that adjusts the opening to increase or decrease pressure.

Nursing responsibilities

Secure all connections. Monitor catheters to prevent kinking. Monitor drainage output. Assess for air leaks. Maintain unit in upright position. Monitor intrathoracic pressure.

Assessing for air leaks

Look at underwater seal. Leak may originate with the patient or the drainage system. For a patient receiving mechanical ventilation with positive end expiratory pressure (PEEP), leaking causes continuous bubbling. Clamp chest tube at the dressing site with a toothless clamp. If bubbling stops, leak is from the lung. If bubbling continues, leak is distal to the clamp. Move clamp incrementally toward the drainage unit. If bubbling stops before the end of the tubing, leak is in the tube so tube must be replaced. If the unit is still bubbling when the very end of the tubing is clamped, the unit has the leak and should be changed.

Indications of patency

Water level in the water seal should fluctuate with breathing, rising with inspiration and falling with expiration, and is an indicator of chest tube patency. If the patient is on mechanical ventilation, this pattern is reversed because breaths are delivered under positive pressure. Fluctuations stop when the lung is fully reexpanded, or when the tube is kinked or compressed.

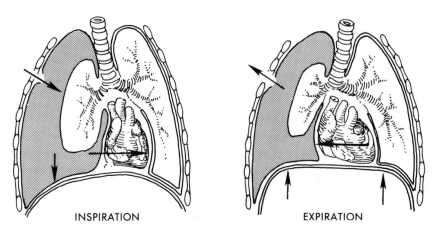

INSPIRATION   EXPIRATION

Figure **25-9**   Open pneumothorax. Collapse of right lung and air in pleural cavity occurs with communication to outside through defect in chest wall. In sucking chest wound, lung volume is greater with expiration. *(From Rosen, et al.:* Emergency medicine, *ed 3, vol 1, St. Louis, 1992, Mosby.)*

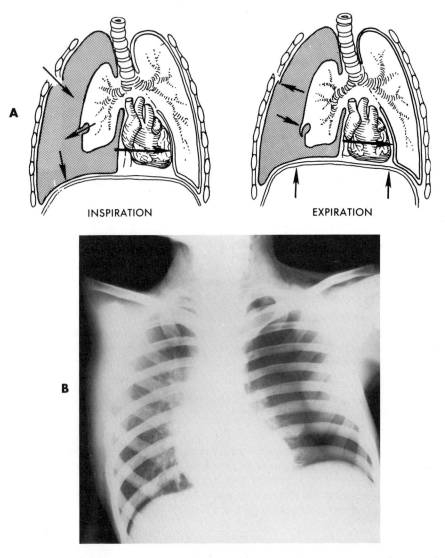

INSPIRATION   EXPIRATION

Figure **25-10**   **A,** Tension pneumothorax. Right pneumothorax under tension, total collapse of right lung, and shift of mediastinal structures to left. **B,** Radiograph of left tension pneumothorax with shift of mediastinal structures to right. Note subcutaneous emphysema in soft tissues of neck. *(From Rosen, et al.:* Emergency medicine, *ed 3, vol 1, St. Louis, 1992, Mosby.)*

escape with expiration. Air continues to accumulate, and intrathoracic pressure increases, forcing thoracic contents away from the injured side. Eventually, the lung on the opposite side, the heart, and great vessels are compressed as mediastinal shift occurs. Auscultation shows decreased or absent breath sounds on the affected side and possibly decreased sounds on the unaffected side as the lung is compressed. If the patient is alert and able to speak, he or she may complain of chest pain, severe shortness of breath, and a feeling of impending doom. Compression of the heart causes cardiac dysrhythmia, decreases diastolic filling, and decreases cardiac output. Vena cava compression impairs venous return to the heart, which worsens diastolic filling and decreases cardiac output. Neck vein distension occurs as venous return is impaired by compression of the heart; however, neck veins may remain flat if concurrent hypovolemia exists. The trachea eventually deviates to the unaffected side as mediastinal shift worsens.

Immediate needle decompression of the affected side is required. A 14- or 16-gauge catheter is inserted into the second intercostal space at the midclavicular line or fifth intercostal space at the anterior axillary line on the injured side. Definitive therapy is chest tube insertion.

Hemothorax. A hemothorax, free blood in the pleural space (Figure 25-11), results from bleeding lung parenchyma, heart and major vessel injury, or injury to internal mammary arteries. The most common cause is an injury to the intercostal arteries, which causes bleeding into the pleural space.[20] In addition to chest pain, shortness of breath, and decreased or absent breath sounds on the affected side, the patient has dullness on chest percussion. Signs and symptoms of hypovolemic shock are often present because of the limited capacity of the pleural space. Treatment includes chest tube insertion, usually size 32F or 36F in an adult, high-flow oxygen by a nonrebreather mask, and large-bore intravenous lines for fluid replacement. Chest drainage

should be carefully monitored to assess the need for possible autotransfusion. If blood return with chest tube insertion is ≥1000 to 1500 ml, or blood loss is >200 to 300 ml/hr, surgical intervention may be indicated.

Autotransfusion. Autotransfusion, collecting and reinfusing the patient's own blood, is a valuable tool during resuscitation of select hypovolemic trauma victims. Blood shed into the thoracic cavity can be easily collected and infused. Significant intrathoracic blood loss (>350 ml) and wounds that are ≤4 to 6 hr old are indications for potential autotransfusion.[1,6] Autotransfusion is also useful when homologous blood is not available, or the patient's religious convictions forbid homologous transfusion. Box 25-5 highlights specific advantages and disadvantages of autotransfusion. Autotransfusion is not appropriate when enteric contamination has occurred, (e.g., ruptured diaphragm).

Autotransfusion requires a chest drainage unit and an autotransfusion device. An anticoagulant may be added before blood collection to prevent clotting during the collection phase and plugging of the blood filter and intravenous line during reinfusion. Anticoagulant Citrate Dextrose Solution-A (ACD-A) and Citrate Phosphate Dextrose (CPD) are the most common anticoagulants used. Serial assessment of laboratory values must be performed to monitor the patient response to autotransfusion and to the anticoagulants.

Pulmonary contusion. Pulmonary contusion is the most common, potentially lethal chest injury seen in North America.[1] Almost 75% of patients with blunt chest trauma have a

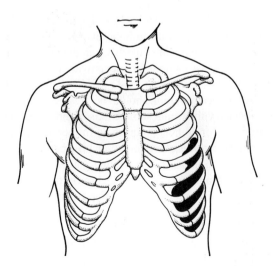

Figure **25-11** Hemothorax. *(From Sheehy SB, Jimmerson CL: Manual of clinical trauma care, ed 2, St. Louis, 1994, Mosby.)*

Box 25-5	**Advantages and Disadvantages of Autotransfusion[2,18]**

Advantages

- Blood is immediately available
- Lower cost compared to banked blood
- No risk of transfusion reaction
- No risk of blood-borne pathogens
- Potential psychologic comfort for the patient
- Normothermic
- Near-normal electrolytes and pH
- Near-normal clotting factors
- Greater oxygen carrying capacity
- RBC half-life near normal

Disadvantages

- Depends on user competence with collection device
- Potential for air embolism exists with reinfusion if air is not removed from collection bag
- Sepsis possible if enteric contamination occurs.
- Coagulopathies may develop because of dilution of clotting factors when the amount of blood transfused is ≥25%-50% of total blood volume
- Citrate toxicity occurs with large doses of citrate
- Blood trauma and hemolysis

pulmonary contusion with mortality about 40%.[33] Contusion occurs when underlying lung parenchyma is damaged, causing edema and hemorrhage. Pulmonary laceration is usually not present. Concussive and compressive forces from blunt trauma are the most common cause of pulmonary contusion. Injury to lung parenchyma worsens progressively over time. Thoracic injuries associated with pulmonary contusion include rib fractures, flail chest, hemopneumothorax, and scapular fractures.[33,11,42]

Injury to the lung parenchyma causes rupture and hemorrhage into pulmonary tissue, alveoli, and small airways. As a result, airways collapse and loss of ventilation and pulmonary shunting occurs followed by hypoxemia. The subsequent inflammatory response impairs gas exchange and worsens the clinical picture. Diagnosis is based on the index of suspicion. Clinical evidence of dyspnea, hemoptysis, hypoxia, and possible chest wall abrasion or ecchymosis may be present. Fifty percent of patients with pulmonary contusion have no physical findings. Auscultation rarely detects abnormalities, but a baseline arterial blood gas test may be helpful.[11] The chest radiograph is usually not helpful during initial evaluation. Computerized tomography (CT) may be used to quantify the contusion because this method is a more sensitive indicator of tissue injury.[6,33,41]

Treatment consists of placing the patient in semi-Fowler's position to facilitate lung reexpansion, suctioning, and chest physiotherapy. Intubation and mechanical ventilation may be required if the patient is hypoxic (PaO_2 <60 on 100% oxygen) or the contusion affects greater than 28% of the lungs, as quantified by a CT scan.[33] In general, intubation and mechanical ventilation is more likely with larger contusions. Intubation may also be required if the patient exhibits signs of shock, has fractured eight or more ribs, is elderly, or has underlying pulmonary disease. Fluids may be restricted if no evidence of hypovolemia exists.

Diaphragmatic injury. Blunt or penetrating trauma may result in diaphragmatic injuries. Blunt injuries result in large radial tears, causing herniation of abdominal contents into the thorax. Herniation may develop slowly with penetrating injuries; sometimes years pass before this occurs.[1] Most injuries occur on the left side of the diaphragm since the right side is protected by the liver. The presence of hemothorax, pneumothorax, or intraabdominal hemorrhage suggests a possible ruptured diaphragm. A nasogastric tube is inserted before obtaining a chest x-ray; the tube is visible in the chest with diaphragmatic rupture. Other signs and symptoms include dyspnea, abdominal or epigastric pain that radiates to the left shoulder (Kehr's sign), bowel sounds in the lower chest, and decreased breath sounds on the affected side. Peritoneal lavage fluid may leak into the chest drainage system. Treatment is surgical repair.

Cardiac and Great Vessel Injuries

Cardiac contusions. A cardiac contusion is a bruise of the heart, usually resulting from blunt trauma to the anterior chest. Common mechanisms of injury include steering wheel impact during a motor vehicle crash, falls, assaults, and direct blows from an object or large animal (e.g., kick from a horse).[5] The myocardium may have a mild contusion or concussion injury or may have a severe injury that mimics an acute myocardial infarction. An echocardiogram differentiates the extent of the injury. A mild injury can have cardiac dysrhythmia; however, the echocardiogram is normal. Extensive myocardial contusion is characterized by dysrhythmia and some evidence of myocardial dysfunction on the echocardiogram.[5]

Signs and symptoms of myocardial contusion and concussion are nonspecific and include chest pain, skin abrasions, and/or ecchymosis to the anterior chest. These signs occur with fractures or other chest wall injuries, so diagnosis is often difficult.[1,5] Not all patients have evidence of chest wall injury.[1,5,6,12] Chest pain associated with myocardial contusion mimics pain that occurs in angina. Unlike anginal pain, however, pain with myocardial contusion does not respond to coronary vasodilators.[6] Contusion is suggested by the patient's history of a significant blunt trauma to the chest. Dysrhythmia seen with myocardial contusion includes sinus tachycardia, atrial fibrillation, atrial flutter, and premature ventricular contractions (PVCs). The most common dysrhythmia is PVCs, which increase with age of the victim.[7]

Serial ECGs and continuous cardiac monitoring are essential. A two-dimensional echocardiography (2-D ECHO) is also recommended. Cardiac isoenzyme analysis has been abandoned as researchers have demonstrated lack of specificity and sensitivity for dysrhythmia development or injury with use of these enzyme values.[5,7] Variable ECG findings occur in myocardial contusion. Specific findings include ST-segment and T-wave changes, a prolonged QT interval, and a right bundle branch block. Echocardiograms are useful for differentiating cardiac dysfunction from other pathologies such as myocardial contusion, pericardial tamponade, valve rupture, and pericardial effusion.[14]

Sequelae following injury include dysrhythmia, valve lesion, and rupture; thromboembolic events; and congestive heart failure.[13] Treatment consists of cardiac monitoring of patients for at least 24 hours. Patients with abnormal ECGs or dysrhythmia should have a 2-D ECHO. Patients with an abnormal echocardiogram should be treated symptomatically. Patients with normal serial ECGs or those who remain asymptomatic for 24 hours require no further treatment.[5,14]

Penetrating cardiac injuries. Person-against-person violence, usually in urban areas, is the leading cause of penetrating trauma in the United States. Most victims of penetrating cardiac injuries arrive in the ED in cardiac arrest or with significant hypotension secondary to cardiac tamponade or hemorrhage.[12,19,35] The right ventricle is the most frequently injured chamber because of its anterior position. Other chambers injured are the left ventricle and right atrium. Gunshot wounds of the heart are significantly more lethal than stab wounds.[19,35] Penetrating injuries are associated with a high mortality (83%), only 20% to 25% of the victims reach the hospital alive. Of those who arrive alive, only 20% are stable.[24] Patients who arrive with stable cardiac injuries have the best chance for survival with early diagnosis and treatment. Patients with injuries to the chest between the midclavicular lines, clavicles, and costal margins should be aggressively evaluated for cardiac involvement.[24]

Immediate thoracotomy in the emergency department is indicated for patients in cardiac arrest.[12,35] Stabilization of the ABCs followed by echocardiography is recommended if the patient has cardiac activity. If the echocardiogram is negative, no further evaluation is indicated. Positive findings indicating tamponade suggest the need for a subxiphoid window. With positive subxiphoid exploration, cardiac surgery is indicated to repair the defect.[6,24,35]

Cardiac tamponade. Cardiac tamponade occurs with rapid accumulation of blood in the pericardial sac, which decreases ventricular filling. As the pericardial sac fills, blood exerts pressure on the ventricles, which impairs ventricular filling and the heart's pumping ability leading to decreased cardiac output. Classic signs of cardiac tamponade are a complex of symptoms called Beck's Triad: hypotension, muffled heart tones, and distended neck veins.

Hypotension is secondary to myocardial compression and decreased cardiac output as more blood accumulates in the pericardium. Muffled heart sounds are caused by the insulating ability of blood in the pericardium, whereas neck vein distension occurs because the heart cannot expand normally to accommodate blood return to the heart. Classic symptoms may not always be evident because of associated injuries such as hypovolemia. As tamponade worsens, the patient exhibits air hunger, agitation, and deterioration in the level of consciousness.[12] Knowing mechanism(s) of injury and location of the wound(s) is crucial for accurate assessment. Gunshot wounds and stab wounds to the chest are the most suggestive for this condition. Hemodynamically unstable patients with injuries to the chest should be immediately evaluated for tamponade. In a stable patient, an echocardiogram and a subxiphoid pericardial window are the diagnostic tools of choice. Pericardiocentesis (Figure 25-12) may be lifesaving for some patients with pericardial tamponade. However, it is not the best diagnostic tool for most patients because of its significant false-positive rate, and risks of secondary injuries such as coronary vessel laceration and dysrhythmia.[12,13,24] Pericardiocentesis may act as a temporizing procedure, performed to improve cardiac function while waiting for surgery. The ECG, chest radiograph, and central venous pressure readings are not reliable diagnostic tools because of inconsistent changes in assessment parameters for each.[12,23,24] Some patients exhibit an unusual rhythm known as electrical alternans (Figure 25-13). Early identification and prompt intervention are essential for patient survival.

Aortic rupture. The majority of victims with aortic rupture caused by blunt trauma die at the scene of the crash; few sur-

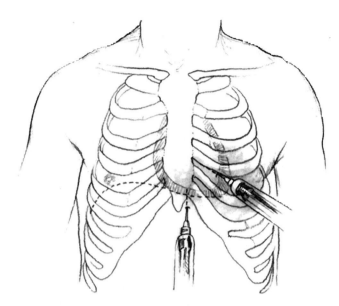

Figure **25-12** Pericardiocentesis for acute cardiac tamponade can be performed via a left subxiphoid or parasternal approach. The subxiphoid route is generally preferred for acute trauma. *(From Davis JH, et al.: Essentials of clinical surgery, St. Louis, 1991, Mosby.)*

vive transport to the hospital. Rapid diagnosis and surgical intervention are essential because half will die in the first 48 hours if left untreated.[4,14,19,37] Traumatic aortic rupture is commonly associated with horizontal or vertical acceleration/deceleration injuries such as high speed motor vehicle crashes and falls from a great height. The most common site of injury involves the area of the aorta just distal to the left subclavian artery, adjacent to the ligamentum arteriosum. The innominate artery at the aortic arch and the aortic valve are also common sites of injury.[18,19,35] Figure 25-14 identifies common sites for aortic disruption.

The patient may complain of chest pain or pain between the scapulae, often described as unrelenting and severe. Other symptoms include dyspnea and hemoptysis. A loud systolic murmur may be heard over the precordium if aortic valve integrity has been lost. Signs of hemorrhagic shock may be present. A discrepancy between blood pressure values in the right and left arms also occurs, depending on the level of the injury. Acute coarctation syndrome can occur as sympathetic fibers in the aorta respond to the stretch stimulus from a torn intima flap or hematoma. Blood pressure and pulse in the upper extremities is elevated, whereas pulses and blood pressure in the lower extremities are decreased or absent.[18]

The most common diagnostic test for aortic disruption is a chest radiograph; the most common finding is mediastinal widening (Figure 25-15). A supine chest radiograph may not adequately demonstrate mediastinal widening. Other chest radiograph findings include the presence of an "apical cap," a displaced esophagus (evidenced by visualization of the naso-

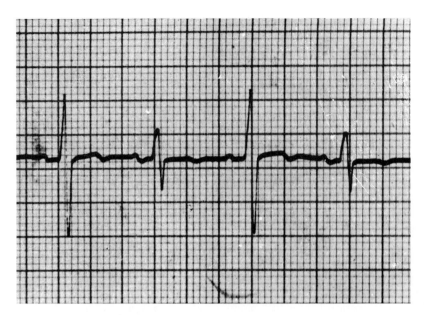

Figure **25-13** Lewis lead ECG shows total electrical alternation of amplitude and configuration of P and QRS complexes. *(From Sotolongo RP, Horton JD:* Am Heart J *101:853, 1981.)*

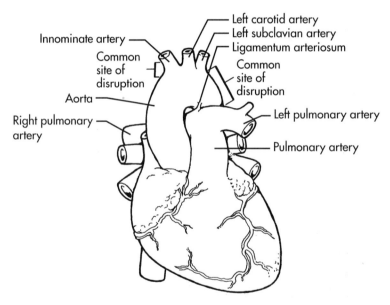

Figure **25-14** Common sites of aortic disruption.

gastric tube), the trachea deviated to the right, obliteration of the aortic knob, fracture of the first or second ribs, depression of the left mainstem bronchus, and massive left pleural effusion.[6,18,35] Radiographic findings are not specific or sensitive enough to pinpoint the injury; up to 28% of victims with aortic rupture have a normal chest radiograph.[35] The diagnostic standard for identification of aortic injury is the aortogram; however, this procedure is not without associated risks. Injection of radiopaque dye may worsen the tear in the aorta and cause complete disruption. Transesophageal echocardiography (TEE), used in some centers across the country, visualizes the aorta from the posterior aspect via the esophagus.

Definitive treatment for aortic disruption is immediate surgical repair. Management in the ED includes insertion of large-bore intravenous catheters and collection of blood for blood type and crossmatch. Some patients require medical management with beta-blockers and antihypertensive agents when associated injuries preclude the safe induction of anesthesia.[4,18]

Esophageal Injury

Injury to the esophagus usually results from penetrating trauma, but may be related to a severe blow to the lower abdomen. Esophageal injuries are rare and often lethal. Com-

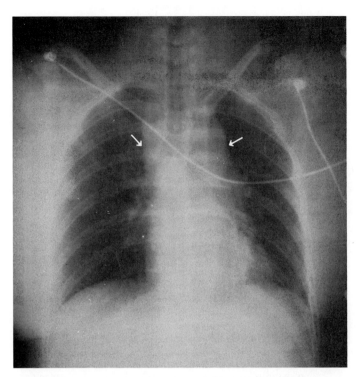

Figure **25-15** Radiograph of chest. Arrows demonstrate widened mediastinum.

Box **25-6** **Changes in Management of Thoracic Trauma**

- Cardiac troponin 1 (cTn1) is a specific marker for myocardial necrosis. Widely accepted for detecting myocardial necrosis following infarction, but has not been sufficiently studied in the trauma patient for widespread use in evaluation of cardiac injury.[5,35]
- Use of petroleum gauze for chest tube dressings has been abandoned in favor of bacteriostatic ointment, dry sterile dressing, and occlusive tape or dry sterile dressing and occlusive tape. Petroleum gauze macerates tissue and predisposes the patient to skin infection.[42]
- Transesophageal echocardiography (TEE) may become the "gold standard" for diagnosis of ruptured aorta. Less invasive, may be performed at the bedside, and less costly than an aortogram. Not widely accepted as a diagnostic tool because of machine and user variability in interpretation of the test.[16] Transthoracic echocardiography (TTE) may be used in place of subxiphoid exploration for identifying cardiac injuries in stable patients with penetrating traumas. The same issues apply to TTE as TEE, in terms of user expertise and interpretation.
- Video-assisted thoracoscopy can reduce nontherapeutic laparotomies, patient morbidity, and costs.[25] The diaphragm may be examined with a video camera through a small opening in the thoracic cavity, similar to laparoscopy.

Box **25-7**

NURSING DIAGNOSIS FOR THORACIC TRAUMA

Ineffective airway clearance
Ineffective breathing pattern
Impaired gas exchange
Decreased cardiac output

mon causes of penetrating injury are iatrogenic events, such as instrumentation during certain procedures.[45] Caustic ingestion, such as alkali or acid; crush injuries; and blast injuries also cause esophageal injury. Regardless of the mechanism, the final result is mediastinitis caused by contamination from saliva and gastric contents. The patient may experience pain and/or shock out of proportion to the apparent chest injury. Pneumothorax or hemothorax without rib fracture may be present. Chest tube drainage may have particulate matter. Diagnosis is confirmed by contrast studies or esophagoscopy. Urgent surgical repair is indicated.

FUTURE TRENDS

Thoracic injuries are challenging, chaotic to manage, and potentially life-threatening. Changes in technology such as TEE have made management easier. With more research, management of chest injuries may change significantly. Box 25-6 highlights some of these current and future changes.

CONCLUSION

The patient with a thoracic injury requires rapid assessment and intervention. The emergency nurse must anticipate potentially lethal thoracic injuries and rapidly intervene. Box 25-7 highlights nursing diagnoses for these patients.

REFERENCES

1. American College of Surgeons: *Advanced trauma life support: Course for physicians,* ed 5, Chicago, 1993, American College of Surgeons.
2. Atrium Medical Corporation: *Managing chest drainage and postoperative autotransfusion* (study guide), Hudson, N.H., 1995, Atrium Medical Corporation.
3. Carroll P: Chest tubes made easy, *RN* 46-55, 1995.
4. Cohn SM, et al.: Exclusion of aortic tear in the unstable trauma patient: The utility of transesophageal echocardiography, *J Trauma Injury, Infect Crit Care* 39:1087-1090, 1995.
5. Daleiden A: Clinical manifestations of blunt cardiac injury: A challenge to the critical care practitioner, *Crit Care Nurs Quart* 17(2):13-23, 1994.
6. Emergency Nurses Association: *Trauma nursing core course,* ed 4, Chicago, 1995, The Association.
7. Fabian TC, et al.: A prospective evaluation of myocardial contusion: Correlation of significant arrhythmias and cardiac output with CK-MB measurements, *J Trauma* 31:653-660, 1991.
8. Flemming AW, Carabello G, Sterling-Scott RP: Esophageal complications. In Mattox KL, editor: *Complications of trauma,* New York, 1994, Churchill Livingstone.
9. Guyton AC, Hall JE: *Textbook of medical physiology,* ed 9, Philadelphia, 1995, WB Saunders.
10. Hills MW, Delpaedo AM, Deane SA: Sternal fractures: Associated injuries and management, *J Trauma* 35(1):55-60, 1993.
11. Horn J: Pulmonary complications. In Mattox KL, editor: *Complications of trauma,* New York, 1994, Churchill Livingstone.
12. Ivatury RR, Rohman M: The injured heart, *Surg Clin North Am* 69(1):93-109, 1989.
13. Ivatury RR, Simon RJ, Rohman M: Cardiac complications. In Mattox KL, editor: *Complications of trauma,* New York, 1994, Churchill Livingstone.
14. Johnson SB, Kearney PA, Smith MD: Echocardiography in the evaluation of thoracic trauma, *Surg Clin North Am* 75(2):193-205, 1995.
15. Kearney KM: Cardiovascular emergencies. In Klein AR, et al., editors: *Emergency nursing core curriculum,* ed 4, Philadelphia, 1994, WB Saunders, pp 53-110.
16. Kearney PA, et al.: Use of transesophageal echocardiography in the evaluation of traumatic aortic injury, *J Trauma* 34:696-703, 1993.
17. Key SP, Merrill WH: Hemothorax. In Cameron JL, editor: *Current surgical therapy,* ed 5, St. Louis, 1995, Mosby.
18. Kosmos CA: Multiple trauma. In Kitt S, et al., editors: *Emergency nursing: a physiologic and clinical perspective,* Philadelphia, 1995, WB Saunders, pp 54-77.
19. Kshettry VR, Bolman RM: Chest trauma: Assessment, diagnosis and management, *Clin Chest Med* 15(1):137-146, 1994.
20. Lewis FR: Chest wall. In Trunkey DD, Lewis FR, editors: *Current therapy of trauma,* ed 2, Toronto, 1986, BC Decker, pp 235-242.
21. LoCicero J, Mattox KL: Epidemiology of chest trauma, *Surg Clin North Am* 69:15-19, 1989.
22. Mattox KL: Indications for thoracotomy: deciding to operate, *Surg Clin North Am* 69:47-57, 1989.
23. Meyer DM, Jessen ME, Grayburn PA: Use of echocardiography to detect occult cardiac injury after penetrating thoracic trauma: a prospective study, *J Trauma: Injury, Infect Crit Care,* 39:902-909, 1995.
24. Nagy KK, et al.: Role of echocardiography in the diagnosis of occult penetrating cardiac injury, *J Trauma: Injury, Infect Crit Care,* 38:859-862, 1995.
25. Ochsner MG, et al.: Prospective evaluation of thoracoabdominal trauma: A preliminary report, *J Trauma* 34:704-710, 1993.
26. Otherson HB, Jr: Cardiothoracic injuries. In Touloukian RJ, editor: *Pediatric trauma,* ed 2, St. Louis, 1990, Mosby.
27. Pate JW: Chest wall injuries, *Surg Clin North Am* 69(1):59-70, 1989.
28. Pate JW: Tracheobronchial and esophageal injuries, *Surg Clin North Am* 69(1):111-123, 1989.
29. Patrick M, et al.: Cardiothoracic trauma. In Howell E, Widra L, Hill MG, editors: *Comprehensive trauma nursing: Theory and practice,* Glenview, Ill., 1988, Scott, Foresman, pp 559-617.
30. Pickard LS, Mattox KL: Chest wall and diaphragm complications. In Mattox KL, editor: *Complications of trauma,* New York, 1994, Churchill Livingstone.
31. Poole GV, et al.: Computed tomography in the management of blunt thoracic trauma, *J Trauma* 35(2):296-302, 1993.
32. Porth CM: *Pathophysiology: Concepts of altered health states,* ed 4, Philadelphia, 1994, JB Lippincott.
33. Prentice D, Ahrens T: Pulmonary complications of trauma, *Crit Care Nurs Quart* 17(2):24-33, 1994.
34. Rielly JP, et al.: Thoracic trauma in children, *J Trauma* 34(3):329-331, 1994.
35. Rosenthal MA, Ellis JI: Cardiac and mediastinal trauma, *Emerg Med Clin North Am* 13(4):887-902, 1995.
36. Rothlin MA, et al.: Ultrasound in blunt abdominal and thoracic trauma, *J Trauma* 34(4):488-495, 1993.
37. Saletta S, et al.: Transesophageal echocardiography for the initial evaluation of the widened mediastinum in trauma patients, *J Trauma: Injury, Infect Crit Care* 39(1):137-142, 1995.
38. Sheehy SB: Chest trauma. In Sheehy SB, editor: *Emergency nursing: Principles and practice,* ed 3, St. Louis, 1992, Mosby.
39. Simon RJ, Ivatury RR: Current concepts in the use of cavitary endoscopy in the evaluation and treatment of blunt and penetrating truncal injuries, *Surg Clin North Am* 75(2):157-174, 1995.
40. Smelcer MG: Respiratory emergencies. In Klein AR, et al.: editors: Emergency nursing core curriculum, ed 4, Philadelphia, 1994, WB Saunders, pp 479-516.
41. Symbas PN: Chest drainage tubes, *Surg Clin North Am* 69(1):41-49, 1989.
42. Tribble RW, Nolan SP: Pneumothorax. In Cameron JL, editor: *Current surgical therapy,* ed 5, St. Louis, 1995, Mosby.
43. Wagner RB, Jamieson PM: Pulmonary contusion: evaluation and classification by computed tomography, *Surg Clin North Am* 69(1):31-40, 1989.
44. Wall MJ, Mattox KL: Thoracic vascular complications. In Mattox KL, editor: *Complications of trauma,* New York, 1994, Churchill Livingstone.
45. Wilson RF: Larynx, trachea, bronchi and lungs. In Trunkey DD, Lewis FR, editors: *Current therapy of trauma,* ed 2, Toronto, 1986, BC Decker, pp 243-246.
46. Ziegler DW, Agarwal NN: The morbidity and mortality of rib fractures, *J Trauma* 37(6):975-979, 1994.

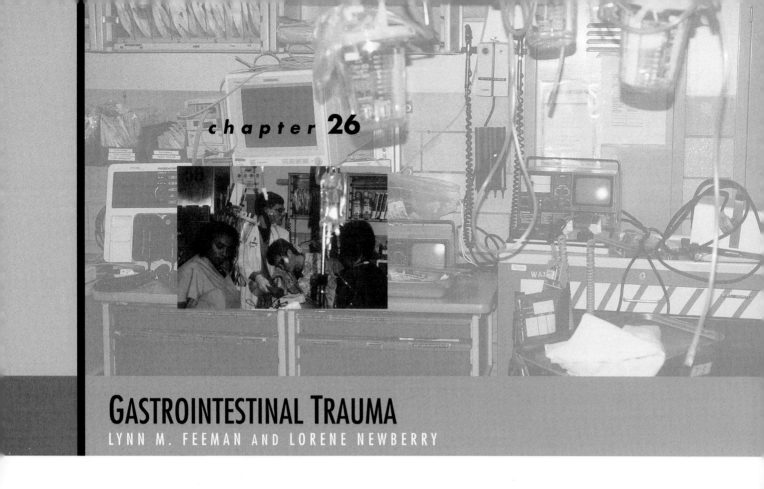

chapter 26

GASTROINTESTINAL TRAUMA

LYNN M. FEEMAN AND LORENE NEWBERRY

Abdominal trauma accounts for approximately 25% of all traumatic injuries. It may occur as an isolated injury or in combination with other injuries. The need for recognition of life-threatening abdominal injuries and rapid surgical intervention cannot be overstated. Abdominal trauma is truly a surgical disease. The role of the emergency nurse is assessment and interventions that focus on the ABCs and rapid movement of the patient to the surgical area.

Two basic mechanisms of injury lead to abdominal trauma: blunt and penetrating. Patterns of injury vary with geographic location of the patient. The incidence of penetrating abdominal trauma is higher in urban centers, but has increased in suburban areas as violence escalates across the country. Injuries secondary to blunt trauma result from diffuse energy over the abdomen that damages abdominal organs but does not injure the abdominal wall. Blunt injuries are the result of motor vehicle crashes, falls, contact sports, or assaults, while penetrating injuries are usually gunshot wounds (GSW) or stab wounds. Gunshot wounds account for 15% of all penetrating wounds to the abdomen, whereas stabbings account for only 2%.[2] Foreign bodies such as pieces of wood or steel and shrapnel injuries from blasts or explosions are also considered penetrating injuries. Between 25% and 33% of all stab wounds penetrate the peritoneal or retroperitoneal cavity. Of these wounds, only 50% to 60% are associated with a major injury.[3] Exploratory laparotomy is required in 76% of all patients with GSW and 33% of patients with stab wounds.[10]

Life-threatening abdominal injuries can occur without any outward sign of injury, so the emergency nurse must have a high index of suspicion for these injuries. Abdominal trauma is suggested when an energy source is applied to the trunk anywhere from the fourth rib to the hips. Inspiration lifts the diaphragm into the thoracic cavity, placing abdominal contents at risk for injury when the chest is injured below the fourth rib. Infants and children, patients under the influence of mind-altering drugs or alcohol, those with an altered level of consciousness, or those with concurrent spinal injuries do not always exhibit abdominal pain, tenderness, or rigidity.

The focus of this chapter is injury to the abdominal organs and abdominal vasculature. In the traditional sense, abdominal trauma is viewed as an injury to the front of the patient (i.e., a blow to the abdomen). However, penetrating injury to the flank also can injure abdominal organs. In blunt trauma, injury to the flank usually damages the kidneys rather than the abdominal organs. Chapter 27 discusses renal trauma in more detail. Trauma in the pregnant patient is discussed in Chapter 33, and pediatric trauma is discussed in Chapter 31.

ANATOMY AND PHYSIOLOGY

Organs in the abdominal cavity include the large and small intestines, liver, spleen, stomach, gall bladder, pancreas, and diaphragm. The spleen and liver are solid organs, whereas the stomach and intestines are hollow organs. Solid organs fracture when injured; hollow organs collapse or rupture. Vascular structures in the abdominal cavity include the aorta, vena cava, hepatic vein, iliac artery, and iliac vein. Most of these structures are located in the peritoneal space. Figures 26-1A and B illustrate location of abdominal contents and gastrointestinal structures. Figure 26-2 shows structures located in the retroperitoneal space.

Peritoneum

The *peritoneum* is the largest serous membrane in the body. The parietal peritoneum lines the abdominal wall, and the visceral peritoneum covers the abdominal organs. The peritoneal cavity is a potential space located between the parietal and visceral peritoneum. Closed in men, in women the peritoneal cavity communicates outside the body through the fallopian tubes, uterus, and vagina. The retroperitoneal space is that area posterior to the peritoneum containing the kidneys and female reproductive organs. The *mesentery* is a double layer of peritoneum that encloses an organ and connects it to the abdominal wall. Mesentery is found in most mobile parts of the intestine. Folds of the

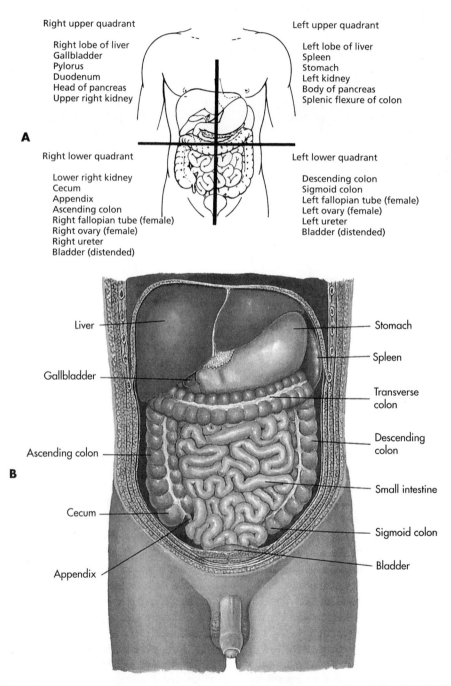

Figure **26-1**   **A,** Abdominal contents. **B,** Gastrointestinal structures. *(**A,** From Stillwell S:* Mosby's critical care nursing reference, *ed 2, St. Louis, 1996, Mosby.* ***B,*** *From Seidel HM et al:* Mosby's guide to physical examination, *ed 3, St. Louis, 1995, Mosby.)*

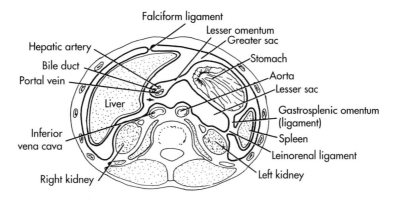

Figure **26-2** Retroperitoneal structures. *(From Snell R, Smith M:* Clinical anatomy for emergency medicine, *St. Louis, 1993, Mosby.)*

mesentery are named the greater and lesser omentum. These folds extend from the stomach to adjacent organs.

Organs

The *stomach* is a hollow organ located in the left upper quadrant, which contains hydrochloric acid and other digestive agents. The pH of gastric fluid is 1. The position of the stomach varies with inspiration into the thoracic cavity. Stomach size changes with consumption of food or liquids. The cardiac sphincter controls entry into the stomach; exit is controlled by the pyloric sphincter. The stomach usually empties within 2 to 6 hours of food ingestion.

The *small intestine* connects to the pyloric sphincter and fills most of the abdominal cavity. Segments include the duodenum, the jejunum, and the ileum. The majority of digestion and absorption occurs here. The pH of the small intestines is between 6.5 and 7.5.

The *large intestine* interfaces with the ileum proximally and exits distally at the rectum. Divisions consist of the ascending colon, transverse colon, descending colon, and the sigmoid colon. Most absorption occurs in the proximal colon.

The *liver,* the largest gland in the body (almost 3% total body weight), is specifically responsible for more than 500 separate metabolic functions including secretion of bile, detoxification of poisons, and storage of glycogen. Box 26-1 lists just a few of the liver's functions. Death occurs in less than 12 hours with complete destruction of the liver; however, only 10% to 20% of the tissue is necessary to sustain life. The liver is extremely vascular. Blood flows through the portal vein at approximately 1000 ml/min, and from the iliac artery at approximately 400 ml/min.

The *gall bladder* is a pear-shaped, hollow sac directly beneath the right lobe of the liver. Its principal function is storage and concentration of bile.

The *pancreas,* located behind the stomach, extends across the posterior abdomen from the duodenum to the spleen. The pancreas has both endocrine and exocrine functions. Exocrine cells produce lipase, amylase, trypsin, and other

---

Box **26-1** **Liver Functions**[5]

Forms and excretes bile; metabolizes old red blood cells
Metabolizes carbohydrates, proteins, and fats
Helps maintain normal blood glucose and energy level
Stores glycogen to create energy reserve
Stores vitamins A, B-12, D, E, K, copper, and iron
Detoxifies drugs and toxins
Acts as flood chamber for blood from the right heart
Inactivates and excretes aldosterone, glucocorticoids, estrogen, progesterone, and testosterone

---

digestive enzymes. Endocrine cells produce insulin, glucagon, and somatostatin.

The *spleen,* a large vascular organ in the left upper quadrant behind the eighth to tenth ribs, is the largest single mass of lymphatic tissue in the body and is essential for defense against bacterial invasion. The spleen is extremely vascular with a blood flow of 200 ml/min, approximately 5% of the cardiac output.[4]

Vascular Structures

The arterial blood supply for the abdominal cavity is the aorta (Figure 26-3). The abdominal aorta lies left of midline in the abdominal cavity and bifurcates into the iliac arteries just above the pelvic brim. Iliac arteries supply arterial blood to the lower extremities. Abdominal organs are supplied by three unpaired arteries originating from the abdominal aorta: the celiac trunk, superior mesentery artery, and inferior mesentery artery. The celiac trunk branches into the hepatic, left gastric, and splenic arteries.

With the exception of the heart and lungs, venous blood returns from the body to the heart through the superior vena cava or inferior vena cava. The inferior vena cava, formed by the union of the two common iliac veins, is the major vein in the abdomen. The superior vena cava is formed when the two brachiocephalic veins unite in the superior mediastinum.

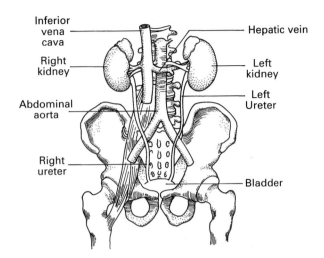

Figure **26-3** Vascular structures in the abdomen. *(From Sheehy SB, Jimmerson CL: Manual of clinical trauma care: the first hour, ed 2, St. Louis, 1994, Mosby.)*

PATIENT ASSESSMENT

Vascular organs like the liver or spleen may lose blood rapidly or leak slowly over time.[3] The patient may come to the emergency department (ED) without specific signs of injury. The nurse should assess the patient carefully and continually reassess the hemodynamic status, level of consciousness, and level of pain. Initial assessment and stabilization begin with maintenance of airway, breathing, and circulation. Critical interventions include oxygenation and intravenous access.

History

The patient with abdominal trauma may not have obvious injuries. Abdominal trauma should be suspected when the patient has a history of a motor vehicle crash or penetrating wounds to the torso or flank. It should also be a consideration in a patient with multisystem trauma and a patient with a history of an injury who has unexplained hypotension or tachycardia. Awake patients may complain of abdominal pain or shoulder pain. Intraabdominal blood irritates the inferior surface of the diaphragm and the phrenic nerve causing referred pain to the shoulder. Called Kehr's sign, this finding should alert the emergency nurse to the possibility of peritoneal bleeding.

Mechanisms of Injury

Injuries from blunt trauma secondary to a motor vehicle crash are influenced by patient location in the vehicle; speed of the vehicle; use of a seat belt, shoulder harness, or air bag; and ejection from the vehicle. Use of seat belts has decreased mortality from injuries but has also led to the identification of injuries caused by the seat belt. "Seat belt syndrome" refers to injuries in the plane of the body where the belt is located, including injuries of the colon, small bowel, stomach, liver, spleen, vascular structures, and the spinal cord, usually the lumbar area.

Injuries secondary to falls vary with the height of the fall, landing surface, and the part of body that hits the ground. Injuries are usually less severe if a person lands on a shock-absorbing surface such as mud, and worse if on concrete. If the injury is due to assault with a blunt object, knowing what the object is, and its size and weight are important.

With penetrating injuries, the weapon must be identified. If it is a gun, knowing the type and caliber, how close the assailant was when firing, and how many shots were fired is helpful. If a knife, stick, or other weapon penetrated the abdomen, the length, width, and composition of the weapon should be determined. Injuries made with wood or other biologic material are more likely to cause infection and complications. The angle of entry suggests the path of the weapon.

Inspection

Bruising, abrasions, and lacerations are assessed. Bruising that mirrors the location of the seat belt may be evident on admission to the ED, but usually does not occur for several hours after the injury. Purplish discoloration of the flanks (Grey Turner's sign) or umbilicus (Cullen's sign) is associated with bleeding into the abdominal wall. Distension may be noted; however, it is not a reliable sign. Two liters of fluid increases abdominal girth by only 0.75 inches. The nurse must note the presence of gunshot wounds or stab wounds. If gunshot wounds are present, the patient's back must be inspected for other wounds.

Old surgical scars are noted. This may help narrow the search for organs that may be injured; for example, if the patient has had a previous splenectomy, this accounts for one less organ that may have been damaged. Previous surgical procedures may have caused adhesions that affect reliability of diagnostic peritoneal lavage (DPL).

Percussion/Auscultation

Percussion of the abdomen can provide helpful information; however, it is usually impossible to hear percussion sounds in the middle of trauma resuscitation. Auscultation can also provide helpful information about the presence or absence of bowel sounds. However, this can take several minutes and is not indicated in the patient who is hemodynamically unstable. Bowel sounds in the chest can be caused by diaphragmatic rupture.

Palpation

The abdomen is palpated carefully for pain, rigidity, tenderness, and guarding, examining all four quadrants. Abdominal masses suggest hematoma of the liver, spleen, or omentum. A sensation of popping bubbles when pressing down suggests injury of the duodenum or distal colon.

Initial Stabilization

Initial stabilization of the patient with abdominal trauma follows the same sequence as any patient with major trauma. Beginning with checking airway, breathing, and circulation, the nurse then inserts bilateral, large-bore intravenous (IV) catheters. Warm crystalloids such as Ringer's lactated or normal saline are infused at a rate adequate to maintain blood pressure. Baseline trauma lab tests are obtained, including CBC, type and crossmatch, and urinalysis. Coagulation studies, serum amylase, liver function tests, and blood chemistries also may be ordered for some patients. A serum pregnancy test should be done on a woman of child-bearing years. A nasogastric tube and urinary catheter should be inserted if the patient does not require immediate transport to surgery.

Diagnostic evaluation of a patient with abdominal trauma is based on the patient's hemodynamic stability. If the patient is or becomes hemodynamically unstable secondary to intraperitoneal injury, transfusion with fluids and/or blood is begun, and the patient is prepared for surgery.

Initial radiographic evaluation of the patient with abdominal trauma includes an AP and lateral chest radiograph. A flat plate of the abdomen and pelvic films may also be done; however, these tests are more effective in identification of bony abnormalities than of life-threatening organ injuries. An ileus and ruptured diaphragm may be detected with these radiographs.

Diagnostic peritoneal lavage is used to determine the presence of peritoneal bleeding in the hemodynamically unstable patient. In penetrating wounds, DPL may be used on a limited basis. A higher rate of false positives occurs for stab wounds. Most patients with gunshot wounds usually require surgery, which obviates the need for DPL.[3] Box 26-2 highlights the indications and contraindications for DPL. DPL is considered negative if newsprint can be read through the fluid; however many institutions analyze specific components of the fluid. Table 26-1 gives parameters for a positive DPL test.

Computerized tomography (CT) is used to evaluate peritoneal and retroperitoneal injury in the stable patient. It also shows skeletal injuries. Solid organ injuries are identified earlier than hollow organ injuries. Oral and IV contrast is used to evaluate abdominal structures. The CT scan cannot differentiate fluid and blood in the peritoneal cavity; therefore, DPL should not be performed if the patient is to have a CT scan. The patient's hemodynamic status should be evaluated before transport for CT in a location remote to the ED.

The primary goal of ultrasound in evaluation of abdominal trauma is to determine the presence of fluid in the abdominal cavity; thereby indicating the need for surgery.[7] Ultrasound is not widely used across the country, but is gaining acceptance in larger centers[11] and has been useful in evaluation of the pregnant trauma patient.[6] A minimum of 70 ml of blood is required for detection with ultrasound.

The range of diagnostic options for evaluation of abdominal trauma has increased with the routine use of CT scans and the introduction of ultrasound. However, the basic principles of patient management have not changed significantly. Immediate surgical intervention is indicated if the patient becomes hemodynamically unstable, has an enlarging abdominal mass without concomitant pelvic or vertebral fractures, or shows a progressive drop in hemoglobin.

Box 26-2 **Diagnostic Peritoneal Lavage**

Indications

Multisystem injury with hemodynamic instability
Blunt abdominal trauma with altered level of consciousness, drugs, or alcohol
Altered sensation from spinal cord injury
Vague abdominal examination

Contraindications

Absolute Contraindication
Obvious need for surgery (i.e., gunshot wound to abdomen)
Relative Contraindications
Previous abdominal surgeries
Pregnancy
Abdominal wall hematoma
Obesity
Distended abdomen

Table 26-1 **Positive DPL Results[4]**

Parameter	Positive results
Hematocrit	≥2 ml/dl
Red blood cell count	≥100,000 cells/mm³
White blood cell count	≥500 cells/mm³
Amylase	≥200 milliunits/ml
Bile	Present
Bacteria	Significant number present

SPECIFIC INJURIES

Penetrating injuries can affect all abdominal structures. Assessment and treatment are usually straightforward. If the abdominal cavity is penetrated or the patient is in shock, surgery is indicated. With blunt trauma, assessment and treatment are more complex because of the presence of multisystem injuries. Abdominal organs injured most often by blunt trauma are the spleen and liver. The colon, vascular structures, stomach, pancreas, and diaphragm also may be injured, but the incidence is lower. The gall bladder is rarely injured by blunt trauma. Management of abdominal trauma in the ED focuses on stabilization of the patient's hemodynamic status, identification of potentially life-threatening injuries, and rapid transport to the surgical suite when indicated. Specific injuries of the abdomen are described below.

Spleen

The spleen is the organ injured most often by blunt trauma. Its small size makes it a difficult target, so it is injured less often with penetrating trauma. Because the spleen is encapsulated, injury may damage only the capsule or may actually fracture the spleen. Table 26-2 summarizes the types of splenic injuries that occur. Splenic injury is suggested when the patient has sustained blunt trauma to the left upper quadrant. When assessing for bruising or pain in the left upper quadrant, Kehr's sign may be present as a result of diaphragmatic irritation by peritoneal blood. Shock and hypotension is present in as few as 30% of patients with splenic trauma.[4]

Not all patients with splenic injury require surgery. Operative management is reserved for unstable patients with splenic injury, gunshot wounds of the spleen, or splenic injuries that violate all layers of the splenic capsule. Stab wounds to the spleen and splenic hematoma are usually observed for changes in physical examination and hemoglobin and hematocrit levels.

Liver

The liver's size and anterior location make it an easy target for blunt and penetrating mechanisms of injury. Overall mortality rate for liver injuries is only 10%.[4] The liver is also encapsulated, so injuries may affect only the capsule or may fracture the liver itself. Table 26-3 presents the types of liver injuries that may occur. Liver injuries are suggested when the patient has a direct blow to the right upper quadrant from the eighth rib to the central abdomen. Clinical indications include pain, bruising over the right upper quadrant, or referred pain to the right shoulder. Hemodynamic instability is almost always present when the liver sustains major damage. Surgical repair of liver injuries is determined by the extent of injury to the liver and the patient's hemodynamic status. More than 50% of adults with liver injury are treated nonoperatively.[9]

Stomach

The stomach is a hollow organ, can be easily displaced, and is rarely injured in blunt trauma. Conversely, size and anterior location increases the risk of a penetrating injury.[4]

Table **26-2** **Splenic Injuries**[8]		
Grade	Category	Description
I	Hematoma	Subcapsular; involves less than 10% surface area; hematoma does not expand
	Laceration	Nonbleeding capsular tear; less than 1 cm deep
II	Hematoma	Subcapsular hematoma covering 10%-50% surface area
		Hematoma does not expand; intraparenchymal hematoma less than 2 cm wide
	Laceration	Capsular tear with active bleeding; intraparenchymal injury 1-3 cm deep
III	Hematoma	Subcapsular hematoma involving more than 50% surface area or one that is expanding; intraparenchymal hematoma less than 2 cm wide or expanding; ruptured subcapsular hematoma with active bleeding
	Laceration	More than 3 cm deep or involving intracellular vessels
IV	Hematoma	Ruptured intraparenchymal hematoma with active bleeding
	Laceration	Segmental laceration or one that involves hilar vessels
		Devascularization of more than 25% of spleen
V	Laceration	Shattered spleen
	Vascular	Hilar vascular injury; spleen is devascularized

Table **26-3** **Liver Injuries**[8]		
Grade	Category	Description
I	Hematoma	Nonexpanding subcapsular hematoma less than 10% of spleen surface
	Laceration	Nonbleeding capsular tear less than 1 cm deep
II	Hematoma	Nonexpanding subcapsular hematoma 10%-50% surface area; less than 2 cm deep
	Laceration	Less than 3 cm parenchymal penetration; less than 10 cm long
III	Hematoma	Subcapsular hematoma more than 50% surface area or one that is expanding; ruptured subcapsular hematoma with active bleeding; intraparenchymal hematoma more than 2 cm
	Laceration	More than 3 cm deep
IV	Hematoma	Ruptured central hematoma
	Laceration	15%-25% hepatic lobe destroyed
V	Laceration	More than 75% hepatic lobe destroyed
	Vascular	Major hepatic veins injured
VI	Vascular	Avulsed liver

Physical signs and symptoms associated with stomach injuries include left upper quadrant pain and tenderness. Diagnosis is based on patient assessment, aspiration of blood via the gastric tube, and the presence of free air on the abdominal radiograph (Figure 26-4). All patients with gastric injury require surgical exploration.

Large and Small Intestine

The intestines are hollow, highly vascular organs approximately 32 feet long and fixed at various points in the peritoneal cavity. Their anterior location, relative lack of protection, vascularity, and fixed points of attachment make the intestines susceptible for blunt and penetrating injuries.[4] Penetrating trauma, particularly stab wounds, can eviscerate the bowel or omentum. Management includes covering the evisceration with saline-soaked pads, establishing IV access, and preparing the patient for surgery.

The intestines are frequently injured by inappropriately worn seat belts.[4] Injury to the intestines usually causes rupture, which spills chemical and bacterial contamination into the peritoneum. Initial signs and symptoms of intestinal injury include tenderness and rigidity. As time progresses and more peritoneal contamination occurs, fever, elevated white count, abdominal distension, and hypoactive bowel sounds occur.

Pancreas

The pancreas, a semisolid organ in the retroperitoneal space well protected by the liver and stomach, is more likely to be injured by penetrating trauma. Pancreatic injury from blunt trauma is unusual, but does occur. Its retroperitoneal location makes DPL an unreliable indicator of pancreatic injury. Elevated serum amylase is also unreliable as an indicator of pancreatic injury—up to 40% of all patients with pancreatic injury initially have a normal serum amylase.[4] An as-

say for pancreatic fraction is proving more reliable; however, this test may not be readily available. Endoscopic retrograde pancreatography (ERP) has been useful in identifying injury to the pancreatic duct.[12] When surgery is required, every effort is made to preserve the pancreas because of essential endocrine and exocrine functions. The majority of patients with pancreatic injury have other injuries, with associated hemorrhage as the major cause of death.

Diaphragm

Diaphragmatic rupture may be due to blunt or penetrating mechanisms. Rupture almost always occurs on the left side because the liver protects the right hemidiaphragm. Rupture should be suspected in all patients with thoracoabdominal injuries. In a diaphragmatic rupture, abdominal contents spill into the thoracic cavity causing respiratory compromise secondary to lung compression. Bowel sounds may be auscultated in the chest cavity. Respiratory function is further compromised by a loss of negative pressure in the chest and an inability of the diaphragm to function normally.[4] Diagnosis is usually confirmed by a radiograph of the chest showing abdominal contents or the gastric tube in the left chest. These patients require immediate surgical repair.

Vascular Structures

Major vascular structures in the abdomen are the abdominal aorta, inferior vena cava, iliac artery, and hepatic veins. Vessels can be injured by blunt or penetrating mechanisms, with injury of major abdominal vessels occurring in between 5% and 10% of patients with blunt abdominal trauma.[4] Disruption of vascular structures causes severe hemorrhage and death if the damage is not repaired. Identification of injuries is often made in the operating room, particularly in an unstable patient. In a stable patient, a CT scan and arteriography may be used. ED management of patients with

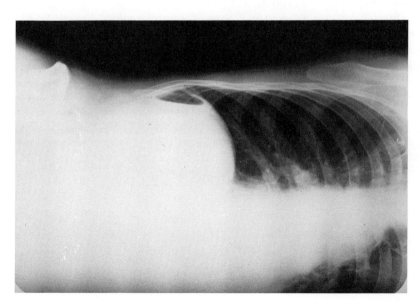

Figure **26-4** Radiograph showing free intraperitoneal air. *(Modified from Rosen P, et al.:* Emergency medicine, *ed 3, St. Louis, 1992, Mosby.)*

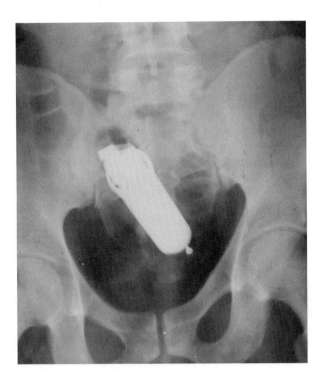

Figure **26-5** Vibrator in rectum. *(From Rosen P, et al:* Emergency medicine, *ed 3, St. Louis, 1992, Mosby.)*

threatening injuries without external evidence of injury. The emergency nurse must assume that an injury is present until the possibility is ruled out. Consideration of mechanisms of injury highlights potential injuries and enhances patient assessment and care. Box 26-3 summarizes nursing diagnoses for the patient with abdominal trauma.

vascular injuries includes establishing IV access and providing rapid transport to the surgical suite.

Foreign Bodies

Another aspect of abdominal trauma is foreign bodies of the stomach and rectum. This may be the result of ingestion, masturbation, autoeroticism, assault, or psychiatric illness. Many patients do not acknowledge the presence of a foreign body during the initial evaluation. Complaints are often vague and relate to pain or discomfort. Diagnosis is usually made using a radiograph. Removal of the foreign body may be done in the ED or may require surgical intervention, depending on the size, shape, and location of the foreign body. Drug-filled condoms or plastic bags may also be swallowed or placed in the rectum. Other foreign bodies include vibrators (Figure 26-5) and live animals.

CONCLUSION

A patient with abdominal trauma presents the care giver with many unique challenges. The patient can have life-

REFERENCES

1. American College of Surgeons: *Advanced trauma life support provider manual,* Chicago, 1988, American College of Surgeons.
2. Cayten CG: Abdominal trauma, *Emerg Med Clin North Am* 2:799, 1984.
3. Feliciano DV: Abdominal trauma. In Shultz, S et al., editors: *Manual of abdominal operations,* ed 9, vol 1, Stamford, Conn., 1990, Appleton & Lange.
4. Feliciano DV, Moore EE, Mattov KL, editors: *Trauma,* ed 3, Stamford, Conn., 1996, Appleton & Lange.
5. Guyton AC, Hall JE: *Textbook of medical physiology,* ed 9, Philadelphia, 1996, WB Saunders.
6. Ma OJ, Mateer JR, DeBehnke DJ: Use of ultrasonography for the evaluation of pregnant trauma patients, *J Trauma* 40(4):665-668, 1996.
7. McKenney MG, et al.: *1,000 consecutive ultrasounds for blunt abdominal trauma, J Trauma* 40(4):607-612, 1996.
8. Moore EE, Malloy KL, Feliciano DV, editors: *Trauma,* ed 2, Norwalk Conn., 1988, Appleton & Lange.
9. Pachter HL, et al.: Stakes of nonoperative management of blunt hepatic injuries in 1995: a multicenter experience with 404 patients, *J Trauma* 40(1):31-38, 1996.
10. Papadopoulos R, Moore EE: Penetrating abdominal wounds. In Callaham ML, editor: *Current therapy in emergency medicine,* Toronto, 1987, BC Decker.
11. Rozycki GS, Shackford SR: Ultrasound, what every trauma surgeon should know, *J Trauma* 40(1):1-4, 1996.
12. Takishima T, et al.: Role of repeat computed tomography after emergency endoscopic retrograde pancreatography in diagnosis of trumatic injury to pancreatic ducts, *J Trauma* 40(2):253-257, 1996.

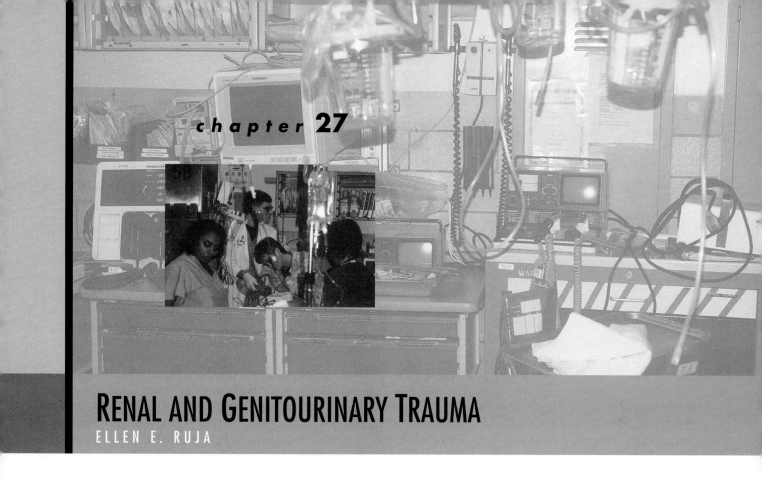

chapter 27

RENAL AND GENITOURINARY TRAUMA

ELLEN E. RUJA

Genitourinary (GU) trauma occurs in approximately 8% to 10% of all trauma patients.[2] The kidney is the GU structure most commonly injured followed by bladder, urethra, and ureter. Genitourinary injury is also common in children but rarely requires surgical management. Trauma to the GU system may be divided into upper urinary tract, lower urinary tract, and genital injuries. Two basic injury mechanism categories exist: blunt and penetrating. Blunt urologic injury, the most common form of trauma, accounts for 70% to 80% of all urologic injuries.[4] The presence of urologic injury should be considered in patients with severe lower abdominal blunt trauma and pelvic fracture. Urinary tract injury should be suspected for all patients with penetrating injuries to the abdomen, chest, or flank until proven otherwise. Prompt diagnosis and management are essential to minimize associated morbidity and mortality rates. This chapter reviews anatomy and physiology, mechanism of injury presentation, investigation, and treatment of genitourinary injuries.

ANATOMY AND PHYSIOLOGY

The genitourinary system consists of the kidneys, ureters, bladder, and urethra. Primary functions include the control of body fluids, regulation of electrolyte concentration, and excretion of metabolic end products. Additional functions include prostaglandin production, renin production, insulin degradation, stimulation of RBC production through production of erythropoietin, and metabolic conversion of vitamin D to an active form.

Kidneys are retroperitoneal organs that lie high on the posterior abdominal wall (Figure 27-1). The right kidney lies inferior and posterior to the liver and posterior to the ascending colon and duodenum. The right kidney is 1 to 2 cm lower than the left. The left kidney lies posterior to the descending colon and is associated with the tail of the pancreas medially and the spleen superiorly. Because of this relationship, major urinary tract trauma is associated with other intraabdominal injuries in approximately 73% of all penetrating trauma cases.[2] Kidneys are enclosed by a strong fibrous capsule and lie within a fatty tissue layer surrounded by Gerota's fascia. The perirenal space allows a large amount of blood to accumulate; however, the fascial layer can effectively tamponade renal bleeding in some cases. Normally, the kidneys are mobile within this area and can move vertically up or down three vertebral spaces (Figure 27-2). The kidney is well protected by the vertebral bodies and the back muscles posteriorly and the abdominal viscera anteriorly.

The pediatric kidney is theoretically at greater risk for injury than the adult kidney because of a relatively larger size, increased lobulation, less thoracic cavity protection, less perirenal fat, and less developed abdominal wall musculature. A child is more likely to undergo traumatic disruption of the ureteropelvic junction than an adult.

Ureters are small muscular tubes that are flexible and mobile. These hollow tubes drain urine from the kidneys to the bladder. Ureters do not contain valves or sphincters; therefore, urine can reflux into ureters from a distended bladder.

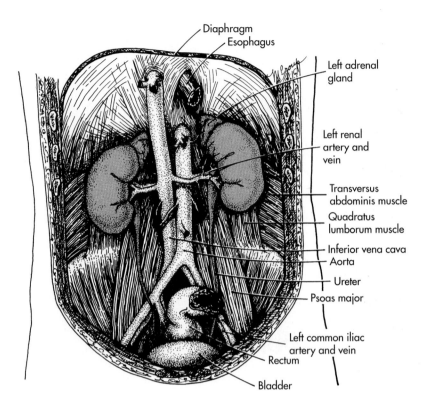

Figure **27-1** The genitourinary tract. *(From Price SA, Wilson LM:* Pathophysiology: clinical concepts of disease processes, *ed 5, St. Louis, 1997, Mosby.)*

They are rarely injured in blunt abdominal trauma because of their deep location in the retroperitoneal space and added protection from the abdominal contents, spine, and surrounding muscles. The blood supply to the ureter comes from the renal artery, aorta, and iliac artery.

The bladder is an extraperitoneal hollow organ located in the pelvis well protected by pelvic bones laterally, urogenital diaphragm inferiorly, and the rectum posteriorly. Until age 6, the bladder is an intraperitoneal organ, lying just beneath the anterior abdominal wall, so it is more vulnerable to external trauma. In the adult, the bladder is covered at the dome by a patch of peritoneum. Blood supply is abundant and mainly derived from the branches of the internal iliac artery. In the male, the prostate gland lies adjacent to the inferior margin and is fixed to the pubis anteriorly by ligaments and inferiorly by the urogenital diaphragm.

The female urethra is short and well protected by the symphysis pubis. In the male patient, the urethra is approximately 20 cm long and lies outside the body. The urogenital diaphragm divides the urethra into posterior and anterior segments (Figure 27-3). The posterior urethra is composed of the prostatic and membranous urethra, extends from the inferior urogenital diaphragm to the bladder neck, and is approximately 3 to 4 cm long. The anterior urethra consists of the bulbous and the pendulous urethra and extends from the external urinary meatus to the urogenital diaphragm.

The penis is composed of three vascular bodies: the paired corpora cavernosa and the corpus spongiosum. These structures are surrounded by deep (Buck's fascia) and superficial fasciae that allow mobility of the penile skin. The testis and epididymis reside in each scrotal compartment. Each testis receives blood via the spermatic cord, and through the testicular artery, the artery to the vas deferens, and the cremasteric artery. Each testis is surrounded by a tough fibrous capsule. The scrotum is covered by a thin layer of skin and receives blood from branches of the femoral and internal pudendal arteries.

PATIENT ASSESSMENT

Rapid diagnosis and treatment of GU trauma can be very difficult since it seldom occurs independently and is often associated with abdominal injuries. For any trauma patient, the most immediate requirements are the airway, breathing, and circulation. Once basic life-support measures are implemented, immediate monitoring of their effectiveness should be instituted.

The first rule of urologic trauma management is to aggressively seek and diagnose urologic injury since many of these injuries are not obvious at the onset. Assessment of GU trauma begins with a brief history including allergies, medications, previous and current illnesses, and known anatomic abnormalities. Preexisting renal abnormalities

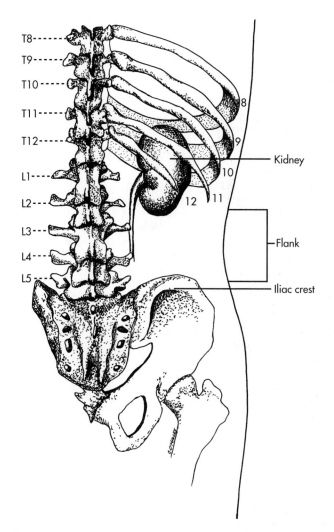

Figure **27-2** Anatomic relationship between kidneys and spine. *(From Neff JA, Kidd PS, editors:* Trauma nursing: the art and science, *St. Louis, 1993, Mosby.)*

may predispose the kidney to severe injury from even minor trauma. Abnormal kidneys occur in 0.1% to 23% of GU trauma cases.[2] Previous injuries to the GU tract may have caused chronic urologic infections and adhesions. Disorders such as chronic renal failure and renal artery stenosis profoundly influence initial treatment and long-term care of GU trauma.

Determining the mechanism of injury, performing a detailed physical examination, and further diagnostic testing complete clinical assessment of the injured patient. Certain mechanisms of injury carry a higher incidence of GU trauma (e.g., victim struck by a car, rapid deceleration incident, and/or penetrating trauma). All clothing is removed for inspection. Several patterns of contusion and bruising are specific to GU injuries. Grey Turner's sign is bruising over the flank and lower back that occurs in retroperitoneal hematoma and is frequently present with pelvic fractures. An edematous and contused scrotum may be seen with straddle in-

juries, pelvic fractures, or dissecting retroperitoneal hematomas. Perineal bruising is a late sign in a fracture of the symphysis pubis or pelvic rami. Fractures of the 11th and 12th ribs (Figure 27-2) have an increased potential of renal injury. Male genitalia are more easily examined than female genitalia. Laceration and avulsion injuries to the penis and scrotum are immediately apparent.

Following observation, the ED nurse auscultates the abdomen for bowel sounds. The absence of bowel sounds, abdominal rigidity, and guarding are not specific to GU injury, but may be indicative of intraperitoneal urine extravasation or renal injuries. The abdomen is palpated gently for the presence of a distended bladder. An empty bladder is not palpable; a full bladder may indicate an inability to void. If the patient cannot urinate, the urinary meatus should be checked carefully for blood. Blood at the meatus is a cardinal sign for anterior urethral injury. A digital rectal examination provides information on the condition of the prostate gland and posterior urethra. A high-riding prostate or boggy mass indicates a posterior rupture of the urethra. Extravasated urine and blood can dislocate the prostate. Percussion of the abdomen may reveal dullness suggesting extravasated urine or blood.

Baseline hematologic, coagulation, and electrolyte panels should be obtained. Hematuria is a strong indication of GU trauma. Radiologic tests are discussed further in this chapter with specific injuries. If the hemodynamic condition remains unstable despite control of external bleeding and fluid replacement, the patient should be prepared for exploratory surgery.

RENAL TRAUMA

Injuries to the kidneys may be limited to minor tissue damage or involve major vascular structures.

Blunt trauma accounts for 70% to 80% of renal injuries, whereas penetrating trauma accounts for only 6% to 14%.[4] Blunt injuries are most commonly caused by a motor vehicle collision; sports injuries, occupational injuries, and assault are less common. An injury from blunt trauma may be explained by three mechanisms: a direct blow to the flank, laceration of renal parenchyma from a fractured rib or vertebrae, or a sudden deceleration that causes shearing resulting in a renal pedicle injury or parenchymal renal damage. Falls from heights are associated with ureteral avulsion at the ureteropelvic junction. Renal injuries are more common than splenic rupture, four times more common than hepatic and intestinal injuries, and ten times more common than injuries to the lung, heart, pancreas, or major vessels. Boys sustain blunt renal injuries more often than girls; however, injuries in females are more severe. The majority of injuries caused by blunt trauma have limited severity and do not require exploration. Between 4% and 25% of blunt injuries are classified as major lacerations or vascular injuries as compared with 40% to 68% of penetrating injuries. Penetrating injuries are typically caused by gunshot or stab wounds,

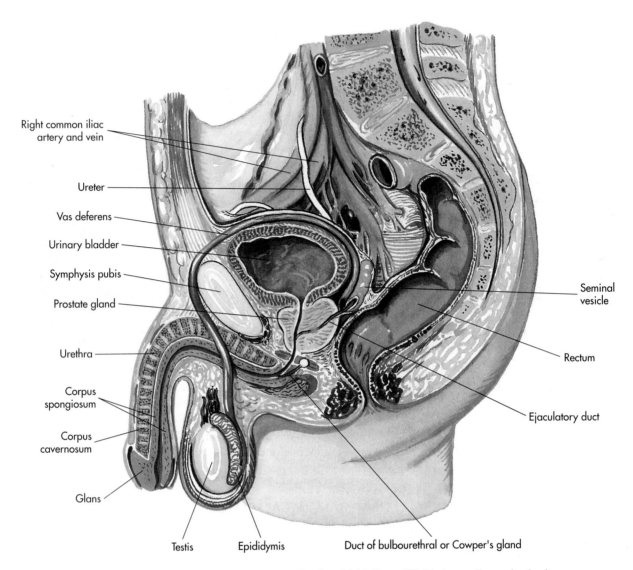

Right common iliac
artery and vein

Ureter

Vas deferens

Urinary bladder

Symphysis pubis

Prostate gland

Urethra

Corpus
spongiosum

Corpus
cavernosum

Glans

Testis   Epididymis

Seminal
vesicle

Rectum

Ejaculatory duct

Duct of bulbourethral or Cowper's gland

Figure **27-3**   The male genital tract. *(From Huether SE, McCance KL:* Understanding pathophysiology, *St. Louis, 1996, Mosby. Modified from Thibodeau GA:* Anatomy & physiology, *St. Louis, 1989, Mosby.)*

with gunshot wounds usually causing more complex injuries. Damage to the kidney may be caused by the bullet, bullet fragment, or blast effect. The majority of penetrating injuries require surgical intervention.

Classification of renal injuries has been established by the Organ Injury Scaling Committee of the American Association for the Surgery of Trauma (see Box 27-1 and Figure 27-4). A more practical staging system divides injuries into contusions, minor lacerations confined to the renal cortex, major lacerations that involve the collecting system, and vascular injuries.

Clinical indicators of blunt renal injury include a history of a direct blow to the flank, lower thoracic, or upper abdomen, and associated intraabdominal injuries. Signs of flank trauma include lower rib fractures, fracture of the lumbar transverse processes, bruising of the body wall, flank

mass, and flank tenderness. Patients may develop microscopic or gross hematuria. Hematuria is the best indicator of renal injury; however, the degree of hematuria does not always correlate with the degree of injury. Seven percent to 14% of patients with major lacerations or vascular injury and 6% to 10% of patients with minor lacerations after penetrating trauma do not have hematuria. Significant renal injury can occur with microhematuria in the absence of hypotension. Hypovolemic shock secondary to a major renal laceration may occur.

Initial radiographic evaluation of penetrating wounds consists of plain radiographs of the kidneys, ureters, and bladder (KUB) to determine path and appearance of the projectile. A flat plate radiograph of the abdomen may reveal loss of normal renal outline, loss of psoas shadow on the affected side, scoliosis away from the kidney, and a flank

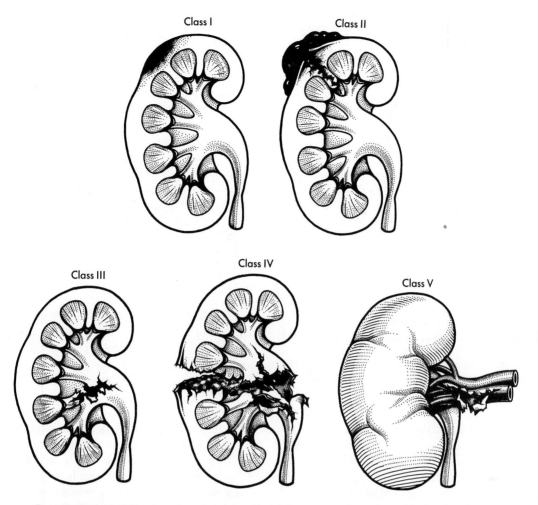

Figure **27-4**   Classification of renal trauma. *Class I,* Renal contusion; *Class II,* cortical laceration; *Class III,* caliceal laceration; *Class IV,* complete renal fracture; *Class V,* vascular pedicle injury. *(From Rosen P et al:* Emergency medicine, *ed 3, St. Louis, 1992, Mosby.)*

mass. Fractures of transverse processes and lower ribs may also be clues that a renal injury has occurred. Indications for radiologic evaluation to stage renal trauma include penetrating injuries proximal to the GU system, and blunt trauma with gross hematuria or microscopic hematuria associated with hypotension.

An intravenous pyelogram (IVP) is the initial examination of choice in patients with penetrating injury who are unstable and require immediate operative intervention. However, an IVP has significant limitations in assessing associated intraabdominal injuries and staging renal injuries. An IVP should not be the initial study in patients with blunt trauma who are hemodynamically stable.

Computed tomography (CT) is the most accurate modality available for staging renal injuries, determining renal pedicle injuries, depicting size and extent of retroperitoneal hematoma, and evaluating associated intraabdominal injuries. Angiography is a sensitive modality for staging renal injuries and for ruling out vascular injuries. This invasive modality does not evaluate other abdominal injuries; there-

fore, angiography is reserved for high-risk patients with an indeterminate CT scan.

Magnetic resonance imaging (MRI) can complement a CT scan in patients with severe renal injury, a preexisting renal abnormality, equivocal CT findings, or when a repeat radiographic follow-up is required. Magnetic resonance imaging replaces CT in patients with an iodine allergy and may be used for initial staging when CT is not available. A patient must be hemodynamically stable before MRI can be used.

Radionucleotide renal scans are particularly helpful in detecting arterial injury; however, minor extravasation is missed, and lacerations are less likely to be seen than in other studies. Ultrasonography is appropriate for cases when mild injury is present or when suspicion of injury is low. This diagnostic modality cannot differentiate a hematoma, laceration, or urine; therefore, CT is more appropriate for a moderate-to-high suspicion of renal injury.

Significant progress in the management of renal trauma during the last three decades has increased the rate of renal

Box **27-1**	**Classification of Renal Injuries. Organ Injury Scaling Committee.**
Grade I	Contusion: microscopic or gross hematuria; normal urologic studies
	Subcapsular hematoma, nonexpanding; no laceration
Grade II	Laceration of renal parenchyma <1 cm; no extravasation
	Perinephric hematoma, nonexpanding
Grade III	Laceration of renal parenchyma >1 cm
	No urinary extravasation; no collecting system involvement
Grade IV	Laceration involving collecting system
	Perinephric and paranephric extravasation
	Thrombosis of segmental renal artery
	Main renal artery or vein injury, hemorrhage controlled
Grade V	Fractured kidney
	Thrombosis of main renal artery
	Avulsion of main renal artery or vein

*Grades I and II are minor; Grades II, IV, and V are major.
From Dixon MD, McAninch JW: *American Urological Association update series, traumatic renal injuries, part I: assessment and management,* Houston, 1991, The Association.

salvage. Surgical exploration is mandatory in patients with gunshot wounds. Vital renal structures are located toward the midline of the abdomen, so penetration through the anterior abdomen has a greater chance for major injury. Management of stab wounds is different than management of gunshot wounds. Peripheral stab wounds, such as flank wounds posterior to the anterior axillary line, are more likely to injure nonvital structures.

Most blunt renal injuries can be treated nonoperatively with bedrest, frequent examinations, serial urine analyses, and analgesics. Controversy still exists about whether surgical or conservative management should be used in hemodynamically stable patients with severe renal injury. Unless immediate exploratory laparotomy is indicated for associated injuries or shock, most hemodynamically stable patients with major renal injuries, penetrating or blunt, can be managed by nonsurgical treatment with delayed intervention as needed. Hemodynamically unstable patients with renal pedicle or ureteral injuries, an expanding retroperitoneal hematoma, falling hemoglobin levels, pulsatile hematoma, extensive extravasation, and nonviable tissue in more than 20% of the kidney may require immediate surgical management.

Early complications related to renal injury include delayed bleeding, urinoma, abscess formation, renal insufficiency, urinary extravasation, and fistula formation. Late complications include arteriovenous fistulas, hydronephrosis, stone formation, chronic pyelonephritis, and pain. Hypertension may occur after a renal artery injury or renal compression injury. Patients may become hypertensive within 24 hours of injury, or onset of hypertension may be delayed up to 10 years following injury. Patients with severe renal injuries require long-term follow-up to examine for hypertension, perinephric cysts, arteriovenous fistulas, stones, and retarded growth in the injured kidney.

Renal pedicle injuries usually occur in a seriously traumatized patient. The majority of renal pedicle injuries occur in children and young adults. The left renal vein is the most commonly injured vessel. The usual mechanism of renal artery occlusion is an intimal tear secondary to an acceleration-deceleration injury. Renal vascular injuries include a vessel injury, renal artery thrombosis, and disruption of the renal artery intimal layer resulting in an aneurysm or thrombosis. No signs or symptoms are specific for renal pedicle injury. Hematuria is absent in one third of cases. Despite immediate diagnosis by CT or IVP, most patients are not candidates for vascular repair because of the high incidence of severe associated injuries. Early diagnosis is essential. Surgical repair of pedicle injury within 12 hours is required to restore blood flow to the ischemic kidney and to salvage renal function. Total avulsion of the renal pedicle is an indication for nephrectomy.

URETERAL INJURIES

Ureteral injuries from trauma are rare. The most common mechanism of ureteral injury is penetrating trauma. A high index of suspicion is necessary to diagnose ureteral injury since no early signs may be evident on initial examination. Blunt trauma usually causes avulsion of the ureteropelvic junction subsequent to major hyperextension of upper lumbar and lower thoracic areas. A penetrating injury may cause partial or complete ureteral transection. With a penetrating lower abdominal injury, careful examination of the wound with the ureter in mind is essential. Physical findings of ureteral injury are nonspecific and usually relate to an associated intraabdominal injury. Only when the ureter is obstructed and produces pain with classic radiation to the groin is diagnosis easy. Microhematuria is seen in 90% of cases.

Diagnosis of ureteral injury is made by IVP and retrograde ureteropyelography. Most patients with a ureteral injury require operative exploration for associated abdominal injuries. Dismembered pyeloplasty with ureteral stenting and a nephrostomy tube is the treatment of choice. Untreated ureteral injury can lead to urinoma, abscess, or stricture.

BLADDER INJURIES

Major bladder trauma is relatively uncommon, accounting for less than 2% of abdominal injuries requiring surgical repair and occurring in only 5% to 10% of patients with pelvic fracture.[2] Rupture of the bladder does not usually occur as an isolated injury and rarely presents without fracture of the pelvis. The mechanism of injury in bladder rupture varies with patient population, amount of urine in the blad-

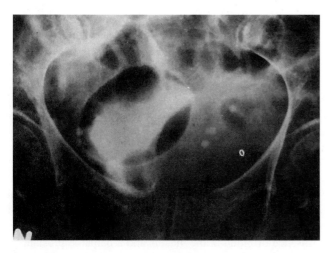

Figure **27-5** Bladder contusion secondary to a pelvic hematoma and pelvic fracture. *(From Sandler CM, et al:* Radiology of the bladder and urethra in blunt pelvic trauma, *Radiol Clin North Am 19:195, 1981.)*

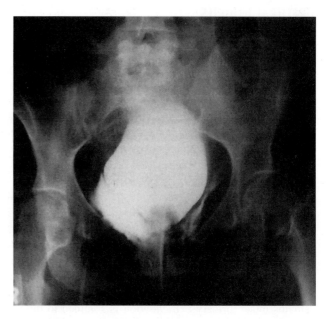

Figure **27-6** Extraperitoneal bladder rupture secondary to pelvic fracture. *(From Gillenwater JY et al:* Adult and pediatric urology, *ed 3, vol 1, St. Louis, 1996, Mosby.)*

der at the time of injury, and location of injury within the bladder. Children are more susceptible to direct force and intraperitoneal rupture because of location. Injury to the bladder base and bladder neck may be caused by direct laceration from a fractured pelvic bone or shearing mechanism.

Bladder injuries may be classified as contusions, extraperitoneal ruptures, intraperitoneal ruptures, and combined injuries. Nonpenetrating bladder injuries account for the majority of injuries. Twenty-five percent are intraperitoneal and usually not associated with a pelvic fracture (Figure 27-5). Injuries are usually caused by a suprapubic blow in the presence of a full bladder. The bladder tends to rupture at the weakest point (i.e., dome or posterior wall of the bladder). Intraperitoneal ruptures involve extravasation of blood and urine into the peritoneal cavity. Fifty-six percent to 78% of bladder ruptures are extraperitoneal, secondary to a bony part rupture or shearing forces associated with pelvic fracture (Figure 27-6). Extraperitoneal bladder rupture involves perforation of the anterolateral bladder with extravasation of blood and urine into the retroperitoneal space. Seventy percent to 83% of blunt bladder injuries are associated with pelvic fracture; however, only 10% of patients with a pelvic fracture have a ruptured bladder.[2] Combined intraperitoneal and extraperitoneal ruptures occur in up to 12% of cases, are associated with severe pelvic injury, and have a high mortality rate.[2]

Blunt lower abdominal trauma is suggested by a patient's history. Most patients with bladder perforation are unable to void, and have suprapubic pain and hematuria. Associated leg fractures are also often found. Hemodynamic instability is common because of extensive blood loss in the pelvis and associated injuries. Gross hematuria and pelvic fractures are present in over 90% of all bladder ruptures.[2] Extravasation

of sterile urine may not lead to signs of peritoneal irritation. Late signs and symptoms are abdominal distension, acute abdomen, and increased blood urea nitrogen and serum creatinine levels.

Radiographic evaluation consists of a retrograde urethrogram and cystogram in all male patients with pelvic fractures associated with gross hematuria, inability to urinate, blood at meatus, perineal swelling, or nonpalpable prostate. Female patients with a pelvic fracture should undergo careful visual inspection of the urethra.

Cystography is the most accurate method of diagnosis. A plain film of the pelvis should be obtained before cystography. Computed tomography can detect bladder rupture but is inferior to cystography. Contrast infused into the bladder is seen as extravasate by CT. A CT scan appears to be no more accurate than standard cystography, but is better than intravenous urography. Only 15% of bladder injuries are identified with IVP.[2]

The usual treatment for bladder ruptures is surgical repair. Intraperitoneal ruptures do not close spontaneously and most extraperitoneal ruptures are associated with bony injuries or other intraabdominal traumas that necessitate surgical exploration. Conservative therapy consisting of catheter drainage, antibiotics, and close clinical observation has been advocated for extraperitoneal tears in cases with minimal bleeding, no sepsis, and maintenance of adequate drainage.

Bladder injuries can lead to urinary ascites, abscess formation, and urinary fistula formation. An overall mortality of 9% reported for bladder rupture is clearly related to the high incidence of severe associated injuries.

URETHRAL INJURIES

A urethral injury should be suspected in any patient with a history of perineal or pelvic trauma. Urethral injuries rarely occur in females. When they do occur, injuries are usually associated with a pelvic fracture, obstetric injury, and anterior vaginal lacerations. Proximal urethral injuries almost invariably occur in men. Three percent to 25% of male patients sustaining a pelvic fracture suffer injury to the posterior urethra. Sixty-five percent experience complete urethral disruption; 34% experience partial urethral tears. Urethral injuries are usually caused by shearing rather than direct laceration. If injury is superior, the prostate may be forced upward by a developing hematoma. In addition, 10% to 20% of patients with bladder rupture caused by pelvic trauma have a concomitant urethral injury.[2] Injuries to the anterior urethra can occur as a result of a straddle injury, or blunt or sharp trauma to the penis caused by passage of a foreign body. Partial transection occurs most often. If Buck's fascia remains intact, urinary extravasation is confined to the penile shaft and perineum. With rupture of Buck's fascia, voiding can cause extensive extravasation along the abdominal wall.

Blunt trauma to the posterior urethra may result in three general types of injuries, which may be either incomplete or complete. With Type I injuries, the urethra is stretched but does not rupture. Type II injuries are disruption of the urethra above the urogenital diaphragm, and Type III injuries are bulbomembranous injuries inferior to the urogenital diaphragm. Injuries to the anterior urethra are classified as contusions or partial or complete lacerations (Figure 27-7).

Clinical symptoms may be variable. Some patients have a classic triad of blood at the urethral meatus, inability to uri-nate, and a distended, palpable bladder. However, many patients with partial urethral tears can void. Other signs and symptoms include pain on micturition, perineal/scrotal/penile hematoma or swelling, hematuria, and a "high-riding" prostate.

A digital rectal examination should be performed in all trauma patients to exclude associated rectal injury. Inability to palpate the prostate has been described as a classic sign of posterior urethral injury. A retrograde urethrogram is the study of choice for evaluation of urethral injuries.

A urethral catheter should not be inserted when urethral injury is suspected. Such a procedure can convert a partial urethral disruption into a complete one, raises the risk of contamination, and increases the risk of further hemorrhage. Absence of blood at the meatus and a palpable prostate on rectal examination are sufficient evidence to allow passage of a urethral catheter. If resistance is encountered, the procedure should be stopped and urethrography performed. With minimal disruption of the urethra, gentle placement of a soft Foley catheter may be the only treatment required. With complete disruption, prompt suprapubic cystostomy drainage of the bladder is mandatory.

Impotence, stricture, and incontinence are the most severe complications of posterior urethral disruption. With anterior urethral injury, stricture formation is the most common complication. Impotence and incontinence are rare with anterior urethral injuries.

GENITAL INJURIES

Testicular and penile injuries are not common. The majority of injuries to the testes are secondary to blunt trauma. Patients with testicular contusions are treated with analgesics, elevation of the scrotum, iced compresses, and bedrest. Occasional lacerations of the scrotum and contents are seen. Penetrating and degloving injuries of the penis can occur in the workplace. Sexually related injuries involving strangulation or amputation of the penis have also been reported. Penetrating injuries mandate exploration and reconstruction. Traumatic amputation may be amenable to microsurgical reanastomosis.

Penile Trauma

Blunt trauma to the erect penis can rupture the tunica albuginea surrounding the corpora cavernosa. A patient typically reports a "cracking or popping sound" during intercourse or sexual play, severe pain, and immediate detumescence. A hematoma with marked edema develops in the penile shaft. The fracture can sometimes be palpated and the defect detected. In 30% of patients, the urethra is lacerated, so urethrography should be considered.[2] In cases without urethral injury, most patients can urinate normally. Occasionally, a hematoma and edema cause external urethral compression leading to urinary retention. Management is controversial. Early surgical repair is associated with a lower risk of persistent penile angulation, a shorter hospital

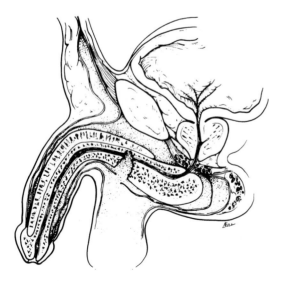

Figure 27-7   Depiction of anterior urethral injury. *(From Neff JA, Kidd PS:* Trauma nursing: the art and science, *St. Louis, 1993, Mosby.)*

stay, and more rapid functional return. Conservative treatment may be warranted in cases with minimal hematoma and no extravasation during a cavernosography. Treatment includes sedation, elevation of the penis, and ice packs.

Other penile injuries may be the result of direct trauma caused by zippers, bites, or knives. Treatment is determined by the severity of the injury.

Testicular Trauma

Blunt trauma to the scrotum can cause a testicular rupture. The patient with a scrotal injury may have acute pain, nausea, vomiting, syncope, and urinary retention. Patients may have large scrotal hematomas that make examination difficult, so sonography is useful. Testicular rupture should be repaired immediately, and in most cases reconstruction is possible. All penetrating testicular injuries should be explored and repaired. Orchiectomy is necessary in some cases.

Avulsion injuries can cause loss of all or part of penile and scrotal skin (Figure 27-8). Industrial or farming accidents are often responsible for such injuries. The penile shaft can be covered with skin grafts, and return of function is expected. Partial scrotal skin loss is managed by primary closure. The scrotum regenerates to accommodate the testicles and spermatic cords. Total skin loss leaves the testicles unprotected; testicles should be temporarily placed in thigh pouches when immediate grafting is not possible.

Straddle Injuries

Straddle injuries occur when a patient falls and takes the brunt of the fall on the perineum. These injuries commonly occur in young patients as they fall onto bicycle bars, motorcycles, and fences. On examination of a female patient, a vulvovaginal laceration with extensive ecchymosis of the perineum may be evident. Straddle injuries are often accompanied by vulvar hematomas that can extend into the retroperitoneal space. Associated urethral injuries and rectal tears should be ruled out. Treatment of straddle injuries involves repair of the laceration with evacuation and drainage of any hematomas. The most common complication in the immediate postoperative period is infection. Sexual dysfunction may also occur.

Foreign Bodies

The medical literature contains numerous case reports of various foreign bodies found in the urethra and bladder. Almost anything small and firm that can be passed into the urethra has been found there, including electric cable, tweezers, spaghetti, pebbles, paper clips, hairpins, and screws. In adults, most foreign bodies are inserted for erotic stimulation. However, psychologic disorders and drug ingestion are other frequent reasons for such activity. Children with foreign bodies in the urethra are usually curious.

Patients may be too embarrassed to admit they inserted or applied any object and usually present when a complication or symptom occurs. The most common reason for consultation is dysuria. Other complaints are suprapubic or perineal pain, urethral discharge, hematuria, difficulty urinating, swelling, or abscess formation.

Clinical diagnosis is based on history and should always be considered in patients with chronic urinary tract infections. Radiographic studies, including plain radiographs, are usually helpful for radiopaque objects. Xeroradiography is effective for detecting nonmetallic foreign bodies traumatically or deliberately introduced into the genital tissues, including objects made of plastic, glass, rubber, cloth, or wood.

Foreign bodies below the urogenital diaphragm can usually be palpated and readily removed endoscopically, whereas foreign bodies above the urogenital diaphragm require greater endoscopic manipulation, perineal urethrostomy, or suprapubic cystotomy.

SUMMARY

Urinary trauma can be readily identified clinically, and the extent of injury ascertained with radiographic imaging.

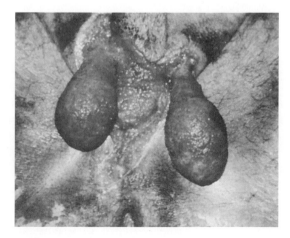

Figure **27-8** Scrotal avulsion injury. *(From Neff JA, Kidd PS: Trauma nursing: the art and science, St. Louis, 1993, Mosby. Courtesy Tucson Medical Center Radiology Department, Tucson, Ariz.)*

Box **27-2**

NURSING DIAGNOSES FOR GU TRAUMA

Altered tissue perfusion
High risk for fluid volume deficit
Pain related to injury
Impaired tissue integrity
Altered patterns of urinary elimination
High risk for infection
High risk for sexual dysfunction
High risk for body image disturbance
Anxiety related to injury

An injured patient with suggested urologic injury has a host of general surgical concerns, particularly in conjunction with pelvic fractures; however, life-threatening concerns related to airway control, ventilation, and hemodynamic status are the first priority. Following treatment of these concerns, organ-specific work-up may proceed. Close cooperation among the health care team is required for optimum outcome. Box 27-2 highlights nursing diagnoses for patients with GU trauma.

REFERENCES

1. Carroll PR, McAninch JW: Staging of renal trauma, *Urol Clin North Am* 16:193, 1989.

2. Feliciano DV, Moore EE, Mattox KL: *Trauma,* ed 3, Stamford, Conn., 1996, Appleton & Lange.

3. Leppaniemi A, et al.: Comparison of high-field magnetic resonance imaging with computed tomography in the evaluation of blunt renal trauma, *J Trauma,* 38(3):420-427, 1995.

4. Peterson NE: Current management of acute renal trauma. In Rous SW, editor: *Urology annual,* Norwalk, Conn, 1991, Appleton & Lange, pp 151-179.

5. Quilan D, Gearhart J: Blunt renal trauma in childhood, *Br J Urol* 66:526-531, 1990.

6. Stern JP, et al: Blunt renal trauma in the pediatric population: indications for radiographic evaluation, Department of Pediatric Urology University of Southern California School of Medicine, Children's Hospital of Los Angeles, *Urology* 44(3):406-410, September 1994.

7. Swischuk LE: Abdominal trauma and hematuria, *Pediatr Emerg Care* 10(3):181-182, June 1994.

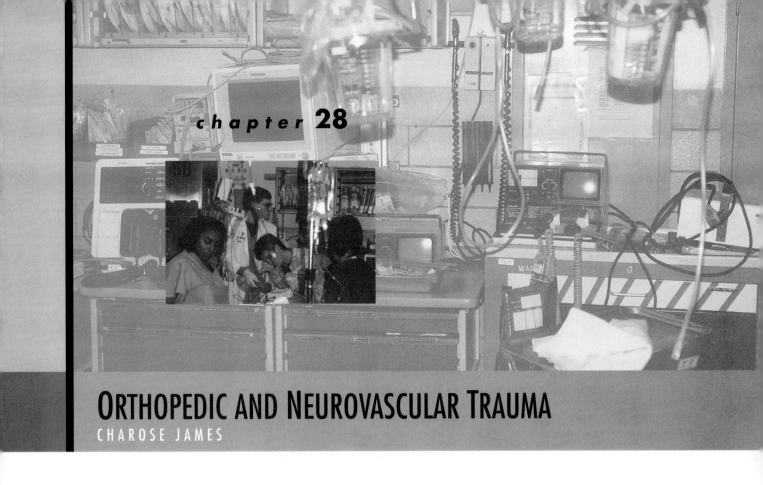

chapter 28

ORTHOPEDIC AND NEUROVASCULAR TRAUMA

CHAROSE JAMES

Approximately 33 million musculoskeletal injuries occur annually, including 20 million fractures, dislocations, and sprains, and approximately 8000 deaths.[25] Primary mechanisms of injury are motor vehicle collisions (MVCs), assaults, falls, sports/recreation, and injuries sustained at work or home.

Musculoskeletal injury is one of the most common types of injury seen in the emergency department (ED) and a significant cause of disability. Bone, soft tissue, and associated neurovascular injuries are rarely emergent unless accompanied by a life-threatening hemorrhage as in certain amputations and pelvic fractures. Fractures and soft tissue injuries are primarily designated as urgent because of potential neurovascular injury with resultant limb disability and pain. Early intervention enhances preservation of limb and function. This chapter focuses on common orthopedic and neurovascular extremity injuries and appropriate therapeutic interventions. Related anatomy and physiology are briefly reviewed.

ANATOMY AND PHYSIOLOGY

The musculoskeletal system and related neurovascular structures consist of bones, joints, tendons, ligaments, muscles, vessels, and nerves. The skeletal system contains 206 bones, which provide support, strength, movement, and protection to the body and organs (Figure 28-1, *A* and 28-1, *B*). Bones also store calcium and are involved in blood cell production.

Bones are characterized by shape as long, short, flat, or irregular, with the shape of a particular bone suited for a

unique function or purpose. The skeleton is composed of two types of bones: cancellous and cortical. Cancellous (spongy) bone is found in the skull, vertebrae, pelvis, and long-bone ends. Cortical (dense) bone is found in the long bones. Bones are supplied by blood vessels, nerves, and lymphatic vessels that nourish bone tissue and allow the bone to repair injuries. The periosteum covers the bones and provides an additional blood supply.

Bone is connected to other bone by stabilizing bands of elastic, fibrous connective tissue called ligaments. Nonelastic fibrous cords that connect muscle to bone are tendons. Dense connective tissue found between the ribs, in the nasal septum, ear, larynx, trachea, bronchi, between vertebrae, and on articulating surfaces is known as cartilage. Cartilage has a limited vascular supply, whereas bone tissue has abundant vascular structures.

Joints are classified as nonsynovial (immovable and slightly immovable) and synovial (freely movable). Synovial joints have two articulating surfaces covered with cartilage and surrounded by a two-layered synovial membrane sac. The entire joint is then encapsulated by dense, ligamentous material. Joints provide mobility and stability, flexion and extension, medial and lateral rotation, and abduction and adduction. Joint movement is enhanced by muscles and ligaments that overlie the joint.

Nerves and arteries lie in close proximity to bones and muscle groups, with arterioles distributed throughout the periosteum to provide nutrients. Nerves provide sensation

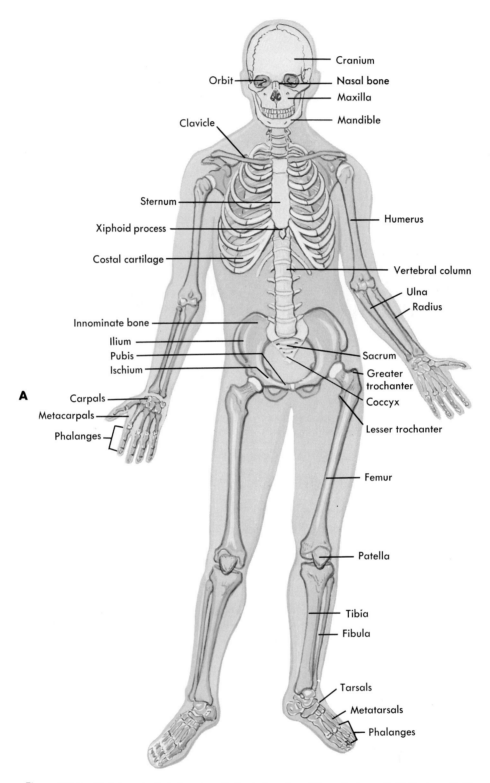

Figure **28-1**   Skeleton. **A,** Anterior view. **B,** Posterior view. *(From Anthony C, Thibodeau G: Text-book of anatomy and physiology, ed 11, St. Louis, 1983, Mosby.)*

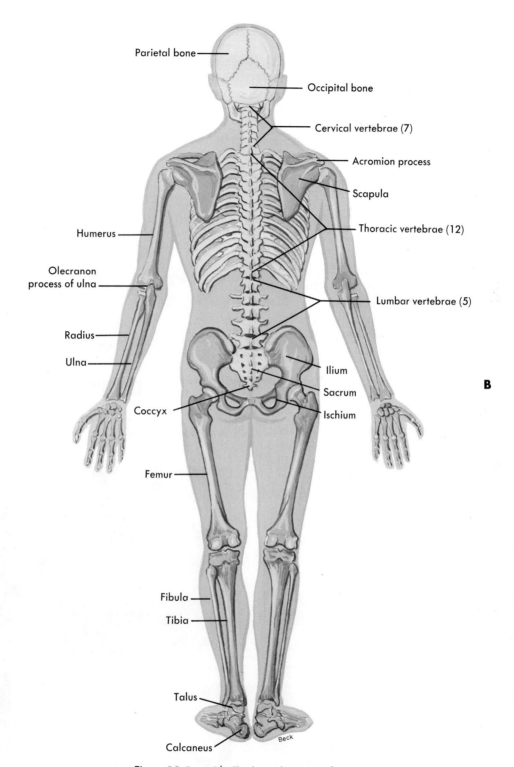

Figure **28-1** cont'd   For legend see opposite page.

and movement. Close proximity of arteries and nerves to bone structures increases the risk for injury with trauma to soft tissue, muscle, bone, or joint.

PATIENT ASSESSMENT

Assessment of orthopedic trauma begins with an assessment of the airway, breathing, and circulation (ABCs). Rapid assessment identifies major injuries of head, cervical spine, chest, and abdomen, and prioritizes essential interventions. Once assured that no life-threatening injury has been left unattended, the nurse assesses and stabilizes any extremity injuries. Box 28-1 highlights essential assessment parameters for orthopedic injuries.

Before immobilization, open fractures should be stabilized and bleeding controlled. Open fractures with obvious bone protrusion or a deep laceration should be rinsed with sterile normal saline to remove gross contamination and covered with a dry sterile dressing. Irrigation of a puncture wound should not occur over a fracture site, since this can force bacteria deeper into the wound. Reduction of an open fracture also forces contaminants into the wound and should not be attempted in a prehospital setting.

To control bleeding, pressure is applied directly to the injury site, edges of the wound, or an adjacent pressure point. A tourniquet should not be used because of potential neurovascular compromise.

Immobilization

Immobilization should be accomplished as soon as possible to minimize further damage or complications secondary to bone fragments and to reduce pain in the injured limb. A splint should include the area above and below the injury. The neurovascular status should be checked before and after immobilization. If neurovascular status is initially compromised, gradual traction may be used to allow return of neurologic or vascular function before splinting. If neurovascular status is compromised after splinting or traction, the splint

should be removed or traction decreased and the splint reapplied. Angulation should be corrected only if it prevents immobilization or if neurovascular compromise is present. Splinting is best accomplished with an assistant to support the limb while the padded splint is placed and wrapped with a noncompressive bandage. Neurovascular status is rechecked after splinting.

Four basic types of splints exist including soft splints, such as pillows; hard splints such as padded board, cardboard, aluminum, or a ladder splint; inflatable air splints (Figure 28-2) or vacuum splints (Figure 28-3); and traction splints, which reduce angulation and provide support (Figure 28-4).

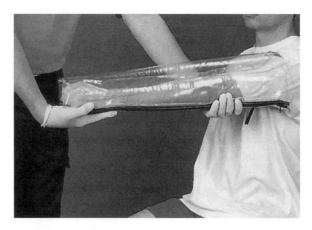

Figure **28-2** Air splint. *(From Stoy WA/CEM:* Mosby's EMT—basic textbook, *St. Louis, 1996, Mosby.)*

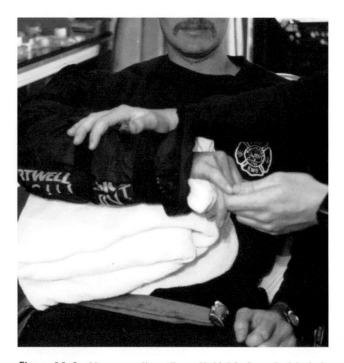

Figure **28-3** Vacuum splint. *(From Kidd PS, Sturt P:* Mosby's emergency nursing reference, *St. Louis, 1996, Mosby.)*

Box **28-1**   **Assessment of Orthopedic Injuries**
Swelling and deformity
Contusion, abrasion, laceration, puncture wound
Bruising
Crepitus
Point tenderness
Neurovascular assessment
*P*ain
*P*ulses
*P*aralysis
*P*aresthesia
*P*allor
Tem*P*erature
Ca*P*illary refill

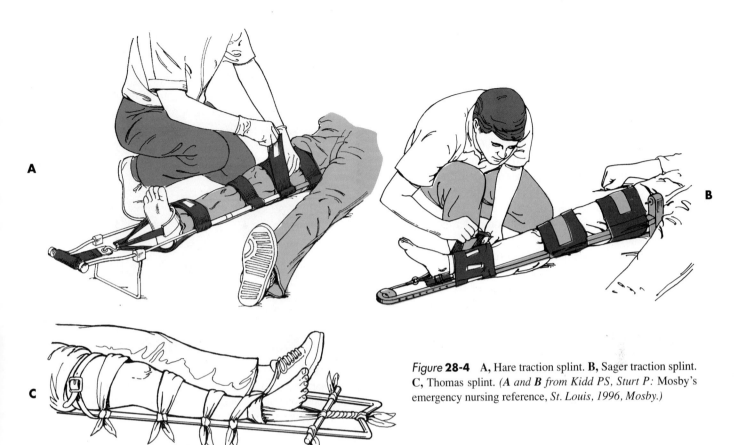

Figure **28-4** **A,** Hare traction splint. **B,** Sager traction splint. **C,** Thomas splint. *(A and B from Kidd PS, Sturt P:* Mosby's emergency nursing reference, *St. Louis, 1996, Mosby.)*

Air splints were used extensively when first developed because they conformed well and provided visualization of the injured extremity. However, an air splint that is not open on the distal end does not allow neurovascular checks without deflating or unzipping the splint. An air splint should be inflated so that a finger can be slipped between the splint and the skin. Excessive pressure in the splint can compromise circulation. Air splints can also stick to the skin, cause irritation, and are difficult to remove with excessive diaphoresis.

Several types of traction splints are available and are usually applied by prehospital providers. The Thomas ring splint, Sager splint, and Hare splint (Figure 28-4) are used for fractures of the midshaft of the femur or upper third of the tibia but should not be used for the hip, lower tibia or fibula, ankle, or femur with associated tibial-fibular fractures.

After immobilization, the limb should be elevated and an ice pack applied to minimize swelling. Caution is advised since overzealous elevation may compromise arterial circulation, and excessive prolonged cold may damage tissues.

The patient should be completely disrobed and examined for anterior injuries and then logrolled to identify posterior injuries while maintaining adequate cervical spine immobilization. Rings should be removed if the injury involves the hand or arm. Elevation and cooling measures should be maintained, and neurovascular status checked periodically.

Careful history should include circumstances of the injury (time and mechanism) and significant medical history including acute and chronic alcohol use, medications, allergies, and tetanus immunization status. Time of last oral intake should be recorded and NPO status initiated if surgical intervention is a possibility.

SOFT TISSUE INJURIES

Soft tissue injuries generally accompany orthopedic trauma; involve skin, muscles, tendons, cartilage, ligaments, veins, arteries, and nerves; and can compromise circulation and function. Injuries to the skin include abrasions, avulsions, contusions, hematomas, lacerations, and puncture wounds (Chapter 17).

Principles of nursing care are generally the same for various soft tissue injuries. Inspection involves checking for wounds, swelling, hematomas, and bleeding, and then assessing neurovascular status. A soft bulky dressing is applied, swelling is minimized with elevation and cooling measures. Radiographs are used to rule out foreign bodies and fractures. Analgesia is administered as prescribed for isolated injuries, and antibiotics for significant, contaminated wounds. Written discharge instructions discuss elevation and cold therapy (i.e., a covered ice bag to the injury for 20 minutes, every 2-3 hours for 24 to 48 hours).

Fingertip Injuries

Fingertip injuries are frequently seen in the ED with the most common types being a crush injury to the distal phalanx, secondary to a heavy object falling on the finger, or the digit being caught in a house or car door. Crush injuries can also be associated with a fracture. If a hematoma forms under the fingernail (subungual hematoma), nail trephination should be carried out by penetrating the fingernail over the site of the hematoma with a nail drill, scalpel, pencil cautery, or superheated paperclip to release blood under the nail and relieve pressure.

A fingertip injury seen with increasing frequency is one caused by a high-pressure paint or grease gun. Injury may occur when a person is cleaning the tip of the gun and a stream of paint or grease is released into the fingertip and into the hand at high pressure. Particular attention to history is crucial since the injury appears as a small pinhole in the fingertip, but is a serious, limb-threatening surgical emergency. Therapeutic intervention requires debridement of the paint- or grease-infected limb under general anesthesia.

Impaling Injuries

Impaling injuries usually result from an industrial accident in which the victim falls onto a sharp, immobile object. Nails from a powered nailgun are also common. Impaled objects are not immediately removed. Surgical removal may be required. Complications from this type of injury include infection and problems specific to the structures impaled. Biologic substances such as wood carry an increased risk of infection.

Gunshot Wounds

Gunshot wounds usually result from hunting or acts of violence. Tissue damage depends on type of weapon and caliber of ammunition used, distance from the weapon, and part(s) of the body injured (Figure 28-5). Tissue, bones, organs, and vessels away from the bullet's unpredictable path may also be injured. Appearance of the entrance wound does not always reflect destruction beneath. An extremity injury may be associated with a truncal injury because of a projectile path through the chest into the arm or through the arm into the chest, or because of multiple bullet wounds. Careful assessment including neurovascular assessment of all the limbs is critical so that details such as other wounds or tetanus immunization status are not overlooked. With gunshot wounds, police may need to document evidence surrounding the wound site or powder burns on the hand. See Chapter 4 for a discussion of evidence collection/preservation.

Tendon and Muscle Rupture

Tendon and muscle ruptures are generally related to sports or recreation although metabolic disease and age may

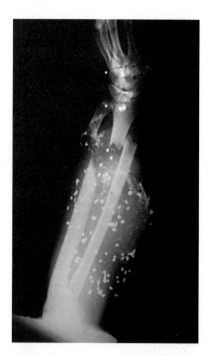

Figure **28-5** Gunshot wound fracture of radius and ulna with extensive soft tissue damage. *(From Ballinger:* Merrill's atlas of radiographic positions and radiologic procedures, *ed 8, St. Louis, 1995, Mosby. Courtesy Sharon A. Coffey, RT.)*

be a causative factor. Runners may experience a quadriceps tear, whereas a biceps tear may occur with minimal effort in middle-aged or older individuals. Surgery may be required to restore function for complete tears. For incomplete injury, rest and ice for 24 to 48 hours followed by heat may be prescribed.

An Achilles tendon rupture may occur in start-and-stop sports in which one steps off abruptly on the forefoot with the knee forced in extension. This causes sharp pain extending from the heel into the back of the leg, sudden inability to use the foot, obvious deformity, and a positive Thompson's sign (Figure 28-6). A compression bandage should be applied and the patient prepared for surgery.

Crush Injuries

Crush injuries frequently occur in industrial settings (e.g., arm caught in the wringer of an industrial washing machine, press, or conveyor; or limbs or trunk caught between equipment). Injury may involve only the distal end of a digit or large areas of the body. Depending on the extent of damage, orthopedic, surgical, neurosurgical, or vascular-surgical intervention may be required.

Complications from crush injuries depend on the mechanism of injury and extent of tissue damage. With significant tissue necrosis (multicompartment), systemic crush syndrome characterized by myoglobinuria, extracellular fluid loss, acidosis, increased potassium, renal failure, shock, and cardiac disruption may occur.

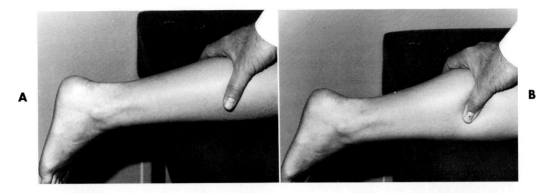

Figure **28-6** Thompson test. **A,** No pressure on gastrocnemius. **B,** Pressure on gastrocnemius and associated plantar flexion. If Achilles tendon is torn, plantar flexion does not accompany pressure. *(From Nicholas JA, Hershman EB, editors:* The lower extremity and spine in sports medicine, *ed 2, vol 1, St. Louis, 1995, Mosby.)*

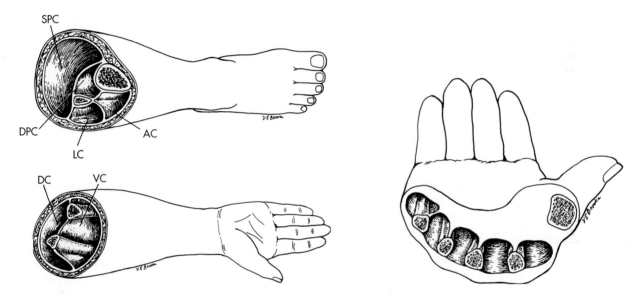

Figure **28-7** Cross section anatomy of calf, forearm, and hand showing fibrosseous compartments. *(From Matsen FA, III:* Compartmental syndromes, *New York, 1980, Grune & Stratton.)*

Compartment Syndrome

Compartment syndrome occurs when swelling and/or compression-restriction causes pressure in the muscle compartment to rise to the point that microvascular circulation is interrupted. The resulting tissue ischemia threatens limb survival. Compression may be caused by severe soft tissue injuries, a fracture, casts, or a pneumatic antishock garment (PASG). Prolonged pressure on a limb, frostbite, or a snake bite can also cause compartment syndrome. Compartment syndrome usually occurs in compartments of the lower leg and forearm (Figure 28-7). Symptoms develop 6 to 8 hours after injury, but may be delayed for 48 to 96 hours.

Symptoms include deep, throbbing pain out of proportion to the original injury, which is not relieved by narcotics; pain with passive flexion; decreased mobility of digits; paresthe-

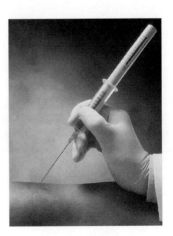

Figure **28-8** Intracompartmental pressure monitor. *(Courtesy Horizon Medical Inc., Santa Ana, Calif.)*

sia; decreased or absent pulses; coolness; pallor; and tense-ness of overlying skin. Pulses may be absent, decreased, or palpable with compartment syndrome.

Irreversible tissue damage occurs within 4 to 6 hours of ischemia; therefore, prompt physician notification is essen-tial. The limb is positioned level with the heart. Neurovascu-lar function is assessed hourly or more often if indicated to identify changes. Diagnosis is made by measuring compart-ment pressure with a syringe or catheter device (Figures 28-8 and 28-9). Pressures greater than 30 to 60 mm Hg require fasciotomy. A high index of suspicion is necessary when caring for injured comatose patients who cannot verbalize increasing pain or paresthesia.

Peripheral Nerve and Artery Injury

The most common causes of peripheral nerve and artery injuries are lacerations, penetrating wounds, fractures, and dislocations. Joints are particularly well innervated and vascularized and are especially prone to nerve or artery damage. Familiarity with major nerves and arteries is nec-essary for assessment of tissue injuries. Table 28-1 summa-rizes major vessels, associated injuries, and assessment findings.

Nerve injury may also occur from compression caused by prolonged PASG use or skeletal traction. Resolution of symptoms depends on the type of injury and length of time before compression is corrected. Partial nerve injury may be caused by a contusion that causes temporary paralysis and sensory deficit. Complete and total disruption of the nerve causes loss of all functions and usually requires surgical re-pair. Nerve evaluation and repair of an isolated injury may be done on an outpatient basis.

Axillary, brachial, radial, and ulnar arteries are the major arteries in the arms. Femoral, popliteal, anterior tibial, poste-rior tibial, and peroneal arteries are major arteries in the leg. High-impact and rapid deceleration mechanisms are most likely to cause arterial injury. Assessment should evaluate pulse quality, skin color and temperature, capillary refill, bleeding, hematoma formation, and presence of bruits. Table 28-2 summarizes the assessment of acute arterial ischemia. Arterial injuries may be difficult to discover; 10% to 15% of significant arterial disruptions still have detectable distal pulses.[7] A Doppler should be used for pulses that are difficult to palpate. Evaluation may require angiography; however, in-jury in association with an open fracture may be evaluated during surgery. Arterial injuries may not require repair if ex-isting collateral circulation prevents ischemia. Complica-tions of undiagnosed arterial disruptions include thrombosis, arteriovenous fistula, aneurysm, false aneurysm, and tissue ischemia with resultant limb dysfunction.

Table **28-1**	**Assessment of Common Peripheral Nerve Injuries**	
Nerve	Frequently associated injuries	Assessment findings
Radial	Fracture of humerus, especially middle and distal thirds	Inability to extend thumb in "hitchhiker's sign"
Ulnar	Fracture of medial humeral epicondyle	Loss of pain perception in tip of little finger
Median	Elbow dislocation or wrist or forearm injury	Loss of pain perception in tip of index finger
Peroneal	Tibia or fibula fracture; dislocation of knee	Inability to extend great toe or foot; may also be associated with sciatic nerve injury
Sciatic and tibial	Infrequent with fractures or dislocations	Loss of pain perception in sole of foot

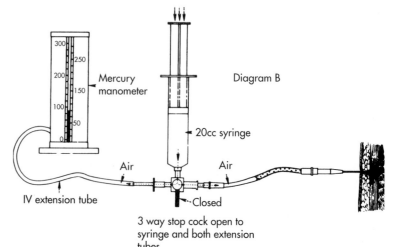

Figure **28-9** Whitesides' method for measuring intra-compartmental pressure. *(From Whitesides TE et al.: Tis-sue pressure measurements as a determinant for the need of fasciotomy, Clin Orthop Rel Res 113:43, 1975.)*

Table 28-2	**The "Five Ps" of Acute Arterial Ischemia**	
	Subjective	Objective
Pain	Aching pain	Tenderness more proximal than numbness
Paralysis	Weakness or "giving out"	Weak extensors and flexors
Paresthesia	Numbness	Decreased to absent sensation, most dense distally
Pallor	White and cold	Pallor (or dusky if has been dependent); coolness gradually decreasing proximally
Pulselessness	Rarely appreciated by patient (pulselessness better replaced by coldness, such as in "poikilothermia")	Better documented by segmental blood pressures or Doppler pulses being absent (pulselessness better replaced by "pressureless" or "Dopplerless" state)

From: Davis et al, editors: *Clinical surgery*, St. Louis, 1987, Mosby.

Strains

A strain is a weakening or overstretching of a muscle at the point of attachment to the tendon. Strains may occur as a result of almost any type of movement, from stepping off a curb and twisting the ankle, to the wrenching force caused by a motor vehicle collision or violent muscle contraction. Strains are most often associated with athletic injuries.

A patient with a *mild* strain complains of local pain, point tenderness, and slight muscle spasms. Therapeutic interventions include a compression bandage, intermittent elevation of the limb above heart level for 12 hours, the application of a cold pack for the same period, and light weight-bearing on the injured part.

With a *moderate* strain, the patient has local pain, point tenderness, swelling, discoloration, and inability to use the limb for prolonged periods. Therapeutic interventions include a compression bandage, elevation and cold pack application for 24 hours; analgesia; and light weight-bearing.

When the strain is *severe,* the patient complains of local pain, point tenderness, swelling, and discoloration. The patient describes a "snapping noise" at time of injury. Therapeutic interventions include a compression bandage or splints, elevation, and cold pack application for 24 to 72 hours; analgesia; and *no* weight-bearing for 48 hours. Surgery may be required if a complete rupture occurs at the tendon-bone attachment site.

Sprains

The mechanism of injury for sprains may be the same as that for a strain, but a sprain is usually the result of more traumatic force. A sprain occurs when a joint exceeds its normal limit and damages ligaments. The patient may have a history of a popping or snapping sound. Sprains often occur in ankles, knees, and shoulders. In children, epiphyseal disruption is more common than ligamentous injury. A *mild* sprain produces slight pain and slight swelling. Therapeutic interventions include a compression bandage, elevation, cold pack application for 12 hours, and light weight-bearing. A *moder-*

ate sprain causes pain, point tenderness, swelling, and an inability to use the limb for more than a brief period. Therapeutic interventions include compression bandage, elevation, cold pack application for 24 hours, and light weight bearing with crutches. A stirrup ankle brace applied to the ankle prevents inversion/eversion but allows flexion and extension. Figure 28-10 shows one brand of stirrup ankle brace.

A *severe* sprain involves torn ligaments, which cause pain, point tenderness, swelling, discoloration, and the inability to use the limb. Therapeutic interventions include a splint or cast, elevation, and cold pack application for 48 hours, and light-to-no weight-bearing with crutches.

Knee Injuries

Knee injuries are a common form of soft tissue injury in which rotational or extraflexion trauma strains or tears the medial meniscus, collateral ligament, or cruciate ligament. Symptoms include swelling, ecchymosis, effusion, pain, and tenderness. Therapeutic interventions include a compression bandage, knee immobilizer, or cylinder cast; elevation of the injured limb; an intermittent cold pack application to the injured area for the first 24 hours; and nonweight bearing with crutch walking. If the injury is a ligament tear, surgical repair within 24 to 48 hours of injury is recommended.

TRAUMATIC AMPUTATIONS

Traumatic amputations occur among farm workers who have accidents associated with heavy farm machinery; in factory workers when a limb is caught by a heavy machine; and in motorcyclists when the motorcycle and driver collide with another vehicle. Other causes include snow blowers and lawn mowers. Arm amputations secondary to one vehicle glancing off another while the arm is out the window have greatly declined, probably in part because of public education but also because of widespread use of car air conditioning.[8] Body parts frequently amputated are digits (fingers, toes), the distal half of the foot (transmetatarsal), the leg (above, at, or below the knee), hand, forearm, arm, ears, nose, and penis.

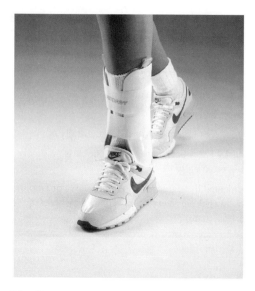

Figure 28-10 Stirrup splint. *(Courtesy Aircast, Inc., Summit, N.J.)*

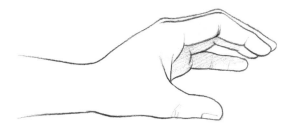

Figure 28-11 Anatomical position of the hand. *(From Davis, et al., editors:* Surgery: a problem-solving approach, *ed 2, vol 2, St. Louis, 1995, Mosby.)*

FRACTURES

A fracture is a disruption or break in the bone. Patients arrive in the ED with angulation, deformity, pain, regional and point tenderness, swelling, immobility, and crepitus. Other findings include bony fragment protrusion, impaired neurovascular status, and occasionally shock.

Fractures are divided into two general categories. With closed or simple fractures, the bone is broken but the skin is intact. Open or compound fractures are characterized by bone protrusion puncture wounds where the bone punctures the skin or a foreign object penetrates the skin and bone causing a fracture.

Open fractures are contaminated and considered a surgical emergency. They are graded by severity and further categorized by wound size, amount of soft tissue damage, injury to the periosteum, and vascular damage. Table 28-3 describes etiology for various types of fractures; Figure 28-12 provides illustrations for each type. A greater potential for shock exists with open fractures since they can cause significant blood loss; closed injuries tamponade and limit blood loss. General nursing care includes IV access for fluid replacement, antibiotics, analgesia, and anesthesia. Wound care includes irrigation with normal saline, covering with a dry sterile dressing, and verification of tetanus immunization status. Wound culture may be ordered before irrigation.

After evaluation of ABCs, specific limb injury assessment should be completed followed by immobilization, elevation, and ice packs. Repeated neurovascular assessments are essential to evaluate changes secondary to swelling. A history should be obtained to determine mechanism of injury. The emergency nurse should be alert for signs of abuse when the injury does not match the history.

When a limb is traumatized, a fracture is generally suggested until proven otherwise by radiologic studies. Radiography should include anterior and lateral views since some fractures are demonstrated from only one angle. Joints above and below the injury should be included.

Open fractures and certain closed fractures require surgical intervention. The patient should be kept NPO and prepared for surgery. Intravenous lines are inserted, with consent obtained before narcotics are administered. Prophylactic broad-spectrum antibiotics are given as soon as possible.

Therapeutic interventions for amputations include stabilization of the ABCs including administration of high-flow oxygen, initiation of two large-bore intravenous lines, control of bleeding, and rapid transportation to a facility for definitive care. The limb should be supported and splinted in a position of anatomic function if the part is partially amputated (Figure 28-11 shows anatomic hand position). A completely amputated stump should be irrigated for gross contamination, dressed, and elevated. Antibiotics, a tetanus booster, and immune globulin as indicated should be initiated in the ED. Tourniquet application should be avoided.

Whenever possible, the amputated part is preserved for reimplantation. The part is cooled by wrapping in saline gauze and placing in a plastic bag or container, then placing on top of crushed ice and water. Distilled water is not used because of its deleterious effect on tissue. *The part must not be placed directly on ice, and iodine must not be used. Also the part must not be frozen.* The limb should be kept in correct anatomic position.

Reimplantation

Occasionally reimplantation is possible. Limiting factors for successful reimplantation are availability of a reimplantation team, amount of damage to the attached and amputated part, and time elapsed since the accident. Sharp cuts have a better outcome than crush/avulsion-type injuries. Muscles can survive 12 hours of cold ischemia; bone, tendon, and skin can survive 24 hours. Warm survival time is much less. Predicted outcome of reimplantation is further determined by age, occupation, motivation, and general physical condition of the victim. Historically, upper-extremity reimplantations are more successful than lower-extremity reimplantations, and children typically have a better outcome.

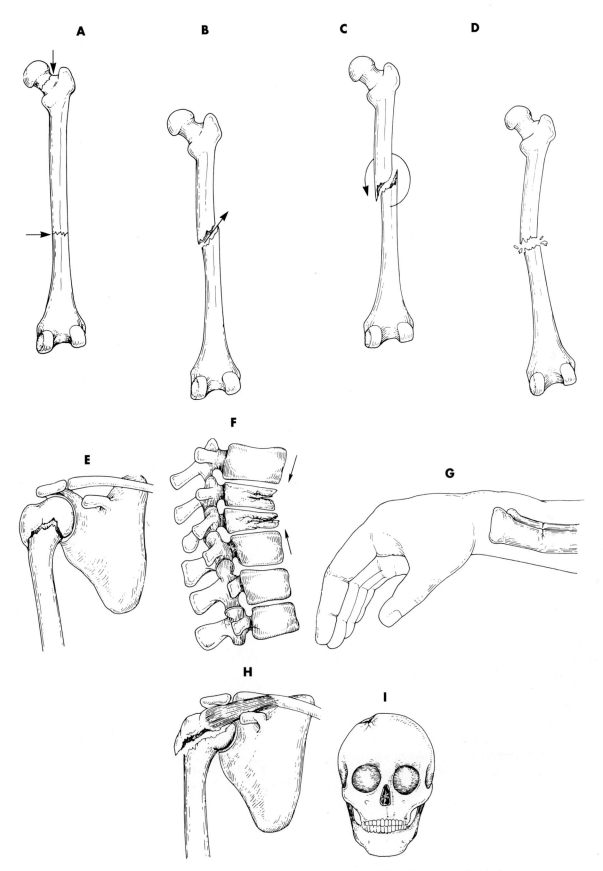

Figure **28-12** Types of fractures. **A,** Transverse fracture. **B,** Oblique fracture. **C,** Spiral fracture. **D,** Comminuted fracture. **E,** Impacted fracture. **F,** Compression fracture. **G,** Greenstick fracture. **H,** Avulsion fracture. **I,** Depression fracture.

Table **28-3**	**Etiology of Different Types of Fractures**
Type	Etiology
Oblique fracture	Twisting force
Spiral fracture	Twisting force while foot is firmly planted
Comminuted fracture	Severe direct trauma causes more than two fragments
Impacted fracture	Severe trauma, causes fractured bone ends to jam together
Compression fracture	Severe force to top of head, sacrum, or os calcis (axial loading) forces vertebrae together
Greenstick fracture	Compression force—usually school-age children
Avulsion fracture	Forceful contraction of a muscle mass—causes a bone fragment to break away at the insertion point
Depressed fracture	Blunt trauma to a flat bone. Usually associated with significant soft-tissue damage

Many complications are associated with fractures. Jagged bone ends may lacerate vital organs, arteries, and nerves causing hemorrhage and neurovascular compromise. Open fractures may lead to serious infections with potential limb dysfunction or limb loss. Long-term complications of fractures include non-union, deformity, disability, avascular necrosis from decreased blood supply, and Volkman's contracture secondary to untreated compartment syndrome.

Fat embolism is a relatively uncommon, but life-threatening, sequela of bone injury, which presents 24 to 48 hours after injury. Seen most often with pelvic, femoral, or tibial fractures, this complication has a high mortality rate. Fracture causes release of fat particles into the blood stream that can embolize to end-organs, particularly pulmonary vasculature. The patient has a sudden onset of tachycardia accompanied by elevated temperature, altered level of consciousness, tachypnea, cough, shortness of breath, cyanosis, petechiae, and pulmonary edema leading to adult respiratory distress syndrome. Immediate therapeutic interventions include high-flow oxygen, support of ABCs, and possible administration of corticosteroid and heparin (Chapter 34).

Fractures occur frequently among children 6 to 16 years old and the elderly. Children's bones are softer and more porous, and therefore more likely to have a partial or greenstick fracture. Epiphyseal or growth plate (Salter-type) fractures may affect future bone growth because of early closure of the epiphyseal plate and resultant limb shortening. Angulation may occur with a partial growth plate fracture, since bone growth continues in the noninjured area. Epiphyseal fractures need close orthopedic follow-up for several months. Another concern with pediatric fractures is bleed-

ing. A child with a femur fracture may lose 300 to 1000 ml of blood, a significant amount given the child's body size.

Elderly patients have brittle bones, are more likely to have problems with balance, and are prone to falls and fractures. These patients can have multiple medical problems that complicate recovery. Planning home care may be difficult for the elderly patient with a fracture who may already be challenged by normal activities of daily living. A cast and crutches cause greater loss of balance and impaired mobility.

Fracture Healing

Bone healing occurs over weeks or can take months (Figure 28-13). Fracture healing is determined by the type of bone, type of fracture, degree of opposition, immobility, and the general state of health. Infection and decreased neurovascular supply hamper healing as does chronic hypoxia. Exercise promotes bone healing. Alterations in healing are described as delayed, malunion (residual deformity), and non-union (failure to unite).

Upper Torso Fractures

Bones in the upper torso that communicate with the upper extremities include the clavicle and the scapula.

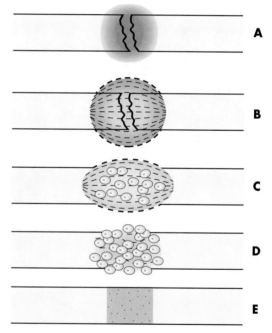

Figure **28-13** Bone healing (schematic representation). **A,** Bleeding at broken ends of the bone with subsequent hematoma formation. **B,** Organization of hematoma into fibrous network. **C,** Invasion of osteoblasts, lengthening of collagen strands, and deposition of calcium. **D,** Callus formation: new bone is built up as osteoclasts destroy dead bone. **E,** Remodeling accomplished as excess callus is reabsorbed and trabecular bone is laid down. *(Redrawn from Long BC, Phipps WJ, Cassmeyer VL: Medical-surgical nursing, St. Louis, 1993, Mosby. In Lewis SM, Collier IC, Heitkemper MM: Medical-surgical nursing, ed 4, St. Louis, 1996, Mosby.)*

Clavicular fracture. Fracture of the clavicle is found in all age-groups (Figure 28-14), but is particularly common in children. A fall on an arm or shoulder such as in contact injury when athletes run into each other, or in a direct frontal impact, is a frequently reported mechanism of injury. Eighty percent of fractures occur in the middle third of the clavicle. Patients complain of pain in the clavicular area with point tenderness, swelling, deformity, and crepitus; the patient will not raise the affected arm and tilts the head toward the side of injury with the chin directed toward the opposite side. Neurovascular status of the arm is assessed, with the arm supported, and the shoulder placed in a figure-eight support (Figure 28-15).

A sling or sling and swathe may be used for an elderly patient. The patient should be instructed to apply a cold pack intermittently to the injured area for 12 to 24 hours, and take only tub or sponge baths. A referral should be given for orthopedic follow-up. Complications include pneumothorax and hemothorax, particularly from the more serious frontal-impact injuries, and brachial plexus injuries.

Scapular fracture. Scapular fractures occur in 1% of all fractures, primarily in young men (Figure 28-16). This injury is usually caused by violent, direct trauma, but may be seen with severe muscle contraction. Common mechanisms of injury include MVCs, falls, and crush injuries. Patients

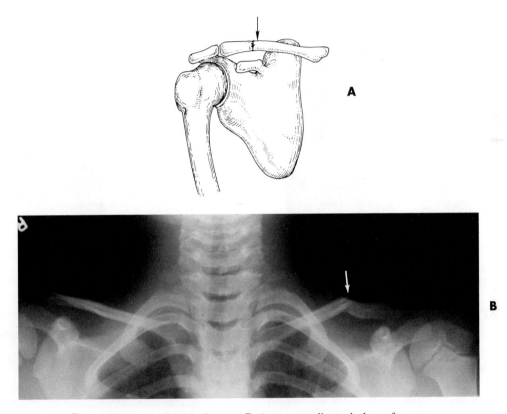

Figure **28-14**   **A,** Clavicle fracture. **B,** Arrow on radiograph shows fracture.

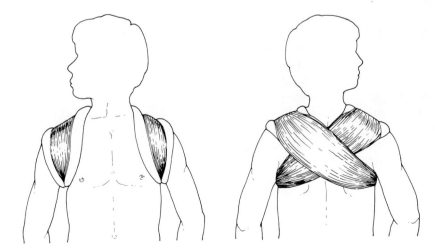

Figure **28-15**   Figure-eight support.

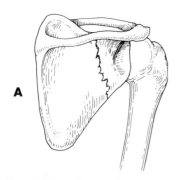

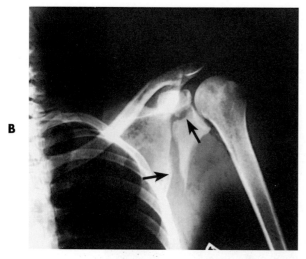

Figure **28-16** **A,** Scapular fracture. **B,** Radiograph. *(B, from Ballinger:* Merrill's atlas of radiographic positions and radiologic procedures, *ed 8, St. Louis, 1995, Mosby. Courtesy Sharon A. Coffey, RT.)*

complain of point tenderness and pain during shoulder movement. Bone displacement and swelling over the injured area may be evident. Therapeutic interventions include assessment of neurovascular status of the affected arm, placement of a compression bandage over the scapula if the bone is not displaced, sling and swath bandage or shoulder immobilizer for 1 to 2 weeks, and application of a cold pack for the first 24 hours. Complications include injuries to underlying ribs or viscera from the force required to cause the fracture.

Upper Extremity Fractures

Shoulder fracture. A shoulder fracture is a fracture of the glenoid, humeral head, or humeral neck (Figure 28-17). Shoulder fractures occur frequently in elderly patients due to a fall on an outstretched arm or direct trauma to the shoulder. When this same mechanism of injury occurs in a younger person, shoulder dislocation usually occurs. Fracture occurs in an elderly person because of the weaker bone structure.

The patient arrives with pain in the shoulder area with point tenderness, immobility of the affected arm, gross swelling, and discoloration. The majority of injuries are im-

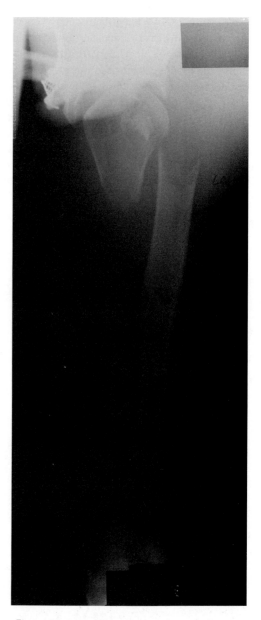

Figure **28-17** Radiograph of shoulder fracture.

pacted or nondisplaced and require only a sling and swath (Figure 28-18) or shoulder immobilizer. A Velpeau version of the sling and swath (with affected hand pointing to the opposite shoulder) may be used. A significantly displaced fracture may require open reduction or skeletal traction but is generally reduced with closed traction. This injury truly complicates activities of daily living and requires extra planning for home care, particularly for an elderly patient living alone. Complications include neurovascular compromise (axillary nerve) and possible adhesive capsulitis or "frozen" (stiff) shoulder.

Upper arm fractures. Fractures of the upper arm (humeral shaft) are commonly seen in children and the elderly (Figure

28-19). This type of fracture results from a fall on the arm, direct trauma, or in association with dislocation of the shoulder and may also occur as a stress injury in weight lifting. The patient complains of point tenderness and significant discomfort. Swelling, inability or hesitancy to use the arm, severe deformity or angulation, and crepitus also occur. Therapeutic interventions include a sling and swath, and assessment for

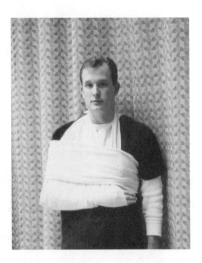

Figure **28-18**   Sling and swath.

other injuries (e.g., chest trauma). The fracture is usually reduced by closed reduction with mild, steady, downward traction. The arm is casted with a "Y-shaped" (sugar-tong) plaster splint applied from the axilla, around the elbow, and back to the shoulder (acromial process). The patient should sit and lean forward during this procedure. The arm may be secured to the chest for additional stabilization. In addition to routine cast care instructions, the patient should be given instructions to exercise the wrist and fingers frequently. Radial nerve damage can accompany fracture of the middle or distal portion of the shaft. Hemorrhage is possible if bleeding is not controlled within moments of the injury.

Elbow fractures. Elbow fractures, (Figure 28-20) seen most often in young children and athletes, usually result from a fall on an extended arm or flexed elbow, such as in a fall from a skateboard. Fractures of the elbow involve the distal humerus or head of the ulna or radius. Supracondylar fractures of the humerus are typically extension injuries and likely to damage the brachial artery. Ulnar head fractures are generally the result of a direct blow and usually comminuted.

Elbow fractures are associated with considerable swelling and potential neurovascular compromise. Initial assessment should be done promptly and at regular 30-minute intervals.[14] If compromise is present, the arm may be flexed at a greater angle. The arm should be splinted as found, and a sling may be applied. When closed reduction is employed,

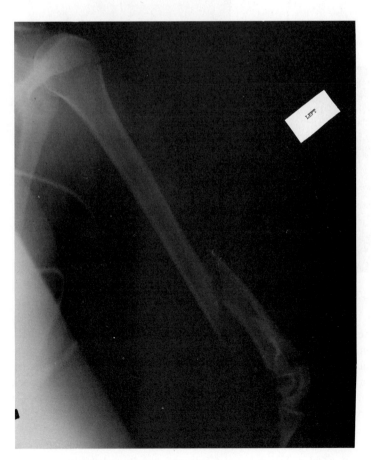

Figure **28-19**   Radiograph of humerus fracture.

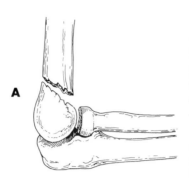

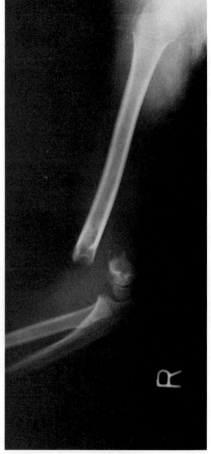

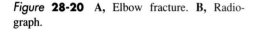

Figure **28-20** **A,** Elbow fracture. **B,** Radiograph.

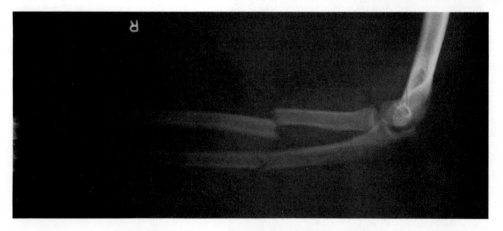

Figure **28-21** Radiograph of fracture of radius and ulna.

the arm is casted and placed in a sling. Radial head fractures may require only sling immobilization. Open reduction and fixation is required for comminuted or intraarticular fractures. Complications associated with elbow fractures are brachial artery laceration, nerve (median, radial, or ulnar) damage, and Volkmann's contracture.

Volkmann's contracture results from ischemia of muscles and nerves. Signs and symptoms include inability to move fingers, severe pain with manipulation, severe pain in fore-

arm flexor muscles even after reduction, pulse deficit, swelling, extremity coolness, cyanosis, and decreased sensation. Temporary therapeutic intervention includes cast removal and extension of the forearm with possible cold pack application. Prompt orthopedic consultation is essential for further therapeutic intervention. Nonintervention leads to atrophy and a claw-like deformity.

Forearm fractures. Forearm fractures include fractures of the radius and ulna. Common in adults and children, forearm fractures usually result from a fall on an extended arm or from a direct blow (Figure 28-21). The patient has pain, point tenderness, swelling, deformity, angulation, and occasional shortening of the extremity. Therapeutic interventions include a splint to immobilize the fracture, and a sling. Many fractures can be manipulated by closed reduction and then casted with the elbow in 90° of flexion. The shoulder and fingers should be free of the cast. If a sling is used, the entire arm and hand should be supported. The hand should not become dependent or droop at the wrist. Complications of forearm fractures include neurovascular compromise leading to Volkmann's contracture.

Wrist and Hand Fractures

Carpal fractures. The scaphoid (Figure 28-22) is the carpal bone most prone to fracture. The patient complains of tenderness over the depression in the wrist on the thumb side of the hand (anatomic snuffbox). A specific navicular view radiograph demonstrates scaphoid fractures best; however, fractures may not appear on radiographs for 2 to 4 weeks. If symptoms are present, a cast is placed regardless of negative radiographs. Complications include avascular necrosis or tissue death from loss of blood supply.

Wrist fractures. Fractures of the wrist include the distal radius, distal ulna, and carpal bones of the hand (Figure 28-23). The most common mechanism is a fall onto an extended arm and open hand, causing swelling and deformity. Fractures of the distal radius and ulna are the most common fracture and typically occur in the elderly. A Colles fracture may also occur in association with a calcaneus and vertebral fracture sustained in a fall from a height. Wrist fractures are generally manipulated with closed reduction and then casted. Some physicians may not prescribe a sling since it can hinder elevation; some prefer a hanging apparatus, such as an IV pole for the first two days of elevation, even for home care.

Metacarpal fractures. Fractures of the metacarpals (Figure 28-24) are common athletic injuries, particularly in contact sports. Striking a person or a wall with a closed fist causes a "boxer's fracture," which is a fracture of the fifth metacarpal. Throwing a baseball may cause the distal attachment of the extensor tendon to tear loose along with a segment of bone, causing an avulsion fracture. Industrial crush injuries to the hand can also fracture metacarpals. If an open fracture occurs, a compression bandage is used to control bleeding. Rings are removed before swelling increases and makes removal difficult. Metacarpal fractures are seldom displaced to any degree and are generally casted in the emergency department.

Phalanx fractures. Fractured phalanges (fingers) are common in all age groups (Figure 28-25). Symptoms are similar to those for carpal and metacarpal fractures, and therapeutic interventions are basically the same. Sometimes a phalanx fracture is associated with a hematoma beneath the fingernail (subungual hematoma) causing severe, throbbing pain. Therapeutic intervention for phalanx fractures is usually splinting the finger. Occasionally, surgical reduction is necessary to realign fractured segments. Subungual hematoma is treated with nail trephination.

Pelvic Fractures

Pelvic fractures (Figure 28-26) occur most frequently in middle-age and elderly adults with mortality of approxi-

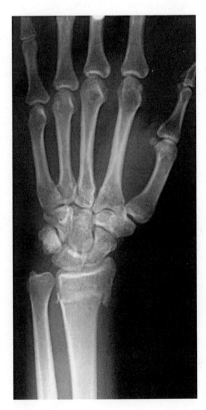

Figure 28-23   Wrist fracture (radius). *(From Ballinger:* Merrill's atlas of radiographic positions and radiologic procedures, *ed 8, St. Louis, 1995, Mosby. Courtesy Keith Shipman, RT.)*

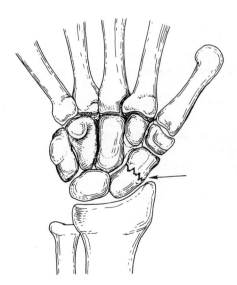

Figure **28-22**   Wrist fracture (carpal).

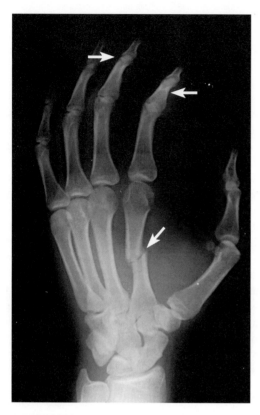

Figure 28-24 Metacarpal fracture. *(From Ballinger:* Merrill's atlas of radiographic positions and radiologic procedures, *ed 8, St. Louis, 1995, Mosby. Courtesy Peter DeGraaf, RT.)*

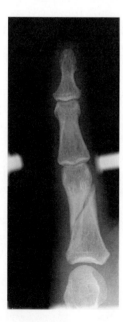

Figure 28-25 Fractured fifth digit. *(From Ballinger:* Merrill's atlas of radiographic positions and radiologic procedures, *ed 8, St. Louis, 1995, Mosby. Courtesy Keith Shipman, RT.)*

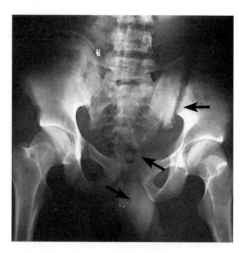

Figure 28-26 Pelvis fracture. *(From Ballinger:* Merrill's atlas of radiographic positions and radiologic procedures, *ed 8, St. Louis, 1995, Mosby. Courtesy Sharon A. Coffey, RT.)*

mately 8% to 10%; however, open pelvic fractures have a much greater mortality. Open fractures into the rectum or vagina comprise approximately 3% of pelvic injuries but have a 40% to 60% mortality.[30] An estimated 65% of patients with pelvic fractures have other injuries. Pelvic fractures coexist in nearly 30% of all multiple trauma injuries.[3] Vehicular trauma, particularly in pedestrians, accounts for almost two thirds of pelvic fractures.[7] Other causes are direct trauma, falls from a height, sudden contraction of a muscle against a resistance, and even doing the splits while waterskiing. Pelvic fractures are classified as stable or unstable, depending on the disruption of the "pelvic ring" (Figure 28-27). A particularly unstable fracture results from vertical-shear force, which causes significant bone and tissue damage. Specific neurovascular structures at risk for injury with pelvic fractures include the iliac artery, venous plexus, and sciatic nerve.

Patients with a pelvic fracture have tenderness over the pubis with compression of iliac wings, paraspinous muscle spasm, sacroiliac joint tenderness, paresis or hemiparesis, pelvic ecchymosis, and hematuria. The patient may also exhibit impending shock as evidenced by tachycardia and hypotension.

Therapeutic interventions include high-flow oxygen, vital signs every 5 minutes, two large-bore intravenous lines for volume replacement titrated to blood pressure and pulse rate, and a possible placement of the PASG. The spine and legs are immobilized with a long board flexing the knees to decrease pain. Patients should be rapidly transported to a hospital so that early radiographic studies, peritoneal lavage, and blood type and crossmatch tests can be performed. Patients with pelvic fractures have a tendency to bleed profusely, so blood should be typed and crossmatched for at least five units. Average blood loss is 2 units with a potential loss up to 4000 ml. A Foley catheter should be inserted cau-

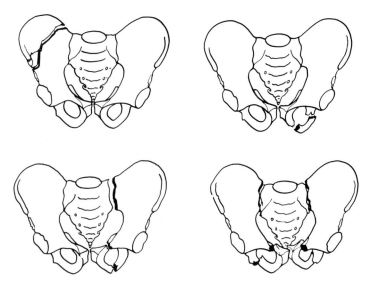

Figure **28-27** Types of pelvic fractures. *(From Sheehy SB, Jimmerson CL:* Manual of clinical trauma care, *ed 2, St. Louis, 1994, Mosby.)*

tiously in a patient with pelvic trauma but should never be used when there is blood at the meatus.

Definitive interventions depend on the severity of the fracture. Unstable, weight-bearing fractures are treated with external fixation devices (possibly applied in the ED) or with open reduction using internal fixation devices. Less severe, non-weight-bearing injuries are treated with bedrest and traction.

Complications from pelvic fractures include bladder trauma, genital trauma, lumbosacral trauma, ruptured internal organs, sepsis, shock, and death. Long-term complications include thrombophlebitis, fat embolism, chronic pain, and loss of function.

Hip Fractures

Hip fractures are common in elderly people and usually result from a fall or minor trauma (Figure 28-28). Hip fracture in a younger person is usually due to major trauma. Fractures of the femoral head, femoral neck (intracapsular), and intertrochanteric region occur. Fractures to the femoral head are rare, and generally occur in a high-speed MVC. Symptoms associated with hip fractures include pain in the groin, hip, or possibly the knee, and severe pain with leg movement, and immobility. However, patients with greater trochanteric fractures can be ambulatory. Extracapsular, trochanteric fractures are associated with pain in the lateral hip, increased shortening of the extremity, and a greater degree of external rotation.

Immediate therapeutic interventions include splinting the hip to a long board or the opposite leg, and checking vital signs frequently. Early immobilization with Bucks traction or surgical intervention is often necessary. Complications of hip fracture include hypovolemia, shock, avascular necrosis with femoral head and neck fractures, and non-union.

Lower Extremity Fractures

Femoral fracture (Figure 28-29). Femoral fractures occur in all age groups, usually secondary to major trauma. The patient has severe pain, inability to bear weight on the injured leg, deformity, swelling, and angulation. The limb shortens from severe muscle spasms, and crepitus over the fracture site may be noted.

Initial therapeutic intervention includes use of a Hare traction, Sager, or Thomas splint for traction on the limb. A long air splint with an enclosed foot or using the other leg as a splint is not recommended, because they do not provide enough stability. Associated injuries such as knee trauma are assessed. Intravenous access is established, ideally in two sites, and vital signs are monitored frequently. If the injury is isolated, analgesia may be considered. The patient should be prepared for traction, pin placement, or surgery.

The greatest complication of femoral fracture is shock secondary to hypovolemia. Blood loss ≥ 2 units into the thigh from a fractured femur is not uncommon and can exceed 3000 ml. Severe muscle spasms can move bone ends causing further soft-tissue injury, muscle damage, and pain. Neurovascular structures that can be damaged include the peroneal and sciatic nerve and popliteal artery.

Knee fractures. Knee fractures may be supracondylar fractures of the femur or intraarticular fractures of the femur or tibia (Figure 28-30). This type of injury occurs in all age groups and is usually the result of automobile, motorcycle, or automobile-pedestrian collisions that cause direct trauma to the knee. Patients complain of knee pain, an inability to bend or straighten the knee (depending on the position of the knee at the time of the accident), swelling, and tenderness. Therapeutic interventions include a long-leg splint or securing one leg to the other. Depending on the extent of injury,

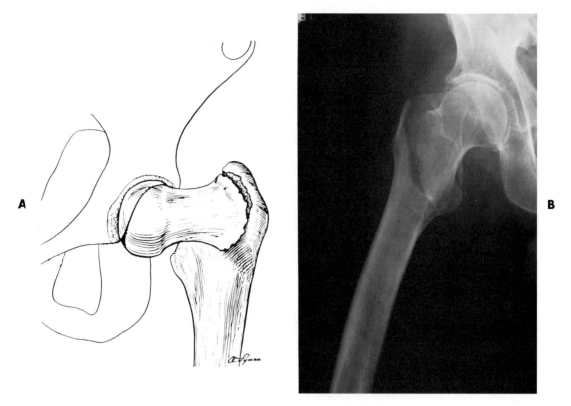

Figure **28-28** **A,** Hip fracture. **B,** Radiograph.

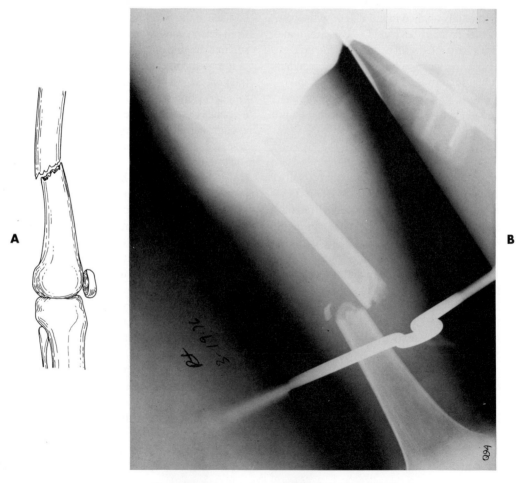

Figure **28-29** **A,** Femur fracture. **B,** Radiograph.

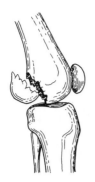

Figure **28-30**   Knee fracture.

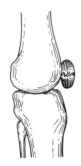

Figure **28-31**   Patellar fracture.

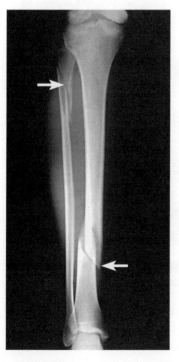

Figure **28-32**   Tibia/fibula fracture. *(From Ballinger PW: Merrill's atlas of radiographic positions and radiologic procedures, ed 8, vol 1, St. Louis, 1995, Mosby. Courtesy Sharon A. Coffey, RT.)*

the patient may require surgical repair. The knee will most likely be casted. The most common complication of knee fractures is neurovascular compromise of the peroneal or tibial nerve or popliteal artery.

Patellar fractures. Patellar fractures are seen in all age groups (Figure 28-31), usually as a result of direct trauma from a fall, or impact with the dashboard, or from an indirect trauma such as a severe muscle pull. The patient complains of pain in the knee, and the fracture can often be palpated. Open fractures can also occur. Therapeutic interventions include covering the open wound and applying a long-leg splint. Radiographs of the affected limb should be obtained to determine the extent of the fracture. If the fracture is nondisplaced, the leg is usually placed in a long-leg cylinder cast. If the fracture is displaced, reduction is attempted to realign fractured parts. The patient may go to surgery for open reduction and pinning as appropriate. The patella is an important part of the knee that aids in leverage and protects the knee joint. Complete disruption of extension warrants surgery.

Tibial and fibular fractures. Tibial and fibular fractures are seen in all age groups (Figure 28-32) and are a result of direct trauma, indirect trauma, or rotational force. The patient has pain in the leg, point tenderness, swelling, deformity, and crepitus. Many tibial and fibular fractures are open. These injuries should be splinted as found; realignment should not be attempted unless neurovascular compromise is present with an open fracture; the wound is covered with a dry sterile dressing. The leg can usually be splinted with a long-leg splint. Open or closed reduction may be necessary; however, the leg is almost always casted. An isolated fibular fracture is unusual. A walking cast is usually applied since the fibula is not a weight-bearing bone. Complications of tibial and fibular fractures include blood loss up to 2 L, infection, soft-tissue damage, neurovascular compromise, compartment syndrome, and Volkmann's contracture.

Ankle fractures. Fractures of the ankle involve the distal tibia, distal fibula, or talus and are seen in all age groups (Figure 28-33). These injuries occur as a result of direct trauma, indirect trauma, or torsion. Open fractures and/or dislocations may also occur (Figure 28-34). The patient complains of pain in the injured area, inability to bear weight on the extremity, point tenderness, swelling, and deformity. After closed reduction, the patient is placed in a walking cast. Depending on the extent of injury, the patient may require open reduction and pinning. The most frequent complication is neurovascular compromise, particularly of the peroneal nerve.

Foot fractures

Tarsal and metatarsal fractures. Fractures of the tarsals and metatarsals (Figure 28-35) occur in all age groups, usually from MVCs, athletic injuries, crush injuries, or direct trauma. Fifth metatarsal fractures can occur with inversion injuries of the foot. The patient complains of pain in the foot and hesitates to bear weight. Therapeutic intervention in-

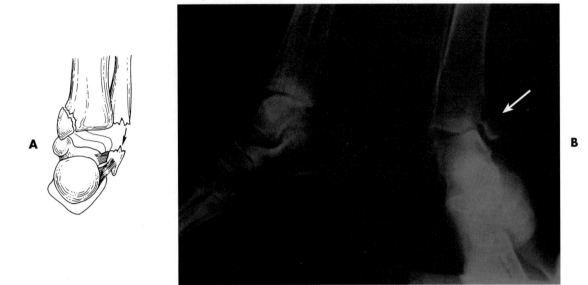

Figure **28-33** **A,** Ankle fracture. **B,** Radiograph.

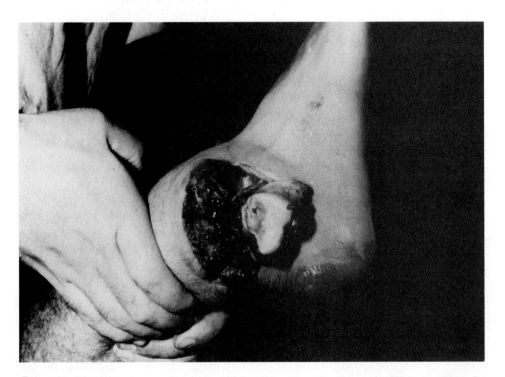

Figure **28-34** Open fracture dislocation of the talus. *(From Davis, et al.:* Clinical surgery, *St. Louis, 1987, Mosby.)*

cludes a compression dressing and soft splint. Minimally displaced fractures are treated with open-toed walking shoes or casts. With significant displacement, open reduction may be required. Crutches may be used to assist with weight bearing or nonweight bearing. Complications from this type of fracture are rare.

Calcaneus fracture. Fractures of the calcaneus are usually seen in young adults secondary to a fall in which the victim lands on the feet (Figure 28-36). The patient complains of pain in the heel, point tenderness, and swelling. Dislocation may also occur. Management includes reduction of the fracture when necessary and application of a below-the-knee, weight-bearing cast. Open reduction is occasionally necessary. Other injuries associated with this injury are lumbosacral compression fracture and Colles fracture.

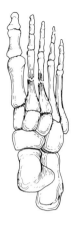

Figure **28-35**   Foot fracture.

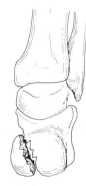

Figure **28-36**   Heel fracture.

Toe (phalangeal) fracture. Fractures of the toes are seen in all age groups (Figure 28-37), caused by kicking a hard object or running into an immovable object. The patient has pain in the toe, swelling, and discoloration. Felt or cotton is placed between the fractured toe and adjacent toe, then both toes are taped together (buddy taped) so the uninjured toe acts as a splint. The patient may bear weight as tolerated and is instructed to wear hard-soled shoes, such as wooden or hard-soled open-toed shoes, that do not put pressure on the toes. Complications are rare, but nail injury may occur.

DISLOCATIONS

Dislocations occur when a joint exceeds its normal range of motion so that joint surfaces are no longer intact. Partial (subluxation) or complete separation of both articulating surfaces can occur. Soft-tissue injuries within the joint capsule and surrounding ligaments; severe swelling; and nerve, vein, and artery damage are observed with dislocations. Diagnosis can often be predicted before radiographs are taken by soliciting information about mechanisms of injury.

In general, dislocations produce severe pain, joint deformity, inability to move the joint, swelling, and point tenderness. A potential for vascular compromise also exists, so the pulse should be assessed carefully. Initial interventions include careful palpation of the joint and splinting the injury as it is found. The dislocation is reduced with analgesia and sedation by the ED physician or orthopedist. Significant se-

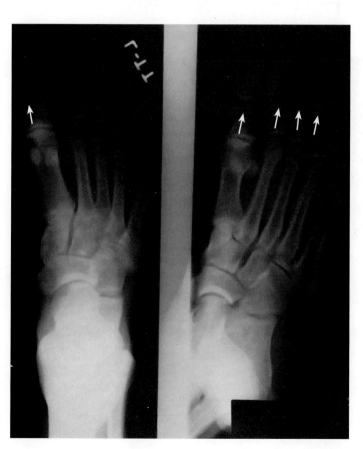

Figure **28-37**   Radiograph of toe fracture.

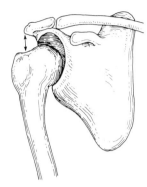

Figure **28-38** Acromioclavicular separation.

dation may be required to reduce dislocations, so the patient should be carefully monitored. Nitrous oxide may also be used. Complications include ischemia, aseptic necrosis, and recurrent dislocations.

Acromioclavicular Dislocation

Acromioclavicular separations (Figure 28-38) are commonly seen in athletes secondary to a fall or force on the point of the shoulder. The patient complains of great pain in the joint area and cannot raise the affected arm or bring the arm across the chest. Deformity, point or area tenderness, swelling, and hematoma over the injury site are also noted. Separation is usually reduced, then the arm and shoulder is

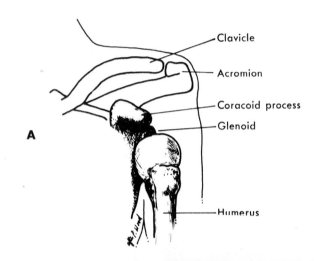

A

- Clavicle
- Acromion
- Coracoid process
- Glenoid
- Humerus

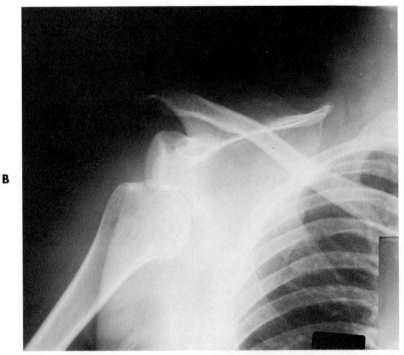

B

Figure **28-39** **A,** Anterior shoulder dislocation. **B,** Radiograph.

immobilized with a sling and swath. Occasionally, the patient requires surgery for open reduction and wiring. The patient may experience painful range of motion following reduction.

Shoulder Dislocation

Dislocations of the shoulder usually occur in children and athletes. Two general categories are anterior and posterior dislocations.

Anterior shoulder dislocations usually occur as an athletic injury when the athlete falls on an extended arm that is abducted and externally rotated. The force pushes the head of the humerus in front of the shoulder joint (Figure 28-39).

Posterior dislocations are rare and usually occur in patients with seizures when the arm is abducted and internally rotated.

In all shoulder dislocations, the patient complains of severe pain in the shoulder area, inability to move the arm, and deformity. Deformity is sometimes difficult to see in posterior dislocation. An estimated 55% to 60% of shoulder dislocations seen in the ED are recurrent. The extremity is placed in the position of greatest comfort, then distal pulses are checked, followed by skin temperature and moisture evaluation, and neurologic status assessment. Radiographs are obtained before the joint is relocated, unless neurovascular compromise has occurred. Once the joint is relocated, it is immobilized with a sling and swath bandage or shoulder immobilizer. Postreduction radiographs are obtained to confirm placement. The patient should be referred to an orthopedic surgeon. Complications from this type of injury are neurovascular compromise of the brachial plexus and axillary artery, and associated fractures.

Elbow Dislocation

Dislocations of the elbow are seen most often in children, teenagers, and young adults. Elbow dislocation is a common athletic injury (Figure 28-40) caused from a fall on an externally rotated arm or when a young child is jerked or lifted by a single arm (known as nursemaid's elbow). The patient complains of pain in the joint, which may feel "locked." Any movement can produce severe pain. Swelling, deformity, and displacement are also noted. The arm is immobilized in the position of greatest comfort. The joint is relocated, then immobilized once radiographs are obtained. The most common complication of this injury is neurovascular compromise to the median nerve or brachial artery.

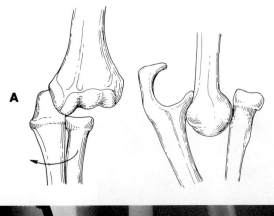

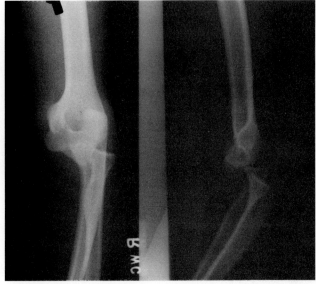

Figure **28-40**   **A,** Elbow dislocation. **B,** Radiograph.

Radial head subluxation (nursemaid's elbow) accounts for about 20% of upper extremity injuries in children, and is seen in ages 6 months to 5 years, most often in 1 to 3 year olds. History of a pull on the arm or a fall is given. The child refuses to use the arm, but does not seem in pain or distress. The injury does not require radiographic studies if the dislocation can be easily relocated with good return of function.

Wrist Dislocation

Dislocation of the wrist is seen most frequently in athletes and in all age groups from a fall on an outstretched hand (Figure 28-41). The patient complains of severe pain in the wrist with swelling, deformity, and point tenderness. The wrist is placed in a splint in the position of comfort, and a cold pack is applied. Radiographic studies are obtained, the joint is relocated, and a cast is applied. Complications in-

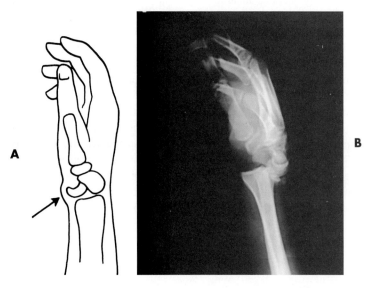

Figure **28-41** **A,** Wrist dislocation. **B,** Radiograph. (**B,** *from Ballinger:* Merrill's atlas of radiographic positions and radiologic procedures, *ed 8, St. Louis, 1995, Mosby. Courtesy Sharon A. Coffey, RT.)*

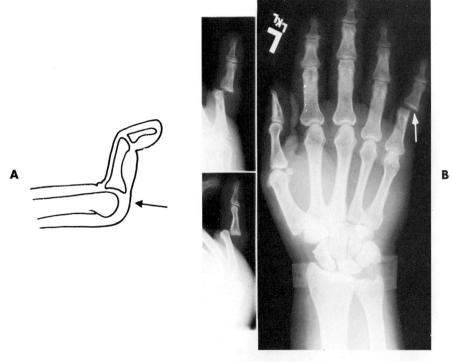

Figure **28-42** **A,** Finger dislocation. **B,** Radiographs.

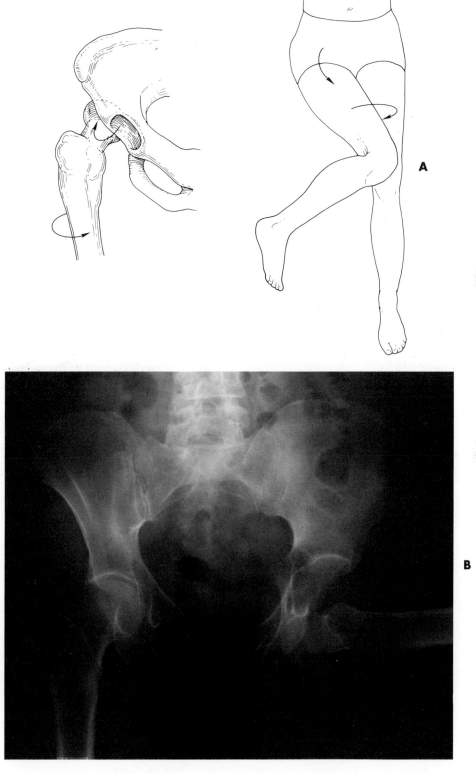

Figure **28-43**   **A,** Hip dislocation. **B,** Radiograph.

clude neurovascular compromise, especially median nerve damage.

Hand or Finger Dislocation

Hand or finger dislocations are usually seen in athletes secondary to a fall on an outstretched hand or finger and may also result from direct trauma to the tip of the finger (Figure 28-42). The patient complains of pain in area of the injury and an inability to move the joint with deformity and swelling. The injury is splinted in the position of comfort and a cold pack applied until radiographs are obtained and relocation is attempted. The injured area is usually splinted to immobilize the joint.

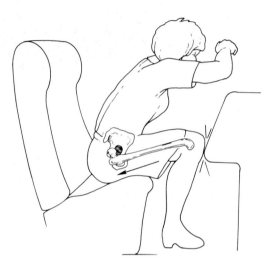

Figure **28-44**   Knee impact with dashboard.

Hip Dislocation

Hip dislocations (Figure 28-43) occur in all age groups secondary to a major trauma where the leg is extended before impact and is common in head-on MVCs when the leg is extended and the foot is on the brake pedal just before impact or when the knee jams into the dashboard (Figure 28-44). Injury also occurs with falls and crush injuries. Dislocation may be anterior or posterior. The patient complains of pain in the hip and knee, and arrives with the hip flexed, adducted, and internally rotated (posterior dislocation) or flexed, abducted, and externally rotated (anterior dislocation). The joint feels locked, and the patient cannot move the leg.

The extremity is splinted in the presenting position or position of greatest comfort. Other injuries are assessed. Necrosis of the femoral head may occur if the joint is not relocated within 6 hours. Once the hip joint is relocated, the patient begins a period of bed rest with traction. Children may be placed in a spica cast. Complications from this type of injury are femoral artery and nerve damage.

Leg Dislocation

Knee dislocation. Knee dislocations (Figure 28-45) are common in all age groups and are usually caused by a major trauma. The patient complains of severe pain in the knee, an inability to move the leg, swelling, and deformity. Immediate therapeutic intervention consists of splinting the limb in the position of comfort or the presenting position. A fractured tibia is frequently associated with knee dislocation. Almost all persons with dislocation of the knee joint have associated, severe damage to the joint capsule.

After reduction, the patient is admitted to the hospital for bed rest with the knee elevated and intermittent cold packs

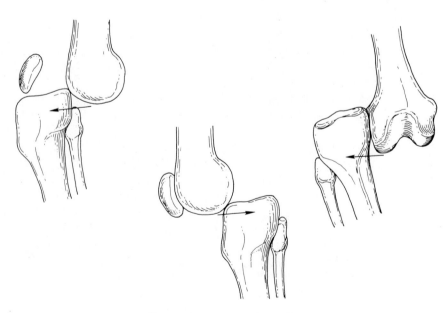

Figure **28-45**   Knee dislocation.

applied for 7 to 10 days, then casted. Complications include peroneal, popliteal, and tibial nerve damage.

Patellar dislocation. Dislocation of the patella (Figure 28-46) occurs in all age groups, usually during athletic events secondary to direct trauma to the lateral aspect of the knee or to rapid rotation on a planted foot. Patients usually have severe pain, keep the affected knee in a flexed position, and are unable to use the knee. Significant tenderness and swelling in the patellar area is evident. The leg is splinted in the presenting position and a cold pack applied. After radiographs, the patella is reduced if spontaneous reduction does not occur with extension of the leg. After relocation, the knee is placed in a compression bandage and knee immobilizer or cylinder cast.

Ankle dislocation. Ankle dislocation (Figure 28-47) is usually due to athletic injury and is commonly associated with a fracture. Such a dislocation results from lateral stress motion when normal range of motion for the ankle is exceeded. Patients complain of severe pain in the ankle, an inability to move the joint, swelling, and deformity. The ankle and foot are splinted in a position of comfort, and an ice pack is applied. The ankle may be relocated by a closed or open method, depending on the degree of injury and associated fractures. Primary complication of this injury is neurovascular compromise including the tibial artery.

Foot dislocation. Dislocations of the foot can occur in all age groups, but this is a rare injury. Injury is often the result of an automobile or motorcycle collision in which a combination of forces have acted at the same time. Foot dislocation is almost always associated with an open wound. The patient complains of severe pain in the foot with point tenderness and an inability to use the foot. Significant swelling and deformity are evident. If present, an open wound is covered with a sterile dressing before a soft splint is applied. Once the foot is relocated, a cast is applied, and the patient is instructed to elevate the limb and apply cold packs for 24 hours. No weight-bearing is permitted.

Toe (metatarsophalangeal) dislocation. Dislocations of the metatarsophalangeal joints (toes) are rare (Figure 28-48). When they do occur, they are often associated with open fractures, which should be reduced immediately since delay can result in an inability to perform closed reduction because of the swelling. The patient complains of pain and point tenderness in the joint area with significant swelling and noticeable deformity. The area should be covered with a bulky dressing to prevent further damage. After radiographs have been obtained, the dislocation is reduced, and then the foot and toes are immobilized.

REDUCTION ISSUES

The goal of reduction of fractures and dislocations is to restore anatomic alignment, allow bone healing, and preserve function. Fractures that do not require anatomic alignment for healing include an impacted fracture of the humeral neck, a fractured clavicle (particularly in children), and a pediatric nonangulated femur. Conversely, reduction is particularly important for intraarticular fractures, especially for weight-bearing bones.

Reduction methods are described as closed or open (surgical). Closed reduction is accomplished by traction-countertraction, angulation, and rotation (i.e., the reverse force of what caused the injury). A fingertrap and weights may be used for forearm reduction (Figure 28-49). Manipulation may require local anesthesia, conscious intravenous sedation or pain medications, or general anesthesia. Reduction should be accomplished as soon as possible after stabi-

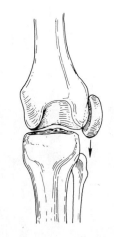

Figure **28-46** Patella dislocation.

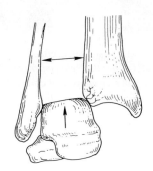

Figure **28-47** Ankle dislocation.

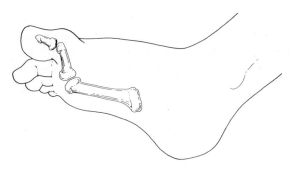

Figure **28-48** Metatarsophalangeal joint dislocation.

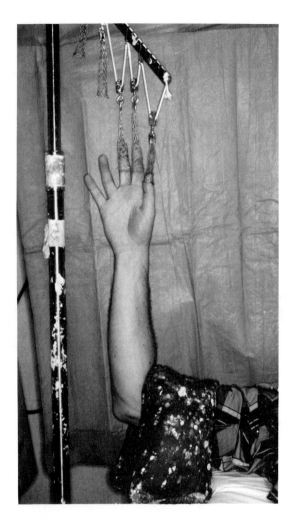

Figure **28-49** Finger traps and distal traction at the elbow to distract and reduce fracture dislocations. *(From Rosen P, et al.:* Emergency medicine: concepts and clinical practice, *ed 3, vol 1, St. Louis, 1992, Mosby.)*

lization of other injuries, since swelling can impede successful reduction. Postreduction radiographs are done after casting to verify acceptable bone alignment.

Open reduction is used for open fractures; multiple injuries; major fractures; and fractures involving intraarticular joints, the epiphysis, or femoral neck. Surgical reduction is also used for soft-tissue entrapment; major nerve, arterial or ligament injuries; pathologic fractures; unsatisfactory/failed closed reduction; or delayed union. Open reduction employs internal fixation or external fixation devices (Figure 28-50).

TRACTION

Skin or skeletal traction may be initiated in the ED. A Hare traction splint may be used until more definitive stabilization is available. Bucks traction uses a wrapped dressing or boot to provide temporary immobilization before surgery for a hip or femur fracture and to reduce muscle spasm.

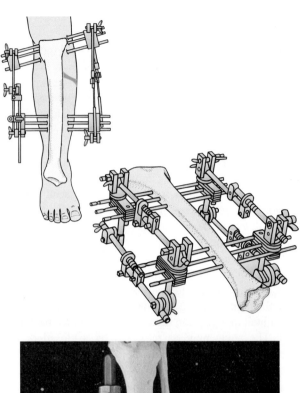

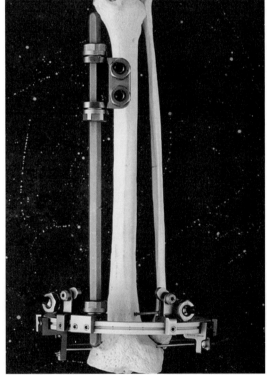

Figure **28-50** External fixator attached to bones of lower extremity. *(From Lewis SM, Collier IC, Heitkemper MM:* Medical-surgical nursing: assessment and management of clinical problems, *ed 4, St. Louis, 1996, Mosby; Courtesy Zimmer, Inc.)*

Traction is set up on a hospital bed that is brought to the ED; this eliminates painful and possibly injurious removal of traction with transfer of the patient from the ED stretcher.

Steinman Pin

Skeletal traction may be applied in the ED with a Steinman pin (Figures 28-51) for temporary reduction of long-bone fractures until open reduction and internal fixation can be done. The pin is a round stainless steel rod drilled perpendicularly into the distal femur or proximal tibia for connection to a stirrup with traction (15 to 40 lbs). Some centers obtain informed consent for this procedure. After pin placement, sterile dressings are placed around insertion sites. Osteomyelitis is a potential complication of pin insertion.

Casts

A brief overview of casting and care of casts is presented here. An orthopedic or medical-surgical text should be consulted for complete description of techniques and types of casts.

Before a cast is applied, any particulate matter is removed and the skin must be totally dry. Any skin abnormalities are documented. Casting equipment includes plaster or fiberglass casting material, stockinette and padding, a bucket of cool-to-warm water, gloves, and a kling or ace bandage if a splint is applied.

After the cast is applied, the patient should remain immobile with the limb placed on a plastic-coated pillow to avoid pressure and indentations for at least 20 minutes to allow the cast to set. A plaster cast generally requires 24 hours or more to dry thoroughly; a fiberglass cast dries in about an hour. Box 28-2 lists aftercare instructions for a patient with a cast.

Compartment syndrome and pressure sores can occur with casts. Symptoms include elevated temperature and continuing pain after several days, which causes insomnia. Interventions include immediate cast removal. Cast removal or a bi-valve procedure is accomplished with an electric cast saw. The saw blade cuts by vibrating rapidly back and forth. The patient should be reassured that the blade does not cut the skin, but heat, vibration, or pressure may be felt. Burns secondary to the blade are rare. After the cast is cut, a cast spreader is used to widen the split and allow removal. Padding beneath the cast should be cut with bandage scissors.

ASSISTED AMBULATION: CRUTCH, CANE, AND WALKER

When fitting a patient for crutches, a cane, or a walker, a measurement is taken with the shoes to be worn for ambulating. The shoes should be sturdy, fit well, and fasten with a tie, buckle, or adherent Velcro.

Box **28-2**   **Aftercare Instructions for Patients with Casts**
Keep cast dry and elevated above heart 24 hours after injury.

Apply cold packs or sealed ice bags over injured area for 30 min every 2 to 3 hours for 1 to 2 days.
See your doctor immediately with:
   a change in temperature of fingers or toes (digits are very cold or very hot);
   a change in color of fingers or toes (they are blue); or
   loss of feeling in fingers or toes.
Wiggle fingers or toes at least once each hour.
See a physician immediately if a foreign object is dropped into the cast.
Do not put anything inside your cast.
If swelling returns or a foul odor is present, see your physician.
Make an appointment to see a private physician or orthopedic physician for follow-up care.

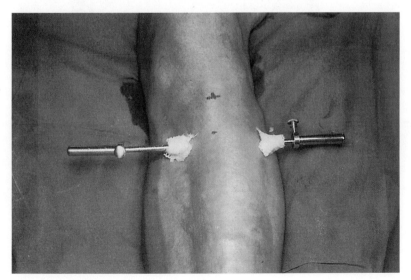

Figure **28-51** The pin is passed through the tibia to project equally medially and laterally. Points are protected with covers. *(From Mills K, Morton R, Page G: Color atlas and text of emergencies, ed 2, London, 1995, Times Mirror International.)*

Axillary Crutches

Axillary crutches should fit so that each armpiece is 2 inches or two finger widths below the axilla with no weight on the axilla. Tips of the crutches should be placed 6 inches to the side and 6 inches to the front. Each handpiece should be fitted so that the elbow is flexed 30°.

Cane

A cane should be fitted so that when it is held next to the heel, the elbow is at a 30° angle of flexion. A cane should be used for minimal support during ambulation, and to assist with balance and stability.

Walker

A walker may be chosen for patients who are unsteady on crutches and who can bear full weight on at least one leg. A walker is measured to fit with the arms bent at 30°. Patients having difficulty ambulating with assist devices may require physical therapy for training, using a wheelchair temporarily until able to ambulate safely. A walker is not ideal for use on stairs.

Gait Training

A three-point gait is used when little or no weight-bearing is desired, making this gait ideal for ED patients. Figure 28-

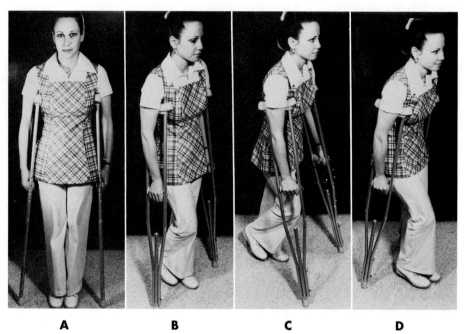

Figure **28-52** Three-point gait. **A,** Standing and balancing. **B,** Holding crutches. **C,** Straightening elbows to carry weight on hands. **D,** Three-point gait. *(Photos by Richard Lazar.)*

A   **B**   **C**   **D**

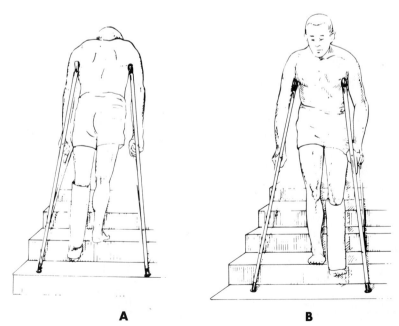

Figure **28-53 A,** Going upstairs and, **B,** going downstairs with crutches. *(From Barber J, Stokes L, Billings D:* Adult and child care, *ed 2, St. Louis, 1977, Mosby.)*

A   **B**

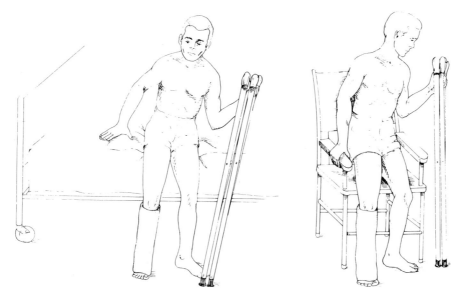

Figure **28-54** Transferring from sitting to standing with crutches. *(From Barber J, Stokes L, Billings D:* Adult and child care, *ed 2, St. Louis, 1977, Mosby.)*

Box **28-3**

NURSING DIAGNOSES FOR ORTHOPEDIC OR SOFT-TISSUE INJURY

Potential alteration in tissue perfusion
Fluid volume deficit
Physical mobility impaired
Potential risk of infection
Impaired skin integrity
Pain

52 shows this gait. Figures 28-53 and 28-54 illustrate movement on stairs and changing from a sitting to standing position using crutches.

CONCLUSION

Advances in surgical and orthopedic treatments have improved outcome for patients with soft-tissue injuries and fractures. However, the best outcome occurs if injury is not sustained. Trauma prevention through education and legislation should be the primary goal of overall trauma management.

The main objective for nursing care of the patient with an orthopedic or soft-tissue injury is to preserve or restore normal neurovascular status and motor function. Attention to these injuries is a secondary priority to ABCs. The emergency nurse must assess and intervene as soon as possible and monitor for developing complications to prevent further harm to the extremity. Box 28-3 summarizes nursing diagnoses for these patients.

REFERENCES

1. Ballinger PW: *Merrill's atlas of radiographic positions and radiologic procedures,* ed 8, vol 1, St. Louis, 1995, Mosby.
2. Birolini D, et al.: Open pelviperineal trauma, *J Trauma* 30:492-495, 1990.
3. Black JM, Matassarin-Jacobs E: *Luckman and Sorensen's medical-surgical nursing,* ed 4, Philadelphia, 1993, WB Saunders.
4. Butler AB, Salmond SW, Pellino TA: *Orthopedic nursing,* Philadelphia, 1994, WB Saunders.
5. Castiglioni A: *A history of medicine,* New York, 1975, Jason Aronson.
6. Cox SA: Pediatric trauma: Special patents/special needs, *Crit Care Nurs Quart,* 17(2):51-61, 1994.
7. Cwinn AA: Pelvis and hip: In Rosen P, et al., editors: *Emergency medicine: concepts and clinical practice,* vol 1, St. Louis, 1992, Mosby, p 658.
8. Duncan G, Meals R: One hundred years of automobile-induced orthopedic injuries, *J Orthop* 18(2):165-169, 1995.
9. Emergency Nurses Association: *Musculoskeletal trauma: trauma nursing core course,* ed 4, 1995, Award Publishers, pp 225-252.
10. Farrell J: *Illustrated guide to orthopaedic nursing,* ed 3, Philadelphia, 1986, JB Lippincott.
11. Fultz J: Extremity trauma. In Kidd PS, Sturt P, editors: *Mosby's emergency nursing reference,* St. Louis, 1996, Mosby, pp 279-311.
12. Geiderman JM: Orthopedic injuries: Management principles. In Rosen P, et al., editors: *Emergency medicine concepts and clinical practice,* vol 1, St. Louis, 1992, Mosby, pp 522-544.
13. Greigheimer EM, Weideman MP: *Physiology and anatomy,* ed 9, 2nd printing, Philadelphia, 1972, JB Lippincott.
14. Harwood-Nuss A, et al.: *The clinical practice of emergency medicine,* ed 2, Philadelphia, 1996, JB Lippincott.
15. Horowitz BR, DeStefano V: Stress fracture of the humerus in a weightlifter, *Orthopedics* 18(2):185-186, 1995.
16. Hussein MK: Kocher's method is 3000 years old, *J Bone Joint Surg* 50(B):669, 1968.
17. Joffe M: Upper extremity. In Shanahan J, editor: *Pediatric emergency medicine concepts and clinical practice,* St. Louis, 1992, Mosby, pp 340-352.
18. Marcus RE, Goodfellow DB, Pfister ME: The difficult diagnosis of posterior tibialis tendon rupture in sports injuries, *Orthopedics* 18(8):715-721, 1995.

19. McGinnis M, Denton JR: Fractures of the scapula: A retrospective study of 40 fractured scapula, *J Trauma* 29:1488, 1989.

20. Mercier LR: *Practical orthopedics,* ed 4, St. Louis, 1995, Mosby.

21. Mills K, Morton R, Page G: *Color atlas and text of emergencies,* ed 2, London, 1995, Times Mirror International.

22. Moehring HD, Voightlander JP: Compartment pressure monitoring during intramedulary fixation of tibial fractures, *Orthopedics* 18(7):631-636, 1995.

23. Neer CS, Rockwood CA: Fractures and dislocations of the shoulder. In Rockwood CA, Green DD, editors: *Fractures in adults,* ed 4, Philadelphia, 1996, JB Lippincott.

24. Nolan BG, Sturt P: Splint application. In Kidd PS, Sturt P, editors: *Mosby's emergency nursing reference,* St. Louis, 1996, Mosby, pp 819-831.

25. Praemer A, Furner S, Rice D: *Musculoskeletal conditions in the United States,* Park Ridge, Ill. 1992, American Academy of Orthopaedic Surgeons.

26. Proehl J: *Adult emergency nursing procedures,* Boston, 1993, Jones and Bartlett.

27. Sanders R, et al.: Management of fractures and soft tissue disruptions, *J Bone Joint Surg* 75(5):778-786, 1993.

28. Schoen DC: *The nursing process in orthopedics,* Norwalk, Conn., 1986, Appleton-Century-Crofts.

29. Stiles NA: High pressure injection injury of the hand: A surgical emergency, *J Emerg Nurs* 20(5):351-354.

30. Strange JM, Kelly PM: Musculoskeletal injuries. In Cardona VD, et al., editors: *Trauma nursing: from resuscitation through rehabilitation,* ed 2, Philadelphia, 1994, WB Saunders, pp 548-586.

31. Zavotsky KE, Banavage A: Management of the patient with complex orthopaedic fractures, *Orthop Nurs* 14(5):53-57.

32. Zigler MK, Parrish RS: An 18 year old male with multiple trauma including an open pelvic fracture, *J Emerg Nurs* 20(4):265-270, 1994.

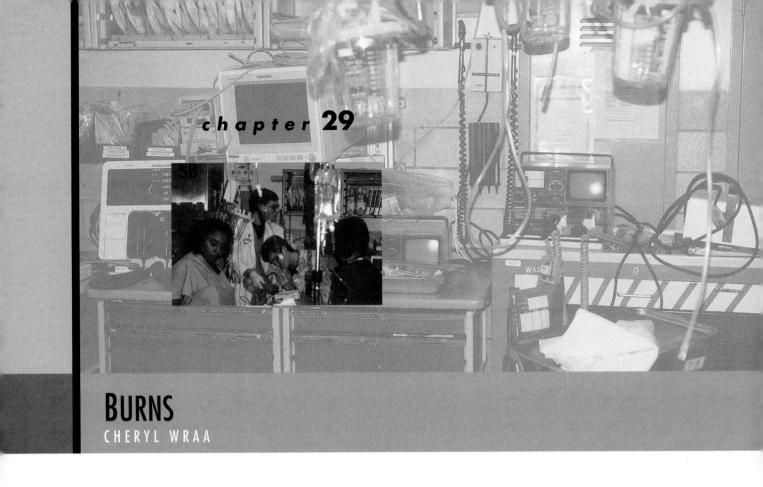

chapter 29

BURNS

CHERYL WRAA

Burn trauma is the fourth leading cause of trauma deaths in the United States. Annually, close to 2.5 million people are treated for burn injuries. Of these 10,000 die and 60,000-100,000 require hospitalization. A significant portion of morbidity and mortality associated with burn injuries results from associated injuries. Pulmonary pathology from inhalation injury is the major cause of burn trauma death. The majority of victims are pediatric, elderly, or disabled. Burn injury and deaths associated with fires are the third leading cause of accidental death in children between the ages of 1 and 14 years.[4,5,6]

More than 90% of all burns are considered preventable. Education, particularly in the school-age population, combined with legislative efforts are helping decrease the number of burn injuries. The American Burn Association has developed very effective public education programs. Legislation has been enacted that requires smoke alarms and sprinkler systems in public buildings, hotels, apartments, and new homes. For the care giver, an accurate classification of injury, timely intervention, and rapid transport to an appropriate facility significantly reduces burn injury mortality and morbidity.[2,7,8]

ETIOLOGY

Not all burns are caused by fire. Tissue damage may be secondary to chemicals, tar, electricity, lightning, or frostbite. The location of exposure and duration of exposure to the source affects outcome, regardless of the specific source of burn injury. Specific mechanisms of burn injury are described below.

Thermal Burns

Thermal injuries comprise 60% of all burns. They may result from flame, flash, steam, or scalding liquid.[2,8] Figure 29-1 is an example of one cause of burn injury.

Scald burns. Scalds from hot liquids are the most common cause of all burns. Exposure to water at 140° F for 3 seconds can cause a deep partial-thickness or full-thickness burn. If water is 156° F, the same burn occurs in 1 second. As a comparison, fresh brewed coffee is about 180° F. Soups and sauces, which are a thicker consistency, remain in contact longer with the skin and cause deeper burns. Immersion burns are usually deep and severe. Even though the water is usually cooler than a scalding liquid, the duration of contact is longer.

Other liquids that cause scalds are cooking oil and grease. When used for cooking, oil and grease may reach 400° F.

Flame burns. Burns from flames are the next most common cause of burns. The actual number of house fires has decreased because of the increased use of smoke detectors. Most flame burns are now caused by careless smoking, motor vehicle crashes, and clothing ignited from stoves or space heaters. Flame burns that occur outdoors are usually secondary to misuse of cooking stoves fueled by white gasoline, use of lanterns in tents, smoking in a sleeping bag, and use of gasoline or kerosene in a charcoal fire.[2]

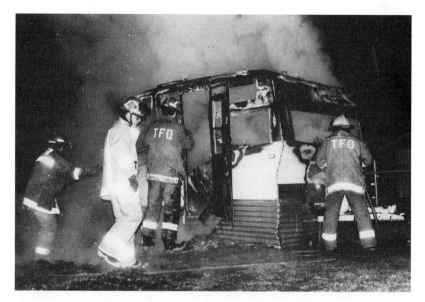

Figure **29-1** Burn injuries occur as a result of exposure to flame and smoke. *(Courtesy Tacoma Fire Department, Tacoma, Wash.)*

Flash burns. These burns are the third most common type of thermal burn. They are caused by explosions of natural gas, propane, gasoline, or other flammable liquids. Their explosion causes intense heat for a very brief time. Flash burns are usually partial thickness, although depth is dependent on the amount and kind of fuel that explodes. Flash burns may be large and are associated with significant thermal upper airway damage.[2]

Contact burns. Contact with a hot object such as metal, plastic, glass, or hot coals results in contact burns. They are usually not extensive but tend to be deep. Persons involved in industrial accidents often have contact burns associated with crush injuries from machine presses or hot, heavy objects. An increase has been seen in toddlers with contact burns secondary to the increased use of wood-burning stoves. The most common injury is to the palm because the child falls with hands outstretched against the stove.[2]

Electrical Burns

As electricity passes through the body and meets resistance of the body tissues, it is converted to heat in direct proportion to the amperage of the current and the electrical resistance of the body parts. It initially passes through the skin, causing an external burn at the entry and exit sites with extensive damage internally between these sites. Nerves, blood vessels, and muscle are less resistant and more easily damaged than bone or fat. The heart, lungs, and brain can sustain immediate damage. The nervous system is particularly sensitive to electrical burns. Damage to the brain, spinal cord, and myelin-producing cells causes devastating transverse myelitis. The smaller the body part through which the electricity passes, the more intense the heat and the less it is dissipated. Consequently, extensive damage can occur in the fingers, hands, forearms, toes, feet, and lower legs. If the path is near or through the heart, damage to the

heart's electrical conduction system can cause spontaneous ventricular fibrillation or other dysrhythmias. Papillary muscle damage may lead to sudden valvular incompetence and cardiac failure. Alternating current (AC) is more likely to induce fibrillation than direct current (DC).

Most lightning injuries do not traverse the body but flow around it, creating a shock wave capable of causing fractures and dislocations. About 70% of patients who survive a lightning strike complain of paresthesias and/or paralysis. Fortunately, both conditions are temporary.[2,8]

Chemical Burns

Chemicals cause a denaturing of protein within the tissues or a desiccation of the cells. The concentration of the chemical and the time of exposure impacts the extent of the burn. Alkali products cause more tissue damage than acids. The chemical can be removed as soon as possible by flushing with copious amount of water. Care must be taken not to expose the care giver to the chemical during this procedure. All fluids used to decontaminate the patient should be contained; the fluid must not be allowed to drain into the general drainage system. Chemical burns may be deceiving as to their depth; appearances can be similar in surface discoloration until tissue begins to slough days later. Therefore, all chemical burns should be considered deep partial thickness or full thickness until proven otherwise. After removal of the chemical, the wounds are managed in the same manner as thermal burns.[2,8]

Frostbite

Frostbite is the actual freezing of tissue secondary to exposure to freezing or below-freezing temperatures. In a cold environment, the body attempts to maintain heat by vasoconstriction of peripheral blood vessels in an effort to reduce heat exchange. The longer the period of exposure, the more the peripheral blood flow is reduced. When the extremities are left unprotected, intracellular and extracellular fluids can freeze, forming crystals that damage local tissues. Blood clots may form that impair circulation to the area.

Signs, symptoms, and classification of frostbite are the same as thermal burns. The affected extremity should be rapidly rewarmed using warm water. Use of excessive heat such as steam is dangerous and may cause unnecessary damage. Dress the rewarmed extremity and immobilize it with a padded splint. As with flame burns, frostbite may be very painful, so pain management is needed.[3,6]

BURN ASSESSMENT

Burn depth and extent are assessed to determine severity of the burn injury. In many cases, final determination is not made for several days.

Depth of Burn

The degree of the burn is described as first, second, or third degree or partial thickness or full thickness (Table 29-1). Identification of the depth of injury may be difficult initially. The depth of the injury may actually increase over

Table **29-1**	**American Burn Association's Classification of Severity of Injury**	
Classification	Characteristics	Treatment facility
Minor	SPT* DPT† <15% TBSA adult DPT <10% TBSA child FT‡ <3% TBSA adult, child (not involving face, hands, feet, or perineum)	Outpatient or inpatient (for 24 hr)
Moderate	DPT 15%-25% TBSA adult DPT 10%-20% TBSA child FT 3%-10% TBSA adult, child (not involving face, hands, feet, or perineum)	Community hospital
Major	DPT >25% TBSA adult DPT >20% child FT >10% TBSA adult, child Burns of face, hands, feet, and perineum Burns complicated by: ■ inhalation injury ■ major associated trauma ■ preexisting illness ■ all major electrical injuries	Burn center

*Superficial, partial-thickness burns
†Deep, partial-thickness burns
‡Full-thickness burns
From American Burn Association, 1983, Miami.

time as edema forms and circulation to the area of injury is compromised. This process usually peaks at 48 hours, so a more accurate determination of depth can be made at 48 to 72 hours. Depth determination is not a priority during the initial resuscitation.

Extent of Burn

Extent of injury for thermal and chemical injuries is assessed by using formulas such as the Rule of Nines (Figure 29-2), the Berkow, or the Lund and Browder (Figures 29-3 and 29-4).[8] For the Rule of Nines, the care giver should remember that the formula must be modified for children. As noted in Figure 29-2, B, the head and neck of an infant represent 18% of the body surface area (BSA), whereas the legs represent 13% for each lower extremity. To correct for age, 1% is subtracted from the head for each year of age, through 10 years, and 0.5% is added to each lower extremity. To estimate scatter burns, the size of the patient's palm is used to represent 1% of the total BSA (TBSA). The palm is visualized over the burned areas. To obtain a more accurate estimate of the extent of burn, both burned and unburned areas are calculated. The two estimates should then be compared. If the total is more or less than 100%, the areas should be reestimated. In electrical injuries, assessing the extent of injury is more difficult because surface damage may be minimal when compared with the underlying damage. When describing an electrical injury, describing the injury anatomically is more important than calculating the percentage of BSA burned.

Severity of Burn

The severity of the burn injury is based on assessment of the extent and depth of injury, as well as the age of the patient, presence of concomitant injuries, smoke inhalation, or preexisting diseases. The American Burn Association's classification of severity for burn injuries are listed in Table 29-2.

Care of patients with burns of different severity is determined by the availability of specialized care facilities. Initial stabilization of a burn patient should be available in any community hospital that has 24-hour emergency capabilities. Patients with minor burns may be treated as outpatients or admitted to the community hospital. Patients with moderate burns may be treated in a community hospital with appropriate staff and facilities to deliver burn care or a specialized burn care facility. Patients with major burns should be cared for in a specialized burn care facility. Transfer agreements with special-care units should be developed in advance to facilitate a timely and uneventful transfer. Box 29-1 summarizes criteria for transfer to a burn center. Any patient with concomitant trauma that poses an increased risk for morbidity or mortality should be treated in a trauma center until stable and then transferred to a burn center as appropriate.

PATHOPHYSIOLOGY

Burn injury occurs when the skin is exposed to more energy than it can absorb. The cause of the burn may vary, but

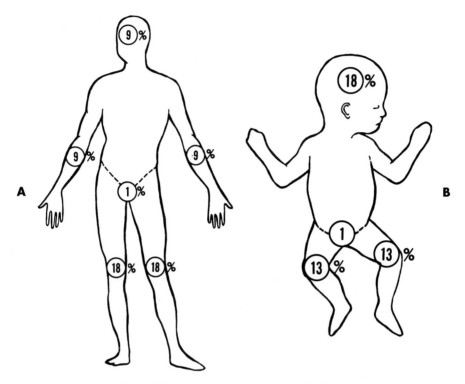

Figure **29-2**   Rule of nines. **A,** Adult. **B,** Child.

Table **29-2** **Classification of Burn Injury**				
Depth of burn	Sensitivity	Appearance	Healing time and results	Treatment
Partial thickness *First degree*				
Epidermal	Hyperalgesia	Erythema	3 to 5 days; no scarring	Moisturizers
Superficial dermal	Hyperalgesia	Blisters, red, moist	6 to 10 days; minimal scarring	Topical antibacterial agents or biologic dressings required
Second degree				
Moderate dermal	Normal algesia	Blisters, pink, moist	10 to 18 days; some scarring	Topical antibacterial agents or biologic dressings required
Deep dermal	Hypoalgesia or analgesia	Blisters, opaque, with less moisture	>21 days; maximal scarring if not excised and grafted	Topical antibacterial agents and early excision and grafting
Full thickness *Third degree*				
Loss of all dermal elements with extension into fat, muscle, and bone	Analgesia	White, opaque, brown, or black, occasionally deep red; very dry, leathery; may or may not have blisters or thrombosed veins	Never heals if area is larger than 3 cm^2; the longer the wound is open, the more hypertrophic the scar	Topical antibacterial agents and early excision and grafting

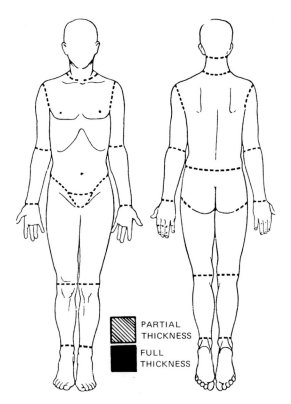

AREA	1 YEAR	1-4 YEARS	5-9 YEARS	10-14 YEARS	Y 15 YEARS	ADULT	2°	3°
Head	19	17	13	11	9	7		
Neck	2	2	2	2	2	2		
Ant. Trunk	13	13	13	13	13	13		
Post Trunk	13	13	13	13	13	13		
R. Buttock	2½	2½	2½	2½	2½	2½		
L. Buttock	2½	2½	2½	2½	2½	2½		
Genitalia	1	1	1	1	1	1		
R. U. Arm	4	4	4	4	4	4		
L. U. Arm	4	4	4	4	4	4		
R. L. Arm	3	3	3	3	3	3		
L. L. Arm	3	3	3	3	3	3		
R. Hand	2½	2½	2½	2½	2½	2½		
L. Hand	2½	2½	2½	2½	2½	2½		
R. Thigh	5½	6½	8	8½	9	9½		
L. Thigh	5½	6½	8	8½	9	9½		
R. Leg	5	5	5½	6	6½	7		
L. Leg	5	5	5½	6	6½	7		
R. Foot	3½	3½	3½	3½	3½	3½		
L. Foot	3½	3½	3½	3½	3½	3½		
TOTAL								

Figure **29-3** Lund and Browder formula. *(From Artz CP, Moncrief JA:* The treatment of burns, *ed 2, Philadelphia, 1979, WB Saunders.)*

the local and systemic responses are similar. To understand the pathophysiology of burns, one must first understand the functions of the skin. It consists of two layers: the epidermis and the dermis. The epidermis, the outer layer of the basement layer of cells, consists of cells that migrate upward to become surface keratin. The dermis, or inner layer, consists of collagen and elastic fibers and contains hair follicles, sweat and sebaceous glands, nerve endings, and blood vessels. The skin is the largest organ of the body and acts as an infection barrier, a vapor barrier, and a heat regulator.[4,7]

Three zones of tissue damage occur at the burn site. First is the central zone of coagulation, an area of irreversible damage. Concentrically surrounding this area is the zone of stasis where capillary and small vessel stasis occurs. The ultimate fate of the burn wound depends on resolution or progression of the zone of stasis. Edema formation and prolonged compromise of blood flow to this area cause a deeper, more extensive wound; therefore, depth and severity of burn wounds may not be known for 3 to 5 days after the initial injury. The third zone of damage is the zone of hyperemia, an area of superficial damage that heals quickly on its own.[2,8]

The body responds to the burn injury with varying degrees of tissue damage, cellular impairment, and fluid shifts.

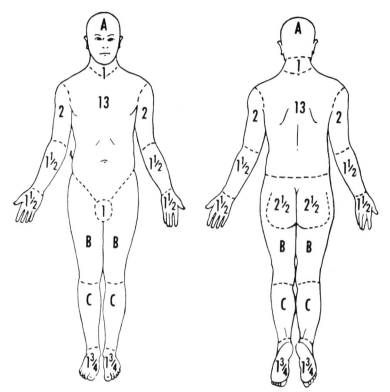

Figure **29-4** Lund and Browder formula. *(From Artz CP, Moncrief JA: The treatment of burns, ed 2, Philadelphia, 1979, WB Saunders.)*

Relative Percentage of Areas Affected by Growth

	Age in Years					
	0	1	5	10	15	Adult
A—½ of head	9½	8½	6½	5½	4½	3½
B—½ of one thigh	2¾	3¼	4	4¼	4½	4¾
C—½ of one leg	2½	2½	2¾	3	3¼	3½

Box 29-1   Criteria for Transfer to a Burn Center

- Partial-thickness and full-thickness burns greater than 10% TBSA in a patient under 10 years or over 50 years of age
- Partial-thickness and full-thickness burns greater than 20% TBSA in other age groups
- Partial-thickness and full-thickness burns involving the face, eyes, ears, hands, feet, genitalia, or perineum or those that involve skin overlying major joints
- Full-thickness burns greater than 5% TBSA in any age group
- Electrical burns, including lightning injury
- Significant chemical burns
- Inhalation injury
- Burn injury in patients with preexisting illness that may complicate management, prolong recovery, or affect mortality
- Children with burns seen in hospitals without qualified personnel or equipment for their care should be transferred to a burn center with these capabilities
- Burn injury in patients who require special social, emotional, or long-term rehabilitative support, including cases of suspected child abuse or neglect

From American Burn Association, 1993.

A brief decrease in blood flow to the affected area is followed by a marked increase in arteriolar vasodilation. Damaged tissues release mediators that initiate an inflammatory response. Histamine, serotonin, prostaglandin derivatives, and the complement cascade are all activated. Release of vasoactive substances combined with vasodilation causes increased capillary permeability and results in intravascular fluid loss and wound edema. For burn injuries of less than 20% TBSA, these actions are usually limited to the burn site. As the affected TBSA goes beyond 20%, local response becomes systemic. Hypoproteinemia resulting from increased capillary permeability aggravates edema in non-burned tissue. Basal metabolic rate (BMR) increases from insensible fluid loss, which along with the fluid shift produces hypovolemia. Capillary permeability increases for 2 to 3 weeks with the most significant changes occurring in the first 24 to 36 hours.[2,4,8]

Initially, blood viscosity increases as a result of a rise in hematocrit as vascular fluid shifts into the interstitium. Because of a marked increase in peripheral resistance, decreased intravascular fluid volume, and increased blood viscosity, cardiac output falls. Capillary leak and depressed cardiac output can depress central nervous system function, causing restlessness, followed by lethargy, and finally coma. Decreased cardiac output, blood volume, and an intense sympathetic response decrease perfusion to the skin, viscera, and renal perfusion. Decreased flow can convert a zone of stasis to zone of coagulation, which increases the depth of the burn. Decreased circulating plasma with increased hematocrit can cause hemoglobinuria, which can lead to renal failure. Immediate hemolysis of red cells occurs, and the life span of the remaining red cells is reduced by approximately 30% of normal. Initially, platelet count and platelet survival time drop drastically. This drop continues for 5 days after the injury, but is followed by an increase in platelets for several weeks.[2,4,8]

Cardiovascular changes begin immediately after a burn. The extent varies depending on size of the burn and the presence of additional injuries. Patients with an uncomplicated burn less than 15% TBSA can usually be treated with oral fluid resuscitation. Burns that surpass 20% TBSA have massive shifts of fluid and electrolytes from the intravascular to the extravascular space. This shift begins to resolve in 18 to 36 hours; however, normal extracellular volume is not completely restored for 7 to 10 days after the burn. If intravascular volume is not replenished, hypovolemic shock occurs. Untreated, the patient dies of cardiovascular collapse. Inadequate treatment leads to renal failure from acute tubular necrosis.

Burn injuries can affect every organ system in the body, causing cerebral perfusion abnormalities, impaired coronary blood supply, renal insufficiency, and acid-base imbalance.[2,7] Realization of these broad effects can enhance management of the burn patient.

Pulmonary Response to Smoke Inhalation

Inhalation injury or smoke inhalation is a syndrome composed of three distinct problems: carbon monoxide intoxication, upper airway obstruction, and chemical injury to the lower airways and lung parenchyma.

Carbon monoxide intoxication is the most common killer of victims of fire. Most people who die in a fire have been overcome by carbon monoxide before they sustain their burn injury. In the body, carbon monoxide has a 200-times greater affinity for hemoglobin than oxygen, which causes inadequate tissue oxygen delivery. Carbon monoxide also combines with myoglobin in muscle cells, which causes muscle weakness. Tissue hypoxia resulting in mental confusion and muscle weakness may be the major reasons for most fire fatalities. Carbon monoxide also combines with the cytochrome oxidase system of the brain and may result in prolonged coma in some fire victims.

Carbon monoxide poisoning is characterized by pink-to-cherry-red skin, tachypnea, tachycardia, headache, dizziness, and nausea. An arterial blood gas sample should be drawn to measure the carboxyhemoglobin level. Levels of up to 15% are rarely associated with symptoms and can be normal for a heavy smoker. Levels of 15% to 40% are associated with varying disturbances such as headache and con-

fusion. Levels greater than 40% can occur in coma. All patients with suspected carbon monoxide poisoning should be placed on 100% oxygen.[4,8]

Upper airway obstruction is the result of intrinsic or extrinsic edema that may lead to airway occlusion at or above the vocal cords (Figure 29-5). This injury is primarily a thermal injury resulting in tissue damage in the posterior pharynx. Actual thermal injury below the vocal cords is rare because the posterior pharynx is such an efficient heat exchange system. True thermal injury below the vocal cords is usually the result of superheated steam where water vapor carries the heat into the lungs. Injuries that occur in an oxygen-enriched atmosphere or one where the person was inhaling explosive gases (e.g., during inhalation anesthesia) also cause true thermal injury below the vocal cords. True thermal injury to the lungs is almost always fatal. Thermal injury to the upper airway is usually associated with facial burns. Edema progresses rapidly, totally occluding the airway in minutes to hours. Management for airway edema is early intubation.

Chemical injury to the lower airways is a common problem with inhalation of smoke. Chemical injury from acids and aldehydes in the smoke may damage the lung parenchyma. These chemicals, attached to carbon particles in the smoke, are heavier than air, so they are readily inhaled and find their way down the bronchi into alveoli. This chemical injury results in hemorrhagic tracheobronchitis, increased edema formation, decreased surfactant levels, and decreased pulmonary macrophage function. This condition leads to rapid development of adult respiratory distress syndrome (ARDS) over 24 to 48 hours. Severe inhalation injury may increase the patient's fluid needs in the first 24 hours by as much as 50% of calculated values.

PATIENT MANAGEMENT

The burn patient may have other injuries in addition to the burn; therefore, the patient should be initially evaluated using the ABC4 survey for trauma. The cervical spine is stabilized while assessing an adequate airway. Assessment of specific burn injuries should then be done. A history is obtained as time and patient condition permit. How did the injury occur? What caused the injury—flame, scald, etc? Was smoke involved? Did injury occur in a confined space? What was the patient doing before the injury? Did the patient have a stroke or myocardial infarction before the injury? Does the patient have any medical problems or allergies? General assessment and intervention for the burn patient are described in this section.

Airway

A high index of suspicion for smoke inhalation is essential for these patients. Burns that occur in small spaces are often associated with smoke inhalation. The oropharynx and vocal cords should be inspected for redness, blisters, and carbonaceous particles. The patient is observed for increasing restlessness, dyspnea, difficulty swallowing, increasing

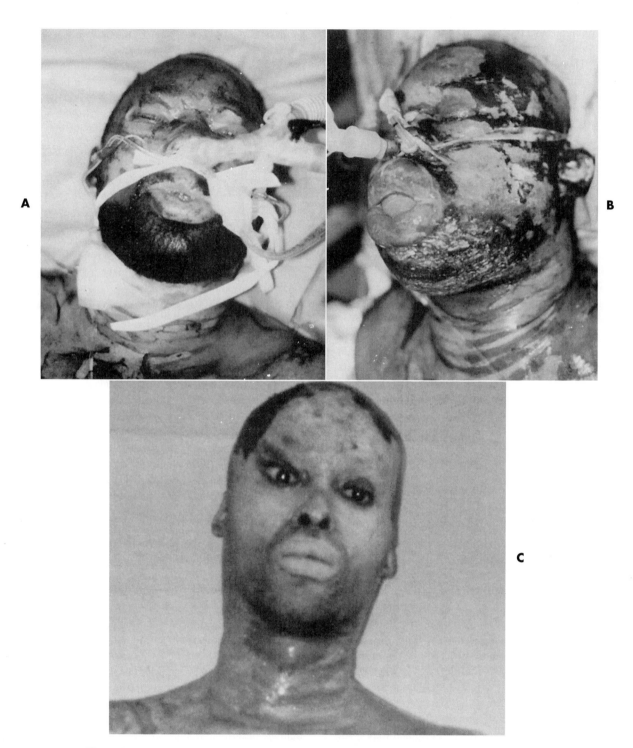

Figure **29-5**   Facial edema. **A,** 4 to 5 hours after burn. **B,** 30 hours after burn, showing distortion of facial features and necessity of intubation before the full extent of burn edema development. **C,** Facial contour 3 months after burn. *(Courtesy Anne E. Missavage, MD, UC Davis Regional Burn Center, Sacramento, Calif.)*

hoarseness, and rapid, shallow respirations. The patient may have increasing difficulty managing secretions with a significant risk for impending airway obstruction. Early intubation is recommended before complete obstruction occurs. Tracheostomies should be avoided initially since edema of the neck makes this procedure difficult.

Breathing

Breathing can be impaired by circumferential full thickness burns of the chest. The burn may limit chest wall excursion and prevent adequate gas exchange. The chest should be visually inspected for tight, leathery eschar that circles the chest. Evidence of breathing compromise includes inadequate chest expansion, restlessness, confusion, decreased oxygenation, decreased tidal volume, and rapid, shallow respirations.

Escharotomy is indicated for circumferential burns that compromise breathing. Surgical incisions are made in the burned tissue on the chest to release the eschar and expose underlying subcutaneous tissue. Improvement in chest wall expansion should occur immediately after the incisions are made. General anesthesia is not required since the incisions are made in a full-thickness burn. Intravenous narcotic analgesia is usually adequate to relieve any pain.

The patient with a burn injury is also at risk for carbon monoxide poisoning. Altered breathing patterns such as decreased respirations or apnea may be evident. The patient may have the characteristic cherry-red skin or may appear slightly cyanotic. Confusion, irritability, or coma may be present. A carboxyhemoglobin level and a chest radiograph are obtained. High-flow oxygen with a nonrebreather mask or bag-valve mask is administered as appropriate. If the patient does not respond after 1 to 1.5 hours of regular oxygen therapy, hyperbaric oxygen therapy may be used.

Adult respiratory distress syndrome may occur in these patients, but is usually not a problem for at least 18 hours after injury. Clinical findings associated with ARDS include decreased oxygenation, increased secretions, rapid respirations, confusion, and increasing patchy infiltrates on the radiograph. Treatment includes intubation and ventilation with positive end expiratory pressure. Bronchodilators may be indicated; however, corticosteroids are not. Giving corticosteroids to patients with burns and smoke inhalation can increase morbidity and mortality. Refer to Chapter 34 for additional information on ARDS.

The burn patient should be assessed for other injuries that can affect breathing, such as pneumothorax, hemothorax, tension pneumothorax, and flail chest. These problems are suggested when a burn injury occurs as a result of a motor vehicle crash or explosion. Additional injuries may be present when a patient has jumped to escape the fire. Preexisting health problems that may affect the patient's respiratory functions, (e.g., chronic obstructive pulmonary disease, asthma) should be noted.

Circulation

The patient with a burn injury is at significant risk for hypovolemia from fluid loss as well as fluid movement from increased capillary permeability and vasodilation. Assess the patient for increased respirations, increased pulse, decreased blood pressure, decreased urine output, diminished capillary refill, restlessness, confusion, and nausea and vomiting. Additional indications of volume compromise include central venous pressure less than 3 cm H_2O, hematocrit greater than 50 mg/dl, presence of an ileus, and urine output less than 0.5 ml/kg/hr.

One or two large-bore intravenous (IV) catheters should be started. A single IV catheter is adequate for a burn less than 40% TBSA. Two are begun if the burn is greater than 40% TBSA or if the patient is to be transferred. Leg veins are avoided because of the increased risk of thrombophlebitis. The IV catheter can be inserted into burned tissue if no other access is available, but this should be considered a last resort. Fluid volume requirements are calculated using an accepted formula such as the Parkland formula or the Baxter formula (Table 29-3). These formulas are a guideline for fluid replacement type and volume and should be adjusted to the patient's response to the fluid. Ideally, fluid resuscitation is adequate if the pulse and blood pressure are within normal limits for age, and urine output is 30 to 50 ml/hr for adults, 20 to 30 ml/hr children, and 1 to 1.5 ml/kg/hr infants.

No formula exists for calculating fluid resuscitation in electrical injuries. An infusion of Ringer's lactated solution is administered at 1 to 2 L/hr in the average adult until the patient shows signs of adequate resuscitation. Urine output should be maintained at 2 to 3 times normal volume to facilitate excretion of myoglobin. Once urine output is established, mannitol may be given to increase urine flow and aid excretion of myoglobin. Significant acidosis may occur; therefore, repeated administration of sodium bicarbonate ($NaHCO_3$) may be required to prevent dysrhythmias. Once fluid therapy corrects the acidosis, this may not be necessary.

Infection

The patient with a burn injury has lost the greatest protection against invasion by various pathogens and must be protected with scrupulous aseptic technique. Gloves, masks, caps, and gowns must be worn. Sterile technique is necessary for all procedures. Wounds are kept covered with clean sheets while other care is provided. If the patient is to be transferred, sterile sheets are used to cover the patient. If treatment is followed by discharge, the nurse should debride the burn, apply a topical antibiotic, and cover the wound with a fluffy dressing. Systemic antibiotics are rarely indicated even in severe burns until infection is confirmed by culture. Exceptions to this guideline may be young children, elderly patients, diabetic patients, or patients with immune compromise.

For minor or moderate burns, tetanus immunization is given if the patient has not been immunized within the past

10 years. In major burns or grossly contaminated burns, tetanus immunization is given if previous immunization has occurred in less than 10 years. If the patient has never been immunized or no clear history of immunization exists, tetanus hyperimmune globulin (Hypertet) and tetanus immunization is given.

Pain Management

Burn wounds are exquisitely painful, especially partial-thickness injuries. The patient may also have pain secondary to other injuries. The patient is probably in pain if restlessness, tachycardia, and tachypnea are evident. Intravenous analgesia is used in burns greater than 15% TBSA. Fluid shifts associated with extensive burns and actual tissue damage impair absorption of intramuscular medications. Morphine should be administered in small, frequent dosages, usually 3 to 5 mg every 20 to 40 minutes. Antianxiety drugs such as diazepam (Valium) or midazolam (Versed) are given if the patient is agitated for no apparent reason and hypoxia and other injuries have been ruled out.

Wound Care

Wound care should be delayed until the patient's condition is stabilized. However, initial management must include removal of jewelry and constrictive clothing. The wounds must be kept covered with clean sheets until more definitive care can be provided. All patients with full-thickness burns are assessed for circulatory problems. Capillary refill and the presence of paresthesia are evaluated, and distal pulses are checked with a Doppler. Burn tissue does not stretch, so swelling beneath burned tissue can compromise circulation

because of the lack of elasticity. If the patient has signs of compromise, escharotomy is indicated. Figure 29-6 illustrates placement of these surgical incisions. Significant bleeding can occur with escharotomy, which can be controlled with an electrocautery unit or small hemostats (Fig-

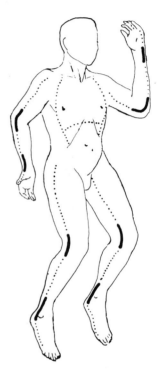

Figure **29-6**   Placement of escharotomies.

Table **29-3**   **Fluid Replacement Formulas**

Formula	Electrolyte solution	Colloid	Water	Rate	Example: 70 kg/45% TBSA (per 24 hr)
Evans	1 ml/kg/% TBSA normal saline (NS)	1 ml/kg/%	2000 ml	½, 1st 8 hr; ½, next 16 hr	3150 ml NS 3150 ml colloid 2000 ml water 8300 ml TOTAL
Brooke	1.5 ml/kg/% TBSA lactated Ringer's solution (LR)	0.5 ml/kg/%	2000 ml	½, 1st 8 hr; ½, next 16 hr	4725 ml LR 1575 ml colloid 2000 ml water 8300 ml TOTAL
Modified Brooke	2-3 ml/kg/% TBSA LR	None	None	½, 1st 8 hr ½, next 16 hr	6300-9450 ml LR
Parkland (Baxter)	4 ml/kg/% TBSA LR	None	None	½, 1st 8 hr; ½, next 16 hr	12,600 ml LR
Hypertonic formula	Rate based on urine output of 30 ml/hr with hypertonic LR (sodium, 250 mEq/L)	None	None	To maintain urine output	Unknown

From Neff JA, Kidd PS: *Trauma nursing,* St. Louis, 1992, Mosby.

ure 29-7). Once the procedure is completed, a topical antibacterial agent is applied to the open wound, a light pressure dressing is applied, and the extremity is slightly elevated.

Thermal burns may be secondary to flame, flash, scalds, or hot objects. Figure 29-8 shows an example of a thermal burn. Thermal burns are cleaned with sterile or clean water using 0.25 strength povidone iodine *(Betadine)* and clean cloths or coarse mesh gauze dressing. The outer covering of blisters larger than a half dollar are broken and removed, except for those on the palms of the hands and the soles of the feet. Hair is shaved from burns and surrounding areas. The

wound is covered immediately with a topical antibacterial agent such as silvadene or bacitracin.

Chemical burns should be immediately irrigated with tap water or saline for at least 5 to 10 minutes to remove the chemical. Clothing and jewelry is removed, and unburned areas adjacent to the burned areas are rinsed. These areas may be injured, but may not hurt, blister, or turn red immediately. If the chemical is dry, it can be brushed from the patient before irrigating. After the wound is thoroughly irrigated, it is treated like a thermal burn. Chemical burns of the eye are an ophthalmologic emergency. The eye must be irrigated thoroughly with copious amounts of water or saline.

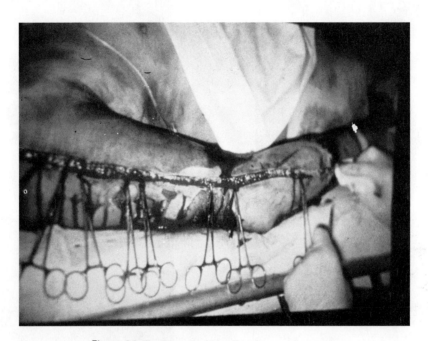

Figure **29-7** Control of bleeding from escharotomy.

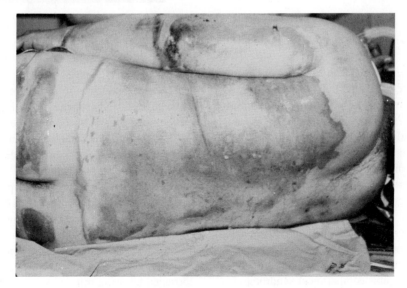

Figure **29-8** Flame burns to back.

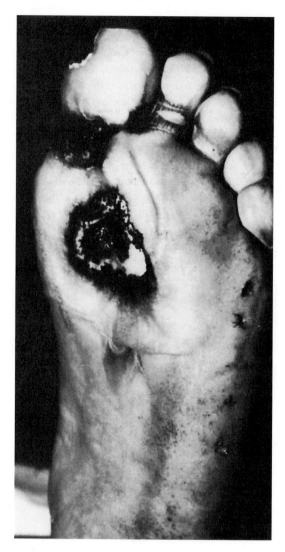

Figure **29-9** Exit wound from direct current. *(From NFNA: Flight nursing, ed 2, St. Louis, 1996, Mosby.)*

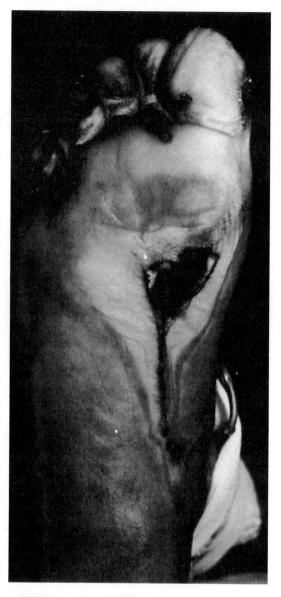

Figure **29-10** Exit wound from alternating current. *(From NFNA: Flight nursing, ed 2, St. Louis, 1996, Mosby.)*

Refer to Chapter 48 for additional discussion of chemical eye injuries.

Electrical injuries are different from thermal or chemical burns. They may have little superficial tissue loss; however, massive muscle injury may be present beneath normal-looking skin (Figures 29-9 and 29-10). These wounds should be cleansed gently with water or saline and 0.25 strength povidone iodine *(Betadine);* they rarely need immediate debridement. Handling and manipulation of these cadaverlike limbs are kept to a minimum. Large patent vessels may be torn leading to massive hemorrhage. Topical agents such as mafenide acetate *(Sulfamylon)* that deeply penetrate tissue are used to cover the wound. Light dressings may be applied to cover these often grotesque wounds; however, dressings must not interfere with assessment for circulatory compromise and possible compartment syndrome.

Electrical injuries of the extremities cause significant damage that leads to tissue swelling. Consequently, these patients are at risk for compartment syndrome. Symptoms associated with this condition include pain, pallor, paresthesia, pulselessness, and paralysis. Fasciotomies are used to relieve compartment syndrome.

Tar or asphalt burns may be deep or superficial depending on the temperature of the tar, which may range from 150° F to more than 600° F. Figure 29-11 shows a tar burn before tar removal. Figure 29-12 shows the same burn after the tar has been removed. Immediate treatment of a tar burn is to cool the tar, but do not try to peel it off the patient's skin. The tar is loosened by using mineral oil, petroleum jelly, or a solvent

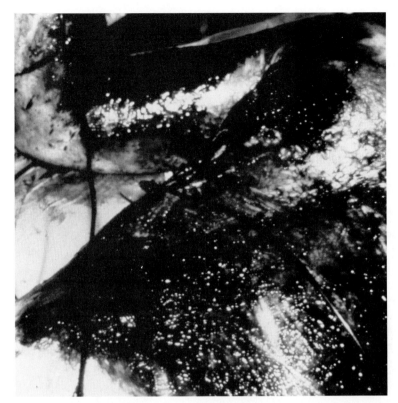

Figure **29-11** Tar burns of chest before removal of tar.

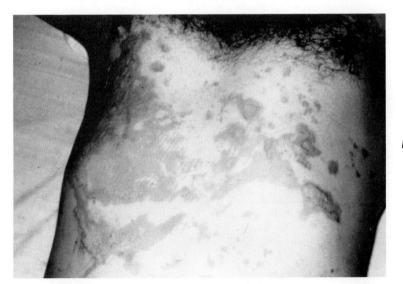

Figure **29-12** Tar burns after removal of tar.

such as *Medi-Sol*. In areas where the burn is not circumferential, oil or ointment is applied, and the burn is covered with a light dressing. Dressings are removed in 4 to 12 hours, oil or ointment reapplied, and a new dressing applied. For areas with circumferential tar, the oil or ointment can be applied with light dressings and changed every 20 to 30 minutes until the tar is removed. Once the tar is removed, the burn is treated like a thermal injury.

Temperature Regulation

The patient with a burn injury has lost a major control mechanism for temperature regulation. This heat loss is worsened by administration of IV fluids, irrigation of burned tissue, and environmental coolness often encountered in the ED. The patient's temperature should be documented as soon as possible after arrival and rechecked within 1 hour. Heat loss is minimized by keeping the patient

Box **29-2**

NURSING DIAGNOSES FOR BURN INJURY

Fluid volume deficit
Impaired gas exchange
Altered tissue perfusion
High risk for hypothermia
High risk for infection
Pain
Body image disturbance

covered, using warmed IV fluids, and increasing room temperature.

CONCLUSION

Burn injury can be devastating to the patient and the family. For the care giver, it can also be visually disturbing. Regardless of how severe the burn may be, a primary survey should be performed of potentially life-threatening injuries. Resuscitation of the burn patient includes evaluation of the burn, replacement of fluid losses, wound care, protection against contamination, maintenance of body temperature, and pain control. Box 29-2 summarizes nursing diagnoses appropriate for the burn patient. A multidisciplinary approach to burn care can reduce mortality and morbidity. Appropriate application of burn center transfer criteria ensures the best outcome for the patient with a major burn injury.

REFERENCES

1. American College of Surgeons: *Advanced trauma life support student manual,* Chicago, 1993, The College.
2. Auerbach P: *Wilderness medicine,* ed 3, St. Louis, 1995, Mosby.
3. Holleran R: *Prehospital nursing: A collaborative approach,* St. Louis, 1994, Mosby.
4. McCloskey K, Orr R: *Pediatric transport medicine,* St. Louis, 1995, Mosby.
5. National Association of Emergency Medical Technicians: *Pre-hospital trauma life support,* ed 3, St. Louis, 1996, Mosby.
6. National Flight Nurses Association: *Flight nurse advanced trauma course student manual,* Park Ridge, Ill, 1995, The Association.
7. National Flight Nurses Association: *Flight nursing: principles and practice,* ed 2, St. Louis, 1996, Mosby.
8. Neff J, Kidd P: *Trauma nursing: The art and science,* St. Louis, 1993, Mosby.

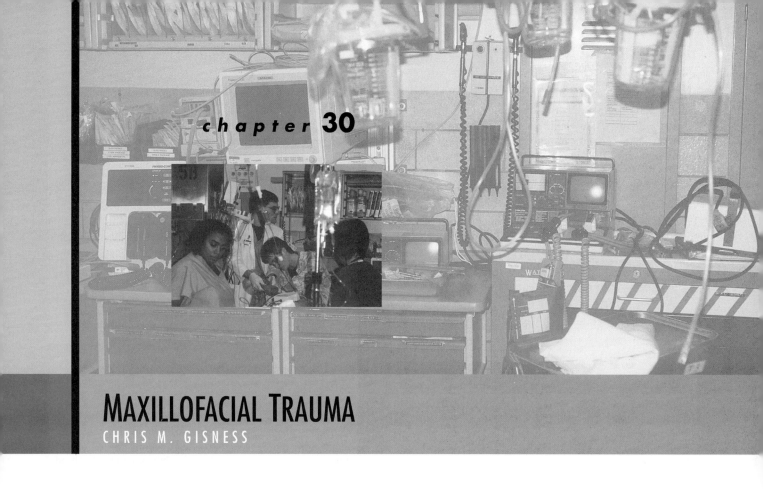

chapter **30**

MAXILLOFACIAL TRAUMA

CHRIS M. GISNESS

Maxillofacial trauma involving injury of the facial bones, neurovascular structures, skin, subcutaneous tissue, muscles, and glands, is a common injury in patients treated in the emergency department (ED). Facial trauma is a complicating factor in management of multiply injured patients. Studies document 20% to 50% incidence of closed head injury associated with significant facial trauma.

Motor vehicle collisions (MVCs) are the most common cause of facial injury in the United States; however, facial trauma from assaults and personal altercations is increasing.[9] Domestic violence is reported as the cause in 10% of all facial fractures.[2] Handguns also cause facial injury. With bullet trajectory above the mandible, intracranial injury should also be considered.[4] Facial injury from falls is common among the elderly and children. In children, skull and facial bone flexibility absorb energy associated with deceleration injuries such as MVCs and falls.[1] Significant energy is required to fracture the maxilla or midface—100 times the force of gravity; consequently patients with midface fractures often have multisystem injuries.[12] Table 30-1 identifies gravitational forces required to fracture various facial bones.

When assessing facial injuries, severe facial injury should not take priority over recognition and treatment of life-threatening injuries. Rapid, thorough assessment using a systematic approach with emphasis on airway, breathing, circulation (ABCs), and cervical spine stabilization is essential.

ANATOMY AND PHYSIOLOGY

Principal facial bones include the frontal, nasal, maxilla, zygoma, and mandible (Figure 30-1). The frontal bone articulates with the frontal process of the maxilla and nasal bone and laterally with the zygoma. The orbital complex is composed of the frontal bone superiorly, zygoma laterally, maxilla inferiorly, and processes of the maxilla and frontal bone medially. Paired nasal bones that form the bridge of the nose articulate with the frontal bone above and maxilla below (Figure 30-2). The nasal cavity is divided by the nasal septum (Figure 30-3); the lateral wall has ridges or concha that affect phonation (Figure 30-4).

The midface, or maxilla, forms the upper jaw, anterior hard palate, part of the lateral wall of the nasal cavity, and part of the orbital floor. Below the orbit, the maxilla is perforated by the infraorbital foramen to allow passage of infraorbital vessels and nerves. Projecting downward, the alveolar process joins the opposite side to form the alveolar arch, which houses upper teeth. Sinus cavities in the midface decrease weight and act as resonating chambers (Figure 30-5).

The zygoma forms the cheek and the lateral wall and floor of the orbital cavity. The zygoma articulates with the maxilla, frontal bone, and zygomatic process of the temporal bone to form the zygomatic arch.

The mandible is a horizontal horseshoe body with two rami, anterior coronoid processes, and posterior condyloid processes.[11] The mandibular notch lies medial to the zygomatic arch and separates the two processes. The mandible articulates with the temporal bone to form the temporo-mandibular joint, whereas the upper body, called the alveolar part, contains lower teeth.

The facial nerve (cranial nerve VII), which provides sensory and motor innervation to the side of the face, originates in the brainstem then divides into six branches to innervate the scalp, forehead, eyelids, facial muscles for expression, cheeks, and jaw (Figure 30-6). Specific functions for each branch are listed in Table 30-2. Other cranial nerves that may be affected by facial trauma are the oculomotor, trochlear, and trigeminal. Function and testing for each are described in Table 30-3.

The parotid gland located adjacent to the anterior ear drains into the oral cavity through the parotid duct (Figure 30-7). These structures are located adjacent to branches of the facial nerve on top of the masseter muscle.[8]

PATIENT ASSESSMENT

An organized approach to patient assessment is essential for identification and stabilization of facial injuries (Table 30-4) with the first priority a clear, secure airway. Damaged facial structures can cause airway obstruction. If displaced, the mandible leaves the tongue without support and occludes the airway. Foreign objects, for example, dentures or

Table **30-1**	Force of Gravity Impact Required for Facial Fracture	
Bone	**Force of gravity (g)**
Nasal bones	30
Zygoma	50
Angle of mandible	70
Frontal-glabellar region	80
Midline maxilla	100
Midline mandible (symphysis)	100
Supraorbital rim	200

From Rosen P et al: *Emergency medicine, ed 3, vol I, St. Louis, 1993, Mosby.*

Table **30-2**	Facial Nerve Branch Functions
Branch	**Function**
Buccal	Wrinkle nose
Cervical	Wrinkle skin of neck
Mandibular	Purse and depress lips
Temporal	Raise eyebrows, wrinkle forehead
Zygomatic	Close eyelids

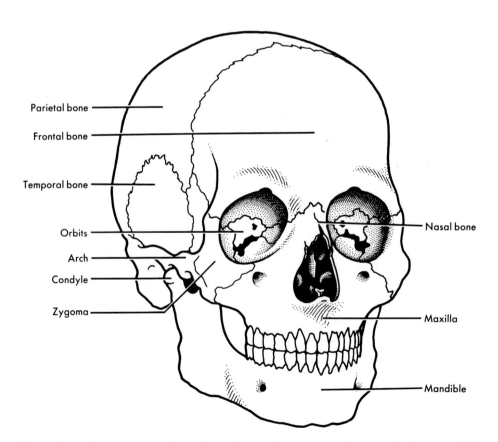

Figure **30-1** Facial skeleton. *(From Rosen P et al:* Emergency medicine, *ed 3, St. Louis, 1992, Mosby.)*

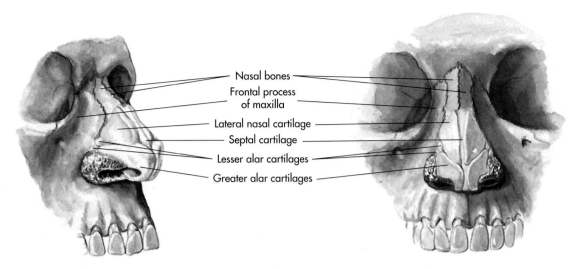

Figure **30-2** Nasal structures. *(From* Mosby's medical, nursing, and allied health dictionary, *ed 4, St. Louis, 1994, Mosby.)*

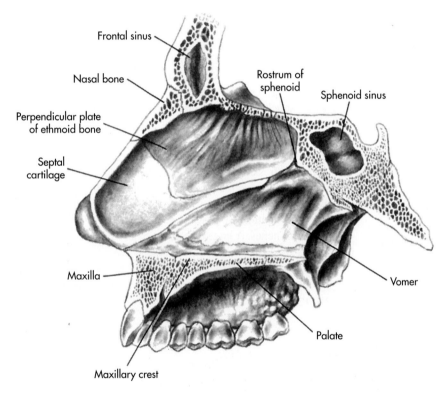

Figure **30-3** Nasal septum. *(From Thompson JM et al:* Clinical nursing, *ed 4, St. Louis, 1997, Mosby.)*

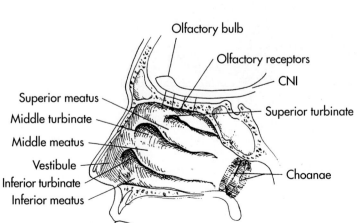

Figure **30-4** Lateral view of the left nasal cavity. *(Modified from Barkauskas VH et al:* Health and physical assessment, *St. Louis, 1994, Mosby.)*

avulsed teeth, also obstruct the airway, whereas fractures of the nasoorbital complex compromise the airway because of hemorrhage. Gunshot wounds to the face cause significant swelling and hematoma formation, which obstruct the airway. When airway compromise is recognized, the chin lift–head tilt method should be used unless cervical spine injury is possible, in which case the jaw-thrust maneuver is indicated. Altered mental status due to alcohol, drugs, or head injury may diminish the gag reflex and leave the airway unprotected. Frequent suctioning of oropharynx and/or nasopharynx is required if bleeding or excessive secretions are present. Tonsil tip suction catheter may be provided for an alert patient to self-suction. Allowing the patient to sit upright or elevating the head of bed promotes drainage; however, the cervical spine must be cleared first.

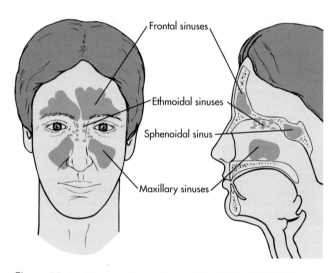

Figure **30-5** Sinuses. *(From Lewis SM, Collier IC, Heitkemper MM: Medical-surgical nursing: assessment and management of clinical problems, ed 4, St. Louis, 1996, Mosby.)*

Excessive bleeding and swelling in the mouth and facial structures, coupled with inability to clear the airway, requires aggressive airway control. Supplemental oxygen and assisted ventilations may be accomplished with a bag-valve-mask. Swelling and facial fractures can make use of a bag-valve-mask difficult with some patients. Oropharyngeal airway can be used in an unconscious patient with obstruction by the tongue. Nasopharyngeal airway can be used in the conscious patient with no nasal or midface fractures.

Orotracheal intubation is preferred in patients with facial injuries; nasotracheal intubation should be avoided. Cribriform plate fractures increase the risk for cerebral penetration by an endotracheal tube. Rapid-sequence induction facilitates intubation and has the added benefit of protecting the patient from increases in intracranial pressure.[13] If rapid-sequence induction is used, equipment to perform surgical airway opening must be available should cricothyroidotomy or tracheostomy be needed. Pulse oximetry should be utilized as an adjunct for monitoring the airway. Cervical spine injury should be considered in all facial trauma patients and plain radiographs or CT scan used to rule out injury.

Once a patent airway is established, the next priority is hemorrhage control. Patients with facial injury rarely develop shock from facial bleeding so hypotension is usually caused by associated injuries in the chest, abdomen, retroperitoneal space, or bones. Facial bleeding can be quickly controlled with direct pressure. An external compression dressing, such as a Barton bandage, wrapped circumferentially, can be used to temporarily control bleeding. Bleeding vessels on the face should be carefully assessed prior to ligation to prevent accidental clamping of facial nerve branches. A large cotton-tip swab can be used to apply direct pressure to bleeding vessels; ice packs and direct nasal pressure usually stop bleeding from the nose. A nasal tampon may be inserted to control anterior bleeding, and a nasal balloon may be used to control posterior bleeding. Se-

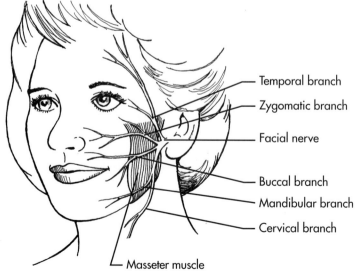

Figure **30-6** Anatomy of the facial nerve.

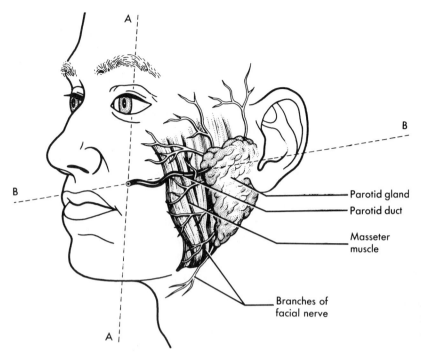

Figure **30-7** Parotid gland and parotid duct with nearby branches of facial nerve. Line *B* demonstrates approximate course of parotid duct from parotid gland, entering mouth at junction of lines *A* and *B*. *(From Rosen P et al:* Emergency medicine, *ed 3, St. Louis, 1992, Mosby.)*

Parotid gland
Parotid duct
Masseter muscle
Branches of facial nerve

Table **30-3**	**Cranial Nerves Involved in Facial Trauma**			
Nerve	Name	Function	Description	Assessment
III	Oculomotor	Motor	Eyeball movement; supplies 5 of 7 ocular muscles	Pupil response; ocular movement to four quadrants
IV	Trochlear	Motor	Eyeball movement (superior oblique)	Same as above
V	Trigeminal	Motor and sensory	Facial sensation; jaw movement	Assessing pain, touch, hot and cold sensations, bite, opening mouth against resistance
VII	Facial	Motor and sensory	Facial expression; taste from anterior two thirds of tongue	Zygomatic branch: have patient close eyes tightly; temporal branch: have patient elevate brows, wrinkle forehead; buccal branch: have patient elevate upper lip, wrinkle nose, whistle

Table **30-4**	**Systematic Assessment for Facial Trauma**
Component	Description
Airway	Assess for open airway; avoid using head-tilt method; consider airway adjuncts; nasopharyngeal airway adjunct is particularly useful with significant edema
Breathing	Ensure adequate breathing; consider supplemental oxygen; noisy breathing suggests obstructed breathing
Circulation	Ensure adequate pulse rate and blood pressure
Cervical spine	Protect cervical spine; assume injury until proven otherwise by cross table lateral radiograph of cervical spine; 10% of patients with severe head trauma have concurrent cervical spine trauma
Control hemorrhage	Use direct pressure whenever possible; protect airway when hemorrhage is present
Neurologic examination	Perform brief neurologic examination; assess for level of consciousness; pupillary response, and accommodation; rate, rhythm, and depth of respiration; and motor movement
Eyes	Evaluate eyes for loss of vision, diplopia (double vision), foreign bodies, penetrating bodies, and hemorrhage
Face	Check for malocclusion, tenderness, asymmetry of infraorbital rim; assess zygomatic arch, anterior wall of antrum, angles of jaw, and lower borders of mandible; check for cerebrospinal fluid leak from nose or face

vere facial trauma such as LeFort II or III fractures requires manual reduction of the face to control bleeding. With closed fractures, bleeding from lacerated arteries and veins in sinus cavities can cause significant posterior pharyngeal bleeding; ligation of arteries and veins is necessary to control blood loss.

Palpate facial structures before edema and hematomas obscure bony landmarks (Figure 30-8) using both hands simultaneously to palpate for step-off irregularities and crepitus of supraorbital ridge and zygoma. Take a bird's-eye view looking down on the face from the eyebrows to compare height of malar eminences, then take a worm's-eye view and look up from below the chin. Gently palpate nasal bones and look intranasally for septal hematoma. Palpate laterally for depressions in the zygomatic arch, then visualize the mouth for gross dental malocclusion. Ask the patient if teeth close and fit together properly, then check ability to completely open the jaw. Upper and lower jaws should be carefully palpated intraorally; gloves should be worn. Check midface stability by attempting to move the upper teeth and hard palate.

Evaluate the facial nerve and branches. Loss of sensation over the lower lip may indicate injury to the inferior alveolar nerve and possible mandibular fracture. Numbness over the upper lip occurs with fracture in the maxilla and injury to the infraorbital nerve. Assess eyes for loss of vision, visual acuity, pupillary reactivity and symmetry, and extraocular movements. Ensure that pupils are on the same facial plane, and assess for enophthalmos and proptosis. Raccoon eyes or periorbital ecchymosis suggests anterior basilar skull fracture, LeFort fracture, or nasoethmoid injury, whereas nasal or ear drainage positive for cerebrospinal fluid (CSF) occurs with cribriform plate fracture or basilar skull fracture. If a bull's eye or halo appears when bloody drainage from the nose or ear is placed on white paper, fluid is considered positive for CSF. Clear fluid positive for glucose or clear fluid that does not crust is CSF. Ruptured tympanic membrane or laceration of the external ear canal also occurs with mandible fractures. Deep lacerations of the cheek should be carefully evaluated for injury to the parotid gland, parotid (Stenson's) duct, and branches of the facial nerve. Diagnostic evaluation for maxillofacial injury includes radiographs, CT, and MRI. Table 30-5 describes various diagnostic tests used to evaluate facial injuries.

SPECIFIC MAXILLOFACIAL INJURIES
Soft Tissue Trauma

For cosmetic purposes, repair of facial lacerations should occur as quickly as possible. Simple lacerations can be cleaned, debrided, and sutured by primary intention within 24 hours of injury. Deeper lacerations and lacerations associated with fractures are conservatively debrided, irrigated, and closed after reduction is completed. Degloving injuries usually involve subcutaneous tissues and underlying skeletal structures.[7] Tissue is considered viable, so excessive debridement should be avoided. Repair of facial lacerations in uncooperative patients is extremely difficult and may injure

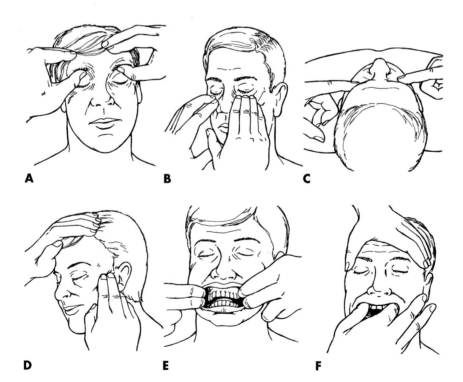

Figure **30-8** Palpation examination techniques for facial injuries. **A,** Palpation for irregularities of supraorbital ridge. **B,** Palpation for irregularities of infraorbital ridge and zygoma. **C,** Comparing height of malar eminences. **D,** Palpation for depression of zygomatic arch. **E,** Visualization of gross dental occlusion. **F,** Maneuver to ascertain motion in maxilla.

other important structures. Delay until the patient is more cooperative results in better outcome. Figure 30-9 illustrates contusions, abrasions, and lacerations of the face.

Lacerations caused by animal or human bites are highly contaminated because of bacteria and debris in the mouth. Human bites should be meticulously cleaned and irrigated; however, controversy surrounds whether wounds should be left open or closed.[12] Extensive or gaping wounds on the face present cosmetic problems so consultation with plastic surgery is recommended. Treatment of animal bites is also controversial. Most experts recommend closing the wound after meticulous irrigation and debridement. Both human and animal bites should be inspected for tooth fragments. Extensive animal bites, usually caused by large dogs, frequently require surgical exploration and repair. A helpful mnemonic for dealing with animal bites is RATS (rabies, antibiotics, tetanus, and soap). Patients with animal and human bites receive prophylactic antibiotics and are immunized for tetanus as appropriate.

Road rash or friction injuries present a unique problem because of potential tattooing or epidermal staining. Debridement should be done within 12 hours to avoid accidental but permanent tattooing from grease and asphalt. Skin should be vigorously scrubbed with mild soap after the area has been injected with local anesthetic. Gunpowder can also

leave permanent discoloration of skin and result in cosmetic disfigurement; therefore black powder fragments embedded in facial skin should be removed by using a local anesthetic and scrubbing with a hard brush or hard bristle toothbrush in the first hour whenever possible.[6] Gunpowder penetrating the skin is very hot and continues to burn epithelial and collagen layers.[10] Removal after 72 hours increases risk for

Table **30-5**	**Radiographic Examination for Maxillofacial Injury**
Test	**Description**
Water's view (posteroanterior)	Single most useful x-ray in maxillofacial injury
	Delineates orbital rim and floor
	Detects blood in maxillary sinus
Towne's view	Mandible condyles-subcondylar regions of orbital floor
Anterior, posterior, & lateral	Skull
	Sinus, roof of orbit
Submental vertex (jughandle)	Zygomatic arch
	Details base of skull
AP & lateral oblique mandible	Condylar, coronoid, body, and symphysis
Occlusal and apical	Palate, symphysis, roots of teeth
CT scan	Provides definitive diagnosis in C-spine injury
	Standard for assessing soft tissue injuries
	Complex facial fractures
MRI	Useful for identifying soft tissue injuries in optic nerve
	Muscle herniation, infraocular and intraocular hematomas, entrapment

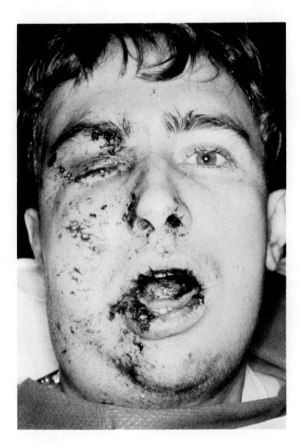

Figure 30-9 Facial injuries. *(From Sheehy SB, Jimmerson CL: Manual of clinical trauma care, ed 2, St. Louis, 1994, Mosby. Courtesy Dr. Daniel Cheney.)*

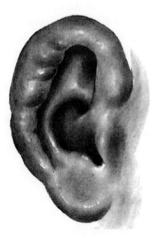

Figure 30-10 Cauliflower ear. *(Modified from Seidel HM et al: Mosby's guide to physical examination, ed 3, St. Louis, 1995, Mosby.)*

permanent discoloration,[7] so dermabrasion may be done after the fifth to seventh day. When glass fragments are visible, tape applied to the face helps pick up glass.

Soft tissue injury from air bags is a newly described event that usually causes minor abrasions of the face, neck, and upper chest.[5] Corneal or scleral injury may also occur but is not a common event. Lacerations of eyebrows and eyelids should be repaired before swelling occurs so borders can be matched. Eyebrows should never be shaved since landmarks are eliminated and the brow is unlikely to grow back. When suturing the brow, hairs are aligned so they slant in a downward and outward direction.

Vermilion-cutaneous and vermilion-mucosal margins are important anatomic landmarks in repair of lip lacerations. Borders must be perfectly aligned to prevent development of step-off deformity of the lip. Tissue loss from the lip requires reconstruction by a plastic surgeon.

Intraoral injuries should be carefully inspected for debris, crushed tissue, and tooth fragments. Injuries should be meticulously cleaned and irrigated. Gaping intraoral lacerations tend to develop ulcerations and become infected, and should be closed. Antibiotics are usually prescribed.

When the tongue is lacerated, the mouth should be carefully inspected for additional lacerations from teeth. Gaping or bleeding lacerations are sutured and antibiotic therapy is indicated. Children are prone to hard and soft palate lacerations, usually from falling with a sharp object in the mouth.

Ear injuries are categorized into three groups: hematomas, lacerations, and avulsions. Hematomas must be properly drained and dressed to prevent a scar deformity that resembles a cauliflower (Figure 30-10). Lacerations may involve skin or skin and cartilage. Wounds require minimal debridement and are usually closed in two layers; however, avulsion injuries of the ear require skin preservation, otherwise grafts from other body sites are required. Antibiotics are prescribed to prevent cartilage infection. Cartilage necrosis can occur if bandages are left unpadded or unchecked for long periods.

Deep cheek lacerations may involve the parotid gland, parotid duct, and branches of the facial nerve, a motor nerve that governs muscles of facial expression. Injury to the temporal branch causes forehead asymmetry, since the patient cannot wrinkle the forehead on the affected side. With injury to the temporal or zygomatic branch, the patient is unable to fully close the eyelids on the affected side. Buccal branch injury prevents the patient from pursing the lips to whistle, and injury to the mandibular branch causes inability to lower or depress the lower lip. At rest, elevation of the lower lip on the affected side occurs. Injury to the facial nerve can be easily missed if the patient is unconscious or has numerous facial dressings. Facial paralysis after blunt facial trauma has a good prognosis for complete recovery if minimal soft tissue damage occurs. Lacerations of the parotid duct or the parotid gland are an infrequent occurrence. Duct cannulation is used to determine patency when injury is suspected.

Nasal Fractures

Nasal fractures are the most common facial fracture because the nose offers the least resistance. The mechanism of injury is usually blunt trauma. Overlooked, nasal injury can lead to permanent deformity and airway obstruction. Clinical findings include swelling, deformity, bleeding, and crepitus (Table 30-6). In children, the nose is more elastic and resistant to fractures; however, dislocations are common. Unrecognized or untreated nasal fractures can lead to abnormal nasal bone growth that affects nasal contour.

Nasal bones are lined with mucoperiosteum, which becomes an open fracture when overlying skin is lacerated.[12] Fractures caused by a frontal blow damage ethmoid and frontal sinuses, lacrimal duct, and orbital margins. If the cribriform plate is affected and the dura torn, cerebrospinal fluid rhinorrhea occurs. The septum should be visualized to rule out septal hematoma, which appears as a bulging, tense bluish mass. Septal hematoma should be emergently drained to prevent airway obstruction and necrosis of septal cartilage, which causes permanent a nasal deformity called saddle deformity.[4]

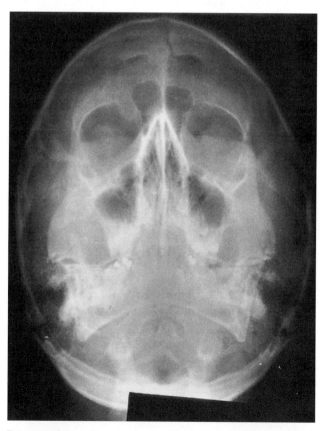

Figure **30-11** Posteroanterior (Water's) radiograph of the paranasal sinuses of a 9-year-old girl. *(From Snell R, Smith M: Clinical anatomy for emergency medicine, St. Louis, 1993, Mosby.)*

Initial interventions focus on bleeding control with direct pressure. Bleeding may be intranasal as well as in the pharynx. Ice compresses applied to the bridge of the nose aid hemostasis and help relieve pain. Anterior or posterior nasal packing may be required to control bleeding. Splinting maintains position, ensures alignment, and prevents further edema and injury. When the fracture involves the nasal mucosa of the lacrimal system, blowing the nose causes intracranial air or subcutaneous emphysema that may later cause localized infection or meningitis.

Maxillary Fractures

Maxillary or midface fractures are the result of significant force and are usually a combination of fractures involving several facial structures. Maxillary fractures are classified as LeFort fractures I, II, and III, that is, lower third, middle third, and orbital complex. Plain radiographs of the face with emphasis on Water's view are used to confirm diagnosis (Figure 30-11) with CT scan used to substantiate the extent of the fractures. Maxillary fractures are rarely seen in children because of the flexibility and pliable nature of their maxillofacial structures.

Patients with maxillary fractures complain of severe facial pain, anesthesia or paresthesia of the upper lip, and some visual disturbances (see Table 30-6). Clinically, the patient has severe facial swelling, ecchymosis, periorbital or orbital swelling, subconjunctival hemorrhage, elongation of the face, epistaxis, malocclusion, and occasionally may exhibit complete airway obstruction.[3] Cerebrospinal fluid may leak from the nose. Figure 30-12 shows technique used to assess for maxillary mobility.

LeFort I, or lower third fracture (Figure 30-13, *A*) is a horizontal fracture in which the body of the maxilla is separated from the base of the skull above the palate but below the zygomatic process attachment. Separation may be unilateral or bilateral. There is a free-floating segment of the upper teeth and lower maxilla; however, the fracture may or may not be displaced. The hard palate and upper teeth are mobile when moved by grasping the alveolar process and anterior teeth.

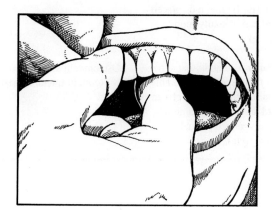

Figure **30-12** Clinical examination for fracture of maxilla.

LeFort II, or middle third fracture (Figure 30-13, *B*), involves the pyramidal area including the central maxilla, nasal area, and ethmoid bones. This portion of the face is a tripod shape with the apex at the nose. Grasping the front teeth and palate causes movement of the nose and upper lip, but no movement of the orbital complex. Significant force is required to fracture this area so the patient should be carefully evaluated for other injuries. The nose, lips, and eyes are usually edematous, with subconjunctival hemorrhage and epistaxis frequently noted. CSF rhinorrhea suggests open skull fracture.

LeFort III, or orbital complex fracture (Figure 30-13, *C*), causes total cranial facial separation. The nose and dental arch move without frontal bone involvement. Massive edema, ecchymosis, epistaxis, and malocclusion are present, and the face has a spoonlike appearance in side profile. Early ocular examination is necessary to prevent unrecognized ocular injuries secondary to extensive swelling. Fractures of the cribriform plate and bleeding from the middle meningeal artery threaten airway patency; cervical spine fracture-dislocation can also occur.[12]

Management of maxillary fractures includes aggressive airway control. Endotracheal intubation may be difficult because of edema and loss of normal anatomic contour, so anticipate cricothyroidotomy or tracheotomy. Excessive secretions and bleeding require frequent suctioning, so allow the patient to use Yankauer suction when appropriate. Position the patient upright and leaning forward (as soon as the cervical spine is cleared) to promote drainage and decrease swelling. Apply ice compresses for pain relief and to decrease swelling, and administer prophylactic antibiotics and tetanus immunization as appropriate.

Zygoma Fractures

Fractures of the zygoma usually occur in two patterns: zygomatic arch fracture and tripod fracture. Fracture of the orbital floor may also be present with zygomatic fractures. Injury is usually caused by blunt trauma to the front and side of the face. With tripod fracture, the zygoma fractures in three places: zygomatic arch, posterior half of the infraorbital rim, and frontozygomatic suture. Step deformity is palpated at the infraorbital rim and frontozygomatic suture area and flattening or asymmetry of the cheek, periorbital edema, circumorbital or subconjunctival ecchymosis, and pain exacerbated by jaw motion are usually present (see Table 30-6).

Entrapment of the inferior rectus muscle causes double vision and asymmetry of ocular levels and anesthesia of the upper lip, cheek, teeth, and gums. The mnemonic TIDES is helpful in determination of zygomatic fractures (Box 30-1). Interventions focus on pain control and decreasing swelling. Plain radiographs with a "jughandle" view demonstrate zygomatic arch fracture (Figure 30-14), whereas CT scans are often needed to demonstrate the extent of a tripod fracture.

Table 30-6	Facial Fractures: Clinical and Radiographic Findings, and Complications for Specific Facial Fractures		
Fracture	Clinical presentation	Radiographic	Complications
Nasoorbital	Symptoms: pain, visual abnormalities Signs: massive periorbital and upper facial edema and ecchymosis, epistaxis, traumatic telecanthus, foreshortening of nose with telescoping; associated intracranial injuries	Views: CT scan Findings: disruption of interorbital space and comminution of nasal pyramid Frontal, zygomatic, orbital, maxillary fractures common	Residual upper midface deformity ("dish face"); telecanthus; frontal sinus-nasolacrimal system pathology with mucocele, mucopyocele, dacryocystitis
Zygoma			
Arch	Symptoms: pain in lateral cheek, inability to close jaw Signs: swelling, crepitus over arch, obvious asymmetry	Views: Water's submentovertex Findings: depression of arch, comminution	Contour irregularities of arch area, flattening of arch
Body "tripod fracture"	Symptoms: pain, trismus, diplopia, numb upper lip, lower lid, bilateral nasal area Signs: swelling, ecchymosis of malar and periorbital areas; palpable infraorbital rim "step-off"; entrapment of extraocular muscles with disconjugate gaze; scleral ecchymosis, displacement of lateral canthal ligament	Views: Water's submentovertex, CT scan Findings: clouding, air/fluid level maxillary sinus, separation of zygomaticomaxillary, zygomaticofrontal, and zygomaticotemporal suture lines	Residual malar deformity, enophthalmos, diplopia, infraorbital nerve anesthesia, chronic maxillary sinusitis
Orbital floor	Symptoms: diplopia, orbital pain Signs: periorbital edema, ecchymosis, enophthalmos, extraocular muscle entrapment, disconjugate gaze; hyphema, subluxation of lens, retinal detachment, rupture of globe with direct eye trauma	Views: Water's, CT scan, tomograms Findings: air/fluid level maxillary sinus, herniated adnexa and/or orbital floor fragments in maxillary sinus	Enophthalmos, diplopia; recurrent orbital cellulitis with implant (alloplastic) extrusion
Mandible			
Condyle	Symptoms: pain at fracture site, referred pain to ear Signs: crepitus, excessive salivation, swelling of condylar region, deviation of jaw toward fracture, cross-bite or open-bite deformity	Views: AP, oblique, Water's, Panorex Findings: nondisplaced, or displaced anteriorly and medially	Ankylosis of TMJ; chronic TMJ
Angle	Symptoms: pain at fracture site, inability to close mouth Signs: swelling at angle of jaw, ecchymosis, crepitus, malocclusion	Views: Panorex, mandibular series Findings: nondisplaced (favorable) or posterior fragment displaced upward and medially (nonfavorable)	Nonunion, malunion, osteomyelitis
Body	Symptoms: pain at fracture site, limitation of movement Signs: swelling, ecchymosis, crepitus, malocclusion	Views: Panorex, mandibular series Findings: nondisplaced (favorable), or posterior fragment displaced upward and medially, anterior fragments rotated lingually (nonfavorable)	Osteomyelitis, infection (tooth in fracture line)

Table 30-6   **Facial Fractures: Clinical and Radiographic Findings, and Complications for Specific Facial Fractures—cont'd**

Fracture	Clinical presentation	Radiographic	Complications
Mandible—cont'd			
Symphysis	Symptoms: pain Signs: malocclusion, frequent association with soft tissue wounds of lower lip, tongue	Views: mandibular series, submentovertex Findings: nondisplaced or lingual rotation of anterior fragments, may be associated with angle or condyle fractures	Residual malocclusion, loss of chin projection, asymmetry; osteomyelitis
Maxilla			
LeFort I (transverse)	Symptoms: pain upper jaw, numb upper teeth Signs: midfacial edema and ecchymosis, epistaxis, malocclusion, mobility of maxillary dentition	Views: Water's, Panorex, CT scan Findings: opaque maxillary sinus, displacement of fragments of alveolus if comminuted; fracture through maxillary sinus and pterygoid plates	Loss of teeth, infection, malocclusion
LeFort II (pyramidal)	Symptoms: pain midface, numb upper lip, lower lid, lateral nasal area Signs: midfacial edema and ecchymosis, epistaxis, malocclusion, mobility of midface, nasal flattening, anesthesia infraorbital nerve territory	Views: Water's, CT scan Findings: opaque maxillary sinuses, separation through frontal process, lacrimal bones, floor of orbits, zygomaticomaxillary suture line, lateral wall of maxillary sinus, and pterygoid plates	Nonunion, malunion lacrimal system obstruction, infraorbital nerve anesthesia, diplopia, malocclusion
LeFort III (craniofacial dysjunction)	Symptoms: pain face, difficulty breathing Signs: "donkey-face" deformity, malocclusion, mobile face, marked facial edema and ecchymosis, epistaxis, CSF rhinorrhea	Views: Water's, CT scan Findings: separation of midthird of face at zygomaticofrontal, zygomaticotemporal, and nasofrontal sutures, and across orbital floors; opaque maxillary sinuses	Nonunion, malunion, malocclusion, lengthening of midface, lacrimal system obstruction

Modified from Trunkey DD, Lewis FR: *Current therapy of trauma*, ed 2, Toronto, 1986, BC Decker.

Orbital Blowout Fractures

Zygoma fractures and orbital blowout fractures can occur independently but are often found in combination. Plain radiographs with Water's view can help distinguish these injuries. Orbital blowout fracture occurs when blunt trauma to the globe causes abrupt rise in orbital pressure. The orbital floor is the weakest part of the bony orbit, so increased pressure causes orbital contents to prolapse into the maxillary sinus.[4] Inferior rectus muscle, inferior oblique muscle, infraorbital nerve, orbital fat, and connective tissue become entrapped in the orbital floor; therefore extraocular movements should be carefully evaluated. The globe may also become entrapped. This fracture often results from sports-related injuries, such as a baseball thrown at the eye, and altercations like fist fights. Golf balls can extend past the protective orbital rim and rupture the globe. If the globe is perforated, manipulation of the eyes or noseblowing can lead to intraorbital air.

Box 30-1   **TIDES Mnemonic for Zygomatic Fractures**

T	Trismus	Tonic contracture of muscles of mastication
I	Infraorbital	Hypoesthesia or anesthesia
D	Diplopia	Double vision
E	Epistaxis	Nosebleed
S	Symmetry absence	Flatness or depression of cheek

Subcutaneous orbital emphysema suggests fracture in the sinus arch. Noseblowing, coughing, sneezing, vomiting, and straining can force air from sinuses through the fracture into the orbital space. Proptosis or bulging of the eye and limitation of extraocular motion may indicate orbital involvement (Figure 30-15). Double vision, pupil

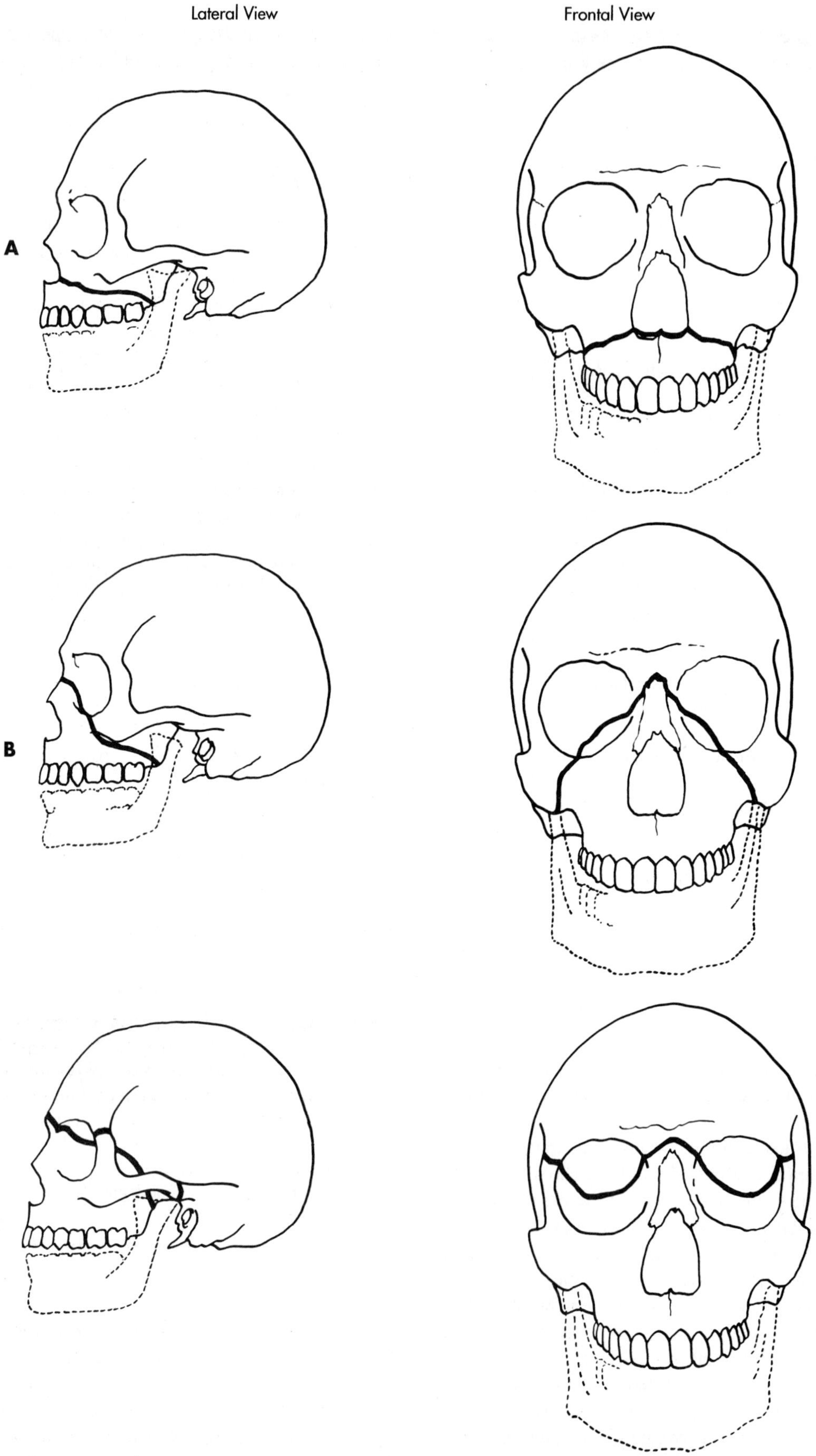
Lateral View
Frontal View
A
B
C

Figure **30-13** **A,** LeFort I facial fracture. **B,** LeFort II facial fracture. **C,** LeFort III facial fracture.

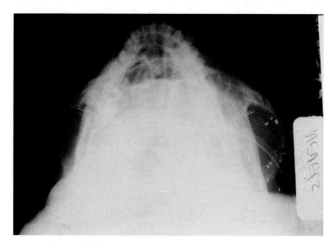

Figure **30-14** Radiograph of zygomatic fracture.

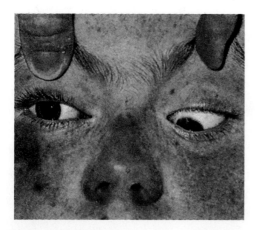

Figure **30-15** Blow-out fracture. *(From Zitelli BJ, Davis HW: Atlas of pediatric physical diagnosis, ed 2, London, 1992, Gower Medical.)*

asymmetry, enophthalmos (sunken appearance), anesthesia of the cheek and upper lip, ptosis or drooping of the lid, and a sunken appearance are clinical manifestations of blowout fracture (see Table 30-6). Globe injury occurs in 10% to 25% of blowout fractures with vision loss noted in 8% of patients.[12] Ophthalmologic consultation is indicated.

Surgical intervention is usually postponed until swelling diminishes. Ice compresses to decrease swelling and relieve pain and elevating the head of the bed are indicated. The patient should be reminded to avoid straining and nose-blowing.[7]

Mandibular Fractures

Mandibular fractures are the second most common facial fracture. Blunt force such as a severe blow to the face during contact sports, altercations, and MVCs, is the usual mechanism of injury. Mandible fractures can be a significant life-threatening injury if loss of bony support displaces the tongue posteriorly and obstructs the airway. Malocclusion is a cardinal symptom for mandible fracture (Figure 30-16). Signs and symptoms vary with fracture site; however, point tenderness and crepitus may be palpated and step-off deformity found. Trismus and decreased range of motion is usually noted. The face may be asymmetric with swelling and ecchymosis. Paresthesias in the lower lip and chin imply injury to the inferior alveolar nerve (see Table 30-6). The oral cavity should be assessed for broken or loose teeth, lacerations, or ecchymosis. Sublingual hematoma can compromise the airway. Inspect ears for tears in the external canal and tympanic membrane.

Mandibular fractures are classified according to the region of the jaw injured. The most common sites for fracture are the angle of the mandible, condyle, and molar and men-

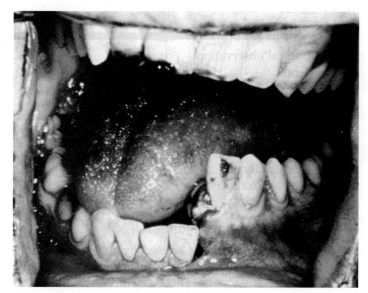

Figure **30-16** Malocclusion caused by fracture. *(From Sheehy SB, Jimmerson CL: Manual of clinical trauma care, ed 2, St. Louis, 1994, Mosby. Courtesy Dr. Daniel Cheney.)*

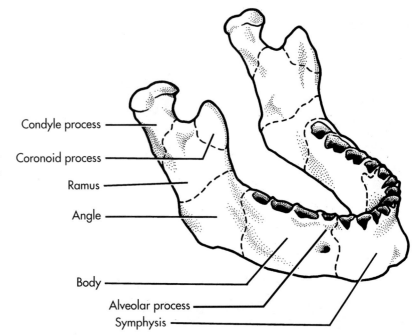

Figure **30-17** Fracture sites of mandible. *(Modified from Rosen P et al:* Emergency medicine, *ed 3, St. Louis, 1992, Mosby.)*

Condyle process

Coronoid process

Ramus

Angle

Body

Alveolar process

Symphysis

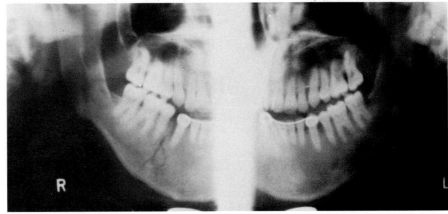

Figure **30-18** Panoramic radiograph of mandible. Note fractures in left angle and right body. (Dental retainer appliance is in place on lower incisors.) *(From Rosen P et al:* Emergency medicine, *ed 3, St. Louis, 1992, Mosby.)*

Box **30-2**

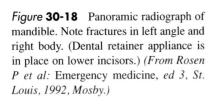

NURSING DIAGNOSES FOR FACIAL INJURIES

Ineffective airway clearance
Pain
Risk for infection
Impaired skin integrity

tal regions, with the symphysis the least common injury site (Figure 30-17). A panoramic radiograph is best for radiographic imaging of the mandible (Figure 30-18). Treatment consists of surgical intervention with open reduction and internal fixation, or wiring jaws, depending on location of the fracture. Nursing care in the ED includes allowing the patient to sit upright as soon as the cervical spine is cleared and applying ice compresses to the face to minimize swelling and relieve pain. Oral saline rinses for the mouth may also be used. Intravenous antibiotics are indicated for open fractures, and repair of lacerations should occur as soon as possible.

SUMMARY

Maxillofacial injuries are a common occurrence in the ED. Special attention should be given to stabilizing the cervical spine, maintaining a patent airway, and controlling hemorrhage. The goal of treatment is life, function, and aesthetics. Box 30-2 identifies priority nursing diagnoses for facial injuries.

REFERENCES

1. Buntain NL: *Management of pediatric trauma,* Philadelphia, 1995, WB Saunders.
2. Colucciello SA: The treacherous and complex spectrum of maxillofacial trauma: etiologies, evaluation, and emergency stabilization, *Emerg Med Rep* 16(7):59, 1995.
3. Crawley WA: Initial assessment and emergency treatment of maxillofacial injuries, *Trauma Q* 9(1):20, 1992.
4. Emergency Nurses Association: *Emergency nursing core curriculum,* ed 4, Philadelphia, 1994, WB Saunders.
5. Huelke DF, Moore JL, Ostrom M: Air bag injuries and occupant protection, *J Trauma* 33(6):894, 1992.
6. Kihtir T, Ivatury RR, Simon RJ et al: Early management of civilian gunshot wounds to the face, *J Trauma* 35(4):569, 1994.
7. Kitt S, Selfridge-Thomas J, Proehl JA et al: *Emergency nursing: a physiologic and clinical perspective,* ed 2, Philadelphia, 1995, WB Saunders.
8. Merriman S, Sargent LA: Anatomy of the face, *Trauma Q* 9(1):9, 1992.
9. Nakhgerany KB, LiBassi M, Esposito B: Facial trauma in motor vehicle accidents: etiological factors, *Am J Emerg Med* 12(2):160, 1994.
10. Pallua N, Schneider W, Berger A: Treatment of traumatic facial tattoos caused by black gunpowder, *Injury* 24(4):227, 1993.
11. Snell RS, Smith MS: *Clinical anatomy for emergency medicine,* St. Louis, 1993, Mosby.
12. Tintinalli et al: *Emergency medicine: a comprehensive study guide,* ed 4, New York, 1996, McGraw-Hill.
13. Wall RM: Rapid sequence intubation in head trauma, *Ann Emerg Med* 22:1008, 1993.

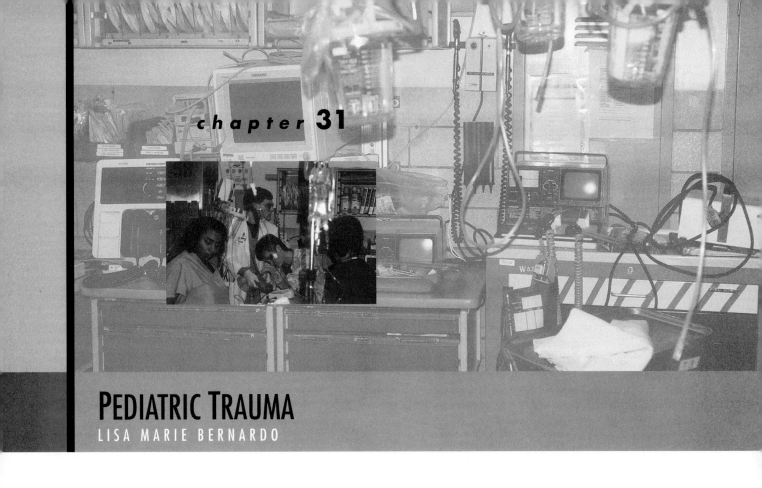

chapter 31

PEDIATRIC TRAUMA
LISA MARIE BERNARDO

Traumatic injury is the leading cause of death in children over 1 year of age. In 1991, 37,529 children and adolescents died in the United States from injuries. Estimated cost exceeded $3 billion.[52] Motor vehicle crashes (MVCs) were the leading cause of death for children and adolescents aged 5 to 19 years, whereas homicide was the leading cause of death for children 0 to 4 years of age and young adults 20 to 24 years of age.[52]

Each year approximately 16 million children are treated in emergency departments (EDs) for traumatic injuries, with an estimated 30,000 permanently disabled.[15] Injury-related morbidity and mortality are greater in minority and poor populations.[15] Direct, estimated costs associated with pediatric trauma in the United States range from $5.1 billion[36] to $7.5 billion.[15]

Frequency and severity of childhood injuries compel the emergency nurse to recognize potentially life-threatening pediatric trauma to reduce trauma-related morbidity and mortality. This chapter highlights anatomic and physiologic differences in pediatric patients, describes patient assessment, essential interventions, and discusses treatment of selected traumatic injuries.

HISTORICAL PERSPECTIVE

Dr. William E. Ladd is considered the pioneer of pediatric surgery.[17] In 1917, he was a medical volunteer who treated thousands of people injured in the collision of two ships in Halifax, Nova Scotia. The burned and injured children had a profound effect on him. He returned to Boston and devoted himself exclusively to the surgical care of children.[17] Dr. Ladd is credited with being the first pediatric surgeon and the originator of pediatric surgery as a specialty.

During the World Wars, surgeons exposed to new techniques in trauma care were not at first interested in the care of pediatric trauma patients. However, pediatric trauma care could not have advanced without their efforts.[63] In the 1960s, pediatric trauma gained recognition as the number of children injured and killed from "accidents" increased. During the late 1980s and early 1990s, pediatric trauma care gathered even more interest. The American Pediatric Surgical Association's Trauma Committee developed guidelines for care of injured children and Emergency Medical Services for Children (EMS-C) grants were implemented. Community groups such as the National Safe Kids Campaign became popular, promoting pediatric injury prevention to the public. Interest in pediatric trauma care—from the prehospital arena through rehabilitation into the prevention phase—continued to grow through ongoing clinical, education, and research endeavors.

EPIDEMIOLOGY

Motor vehicle crashes (MVCs) are the leading cause of death among children aged 5 years through 19 years.[52] Fatalities are evenly distributed among both genders through age 14 years, after which time young men are two to three times more likely to die from MVCs.[52] Unfortunately, alcohol has been involved in almost half of all adolescent fatalities from MVCs.[23] Among 295 injured patients aged 10 to 21 years treated at four EDs, 14 of 125 patients age 17 to 21 years tested positive for alcohol.[39]

An estimated 35% of young children are not restrained in motor vehicles.[44] Among a probability sample of police-reported MVCs for a 1-year period involving children aged 0 through 14 years, optimal restraint usage was found in only 40% of the sample.[31] Car seats were used for 76% of the infants, and only 41% of toddlers.[31] Adolescents aged 10 through 14 years have the highest percentage of unuse of restraints (43%).[31] As unrestrained passengers, young children are thrown about the vehicle, suffering injuries to the head, chest, abdomen, and extremities. They can be pinned beneath the dashboard, impaled on the gearshift, and bounced against doors, seats, and other passengers. Children held on the lap of an adult can be crushed between the adult and point of impact, for example, the dashboard, steering column, or front seat. Unrestrained children have a greater chance of ejection through the windshield, side windows, or rear windows. Head injuries are the leading cause of death among unrestrained children, followed by chest injuries secondary to ejection.[64]

Children riding in the back of pickup trucks can sustain serious injury or death; adolescents aged 10 through 19 years represent more than half the deaths, with males predominating.[10] Most noncollision deaths related to pickup trucks are due to falls during sudden acceleration, deceleration, or swerving; however, ejection causes greater injury severity.[10] Children riding in the back of cars with an open hatchback can be thrown into oncoming traffic, stationary objects such as trees, moving objects, or the road.

Children aged 4 to 9 years restrained with a lap belt and shoulder harness are susceptible to certain injuries. Young children have a shorter sitting height than adults, with a higher center of gravity above the lap belt. Greater proportion of body mass is located above the safety belt, which may cause more forward motion and increase risk for head and neck injury. Children can jackknife over restraints, causing an airway or hanging injury. Similarly, a child can "submarine" under the restraint system, leading to neck and airway injuries. The lap belt itself can also cause injuries. During sudden deceleration, children are thrown forward with full body weight going into the lap belt. Resulting injuries include lumbar spine fractures, small bowel injuries, and abdominal bruising.

Infants and children up to 4 years or 40 lb must be restrained in an infant or child safety seat. Infants less than 26 inches long and less than 20 lb who are unable to sit upright must be secured in the child safety seat at a semireclined angle in a rear-facing position.[58] Children over 20 lb must be restrained in a toddler/convertible seat in a forward-facing position.[58] Injuries occur to toddlers restrained in car safety seats if harnesses are not connected, car seats used are not designed for vehicular use, or the car seat itself is not fas-

tened in the vehicle.[20] Injuries include head injuries, brain hemorrhages, and femoral fractures.[20] High cervical spine injuries have been reported in very young children in forward-facing child safety seats, probably because of the higher fulcrum of cervical spine (C2) movement,[64] which causes hyperflexion and hyperextension during rapid deceleration.

Although air bags have prevented many deaths, they have also contributed to the deaths of eight infants and young children during MVCs.[4] During rapid deceleration prior to impact, the unrestrained front seat child passenger is propelled against the dashboard where the airbag will deploy. Airbag deployment propels the child against the vehicle's inner structures, causing injury or death.[4] Infants riding in rear-facing child safety seats should never ride in the front seat of a car or truck with a passenger-side air bag. Children should ride in the rear seat secured in a child safety seat. If the vehicle does not have a rear seat, children should be positioned as far from the air bag as possible.[4]

Children and adolescents sustain injuries as passengers or operators of all-terrain vehicles (ATVs), snowmobiles, farm equipment, and riding lawnmowers. Young children riding as passengers can be crushed by the adult driver on impact with a stationary or moving object. Older children not the appropriate size or weight to operate such vehicles can flip the vehicles onto themselves and sustain serious multisystem injuries.

Homicide is the leading cause of death among children aged 0 through 4 years and young adults aged 20 through 24 years.[52] Homicide rates are nearly five times higher among African-American youth when compared to white youth.[29] For children up to 4 years of age, homicide is due to physical violence, 10% due to firearms. Among adolescents 15 through 19 years of age, firearm homicides increase to almost 70% of the total.[29]

Suicide rates have more than doubled over recent years for adolescents aged 10 through 19 years, with suicide rates higher for males and whites when compared to females and nonwhites.[27] Unsuccessful suicide attempts are estimated as eight times more common than successful attempts.[29]

Estimates suggest half of all American homes contain firearms, translating to 200 million firearms, with 60 million handguns.[11] Societal factors such as use of firearms in the media foster gun play among the pediatric and adolescent population. Impulsive behavior, poor judgment, and active imaginations[11] contribute to the lure of firearms for these individuals. In one pediatric trauma center, penetrating trauma increased over a 7-year period from 20% to 35% with an increase from 45% to 66% in the 12- to 15-year age group.[24]

Among 5233 families who attended 29 pediatric practices in seven different states, gun ownership was reported by 37%, with rifles (26%), handguns (17%), and powder firearms (32%) the most prevalent.[60] Of 823 handguns and 1327 rifles possessed by these families, 13% and 1%, respectively, were kept unlocked and loaded.[60] Handgun ownership is associated with a rural domicile, living in a single-family dwelling, adult males living in the home, less than two preschool children in the family, and at least 12 years of maternal education.[60] Rifle ownership was associated with a rural domicile, living in a single-family dwelling, adult males living in the home, a white mother, and no preschool children at home.[60]

A 4-year review of Connecticut death certificates and hospital discharge data for firearm-related injuries among individuals from birth through 19 years reported 219 firearm-related deaths.[74] Sixty-eight percent were homicides, 25% suicides, and 6% unintentional; 91% of the deaths occurred in males. Adolescents aged 15 through 19 years accounted for the most homicides (81%) and suicides (93%), with the majority (78%) of homicides in urban areas. Similarly, there were 533 hospitalizations for gunshot wounds, 41% assaults, 39% unintentional, and 1% suicide. Males (93%) were most likely to be hospitalized, with 15- to 19-year-olds accounting for 87% of the assaults in these predominantly urban (76%) youth.

Penetrating injuries from firearms are devastating and occur in all body regions. Entrance and exit wounds may be present. Damage to internal structures is related to the number of bullets that enter the body, type of bullets, type of firearm, and distance from which the firearm was fired. Firearms may be traditional urban weapons, military weapons, or recreational pellet guns. Box 31-1 highlights ways to avoid firearm injuries.

Penetrating injuries from pellet guns can be innocuous; however, in two case studies, serious morbidity and mortality were reported from thoracic penetration by pellets.[16] Such pellet injuries should create a high index of suspicion because modern pellet missiles can reach velocities near those of low-powered rifles. Their characteristics resemble those of a .22-caliber bullet.[16]

Penetrating injuries are also caused by knives and other sharp objects. Young children running with toys or objects in their mouths are susceptible to oropharyngeal and upper airway penetration. A penetrating object causes entrance and exit wounds and can be impaled in the body.

Falls, a common occurrence in the pediatric population, are the most common cause of trauma-related hospitalization and head injury.[3] The highest incidence of falls occurs in the young and the elderly. Boys fall more often than girls.[2] Young children are most frequently injured in falls in the home. Poor home upkeep, windows that do not lock, and windows without screens are contributing factors. Children fall from varying heights. They also fall while running, playing, and participating in sports. Injuries sustained from falls vary from mild to severe single-system or multisystem trauma.

Walker-related injuries were studied in one prospective 3-year study conducted in a Virginia pediatric ED. Sixty-five infants less than 1 year of age accounted for 95% of the injuries.[7] Stairway falls occurred in 46 (71%) infants, tip-overs in 14 (21%), and burns in 3 (5%). The head and neck area accounted for 97% of the injuries. Nineteen (29%) of infants sustained serious injuries, that is, skull fractures, intracranial hemorrhage, full-thickness burns, cervical spine fractures, and death.[7]

In a study of 70 children falling 10 feet or more, the majority were boys. Most falls occurred at home during the summer months, usually from an open window.[41] Injuries most frequently involved the head and skeletal system. Among 69 children less than 5 years of age presenting to a pediatric ED for stairway-related falls, median age was 2 years. Isolated head and neck injuries accounted for 90% of identified injuries.[8] Fifteen (22%) children sustained serious injuries, including concussion, skull fracture, cerebral contusion, subdural hematoma, and a C2 fracture.[8] Three infants carried by an adult sustained significant head injuries.

In a 2-year study at a university trauma center, 61 children were injured in falls, with 1 fatality. Children less than 4 years of age accounted for 54% of falls, involving more boys than girls.[40] For children less than 13 years of age, falls from a window were the most common mechanism of injury, followed by jumping from a bed or other low height during rough play and falls down the stairs. Remaining falls were from heights greater than 10 feet, for example, trees or buildings.[40]

Pedestrian injuries are the second leading cause of death in children aged 5 through 9 years, and the fourth leading cause of death in children aged 10 through 14 years.[52] As pedestrians, children are struck by moving vehicles while playing, walking, running, crossing the street, or entering or exiting a school bus. Most injuries occur in the afternoon and early evening hours on urban streets. Lower socioeconomic status has also been implicated in pedestrian MVCs.

Among 345 pedestrians aged 0 through 14 years treated in a multihospital system over a 2-year period, 53% of injuries occurred midblock (median age = 6 years), 28% at intersections (median age = 10 years), 11% in driveways (median age = 2 years), and 8% in parking lots (median age = 4 years).[1] A New Zealand case control study of 53 children hospitalized or killed in driveway-related pedestrian injuries over a 2-year period was undertaken. Risk factors for driveway-related pedestrian injuries are absence of physical separation of the driveway from the children's play area and

---

Box 31-1	**Ways to Avoid Firearm Injuries**

Remove guns from the home or keep guns locked and unloaded
Store ammunition separate from guns
Limit toy gun play and video games that promote shooting
Observe children for early indicators of aggressiveness
Advocate for appropriate legislation to restrict gun availability

From Webster D, Wilson M: Gun violence among youth and the pediatrician's role in primary prevention, *Pediatrics* 94:617, 1994.

homes with shared driveways.[55] Children sustain a triad of injuries known as *Waddell's triad* when struck by a vehicle. Injuries include thoracic abdominal injuries from striking the bumper; extremity injury from hitting the car and ground; and head injury from landing on the ground.[25] If the child's shoes are knocked from the body, the vehicle's speed is estimated at 40 mph.[64]

Bicycle-related accidents result in fatal and nonfatal injuries. Head injuries are the most frequent and most fatal injuries associated with bicycle-related crashes. Among 2333 children aged 0 through 14 years reported to the National Pediatric Trauma Registry over a 3-year period because of bicycle-related injuries, 54% sustained head injuries.[33] Factors associated with head injury after adjusting for age, gender, and motor vehicle involvement were preexisting mental disorders, lack of helmet use, and riding on roads.[33] Head injuries were also associated with intensive care unit stays, complications, fatalities, and impairments at discharge. Other injuries associated with bicycle crashes are long bone fractures, abdominal injuries, thoracic injuries, and facial injuries. Helmet use significantly reduces morbidity and mortality associated with bicycle-related head injuries.

Children can sustain injuries from skateboards. Younger children use skateboards near their homes. Children have a high center of gravity, which limits their ability to break a fall.[12] The American Academy of Pediatrics recommends that children less than 5 years of age not use skateboards because they do not have a well-developed neuromuscular system, have poor judgment, and cannot protect themselves from injury. Skateboards should not be ridden in traffic. Proper protective wear, including helmets, elbow pads, and knee pads, should be worn.

ANATOMY AND PHYSIOLOGY

Children differ from adults developmentally, anatomically, and physiologically. Recognizing differences and implementing appropriate interventions to support these differences can result in increased survivability of the pediatric trauma patient.

Respiratory System

Crucial anatomic and physiologic differences exist between the adult and pediatric airway. The child's oropharynx is relatively small, so the airway is easily obstructed by the large tongue. The U-shaped epiglottis protrudes into the pharynx, and the tonsils and adenoids are often enlarged. Vocal cords are short and concave, with the larynx relatively cephaloid and easily collapsible if the head is hyperflexed or extended. In a child less than 10 years of age, the narrowest portion of the airway is the cricoid cartilage.[6] Lower airways are smaller and supporting cartilage is less developed in infants and small children, so airways are easily obstructed by mucus and edema.[6]

Ribs are pliable and do not provide adequate support for the lungs; therefore blunt trauma to the chest causes pul-

monary contusions rather than rib fractures. If rib fractures are present, a high index of suspicion for severe internal trauma should be raised. The mediastinum is more mobile, causing greater susceptibility to great-vessel damage. Retractions are more likely when the child is in respiratory distress. Retractions can be suprasternal, supraclavicular, infraclavicular, intercostal, or substernal. Breathing is primarily diaphragmatic or abdominal in children less than 7 or 8 years of age. Crying children are more prone to swallowing air, which causes gastric distention and hampers respiratory excursion. A thin chest wall transmits breath sounds easily, so accurate respiratory assessment may be difficult. Respiratory rates are higher in children because of higher metabolic rates. Oxygen consumption in infants is 6 to 8 ml/kg/min compared to 3 to 4 ml/kg/min in adults, so hyperemia can occur rapidly.[6]

Cardiovascular System

The child's estimated blood volume is 80 ml/kg, regardless of age or size.[42] Although this absolute blood volume is small, it is larger than an adult's on a ml/kg basis. Seemingly small amounts of blood loss can impair perfusion and decrease circulating blood volume. Because of their large cardiac reserve and catecholamine response, children can maintain a high to normal blood pressure even with significant blood loss. Hypotension is not observed until the child has lost 20% to 25% of his or her circulating blood volume.[42] Falling blood pressure is a *late* sign of hypovolemia in children and signals imminent cardiac arrest. The best assessment for cardiac perfusion is capillary refill—normal is less than 2 seconds. Other assessment factors are presence of bradycardia or tachycardia, and decreased urinary output.

Children have a higher metabolic rate and oxygen requirements that require higher cardiac output per kilogram.[61] Tachycardia is the first response to decreased oxygenation. When tachycardia fails to increase oxygen delivery, tissue hypoxia and hypercapnia occur, followed by bradycardia.[68] Bradycardia is a *late* sign of cardiac decompensation.

Children can have a variety of congenital heart defects that may impair circulatory status (tetralogy of Fallot, truncus arteriosus, and large ventricular septal defects). If a child has had a Blalock-Taussig shunt, blood pressure readings are unattainable in the arm from which the subclavian artery was used (that arm is perfused by collateral circulation). Children may also have functional or nonfunctional heart murmurs. Finally, dextrocardia (heart on the right side) or situs inversus (transposition of all thoracic and abdominal organs) may be present.

Neurologic System

An infant's head is larger in proportion to the rest of the body than an adult's. The skull is more malleable, providing less protection to the brain. The posterior fontanelle closes at 4 months of age, anterior fontanelle at approximately 9 to

18 months.[61] Although open fontanelles allow for release of increased intracranial pressure (ICP), they may allow direct injury to the brain or may cause extensive bleeding. Infants bleed significantly from a scalp laceration because of the large surface area and increased vascularity. Finally, a young child has a higher center of gravity, which, together with the larger head, makes the child prone to head injuries.

Cerebral tissues are thin, soft, and flexible compared with those of adults. This difference makes brain tissues more easily damaged, especially from shearing injuries. Sulci are still deepening during childhood, and myelinization is still occurring.

Several features make the juvenile cervical spine vulnerable to injury. Vertebrae themselves are not likely to fracture; however, the cord is at greater risk.

- A heavy head on a small body makes the child susceptible to flexion-extension injury.
- Spinal mobility is greater because of lax spinal ligaments.
- Cervical musculature is undeveloped.
- Horizontal facet joints in cervical vertebrae (C1-3) can result in subluxation from minimal force.
- Immature vertebral joints at C2-4 may not withstand flexion-rotation forces.
- Higher fulcrum of cervical movement at C2-3 is more susceptible to cervical spine injuries.

Gastrointestinal and Genitourinary Systems

Younger children have protuberant abdomens because of underdeveloped abdominal musculature, which leaves abdominal organs vulnerable to blunt trauma. A younger child's small size means the abdominal organs are in close proximity to each other, so multiple organ injury can occur.[66] A pliable rib cage does not afford adequate protection to abdominal organs and can predispose children to further internal injuries. Though partially protected by the rib cage, the liver is still vulnerable to injury because of its large size and fragility.

Renal injuries occur because the relatively large kidneys are not protected because there is less perinephric fat; abdominal muscles are weak; and the rib cage is elastic.[46] Rapid deceleration can lead to kidney injury since the kidney is relatively mobile within the retroperitoneum.[46]

There is a 10% incidence of preexisting kidney abnormalities in children with genitourinary trauma.[38] Congenital abnormalities such as hydronephrosis, horseshoe kidneys, and ectopic kidneys make the child more susceptible to renal trauma.[38,46] Many congenital anomalies are not diagnosed until abdominal trauma has occurred. Greater spinal elasticity makes ureteral tearing injury possible, but rare. Ureteral injuries are suspected with penetrating trauma to the abdomen or flank area. A full bladder becomes an abdominal organ, and is less protected. In girls, the bladder neck is also less protected. Tissues of a prepubescent girl are more rigid because of lack of estrogen; they do not become more pliable until adolescence, when estrogen is released. Serious internal injuries may result from what appears to be mild external trauma.[38]

Musculoskeletal System

Periosteum in a growing child is stronger, thicker, and more osteogenic than in an adult,[45] so bones bend instead of break. Consequently greenstick or incomplete fractures are common in children. Bone osteogenicity allows rapid callus formation, permitting bones to heal quickly. Even though bone is strong, fractures occur more frequently than muscle sprains or ligament tears, because these structures are stronger than the bones themselves.

Another unique feature of the pediatric musculoskeletal system is presence of an epiphyseal or growth plate. This area of bone is responsible for new longitudinal bone growth, and is found between the epiphysis and metaphysis. The growth plate is cartilaginous and does not ossify until puberty; therefore a growth plate fracture can be present without radiographic evidence.[70]

Integumentary System

Children have a larger ratio of body surface area to weight, which makes them prone to convective and conductive heat loss. Infants less than 6 months of age do not have fine-motor coordination to shiver and are unable to keep themselves warm. Nonshivering thermogenesis occurs where brown fat is broken down to produce warmth. Oxygen consumption increases and decompensation occurs.[61] Children have less subcutaneous fat for insulation and can lose heat through radiation, convection, conduction, and evaporation. Therefore external heat sources must be readily available to help injured children maintain thermoregulation.

PATIENT ASSESSMENT

EDs should be equipped with the personnel and supplies necessary to treat the injured child effectively and efficiently. Equipment should be readily available and should be prepared before arrival. Table 31-1 provides a quick reference for emergency equipment for the pediatric patient.

Initial assessment and stabilization of the pediatric trauma patient requires knowledge of developmental and physiologic differences among infants, children, and adolescents. Injured children are frightened—strange, painful things are happening. The patient may feel he or she is being punished for a real or imagined wrongdoing. Talking with the child in language he or she understands is essential for relieving anxiety and developing trust.

Initial assessment consists of the primary and secondary assessment. During primary assessment, airway-cervical spine, breathing, circulation, and disability (neurologic status) are assessed. Life-threatening injuries are identified and treated. Table 31-2 describes the primary survey in preferred order. During secondary assessment, all other body systems are assessed and other injuries are treated. Table 31-3 details

Table 31-1   Quick Reference to Pediatric Emergency Equipment[a]

Equipment	Premature	Neonate	6 mos	1 Y	2 Y	3 Y	4 Y	5 Y	6 Y	7 Y	8 Y	9 Y	10 Y	11-18Y
Airway														
Oral airway[b] (size)	Infant	Infant/small	Small	Small	Small	Small	Med	Med	Med	Med	Med/Lg	Med/Lg	Med/Lg	Large
Endotracheal tube[c] (mm)	2.5-3.0	3.0-3.5	3.5-4.0	4.0-4.5	4.0-4.5	4.0-4.5	5.0-5.5	5.0-5.5	5.5-6.0	5.5-6.0	6.0	6.0	6.0	7.0 C
C = cuffed											6.5 C	6.5 C	6.5 C	8.0 C
Laryngoscope blade[b] s = straight c = curved	0 s	1 s	1 s	1 s	1 s	1 s	2 s/c	2 s/c	2 s/c	2 s/c	2-3 s/c	2-3 s/c	2-3 s/c	3 s/c
Suction catheter[c] (French)	5	6	6	8	8	8	10	10	10	10	10	10	10	12
Breathing														
Face mask[b] (size)	Premie NB	NB	NB	Ped	Ped	Ped	Ped	Ped	Ped	Ped	Ad	Ad	Ad	Ad
Bag-valve device[b] (size)	Inf	Inf	Inf	Ped	Ped	Ped	Ped	Ped	Ped	Ped/Ad	Ad	Ad	Ad	Ad
Chest tube[b] (French)	10-14	12-18	14-20	14-24	14-24	14-24	20-32	20-32	20-32	20-32	28-38	28-38	28-38	28-38
Circulation														
Over-the-needle catheter[d] (gauge)	22-24	22-24	22-24	20-22	20-22	20-22	20-22	18-22	18-20	18-20	16-20	16-20	16-20	14-18
Intraosseous device (gauge)	18	15	15	15	15	15	15	15	—	—	—	—	—	—
Gastrointestinal/ Genitourinary														
Nasogastric tube[e] (French)	5 feeding tube	5 feeding tube	8	8	10	10	10	10	10	12	12	12	12	14-16
Urinary catheter[b] (French)	5 feeding tube	5-8 feeding tube	8	10	10	10	10-12	10-12	10-12	10-12	12	12	12	12-18

From Bernardo L, Bove M: *Pediatric emergency nursing procedures,* Boston, 1993, Jones & Bartlett.

[a]This reference demonstrates suggested sizes only. Always consider each child's size and health condition when selecting appropriate equipment for procedures.

[b]Committee on Trauma: *Advanced trauma life support student manual,* Chicago, 1989, American College of Surgeons.

[c]Motoyama E: Endotracheal intubation. In Motoyama E, Davis P, editors: *Smith's anesthesia for infants and children,* St. Louis, 1990, Mosby.

[d]Chameides L, editor: *Textbook of pediatric advanced life support,* Dallas, 1988, American Heart Association, Academy of Pediatrics.

[e]Skale N: *Manual of pediatric nursing procedures,* Philadelphia, 1992, JB Lippincott.

Table 31-2 Primary Survey of the Pediatric Trauma Patient

Component	Actions
Airway	Assess for patency; look for loose teeth, vomitus, or other obstruction; note position of head.
	Suspect cervical spine injury with multiple trauma; maintain neutral alignment during assessment; evaluate effectiveness of cervical collar, cervical immobilization device (CID), or other equipment used to immobilize the spine.
	Open cervical collar to evaluate neck for jugular vein distention and tracheal deviation.
Breathing	Auscultate breath sounds in the axillae for presence and equality.
	Assess chest for contusions, penetrating wounds, abrasions, or paradoxic movement.
Circulation	Assess apical pulse for rate, rhythm, and quality; compare apical and peripheral pulses for quality and equality.
	Evaluate capillary refill; normal is less than 2 seconds.
	Check skin color and temperature.
	Note open wounds or uncontrolled bleeding.
Disability	Assess level of consciousness; check for orientation to person, place, and time in the older child.
	In a younger child, assess alertness, ability to interact with environment, and ability to follow commands. Is the child easily consoled and interested in the environment? Does the child recognize a familiar object and respond when you speak to him or her?
	Check pupils for size, reactivity, and equality.
Expose	Remove clothing to allow visual inspection of entire body.

Table 31-3 Secondary Survey of the Pediatric Trauma Patient

Component	Actions
Head, eye, ear, nose	Assess scalp for lacerations or open wounds; palpate for stepoff defects, depressions, hematomas, and pain.
	Reassess pupils for size, reactivity, equality, and extraocular movements; ask the child if he or she can see.
	Assess ears and nose for rhinorrhea or otorrhea.
	Observe for raccoon eyes (bruising around the eyes) or Battle's sign (bruising over the mastoid process).
	Palpate forehead, orbits, maxilla, and mandible for crepitus, deformities, stepoff defect, pain, and stability; evaluate malocclusion by asking child to open and close mouth; note open wounds.
	Inspect for loose, broken, or chipped teeth as well as oral lacerations.
	Check orthodontic appliances for stability.
	Evaluate facial symmetry by asking child to smile, grimace, and open and close mouth.
	Do not remove impaled objects or foreign objects.
Neck	Open cervical collar and reassess anterior neck for jugular vein distention and tracheal deviation; note bruising, edema, open wounds, pain, and crepitus.
	Check for hoarseness or changes in voice by asking child to speak.
Chest	Obtain respiratory rate; reassess breath sounds in anterior lobes for equality.
	Palpate chest wall and sternum for pain, tenderness, and crepitus.
	Observe inspiration and expiration for symmetry or paradoxic movement; note use of accessory muscles.
	Reassess apical heart rate for rate, rhythm, and clarity.
Abdomen/pelvis/ genitourinary	Observe abdomen for bruising and distention; auscultate bowel sounds briefly in all four quadrants; palpate abdomen gently for tenderness; assess pelvis for tenderness and stability.
	Palpate bladder for distention and tenderness; check urinary meatus for signs of injury or bleeding; note priapism and genital trauma such as lacerations or foreign body.
	Have rectal sphincter tone assessed, usually by physician.
Musculoskeletal	Assess extremities for deformities, swelling, lacerations, or other injuries.
	Palpate distal pulses for equality, rate, and rhythm; compare to central pulses.
	Ask child to wiggle toes and fingers; evaluate strength through hand grips and foot flexion/extension.
Back	Logroll as a unit to inspect back; maintain spinal alignment during examination; observe for bruising and open wounds; palpate each vertebral body for tenderness, pain, deformity, and stability; assess flank area for bruising and tenderness.

the secondary survey. Throughout the initial assessment and stabilization process, airway, breathing, and circulation are continually reassessed.

History

History allows the trauma team to prepare for the patient and anticipate interventions that may be required. However, this information is not always available since the injury may not have been witnessed. The awake, nonverbal child also cannot relate the circumstances surrounding the injury. Such situations require special attention, as child neglect or abuse may be involved (see Chapter 51). Information related to mechanism of injury is found in Table 31-4. In all injuries it is important to ascertain if loss of consciousness occurred.

The AMPLE mnemonic (Box 31-2) is helpful for organizing and obtaining an adequate patient history. This information may be obtained from the parent, family member, or awake older child or adolescent. In addition to this information, it is important to determine the need for vision or hearing aids, such as eyeglasses, contact lenses, or hearing aids. These may or may not be with the child on arrival.

Initial Stabilization

Airway/cervical spine. The tongue is the most common cause of airway obstruction in the child. First, relieve airway obstruction by opening the airway, using the jaw-thrust technique to prevent hyperextension of the cervical spine. Suction the oropharynx with a tonsil suction device if vomitus, blood, or loose teeth are present.

Place an oropharyngeal airway to help maintain airway patency in the child with altered level of consciousness who does not have an intact gag reflex. Oropharyngeal airways are measured from the corner of the mouth to the tragus of the ear. An oropharyngeal airway that is too small or too large will obstruct the airway. Use a tongue depressor to insert the airway directly. Do not rotate 90 degrees as in the adult patient because oropharyngeal tissues can be damaged and the tongue inadvertently pushed posteriorly, causing an obstruction. A nasopharyngeal airway may be used for airway patency if there is no evidence of head trauma. This airway is measured from the naris to the tragus of the ear.

In a child who requires continuous airway maintenance, rapid-sequence endotracheal intubation is necessary. This procedure must be undertaken by a health care professional skilled in pediatric intubation. Rapid-sequence intubation involves administration of medications to produce unconsciousness, analgesia, paralysis, and intracranial pressure control during the intubation attempt.[43] The orotracheal route is preferred because the nasotracheal route can be difficult or contraindicated in severe facial trauma or basilar skull fracture.

Prior to the intubation attempt, cardiac and pulse oximetry monitoring devices are placed on the child. Desired medications are administered and the child's lungs ventilated with 100% oxygen. Table 31-5 lists drugs used for rapid-sequence induction. Once the trachea is intubated, auscultate breath sounds over the trachea, bilateral anterior aspect of the chest, and epigastrium. Listen high in the axilla because breath sounds are easily transmittable across the thin chest wall. Correct endotracheal tube placement is determined through auscultation of equal, bilateral breath sounds in all fields, observation of condensation in the endotracheal tube, and assessment of end tidal CO_2 measurements. Final confirmation is by chest radiograph.

Right mainstem bronchus intubations are a common complication with pediatric intubation, therefore bilateral chest wall movement should be observed during ventilation with a

Box **31-2**	**AMPLE Mnemonic**
A	Allergies
M	Medications
P	Past health history
L	Last meal eaten
E	Events leading to the injury

Table **31-4** History Based on Mechanism of Injury

Mechanism of injury	History
Pedestrian MVC	Speed of vehicle; distance child thrown; run over or struck by vehicle; where child was struck (right or left side)
Passenger MVC	Restrained or unrestrained; position in vehicle; ejection from vehicle; extrication time; scene fatalities; site of impact (rear, head on); crash scene (stationary or moving vehicle); vehicle speed at impact
Bicycle crash	Speed of bicycle; helmet use; crash into stationary object or moving vehicle
Fall	Height of fall; landing surface; body area striking ground first
Gunshot wound (GSW)	Bullet caliber; number of shots fired; type of firearm; range; suicide or homicide, i.e., presence of a suicide note or death threats; entrance and/or exit wounds
Stab wound (SW)	Penetrating object, i.e., knife; entrance and/or exit wounds; object still in place

Table 31-5	Medications for Rapid-Sequence Intubation		
Medication	**Dose range**	**Indications**	**Comments**
Atropine	0.1 mg/kg minimum 0.5 mg/kg maximum	Prevent bradycardia	Elect not to use if child is tachycardic
Lidocaine	1 mg/kg	Decrease intracranial pressure; decrease vagal stimulation	
Sedation			
Fentanyl	2 μg/kg	Sedation	May cause hypotension
Midazolam (Versed)	0.035 mg/kg 0.2 mg/kg maximum	Sedation	May cause hypotension; give over 2 minutes
Thiopental (Pentothal)	3-5 mg/kg	Decrease intracranial pressure	May cause respiratory depression and hypotension
Paralysis			
Vecuronium	0.1 mg/kg to 0.2 mg/kg	Paralyzation	Causes apnea; must be able to manually ventilate patient's lungs; administer *after* sedation

Modified from Holleran RS: *Prehospital nursing: a collaborative approach,* St. Louis, 1994, Mosby.

bag-valve-mask device set at 100% oxygen. Movement is best assessed by standing at the foot of the bed watching the child's chest rise and fall during ventilation. After endotracheal tube placement is confirmed by auscultation, a chest radiograph must be obtained. In the meantime, the tube must be securely taped with benzoin and adhesive tape. The tube should not press on the corner of the mouth, or nares with nasotracheal intubation, due to the potential for tissue breakdown. Frequent suctioning may be necessary if aspiration is suspected or injury to the airway or lung tissue occurred.

Children are diaphragmatic breathers so compression on the diaphragm impedes lung expansion. A gastric tube is inserted to relieve gastric distension. The tube is inserted nasally if there are not signs of a basilar skull fracture. Once the tube is inserted it is taped to the child's face and connected to low intermittent suction.

Cricothyrotomy and tracheostomy are reserved for severe cases of airway instability from facial, head, and neck trauma. Fortunately, they are rarely required in children.

Spinal precautions are initiated in the multiply-injured child, including application of a rigid collar, cervical immobilization device (CID), and an immobilization board. A modified backboard with a recessed area for the child's large occiput is strongly recommended; however, such backboards may be difficult to find.[67] Care must be taken to prevent cervical spine flexion from the cervical collar or backboard. Movement can worsen a spinal cord injury and compromise the airway. Immobilization devices remain intact until radiographic and clinical evidence demonstrate spinal cord injury is not present.

When a cervical collar is applied, the appropriate size must be used. A collar that is too large pushes the jaw backward and causes an airway obstruction, and the child can move the head from side to side, which prevents cervical spine control. A collar that is too small does not provide appropriate alignment and may cause airway compromise because it is too tight around the neck. A cervical collar fits properly if the chin rests securely in the chin holder, the collar is beneath the ears, and not covering the upper part of the sternum.

Infants and young children may arrive in the ED secured in their car safety seat. Such children can be immobilized in the car seat if they have a patent airway, effective respirations, and adequate circulation; they were in the car safety seat at the time of the injury; the car seat is intact; and child immobilization equipment is not available.[72] To immobilize the child in the car safety seat, place towel or washcloth rolls on either side of the child's neck and secure with tape. Tape should reach from one side of the car safety seat across the child's forehead to the other side. Small towels can be secured between the child's body and car seat to allow additional immobilization.[32]

Cervical spine radiographs from C1 through T1 are obtained in the anterior-posterior and lateral views to evaluate for vertebral fractures. The radiograph is assessed for vertebral symmetry, alignment, and spacing. If there is no radiographic evidence of cervical spine injury and the child has normal neurologic findings, spinal immobilization can be removed.

Breathing. Supplemental oxygen is administered to any child with multiple trauma. The child breathing spontaneously who has effective air exchange can receive humidified oxygen with a nasal cannula, partial nonrebreather face mask, or nonrebreather face mask.

A nasal cannula can be set at 4 to 6 L/min of oxygen; higher flow rates irritate the nasopharynx. A cannula is used in children with minimal oxygen requirements. With infants and young children, secure the cannula in the nares then start oxygen flow, because oxygen flow may frighten the child. A partial rebreathing mask set at a flow rate of 10 to 12 L/min delivers an inspired oxygen concentration of 50% to 60%.

Nonrebreather oxygen masks are used for a child with a greater oxygen requirement, and are also set at a flow rate of 10 to 12 L/min. A properly fitting face mask fits snugly on the face, covering the nose and mouth without covering eyes or cheeks. Young children who do not accept a face mask may cooperate if told it is a "space mask like astronauts use" or other suggestions that engage the child's imagination.

In the child who is not breathing spontaneously or effectively, ventilations are assisted with a bag-valve-mask device set at 15 L/min, which allows delivery of 90% oxygen at best.[67] A bag-valve-mask device must have a minimum volume of 450 ml, be self-refilling, and available in both pediatric and adult sizes.[22] Bag-valve devices are equipped with pop-off valves, which can be utilized when great resistance is met during ventilation attempts. When assisting ventilations with a bag-valve-mask device, the bag is squeezed until enough air volume is delivered to allow easy rise and fall of the chest. Care must be taken not to ventilate with too great a force, since a pneumothorax can occur as a result of the high volume.

A pulse oximeter is applied to the child's finger, ear lobe, or toe to determine oxygen saturation. Pulse oximetry readings should be 95% or more.

Chest tubes are inserted if there is indication of hemothorax, pneumothorax, or hemopneumothorax. Local anesthetic (and preferably sedatives) should be administered before insertion of chest tubes.

Circulation. Continuous cardiopulmonary and blood pressure monitoring devices are connected to the child. Vital signs are measured every 5 minutes until the child's condition stabilizes. Blood pressure readings should be evaluated against other vital signs. A properly fitting blood pressure cuff fits two thirds of the upper arm. A cuff that is too small gives false high readings, whereas a cuff that is too large gives false low readings. Apply direct pressure to open, bleeding wounds. Tourniquets are not recommended because direct tissue damage may occur.

Two large-bore intravenous catheters are inserted, preferably in the antecubital fossae, for venous access and fluid replacement. Catheter size is determined by the size of the child's veins. After the catheter is secured, obtain blood for laboratory analyses, then initiate crystalloid fluid replacement.

If peripheral venous access is not established after three attempts, alternate methods of access are employed. Intraosseous route should be considered in children less than 6 years of age. Bones in older children are calcifying, which makes intraosseous access difficult, so access to a central line through the jugular, subclavian, or femoral vein by an experienced physician is the next possibility. Venous cut-down in the saphenous or brachial vein is the last choice. Central venous pressure monitoring or arterial pressure monitoring is reserved for severely injured children and should be performed only under controlled circumstances by experienced personnel.

Crystalloid fluid replacement is initiated with lactated Ringer's solution, which should be warmed if large volumes will be administered. Stopcocks connected to IV tubing allow easy administration of fluid boluses. Crystalloids are infused at a maintenance rate based on estimated weight. If the child is hemodynamically stable or has a head injury, infusion rate may be decreased, usually to two-thirds maintenance rate. Excessive fluid administration in the child with a head injury may increase intracranial pressure (ICP).

Hypovolemic shock is suspected in the child with tachypnea, tachycardia, decreased level of consciousness, decreased urinary output, and prolonged capillary refill. Fluid bolus of 20 ml/kg lactated Ringer's solution is rapidly administered with effectiveness observed almost immediately. If there is no improvement, another bolus can be administered, followed by a third bolus, and warm O-negative blood at 10 ml/kg if there is no improvement after the third fluid bolus.[57]

Routine blood tests include complete blood count (CBC) and differential, electrolytes, blood urea nitrogen (BUN), creatinine, glucose, and type and screen. If abdominal trauma is suspected, amylase, lipase, and liver enzymes may be obtained. In suspected cardiac or muscle damage, creatine phosphokinase levels are also obtained. Other blood tests include prothrombin time, partial thromboplastin times, toxicology screening, and arterial blood gases. Urine may be sent for complete urinalysis and toxicology testing. Pregnancy testing should be considered in the postmenarcheal female.

Pneumatic antishock garments (PASG) are not routinely used in pediatric trauma, because they have been associated with compromised blood flow to the extremities.[73] They can be used as a splint for pelvic fractures or femur fractures when other forms of splinting are not available.

An indwelling urinary catheter is placed if there is no sign of genitourinary trauma, that is, no blood at the meatus. A urimeter on the urine collection bag allows careful monitoring of urinary output. Decreased output can indicate fluid overload. Hematuria indicates genitourinary trauma; however, the first urine specimen may test negative for blood because of urine in the bladder before the injury. Therefore a subsequent urine specimen may be necessary. Normal urinary output for children less than 1 year of age should approach 2 ml/kg/hr; for children more than 1 year of age, 1 ml/kg/hr is optimal.[75]

Disability. Serial neurologic assessments are necessary to identify changes in mental status. Changes in level of consciousness can indicate hypovolemia or increased ICP. Early signs of increased ICP are vomiting and irritability. In the infant, a bulging fontanelle is a *late* sign of increasing ICP.

In older children, the first sign of increased ICP is disorientation to time, place, and familiar persons, then to self.

This description is not applicable to the younger child, who has no concept of time or place. The Glasgow coma scale, although appropriate for adults and older children, is not appropriate for infants and preverbal children. The pediatric coma scale is a more reliable measurement of neurologic status in these age groups (Table 31-6). Children should be given developmentally appropriate neurologic tests. A preschool-age child is not able to give the time of day, day of the week, or name of the President of the United States. However, this child may recognize the Power Rangers, Lion King, or a picture of Mister Rogers.

In a child with a severe head injury, hyperventilation with 100% oxygen is initiated to keep $PaCO_2$ between 30 to 34 mm Hg; $PaCO_2 \leq 28$ mm Hg can lead to brain ischemia. Recent studies suggest hyperventilation may not be as effective as previously indicated. However, more research is necessary in the pediatric population. Mannitol may be administered at 1 g/kg to decrease cerebral swelling.

Expose. The child's temperature is recorded initially and again during initial stabilization to detect and treat hypothermia. Common temperature measurement routes are tympanic, oral, rectal, and bladder. In one study comparing rectal and tympanic membrane temperatures in injured children, an 85% correlation was found, with the rectal temperatures an average of 0.3°C higher.[9] There is some question of accuracy in children less than 2 years of age, so caution should be used. Passive warming measures include increasing ambient temperature using overhead lights and applying warm blankets. Active warming measures include administration of warm intravenous fluids and blood products.

Musculoskeletal. Frequent monitoring of the neurovascular status of an injured extremity is necessary to identify impairment of circulation or possible compartment syndrome. An injured extremity can be splinted for protection and comfort until definitive care is provided. Once the extremity has been splinted or casted, frequent reevaluation is necessary because edema may develop and impede circulation.

Additional interventions. Additional interventions undertaken during emergency treatment of the injured child include radiologic testing, medication administration, management of pain, and provision of emotional support.

Radiologic testing. Along with cervical spine radiographs, other radiographic testing may be undertaken relative to the suspected injuries. An abdominal series may be indicated in a child with a history of abdominal trauma, whereas chest and spinal films may be indicated in the child with multiple injuries. Intravenous pyelogram (IVP) may be performed if renal trauma is suspected. Specific radiographs with varying views of injured extremities prior to definitive treatment may also be done. Radiographs may be obtained in the trauma room or the child may be transported to the radiology department. In either case, a nurse should remain with the child to explain the procedures and monitor the child's condition.

Computed tomography (CT) is indicated in children with head, chest, spinal, or abdominal trauma. Xenon testing may be indicated in the child with a severe head injury. Again, a

Table **31-6**	**Pediatric Coma Scale***			
	Score	Age over 1 year		Less than 1 year of age
Eye opening	4	Spontaneously		Spontaneously
	3	To verbal command		To shout
	2	To pain		To pain
	1	No response		No response
Best motor response	6	Obeys		
	5	Localizes pain		Localizes pain
	4	Flexion withdrawal		Flexion withdrawal
	3	Flexion-abnormal (decorticate rigidity)		Flexion-abnormal (decorticate rigidity)
	2	Extension (decerebrate rigidity)		Extension (decerebrate rigidity)
	1	No response		No response
		Age over 5 years	**Age 2-5 years**	**Age 0-23 months**
Best verbal response	5	Oriented and converses	Appropriate words and phrases	Smiles, coos
	4	Disoriented and converses	Inappropriate words and phrases	Cries appropriately
	3	Inappropriate words	Cries and/or screams	Cries, screams
	2	Incomprehensible sounds	Grunts	Grunts
	1	No response	No response	No response
Total				

Modified from Wong DL: *Whaley & Wong's essentials of pediatric nursing,* ed 5, St. Louis, 1997, Mosby.
*Modification of Glasgow coma scale

nurse must accompany the child for continuous monitoring and must have appropriate equipment readily available in case there is a change in the child's status. Angiography may be necessary in the child with vessel injury.

Medications. Antibiotics may be administered in the child with large, open contaminated wounds, open fractures, or arterial injury. Tetanus prophylaxis is also necessary. It is important to determine the status of the child's immunization to ensure appropriate prophylaxis.

Management of pain. Pain management is of utmost importance when treating the injured child; however, it is often neglected. Never tell a child he or she does not have pain or that it does not hurt. This kind of statement will cause the child to mistrust his or her caregiver. Analgesics may be administered once all injuries are identified and the child is determined to be physiologically and neurologically intact. Pharmacologic management of pain includes narcotic and nonnarcotic analgesics. Nonpharmacologic management of pain includes comfort measures such as distraction techniques, progressive relaxation, positive self-talk, and deep breathing exercises. Allowing an infant to suck a pacifier promotes comfort, whereas allowing a toddler to hold a transitional object, that is, a blanket or toy, promotes security. The awake child may be able to use a pain scale to rate the pain. Reevaluation is necessary after any interventions.

Emotional support. The injured child has a number of fears—mutilation, losing control, getting in trouble with his or her parents for engaging in a forbidden activity, death, disfigurement, and pain. It is the responsibility of the emergency nurse to help the child cope effectively with those fears during the trauma resuscitation.

Assign one nurse as the child's support person. When the child has cervical and spinal immobilization, the nurse should stand at the child's side and down from his or her face, about chest level, so the child is able to see the nurse. Standing directly over the child's face is frightening, especially when different faces keep appearing and reappearing. Hold the child's hand or stroke his or her hair to provide tactile comfort. Talk softly and slowly, using words he or she can understand, that is, "The doctor is going to listen to your heartbeat," "You will feel a pinch in your right arm. You can scream, but you must keep your right arm still." Avoid words such as "take" or "cut out" because they imply mutilation. Use words such as "make it better." If the child requires general anesthesia, avoid telling the child he or she will "be put to sleep." If the child had a pet that was "put to sleep," this statement may create death fears. Instead, tell the child he or she will get "special medicine to help you take a short nap." The child understands "nap" is a short time. Tell the child what will happen before it happens. Children do not like surprises any more than adults do. Prepare them by using feeling terms, that is, "This will feel cold; this will feel heavy; this will smell sweet." If a procedure will hurt, tell the child. Lying will only cause him or her to mistrust you.

Children cope in a variety of ways. Because young children are mobile, crying and kicking are ways for them to cope. To them, being restrained may mean not being alive. School aged children and adolescents cope by seeking information;[54] they may ask the same questions over and over again. Be patient. Scolding or threatening the child is fruitless and will only increase fear and resistance.

Children with severe mutilating injuries should be shielded so the deformity is not readily visible to the child. Refrain from discussing how horrible the injury is in front of the child. Children's reported fantasies are worse than reality, so the child will imagine terrible things. It is not known how much information unconscious children remember. Avoid talking about other family members or the child's condition in his or her presence. Talk to the child who is comatose or unresponsive just as if he or she were awake.

The presence of a supportive parent does wonders for a frightened child. Have parents see the child as soon as possible after stabilization is complete. Explain to the parents beforehand what they will see and why. Explanations prevent any surprises. Parents may need permission to touch or talk to their child, so encourage them to do so.

Controversy exists as to whether parents should be present during resuscitations. If the parents are present, one nurse must stay with them and explain what is happening to their child. The Emergency Nurses Association advocates parental presence during resuscitation. Such presence may be beneficial to the child as well as family members. A designated emergency nurse or social worker can stay with the family and explain treatment that is taking place.

While parents are waiting to see their child, a social worker or an emergency nurse should keep them apprised of the situation and serve as a support person. If the decision is made to transfer the child to another facility, parents should see their child before his or her departure. If the child dies before parents arrive at the accepting institution, they feel guilt because they were not able to see the child or agreed to the transfer. When the child leaves, say "Mommy will see you later" rather than "goodbye" because "goodbye" implies that they may never see each other again.

SPECIFIC CONDITIONS
Head Injuries

Seventy percent of injury-related deaths in children are due to head trauma. The rate of head injury is approximately 200 per 100,000 population.[69] Head injury often results from blunt trauma due to MVCs, bicycle crashes, falls, and child maltreatment. Children are susceptible to brain injury due to their larger head-to-body ratio, thin cranial bones, and less myelinated brain. These factors leave the brain relatively unprotected and vulnerable to injury.[35,57] The thinner cranium allows injury forces to be transmitted directly to the brain itself.[69] Unmyelinated brain tissue in infants and young children appears to be more susceptible to shearing forces as compared to older children and adults.[69] Furthermore, cranial sutures remain open in early infancy, and the anterior fontanelle is open until 18 months. These features increase the child's susceptibility to head injury, but they also serve as an outlet for swollen cerebral tissues, allowing greater tolerance for increases in intracranial pressures.

Mild to moderate head injuries (Glasgow Coma Scale [GCS] 13 to 15) are more common than severe head injuries, accounting for 90% of admissions. In contrast, severe head injuries (GCS ≤8) account for approximately 5% of admissions.[18] Brain injuries are divided into primary and secondary phases. Primary injury results from mechanical damage from traumatic forces applied to the brain where the brain contacts the interior skull or foreign bodies that cause direct brain injury.[18] Diffuse axonal injury, skull fractures, contusions, and hemorrhage result. Secondary injury occurs from the resultant changes in the brain caused by the initial injury, for example, cerebral edema, hypoxia, increased intracranial pressure, and decreased cerebral blood flow.[18]

Mild to moderate head injury. Mild to moderate head injury may cause persistent vomiting, posttraumatic seizure, and loss of consciousness. Posttraumatic seizures or loss of consciousness indicate that force applied to the head was severe enough to cause transient neurologic dysfunction.[30] Hemotympanum, cerebrospinal fluid (CSF) otorrhea, or CSF rhinorrhea indicate a basilar skull fracture, whereas orbital bruising (raccoon eyes) or mastoid bruising (Battle's sign) indicates significant cranial injury.[30] Focal neurologic signs suggest severe injuries (Table 31-7).

Children with mild to moderate head injuries must receive serial neurologic evaluations to determine if intracranial pressure is increasing. Serial evaluations include measurement of level of consciousness, pupillary response, motor and sensory response, and vital signs. Making a game of the assessment may elicit the cooperation of the young, awake, and frightened child. Having the awake child touch the nose and move the heels down the shins tests cerebellar function, while having the child squeeze the nurse's fingers and "push on the gas pedal" tests motor strength. The awake

infant and toddler should be able to focus on and reach for a toy or object. This child should recognize the parent and be easily consoled. Any changes in the child's level of consciousness should be reported immediately to avoid subsequent deterioration and possible brainstem herniation from increased intracranial pressure. A CT scan without contrast may be obtained if intracranial pathology is suspected. Skull radiographs may be obtained to detect the location and extent of skull fractures in infants and young children. Toxicology screening should be considered in children with an altered level of consciousness.

In general, children with a head injury are admitted to the hospital for observation if they have any neurologic deficits, seizures, vomiting, severe headache, fever, prolonged loss of consciousness, skull fracture, altered level of consciousness, or suspected child maltreatment.[69]

Children with mild head injuries may be discharged home if parents or guardians understand the required home care. Parents should be instructed to return to the ED if the child has persistent vomiting, changes in vision, unequal pupil size, persistent headache or drowsiness, changes in level of consciousness, unequal strength or gait, or seizures. Parents should awaken the child every few hours to evaluate for changes in level of consciousness. They may also observe for nose or ear drainage on the pillow and should contact the ED if this is observed. Acetaminophen may be administered for headache. Be sure parents understand that the child may sleep, that sleeping is not an indication of a problem.

Infants with skull fractures may be admitted for 24-hour observation. Infants may have skull fractures that occur in one of the suture lines. These diastatic fractures occur most commonly in the lamboid suture.[69] Such fractures should create a high index of suspicion for epidural hematomas. A complication of these fractures is the fracture can "grow." Growing skull fractures are usually observed in infants and young children less than 3 years of age and are thought to result from cerebral tissue or arachnoid membrane herniation through a dural laceration.[30] A pulsatile mass may be felt and surgery may be indicated. Therefore infants and young children with this fracture must receive follow-up treatment. Infants can sustain significant blood loss from scalp lacerations, so they require close observation for the development of hypovolemic shock.

One study found children hospitalized for mild to moderate head injury also had more functional disabilities as compared to previous reports, probably because previous studies focused on clinical outcomes rather than functional outcomes. Children may exhibit minor limitations that are not clinically obvious but that affect daily function and performance.[21] Therefore early aggressive management of the child with a head injury is initiated to improve functional outcome.

Severe head injury. Severe head injury is characterized by a decreased level of consciousness, posturing, combative behavior, and abnormal neurologic findings. In shaken baby

Table **31-7**	**Focal Neurologic Signs and Suspected Injuries**
Neurologic sign	**Suspected injury**
Monoparesis/hemiparesis	Structural injury to the motor cortex
Visual dysfunction	Injury to optic nerves or occipital cortex
Cranial nerve abnormalities	Basilar skull fracture
Vestibulocochlear nerve dysfunction	Basilar skull fracture

From Jaufmann B: Central nervous system injuries. In Ford E, Andrassy R, editors: *Pediatric trauma: initial assessment and management*, Philadelphia, 1994, WB Saunders.

syndrome, retinal hemorrhaging, seizures, and a decreased level of consciousness may be observed (see Chapter 51).

In severe head injuries, the airway is secured using rapid-sequence intubation, then hyperventilation is initiated. A quick neurologic assessment should be completed prior to administration of paralytic and sedative agents. Because CO_2 is a potent vasodilator, the $PaCO_2$ should be maintained at 30 to 34 mm Hg to allow adequate cerebral blood flow. A $PaCO_2 \leq 28$ mm Hg may cause cerebral ischemia due to excessive vasoconstriction. SaO_2 should be maintained at $\geq 90\%$ with mean arterial pressure maintained slightly higher than age-appropriate norms. Intravenous crystalloids such as normal saline or lactated Ringer's solution are administered, preferably at one half to two thirds maintenance requirements. Glucose-containing fluids are avoided due to potential for cerebral edema. Mannitol 1 g/kg may be infused to remove fluid from the interstitial spaces. Phenobarbital or phenytoin may be administered to prevent seizures.

Oculovestibular response may be assessed using the caloric response with iced saline solution, provided tympanic membranes are intact. Doll's eye maneuver can be performed provided cervical spine is free of injury. Babinski's reflex may be present with severe brain injury, and hyperreflexia may also be noted.[69] Laboratory analyses, including type and cross-match, toxicologic testing, and clotting times (PT/PTT) should be performed in the event surgery is required. A CT scan without contrast is usually done to determine location and extent of the injury. Operative management may be indicated, with admission to an intensive care unit for ongoing nursing and medical care.

Generally children have better outcomes than adults with a head injury, probably due to a multitude of factors unclear at this time.[69] Neurologic deficits are the most common complications of head injury and are relative to the area of brain injury. For example, frontal brain injury results in cognitive deficits. Children may require rehabilitation for speech, motor, and cognitive improvements. Among 95 children hospitalized for head injury, compared with the general population, limitations in physical health, behavioral problems, and special education requirements were more likely to occur.[21]

Spinal Cord Injuries

Spinal cord injuries are relatively uncommon in the young pediatric population. When they do occur, rapid acceleration-deceleration forces and hyperflexion-hyperextension forces are suspected. Children less than 8 years of age are susceptible to cervical spine injuries because of their larger head size, weaker neck muscles and ligaments, and horizontal facets.[57] The cervical musculature does not provide complete support until puberty, so young children have lax intraspinal ligaments and capsules, and more horizontal facet joints. These features can lead to pseudosubluxation of the cervical spine.[59] Once the child reaches 8 years of age, the spine is essentially similar to an adult spine. High cervical fractures can

occur because the fulcrum of cervical mobility is at C2-3, as compared to C5-6 or C6-7 in the adult.[35]

Because of laxity of the pediatric spine, spinal cord injury without bony abnormality can occur. This phenomenon, known as *spinal cord injury without radiographic abnormalities* (SCIWORA),[48,49] occurs because of the inherent elasticity of the pediatric spine, which allows transient displacement of the cerebral column by flexion-extension or acceleration-deceleration forces.[51] As the head is hyperflexed or hyperextended, the spinal cord stretches, which leads to injury or transection. The spinal cord then returns to normal length and vertebrae to normal alignment. The child may exhibit signs of spinal cord injury, such as numbness, tingling, or weakness; however, subsequent radiographs show no evidence of bony abnormality. Although SCIWORA is most often diagnosed at the cervical level, thoracic SCIWORA is also possible. One review of reported literature demonstrates an approximate 35% incidence of SCIWORA in children with traumatic myelopathy.[51] Most children younger than 8 years of age experience SCIWORA at a higher level of spinal involvement with greater severity of injury as compared to older children.[51] Among seven children with SCIWORA who received MRI testing, ligamental and disk injuries and cord disruption were found. Findings support the hypothesis that self-reducing transient subluxation or distraction of the pediatric spine accounts for neurologic injury.[19] Furthermore, MRI findings of abnormalities such as major cord hemorrhage were consistent with permanent complete cord injuries. Likewise, normal MRI spinal cord findings were associated with complete neurologic recovery.[19]

Signs and symptoms of spinal cord injury are the same in the child as in the adult. Numbness, tingling, weakness, and spasticity or flaccidity may be observed. Priapism and perianal wink may also be demonstrated. The child may complain of pain in the back or neck and may be tender upon palpation. The awake child with a spinal cord injury may feel helpless and afraid, so continuous reassurance is essential.

Spinal injuries must always be suspected in multiply injured children. Complete spinal immobilization is maintained until it is clinically determined that spinal cord injury is not present. Children with high spinal cord injuries should be intubated and their lungs mechanically ventilated, whereas children with lower cervical injuries should be closely observed for changes in their respiratory status. Intravenous fluids should be administered at one half to two thirds maintenance requirements. High-dose steroids should also be administered. Current recommendations are methylprednisolone (30 mg/kg) followed by 5.4 mg/kg/hr for 23 hours if injury occurred within 8 hours.[62] It is important to note there is limited research in children less than 13 years of age. Lateral, anterior-posterior, and open mouth (odontoid) radiographic views of the cervical spine are obtained. Anterior-posterior views of the thoracic or lumbar spine are obtained as needed. Serial neurologic assessments are performed to determine if cord swelling is progressing.

Unconscious children with suspected spinal cord injury should remain immobilized until they are awake and able to complete a neurologic examination. Advanced diagnostic tests, such as somatosensory evoked potentials (SSEPs), may be indicated to determine the presence or extent of spinal cord injury. Operative management may be needed for children with vertebral fractures or dislocations.

Complications or sequelae of spinal cord injury range from mild neurologic deficits to complete hemiplegia, paraplegia, or quadriplegia. Autonomic areflexia, bowel and bladder incontinence, and ventilator dependence occur relative to the level of the cord lesion. Rehabilitation is indicated to assist the child to maximize his or her potential for recovery.

Thoracic Injuries

Thoracic injuries are most often the result of blunt trauma. With infants and young children these injuries are most likely caused by falls, whereas older children sustain these injuries in MVCs as pedestrians or passengers.[53] Penetrating chest trauma may be seen in adolescents as a result of violent activities. Common thoracic injuries in the pediatric population are pulmonary contusion, cardiac contusion, and pneumothorax.

Children are susceptible to transmission of blunt forces to underlying thoracic structures (heart, lungs, great vessels) because their soft cartilage and developing bones make the thorax pliable.[53] When rib fractures occur, a high index of suspicion for severe blunt forces should be maintained. Similarly, when flail segments are present, severe parenchymal pulmonary injury should be suspected.[53] The mediastinum is easily displaced by air or fluid. Mediastinal shift compromises venous return, cardiac output, and lung volume.[53]

Rib fractures. Rib fractures are associated with chest pain, tenderness on palpation, and respiratory distress. Flail segments lead to paradoxic chest wall movement during respiration. Changes in pulse oximetry and respiratory rate and effort may be noted. Children should receive oxygen via face mask, and analgesics for pain relief. A chest radiograph is obtained to determine location and extent of fractures. External immobilization (splinting) of the chest is not necessary because remodeling of the chest wall occurs rapidly without subsequent deformity.[53] Evaluate carefully for spleen or liver injury with lower rib fractures.

Pneumothorax/hemothorax. Pneumothorax may be open, closed, or tension. Clinical signs and symptoms vary with severity of the injury and include respiratory distress, air hunger, decreased or absent breath sounds on the affected side, and anxiety. In a tension pneumothorax tracheal deviation away from the affected side and jugular vein distention are often observed. Hemothorax can result from severe blunt or penetrating chest trauma. The child may have hypovolemic shock, decreased or absent breath sounds on the affected side, and respiratory distress.

Pneumothoraces are treated relative to severity. Chest radiographs confirm the presence of air in the pleural space, but should not delay treatment in a symptomatic child. Children in no acute distress with a small pneumothorax receive supplemental oxygen and are observed to determine if the pneumothorax is worsening. Large pneumothoraces require needle decompression and chest tube placement. The needle is inserted at the fourth intercostal space midaxillary line, followed by chest tube placement with water seal suction. In tension pneumothoraces, chest radiographs are not obtained prior to needle insertion, because this situation is life threatening. Following needle decompression, chest tubes are inserted and a chest radiograph is obtained. Similarly in hemothoraces, chest radiographs may be delayed until the chest tubes are inserted. Autotransfusion should be considered for these patients when there are no contraindications, for example, enteric contamination, wound greater than 6 hours old. Surgical intervention is indicated if ongoing blood loss into the chest drainage system is greater than 100 ml/kg/hr or if the immediate blood loss is greater than 20% of the child's estimated circulating blood volume.[53]

Pulmonary contusion. Pulmonary contusions should be suspected in children with respiratory distress after blunt chest trauma who do not have abnormal radiographic findings. Pulmonary contusion is usually not diagnosed until after admission to the hospital. Signs and symptoms include increasing respiratory distress, hemoptysis, and decreased pulmonary function. Chest radiographs show changes from the initial film. The ED management of these patients begins with supplemental oxygen. Endotracheal intubation and subsequent ventilation with positive end-expiratory pressure (PEEP) is usually reserved for severe injuries. Fluids may be limited if the child is not hypovolemic.

Tracheobronchial injury. Tracheobronchial rupture, while rare, can occur with blunt or penetrating forces to the neck and chest. The child may have respiratory distress, subcutaneous emphysema, and cyanosis. Severe tracheobronchial rupture causes massive subcutaneous emphysema, persistent air leak, mediastinal air, tension pneumothorax, and failure of the lung to expand following chest tube insertion.[53] Airway management with endotracheal intubation or tracheostomy is imperative. Chest tubes may also be inserted. Operative management is necessary for definitive treatment.

Diaphragmatic injury. Diaphragmatic rupture usually occurs following blunt trauma. The left side is most often affected because the liver protects the right side. Signs and symptoms include respiratory distress, abdominal or chest pain, abdominal tenderness and decreased breath sounds on the affected side, and decreased or absent bowel sounds.[53] Bowel sounds may be heard on the affected side. Diaphragmatic rupture requires operative management and repair.

Cardiac injury. In general, cardiac injuries are suspected in children with chest bruising, upper body cyanosis, unexplained hypotension, and dysrhythmias.[56] Injuries include cardiac tamponade, myocardial contusion, and great vessel injuries. Cardiac injuries are managed relative to severity and include initial and ongoing evaluations of ECGs, cardiac enzymes, and echocardiographic studies.

Abdominal Injuries

Blunt force is the most common cause of abdominal trauma in children, with subsequent hemorrhaging a common cause of traumatic death. Because of the child's smaller abdomen, injuries can occur to multiple organs. The spleen is the most commonly injured abdominal organ, followed by the liver.[57] Injuries to the pancreas and intestinal tract also occur. Trauma can result from bicycle injuries where the child's abdomen is struck by the bicycle's handlebars. Sledding, MVCs, altercations, falls, child maltreatment, and sports activities are other mechanisms of injury. Penetrating abdominal trauma is increasing as a result of the rise in violent crimes.

The alert child who sustains abdominal trauma may complain of tenderness with palpation. Abdominal distention, abrasions, or contusions may be noted. Signs of hypovolemic shock may be present internal hemorrhaging. Absence of bowel sounds does not confirm an abdominal injury; an ileus can occur because the child is crying, swallowing air, or frightened.[65] Elevated liver enzymes (SGPT and GGPT) may be noted with liver injuries; however, these are not specific to the liver. Tenderness in the left upper quadrant is associated with splenic injury. Pain in the left shoulder may be elicited with abdominal palpation (Kehr's sign). Elevation of serum amylase and lipase levels indicates possible pancreatic injury. A tender mass in the epigastric region may also be palpated.[65] Free air may be noted on radiographs in cases of injury to the gastrointestinal tract. Computed tomography can identify specific injuries to each abdominal organ.

All children who sustain high-velocity abdominal trauma, that is, GSWs, should undergo surgical exploration to ensure that all injuries are identified and treated appropriately. Low-velocity injuries, that is, stab wounds, are treated according to the child's condition. Cutaneous wounds are cleaned and irrigated, whereas deep wounds may require surgical repair. In both instances, the child is admitted for further observation.

Children with blunt abdominal trauma are treated according to their hemodynamic stability. A hemodynamically stable child may have a CT scan with contrast to determine the extent of the injuries. This is preferred over diagnostic peritoneal lavage (DPL) because of accuracy in detecting specific abdominal injuries. Many injuries are treated conservatively with serial reevaluation; however, surgical intervention is indicated if hemorrhaging or peritonitis are suspected. The hemodynamically unstable child who does not respond to fluid and blood boluses must be prepared for immediate surgery.

Children with splenic injuries who are hemodynamically stable are admitted to the hospital and managed with bed rest and frequent serial reevaluation. Large liver lacerations may result in significant blood loss and require immediate surgical repair, whereas smaller lacerations without signs of hypovolemia can be managed conservatively. Pancreatic injuries to the tail of the pancreas involving major ductal structures are usually managed with a distal pancreatectomy.[26] Perforation of the intestines requires surgical intervention.

Genitourinary Emergencies

Genitourinary (GU) injuries frequently occur in the second decade of life and usually result from blunt trauma.[28] Injuries can result from pedestrian or passenger MVCs, sledding, sports activities, falls, and altercations. While most GU injuries are minor, recent increases in violent crime have led to more serious penetrating injuries. Blunt trauma is responsible for approximately 80% of all renal injuries; the remaining 20% are due to gunshot wounds. Ureteral injuries are most commonly due to gunshot wounds; knife wounds are the next most common cause.[13] Bladder and urethral injuries result mostly from blunt trauma and are often associated with pelvic fractures. Approximately 40% of GU injuries are associated with abdominal, musculoskeletal, and central nervous system injuries.[28]

Injuries to female genitalia can result from falls, straddle-type injuries (i.e., falls on picket fences or diving boards), and sexual abuse or assault. Testicular trauma can also result from straddle-type injuries. The majority of testicular injuries occurs in adolescents who are struck in the scrotum while playing sports or during an altercation.[13] The most common cause of penile injuries is direct forces such as zipper injuries and trauma from toilet seats. Infants can sustain a tourniquet injury from threads, bands, rings, or human hair lodged in the coronal groove forming a constricting ring and lacerating the penile shaft. Degloving injuries and penile amputations are not common in children.[13] Sexual abuse must be considered in any child with genital trauma and when injuries are inconsistent with the history.

The child's GU system is more vulnerable to certain injuries than an adult's. Larger kidneys with less perinephric fat and a mobile bony rib cage offer less protection to the kidney. Preexisting abnormalities such as Wilms' tumor, ectopic kidneys, and hydronephrosis predispose children to renal trauma. Ureteral injuries occur in children as a result of greater elasticity and torso mobility. The bladder is located in the abdomen and is less protected when full. A full bladder can rupture between a seatbelt and the pelvis or vertebral column as a result of deceleration injury.[13] The bladder neck, especially in female children, is less protected. Males are more vulnerable to urethral injuries as a result of the length and position of the urethra.[28] Tissues of prepubescent girls are smaller and considerably more rigid than those of the adolescent or adult, thus increasing the risk of tearing with either blunt or penetrating trauma. Prepubescent girls also have a thin vesicovaginal septal wall. Serious internal injury can result from both penetrating and blunt trauma.[14]

Renal injury. Symptoms of renal trauma include abdominal, back, or flank tenderness. Physical signs include localized abrasions or lacerations and hematuria. Degree of hematuria does not correlate with degree of injury. Little or no hematuria may occur in serious injuries such as a renal pedicle or parenchymal injury and gross hematuria may result from a minor renal injury.[13] Renal injury should be considered in children who sustain fractures to the lower ribs or the transverse process of the vertebrae. If severe hemorrhaging occurs, a child may display signs of hypovolemic shock.

Once the child's condition is stabilized, a urine specimen is obtained. The awake, stable child may be able to provide a urine specimen by voiding spontaneously. The unstable child may require an indwelling bladder catheter unless contraindicated. Some authors believe that insertion of a urinary catheter in males less than 5 years of age may be harmful and should be avoided if at all possible.[34] If a urethral injury is suspected, a retrograde urethral contrast study should be performed prior to catheterization.[28] A CT scan with contrast dye is usually obtained. Treatment is specialized relative to the type of injury, and may range from observation and bed rest to surgical exploration. Indications for surgical exploration are expanding or uncontained hematoma; major segments of nonviable renal parenchyma; and ureteropelvic junction disruption.[13] If renal pedicle injury is found, repair of renal vessels must be performed within 12 to 18 hours.[28]

Ureteral injury. Ureteral injuries are rare, so recognition may be delayed unless the possibility for this injury is entertained. Hematuria or a urinary leak may be present, and flank mass and iliac pain may also occur. Symptoms may not be noted until 7 to 10 days after the initial injury. Urine may appear at entrance or exit wounds or on surgical dressing. If no wound is present, signs of retroperitoneal abscess may occur, that is, chills, fever, lower abdominal pain, palpable mass, pyuria, and frequency. Surgical repair is indicated for ureteral injuries; a ureteral stent may be required.

Bladder injury. Symptoms of bladder injuries vary with sustained injury. Suprapubic tenderness, urgency to void, inability to void, hematuria, and palpable abdominal mass may be observed with a ruptured bladder. Children with an extraperitoneal rupture may be able to pass small amounts of sanguineous urine but will have significant discomfort. Retrograde cystogram before Foley catheterization is recommended in male patients because of the incidence of urethral injuries.[62] If severe hemorrhaging is present, signs of shock will be observed. Most bladder contusions are minor and managed conservatively with observation and reevaluation. Large extraperitoneal injuries and intraperitoneal bladder ruptures require surgical repair and suprapubic diversion.

Urethral injury. There is a high association between pelvic fractures and urethral injury. Blood at the urinary meatus is noted in the majority of children with these injuries. If such blood is noted in boys or girls, blood is observed in the scrotum, or the prostate is abnormally positioned or abnormally mobile, a urethral injury is highly likely and a retrograde urethrogram is indicated.[34] It is imperative that no attempt be made to insert a urinary bladder catheter. The child may have a partial urethral tear. Inserting a catheter may convert a partial tear to a complete tear. Other signs of urethral injuries include inability to void, sensation to void, and ecchymoses in the scrotum, penis, or perineum. A high-riding prostate resulting from a large associated pelvic hematoma may be noted on rectal examination.[13]

Partial urethral tears are managed conservatively with a suprapubic catheter or an indwelling urethral catheter inserted under fluoroscopy. Complete urethral tears require surgical repair.

Female genital injury. A girl sustaining genital trauma may have hymenal tears, vaginal bleeding or hematoma, tears of the perineal body, inability to urinate, gross hematuria, abnormal sphincter tone, or rectal bleeding.[14] Abrasions, contusions, and lacerations may be noted with superficial, moderate, or severe genital trauma. Lower abdominal and perineal pain, abdominal tenderness and guarding, and signs of hypovolemia may be present with severe injuries.[14]

Girls with superficial genital injuries usually do not require hospitalization; injuries are managed with sitz baths, good perineal cleansing, and bacteriostatic ointment. Deep tears may be sutured under anesthesia. Moderate perineal injuries with signs of internal extension require examination under anesthesia and subsequent repair. Severe injuries require hemodynamic stabilization and surgical exploration and repair.[14]

A child should never be restrained for a genital examination. The exam can be attempted by having the child sit on the parent's lap. Comfort measures and explanation of procedures should be done throughout the examination. If the child is unable to cooperate, the exam is performed under general anesthesia. Children who are hearing impaired or require a translator should have an interpreter other than a family member present during the examination. In suspected sexual abuse or assault, proper evidence collection must be initiated.

Penile injury. Minor direct penile injuries can be treated in the ED. Parents require reassurance and instructions on observing the child as he voids. Warm soaks or baths are helpful. Zipper injuries are treated by sedating the child, then cutting the median bar of the zipper with a pair of wire cutters so the two halves of the zipper fall apart. Significant edema may be present, so parents require reassurance the edema will subside. Tourniquet injuries require release of the constricting band. If the band cannot be released in the ED once adequate sedation has been administered, operative management with general anesthesia may be warranted.

Musculoskeletal Injuries

Musculoskeletal injuries are common occurrences in the pediatric population. Long bone fractures occur from falls, sports activities, and motor vehicle and pedestrian crashes. Children's bones are more porous, and the periosteum is strong and thick, which causes bone to bend as with greenstick fractures. The active periosteum allows quicker fracture healing but may impede fracture reduction.[47] Ligaments are strong, which accounts for the prevalence of fractures rather than ligamentous injury.

The most unique feature of the child's musculoskeletal system is the epiphyseal growth plate (physis) located at the articulating ends of bones between the epiphysis and metaphysis.[50] The epiphyseal growth plate is responsible for longitudinal bone growth, so injury may result in growth disturbance or arrest. In general, growth is completed in boys by age 16 years, in girls by 14 years of age. Children sustaining injuries near the physis should have appropriate follow-up to detect limb-length discrepancies and angular deformities.[47] Growth plate fractures are categorized with the Salter-Harris classification (Table 31-8).

Signs of musculoskeletal trauma include point tenderness, soft tissue swelling, discoloration, limitations in range of motion, loss of function, altered sensory perception, and changes in pulses, temperature, or capillary refill distal to the injury.[50] An obvious deformity may be noted or an open fracture may be observed. The child may complain of pain and may splint the injured extremity, such as holding the broken arm with the other hand.

Musculoskeletal trauma is rarely life threatening, so the child's airway, breathing, circulation, and neurologic status are usually intact. The injured extremity is elevated and ice is applied. A splint or sling and swath can be applied, provided neurovascular status is assessed before and after splint application. A sterile dressing is applied to any open fracture. Prophylactic antibiotics are usually given for open fractures, and tetanus prophylaxis is administered. Analgesics may be required.

Radiographs are obtained to include the joint above and below the injury. Comparative views of the injured and uninjured extremities may be obtained. Such radiographs allow for detection of previous fractures that may not have been reported by the family. Child maltreatment should be investigated in nonambulatory children with spiral fractures in the lower extremities, toddlers with femur fractures, young children with multiple fractures, or in circumstances where the injury does not match the history.

Most children require a simple cast when the fracture is nondisplaced. Following application of the cast, the child is discharged from the ED. Parents or guardians are given discharge instructions to observe for swelling of the toes or fingers, odor from the cast, and changes in skin color and temperature. Parents should contact the ED with any of these complaints or if the child complains of sharp pain or numbness. If there is too much swelling to allow for application of a cast, the child is discharged with a splint, and the cast is applied after swelling subsides.

The fracture can be displaced and require manipulation to realign the fractured bone(s). In such situations, the ED physician or orthopedic surgeon may attempt a closed reduction in the ED. Conscious sedation is administered using such medications as midazolam, fentanyl, or ketamine. The nurse must carefully monitor the child for adverse effects to the sedation. Once the fracture is reduced, sedatives are stopped, the cast is applied, and postreduction radiographs are obtained. If reduction is not successful, the child may require open reduction and internal fixation in the operating room.

Treatment for femoral fractures varies with age. Infants are placed in spica casts, often in the ED. Reamed and nonreamed intramedullary rodding used in older children allows early mobilization. Tibial skeletal traction, external fixation, and plating techniques are also used depending on the type of fracture and the child's age. Children with

---

Table **31-8** **Salter-Harris Classification, Fracture Descriptions, and Outcome**

Type	Description of fractures	Treatment and outcome
Type I	Horizontal separation of epiphysis and metaphysis; point tenderness; radiographs may be normal; mild soft tissue swelling produced by shearing forces	No disturbance in growth if properly diagnosed; favorable prognosis; treated with closed reduction and casting
Type II	Separation of epiphysis and metaphysis with some avulsion of the metaphysis produced by shearing forces	No disturbance in growth if properly diagnosed; favorable prognosis; treated with closed reduction and casting
Type III	Produced by intraarticular shearing forces; intraarticular fracture; fracture extends through epiphyseal plate into the metaphysis	Angular deformities may occur; requires good reduction; variable-poor prognosis
Type IV	Fracture starts at the articular surface and extends through the epiphysis, epiphyseal plate, and metaphysis; intraarticular fracture produced by shearing forces	Open reduction and external fixation is needed; variable-poor prognosis; angular deformity may result
Type V	Epiphyseal plate is crushed without fracture or displacement; radiographic diagnosis virtually impossible, produced by crushing forces	Poor prognosis, even when correctly identified and treated

From Bernardo LM, Trunzo R: Pediatric trauma. In Kitt S, Selfridge-Thomas J, Proehl J et al, editors: *Emergency nursing: a physiologic and clinical perspective*, ed 2, Philadelphia, 1995, WB Saunders.

Box **31-3**

NURSING DIAGNOSES FOR THE PEDIATRIC TRAUMA PATIENT

Ineffective airway clearance
Ineffective breathing pattern
Impaired gas exchange
Decreased cardiac output
Fluid volume deficit
Pain
Fear
Anxiety
Altered family processes

pelvic fractures require admission to the hospital and subsequent bed rest. Unstable pelvic fractures may require application of an external fixation device, which is an operative procedure.

SUMMARY

Pediatric trauma patients provide a unique challenge for the emergency nurse. Ability to identify potentially life-threatening conditions is essential. Box 31-3 highlights nursing diagnoses appropriate for these patients. Emergency nurses are in a unique position to offer anticipatory guidance to families concerning prevention of injuries. Becoming actively involved in trauma prevention and safety education is another way for nurses to promote safety. Talking with school groups about safety (wearing bicycle helmets, safe water play, wearing safety belts) enhances the image of emergency nursing and educates children and their families. Become politically aware and support legislators who favor trauma legislation.

Emergency nurses can become involved in other organizations, such as the National Safe Kids Campaign, and Emergency Nurses Cancel Alcohol Related Emergencies (ENCARE). The Emergency Nurses Association has resources related to injury control and prevention. Emergency nurses can minimize the effects of pediatric trauma by providing quality patient care to injured children and their families. Participating in injury prevention activities helps reduce the incidence of pediatric trauma and enhances the professional image of nursing.

REFERENCES

1. Agran P, Winn D, Anderson C: Differences in child pedestrian injury events by location, *Pediatrics* 93(2):284, 1994.
2. Bernardo LM, Kelley SJ: Care of the multiply-injured child. In Kelley SJ, editor: *Pediatric emergency nursing,* ed 2, Norwalk, Conn, 1994, Appleton & Lange.
3. Bernardo LM, Trunzo R: Pediatric trauma. In Kitt S, Selfridge-Thomas J, Proehl J et al, editors: *Emergency nursing: a physiologic and clinical perspective,* ed 2, Philadelphia, 1995, WB Saunders.
4. Centers for Disease Control: Air-bag—associated fatal injuries to infants and children riding in front passenger seats—United States, *MMWR* 44(45):845, 1995.
5. Chadwick D, Chin S, Salerno C et al: Deaths from falls in children: how far is fatal? *J Trauma* 31(10):1353, 1991.
6. Chameides L, Hazinski M: *Textbook of pediatric advanced life support,* Dallas, 1994, American Heart Association, American Academy of Pediatrics.
7. Chiaviello C, Christoph R, Bond G: Infant walker-related injuries: a prospective study of severity and incidence, *Pediatrics* 93(6):974, 1994.
8. Chiaviello C, Christoph R, Bond G: Stairway-related injuries in children, *Pediatrics* 94(5):679, 1994.
9. Clemence B, Hogue B, Schenkel K et al: The comparison of tympanic and rectal temperatures in moderately and severely injured children, Unpublished manuscript, 1996.
10. Committee on Injury and Poison Prevention: Children in pickup trucks, *Pediatrics* 88(2):393, 1991.
11. Committee on Injury and Poison Prevention: Firearm injuries affecting the pediatric population, *Pediatrics* 89(4):788, 1992.
12. Committee on Injury and Poison Prevention: Skateboard injuries, *Pediatrics* 85(4):612, 1995.
13. Corriere J: Urinary tract injuries. In Ford EG, Andrassy RJ, editors: *Pediatric trauma,* Philadelphia, 1994, WB Saunders.
14. Davis H: Child abuse and neglect. In Zitelli B, Davis H, editors: *Atlas of pediatric physical diagnosis,* ed 2, St. Louis, 1991, Mosby.
15. Division of Injury Control, Center for Environmental Health and Injury Control, Centers for Disease Control: Childhood injuries in the United States, *Am J Dis Child* 144:627, 1990.
16. Fernandez L, Radhakrishnan J, Gordon R et al: Thoracic BB injuries in pediatric patients, *J Trauma* 38(3):384, 1995.
17. Goldbloom R: Halifax and the precipitate birth of pediatric surgery, *Pediatrics* 77(5):764, 1986.
18. Goldstein B, Powers K: Head trauma in children, *Pediatr Rev* 15(6):213, 1994.
19. Grabb P, Pang D: Magnetic resonance imaging in the evaluation of spinal cord injury without radiographic abnormality in children, *Neurosurg* 35(3):406, 1994.
20. Graham C, Kittredge D, Stuemky J: Injuries associated with child safety seat misuse, *Pediatr Emerg Care* 8(6):351, 1992.
21. Greenspan A, MacKenzie E: Functional outcome after pediatric head injury, *Pediatrics* 94:425, 1994.
22. Guidelines for cardiopulmonary resuscitation and emergency cardiac care, *JAMA* 268(16):2262-2275, 1992.
23. Guyer B, Ellers B: Childhood injuries in the United States, *Am J Dis Child* 144:649, 1990.
24. Hall J, Reyes H, Meller J et al: The new epidemic in children: penetrating injuries, *J Trauma* 39(3):487, 1995.
25. Halpern J: Mechanisms and patterns of trauma, *J Emerg Nurs* 15:380, 1989.
26. Harlow K, Ford E: Abdominal injury. In Ford EG, Andrassy RJ, editors: *Pediatric trauma,* Philadelphia, 1994, WB Saunders.
27. Holinger P: The causes, impact, and preventability of childhood injuries in the United States: childhood suicide in the United States, *Am J Dis Child* 144:670, 1990.
28. Hoover D, Belinger M: Genitourinary trauma. In Ehrlich F, Heldrich F, Tepas J, editors: *Pediatric emergency medicine,* Rockville, Md, 1987, Aspen.
29. Horowitz JR, Andrassy RJ: Considerations unique to children. In Ford EG, Andrassy RJ, editors: *Pediatric trauma,* Philadelphia, 1994, WB Saunders.
30. Jaufmann B: Central nervous system injuries. In Ford E, Andrassy R, editors: *Pediatric trauma: initial assessment and management,* Philadelphia, 1994, WB Saunders.
31. Johnston C, Rivara F, Soderberg R: Children in car crashes: analysis of data for injury and use of restraints, *Pediatrics* 93(6):960, 1994.

32. Lang S: Procedures involving the neurological system. In Bernardo L, Bove M, editors: *Pediatric emergency nursing procedures,* Boston, 1993, Jones & Bartlett.

33. Li G, Baker S, Fowler C et al: Factors related to the presence of head injury in bicycle-related pediatric trauma patients, *J Trauma* 38(6):871, 1995.

34. Lobe T, Gore D, Swischuk L: Urinary tract injuries. In Buntain W, editor: *Management of pediatric trauma care,* Philadelphia, 1995, WB Saunders.

35. Ludwig S, Loiselle J: Anatomy, growth and development: impact on injury. In Eichelberger M, editor: *Pediatric trauma,* St. Louis, 1993, Mosby.

36. Malek M, Chang B, Gallagher S et al: The cost of medical care for injuries to children, *Ann Emerg Med* 20(9):997, 1991.

37. Manley L: Procedures involving the airway. In Bernardo L, Bove M, editors: *Pediatric emergency nursing procedures,* Boston, 1993, Jones & Bartlett.

38. Marsden C, Jackimczyk K: Genitourinary trauma. In Reisdorff E, Roberts M, Wiegenstein J, editors: *Pediatric emergency medicine,* Philadelphia, 1993, WB Saunders.

39. Meropol S, Moscati R, Lillis K et al: Alcohol-related injuries among adolescents in the emergency department, *Ann Emerg Med* 26(2):180, 1995.

40. Mosenthal A, Livingston D, Elcavage J et al: Falls: epidemiology and strategies for prevention, *J Trauma* 38(5):753, 1995.

41. Musemeche C, Barthel M, Cosentino C et al: Pediatric falls from heights, *J Trauma* 31:1347, 1991.

42. Nakayama D: *Pediatric surgery: a color atlas,* Philadelphia, 1991, Lippincott.

43. Nakayama D, Wagner T, Venkataraman S et al: The use of drugs in emergency airway management in pediatric trauma, *Ann Surg* 216(2):205, 1992.

44. National Center for Statistics and Analysis, National Highway Traffic Safety Administration: *National occupant protection use survey: controlled intersection study,* Research note, Washington, DC, May 1995, US Department of Transportation, National Highway Traffic Safety Administration.

45. Neudstadt J: Pediatric skeletal injuries, *Trauma Q* 8(3):11-21, 1992.

46. O'Connor K, Gribbons M: Pediatric renal injuries, *Trauma Q* 8(3):79-90, 1992.

47. Olney B, Toby E: Musculoskeletal injuries. In Buntain W, editor: *Management of pediatric trauma care,* Philadelphia, 1995, WB Saunders.

48. Pang D, Pollack I: Spinal cord injury without radiographic abnormality in children—the SCIWORA syndrome, *J Trauma* 2(9):654, 1989.

49. Pang D, Wilberger J: Spinal cord injury without radiographic abnormalities in children, *J Neurosurg* 57:1114, 1982.

50. Phelan A: Musculoskeletal trauma. In Kelley SJ, editor: *Pediatric emergency nursing,* ed 2, Norwalk, Conn, 1994, Appleton & Lange.

51. Pollack I, Pang D: Spinal cord injury without radiographic abnormality (SCIWORA). In Pang D, editor: *Disorders of the pediatric spine,* New York, 1995, Raven Press.

52. Ray L, Yuwiler J: *Child and adolescent fatal injury databook,* San Diego, 1994, Children's Safety Network.

53. Reynolds M: Pulmonary, esophageal, and diaphragmatic injuries. In Buntain W, editor: *Management of pediatric trauma care,* Philadelphia, 1995, WB Saunders.

54. Ritchie J, Caty S, Ellerton M: Coping behaviors of hospitalized preschool children, *Matern Child Nurs J* 17:153, 1988.

55. Roberts I, Norton R, Jackson R: Driveway-related child pedestrian injuries: a case-control study, *Pediatrics* 95(3):405, 1995.

56. Roberts S, Holder T, Ashcraft K: Cardiac and major thoracic vascular injuries. In Buntain W, editor: *Management of pediatric trauma care,* Philadelphia, 1995, WB Saunders.

57. Schafermeyer R: Pediatric trauma, *Emerg Med Clin North Am* 11(1):187, 1993.

58. Schoettle B: Car seat update, *J Pediatr Health Care* 5(3):160, 1991.

59. Scully T, Luerssen T: Spinal cord injuries. In Buntain W, editor: *Management of pediatric trauma care,* Philadelphia, 1995, WB Saunders.

60. Senturia Y, Christoffel K, Donovan M: Children's household exposure to guns: a pediatric practice-based survey, *Pediatrics* 93(3):469, 1994.

61. Soud T, Pieper P, Hazinski M: Pediatric trauma. In Hazinski M, editor: *Nursing care of the critically-ill child,* ed 2, St. Louis, 1992, Mosby.

62. Strange GR, Ahrens W, Lelyveld S et al: *Pediatric emergency medicine: a comprehensive study guide,* New York, 1996, McGraw-Hill.

63. Stylianos S, Harris B: The history of pediatric trauma care. In Buntain W, editor: *Management of pediatric trauma care,* Philadelphia, 1995, WB Saunders.

64. Templeton J: Mechanisms of injury: biomechanics. In Eichelberger M, editor: *Pediatric trauma,* St. Louis, 1993, Mosby.

65. Tepas J: Abdominal injury. In Ehrlich F, Heldrich F, Tepas J, editors: *Pediatric emergency medicine,* Rockville, Md, 1987, Aspen.

66. Tepas J: Hemorrhagic shock in the child, *Trauma Q* 8(3):69, 1992.

67. Todres I: Pediatric airway control and ventilation (part 2), *Ann Emerg Med* 22(2):440, 1993.

68. Vaughan VC, Litt IF: Developmental pediatrics. In Behrman R, Vaughan V, editors: *Nelson textbook of pediatrics,* ed 15, Philadelphia, 1996, WB Saunders.

69. Ward J: Craniocerebral injuries. In Buntain W, editor: *Management of pediatric trauma care,* Philadelphia, 1995, WB Saunders.

70. Ward T, Davis H, Hanley E: Orthopedics. In Zitelli B, Davis H, editors: *Atlas of pediatric physical diagnosis,* ed 2, St. Louis, 1991, Mosby.

71. Webster D, Wilson M: Gun violence among youth and the pediatrician's role in primary prevention, *Pediatrics* 94:617, 1994.

72. Widner-Kolberg M: Immobilizing children in car seats—why, when, and how, *J Emerg Nurs* 17(6):427, 1991.

73. Yurt: Triage, initial assessment, and early treatment of the pediatric trauma patient, *Pediatr Clin North Am* 39(5):1083, 1992.

74. Zavoski R, Lapidus G, Lerer T et al: A population-based study of severe firearm injury among children and youth, *Pediatrics* 96(2):278, 1995.

75. Ziegler M: Major trauma. In Fleisher G, Ludwig S, editors: *Textbook of pediatric emergency medicine,* ed 2, Baltimore, 1988, Williams & Wilkins.

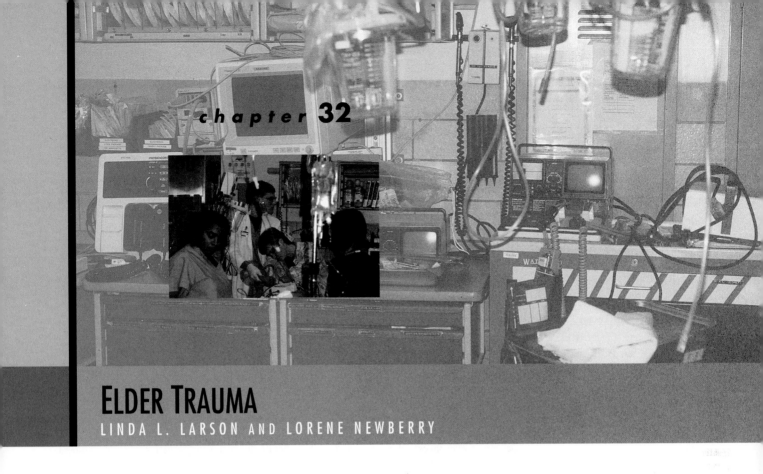

chapter 32

ELDER TRAUMA

LINDA L. LARSON AND LORENE NEWBERRY

Elders or geriatrics are individuals over age 65,[8] a definition that follows government statistics and matches when Medicare benefits begin. In 1991, 31.8 million people or 12.6% of the U.S. population were over age 65.[11] Factors that contribute to the expanding elder population include increasing life expectancy and improved health care.

More individuals live to age 65; the number of individuals between 75 and 84 years of age is currently 13 times greater than in 1900. The number of individuals 85 years of age and older is 24 times greater than in the same period and is the fastest-growing segment of the population today. Birthday celebrations for centenarians are increasingly common. Women in every age group have a lower probability of dying than men. Three quarters of men over 65 are still married, whereas more than half of older women are widows.

PHYSIOLOGIC CHANGES

Aging is progressive, predictable, and inevitable—evolution of life from birth until death. Progressive deterioration of hemostatic control mechanisms causes slower reactions to stimuli and longer recovery periods. Organ reserves diminish to the point that any stress causes more extensive injury with less ability to compensate.

Nervous System

The brain shrinks with age but the dura adheres tightly to the skull.[7] Progressive loss of brain volume occurs as the brain shrinks, and cerebrospinal fluid (CSF) production decreases. Consequently, space around the brain increases, which may decrease incidence of contusions. However, stretching of dural connections increases the risk of bleeding.[2] The brain is also at greater risk for ricochet or coup-contrecoup injuries due to increased freedom of movement within the cranial vault.

Age-related changes in the autonomic nervous system, primarily the baroreflex, affect the elder person's ability to respond to injury. The problem may lie in the baroreceptor or α-adrenergic and/or β-adrenergic response. Normally the baroreflex increases peripheral vascular resistance, heart rate, blood pressure, and ultimately, cardiac output. In elders, heart rate and blood pressure do not always increase with stimulation of the baroreflex.

Thermoregulation decreases in elders, which increases their risk for hypothermia and hyperthermia. Decrease in lean body mass, decreased muscle activity, less efficient shivering, and 50% reduction in glucose-induced thermogenesis make maintenance of normal body temperature difficult. Problems in thermoregulation are associated with inability to regulate body fluid. Vasopressin secretion may be inhibited by inadequate release of stimulating hormones. The elderly also experience less thirst with water deprivation, so water consumption may not be adequate. Table 32-1 summarizes variances in assessment of the nervous system in older patients.

Respiratory System

Healthy elderly patients also experience increased calcification of the trachea, decreased elasticity, and stiffening of

Table 32-1	Gerontologic Differences in Assessment: Nervous System	
Component	Changes	Differences in assessment findings
Central nervous system		
Brain	Reduction in cerebral blood flow and metabolism	Alterations in selected mental functioning
	Decrease in efficiency of temperature-regulating mechanism	Decrease in body temperature, impairment of ability to adapt to environmental temperature
	Decrease in neurotransmitter content, disruption in integration as result of loss of neurons	Repetitive movements, tremors
	Decrease in oxygen supply, changes in basal ganglia caused by vascular changes	Changes in gait and ambulation (e.g., extrapyramidal, parkinson-like gait); diminished kinesthetic sense
Peripheral nervous system		
Cranial and spinal nerves	Loss of myelin and decrease in conduction time in some nerves	Decrease in reaction time in specific nerves
	Cellular degeneration, death of neurons	Decrease in speed and intensity of neuronal reflexes
Functional divisions		
Motor	Decrease in muscle bulk	Diminished strength and agility
	Decrease in electrical activity	Decrease in reactions and movement time
Sensory	Decrease in sensory receptors caused by degenerative changes and involution of fine corpuscles of nerve endings	Diminished sense of touch; inability to localize stimuli; decrease in appreciation of touch, temperature, and peripheral vibrations
	Decrease in electrical activity	Slowing of or alteration in sensory reception
	Atrophy of taste buds	Signs of malnutrition, weight loss
	Degeneration and loss of fibers in olfactory bulb	Diminished sense of smell
	Degenerative changes in nerve cells in vestibular system of inner ear, cerebellum, and proprioceptive pathways in nervous system	Poor ability to maintain balance, widened gait
Reflexes	Possible decrease in deep tendon reflexes	Below-average reflex score
	Decrease in sensory conduction velocity as result of myelin sheath degeneration	Sluggish reflexes, slowing of reaction time
Reticular formation		
Reticular activating system	Modification of hypothalamic function, reduction in stage IV sleep	Increase in frequency of spontaneous awakening together with tiredness, interrupted sleep, insomnia
Autonomic nervous system		
SNS and PSNS	Morphologic features of ganglia, slowing of ANS responses	Orthostatic hypotension, systolic hypertension

From Lewis SM, Collier IC, Heitkemper MM: *Medical-surgical nursing: assessment and management of clinical problems,* ed 4, St. Louis, 1996, Mosby.
ANS, Autonomic nervous system; *PSNS,* parasympathetic nervous system; *SNS,* sympathetic nervous system.

the rib cage, which decrease pulmonary function.[7] Increased residual lung volume and decreased alveolar surface area lead to slightly elevated PCO_2 levels. The work of breathing is complicated by structural changes in the chest that decrease overall pulmonary reserve and may cause more complications in the injured elder such as atelectasis, pneumonia, or adult respiratory distress syndrome. Table 32-2 identifies age-related differences in assessment of the respiratory system.

Cardiovascular System

Changes in the peripheral vascular system decrease arterial compliance, increase blood pressure, and decrease ventricular filling.[7] There is a 50% decline in ventricular filling from age 20 to 80. Peripheral vascular resistance increases 1% per year. Intracellular calcium levels remain higher for a longer period in the elderly, which changes the action potential and electrical activity of the heart in

Table **32-2**	**Gerontologic Differences in Assessment: Respiratory System**
Changes	Differences in assessment findings
Structure	
↓ Elastic recoil ↓Chest wall compliance ↑ Anteroposterior diameter ↓ Functioning alveoli	Barrel chest appearance; ↓ chest wall movement; ↓ respiratory excursion; ↓ vital capacity; ↑ functional residual capacity; diminished breath sounds particularly at lung bases; ↓ PaO_2 and SaO_2; normal pH and $PaCO_2$
Defense mechanisms	
↓ Cell-mediated immunity ↓ Specific antibodies ↓ Cilia function ↓ Cough force ↓ Alveolar macrophage function	↓ Cough effectiveness; ↓ secretion clearance; ↑ risk of upper respiratory infection, influenza, or pneumonia; respiratory infections may be more severe and last longer
Respiratory control	
↓ Response to hypoxemia ↓ Response to hypercapnia	Greater ↓ in PaO_2 and ↑ in $PaCO_2$ before respiratory rate changes. Significant hypoxemia or hypercapnia may develop from relatively small incidents. Retained secretions, excessive sedation, or positioning that impairs chest expansion may substantially alter PaO_2.

From Lewis SM, Collier IC, Heitkemper MM: *Medical-surgical nursing: assessment and management of clinical problems,* ed 4, St. Louis, 1996, Mosby.

Table **32-3**	**Gerontologic Differences in Assessment: Cardiovascular System**
Changes	Differences in assessment findings
Chest wall	
Senile kyphosis	Altered chest landmarks for palpation, percussion, and auscultation; distant heart sounds
Heart	
Myocardial hypertrophy, increase in collagen and scarring, decrease in elasticity	Decrease in cardiac reserve, slight decrease in HR
Downward displacement	Difficulty in isolating apical pulse
Decrease in CO, HR, SV in response to exercise or stress	Slowed, decreased response to stress; slowed recovery from activity
Cellular aging changes and fibrosis of conduction system	Decrease in amplitude of QRS complex and lengthening of PR, QRS, and QT intervals; left axis deviation; irregular cardiac rhythms
Valvular rigidity from calcification, sclerosis, or fibrosis, impeding complete closure of valves	Systolic murmur (aortic or mitral) possible without indication of cardiovascular pathology
Blood vessels	
Arterial stiffening caused by loss of elastin in arterial walls, thickening of intima of arteries, and progressive fibrosis of media	Elevation in systolic and possibly diastolic BP (e.g., 160/90) possible widened pulse pressures; more pronounced arterial pulses; pedal pulses often not detectable; color and temperature changes in extremities; loss of hair on lower legs
Increase in tortuosity and varicosities of veins	Ulcerated, inflamed, painful, or cordlike varicosities

From Lewis SM, Collier IC, Heitkemper MM: *Medical-surgical nursing: assessment and management of clinical problems,* ed 4, St. Louis, 1996, Mosby.
BP, Blood pressure; *CO,* cardiac output; *HR,* heart rate; *SV,* stroke volume.

relation to mechanical activity. Inotropic response to catecholamines and cardiac glycosides decreases and refractoriness to electrical stimulation increases. Gerontologic differences in cardiovascular assessment are summarized in Table 32-3.

Renal System

Renal perfusion decreases by 50% and renal mass decreases 25% to 30%, mostly in the renal cortex.[7] As the number of nephrons with long Henle's loops into the cortex decreases, glomerular filtration rate decreases and BUN and

Table **32-4** **Gerontologic Differences in Assessment: Urinary System**	
Changes	Differences in assessment findings
Kidney	
Decrease in amount of renal tissue	Less palpable
Decrease in number of nephrons and renal vascular bed; thickened basement membrane of Bowman's capsule and glomeruli	Decrease in creatinine clearance, increase in BUN level
Decrease in function of Henle's loop and tubules	Alterations in drug excretion; nocturia; loss of normal diurnal excretory pattern because of decreased ability to concentrate urine; less concentrated urine
Ureter, bladder, and urethra	
Decrease in elasticity and muscle tone	Palpable bladder after urination because of retention
Weakening of urinary sphincter	Stress incontinence (especially during Valsalva maneuver), dribbling of urine after urination
Decrease in bladder capacity and sensory receptors	Frequency, urgency, nocturia, overflow incontinence
Estrogen deficiency leading to thin, dry vaginal tissue; prostatic enlargement; uninhibited bladder contractions	Stress incontinence, dribbling

From Lewis SM, Collier IC, Heitkemper MM: *Medical-surgical nursing: assessment and management of clinical problems,* ed 4, St. Louis, 1996, Mosby.
BUN, Blood urea nitrogen.

Table **32-5** **Gerontologic Differences in Assessment: Musculoskeletal System**	
Changes	Differences in assessment findings
Muscle	
Decreased number and diameter of muscle cells, replacement of muscle cells by fibrous connective tissue	Decreased muscle strength and bulk, abdominal protrusion, muscle flabbiness
Loss of elasticity in ligaments and cartilage	Decreased fine motor activity, decreased agility
Decrease in oxidate activity from reduction in glycolytic enzymes	Slowed reaction times, slowing of most muscle reflexes, slowing of impulse conduction along motor units, easy fatigability
Joints	
Erosion of articular cartilage, possible direct contact between bone ends	Manifestations of osteoarthritis, joint stiffness, possible crepitation on movement of joints, pain with range-of-motion movements
Overgrowth of bone around joint margins (osteophytes)	Heberden's nodes in fingers (especially in women), limited mobility in affected joints
Loss of water from disks between vertebrae, narrowing of joint vertebral spaces	Loss of height, kyphosis, back pain
Bone	
Decrease in bone mass	Dowager's hump (kyphosis)

From Lewis SM, Collier IC, Heitkemper MM: *Medical-surgical nursing: assessment and management of clinical problems,* ed 4, St. Louis, 1996, Mosby.

creatinine levels increase. Elderly persons also have decreased renin, angiotensin, and aldosterone levels, which ultimately leads to inability to regulate fluid and electrolyte
balance. Table 32-4 describes age-related differences in the
assessment of the urinary system.

Musculoskeletal System

Muscle weight relative to total body weight decreases
with aging. Bone reabsorption increases with decreased
bone remodeling and decreased bone density. Bone loss occurs more rapidly in women than in men. Loss of water content makes cartilaginous structures stiffer and more susceptible to injury. Assessment of the musculoskeletal system in
older patients is addressed in Table 32-5.

Gastrointestinal System

Peristalsis decreases significantly with aging so elders are
prone to constipation.[1] Decreased blood flow to the rectum
contributes to this problem and may affect the healing of
rectal injuries. Diminished intestinal enzymes affect digestion and electrolyte balance. Changes in appetite can lead to
poor eating habits and malnutrition, which affect wound

healing. Assessment findings related to aging and the gastrointestinal system are listed in Table 32-6.

Integumentary System

Dermal thickness decreases as much as 20% with age[5]
with significant loss of vascularity and proliferative ability.
Dermatologic changes affect wound healing and thermoregulation and decrease the barrier against bacterial invasion.
Additional information on age-related changes in the integumentary system is presented in Table 32-7.

EPIDEMIOLOGY OF TRAUMA

"Trauma is the seventh leading cause of death in persons
over 65 years of age . . ."[2] Etiology includes motor vehicle
collisions, falls, burns, and penetrating trauma. Motor vehicle collisions involving the elderly are more likely to occur
when split-second decisions or reactions to a specific hazard
are required, for example, at intersections, rights of way, or
traffic signs. Box 32-1 identifies factors that may play a role
in these crashes.

Elderly persons have one of the highest rates for pedestrian
accidents, representing 46% of all pedestrian fatalities.[4]

Table 32-6 Gerontologic Differences in Assessment: Gastrointestinal System

Changes	Differences in assessment findings
Mouth	
Loss of teeth	Presence of dentures, difficulty chewing
Decreased taste buds, decreased sense of smell	Diminished sense of taste (especially salty and sweet)
Decreased volume of saliva	Dry oral mucosa
Atrophy of gingival tissue	Poor-fitting dentures
Esophagus	
Decreased tone and motility	Complaints of pyrosis (heartburn), dysphagia, eructation
Abdominal wall	
Thinner and less taut	More visible peristalsis, easier palpation of organs
Decrease in number and sensitivity of sensory receptors	Less sensitivity to surface pain
Stomach	
Decreased acid secretion, atrophy of gastric mucosa, hypochlorhydria	Food intolerances, signs of anemia as result of vitamin B_{12} malabsorption
Small intestines	
Decreased secretion of most digestive enzymes, decreased motility	Complaints of indigestion
Liver	
Increased size and lowered position	Easier palpation
Large intestine, anus, rectum	
Decreased anal sphincter tone and nerve supply to rectal area	Fecal incontinence
Decreased muscular tone, decreased motility	Flatulence, abdominal distention, relaxed perineal musculature
Increase in transit time	Constipation, fecal impaction

From Lewis SM, Collier IC, Heitkemper MM: *Medical-surgical nursing: assessment and management of clinical problems,* ed 4, St. Louis, 1996, Mosby.

Table 32-7	**Gerontologic Differences in Assessment: Integumentary System**
Changes	**Differences in assessment findings**

Skin

Decreased subcutaneous fat, muscle laxity, degeneration of elastic fibers, collagen stiffening	Increased wrinkling, sagging breasts and abdomen, redundant flesh around eyes, slowness of skin to flatten when pinched together (tenting)
Decreased extracellular water, surface lipids, and sebaceous gland activity	Dry, flaking skin with possible signs of excoriation caused by pruritus
Less active apocrine and sebaceous gland activity	Dry skin with minimal to no perspiration
Increased capillary fragility and permeability	Evidence of bruising
Increased melanocytes in basal layer with pigment accumulation	Senile lentigines on face and back of hands
Diminished blood supply	Decrease in rosy appearance of skin and mucous membranes; cool to touch; diminished awareness of pain, touch, temperature, and peripheral vibration
Decrease in proliferative capacity	Diminished rate of wound healing

Hair

Decreased melanin and melanocytes	Graying hair
Decreased oil	Dry, coarse hair; scaly scalp
Decrease in density of hair follicles	Thinning and loss of hair; loss of hair in outer one half or one third of eyebrow
Cumulative androgen effect; decreasing estrogen levels	Facial hirsutism; baldness

Nails

Decreased peripheral blood supply	Thick, brittle nails with diminished growth
Increased keratin	Ridging
Decreased circulation	Prolonged return of blood to nails on blanching

From Lewis SM, Collier IC, Heitkemper MM: *Medical-surgical nursing: assessment and management of clinical problems,* ed 4, St. Louis, 1996, Mosby.

Box 32-1	**Potential Factors in Motor Vehicle Crashes Involving Elderly Persons**

Slowed reaction time
Decreased peripheral vision
Impaired hearing
Loss of motor strength
Arthritis
Dementia
Attention deficits
Concurrent medical conditions
Prescription drugs

Auto-pedestrian collisions may result from decreased mobility, diminished vision, hearing loss, and slowed reaction times. Skeletal changes caused by osteoporosis limit upward gaze and can make visualization of traffic lights or signs difficult.[2] In the United States, crossing time for intersection lights is set at a standard 4 ft/sec.

Mobility may be one of the most significant problems facing the elderly. Limited mobility is a major factor in increased incidence of falls and injury. One in three elderly persons falls each year.[9,10] Five percent of falls in institutionalized or community-dwelling adults cause fractures, an additional 5% to 10% cause restricted activity for days or weeks due to hematomas, sprains, or dislocations. Up to 25% of all elders who have previously fallen admit to restricting their activities due to fear of additional falls and injury. Factors leading to falls in the elderly may be environmental or physiologic (Box 32-2). The elderly also have an increased risk for head injury, fractured mandibles, and ruptured globes. Loss of teeth leads to mandibular instability and increased incidence of fractures. Thinning of the limbus increases the risk for globe rupture.

Decreased reaction time, preexisting health problems, and altered sense of hearing, vision, and smell place elders at greater risk for burn injuries. Elderly persons do not tolerate burn injuries as well as younger patients because of diminished cardiac, pulmonary, and metabolic reserves. Mortality is reported between 33% and 40%, depending on the percent of body surface involved. A general rule of thumb in elderly burn patients is that the percent of body surface area burned is roughly equivalent to mortality.

Other areas of injury in the elderly are penetrating trauma and abuse. Mortality from penetrating injuries is higher in

---

Box **32-2**	**Factors That Contribute to Falls in the Elderly**

Environmental	**Physiologic**
Throw rugs	Musculoskeletal weakness
Staircases	Arthritis
Changes in floor surface	Poor balance
Furniture out of place	Impaired proprioception
Animals	Syncope
Lack of assist devices, i.e.,	Dizziness
handrails, walkers, canes	Vertigo
	Hypoglycemia
	Postural hypotension
	Anemia
	Medications

Box **32-3**

NURSING DIAGNOSES FOR THE ELDERLY TRAUMA PATIENT

Fluid volume deficit
Fluid volume excess
Impaired gas exchange
Decreased cardiac output
Ineffective breathing pattern
Anxiety
Fear

---

the elderly patient than in younger age groups, 17.3% compared to 4.7%.[3] Increased mortality is the result of diminished patient reserves and increased incidence of complication. Elderly suicide patients tend to use guns more often than substance ingestion, so they are usually more successful in their attempts. Increased violence across the country may lead to an increased number of elderly patients with penetrating trauma. Elder abuse has also increased over the past decade. Refer to Chapter 53 for more discussion on this disturbing health problem.

INJURIES

Injuries in the elderly are similar to injuries in younger patients. Differences relate to frequency of specific injuries and absence of significant hemodynamic changes in response to blood loss. Physiologic changes of aging and medications such as β-blockers affect elders' ability to respond to blood loss. Elder trauma patients can be in profound cardiogenic shock with minimal changes in vital signs. Some centers suggest early invasive hemodynamic monitoring for the severely injured elder. Fluid should be administered cautiously because of potential fluid overload and decreased cardiac reserve, which can lead to pulmonary edema.

The most common injury in the elderly patient is fractures. With decreased bone density, less stress is required to break bones. Older patients are particularly prone to long-bone fractures resulting from osteoporosis. Early stabilization is recommended to decrease potential pulmonary complications. Significant retroperitoneal bleeding can occur with minor pelvic or hip fractures. Careful assessment and monitoring are essential to minimize associated complications.

Delayed wound healing is a problem in elderly patients with lacerations, surgical incisions, or burn injuries. Geriatric patients are at risk for infectious complications due to changes in skin and the immune system. Tetanus prophylaxis is not always adequate in the elderly. Elderly women in rural areas, particularly those who never worked outside the

home, may have never received or completed tetanus immunization. Elderly men are more likely to have served in the military, where they would have received tetanus immunization.

SUMMARY

The elderly trauma patient presents an assessment challenge for the emergency nurse. Knowledge of physiologic changes of aging is essential for management of these patients. Geriatric patients also require awareness of their worth as individuals and their right to make their own health care decisions. Box 32-3 summarizes potential nursing diagnoses for the elderly trauma patient.

REFERENCES

1. Beck JC, editor: *Geriatric review syllabus: a core curriculum in geriatric medicine,* New York, 1991, American Geriatrics Society.
2. Feliciano DV, Moore EE, Mattox KL: *Trauma,* ed 3, Stamford, Conn, 1996, Appleton & Lange.
3. Finelli F, Jonsson J, Champion HR et al: A case controlled study of major trauma in geriatric patients, *J Trauma* 29:541, 1989.
4. Jones J, Dougherty J, Schelble D et al: Emergency department protocol for the diagnosis and evaluation of geriatric abuse, *Ann Emerg Med* 17:1006, 1988.
5. Kaminer MS, Gilchrest BA: Aging of the skin. In Hazzard WR et al, editors: *Principles of geriatric medicine and gerontology,* New York, 1994, McGraw-Hill.
6. Lewis SM, Collier IC, Heitkemper MM: *Medical-surgical nursing: assessment and management of clinical problems,* ed 4, St Louis, 1996, Mosby.
7. McCance KL, Huether SE: *Pathophysiology: the biologic basis for disease in adults and children,* ed 2, St Louis, 1994, Mosby.
8. Reuben DB, Yoshikawa TT, Besdine RW, editors: *Geriatric review syllabus supplement: a core curriculum in geriatric medicine,* New York, 1993, American Geriatrics Society.
9. Sattin RW, Lambert-Huber DA, DeVito CA et al: The incidence of fall injury events among the elderly in a defined population, *Am J Epidemiol* 131:1028, 1990.
10. Tinnetti ME, Speechley M, Ginter SF: Risk factors for falls among elderly persons living in the community, *N Engl J Med* 319:1701, 1988.
11. US Senate Special Committee on Aging, American Association of Retired Persons, Federal Council on Aging, and US Administration on Aging: *Aging America, trends and projections,* FCOA Pub No 91-28001, Washington, DC, 1991, US Department of Health and Human Services.

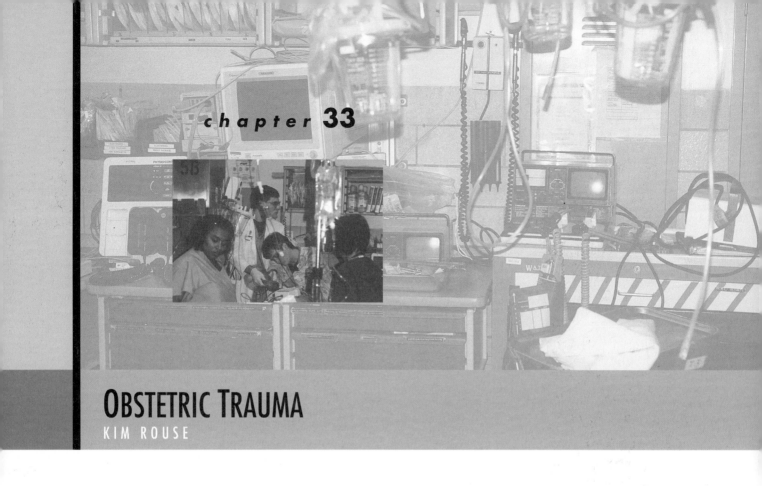

chapter 33

OBSTETRIC TRAUMA

KIM ROUSE

Actual incidence of obstetric trauma is unknown, but trauma has been estimated to occur in 6% to 7% of all pregnancies.[1,36] Most obstetric trauma involves minor injury,[26] with falls the most common cause.[12,20] Significant trauma is reported in 1 of 12 pregnant women. Life-threatening injuries that require intensive care have been estimated in three to four gravid patients per 1000 deliveries.[4,26] Motor vehicle collisions (MVCs) are the leading cause of nonobstetric death for women during their reproductive years. Head injury and hemorrhagic shock account for most maternal deaths from trauma.[44]

Fetal death is most often caused by maternal death but can occur after minimal maternal injury.[37] Abruptio placentae and maternal shock are other common causes of fetal demise.

The leading mechanisms of obstetric trauma are blunt and penetrating injuries. Blunt injuries occur secondary to MVCs, falls, and assaults. Literature reports a 5.5% to 17% incidence of physical abuse during pregnancy, with severity and frequency on the increase.[31] Penetrating injuries include gunshot wounds and stab wounds.

ANATOMY AND PHYSIOLOGY

Initial assessment and management of the pregnant trauma patient is often provided by prehospital and emergency personnel. Optimal outcome for mother and fetus is based on sound knowledge of maternal anatomy and physiology, and implications for interventions.

Uterine

The uterus grows from 7 cm and 70 g to a 36-cm and 1100-g walled organ. As the uterus grows, the wall becomes thinner. Until 12 weeks of pregnancy, the uterus remains a small self-contained intrapelvic organ, protected from abdominal injury by the bony pelvis. The uterus becomes an intraabdominal organ as it enlarges and ascends, encroaching on the peritoneal cavity and confining the intestines to the upper abdomen. Figure 33-1 shows uterine size for various gestation periods. During the second trimester, the uterus is susceptible to abdominal injury, while the fetus remains small and relatively cushioned by large amounts of amniotic fluid. By the third trimester, the uterus is large and thin walled. During the last 2 to 8 weeks of gestation, the fetus descends and the fetal head engages in the pelvis. The fetus occupies most of the space as the head becomes fixed in the pelvis.[30] Maternal pelvic fractures during this period are frequently associated with fetal skull fractures and intracranial hemorrhage.

Uterine blood flow increases from 60 ml/min to 600 ml/min during the third trimester. Total maternal circulating blood volume passes through the uterus approximately every 8 to 11 minutes.[34] Uterine blood flow has no autoregulation and depends solely on maternal perfusion pressure; therefore uterine injury may be a major source of blood loss.

By the third trimester, the uterus and placenta have reached maximum vasodilation and cannot increase blood flow in response to decreased perfusion. During maternal

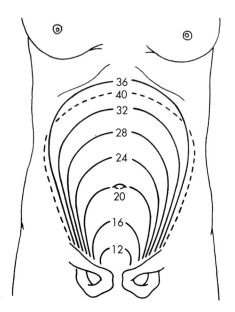

Figure **33-1** Uterine size at various weeks of gestation. *(From Buchsbaum HJ, editor:* Trauma in pregnancy, *Philadelphia, 1979, WB Saunders.)*

stress or injury, catecholamines are released by the sympathetic nervous system. Potent α-adrenergic properties of catecholamines cause marked uteroplacental constriction and decreased perfusion, which lead to fetal distress.

Cardiovascular

Anatomically, the heart is elevated and rotated forward by the ascending diaphragm pushed up by the enlarging uterus, causing a 15-degree left axis deviation that can lead to electrical changes considered normal changes of pregnancy. The electrocardiogram may show a flattened or inverted T wave in lead III and Q waves in III and aV$_F$. Ectopic beats are also common during pregnancy.

Cardiovascular physiology is profoundly altered during pregnancy. Maternal blood volume increases by the tenth week of gestation, increases 40% to 50% by the twenty-eighth week, and remains at that level until delivery. Uterine blood flow increases by 600 ml/min by the end of pregnancy. Increased blood flow and volume increase maternal cardiac output by 1 to 1.5 L/min. At 20 weeks' gestation or more, cardiac output (CO) may be decreased by compression of the vena cava and aorta by the fetus when the mother is in a supine position. This event is called inferior vena cava syndrome or supine hypotensive syndrome. The uterus at 20 weeks has grown and risen to the level of the inferior vena cava. Compression of the vena cava by the uterus may decrease CO by 28% and systolic blood pressure (BP) by 30 mm Hg. Sequestering blood in the venous system may decrease perfusion to the uterus. Displacing the gravid uterus to the left by placing the pregnant patient in the left lateral decubitus position can release aortocaval compression.

When spinal injury is suspected, maintain spinal immobilization and tilt the backboard 15 degrees or manually displace the uterus to the left.

Resting heart rate increases until the second trimester and remains 10 to 20 beats per minute above baseline. Systolic and diastolic pressures decrease in the first trimester and level off during the second trimester. A decrease of 15 mm Hg for systolic and diastolic pressure is normal. A gradual increase to prepregnant levels occurs at the end of the third trimester.[39]

Hemodynamic measures may be misleading. Signs of shock, that is, tachycardia and hypotension may be normal physiologic changes of pregnancy. Conversely, normal findings may mask an underlying shock state. Hypervolemia of pregnancy enables a woman to tolerate acute blood loss up to 10% to 20% or gradual loss of 35% (1500 ml) without a change in vital signs.[7]

Catecholamine release caused by maternal hypovolemia vasoconstricts peripheral and uterine vascular beds, shunting blood to vital maternal organs. A 20% reduction of uterine blood flow can occur without obvious change in maternal blood pressure. Uterine hypoperfusion and fetal hypoxia may occur before evidence of maternal shock. Fetal mortality up to 85% has been associated with maternal shock.[9]

Gravid women in shock may not have the cool, clammy skin typical of shock because of maternal vasodilation in the first and second trimester. Vasoconstriction in response to stress occurs predominately in the third trimester.[29]

Decreased central venous pressure (CVP) may be normal during pregnancy. Serial CVP readings rather than isolated readings are valuable in measuring a trend of response to fluid resuscitation.[7] Adequate and appropriate fluid delivery is necessary to restore maternal and uteroplacental perfusion. Lactated Ringer's is the recommended fluid of choice.[7] Blood transfusions should be given with Rh-compatible blood. In cases of impending shock, only O negative or type specific blood is acceptable. Vasopressors are generally discouraged in initial management of traumatic shock with the exception of cardiogenic shock in cardiac contusion and neurogenic shock in spinal cord injury.[7]

Hematologic

Dilutional anemia in pregnancy is caused by the disproportional increase of plasma volume when compared to erythrocyte volume. Plasma volume increases by 45% to 50% whereas red blood cell (RBC) mass increases only 18% to 30%. Dilutional states can reduce hematocrit level from 31% to 35% and hemoglobin to 11.0 g, changes termed "physiological anemia of pregnancy."[34]

Platelet levels may be normal or slightly decreased. Physiologic leukocytosis occurs during the second and third trimester. An increase in white blood cells (WBC) of 18,000 may occur by term and rise even higher during stress or labor. Sedimentation rate also increases during pregnancy.

Cautious interpretation of lab values is required; increased levels may mask or falsely indicate an infectious process.

Fibrinogen levels start to rise in the third month and double by term. Normal levels may indicate disseminated intravascular coagulapathy (DIC). An increase in clotting factors VII, VIII, IX, and X produces hypercoagulability and the potential for thromboembolic risk, that is, deep vein thrombosis or pulmonary embolism, especially when the gravid woman is inactive.

Pulmonary

Significant anatomic and physiologic alterations occur in the pulmonary system during pregnancy. Capillary engorgement of the mucosal lining of the respiratory tract predisposes gravid women to nosebleeds and airway obstruction. Gentle suction and gentle intubation may be necessary to control epistaxis and prevent airway compromise.

The diaphragm elevates as the uterus enlarges, up to 4 cm elevation with associated flaring of the ribs.[34] During the third trimester, chest tubes, when needed, should be inserted in the third or fourth intercostal space to avoid diaphragm injury.[11,23]

Diaphragm elevation reduces pulmonary functional reserve capacity by 20% at the end of pregnancy. Reduction is associated with increased maternal oxygen consumption and a diminished oxygen reserve. Maternal tidal volume and minute ventilations increase 30% to 40% by late pregnancy.[39,40] Respiratory rates increase by 15%. Arterial $PaCO_2$ decreases to approximately 30 mm Hg by the end of the second trimester and remains at this level until delivery. PaO_2 levels increase to 101 to 104 mm Hg.[14]

The maternal respiratory center is especially sensitive to minute changes in $PaCO_2$ levels. Partially compensated respiratory alkalosis occurs during pregnancy, although a normal serum pH is maintained by increased renal excretion of bicarbonate.[39] Diminished maternal oxygen reserve makes the gravid uterus vulnerable to hypoxia. Maternal hypoxia affects fetal oxygenation, so fetal compromise may occur. Fetal heart rate changes are frequently the first indicator of maternal hypoxia. Maternal trauma requires measurement of arterial blood gas (ABG) levels to determine hypoxia and acidosis.[7] Supplemental oxygen at 100% is essential until maternal and fetal hypoxia is ruled out or resolved.

Gastrointestinal

Various anatomic and physiologic gastrointestinal (GI) changes occur during pregnancy. The small bowel is pushed up by the uterus into the upper abdomen and the large bowel moves posteriorly. Diminished bowel sounds may be a normal finding in pregnancy or indicate intraperitoneal injury. Stretching of the abdominal wall by uterine growth can impair maternal sensitivity to peritoneal irritation, so muscle guarding, rigidity, or rebound tenderness may be dulled or absent.

Progesterone has a smooth-muscle effect on the GI tract, reducing motility and tone while relaxing the gastric sphincter. Gastric emptying is delayed and gastroesophageal reflux occurs frequently, increasing the risk of aspiration. Assume all gravid trauma patients have a full stomach, so a nasogastric tube should be promptly inserted to minimize risk of aspiration.

Genitourinary

Maternal susceptibility to traumatic bladder injury increases as the bladder moves from a pelvic organ to an intraabdominal position by 12 weeks' gestation.[7] Urinary frequency increases in the third trimester from bladder compression by the uterus. Dilation of the ureters (right greater than left), renal calyces, and pelvis from compression by the ovarian plexus may result in urinary stasis.[40] Glomerular filtration rate increases by approximately 30% and blood urea nitrogen (BUN) and creatinine decrease.

Musculoskeletal

The pelvis becomes more flexible during pregnancy in preparation for fetal delivery. Hormonal changes loosen ligaments of the symphysis pubis and sacroiliac joints. By 7 months' gestation, there is considerable widening of the pelvis.[29] An unsteady gait caused by the widening pelvis and a heavy abdomen predisposes the gravid female to falls.

Neurologic

Changes in the central nervous system (CNS) related to pregnancy are abnormal findings. Preeclampsia occurs after 20 to 24 weeks' gestation and is characterized by hypertension, proteinuria, and edema. CNS irritability can lead to eclampsia, which is marked by seizure activity. Hypoxia from seizure activity places the mother and fetus at risk.[29] Altered mentation, seizures, and hypertension may also indicate head injury[7]; therefore meticulous neurologic assessment of the pregnant trauma patient is essential.

Endocrine

The pituitary gland doubles in size and weight by term and requires a greater blood supply. Hypoperfusion causes ischemia and can lead to pituitary necrosis. Hemorrhage within the gland may occur with reperfusion. Sheehan's syndrome, necrosis of the anterior pituitary gland, produces long-term complications related to decreased hormone levels. Aggressive and rapid treatment of shock are required to prevent these serious complications.

PATIENT ASSESSMENT

Anatomic and physiologic changes during pregnancy can obscure the mother's response to trauma. Maternal compensatory mechanisms preserve vital maternal functions at the expense of the fetus. Fetal survival depends on adequate gas exchange and uterine perfusion. Rapid and efficient assessment and correct intervention of abnormalities provide optimal maternal-fetal outcome.

Maintenance of cervical spine immobilization is necessary when neck injury is suspected until the neck is clinically and radiographically cleared. A lateral backboard tilt of 15 degrees maintains immobilization and deflects the uterus from the vena cava. Repositioning the airway by chin-tilt or jaw-thrust maneuvers may be enough to establish patency and should not interfere with cervical immobilization. Use oral or nasal airways because the mother is predisposed to nasopharyngeal bleeding that may lead to further obstruction. Early orotracheal or nasotracheal intubation prevents further trauma or obstruction.

All trauma patients need supplemental oxygen. Injury can exacerbate existing pulmonary alterations related to pregnancy such as decreased pulmonary reserve, increase maternal oxygen consumption, and compromise the mother and fetus. Oxygen is critical for fetal survival because of fetal inability to tolerate hypoxia.

Assessment and intervention for external and internal hemorrhage is necessary to ensure maternal-fetal survival. Apply direct pressure to sites of uncontrolled external bleeding. The mother can lose 1500 ml of blood before signs of shock are evident. Retroperitoneal and uteroplacental injury can be sources of occult blood loss. Venous access with two large-bore catheters and aggressive fluid volume replacement optimize maternal blood volume and oxygen-carrying capacity.[7] Initiate blood replacement with Rh-compatible blood if crystalloids do not stabilize circulatory status. Aortocaval compression may occur by 20 weeks' gestation; displacing the uterus to the left may increase cardiac output by 20%.

Insertion of an arterial line and/or central venous line provides accurate monitoring of circulation and the response to treatment and may be used in some centers. Assessment of neurologic defects should include consideration of eclampsia.

Secondary assessment involves identification of other injuries. A thorough history includes standard trauma history and obstetric history, including last menstrual period (LMP), expected date of confinement (EDC), parity, problems and complications of current or past pregnancies, presence of uterine contractions, and current fetal activity.[6] Specific obstetric assessment in the secondary survey includes the abdomen, uterus, and fetus.

Abdomen

The abdomen may be difficult to assess because of blunted signs of intraperitoneal irritation. Severe occult intraabdominal hemorrhage may occur without signs of impending shock. Liver and splenic injury occur in up to 25% of severe MVCs. The most common cause of intraperitoneal hemorrhage in gestational trauma is splenic rupture.[25]

Inspect the abdomen for signs of injury, including ecchymosis, abrasions, and contusions. Note the shape and contour of abdomen. Irregularity or deformity may indicate uterine rupture. Inspect for fetal movement. Palpate for masses and abdominal tenderness. Remember abdominal rigidity, guarding, and rebound tenderness may be blunted by the stretched abdominal wall.

Diagnostic peritoneal lavage (DPL) has been safely and accurately performed to detect intraperitoneal hemorrhage in obstetric trauma.[8,9,43] Ultrasonography (US) is also beneficial in determining intraabdominal injury and fetal status.[2,4] A recent study used only sonography to assess for intraabdominal injury and the need for laparotomy. Need for immediate or conclusive laparotomy was correctly diagnosed by US with an accuracy level of 99.4% and a sensitivity of 92.8%.[2]

Fetus and Uterus

Simultaneous assessment of the fetus and uterus should occur early in the secondary survey. Signs of abdominal pain, uterine tenderness, or contractions may indicate uteroplacental injury and potential for maternal-fetal compromise.

Determining gestational age is critical and guides fetal assessment and intervention. The best indicator of gestational age is LMP. If the woman is unsure or unresponsive, she is assumed pregnant until a negative human chorionic gonadotropin (HCG) is documented. Normal gestation is 40 weeks; however, the uterus is usually palpable by 12 to 14 weeks' gestation. The fundus generally reaches the umbilicus by 20 weeks' gestation. Fundal height just below the xiphoid indicates a term fetus. An estimate of gestational age of a single fetus can be accomplished by measuring fundal height. A measurement midline from the symphysis pubis to the top of the uterus correlates gestational age with the height of the fundus in centimeters. A fundal height of 25 cm corresponds with gestational age of 25 weeks. Fetal viability is generally considered to be 24 to 25 weeks' gestation, although viability has occurred earlier with advanced neonate resuscitation and treatment in a neonatal ICU. Serial fundal measurements are beneficial because increase in fundal height may indicate occult intrauterine bleeding or uterine injury.

Evaluation of fetal well-being begins with a baseline fetal heart tone (FHT) on arrival at the ED. Fetal heart tones are audible by Doppler by the tenth to twelfth gestational week. Normal FHT ranges from 120 to 160 beats/min. Fetal bradycardia is FHT of less than 110 beats/min and indicates serious fetal stress and decompensation. Sustained fetal tachycardia greater than 160 beats/min also indicates fetal distress. Significant FHT patterns such as variability or late deceleration are ominous signs of fetal distress. Intermittent monitoring of FHT for the previable fetus is acceptable. Early continuous monitoring should be initiated for the viable fetus.[7] Studies suggest a minimum of 4 hours of cardiotocographic monitoring in the absence of uterine tenderness, vaginal bleeding, fetal distress, or serious maternal injury.[37] One study suggests 24 to 48 hours of continuous fetal monitoring.[8]

Another indicator of fetal well-being is fetal movement. A US can determine fetal cardiac activity, body movement, placental location, estimated gestational age, and volume of amniotic fluid. Fetal death may also be diagnosed by US.

Uterine and fetal assessment includes inspection of the perineum for blood or amniotic fluid. The presence of amniotic fluid is most accurately identified by microscopic procedure. A fern pattern appears on the slide if the specimen contains amniotic fluid.

In the absence of blood or urine, nitrazine paper can be used to differentiate amniotic fluid from vaginal fluid. Normal vaginal fluid has a pH of 4.5 to 5.5, amniotic fluid a pH of 7.0 to 7.5, which turns nitrazine paper blue. Kleihauer-Betke staining is used to determine the presence of fetal blood in perineum. A general pelvic exam identifies crowning, fetal presentation, blood, and fluids. The necessity of a speculum exam is determined by the trauma physician and may be deferred to the attending obstetrician. Direct visualization allows assessment of cervical dilation, locates source of blood or fluids, and identifies uterine or fetal injury. Bimanual exam is avoided unless delivery is imminent or genital tract injury is present.[7] Foley catheter placement is indicated to empty the bladder. Return of blood or hematuria suggests GU injury.

Diagnostics

Cardiotocography. Fetal monitoring should begin immediately but should not interfere with maternal resuscitation and stabilization. Initial FHT may be determined by intermittent doptone; however, the obstetric trauma patient requires continuous fetal monitoring. Cardiotocography consists of continuous electronic monitoring of FHT, patterns, and uterine contractions. An external transducer registers motion of fetal heart valves and a second transducer monitors uterine contraction. Signals are interpreted as electrical impulses and recorded as fetal monitor tracings. Figure 33-2 shows a normal tracing for fetal heart rate. Box 33-1 summarizes FHT changes that indicate fetal distress, and Figure 33-3 shows the types of deceleration in fetal heart rate. Controversy exists about the length of time for fetal monitoring.

A minimum of 4 hours is recommended in the absence of FHT abnormalities or maternal complications, 24-hour monitoring is suggested with FHT abnormalities until fetal well-being is established.[37] Fetal monitoring should be performed by a clinician skilled in use of equipment, interpretation, and requisite intervention.[5]

Laboratory. Laboratory studies include standard trauma profiles; however, results should be interpreted cautiously because of hematologic changes with pregnancy. Standard lab studies include complete blood count, serum electrolytes, amylase, coagulation profile, arterial blood gas, type and screen or type and cross, toxicology screen, and a urine analysis. Hospital policy and the attending physician determine the need for hepatitis B and HIV screening. HCG levels should be obtained for all women of childbearing age if LMP is unknown or greater than 4½ weeks prior to admission. Special attention to antibody screening is needed for Rh immune status because maternal Rh sensitization may occur when an Rh-negative mother carries an Rh-positive fetus. Administration of Rh (D) immune globulin can prevent maternal sensitization.

Radiographic evaluation. Radiodiagnostic procedures necessary for trauma evaluation should not be omitted in the pres-

---

Box **33-1**   **Fetal Monitoring Indicators of Fetal Distress**
Decreased variability in rate
Rate decelerations
Tachycardia greater than 160 beats/min
Bradycardia less than 110 beats/min
Uterine activity greater than eight contractions per hour

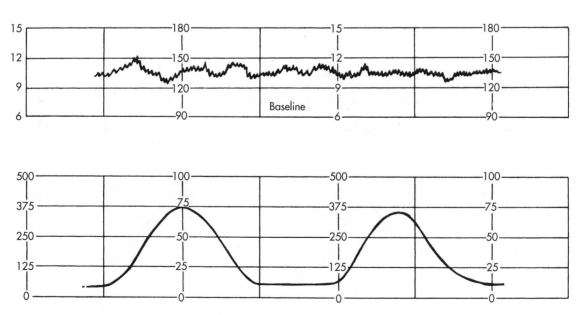

Figure **33-2**   Tracing of normal fetal heart rate. (*From AJN:* AJN/Mosby nursing boards review for the NCLEX-RN examination, *ed 10, St. Louis, 1997, Mosby.*)

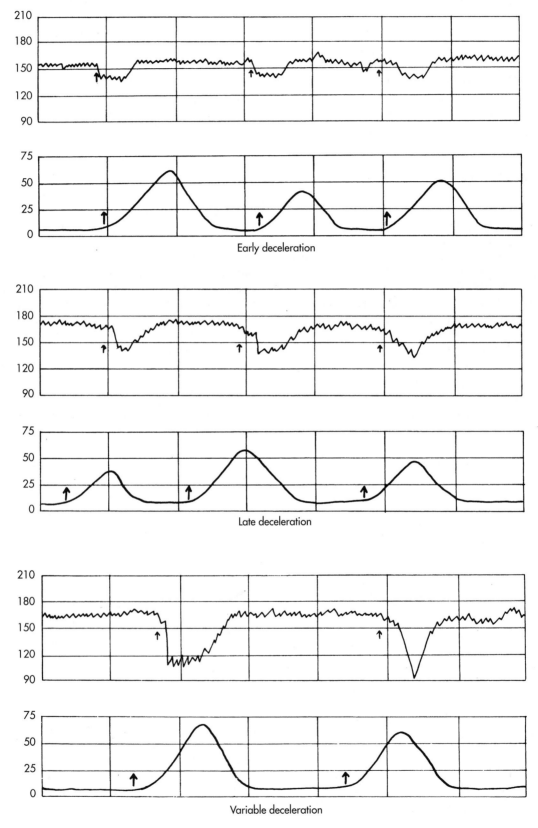

Figure **33-3**   Types of deceleration in fetal heart rate. *(From AJN:* AJN/Mosby nursing boards review for the NCLEX-RN examination, *ed 10, St. Louis, 1997, Mosby.)*

ence of a gravid uterus. Studies should be performed with a vigilant attempt to minimize fetal irradiation and limit radiation risks to decrease potential fetal injury. Radiographic studies are determined by clinical exam and physician suspicion of injury.

Lethal effects of radiation are greatest during the first week after conception. With successful implantation of the embryo, there is a low probability of teratogenic or growth-retarding effects.[32]

Major organogenesis occurs at 2 to 7 weeks' gestation. Radiation risks to the embryo include teratogenic, growth-retarding, lethal, and postnatal neoplastic effects. There is decreased radiosensitivity for multiple organ teratogenesis from 8 to 40 weeks' gestation; however, growth retardation, functional abnormalities, and postnatal neoplastic effects may occur.[32]

Minimal risk is documented with fetal radiation exposure less than 5 to 10 rad; however, teratogenic or mutagenic effects are possible at 10 rad.[13,25,32] Increasing fetal injury occurs at 15 rad exposure.[25,33] Indirect radiation exposure when the primary beam borders are more than 10 cm from the uterofetal area is considered insignificant.[32] Since the fetus is greater than 10 cm from the primary border of a cervical spine radiograph, fetal exposure is considered negligible. Increased radiation exposure occurs from a CT scan. Shielding the uterus minimizes fetal exposure; however, direct CT scan of the lower abdomen and pelvis produces a 3 to 5 rad dose.[33] Table 33-1 shows radiation doses for various diagnostic tests.

Every effort should be made to minimize fetal risk. An expert radiology technician can avoid duplicate films, shield the uterus whenever possible, and perform only essential radiodiagnostics. Counseling with the obstetrician or a geneticist may be beneficial when fetal radiation exposure is a concern.[42]

Diagnostic peritoneal lavage. DPL can effectively assess abdominal injury for hemoperitoneum and is considered safe and accurate for the gravid trauma patient. DPL does not assess retroperitoneal or intrauterine injury.[8] Indications for DPL after blunt trauma are abdominal signs and symptoms, altered level of consciousness, unexplained shock, severe thoracic injuries, and multiple or major orthopedic injuries.[43]

Before the procedure, insert an indwelling urinary catheter and orogastric or nasogastric tube to decompress the bladder and stomach and prevent complications. The peritoneal catheter is inserted with direct visualization using the open technique to avoid the gravid uterus. An intraumbilical incision may be used during the first trimester; however, the supraumbilical route is performed in later trimesters. Box 33-2 highlights positive findings in DPL. Further diagnostics are required to locate source and extent of injury. Immediate, delayed, or deferred laparotomy is determined by maternal and fetal condition.

INJURIES
Blunt Trauma

Blunt abdominal trauma may cause minor or severe life-threatening trauma to the mother and fetus. The most common causes of abdominal trauma are MVCs, falls, and assaults. Falls are the most common cause of minor injury. Hormonal changes soften joints and relax pelvic ligaments, which produces increasing instability in balance and gait. These changes in combination with the protruding abdomen and easy fatigue increase the mother's susceptibility to falls. Eighty percent of falls occur during the third trimester.[46]

Physical abuse has been reported in 5.5% to 17% of pregnancies.[31] A recent study reports an abuse rate during pregnancy of 20.6% for teens and 14.2% for adult women. Adult women sustain more severe emotional and physical abuse.[35] Many assaults are the result of domestic violence with a potential for repeat attacks. Any woman entering the ED with unexplained injury should be screened for abuse. Direct battery to the gravid abdomen may cause uterine injury.[16]

Table **33-1**	**Absorbed Radiation Doses to Unshielded Gravid Uterus**
Diagnostic study	Dose range (Rads)
Cervical spine	Negligible
Chest anterior-posterior view	0.0003-0.0043
Pelvis anterior-posterior view	0.142-0.486
Abdomen anterior-posterior view	0.133-0.451
Intravenous pyelogram	0.202-0.815
Spine anterior-posterior view	0.154-0.527
Femur	0.0016-0.012
Cystography	0.135-0.441
Computed tomography	
Head	<0.05
Thorax	<1.0
Upper abdomen	<3.0
Lower abdomen/pelvis	3-9
Upper gastrointestinal series	0.001-1.23
Barium enema	0.005-9.23

From Lavery P, Staten-McCormick M: Management of moderate to severe trauma in pregnancy, *Obstet Gynecol Clin North Am* 22(1):76, 1995.

Box **33-2**	**Positive DPL Results**

Aspiration ≥10 ml free blood
Grossly bloody lavage fluid
RBC count >100,000/mm³
WBC count >500/mm³
Amylase >175
Presence of bile or bacteria

Injury to the abdomen may result from the direct force of hitting the dashboard or steering wheel or as a result of organ displacement and hemorrhage from a coup-contrecoup event.[31] Injury to the uterus can cause severe complications for the fetus, including premature labor, abruptio placentae, uterine rupture, fetal head injury, and fetal-maternal hemorrhage.

Premature uterine contractions. The most frequent complication of obstetric trauma is uterine contractions[38,46] stimulated by release of prostaglandins from damaged myometrial and decidual cells. Amounts of uterine damage and released prostaglandins along with fetal age determine labor progression.[38] Usually contractions are self-limiting and tocolysis is not indicated. Tocolysis refers to the pharmacologic suppression of contractions. Continued contractions may indicate other uterine complications such as abruptio placentae.[38] Tocolysis may be effective in halting preterm labor of the injured but hemodynamically stable gravida. Pharmacology is determined by physician discretion.

Adequate fluid volume replacement and positioning the mother in the left lateral tilt position can minimize uterine irritability.[25] Cardiotocographic monitoring should be initiated early to assess uterine activity and fetal response.

Abruptio placentae. Most fetal deaths from blunt maternal trauma are due to placental abruption, with a reported incidence in severe trauma ranging from 6.6% to 66%.[18,37] Minor trauma associated with abruption is documented in 2% to 4%.[15,38] Abruptio placentae is premature, partial, or complete separation of the placenta from the uterine wall (Figure 33-4). Blunt force produces deformation of the elastic uterus, causing the placenta, which is relatively inelastic, to shear away from the uterine lining. The injury may be exacerbated by increased intraamniotic pressure.[37,39] All maternal-fetal gas exchange occurs across the placenta, therefore separation of the placenta from the uterus decreases oxygen delivery and increases carbon dioxide accumulation in fetal circulation. Fetal insult or fetal death may occur with abruption.[39] A separation greater than 50% usually results in fetal death.[7] Release of thromboplastin (plasminogen activator) with acute placental separation can lead to disseminated intravascular coagulation (DIC).[7]

Classic signs and symptoms of abruption include vaginal bleeding, uterine tenderness, and abdominal pain. Presenting signs and symptoms may also be vague or absent. Other indications of abruption include uterine contractions, maternal shock, increasing fundal height, and fetal distress.[6] Vaginal bleeding may be absent with concealed retroplacental bleeding. Fetal distress may be the first indication of uteroplacental injury and potential abruption. Risk for abruptio placentae is usually immediately after injury.[24,25,37] Immediate fetal monitoring should occur and continue for a minimum of 4 hours in a mother at greater than 20 weeks' gestation, more if maternal-fetal condition warrants. A small abruption may be compatible with fetal survival; however, a viable fetus in distress requires immediate surgical delivery.

Uterine rupture. Rupture of the uterus is an uncommon catastrophic injury resulting from blunt abdominal trauma. Uterine rupture occurs in mid to late pregnancy with a reported incidence less than 0.6%.[39] Previous cesarean section is a predisposing factor; rupture occurs at the healed incision site. Rupture of the posterior aspect of the uterus usually occurs in an unscarred uterus and is likely to involve bladder injury.[7] Increased maternal blood volume and perfusion increases the risk for maternal hypovolemic shock with uterine rupture. Maternal death occurs in less than 10% of cases and is usually associated with other injuries. Fetal mortality is almost 100%.[39] Rarely can the uterus be repaired, so hysterectomy is indicated for almost all patients with uterine rupture.

Direct fetal injury. Blunt trauma infrequently results in direct fetal injury with fetal skull fractures and intracranial hemorrhage the most common injuries noted. Injuries usually occur in association with maternal pelvic fractures. Later in pregnancy when the head is engaged in the pelvis, the fetal skull may become trapped and injured by the fractured pelvis.[37] Compression of the fetal skull may occur between the maternal spine and restraining lap belt or a striking object.[37,40] Other fetal fractures include clavicle and long-bone injury.

Figure **33-4** Abruptio placentae. Premature separation of normally implanted placenta. (*Courtesy Ross Laboratories, Columbus, Ohio.*)

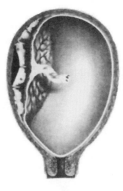
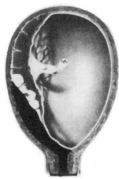
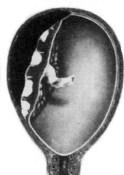

Partial separation (concealed hemorrhage)   Partial separation (apparent hemorrhage)   Complete separation (concealed hemorrhage)

Penetrating Injury

Increasing size and position make the gravid uterus susceptible to penetrating trauma. Gunshot wounds to the abdomen are more common than stab wounds. The degree of injury depends on the type, caliber, and range of weapon.[48] Maternal visceral organs are frequently shielded by uterine muscle, amniotic fluid, and fetal mass. Approximately 19% of pregnant women who sustain uterine gunshot wounds have visceral injuries.[3] Upper abdominal wounds involve bowel perforation or retroperitoneal injuries caused by compartmentalization by the gravid uterus. Lower abdominal entry wounds cause direct injury to the fetus. Indirect injury to the fetus may be caused by trauma to the cord, placenta, or membrane.[11] Fetal injury is reported as 59% to 89% with mortality from 47% to 71%.[3]

Stab wounds have a better prognosis for the mother and fetus. Visceral organs may slide away from the penetrating object so fewer organs are injured. Surgical exploration is usually required in cases of upper abdominal trauma from a bullet or stab wound. Recent literature supports conservative management of lower abdominal injuries if the patient is stable, there is no evidence of GI or GU trauma, and the bullet can be radiographically located in the uterine cavity.[11] Diagnostic options include local exploration of wounds, DPL, ultrasonography, and CT of the abdomen. Exploratory laparotomy remains the most reliable means to identify and treat penetrating abdominal injury; however, management should be individualized for the maternal-fetal condition.[11]

Maternal-Fetal Hemorrhage

Maternal-fetal hemorrhage (MFH) is transplacental fetal hemorrhage into the maternal bloodstream. MFH may occur to some degree in normal pregnancies.[25] Incidence after trauma varies and has been documented in up to 28% to 30% of the cases.[38,41] Anterior placental location has been associated with MFH.[37,38] However, Goodwin and Brun[15] did not find placental location helpful in predicting MFH. Uterine tenderness appears to be the only symptom frequently associated with MFH.[15,37,38] The general assumption is that MFH is less likely to occur before 12 weeks' gestation due to protection by the pelvis,[37] although some studies indicate equal frequency at every gestational age.[15,41]

Severe fetal complications do not usually follow MFH although some fetal risk is involved.[38] Fetal complications include fetal hemorrhage, neonatal anemia, paroxysmal atrial tachycardia, and intrauterine fetal death.[37] Massive fetal bleeding may lead to fetal anemia and death. Intravascular transfusion has been successful in treating fetal anemia.[25] The primary result of MFH is maternal isoimmunization when the mother is Rh negative. Figure 33-5 illustrates Rh sensitization. The Kleihauer-Betke (KB) acid elution assay can detect MFH and estimate the amount of fetal hemorrhage. The exact volume needed to sensitize the mother is unknown; however, minute amounts have caused Rh sensitization in some women. Unfortunately the KB test may not

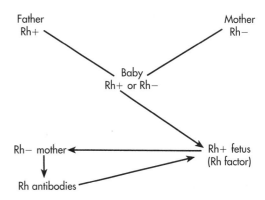

Figure **33-5**   Rh sensitization. *(From AJN:* AJN/Mosby nursing boards review for the NCLEX-RN examination, *ed 10, St. Louis, 1997, Mosby.)*

detect small amounts.[15] Therefore an Rh-negative mother with MFH should be treated with Rh immune globulin (RhoGam).[41] Goodwin and Brun[15] suggest all Rh-negative women receive full dose RhoGam following trauma despite probable negative KB assay. Serial KB tests are suggested for all positive KB stains to detect further bleeding.[15,41]

Burns

Most burn injuries in pregnant women occur in the home, with the extremities, face, and neck burned most often.[41] Fortunately the majority of these burn injuries are minor. Less than 1% of burned pregnant women require hospitalization for severe burns.[7] Pregnancy does not appear to affect maternal outcome; however, fetal outcome is affected by maternal condition. Total body surface area (TBSA) involved and severity of burn are associated with maternal outcome, premature delivery, and fetal death. A TBSA burn of 30% is predictive of premature labor.[41] Fetal survival is negligible with a 60% TBSA maternal burn. Primary concerns include premature contractions and intrauterine fetal death.[41] Fetal mortality results from hypoxia, hyponatremia, sepsis, and prematurity.[7] Spontaneous abortion usually occurs within the first week after the burn event. Delivery of a healthy term infant is probable with fetal survival over 1 week.

Severe burns require treatment at a burn center. Aggressive and appropriate fluid resuscitation, electrolyte therapy, supplemental oxygen, ventilation, and prevention of infection are critical. Sterile, dry dressings should be applied. Avoid wet or cool dressings.[7] Antibiotics should be used if necessary; however, silver sulfadiazine cream should be avoided because of possible development of fetal kernicterus.

Electrical Injury

There are a few reported cases of electrical injury during pregnancy; however, fetal mortality has been associated with minor electrical shock. Most electrical accidents occur at home. Alternating current (AC) found in the home follows a hand-to-foot route. Therefore the fetus lies in the direct path of the current. Fetal injury may result from cardiac conduction changes or uteroplacental lesions. If the fetus survives, oligohydramnios or growth retardation may develop.[28] Pregnant women should report all incidents of electrical shock to the obstetrician. Baseline fetal monitoring and close, frequent follow-up are necessary to evaluate fetal well-being.

SPECIAL CONSIDERATIONS
Cardiac Arrest

Objectives for cardiopulmonary resuscitation during pregnancy are to sustain circulation and perfusion for both patients—the mother and fetus. Basic and advanced life support should be initiated early and performed with slight variations. The maternal heart is located cephalad and laterally rotated, therefore compressions should be slightly higher on the sternum. Prompt, gentle intubation may reduce the risk of nasoesophageal or oroesophageal bleeding and aspiration.[46] In the presence of maternal hypoxia and acidemia, vasoconstriction occurs in the uteroplacental vascular bed. Monitoring ABGs and serum pH is vital to determine maternal acidosis and response to treatment.[27] Renal excretion of sodium bicarbonate increases during pregnancy; therefore bicarbonate administration should be guided by ABG results. Aggressive ventilation with supplemental oxygen and fluid loading are necessary for resuscitation. Vasopressors should be used with caution because of uteroplacental vasoconstriction and deleterious effects on the fetus. External defibrillation is not contraindicated during pregnancy. Direct current (DC) has successfully been used without fetal dysrhythmia in all three trimesters.[34]

Later in pregnancy, supine hypotension may occur from compression of the inferior vena cava, abdominal aorta, and pelvic veins by the gravid uterus. Cardiac output and venous return may be significantly reduced. Displacing the uterus to the left during chest compressions minimizes this effect and increases cardiac output. After 15 minutes of aggressive resuscitation, thoracotomy and open chest cardiac massage should be considered. Resuscitation efforts focus solely on the mother when gestation is less than 24 weeks. With gestation greater than 24 weeks, fetal viability and survival must be considered. Perimortem cesarean section promotes survival of the mother and fetus. There are documented cases of maternal recovery with return to the preresuscitation state following cesarean delivery.[27] Once the need for perimortem cesarean section is determined, the procedure must be performed quickly, with a neonate resuscitation team immediately available.

Perimortem Cesarean Section

The injured mother may require emergency delivery of a viable fetus. Indications for cesarean delivery include fetal distress, placental abruption, uterine rupture, unstable pelvic or lumbosacral fracture during labor,[25] or impending maternal death.

A perimortem cesarean section (PMCS) is the delivery of the neonate before maternal death. Fetal survival depends on the interval between maternal arrest and fetal delivery, gestational age, fetal condition, and cause of maternal arrest.[45] Gestational age is best determined by LMP. Measurement of fundal height can also estimate fetal age. A fundus above the umbilicus suggests a viable fetus greater than 24 weeks' gestation.

The interval between maternal arrest and fetal delivery is the most important factor predictive of fetal survival. Most infants that survive are delivered within 5 minutes of maternal arrest.[21,45] As the interval increases, neonatal survival decreases. The longest interval infant survivor documented was delivered 25 minutes post–maternal arrest.[22] PMCS should be initiated while maternal CPR is performed to ensure uteroplacental perfusion. The "4 minute rule" (PMCS should be initiated within 4 minutes after maternal cardiac arrest and the infant delivered by the fifth minute), promotes best maternal and fetal outcome. Maternal recovery may occur after cesarean section because of release of aortocaval compression, increased cardiac output, and increased tissue perfusion.

Fetal condition should be determined early during maternal arrest. Evidence of fetal heart tones is an indication for PMCS. Strong and Lowe[45] recommend PMCS regardless of fetal viability due to potential neonatal or maternal survival.

Cause of maternal arrest is a factor in infant survival. Neonates from a chronically ill mother have a poor chance of survival, whereas acute maternal arrest in a previously healthy mother implies a greater chance of infant survival.[21,45]

Attempt to obtain consent for PMCS. However, this effort should not interfere or delay intervention. Risk for legal liability is present but minimal, whereas not performing PMCS in the presence of a viable fetus may be considered negligent.

Neonatal Resuscitation

Emergency delivery of a neonate is performed because of maternal or fetal stress or both. Compromised fetal condition secondary to the maternal arrest or other stressors may necessitate aggressive resuscitation. A neonatal team skilled in assessment and treatment of the newborn should be prepared and have the necessary equipment. Assessment and resuscitation should be performed simultaneously in a stepwise fashion. Drying, warming, suction, and tactile stimulation are the first interventions. Oxygen is needed by a compromised neonate when minimal respiratory effort is made with an adequate heart rate. The neonate requires only bag-valve-mask ventilation with 100% oxygen. Chest compressions should be initiated when the neonate is bradycardic or heart rate is absent. Intubation and medications are the final steps of neonate resuscitation. APGAR scoring is calculated at 1 minute after delivery and repeated in 5 minutes to determine success of resuscitative efforts; however, determining APGAR should not interfere with neonatal resuscitation. Box 33-3 summarizes neonatal CPR.

Box 33-3	Neonatal Resuscitation

Airway

"Sniffing" or neutral position

Endotracheal intubation if needed

Ventilation

Oxygen

Preferred method: simple face mask held firmly on face using 5 to 10 L/min flow

May use standard oxygen tubing and a flow rate of 5 to 10 L/min to direct blow-by oxygen towards the neonate's nares

Bag-valve-mask ventilation

Rate: 40 to 60 breaths/min

Adequate ventilation is assessed by chest wall movement and auscultation of bilateral breath sounds

Bag-valve volume for full term neonate: at least 450 to 750 ml

Compressions

Acceptable methods in newborns

Thumb technique (preferred method): two thumbs on the lower third of the sternum with hands encircling the body and fingers supporting the back

Two-finger technique: two fingers, using the tips of the fingers to compress the lower third of the sternum and the other hand to support the back (unless on a firm surface)

Compression to ventilation ratio

3:1 ratio (three compressions to one ventilation)

Results in 90 compressions and 30 ventilations/minute

Important to allow for adequate ventilation between compressions

Compression depth: Depress the sternum ½ to ¾ inch

Modified from Emergency Cardiac Care Committee and Subcommittees, American Heart Association: Guidelines for cardiopulmonary resuscitation and emergency cardiac care, *JAMA* 268:2276, 1992.

Patient Transport

Prehospital care and transport of the pregnant woman are influenced by several factors. As in any trauma patient, the initial focus is on spinal integrity, BLS assessment, and emergency interventions. Supplemental oxygen benefits the mother and the fetus, because the pregnant woman is at higher risk for respiratory compromise than a nonpregnant woman and the fetus is unable to tolerate hypoxia. Application of supplemental oxygen throughout transport is required until respiratory status is evaluated. Intravenous access is needed for fluid replacement to treat maternal hypovolemia and ensure uterine perfusion. To avoid serious maternal-fetal complications, appropriate maternal positioning during transport is vital. The left lateral decubitus position is advocated to avoid aortocaval compression in gestation greater than 20 weeks. If spinal immobilization is needed, a cervical collar and backboard with a lateral tilt of 15 degrees should maintain immobilization and minimize compression.[22]

Use of the pneumatic antishock garment (PASG) is controversial. Inflating the abdominal compartment may theoretically compress the inferior vena cava and increase the potential for supine hypotension. If the PASG is used, avoid inflation of the abdominal compartment and inflate only the leg compartments.[25]

Seat Belts

MVCs are one of the most common causes of maternal injury or mortality. Ejection from the vehicle with resulting head trauma accounts for most maternal deaths.[9,10,17] Fetal death rates are highest when the mother is ejected.[9] Combined lap and shoulder restraints, that is, three-point restraints, reduce maternal ejection and the risk of fetal injury.[17] Lap belts without shoulder harnesses decrease ejection from the vehicle; however, intraabdominal injuries may result from the lap restraint. Mesenteric tears, small bowel perforations, and lumbar vertebral fractures are reported in nonpregnant patients.[17,19] The small bowel is elevated during pregnancy, so the protuberant uterus is exposed. There is increased potential for uterine or fetal injury from the lap belt. The two-point shoulder harness without lap restraint does not prevent ejection. Literature reports no significant statistical difference in the effectiveness of seat belts to prevent fetal injury or loss. However, *proper* use of three-point restraints is advocated to reduce maternal mortality and fetal risk.[9,47] The lap belt should be worn snugly across the pelvis below the abdomen and uterus; the shoulder harness should be worn in the normal position across the chest and between the breasts.

SUMMARY

Obstetric trauma, although rare, can be a catastrophic event. Two patients, the mother and the fetus, must be considered during the assessment and treatment of the obstetric patient. Clinical management requires a team approach. The emergency physician, emergency nurse, trauma surgeon, obstetrician, perinatologist, labor and delivery nurse, and neonatal nurse may be key members of the trauma team during resuscitation of an obstetric trauma patient.

Optimal fetal outcomes are the result of maternal survival. Aggressive resuscitation and stabilization of the mother promotes the best maternal and fetal outcomes. Box 33-4 highlights nursing diagnoses for the obstetric trauma patient.

Box **33-4**

NURSING DIAGNOSES FOR THE PREGNANT TRAUMA PATIENT

Fluid volume deficit

Risk for impaired gas exchange

Altered tissue perfusion

Anxiety

Fear

Risk for aspiration

Risk for infection

Concern for maternal and fetal condition produces elevated stress levels in the patient and family. Emotional care should not be forgotten. Reassurance is indispensable during trauma intervention.

Prevention efforts may decrease the incidence and severity of obstetric trauma. Public and private education about proper use of seat belts may reduce maternal and fetal injury. Violence, especially domestic violence, should be assessed in the ED. Appropriate intervention may prevent a repeat attack and avoid maternal injury. Education that fetal condition basically depends on maternal condition may help the mother choose actions that promote fetal well-being.

REFERENCES

1. Baker D: Trauma in the pregnant patient, *Surg Clin North Am* 62:275, 1982.
2. Bode PJ, Niezen RA et al: Abdominal ultrasound as a reliable indicator for conclusive laparotomy in blunt abdominal trauma, *J Trauma* 34(1):27, 1993.
3. Buchsbaum HJ: *Trauma in pregnancy,* Philadelphia, 1979, WB Saunders.
4. Drost TF, Rosemurgy AS, Sherman HF et al: Major trauma in pregnant women: maternal fetal outcome, *J Trauma* 30(5):574, 1990.
5. Emergency Nurses Association: *The obstetrical patient in the ED: position statement,* Park Ridge, Ill, 1993, The Association.
6. Emergency Nurses Association: Trauma and pregnancy. In: *Trauma nursing core course,* ed 4, Park Ridge, Ill, 1995, The Association.
7. Esposito TJ: Trauma during pregnancy, *Emer Med Clin North Am* 12(1):167, 1994.
8. Esposito TJ, Gens DR et al: Evaluation of blunt abdominal trauma occurring during pregnancy, *J Trauma* 29(12):1628, 1989.
9. Esposito TJ, Gens DR, Smith LG et al: Trauma during pregnancy: a review of 79 cases, *Arch Surg* 126:1073, 1991.
10. Evans L: Restraint effectiveness, occupant ejection from cars and fatality reductions, *Accid Analys Prevent* 22:167, 1990.
11. Franger AL, Buchsbaum HJ, Peaceman AM: Abdominal gunshot wounds in pregnancy, *Am J Obstet Gynecol* 160(5):1124, 1989.
12. Galen LH: Trauma in pregnancy. In Friedman E, Acker DB, Sachs BP, editors: *Obstetrical decision making,* ed 2, Ontario, 1987, BC Decker.
13. Gerber-Smith L: Assessment and initial management of the pregnant trauma patient, *J Trauma Nsg* 1(1):8, 1994.
14. Gerber-Smith L: The pregnant trauma patient. In Cardona VD, Hurd PD, Mason PJB et al, editors: *Trauma nursing: from resuscitation through rehabilitation,* ed 2, Philadelphia, 1994, WB Saunders.
15. Goodwin TM, Brun MT: Pregnancy outcome and fetomaternal hemorrhage after noncatastrophic trauma, *Am J Obstet Gynecol* 162:665, 1990.
16. Haycock CE: Injury during pregnancy: saving both mother and fetus, *Consultant* 22(1):269, 1982.
17. Hendey GW, Votey SR: Injuries in restrained motor vehicle accident victims, *Ann Emerg Med* 24(1):77, 1994.
18. Higgins S, Garite T: Late abruptio placenta in trauma patients: implications for monitoring, *Obstet Gynecol* 63(suppl):105, 1984.
19. Huelke DF, Snyder RG: Seatbelt injuries: the need for accuracy in reporting of cases, *J Trauma* 15:20, 1975.
20. Johnson JD, Oakley LE: Managing minor trauma during pregnancy, *JOGNN* 20(5):379, 1991.
21. Katz VL, Dotters DJ, Droegmuller W: Perimortem cesarian delivery, *Obstet Gynecol* 68(4):571, 1986.
22. Katz VL, Hansen AR: Complications in the emergency transport of pregnant women, *Southern Med J* 83(1):7, 1990.
23. Kendrick JM, Powers PH: Perioperative care of the pregnant surgical patient, *AORN J* 60(2):205, 1994.
24. Kettel LM, Branch DW, Scott JR: Occult placental abruption after maternal trauma, *Obstet Gynecol* 71(3):449, 1988.
25. Lavery JP, Staten-McCormick M: Management of moderate to severe trauma in pregnancy, *Obstet Gynecol Clin North Am* 22(1):69, 1995.
26. Lavin JP, Polsky S: Abdominal trauma during pregnancy, *Clin Perinatal* 10:423, 1983.
27. Lee RV, Rodgers BD et al: Cardiopulmonary resuscitation of pregnant women, *Am J Med* 81:311, 1986.
28. Leiberman JR, Mazor M et al: Electrical accidents during pregnancy, *Obstet Gynecol* 67(6):861, 1986.
29. Manley LK: Trauma in pregnancy. In Neff JA, Kidd PS, editors: *Trauma nursing: the art and science,* St. Louis, 1993, Mosby.
30. Maull KI, Pedigo RE: Injury to the female reproductive system. In Moore EE, Mattox KL, Feliciano DV, editors: *Trauma,* ed 2, Norwalk, Conn, 1991, Appleton & Lange.
31. McFarlane J, Parker B et al: Assessing for abuse during pregnancy: severity and frequency of injuries and associated entry into prenatal care, *JAMA* 267:3176, 1992.
32. Mossman KL, Hill LT: Radiation risks in pregnancy, *Obstet Gynecol* 60(2):237, 1982.
33. Neufeld JD: Trauma in pregnancy, what if. . . ? *Emerg Med Clin North Am* 11(1):207, 1993.
34. Neufeld JD, Marx JA: Trauma in pregnancy. In Rosen P, Baker FJ, Barkin RM et al, editors: *Emergency medicine: concepts and clinical practice,* ed 3, St. Louis, 1992, Mosby.
35. Parker B, McFarlane J, Soeken K: Abuse during pregnancy: effects on maternal complications and birth weight in adult and teenage women, *Obstet Gynecol* 84(3):323, 1994.
36. Patterson RM: Trauma in pregnancy, *Clin Obstet Gynecol* 27(1):32, 1984.
37. Pearlman MD, Tintinalli JE: Evaluation and treatment of the gravida and fetus following trauma during pregnancy, *Obstet Gynecol Clin North Am* 18(2):371, 1991.
38. Pearlman MD, Tintinalli JE, Lorenz RP: A prospective study of outcome after trauma during pregnancy, *Am J Obstet Gynecol* 162(6):1502, 1990.
39. Pearlman MD, Tintinalli JE, Lorenz RP: Blunt trauma during pregnancy, *N Engl J Med* 323(23):1609, 1990.
40. Pimentel L: Mother and child: trauma in pregnancy, *Emerg Med Clin North Am* 9(3):549, 1991.
41. Rayburn W, Smith B et al: Major burns during pregnancy: effects on fetal well-being, *Obstet Gynecol* 63(3):392, 1984.
42. Rose PG, Strohm PL, Zuspan FP: Fetomaternal hemorrhage following trauma, *Am J Obstet Gynecol* 153(8):844, 1985.
43. Rothenberger DA, Quattlebaum FW et al: Diagnostic peritoneal lavage for blunt trauma in pregnant women, *Am J Obstet Gynecol* 129(5):479, 1977.
44. Rothenberger D, Quattlebaum FW, Zabel J et al: Blunt maternal trauma: a review of 103 cases, *J Trauma* 18:173, 1978.
45. Strong TH, Lowe RA: Perimortem cesarian section, *Am J Emerg Med* 7(5):489, 1989.
46. Williams JD, McClain et al: Evaluation of blunt abdominal trauma in the third trimester of pregnancy: maternal and fetal consideration, *Obstet Gynecol* 75(1):33, 1990.
47. Wolf ME, Alexander BH et al: A retrospective cohort study of seatbelt use and pregnancy outcome after a motor vehicle crash, *J Trauma* 34(1):116, 1993.
48. Zerbe M: Clinical management of the pregnant trauma victim, *AACN* 1(3):479, 1990.

unit V

MEDICAL AND SURGICAL EMERGENCIES

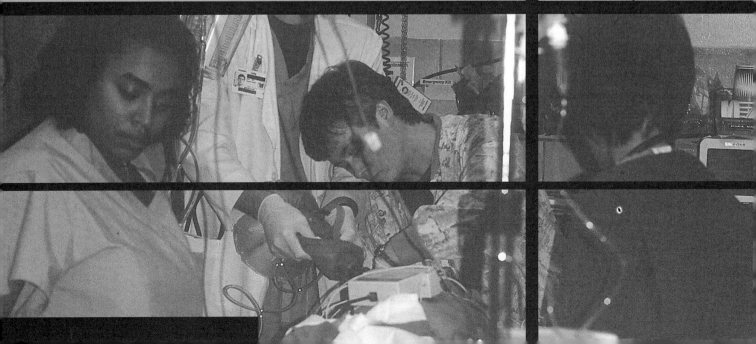

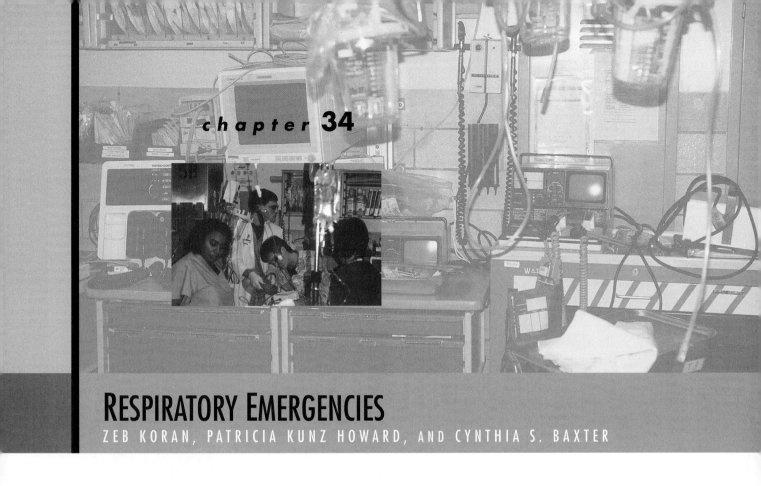

chapter 34

RESPIRATORY EMERGENCIES

ZEB KORAN, PATRICIA KUNZ HOWARD, AND CYNTHIA S. BAXTER

Respiratory emergencies may present as a minor problem, such as upper respiratory infection, or impending respiratory arrest caused by epiglottitis. Rapid assessment and intervention are essential to prevent escalation of respiratory compromise. Respiratory distress is caused by impaired oxygenation or ventilation, so respiratory distress is an emergent condition, regardless of etiology.

This chapter focuses on common respiratory emergencies including asthma, bronchitis, emphysema, pulmonary edema, pulmonary embolus, near-drowning, and spontaneous pneumothorax. Respiratory emergencies that occur more often in the pediatric population, that is, croup, epiglottitis, and bronchiolitis are addressed in the chapter on pediatric emergencies (see Chapter 50), whereas tuberculosis is included in the discussion of infectious diseases (see Chapter 42). Anatomy and physiology of the respiratory system are included to facilitate understanding of these potentially life-threatening conditions.

ANATOMY AND PHYSIOLOGY

Anatomic structures of the pulmonary system include the oral cavity, epiglottis, trachea, bronchi, and lungs (Figure 34-1). Ciliated epithelium located from proximal trachea to terminal bronchioles traps dust particles and other debris, preventing contamination of the lower airways. Goblet cells secrete mucus, which keeps airways moist, and also trap debris that might otherwise enter alveoli. The airway distal to the larynx is considered sterile because of these and other protective mechanisms such as coughing and alveolar macrophages.[5] Upper airways have C-shaped cartilaginous rings that prevent airway collapse. Rings gradually disappear in the lower branches and are replaced by smooth muscle in bronchioles. The functional unit of the pulmonary system is the alveolus, which interacts with adjacent capillaries to ensure oxygen transport from alveolus into blood (Figure 34-2). Alveoli remain open because of the presence of surfactant, a detergent-like substance that reduces surface tension within the alveoli.

Respiration is divided into pulmonary ventilation, diffusion of oxygen and carbon dioxide across the alveolar capillary membrane, transport of oxygen and carbon dioxide to and from cells, and regulation of ventilation. Pulmonary ventilation refers to flow of air between the atmosphere and alveoli. Figure 34-3 illustrates movement of the chest wall during respiration. Negative intrathoracic pressure is the impetus for movement of air into the lungs, whereas flow out of the lungs occurs passively.

Normal gas exchange in the lung depends on adequate ventilation and perfusion (Figure 34-4). Imbalance in either area creates a ventilation/perfusion ($\dot{V}/\dot{Q}$) mismatch. Figure 34-5 illustrates the effect of inadequate ventilation, as well as the consequences of poor perfusion. Extreme imbalance between ventilation and perfusion shunts blood to the arterial system without benefit of oxygenation (Figure 34-6). Congenital heart conditions such as patent ductus arteriosus are a common cause of shunts. Consolidated pneumonia and pulmonary embolus also lead to shunting.

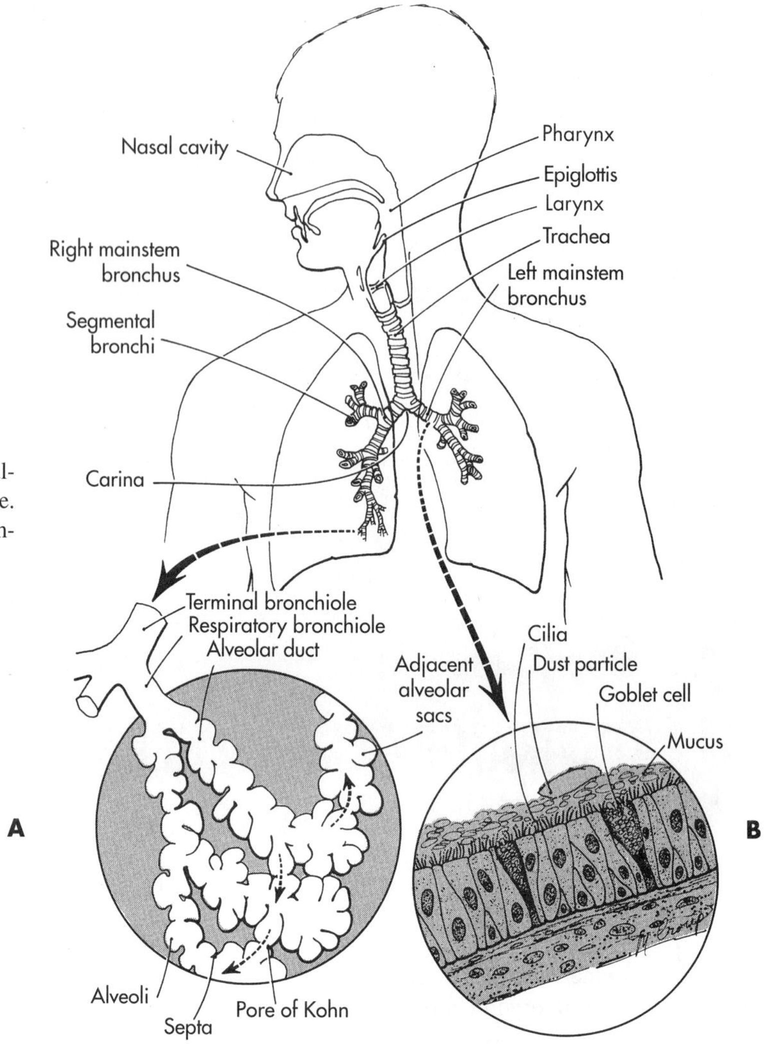

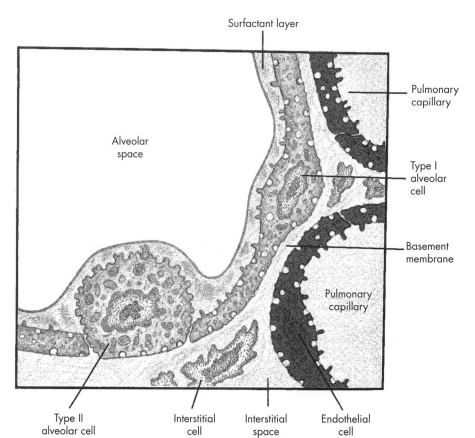

Figure **34-1** Structures of the respiratory tract. **A,** Pulmonary functional unit. **B,** Ciliated mucous membrane. *(From Price SA, Wilson LM:* Pathophysiology: clinical concepts of disease processes, *ed 5, St. Louis, 1997, Mosby.)*

Nasal cavity

Pharynx
Epiglottis
Larynx
Trachea

Right mainstem bronchus

Left mainstem bronchus

Segmental bronchi

Carina

Terminal bronchiole
Respiratory bronchiole
Alveolar duct

Adjacent alveolar sacs

Cilia
Dust particle
Goblet cell
Mucus

A

Alveoli

Septa

Pore of Kohn

B

Figure **34-2** Alveolar wall and space. *(From Thompson JM et al:* Mosby's clinical nursing, *ed 4, St. Louis, 1997, Mosby.)*

Surfactant layer

Pulmonary capillary

Alveolar space

Type I alveolar cell

Basement membrane

Pulmonary capillary

Type II alveolar cell

Interstitial cell

Interstitial space

Endothelial cell

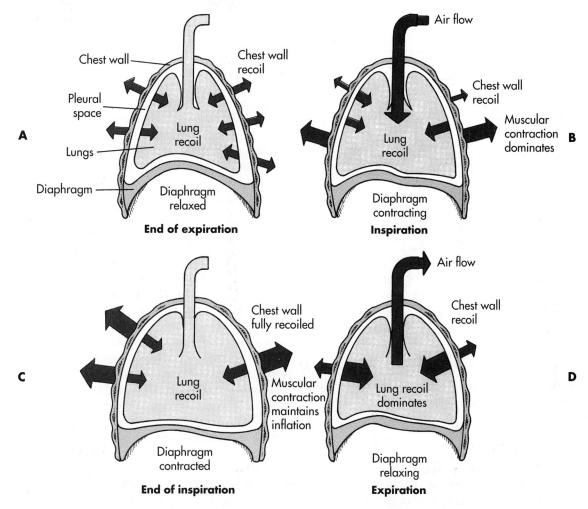

Figure **34-3** Interaction of forces during inspiration and expiration. **A,** Outward recoil of the chest wall equals inward recoil of the lungs at the end of expiration. **B,** During inspiration, contraction of respiratory muscles, assisted by chest wall recoil, overcomes tendency of lungs to recoil. **C,** At the end of inspiration, respiratory muscle contraction maintains lung expansion. **D,** During expiration, respiratory muscles relax, allowing elastic recoil of the lungs to deflate the lungs. *(From Huether SE, McCance KL:* Understanding pathophysiology, *St. Louis, 1996, Mosby.)*

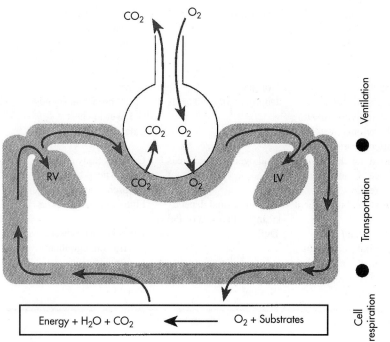

Figure **34-4** Normal gas exchange in the respiratory process. RV, right ventricle; LV, left ventricle. *(From Price SA, Wilson LM:* Pathophysiology: clinical concepts of disease processes, *ed 5, St. Louis, 1997, Mosby.)*

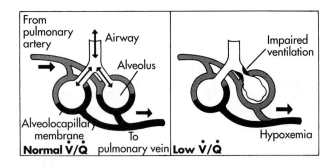

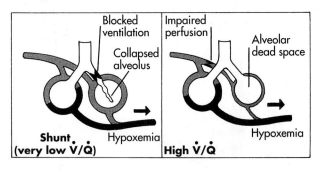

Figure **34-5** Ventilation-perfusion abnormalities. *(From Huether SE, McCance KL:* Understanding pathophysiology, *St. Louis, 1996, Mosby.)*

Cellular oxygenation depends on transport of adequate oxygen to cells, the affinity of hemoglobin for oxygen, and the ease with which hemoglobin releases oxygen to cells. Hemoglobin's affinity for oxygen is described by the oxygen-hemoglobin dissociation curve (Figure 34-7). If the curve shifts to the left, hemoglobin picks up oxygen more easily in the lungs, but does not easily release oxygen to tissues.[3] When the curve shifts to the right, oxygen uptake by hemoglobin is less rapid, but oxygen delivery to cells is easier.[3] Conditions that affect oxygen dissociation are temperature, acid-base balance, and PCO_2 levels.

PATIENT ASSESSMENT

Assessment of the patient with a respiratory emergency begins with evaluation of airway, breathing, and circulation (ABCs). Once the ABCs are assured, assess for objective findings such as flaring of nostrils, cyanosis, pallor, decreasing level of consciousness, and dyspnea. Assess level of consciousness, vital signs, use of accessory muscles, and breath sounds. The presence of barrel chest and clubbed fingers suggests chronic obstructive pulmonary disease (COPD), cardiovascular abnormalities, valvular heart disease, or congenital defects; however, these can be normal findings in patients living at high altitudes or in some elderly patients. Physical examination of the chest varies with condition. Table 34-1

Table 34-1	Chest Examination Findings in Common Pulmonary Problems			
Problem	Inspection	Palpation	Percussion	Auscultation
Chronic bronchitis	Barrel chest; cyanosis	↓ Movement ↑ Fremitus	Hyperresonant or dull if consolidation	Crackles; rhonchi; wheezes
Emphysema	Barrel chest; tripod position; use of accessory muscles	↓ Movement	Hyperresonant or dull if consolidation	Crackles; rhonchi; diminished if no exacerbation
Asthma: In exacerbation	Prolonged expiration; tripod position; pursed lips	↓ Movement ↓ Fremitus if hyperinflation	Hyperresonance sounds	Wheezes; ↓ breath sounds (silent chest) ominous sign if no improvement (severely diminished air movement)
Not in exacerbation	Normal	Normal	Normal	Normal
Pneumonia	Tachypnea; use of accessory muscles; duskiness or cyanosis	Unequal movement if lobar involvement; ↑ fremitus over affected area	Dull over affected areas	Early: bronchial sounds lower in chest Later: crackles; rhonchi
Atelectasis	No change unless involves entire segment, lobe	If small, no change; if large, ↓ movement; ↑ fremitus	Dull over affected areas	Crackles (may disappear with deep breaths); absent sounds if large
Pulmonary edema	Tachypnea; labored respirations; cyanosis	↓ Or normal movement	Dull or normal depending on amount of fluid	Fine or coarse crackles
Pleural effusion	Tachypnea; use of accessory muscles	↓ Movement; ↑ fremitus above effusion; absent fremitus over effusion	Dull	Diminished or absent over effusion; egophony over effusion
Pulmonary fibrosis	Tachypnea	↓ Movement	Normal	Crackles

From Lewis SM, Collier IC, Heitkemper MM: *Medical-surgical nursing: assessment and management of clinical problems,* ed 4, St. Louis, 1996, Mosby.

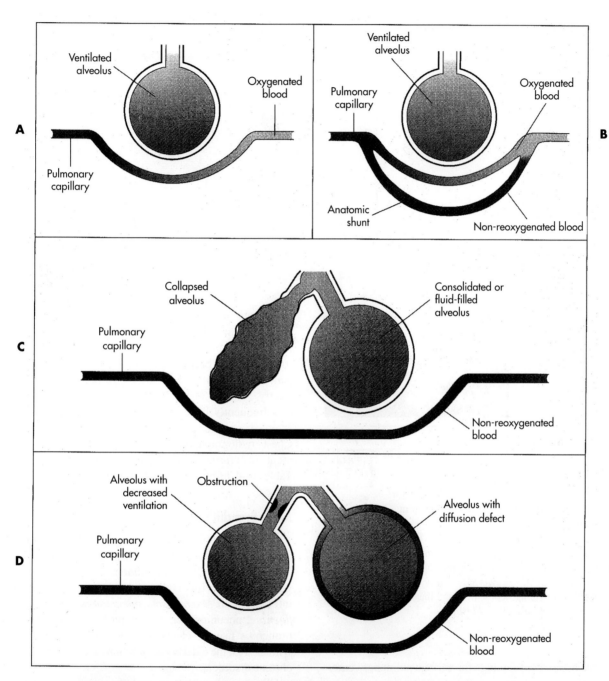

Figure **34-6** Pulmonary shunting. **A,** Normal alveolar-capillary unit. **B,** Anatomic shunt. **C,** Types of capillary shunts. **D,** Types of shuntlike effects. *(Modified from Des Jardins T: Cardiopulmonary anatomy and physiology: essentials for respiratory care, ed 2, Albany, NY, 1993, Delmar Publishers. In NFNA: Flight nursing, ed 2, St. Louis, 1996, Mosby.)*

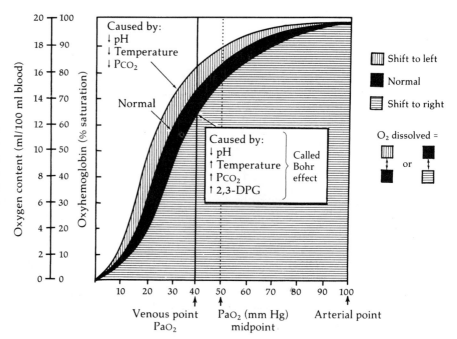

Figure **34-7** Oxygen-hemoglobin dissociation curve. Effects of acidity and temperature changes are shown. *(Modified from Guenter CA, Welch MH: Pulmonary medicine, Philadelphia, 1977, Lippincott. In Thompson JM et al: Mosby's clinical nursing, ed 4, St. Louis, 1997, Mosby.)*

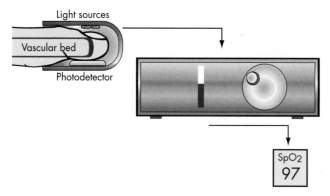

Figure **34-8** A pulse oximeter passes light from a light-emitting diode through a vascular bed to a photodetector. The oximeter compares the amount of light emitted with the amount absorbed and calculates the SpO₂. The oximeter displays the SpO₂ as a digital reading. *(Redrawn from Principles of pulse oximetry, Nillcor Inc., Haywood, CA. In Lewis SM, Collier IC, Heitkemper MM: Medical-surgical nursing: assessment and management of clinical problems, ed 4, St. Louis, 1996, Mosby.*

lists these assessment findings for various pulmonary emergencies.

Obtain historical information related to the onset of symptoms, preexisting conditions, smoking history, and presence of orthopnea or nocturnal dyspnea. Tobacco smoke decreases the efficacy of pulmonary mucosa, cilia, and alveolar macrophages. Table 34-2 highlights tobacco's effects on the respiratory system. Determining the patient's occupation can provide helpful information because certain occupations have an increased incidence of pulmonary diseases (Table 34-3).

Nursing interventions include frequent assessment of oxygen saturation, vital signs, and cardiac rhythm. Early identification and treatment of hypoxia can prevent ventricular dysrhythmias related to myocardial ischemia. Oxygen saturation is monitored using noninvasive pulse oximetry (Figure 34-8). Patients with respiratory emergencies frequently have decreased oxygen saturation. Administer oxygen in cases of decreased oxygen saturation. Chest radiograph, complete blood count, and measurement of arterial blood gases should also be obtained. Table 34-4 provides normal arterial and venous blood gas values.

Acute Bronchitis

Acute bronchitis occurs in all age groups and is more common during cold and flu seasons. Acute inflammation from infectious agents such as influenza, parainfluenza, adenovirus and rhinovirus is the most common cause. Secondary infection with *Mycoplasma pneumoniae, Haemophilus influenzae,* pneumococci, and streptococci also occurs. Acute bronchitis usually clears independently except in patients with COPD, the elderly and debilitated, or patients with other chronic disorders.

Clinical manifestations include recent upper respiratory infection such as sore throat, stuffy nose, and cough. Cough is initially dry, hacky, and nonproductive and most troublesome at night, usually interrupting sleep. Exposure to cold, deep breath, talking, and laughing, may also cause coughing. Within days, sputum production is evident and a retrosternal scratchy feeling is present. Dyspnea is not present unless there is underlying cardiopulmonary disease. Inflammation and hypersensitivity may occur.

Table **34-2**	Effects of Tobacco Smoke on the Respiratory System		
Area of defect	**Acute effects**	**Long-term effects**
Respiratory mucosa		
Nasopharyngeal	↓ Sense of smell	Cancer
Tongue	↓ Sense of taste	Cancer
Vocal cords	Hoarseness	Chronic cough, cancer
Bronchus and bronchioles	Bronchospasm, cough	Chronic bronchitis, asthma, cancer
Cilia	Paralysis, sputum accumulation, cough	Chronic bronchitis, cancer
Mucous glands	↑ Secretions, ↑ cough	Hyperplasia and hypertrophy of glands, chronic bronchitis
Alveolar macrophages	↓ Function	Increased incidence of infection
Elastin and collagen fibers	↑ Destruction by proteases, ↓ function of antiproteases (α_1-antitrypsin), ↓ synthesis and repair of elastin	Emphysema

From Lewis SM, Collier IC, Heitkemper MM: *Medical-surgical nursing: assessment and management of clinical problems,* ed 4, St. Louis, 1996, Mosby.

Chest radiographs may be normal or show signs of inflammation. Scattered wheezing, and a mild or elevated fever may also be present. Management includes bed rest, humidification, cough preparations to allow sleep, antibiotic for secondary infection, especially with underlying pulmonary disease, and forcing fluids. Prognosis is good with self-limiting acute bronchitis but may progress to pneumonia with underlying pulmonary disease.

Chronic Bronchitis

Chronic bronchitis occurs more frequently in middle-age men, is uncommon in nonsmokers, and involves excessive, chronic production of mucus. Direct correlation exists between the amount and duration of cigarette smoking and the severity of the bronchitis. The size and work of goblet and mucus gland cells increase, causing peripheral mucus plugs, inflammation of bronchiole walls, and loss of cilia without a decrease in peak expiratory flow rates. Resistance is contained in smaller (less than 2 mm) airways, which causes a mismatch of $\dot{V}/\dot{Q}$ ratio and hypoxemia. In advanced stages, emphysema, increased pulmonary vascular resistance, right ventricular failure, increased airway obstruction, and polycythemia predispose the patient to thrombi and emboli. Table 34-5 highlights clinical differences between chronic bronchitis and emphysema.

Chronic bronchitis is diagnosed when cough with increased sputum production occurs at least 3 consecutive months each year for 2 successive years. The cough may become purulent. Dyspnea indicates obstruction but has a slow onset unless there is acute exacerbation. In the advanced stages, prolonged expiration with wheezing and dyspnea at rest resembles emphysema. A chest radiograph is insignificant in uncomplicated chronic bronchitis but in the late stages reveals hyperinflation. Pulmonary function tests are normal in the early stages, but chronic obstructive changes increase residual volume, indicating small airway obstruction.

Management for chronic bronchitis, as for COPD in late stages, may include bronchodilators, nebulized inhalers, and steroids. Antibiotics are not used unless obvious infection is present. Unless these patients stop smoking, the majority progress with COPD. The course of chronic bronchitis is cough with expectoration for years.

Pneumonia

Pneumonia results from an acute bacterial, viral, or fungal infection and may be preceded by upper respiratory tract infection, ear infection, or eye infection, or can occur as the primary illness, without precipitating causes. Pneumonia occurs primarily in young children, the elderly, and debilitated individuals. Approximately 1% of the American population will have pneumonia during their lifetime.[5]

Pneumonia may be classified according to causative organism (pneumococcal or streptococcal) or according to location (bronchial or lobar). Figure 34-9 illustrates types of pneumonia. Persons who are bedridden, have rib fractures, or an underlying cardiac or pulmonary disorder have an increased risk for pneumonia. Pneumonia is more likely to occur in those who have had a previous episode of pneumonia. Other causes include smoking, diabetes mellitus, exposure to extreme changes in environmental temperature, steroids, or immunosuppressive therapy. Pneumonia is often seen in persons who abuse alcohol or drugs, and thus have a tendency to aspirate. Box 34-1 highlights factors that predispose persons to pneumonia.

Patients have elevated temperature (39° C to 40° C), diaphoresis, and may complain of chest pain, which is often referred diaphragmatically and mistaken for gastrointestinal disorders. Productive cough, tachypnea, tachycardia, cyanosis, and apprehension may occur. Pleuritic chest pain is frequently noted. Breath sounds are present, but are diminished over the area of pneumonia. Rales also occur. Abdominal distention, vomiting, and headache have also been reported.

Table 34-3 Occupational Lung Diseases

Disease	Agents/Industries	Description	Complications
Asbestosis	Asbestos fibers present in insulation, construction material (roof tiling, cement products), shipyards, textiles (for fireproofing), automobile clutch and brake linings	Disease appears 15-35 yr after first exposure; interstitial fibrosis develops; pleural plaques, which are calcified lesions, develop on pleura; dyspnea, basal crackles, and decreased vital capacity are early manifestations	Bronchogenic carcinoma, especially in cigarette smokers; mesothelioma (rare type of cancer affecting pleura and peritoneal membrane)
Berylliosis	Beryllium dust present in aircraft manufacturing, metallurgy, rocket fuels	Noncaseating granulomas form; acute pneumonitis occurs after heavy exposure; interstitial fibrosis can also occur	Progress of disease possible after removal of stimulating inhalant
Bird fancier's, breeder's, or handler's lung	Bird droppings or feathers	Hypersensitivity pneumonitis is present	Progressive fibrosis of lung
Byssinosis	Cotton, flax, and hemp dust (textile industry)	Airway obstruction is caused by contraction of smooth muscles; chronic disease results from severe airway obstruction and decreased elastic recoil	Progression of chronic disease after cessation of dust exposure
Coal worker's pneumoconiosis (black lung)	Coal dust	Incidence is high (20%-30%) in coal workers; deposits of carbon dust cause lesions to develop along respiratory bronchioles; bronchioles dilate because of loss of wall structure; chronic airway obstruction and bronchitis develop; dyspnea and cough are common early symptoms	Progressive, massive lung fibrosis; increased risk of chronic bronchitis and emphysema with smoking
Farmer's lung	Inhalation of airborne material from moldy hay or similar matter	Hypersensitivity pneumonitis occurs; *acute* form is similar to pneumonia, with manifestations of chills, fever, and malaise; *chronic,* insidious form is type of pulmonary fibrosis	Progressive fibrosis of lung
Siderosis	Iron oxide present in welding materials, foundries, iron ore mining	Dust deposits are found in lung	
Silicosis	Silica dust present in quartz rock in mining of gold, copper, tin, coal, lead; also present in sandblasting, foundries, quarries, pottery making, masonry	In *chronic* disease, dust is engulfed by macrophages and may be destroyed, resulting in fibrotic nodules; *acute* disease results from intense exposure in short time; within 5 yr, it progresses to severe disability from lung fibrosis	Increased susceptibility to tuberculosis; progressive, massive fibrosis; high incidence of chronic bronchitis
Silo filler's disease	Nitrogen oxides from fermentation of vegetation in freshly filled silo	Chemical pneumonitis occurs	Progressive bronchiolitis obliterans

From Lewis SM, Collier IC, Heitkemper MM: *Medical-surgical nursing: assessment and management of clinical problems,* ed 4, St. Louis, 1996, Mosby.

Table **34-4**	**Normal Arterial and Venous Blood Gas Values***		

	Arterial blood gases		
Laboratory value	Sea level BP 760 mm Hg	1 Mile above sea level (5280 ft) BP 629 mm Hg	Mixed venous blood gases
pH	7.35-7.45	7.35-7.45	pH 7.34-7.37
PaO_2	80-100 mm Hg	65-75 mm Hg	PVO_2 38-42 mm Hg
SaO_2	>95%†	>95%†	SVO_2 60-80%†
$PaCO_2$	35-45 mm Hg	35-45 mm Hg	$PVCO_2$ 44-46 mm Hg
HCO_3	22-26 mEq/L	22-26 mEq/L	HCO_3 24-30 mEq/L

From Lewis SM, Collier IC, Heitkemper MM: *Medical-surgical nursing: assessment and management of clinical problems,* ed 4, St. Louis, 1996, Mosby.
BP, barometric pressure; *PVO₂,* partial pressure of oxygen in venous blood; *SVO₂,* venous oxygen saturation.
*Assumes patient is ≤60 years of age and breathing room air.
†The same normal values apply when SaO₂ and SVO₂ are obtained by oximetry.

Table **34-5**	**Comparison of Emphysema and Chronic Bronchitis***	

	Emphysema	Chronic bronchitis
Clinical features		
Age	30-40 yr (onset) 60-70 yr (disabling)	20-30 yr (onset) 40-50 yr (disabling)
Body build	Thin	Tendency toward obesity
Health history	Generally healthy, occasional insidious dyspnea, smoking	Recurrent respiratory tract infections, smoking
Weight loss	Often marked	Absent or slight
Dyspnea	Slowly progressive and eventually disabling	Variable, relatively late
Sputum	Scanty, mucoid	Copious, mucopurulent
Cough	Negligible	Considerable
Chest examination	Marked increase in AP diameter, quiet or diminished breath sounds, limited diaphragmatic excursion	Slight to marked increase in AP diameter scattered crackles, rhonchi, wheezing
Cor pulmonale	Rare except terminally	Frequent with many episodes
Diagnostic study results		
ABGs	Near normal, mild ↓ PaO_2, normal or ↑ $PaCO_2$	↓ PaO_2, ↑ $PaCO_2$
Chest x-ray	Hyperinflation, flat diaphragm, attenuated peripheral vessels, small or normal heart, widened intercostal margins	Cardiac enlargement, normal or flattened diaphragm, evidence of chronic inflammation, congested lung fields
Lung volumes		
Total lung capacity	Increased	Normal or slightly increased
Residual volume	Increased	Increased
Vital capacity	Decreased	Decreased
FEV_1	Decreased	Decreased
FEV_1/FVC	Decreased (<70%)	Decreased (<70%)
Hematocrit and hemoglobin	Normal until late in disease	Increased
Pathology		
	Panlobular emphysema	Centrilobular emphysema

From Lewis SM, Collier IC, Heitkemper MM: *Medical-surgical nursing: assessment and management of clinical problems,* ed 4, St. Louis, 1996, Mosby.
ABGs, Arterial blood gases; *AP,* anteroposterior; *FEV₁,* forced expiratory volume in 1 second; *FVC,* forced vital capacity.
*Most persons with COPD have features of both pulmonary emphysema and chronic bronchitis.

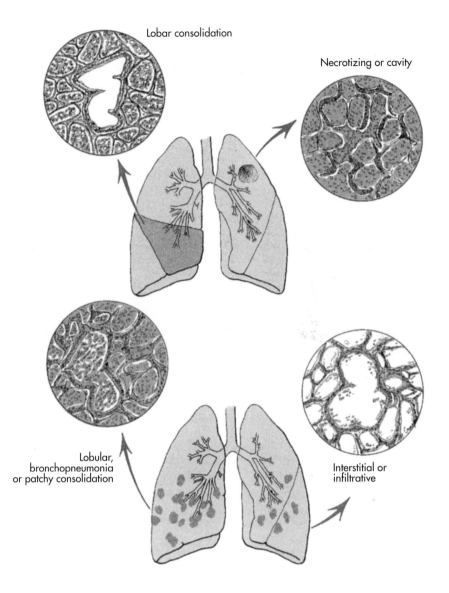

Figure **34-9** Types of pneumonia: lobar—entire lobe consolidated, exudate chiefly intraalveolar, *pneumococcus* and *Klebsiella* are common infecting organisms; necrotizing—granuloma may undergo caseous necrosis and form cavity, fungi and tubercle bacillus infections are common causes; lobular—patchy distribution, fibrinous exudate chiefly in bronchioles, *Staphylococcus* and *Streptococcus* are common infecting organisms; interstitial—perivascular exudate and edema between alveoli, caused by virus or mycoplasmal infection. *(From Price SA, Wilson LM:* Pathophysiology: clinical concepts of disease processes, *ed 5, St. Louis, 1997, Mosby.)*

Table 34-6 compares symptoms and characteristics of various types of pneumonia.

Therapeutic interventions for ED patients with pneumonia include administering humidified oxygen and antibiotics, and controlling fluid and electrolyte balance. Diagnostic assessment includes sputum culture and gram stain, chest radiograph, and complete blood count (CBC). Pulse oximetry should be assessed and arterial blood gas values obtained for most patients.

Asthma

Asthma, as defined by the National Asthma Education Program,[6] is a "disease characterized by airway obstruction that is reversible (at least to a significant degree), airway inflammation and increased airway responsiveness to a variety of stimuli." One in 20 Americans, or approximately 10 million people, are affected by asthma. Asthma can be controlled, not cured, and has an unpredictable course with increasing prevalence and hospitalization. Onset occurs before age 10 in 50% of patients, and there is positive family history in more than one third of asthmatic patients.

Development of airway inflammation and hyperresponsiveness occurs in response to immunologic or nonimmunologic stimuli or triggers (Box 34-2). Immunologic triggers cause a humoral immune response with complex multicell activation, including mast cells, eosinophils, and IGE antibodies (Figure 34-10). Inflammatory mediators cause smooth muscle contraction, vasodilation, mucosal edema, increased mucus secretion, and macrophage eosinophil infiltration. Acetylcholine directly increases airway resistance and bronchial secretions. This cholinergic response further stimulates histamine and inflammatory mediator release excluding IGE antibodies.

Nonimmunologic triggers stimulate the autonomic nervous system and cause mast cell and inflammatory mediator response. The pathway of emotional triggers is through the

Box 34-1	Factors Predisposing to Pneumonia

Smoking
Air pollution
Altered consciousness: alcoholism, head injury, seizures,
 anesthesia, drug overdose
Tracheal intubation (endotracheal intubation,
 tracheostomy)
Upper respiratory tract infection
Chronic diseases: chronic lung disease, diabetes
 mellitus, heart disease, uremia, cancer
Immunosuppression drugs (corticosteroids, cancer chemother-
 apy, immunosuppressive therapy after organ transplant)
HIV
Malnutrition
Inhalation or aspiration of noxious substances
Debilitating illness
Bed rest and prolonged immobility
Altered oropharyngeal flora

From Lewis SM, Collier IC, Heitkemper MM: *Medical-surgical nursing: assessment and management of clinical problems,* ed 4, St. Louis, 1996, Mosby.
HIV, Human immunodeficiency virus.

Box 34-2	Triggers of Acute Asthma Attacks

Allergen inhalation
 Animal danders
 House dust mite
 Pollens
 Molds
Air pollutants
 Exhaust fumes
 Perfumes
 Oxidants
 Sulfur dioxides
 Cigarette smoke
 Aerosol sprays
Viral upper respiratory infection
Paranasal sinusitis
Exercise and cold, dry air
Drugs
 Aspirin
 Nonsteroidal antiinflammatory
  drugs
 β-adrenergic blockers

Occupational exposure
 Metal salts
 Wood and vegetable
  dusts
 Industrial chemicals
  and plastics
 Pharmaceutical agents
Food additives
 Sulfites (bisulfites and
  metabisulfites)
 Tartrazine
Menses
Gastroesophageal reflux
Emotional stress

From Lewis SM, Collier IC, Heitkemper MM: *Medical-surgical nursing: assessment and management of clinical problems,* ed 4, St. Louis, 1996, Mosby.

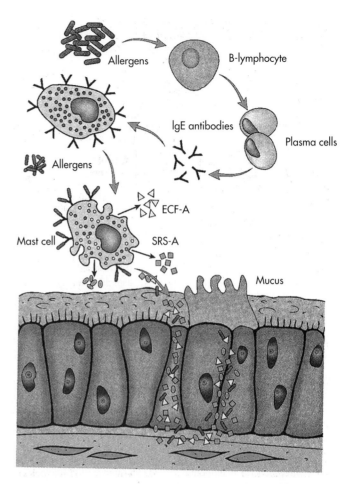

Figure **34-10** Early phase response in asthma is triggered when
an allergen or irritant cross-links IgE receptors on mast cells, which
are then activated to release histamine and other inflammatory mediators. *(From Lewis SM, Collier IC, Heitkemper MM:* Medical-
surgical nursing: assessment and management of clinical problems,
ed 4, St. Louis, 1996, Mosby.)

may be the only trigger for some patients and is usually limited to the early phase. Gastroesophageal reflux, a common
condition associated with asthma, involves esophageal
spasm with reflux of gastric acid causing spasm of nearby
bronchial and esophageal structures.

Immunologic and nonimmunologic triggers cause increased mucus production, airway hyperresponsiveness, airway narrowing, and chronic inflammatory airway changes.
Reaction phases in response to asthma triggers are early and
late. Early phase reaction involves rapid bronchospasm and
late phase reaction involves inflammatory epithelial lesions,
increasing mucosal edema, and increased secretions. Complex interactions among cells in the lungs cause a chronic inflammatory process that irritates airways. Acute exacerbation involves airway obstruction from spasm, inflammation,
and mucus plugging.

Morphologic changes of lung tissue from asthma include
bronchial infiltration with inflammatory cells; vascular dilation, edema, and epithelial damage and detachment; smooth

parasympathetic nervous system and stimulation of the hypothalamus. Aspirin sensitivity causes asthma through reaction to prostaglandin synthesis. Exercise-induced asthma
occurs after 10 to 20 minutes of vigorous exercise through
airway cooling secondary to decreased warming, reduced
humidification, and increased respiratory rates. Exercise

Table 34-6 Comparison of Types of Pneumonia

Causative agent	Characteristics	Clinical manifestations and complications
Gram-positive bacterial pneumonias		
Pneumococcal pneumonia (*Streptococcus pneumoniae*)	URI usually preceding; usual involvement of 1 or more lobes; incubation period of 1-3 days; peak incidence in winter and spring; damage to host by overwhelming growth of organism; necrosis of lung tissue (unusual); chest x-ray shows lobar infiltration; nasopharyngeal carriers; frequent finding of herpes labialis in association with pneumonia; risk factors of chronic heart or lung disease, diabetes mellitus, cirrhosis	Abrupt onset, elevated temperature, tachypnea, chills and rigor, productive cough (often bloody, rusty, or green), nausea, vomiting, malaise, myalgia, weakness, pleuritic chest pain, atelectasis, lung abscess (rare), pleural effusions (25%-50%), empyema, metastatic infection (meninges, joints, heart valves), bacteremia (25%)
Staphylococcal pneumonia (*Staphylococcus aureus*)	Acquisition via hematogenous route or via aspiration into lungs; nasopharyngeal carriers (35%-50% of population); necrotizing infection causing destruction of lung tissue; chest x-ray shows bronchopneumonia; risk factors of chronic lung disease, leukemia, other debilitating diseases; influenza infection (10-14 days earlier) often preceding; drug abusers, diabetics, patients on long-term hemodialysis at risk as carriers; occurrence more frequent in hospitalized patients than in persons in community; prolonged antibiotic therapy usually necessary; high mortality rate in chronically debilitated patients, newborns	Abrupt onset, chills, high fever, productive cough with sputum (often bloody and purulent), tachypnea, progressive dyspnea, pleuritic chest pain, empyema, pleural effusions, lung abscess
Streptococcal pneumonia (*Streptococcus pyogenes*)	Occurrence in military populations after influenza epidemics and sporadically in community; often associated with strep throat; occurrence most frequent in winter; transmission to lung by inhalation or aspiration; destruction of lung tissue; chest x-ray shows bronchopneumonia	Fever (usually >102.2° F [39° C]), chills, cough, pharyngitis, hemoptysis, pleuritic chest pain, dyspnea, myalgia, empyema (common), pleural effusions, bacteremia, mediastinitis, pneumothorax, bronchiectasis
Anthrax pneumonia (*Bacillus anthracis*)	Association with agricultural or industrial exposure (e.g., individuals working with animal hair or contaminated animal hides or bones); transmission to lung via inhalation; formation of spores; ingestion and transport of spores to hilar lymph nodes (site of multiplication of bacteria) by alveolar macrophages; hemorrhagic pneumonitis possible	Early manifestations: insidious onset (2-4 days), mild fever, myalgia, malaise, fatigue, nonproductive cough Later manifestations: dyspnea, profuse diaphoresis, cyanosis
Gram-negative bacterial pneumonias		
Friedländer's pneumonia (*Klebsiella pneumoniae*)	Most common gram-negative pneumonia acquired outside hospital; alcoholics, diabetics, persons with chronic lung disease, and postoperative patients at risk; transmission to lungs via aspiration of oropharyngeal organisms; chest x-ray shows lobar consolidation; rapid progression to lung abscess possible; high mortality and morbidity rates	Sudden onset, fever, cough, purulent sputum, hemoptysis, malaise, pleuritic chest pain, extensive lung necrosis, lung abscess, empyema, pericarditis, meningitis

From Lewis SM, Collier IC, Heitkemper MM: *Medical-surgical nursing: assessment and management of clinical problems,* ed 4, St. Louis, 1996, Mosby.
GI, Gastrointestinal; *GU,* genitourinary; *HIV,* human immunodeficiency virus; *URI,* upper respiratory tract infection.
*Organism has characteristics of both bacteria and viruses.

Table **34-6** **Comparison of Types of Pneumonia—cont'd**		
Causative agent	**Characteristics**	**Clinical manifestations and complications**
Gram-negative bacterial pneumonias—cont'd		
Pseudomonas pneumonia *(Pseudomonas aeruginosa)*	Most common gram-negative hospital-acquired pneumonia; predisposition from endotracheal intubation, intermittent positive-pressure breathing treatments, suctioning, respiratory therapy equipment; high mortality rate in critically ill patients; chest x-ray shows nodular bronchopneumonia; persons with chronic lung disease, debilitating diseases, tracheostomies, cancer, and kidney transplants or those taking immunosuppressive drugs or broad-spectrum antibiotics at risk; high mortality rate (50%-90%)	High fever, cough, copious sputum, hypoxia, cyanosis, lung abscess
Influenza pneumonia *(Haemophilus influenzae)*	Increase in incidence; transmission to lung by endogenous aspiration; chest x-ray shows bronchopneumonia in multiple lobes or lobar consolidation; alcoholics and persons with chronic lung disease, recent viral infections, and immune deficiencies at risk; high mortality rate, especially in older adult patients	Usually gradual onset, sometimes abrupt; fever; chills; cough; purulent sputum; hemoptysis; sore throat; dyspnea; nausea and vomiting; pleuritic chest pain; pleural effusions; lung abscess (common); empyema (common)
Legionnaires' disease *(Legionella pneumophila)*	Occurrence in outbreaks or sporadic; transmission to lung from airborne organisms; proliferation of organisms in water reservoirs (e.g., air-conditioning cooling towers); cigarette smokers and persons with serious underlying diseases (e.g., chronic lung or heart conditions) at increased risk; erythromycin effective	Myalgia (initially), headache (initially), fever, chills, nonproductive cough, pleuritic chest pain, nausea and vomiting, diarrhea, mental confusion, respiratory failure (major complication), healing with fibrosis common
Anaerobic bacterial pneumonias		
Anaerobic streptococci Fusobacteria *Bacteroides* species	Transmission to lung usually by aspiration of oropharyngeal secretions but occasionally via blood from GI or GU tract or wound infections; three or four anaerobes usually causing infections; persons with poor dental hygiene, periodontal disease, and history of altered consciousness at risk; chest x-ray often shows lung abscess, empyema, necrotizing pneumonia	Similar to pneumococcal pneumonia, except for insidious onset; foul-smelling sputum; necrotizing pneumonitis (aspiration induced); lung abscess; empyema
Mycoplasma pneumonia		
Mycoplasma pneumonia *(Mycoplasma pneumoniae)**	Transmission from person to person by respiratory droplets; incubation period of 9-21 days; involvement of epithelial lining of respiratory system; common in children, military populations, college-age groups; increase in cold agglutinin titer in serum or complement fixation with negative bacterial culture; chest x-ray shows interstitial pneumonia, often bilaterally	Gradual onset; URI, including fever (low-grade), nasal congestion; pharyngitis; lower respiratory tract involvement (e.g., bronchitis, bronchiolitis); headache; malaise; cough (initially usually nonproductive); maculopapular rashes

Continued

Table 34-6 Comparison of Types of Pneumonia—cont'd

Causative agent	Characteristics	Clinical manifestations and complications
Viral pneumonias		
Influenza viruses Adenovirus Parainfluenza viruses Respiratory syncytial virus	Influenza A most common in civilian adults; responsible for about one half of all pneumonias; peak incidence in winter; transmission from person to person by respiratory droplets; usually self-limiting; symptomatic treatment; adverse effect on many respiratory defense mechanisms, predisposing patients to secondary bacterial pneumonia; chest x-ray shows interstitial pneumonia	Fever, chills, headache, myalgia, anorexia, sneezing, nasal congestion, cough (initially nonproductive)
Protozoan pneumonia		
Interstitial plasma cell pneumonia (*Pneumocytis carinii*)	Opportunistic infection; persons with immunosuppression (e.g., recipients of organ tranplants, patients with HIV infection, and those with hematologic malignancies) at highest risk; presentation similar to other atypical pneumonias	Cough (usually nonproductive), fever, night sweats, dyspnea (may be only with exertion)

From Lewis SM, Collier IC, Heitkemper MM: *Medical-surgical nursing: assessment and management of clinical problems,* ed 4, St. Louis, 1996, Mosby.
GI, Gastrointestinal; *GU,* genitourinary; *HIV,* human immunodeficiency virus; *URI,* upper respiratory tract infection.
*Organism has characteristics of both bacteria and viruses.

muscle hypertrophy; subepithelial fibrosis; and mucous gland hypertrophy. Radiographs of patients dying from asthma show air trapping caused by mucous plugs containing detached epithelium and eosinophils, with thickened bronchial walls infiltrated by inflammatory cells.

Diagnosis is based on careful history, exam, and lab studies. History includes symptoms, patterns, usual triggers, family history, and allergic background. Physical exam may reveal upper airway rhinitis, sinusitis, and/or nasal polyps. Wheezes and prolonged expiratory phase may be noted, with flexural eczema a common finding. CBC with differential may reveal increased eosinophils. Nasal smears or sputum specimens should also be obtained. Chest radiograph may show increased hilar or basilar infiltrates or areas of atelectasis secondary to mucus plugging and alveolar collapse.

Seventy-five percent to 85% of asthmatic patients have positive skin reaction, so allergy testing is indicated. Inhaled allergens are important triggers, particularly for patients less than 30 years of age. Food allergens are not common triggers. Sinusitis and allergic rhinitis with postnasal drip are common triggers and may necessitate sinus radiographs. Polyps are associated with asthma in patients more than 40 years of age.

Viral, occupational exposures, and gastroesophageal (GE) reflux are more common triggers in older adults and can be identified by careful history. Gastroesophageal reflux is associated with nocturnal exacerbations that respond poorly to

Box 34-3 Occupations and Agents Associated With Asthma

Occupation	Agent
Animal workers	Dander, urine protein
Dairy farmers	Storage mites
Bakers	Flour
Carpenters	Wood dust
Electroplating, plastics	Nickel salts
Welding	Stainless steel fumes
Manufacturing	Antibiotics
Hospital workers	Disinfectants

From National Asthma Education Program: *Guidelines for the diagnosis and management of asthma: speaker's kit,* 1992, National Heart, Lung, and Blood Institute.

nebulized therapy. GI workup is indicated when GE reflux is suspected.

Occupational asthma initially presents with rhinitis and/or eye irritation along with evening or nocturnal cough. Coughing, wheezing, and dyspnea progress with continued exposure but symptoms decrease on days off work. Smokers have a higher incidence of occupational asthma than nonsmokers, secondary to increased airway irritation. Occupations and agents associated with asthma are listed in Box 34-3.

The hallmark of asthma diagnosis is spirometry before and after bronchodilator therapy to document reversibility

Table **34-7**   **Asthma Severity Classification**

Variables	Mild	Moderate	Severe
Symptom frequency	<1 hr, 1-2 times/wk	>1-2 times/wk lasting several days, occasional ED visits	Daily signs and symptoms
Activity intolerance	<½ hr of wheezing or cough with activity	Moderate activity intolerance	Marked limitation
Nocturnal asthma	<1-2 times/mo	2-3 times/wk	Almost every night
School-work	Attendance rarely affected	Attendance affected	Poor attendance
PEFR	>80% best	60%-80% best	<60% best
	<20% daily variations	20%-30% daily variations	>30% daily variations

of airway narrowing, usually by peak expiratory flow rates. Peak expiratory flow rate (PEFR) is the greatest flow velocity produced during forced expiration after fully expanding lungs during inspiration. Peak expiratory flow measurement is simple, portable, and quantitative; however, lung volumes are not measured and measurement is effort dependent. Bronchoprovocation may be utilized with histamine, methacholine, or exercise. The lower the dose that causes a 20% fall in forced expiratory volume, the more severe the disease.

Clinical manifestations include cough, wheezing, prolonged expiratory time, and reduced peak expiratory flow. Increased work of breathing and use of accessory muscles may also be present. Arterial blood gas values initially have reduced PaO_2 and $PaCO_2$ from hyperventilation. $PaCO_2$ eventually rises, which indicates further $\dot{V}/\dot{Q}$ mismatching. Fine crackles may be heard with opening and closing of distal air sacs in response to mucus plugging and atelectasis. Breath sounds may be diminished in lower lobes. Decreased air sounds, decreased oxygen saturation, decreased respiratory effort, and decreased level of consciousness are signs of impending failure that require immediate intervention. Asthma is classified according to severity; however, asthma is a chronic state with exacerbations ranging from mild to severe (Table 34-7). Severity can be assessed by examining medications required to control symptoms, need for prednisone, prior intubation, recent hospitalizations, spirometric indices of air flow obstruction, occurrence of night symptoms, and number of ED visits.

Management goals are to maintain near-normal pulmonary function and exercise levels, prevent chronic symptoms and acute exacerbations, and avoid adverse effects of medications. Therapy includes objective measurement of lung function, environmental control, avoidance of triggers, select drugs, and comprehensive patient education.

Peak expiratory flow rate (PEFR) provides objective data for management, documents personal best and daily variations, detects impending exacerbation, guides medicine therapy, and helps identify triggers. To correctly obtain peak expiratory flow measurements the patient should stand, if able, take a deep breath, and forcefully blow out all inspired air. The highest of three readings is recorded. A diary of peak expiratory flow measurements, along with documentation of viral infections, weather, medicine changes, environments, and other possible trigger exposures aids in management of asthma.

Avoidance and environmental control of allergens such as dust mite antigen, animal dander, pollens, and molds can greatly reduce symptoms. Encasing pillows and mattresses in vinyl and washing bedding every week in water temperatures greater than 130° F, along with carpet removal or antimite treatment, reduces dust mite allergen. Keeping cats and dogs outside the house reduces dander allergen and outdoor pollens and mold. Asthma patients should remain inside with air conditioning during early morning and midday hours to further reduce exposure.

Drugs for asthma reduce contraction and spasm of bronchial smooth muscle, airway inflammation, mucosal edema, and airway hyperreactivity. Medications are given PO, IV, SQ, and inhaled (Table 34-8 and Box 34-4). Several forms of aerosolized therapy are used (Table 34-9). Advantages of aerosol therapy include smaller drug amounts, rapid onset of action, direct delivery to respiratory system, fewer side effects, and painless, convenient administration. Table 34-10 highlights over-the-counter drugs used for management of asthma.

Asthma education and clinician-patient communication are primary concerns when treating and controlling asthma. Asthma education should convey clinician-patient partnership, the concept of asthma as a chronic but controllable disease, the role of environmental control and use of medication, the importance of objective PEFR measurements, specific individualized guidelines for managing acute exacerbations, and when to call for help. Action, indication for use, and side effects of each medication should be provided orally and in written form in easy-to-understand language. More in-depth information can be added for individuals with specific learning needs. Detailed, written instructions are given to outline a plan for continuing care that is indi-

Table **34-8**   **Common Pulmonary Drugs**

Medication	Actions	Strength/dosage	Side effects/comments/precautions
Bronchodilators			
Sympathomimetics Epinephrine (Adrenalin)	Stimulates β-receptors for bronchodilation	Epi: 1:100 (1%) neb 0.25-0.5 ml QID or q 20-30 min for 3 doses (0.3 mg/max)	Unwanted SE: tremor, palpitations, increased blood pressure, headache, nervousness, dizziness, and nausea because both α and β are stimulated
Racemic epi (Micronefrin, Asthma nefrin)		Racemic: 2.25% neb; 0.25-0.5 ml	Racemic has ½ cardiac effects of epinephrine Rapid onset, short duration of action Monitor for rebound effect 2-4 hours after treatment
Terbutaline (Brethaire, Brethine)	As above	Brethaire metered-dose inhaler (MDI) 0.2 mg/puff, 2 puffs q 4-6 hr Brethine SQ 1 mg/ml, 0.1 mg/kg/q 2-6 hr, 0.3 mg max	4-6 hour duration β-2 specific so less cardiac effects Peak 30-60 min Onset 5-15 min
Albuterol (Proventil, Ventolin)	As above	Neb: 0.5%, 2.5-5.0 ml TID/QID MDI: 90 µg/puff, 2 puff TID/QID Tab: 2 and 4 mg tabs, 2-4 mg TID/QID Extended release tabs (Repetabs): 4 mg/tab, q 12 hr Spinhaler: 200 µg/cap, 1 cap q 4-6 hr	As above
Isoetharine (Bronkosol, Bronkometer)	As above	Neb: 1.0% 0.25-0.5 ml QID MDI: 340 µg/spray, 1-2 puffs QID	β-2 specific Short duration of action Rapid onset Minimal β-1 or cardiac stimulation
Salmeterol zinafoate (Serevent)	As above	MDI: 35 µg/puff, 1-3 puffs q 12 hr	Not for use in acute bronchospasm and asthma attacks because of long onset of action Onset 20-30 min Peak 2-3 hr Duration 8-12 hr Side effects are cough with administration and same as albuterol, especially when given with albuterol for control of acute symptoms
Zanthines	Smooth muscle dilation, CNS stimulation, and cerebral vasoconstriction, vasodilation of periphery and cardiac vessels, cardiac stimulation, and diuresis	Dosage depends on age, previous theophylline therapy, acute or chronic situation Dosage altered with: *increased serum levels*—barbiturates, calcium channel blockers, cimitidine, zantac, corticosteroids, ephedrine, viral infections, pneumonia; *decreased serum levels*—barbiturates, β-agonist, rifampin, phenytoin, cigarette smoking	Levels: <5 µg/ml—no effects 10-20 µg/ml—therapeutic range >20 µg/ml—nausea >30 µg/ml—cardiac dysrhythmias >40-45 µg/ml—seizures Dosages decreased with children, liver failure, and CHF

Table 34-8   Common Pulmonary Drugs—cont'd

Medication	Actions	Strength/dosage	Side effects/comments/precautions
Bronchodilators—cont'd			
Theophylline anhydrous (100% theophylline—Theodur, Respbid, Solphyllin, Bronkodyne)	As above	Oral or IV rapid onset load: 5-6 mg/kg Each 0.5 mg/kg increase will increase serum level by 1 µg/ml	Side effects: CNS—headache, anxiety, restlessness, dizziness, insomnia, tremor, seizures GI—abdominal pain, nausea/vomiting, anorexia, diarrhea, GE reflux
Aminophyline (79% theophylline)		Chronic therapy load: 16 mg/kg per 24 hr or 400 mg/24 hr, whichever is less	Resp—increased respiratory rate CV—palpitations, SVT, ventricular dysrhythmias, hypotension Renal—diuresis (increase hydration to prevent thick secretions) Food/drug interactions: Increased levels with caffeine (tea, cola, chocolate), and charbroiled foods, increased protein and decreased carbohydrate diets
Parasympatholytics/Anticholinergics			
Atropine Ipratropium (Atrovent)	Antimuscarinic action: blocks acetylcholine by occupying receptor site and blocks PSNS bronchoconstriction effect, inhibits mast cell release (decreased mucus and chemotaxis), blocks cough receptors	Neb: 0.2% (1 mg/0.5 ml), 0.025 mg/kg TID/QID MDI: 18 µg/puff, 2 puff QID	Side effects: 0.5 mg—dryness of mouth and eyes 2.0 mg—pupil dilation, increased heart rate, blurred vision 5.0 mg—slurred speech, impaired swallowing and urination, flushed skin >5.0 mg—CNS excitement Onset 15 min Peak ½ to 1 hr for atropine and 1-2 hr for ipratropium Duration 3-4 hr for atropine and 4-6 hr for ipratropium
Corticosteroids			
	Decreased inflammation of inflamed epithelial cells in asthma		Systemic side effects are related to dose and minimal compared to systemic administration but can occur with >800 µg/day, >400 µg/day in children Side effects topical under 800 µg/day: oropharyngeal fungal infections, hoarseness, cough, and can be eliminated or reduced with use of spacers and rinsing mouth after each puff Can be used intranasally to prevent allergic rhinitis or decrease signs and symptoms; must be figured into overall total daily dose

Continued

Table **34-8** **Common Pulmonary Drugs—cont'd**			
Medication	Actions	Strength/dosage	Side effects/comments/precautions
Corticosteroids—cont'd			

Inhaled corticosteroids
  Dexamethasone (Decadron Respinhaler)
  Beclomethasone (Beclovent, Vanceril)
  Triamcinolone (Azmacort)
  Flunisolide (Aerobid)
	As above	MDI (μg/puff) AND dose
		Dexamethasone (84) 3 puffs TID/QID
		Beclomethasone, etc—(42) 2 puffs TID/QID
		Triamcinolone (100) 2 puffs TID/QID
		Flunisolide (250) 2 puffs TID/QID
			As above

Oral corticosteroids
  Outpatient: prednisone
 	
  Inpatient: methylprednisone
	As above	Short bursts for 3 days may be all that is needed, >5 days need to taper reduction of doses, 1-2 mg/kg/day in single or divided doses
		1-2 mg/kg/dose q 6 hr, length depends on severity, dose tapered off
			Side effects:
			Increased appetite, mood swings, fluid retention, increased WBC, hypertension (fluid retention), ulcer, gastritis, increased serum glucose
			Long term SE:
			Osteoporosis, myopathy of striated muscle, cataract formation, immunosuppression, suppression of HPA axis

Antiasthmatics
  Cromolyn (Intal)
  Nedocromil (Tilade)
	Inhibition of mast cell degranulation—blocks release of chemical mediators of inflammation (can prevent late phase reaction of asthma)	MDI:
		Cromolyn: 0.8 mg/puff, 2 puffs QID
		Nedocromil: 1.75 mg/puff, 2 puffs QID
		NEB:
		Cromolyn: 20 mg/amp, 1 amp QID
			Comes in intranasal, ophthalmic, and oral preparations
			Side effects: minimal, seen mostly with inhaled powder form—cough, bronchospasm
			Does not treat acute attacks of bronchospasm
			Peak 5-30 min
			Duration 4-6 hr

vidualized to each patient's capability. Correct use of spacers, inhalers, and PEFR meters must be assessed. Teach patients to check medication levels in MDI canisters by simply placing in a cup of water (Figure 34-11). If the canister floats sideways on top of the water, it is empty, whereas a full canister sinks. Dispel common misconceptions about asthma: for example, asthma is NOT an emotional or psychiatric disease; activity and exercise should be included in plan of care (not decreased); asthma medication is NOT addictive; inhaled, oral, or IV corticosteroids are NOT the same as anabolic steroids; medication DOES NOT lose effectiveness with increased or continuous use; and episodes are NOT sudden and without warning but can be predicted by identifying triggers and PEFR measurements.

Ongoing research is comparing the benefits of theophylline with known side effects. Foley[2] cites a small study that confirms the benefits of theophylline in moderate doses in patients with acute bronchospasm of COPD and asthma with minimal side effects within therapeutic range. Magnesium sulfate for the treatment of acute bronchospasm of asthma is based on the theory that magnesium acts as a calcium channel antagonist, blocks uptake of calcium in bronchial smooth muscle, and causes bronchial relaxation. Recent studies suggest magnesium may be beneficial for patients with acute, severe asthma when conventional therapy does not control exacerbation; however, more extensive study is required.

Emphysema

Emphysema refers to permanent abnormal enlargement of air spaces distal to terminal bronchioles and associated destructive changes of the alveolar wall. Asthma is characterized by simple overdistention without alveolar destruction. Three types of emphysema are categorized according to area of lung tissue involved. There are 25,000 acini, or airways distal to terminal bronchiole/conducting airway, and

---

Box **34-4**   **Common Cough and Cold Agents Used With Asthma Medications**

Adrenergic nasal decongestants

Oral: phenylephrine (Neosynephrine, Coricidin) pseudoephedrine (Sudafed)

Topical: oxymetazoline (Afrin)

Cause vasoconstriction

Side effects include increased blood pressure and heart rate, especially with oral prep.

Side effects with topical administration include necrosis of nasal septum with prolonged use—use only during acute episodes and no more than 3 days BID per month.

Antihistamine drying agents

Diphenhydramine (Benadryl)

Clemastine (Tavist)

Promthazine (Phenergan)

Terfenadine (Seldane)

Axtemizole (Hismanal)

Block H1 receptors of bronchopulmonary smooth muscle and blood vessels

Sedative and anticholinergic effects: drowsiness and dryness of mouth and eyes

Expectorants

Guaifenesin (Robitussin, etc.)

Iodinated glycerol (Organidin)

SSKI (Potassium iodide)

Aid in mucus clearing by mucolytic or stimulant action; major use in bronchitis

Iodides associated with hypersensitivity reactions

Antitussives

Codeine (Robitussin AC, etc.)

Hydrocodone (Tussionex, Triaminic expectorant DH)

Dextromethorphan (Formula 44D, Robitussin DM, etc.)

Control cough; use only with dry hacking cough, do not use with productive cough

Use of products that have cough suppression with expectorant and antihistamine with expectorant is questionable

---

3 million alveoli. *Centrilobular emphysema* occurs in the center of lobules and corresponds to enlargement of respiratory bronchioles, is associated with chronic bronchitis, rarely occurs in nonsmokers, and involves upper lung fields. *Panlobular emphysema* is less common, occurs throughout the lung but primarily in lower and anterior fields, has less correlation with smoking, and is more associated with familial α-1 antiprotease deficiency. Entire acini and many bullae (airspaces less than 1 mm in diameter in distended state) are involved. *Bullous emphysema* is characterized by isolated emphysemic changes in bullae with absence of generalized emphysema.

There is a definite relationship between smoking, chronic bronchitis, and emphysema; however, all smokers do not de-

---

Correct Use of a Metered-Dose Inhaler

Using a metered-dose inhaler (MDI) is a good way to take asthma medicines. There are few side effects because the medicine goes right to the lungs and not to other parts of the body. It takes only 5 to 10 minutes for the medicine to have an effect compared to liquid asthma medicines, which can take 1 to 3 hours. Inhalers can be used by all asthma patients age 5 and older. A spacer or holding chamber attached to the inhaler can help make taking the medicine easier. These devices are helpful to people having trouble using an inhaler.

The inhaler must be cleaned often to prevent buildup that will clog it and reduce how well it works.
- The guidelines that follow will help you use the inhaler the right way.
- Ask your doctor or nurse to show you how to use the inhaler.

Using the Inhaler
1. Remove the cap and hold the inhaler upright.
2. Shake the inhaler.
3. Tilt your head back slightly and breathe out.
4. Use the inhaler in any one of these ways.
   (A is the best way, but C is okay if you are having trouble with A or B).
   A. Open mouth with inhaler 1 to 2 inches away
   B. Use spacer
   C. In the mouth

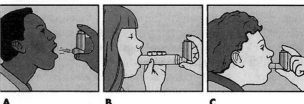

A   **B**   **C**

5. Press down on the inhaler to release the medicine as you start to breathe in slowly.
6. Breathe in *slowly* for 3 to 5 seconds.
7. Hold your breath for 10 seconds to allow the medicine to reach deeply into your lungs.
8. Repeat puffs as prescribed. Waiting 1 minute between puffs may permit the second puff to go deeper into the lungs.

Note: Dry powder capsules are used differently. To use a dry powder inhaler, close your mouth tightly around the mouthpiece and inhale very fast.

Cleaning
1. Once a day clean the inhaler and cap by rinsing it in warm running water. Let it dry before you use it again. Have another inhaler to use while it is drying.
2. Twice a week wash the plastic mouthpiece with mild dishwashing soap and warm water. Rinse and dry well before putting it back.

Checking How Much Medicine Is Left in the Canister
1. If the canister is new, it is full.
2. An easy way to check the amount of medicine left in your metered dose inhaler is to place the canister in a container of water and observe the position it takes in the water.

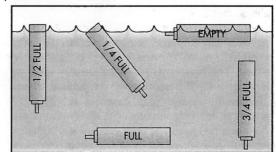

Figure **34-11** Correct use of a metered-dose inhaler. *(From Teach your patients about asthma: a clinician's guide, National Asthma Education Program, NIH Publication No. 92-2737, October 1992.)*

Table 34-9   Forms of Aerosolized Therapy[7]

Types	Description	Indications
Nebulizers (ultrasonic, small particle, and small volume)	Drug solution in liquid reservoir chamber is shattered into suspension by aerosol and/or acoustic energy with varying particle size.	Unable to cooperate or disoriented Incapable of inspiratory hold Reduced tidal volume Tachypneic or unstable respiratory pattern Achieves better distribution of drug to lower airways
MDI (metered-dose inhalers)	Suspension of drug (micronized powder or liquid) in chlorofluorocarbon liquid propellant (freon)	Able to follow instructions Capable of inspiratory hold Stable respiratory pattern Needs drug available in MDI form Requires timing and coordination of inspiration and delivery of drug
Auxiliary devices	Spacers—increase vaporization of particles and increased lung penetration, decreased loss of drug in air or mouth, simplify coordination (puff then inhale vs puff and inhale during midpuff with MDI). Breath actuated devices—aimed at reducing coordination and grip strength problems (elderly, arthritic)	Spacers— Increase delivery of drug Decrease coordination requirements with MDI Breath actuated devices— Reduce coordination and grip strength requirements for use with MDI
Dry powder inhalers	Powdered drug to be inhaled to cause aerosolization of solid particles	Poor MDI coordination Sensitive to CFC propellants in MDI Capable of high inspiratory volumes May cause bronchospasm in hyperreactive airways

Table 34-10   Nonprescription Combination Asthma Drugs

Drug product	Ingredients		
	Sympathomimetic	Xanthine	Other
Amodrine	Ephedrine	Aminophylline	Phenobarbital
Asthma Nefrin inhalant	Epinephrine	—	Chlorobutanol
Bronkaid tablets	Ephedrine	Theophylline	Guaifenesin
Bronkaid mist	Epinephrine	—	Ascorbic acid, alcohol
Bronkotabs	Ephedrine	Theophylline	Guaifenesin, phenobarbital
Primatene M tablets	Ephedrine	Theophylline	Pyrilamine
Primatene P tablets	Ephedrine	Theophylline	Phenobarbital
Primatene Mist	Epinephrine	—	Ascorbic acid, alcohol
Tedral	Ephedrine	Theophylline	Phenobarbital
Vaponefrin inhalant	Epinephrine	—	Chlorobutanol
Verquad	Ephedrine	Theophylline	Guaifenesin, phenobarbital

From Lewis SM, Collier IC, Heitkemper MM: *Medical-surgical nursing: assessment and management of clinical problems,* ed 4, St Louis, 1996, Mosby.

velop emphysema, so some genetic or familial trait may predispose patients. A small minority of patients have a genetic deficiency of serum α-1 antiprotease, otherwise known as antitrypsin, which inhibits protease that digests proteins such as elastic and collagen fibers of the lung. Protease is present in macrophages and polymorphonuclear leukocytes released during inflammatory processes. Protease-antiprotease imbalance infection or respiratory irritants such as smoke and pollutants inactivate inhibitors.

The end result is destruction of elastic properties of the lung and loss of natural recoil and support. During expiration, increased intrathoracic pressure causes collapse and premature closure of airways, and decreased support of the lung causes large residual volumes and decreased flow rates during expiration. Inspiratory rates are normal unless there is airway obstruction from chronic bronchitis, airtrapping, and overdistended airspaces. Eventually, the area for gas exchange at the alveolar capillary membrane decreases because of destruction of alveolar wall, so $\dot{V}/\dot{Q}$ mismatch occurs with patchy emphysemic changes, increased physiologic dead space, and abnormal arterial blood gases.

Early manifestations include signs of chronic bronchitis and may not be specific. Dyspnea on exertion occurs first, progressing to dyspnea at rest. Primary emphysema presents with dyspnea without cough or expectoration. The severity of dyspnea does not correlate with the severity of the destructive changes in the lung. Increasing dyspnea indicates increasing airway obstruction. In advanced stages, the patient may have increased anteroposterior (A-P) diameter of the chest, dorsal kyphosis, elevated ribs, flare at the costal margin, and widening of the costal angle, that is, barrel chest. Breath sounds are decreased with expiratory wheezes. Chest radiographs may show depression and flattening of the diaphragm, indicating hyperinflation of lungs. Decreased vascular markings, hyperlucency, deeper space between sternum and heart, and increased A-P diameter may also be present. Pulmonary function tests reveal hyperinflation, increased residual volume, reduction in vital capacity, and increased total lung capacity with decreased expiratory flow rates. Reduction in diffusion capacity differentiates emphysema from asthma or bronchitis. Arterial blood gases are normal in mild cases with decreased PaO_2 the most common change, in advanced stages or acute exacerbation $PaCO_2$ is elevated. Chest auscultation usually finds hyperresonance in all fields.

The cause of emphysema is variable and may include an annual decline in expiratory flow rates. Progression varies, but increased obstruction correlates with increased severity. ED management includes pulse oximetry, oxygen therapy, bronchodilators, and steroids. Decreased oxygen saturation should be addressed immediately.

Chronic Obstructive Pulmonary Disease

COPD is a group of conditions associated with chronic obstruction of air flow, which can result from chronic bronchitis, emphysema, and asthma. Fifteen million Americans have COPD, making it the second most common disability in the United States. There are many pathways to the final common state of COPD, with frequent overlapping of asthma, bronchitis, and emphysema.

Cessation of smoking may prevent progression to COPD in smokers. Early changes with chronic bronchitis are reversible when limited to small airways. Structural changes with emphysema are not reversible, so further insults must be avoided. Outpatient management includes avoiding irritants, good bronchial hygiene (adequate hydration, humidification, and postural drainage), bronchodilators, expectorants, and mucolytics. Nebulized therapy is as effective as IPPB treatments, whereas anticholinergic bronchodilators may have better results. Corticosteroids are used sparingly, although infections should be treated aggressively. Viral and bacterial infections play a major role in exacerbations of COPD and contribute to disability. Preventive measures include pneumococcal and viral immunizations. Antibacterial prophylaxis may be used for bacterial prone patients, although resistant organisms have made this practice questionable. Changes in cough and sputum production and characteristics require prompt antibiotic therapy. Proper education, patient compliance, adequate nutrition, and exercise are important parts of therapy. In advanced disease, chronic respiratory failure with severe hypoxemia and hypercapnia are present, so serum CO_2 levels no longer provide the drive for respiration. Hypoxia, or low serum O_2, is the drive for respiration. Chronic oxygen delivery is necessary if PaO_2 falls below 55 and high-flow oxygen should not be withheld if the patient is in respiratory failure. ED management includes oxygen therapy, nebulized inhalers, bronchodilators, and steroids. Low-flow oxygen may be administered with nasal cannula or venturi mask.

Pulmonary Embolus

Signs and symptoms of pulmonary embolus are frequently confused with those of myocardial infarction, pneumothorax, rib fractures, or other phenomena with the chief complaint of chest pain. Consequently, pulmonary embolus is extremely difficult to diagnose in the emergency care setting. Pulmonary embolus is one of the four leading causes of death in the United States and the most common form of death among hospitalized patients. Sixty percent of deaths from pulmonary embolism occur within 30 minutes of embolus formation.

Pulmonary embolus commonly results from trauma to the lower extremities or pelvis, surgery, long-bone fractures, or immobility, but is seen occasionally with obesity, decreased peripheral circulation, congestive heart failure, or thrombophlebitis. Cardiac diseases such as congestive heart failure or myocardial infarction may cause pulmonary emboli. Pulmonary emboli may also appear in conjunction with acute infections, blood dyscrasias, childbirth (amniotic fluid emboli), scuba diving (air emboli), oral contraceptives, cigarette smoking, neoplasms, and central venous catheter insertion.

The most common source of pulmonary embolism is deep leg veins. Venous thrombi form from stasis of blood, damage to epithelium of the vessel wall, or secondary to alterations in coagulation. The clot is dislodged and travels through the venous system and right side of the heart, finally lodging in a pulmonary vessel, obstructing blood flow and decreasing perfusion to a portion of the lungs (Figure 34-12). Lack of perfusion to an area of the lung with continued respirations leads to a disproportionate amount of blood when compared with oxygen in the bloodstream, that is, ventilation/perfusion mismatch. If the embolism lodges in a large pulmonary vessel, pulmonary vascular resistance in-

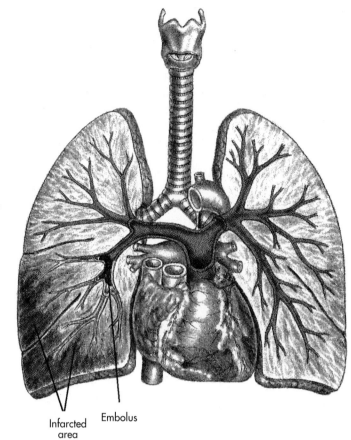

Figure **34-12** Pulmonary embolism. *(From Wilson SF, Thompson JM: Mosby's clinical nursing series: respiratory disorders, St. Louis, 1990, Mosby.)*

Infarcted area   Embolus

creases and cardiac output is decreased. Microscopically, the embolism causes the body to react by releasing serotonin, histamines, prostaglandins, and catecholamines that trigger bronchospasms and vaso-constriction. The production of surfactant ceases and alveoli collapse.

Pulmonary embolus is usually underdiagnosed. Signs and symptoms of pulmonary embolus can be nonspecific and lead the emergency nurse to think of other reasons for the signs and symptoms. Common signs and symptoms include shortness of breath, tachypnea, tachycardia, and sudden onset pleuritic chest pain that increases with respirations. The patient may have a cough, hemoptysis (from alveolar damage), diaphoresis, syncope, fever, and crackles. Petechiae (most often on the chest) also occur, but are more common with fat emboli. If the embolism occludes a large vessel, symptoms may be more severe and include anxiety, hypotension, and signs of right ventricular failure.

Diagnosis of pulmonary embolism is primarily made from arterial blood gas values and lung scan or pulmonary angiogram. Figure 34-13 shows a lung scan positive for pulmonary embolus. Decreased PO_2 and decreased PCO_2 are highly suggestive of pulmonary emboli in the presence of other symptoms. Chest radiographs are obtained, but are usually normal. Baseline laboratory studies are completed to rule out other sources of respiratory distress. ECG changes

significant for a pulmonary embolism include new onset right bundle branch block and right axis deviation with peaked P waves in limb leads and depressed T waves in right precordial leads (V_{1-3}).

Management of the patient with pulmonary embolism includes variable oxygen administration, from low-flow oxygen by nasal cannula to intubation, depending on patient needs. Analgesics may be administered intravenously if the patient is extremely uncomfortable. Intravenous fluids and vasopressors should be used to maintain pressure. Intravenous anticoagulants are initiated to prevent further clot formation. Weight-based heparin protocols are the preferred anticoagulant for these patients. Oral anticoagulants are usually not started in the ED. Thrombolytic therapy may be started to break up existing emboli. The recommended dose for recombinant alteplase (Activase) is 100 mg over 2 hours with heparin infusion near the end of the infusion or immediately after.

Pulmonary Edema

Pulmonary edema is not a primary disease process, but the result of an acute event. Pulmonary edema may be cardiogenic or noncardiogenic. Cardiogenic pulmonary edema occurs with inadequate left ventricular pumping that leads to increased fluid pressure (Box 34-5). Increased left ventricular pressure

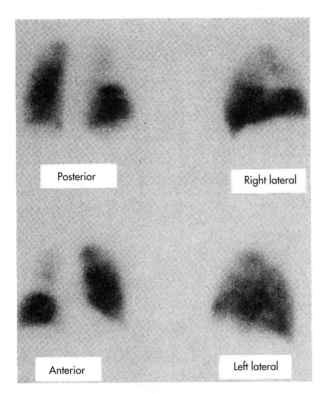

Posterior   Right lateral

Anterior   Left lateral

Figure **34-13** Lung scan showing pulmonary embolism. Note decreased perfusion of right upper lobe indicative of pulmonary embolism. *(From Thompson JM et al:* Mosby's clinical nursing, *ed 4, St. Louis, 1997, Mosby. Courtesy R. Keith Wilson, MD, Baylor College of Medicine, Houston, Texas.)*

Box 34-6   Conditions Predisposing to Acute Respiratory Distress Syndrome

Infectious causes
Gram-negative sepsis
Bacterial pneumonia
Viral pneumonia
Pneumocystis carinii
Tuberculosis

Aspiration
Gastric
Fresh and salt water
   (drowning)
Ethylene glycol
Hydrocarbon fluids

Shock
Septic
Traumatic
Hemorrhagic

Trauma
Generalized
Fat embolism
Lung contusion
Multiple major fractures
Head injury
Burns

Metabolic disorders
Pancreatitis
Uremia
Diabetic ketoacidosis

Inhaled toxic agents
Oxygen
Smoke
Toxic gases

Hematologic disorders
Massive blood transfu-
   sion
Disseminated intravas-
   cular coagulation
Transfusion reaction
Postcardiopulmonary bypass
   or resuscitation

Immunologic reactions
Drug allergy
Anaphylaxis

Drug-related
Dextran 40
Heroin
Methadone
Salicylates
Thiazides
Propoxyphene
Colchicine

Other
Radiation pneumonitis
Amniotic fluid emboli
Increased intracranial
   pressure
High altitude
Fluid overload
Eclampsia
Goodpasture's syndrome
Drug overdose
Bowel infarction
Dead fetus

From Lewis SM, Collier IC, Heitkemper MM: *Medical-surgical nursing: assessment and management of clinical problems,* ed 4, St. Louis, 1996, Mosby.

Box 34-5   Cardiogenic Pulmonary Edema

Inefficient pumping of left ventricle
   Fluid pressure increases in left ventricle
   Left atrium inhibited from pumping efficiently
   Increased alveolar-capillary membrane pressure
   Fluid in alveoli

---

inhibits left atrium emptying, so that blood backs up into alveolar-capillary membranes and pulmonary capillary filtration increases. Fluid from the pulmonary circulation floods the alveolar-capillary membrane and fills alveolar spaces normally containing air. The end result is increased fluid in the lungs. Potential causes of cardiogenic pulmonary edema include myocardial infarction and congestive heart failure.

Excessive extracellular fluid volume can result in pulmonary edema as increased pressure at the arterial capillary membranes pushes fluid into surrounding tissues. Fluid shifts across the alveolar-capillary membrane into the alveoli, resulting in pulmonary edema.

Fluid overload inhibits left ventricular pumping so excess fluid backs up into left atrium with the same effect as car-

diogenic pulmonary edema (Figure 34-14). Excessive fluid volume may be caused by increased sodium intake, such as with packaged foods, abuse of tap water enemas, or overload of intravenous fluids high in sodium. Renal disorders and cirrhosis can also cause fluid overload.

Noncardiogenic pulmonary edema, or acute respiratory distress syndrome (ARDS), is the result of primary damage to the alveolar-capillary membrane. Loss of integrity increases membrane permeability, which causes fluid and protein accumulation in interstitial spaces that eventually floods the alveoli, causing significant fluid accumulation in the lungs. Figure 34-15 illustrates pathophysiology of ARDS. A multitude of conditions, for example, trauma, sepsis, and fluid overload, predispose patients to ARDS (Box 34-6).

Patients with pulmonary edema exhibit cardiovascular and respiratory symptoms. Cardiovascular symptoms result from

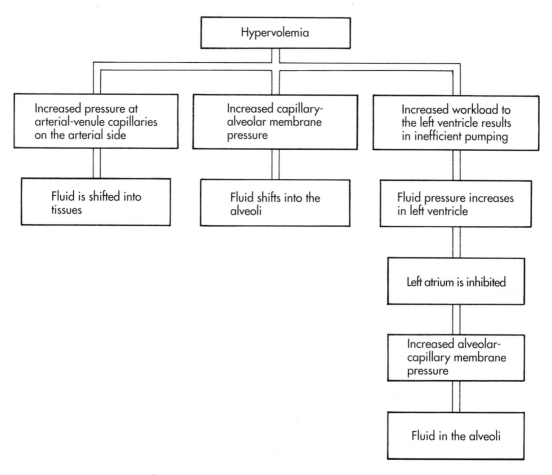

Figure **34-14** Hypervolemia and pulmonary edema.

generalized fluid overload. Poor left ventricular functioning is generally followed by poor right ventricular functioning, which leads to heart failure with engorged neck veins, sacral edema when the patient is sitting with legs not in a dependent position, lower extremity pitting edema, weight gain, rapid, bounding pulse, and S_3-S_4 heart sounds. If the pulmonary edema is untreated, the pulse eventually becomes weak and thready as the condition worsens. The skin is cool, pale, and moist and may appear cyanotic or mottled in some patients. Blood pressure initially increases in an attempt to pump extra fluid but decreases as the condition worsens.

Respiratory symptoms occur as increased alveolar fluid impairs oxygen exchange across the alveolar-capillary membrane. The patient develops dyspnea, and respiratory rate increases in an effort to increase oxygenation. Increased respiratory rate decreases PCO_2, causing respiratory alkalosis. As the condition worsens, metabolic acidosis occurs in an effort to rid the body of metabolic waste products. Respiratory effort becomes labored as the patient becomes fatigued. Fluid causes crackles and productive cough with frothy, white sputum. Sputum has a pink tinge in fulminant pulmonary edema. Cyanosis may be present and oxygen saturation decreased as hypoxia increases. Bronchospasms may develop, causing

wheezing, rales, and rhonchi. Chest radiographs usually show bilateral interstitial and alveolar infiltrates.

Treatment focuses on improving oxygenation through administration of high-flow oxygen (nonrebreather mask or intubation), improvement of cardiac function, and decreasing cardiac workload. Bronchodilators may be given through aerosol inhalation treatments to decrease bronchospasms. Positive end-expiratory pressure (PEEP) is indicated when hypoxia continues despite aggressive oxygen therapy. Some experimental treatments under investigation include extracorporeal carbon dioxide removal ($ECCO_2R$), surfactant removal, and inhaled nitrous oxide therapy.[1,8] Most patients with hypoxemia refractory to maximum ventilation have a poor prognosis because of secondary multiple system organ failure. Patients who require mechanical ventilation have a 50% mortality rate.[9]

Heart rate increases in an attempt to manage excess fluid; however, this leads to decreased filling time and decreased contractility. Digoxin is given (0.125 to 0.25 mg IVP) to increase contractility and decrease heart rate. Dobutamine (2 to 30 μg/kg/min) is given intravenously to increase contractility and reduce peripheral vascular resistance. Dopamine (1 to 20 μg/kg/min) is indicated for hemodynamically significant hy-

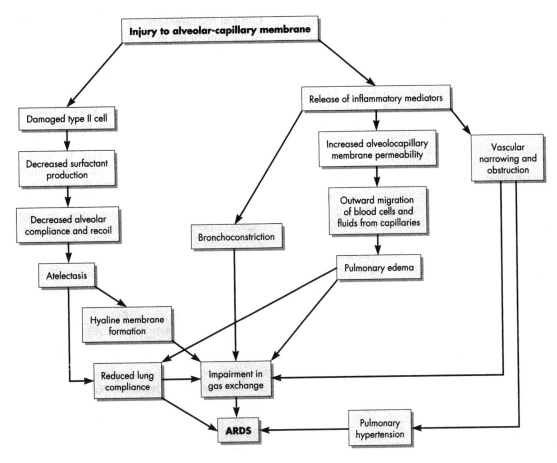

Figure **34-15** Pathophysiology of acute respiratory distress syndrome (ARDS). *(From Lewis SM, Collier IC, Heitkemper MM:* Medical-surgical nursing: assessment and management of clinical problems, *ed 4, St. Louis, 1996, Mosby.)*

potension. Nitroprusside (0.1 to 5.0 μg/kg/min) decreases afterload by vasodilation. Cardiac workload is also decreased through diuretic therapy (furosemide, bumetanide) and positioning the patient in high Fowler's position with the legs dependent. Dependent leg position results in venous distention in lower extremities or pooling of blood, which decreases circulatory volume. Intravenous morphine increases venous pooling and decreases preload—pressure in left ventricle at end of diastole. Preload is the result of blood volume in the left ventricle. In pulmonary edema, treatment is given to decrease volume so backflow into the atria is decreased and to increase strength of contraction by preventing overstretch of muscle fibers (Starling's law). Nitroglycerin may be administered to increase venous distention and venous pooling, which decrease blood return to the heart. Other interventions include Foley catheter to monitor urine output and effects of diuretics, and administration of dopamine or dobutamine if hypotension occurs.

Spontaneous Pneumothorax

Spontaneous pneumothorax occurs in individuals without underlying pulmonary disease, most often tall, thin males 20 to 40 years of age who smoke. Increased negative pressure at the apex of the lung increases risk for spontaneous pneumothorax in tall, thin individuals.[9] Pneumothorax occurs with rupture of a bleb, bulla, or weakened pleura, usually because of underlying pulmonary conditions such as COPD or pulmonary fibrosis. Patients with COPD on positive pressure ventilation are at increased risk for spontaneous pneumothorax because of changing pressures in the thoracic cavity. Iatrogenic pneumothorax is the result of invasive procedures such as insertion of a subclavian catheter.

Patients have dyspnea and chest pain on the affected side. Subcutaneous emphysema may be present with cyanosis, hypotension, and severe dyspnea if the pneumothorax is large. Oxygen saturation should be carefully monitored. Interventions are determined by the clinical presentation and degree of collapse. Asymptomatic patients with less than 20% pneumothorax may be observed on an inpatient or outpatient basis.[9] Other treatment options include needle aspiration and tube thoracostomy.

Table **34-11**	**COHb Levels and Symptoms**
COHb level	Symptoms
5%-10%	Can be asymptomatic or have mild headache, vertigo
10%-20%	Headache, nausea, vomiting, loss of coordination, may appear flushed, dyspnea
20%-30%	Confusion, lethargy, ST depression, visual disturbances
40%-60%	Coma, seizures, ectopy
60%	Death

Table **34-12**	**Age-Related Risk Factors in Drowning and Near-Drowning**
Age group	Risk factors
Children	Lack of supervision, abuse, neglect, inability to swim, no recognition of dangers of rivers and lakes
Adolescents	Risk-taking, peer pressure, poor swimming skills, alcohol consumption, no recognition of dangers of rivers and lakes, underlying medical conditions such as seizures
Adults	Risk-taking, alcohol consumption, poor swimming skills, underlying medical conditions

Smoke Inhalation

Inhalation injury occurs from inhalation of superheated toxic gases. Products of combustion contain toxic gases such as carbon monoxide, the most common by-product of combustion. Other toxic gases include hydrogen cyanide, from burning synthetic materials such as polyurethane, and hydrogen chloride, a by-product of wall and floor coverings. The degree of injury correlates with the type of noxious gas inhaled, length of exposure, and the mass of inhaled gas. Two prevalent physiologic effects of inhalation injury are caused by thermal damage and toxic fumes.

Obtaining a careful history is essential when caring for the patient with potential inhalation injury. Patients who have carbonaceous sputum, singed facial or nasal hair, or burns of the neck or face should be carefully evaluated for inhalation injury. Hoarseness, wheezing, dyspnea, and restlessness may also be present. Early ventilation is recommended. Upper airway obstruction may result from edema caused by inhalation of superheated air. Other changes associated with inhalation injury include direct mucosal injury, ciliary damage, and ineffective gas exchange.

Carbon monoxide poisoning. Carbon monoxide poisoning is a frequent result of smoke inhalation, and the leading cause of poisoning death in the United States. Carbon monoxide (CO) affinity for hemoglobin is 200 times greater than oxygen, so oxygen is displaced from hemoglobin. Without a mechanism for oxygen transport, tissue becomes hypoxic. Carboxyhemoglobin (COHb) levels greater than 10% indicate smoke inhalation; however, smokers or individuals exposed to automobile exhaust can have baseline COHb levels of 10% to 15%.[4] Fetal hemoglobin binds even more quickly with CO, so the fetus is at greater risk for injury from smoke inhalation.[4] As COHb levels increase, symptoms worsen (Table 34-11).

Initial interventions are directed toward protecting and maintaining a patent airway and support of the patient's hemodynamic status. COHb half-life is 4 to 5 hours with room air, but can be decreased to 90 minutes with administration of 100% oxygen. Hyperbaric oxygenation is indicated for patients with COHb levels of 40%, pregnant patients, and patients with neurologic symptoms.[9]

Smoke poisoning. Smoke poisoning refers to inhalation of toxic gases such as cyanide, hydrogen chloride, phosgene, ammonia, and sulfur dioxide. Pulmonary endothelial cells are injured, epithelial cilia are destroyed, and mucosal edema occurs. Surfactant production decreases, followed by atelectasis.[9] Clinically, the patient develops pulmonary edema, usually within 24 to 48 hours of the initial injury. Clinical interventions focus on presenting symptoms and include humidified oxygen, vigorous pulmonary toilet, and bronchodilators. Intubation and mechanical ventilation are indicated if severe pulmonary edema occurs.

Near-Drowning

Drowning is the third leading cause of accidental death in the United States; approximately 4500 people die of submersion each year.[9] The highest incidence occurs in adolescents aged 15 to 19 years and children less than 4 years of age. Drowning occurs in males five times more often than in females. Risk factors associated with drowning and near-drowning include alcohol, poor swimming skills, and hypothermia. Table 34-12 identifies risk factors associated with various age groups.

Drowning is the result of aspiration of fresh or salt water; however, approximately 10% of all drowning victims do not aspirate. Victims who do not aspirate become hypoxic and asphyxiate due to laryngospasm and glottic closure. Freshwater and salt water drowning both lead to profound hypoxia, the cause of death in all drowning victims. Hypoxemia can occur with aspiration of small amounts of fluid, as little as 2.2 ml/kg.[9] Aspiration of water floods alveoli and impairs gas exchange due to loss of surfactant. Hypertonic salt water pulls fluid from circulating plasma into alveoli, producing intrapulmonary shunt. Freshwater affects the surface tension of surfactant so that alveoli become unstable. Protein and fluid shift from the intravascular space into the alveoli because of damage to alveolar membrane. Subsequent inadequate alveolar ventilation leads to intrapul-

NURSING DIAGNOSES FOR RESPIRATORY EMERGENCIES

Ineffective airway clearance
Impaired gas exchange
Altered tissue perfusion
Fluid volume excess

monary shunt, which worsens existing hypoxia. Pulmonary injury is worsened by contaminants such as chlorine, algae, sand, and mud.

Clinically, patients can have respiratory distress, bronchospasm, loss of consciousness, pulmonary edema (cardiogenic and noncardiogenic), hypothermia, poor perfusion, hypotension, dysrhythmias, metabolic acidosis, electrolyte abnormalities, and associated injuries such as spinal cord damage. Spinal cord injuries are more common in adolescents and young adults injured when diving or falling head first into water. Outcome is determined by age, length of submersion, type of fluid, fluid temperature, and associated injuries. Submersion injury in cold, icy waters is associated with better neurologic recovery. The earlier the victim regains consciousness, the greater the likelihood of return to the prior level of function. Most patients who are alert and conscious on arrival survive without neurologic deficits.[9] Survival with intact neurologic function has been reported in 24% of children who required CPR and presented with a Glasgow Coma Scale of 3 after near-drowning.

ED management involves maintenance of a patent airway in conjunction with stabilization of the cervical spine. Administer supplemental oxygen and assess oxygenation and ventilatory status. Intubation and mechanical ventilation are indicated when supplemental oxygen cannot maintain adequate oxygen saturation. Warm hypothermic patients slowly, 1 to 2° C per hour. Fluid resuscitation with isotonic solutions may be indicated for noncardiogenic pulmonary edema. Diagnostic studies include CBC, electrolyte measurements, arterial blood gas values, and chest radiographs. Insert a nasogastric tube to decompress stomach and minimize the risk for aspiration and a Foley catheter to monitor output. Diuretic therapy, intracranial pressure monitoring, and neuromuscular paralyzing agents may be indicated for some patients. Prophylactic antibiotics and steroids are not recommended.

SUMMARY

Respiratory emergencies may be subtle or obvious. The ability to manage obvious cases of respiratory distress and to identify subtle cases of impending respiratory crisis is a hall-

mark of an effective emergency nurse. Without essential interventions, respiratory emergencies can progress to respiratory arrest and death. Box 34-7 identifies nursing diagnoses applicable to patients with a respiratory emergency.

REFERENCES

1. Chillcott S et al: ECCO$_2$R: an experimental approach to treating ARDS, *Crit Care Nurse* 15(2):50, 1995.
2. Foley J: Drug update, *J Emerg Nurs* 18(1):63, 1992.
3. Guyton AC, Hall GE: *Textbook of medical physiology,* ed 9, Philadelphia, 1995, WB Saunders.
4. Kitt S, Selfridge-Thomas J, Proehl J et al: *Emergency nursing: a physiologic and clinical perspective,* ed 2, Philadelphia, 1995, WB Saunders.
5. Lewis SM, Collier IC, Heitkemper MM: *Medical-surgical nursing: assessment and management of clinical problems,* ed 4, St. Louis, 1996, Mosby.
6. National Asthma Education Program: *Guidelines for the diagnosis and management of asthma: speaker's kit,* 1992, National Heart, Lung, and Blood Institute.
7. Rau JL: *Respiratory care pharmacology,* ed 4, St. Louis, 1994, Mosby.
8. Sinski A et al: Surfactant replacement in adults and children with ARDS: an effective therapy? *Crit Care Nurse* 14(6):54, 1994.
9. Tintinalli JE, Ruiz E, Krome RL: *Emergency medicine: a comprehensive study guide,* ed 4, New York, 1996, McGraw-Hill.

SUGGESTED READING

Black JM, Matassarin-Jacobe E, editors: *Luckman and Sorensen's medical-surgical nursing: a psychophysiologic approach,* ed 4, Philadelphia, 1993, WB Saunders.
Burton G et al: *Respiratory care: a guide to clinical practice,* ed 4, Philadelphia, 1991, JB Lippincott.
Caine RM: Burn injuries. In Clochesy J, Breu C, Cardin S et al: *Critical care nursing,* Philadelphia, 1996, WB Saunders.
Demling RH: Smoke inhalation injury. In Shoemaker W, Ayres S, Grenvik A et al: *Textbook of critical care,* ed 3, Philadelphia, 1995, WB Saunders.
Emergency Nurses Association: *Emergency nursing core curriculum,* ed 4, Philadelphia, 1994, WB Saunders.
Farzan S: *A concise handbook of respiratory diseases,* ed 2, 1985, Prentice-Hall.
Goodwin S, Boysen P, Modell J: Near drowning: adults and children. In Shoemaker W, Ayres S, Grenvik A et al: *Textbook of critical care,* ed 3, Philadelphia, 1995, WB Saunders.
Hammer J: Challenging diagnosis: adult respiratory distress syndrome, *Crit Care Nurse* 15(5):46, 1995.
Howder C: Antimuscarinic and B2-adrenoceptor bronchodilators in obstructive airway disease, *Respir Care* 38(12):1364, 1993.
Janson-Bjerklie S: Clinical markers of asthma severity and risk: importance of subjective as well as objective factors, *Heart Lung* 21(3):265, 1992.
Keen JH: Drug update: intravenous magnesium sulfate for acute asthma, *J Emerg Nurs* 21(1):44, 1995.
Mackey D: Pulmonary emergencies. In Kitt S, Selfridge-Thomas J, Proehl JA et al, editors: *Emergency nursing: a physiologic and clinical perspective,* ed 2, Philadelphia, 1995, WB Saunders.
McGillis H: Comprehensive program to improve care leads to reduced ED use by patients with asthma: one hospital's experience, *J Emerg Nurs* 22(1):18, 1992.
Rachelefsky G: Asthma update: new approaches and partnerships, *J Pediatr Health Care* 9(1):12, 1995.
Scanlon C et al: *Egan's fundamentals of respiratory care,* ed 6, St. Louis, 1995, Mosby.

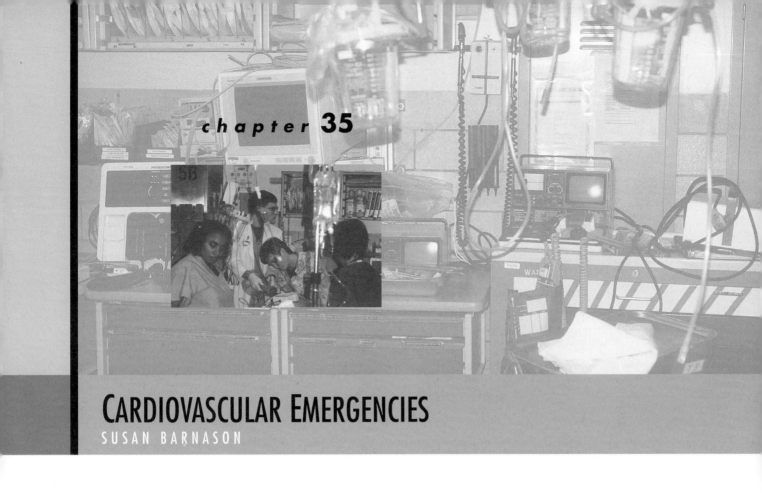

chapter 35

CARDIOVASCULAR EMERGENCIES
SUSAN BARNASON

Cardiovascular emergencies affect the heart and great vessels. The event may be subtle or obvious, caused by progressive disease development or a sudden traumatic event. Emergencies secondary to trauma are described in Chapter 25. Cardiovascular emergencies in children are discussed in Chapter 50. This chapter describes cardiovascular emergencies caused by progressive disease development and/or a sudden nontraumatic cardiac event.

ANATOMY AND PHYSIOLOGY

The heart is a four-chambered, muscular structure with valves between each chamber to prevent back flow with pumping action of the heart (Figure 35-1). The heart works in synchrony as a two-pump system. Deoxygenated blood from the venous system enters the right atrium through the inferior and superior vena cavae. Blood is pumped into the pulmonary vasculature from the right ventricle. After oxygenation, blood returns to the left atrium via the pulmonary veins. The left ventricle then pumps blood to the body via the arterial system. Figure 35-2 illustrates blood flow through the heart. The left side of the heart is the stronger side, with the ability to pump 4 to 8 L of blood per minute. Oxygenation of the heart muscle is provided by blood from the right and left coronary arteries. Arteries arise from the right and left sinuses of Valsalva of the aortic valve. Coronary arteries lie on the surface of the heart and fill during ventricular diastole.

The heart is surrounded by a fibrous, fluid-filled sac called the pericardium. Pericardial fluid lubricates the heart and prevents friction with contraction. The heart is divided into three distinct layers, the epicardium, myocardium, and endocardium. Epicardium serves as the visceral surface of the pericardium. Myocardium, the thickest portion of the heart, is composed of concentric rings of muscle fibers. Contraction of concentric rings facilitates blood flow up and out of the ventricles. The endocardial layer is a smooth tissue that is the inner layer of the atria and ventricles. Endocardium also functions as the surface of the heart valves.

One of the unique characteristics of cardiac tissue is automaticity or intrinsic ability to initiate electrical activity. Figure 35-3 shows the heart's electrical conduction system. The sinoatrial (SA) node has the highest rate of automaticity, spontaneously depolarizing 60 to 100 times per minute. Impulses generated by the SA node are carried to the atrioventricular (AV) node by intraatrial tracts, that is, Bachmann, Bundle, Wenckebach's, and Thorel's tracts. Electrical stimulation of heart muscle at the level of the atria causes the mechanical event of atrial contraction. At the AV node, slight delay in impulse transmission allows completion of atrial contraction prior to ventricular stimulation. From the AV node, the electrical impulse is carried to the ventricles by the right and left bundle branches of the His bundle. Bundles terminate with Purkinje fibers, which deliver the impulse to the ventricular muscle, causing ventricular contraction.

Mechanical events of the cardiac cycle are called diastole and systole. Approximately 60% of the cardiac cycle is dias-

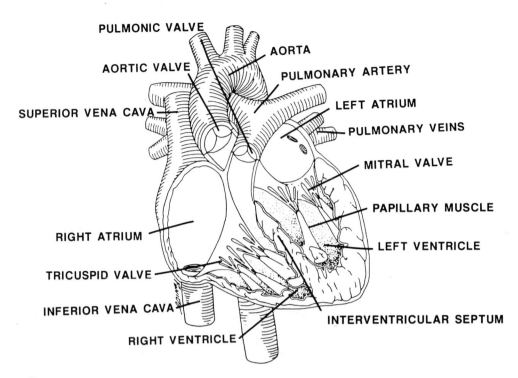

Figure **35-1** Anatomy of the heart. *(From Lounsberry P, Frye SJ:* Cardiac rhythm disorders: a nursing process approach, *ed 2, St. Louis, 1992, Mosby.)*

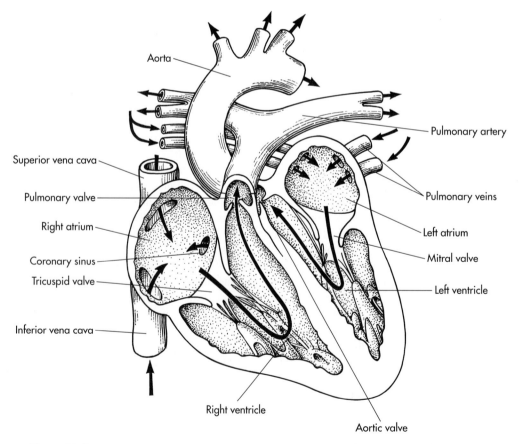

Figure **35-2** Circulation of blood through the heart. Arrows indicate direction of flow. *(From Atkinson LJ, Fortunato NM:* Berry & Kohn's operating room technique, *ed 8, St. Louis, 1996, Mosby.)*

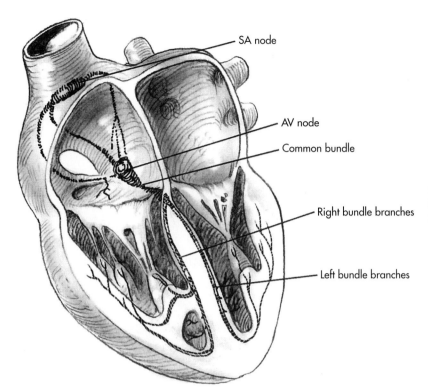

Figure **35-3** Conduction system of the heart. *(From Davis JH, Drucker WR et al:* Clinical surgery, *vol 1, St. Louis, 1987, Mosby.)*

tole, the time when the ventricles are filling. Diastole is also the time when aortic and pulmonic valves close. Mitral and tricuspid valves open during this time. Electrically, this corresponds to electrical stimulation and mechanical contraction of the atria. With atrial contraction and opening of AV valves, pressure in the atria is higher than pressure in the ventricles. Therefore blood flows from an area of greater pressure to an area of lesser pressure (Figure 35-4). The systolic phase of the cardiac cycle corresponds with ventricular contraction and opening of pulmonic and aortic valves. During contraction, AV valves close and chordae tendineae contract to prevent regurgitation. Figure 35-5 depicts the relationship between electrical and mechanical components of the cardiac cycle.

Pressures within the cardiovascular system affect cardiac output because of the effect on preload and afterload. Afterload refers to pressure in the arterial system, which opposes blood flow from the left ventricle. Preload refers to blood volume coming into the right side of the heart. Figure 35-6 illustrates the effect of these pressures on cardiac filling.

Cardiac activity is regulated by branches of the autonomic nervous system. Specific effects of each branch are described in Table 35-1. Receptors in the heart and great vessels respond to signals from the sympathetic nervous system (Table 35-3). Stimulation affects heart rate, contractility, automaticity, conduction, and vascular smooth muscle. These receptors prepare the body to fight or flee perceived threats, including loss of blood volume.

Table **35-1**	**Parasympathetic and Sympathetic Stimulation of the Heart**	
Nerve activation	**Cardiac effect**	**Clinical manifestations**
Parasympathetic	Slows SA node discharge	Symptomatic bradycardia
	Slows AV node conduction and increases refractoriness	Transient heart block
Sympathetic	Heart rate increases	Tachycardia
	Enhances AV node function	Hypertension
	Shortens His-Purkinje and ventricular muscle refractoriness	Increased cardiac output
	Increased ventricular contraction	
	Increased peripheral vascular resistance	

SPECIFIC CARDIOVASCULAR EMERGENCIES

Specific emergencies discussed are cardiac arrest, dysrhythmias, myocardial infarction, abdominal aortic aneurysm, and hypertensive crisis.

Cardiac Arrest

Sudden cardiac arrest can be defined as nontraumatic, nonviolent, and unexpected sudden cardiac arrest within 6

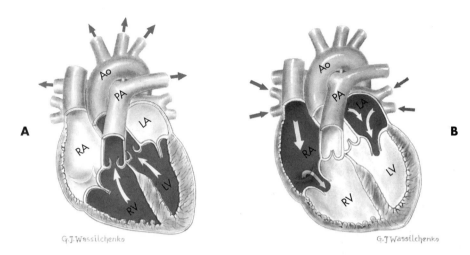

Figure **35-4**   Blood flow during (**A**) systole, and (**B**) diastole. *(From Canobbio MM:* Mosby's clinical nursing series, vol *1,* cardiovascular disorders, *St. Louis, 1990, Mosby.)*

hours of previously witnessed, usual state of normal health.[1] Annually, approximately 500,000 persons experience sudden cardiac arrest, with 80% dying immediately. Common causes of sudden cardiac arrest are ventricular tachycardia (VT) and ventricular fibrillation (VF).[6] These lethal dysrhythmias are usually a late complication of myocardial infarction, but they may also be associated with aneurysm rupture, cardiomyopathies, rheumatic heart disease, mitral valve prolapse, and cardiac surgery. Sudden cardiac arrest can also be associated with other conditions and/or events. Table 35-2 presents etiologic factors associated with other causes of cardiopulmonary arrest.

In young patients, age 14 to 21 years, approximately 30% of sudden cardiac deaths are related to cardiac conditions. Specifically, hypertrophic cardiomyopathy, which results in left ventricular outflow obstruction or myocardial ischemia secondary to small intramural vessels, may potentiate lethal dysrhythmias. Other etiologic factors associated with sudden cardiac arrest in the young may include congenital coronary artery anomalies, myocarditis, idiopathic concentric left ventricular hypertrophy, Marfan's syndrome, mitral valve prolapse, aortic stenosis, idiopathic long QT syndrome, and miscellaneous causes, for example, Wolff-Parkinson-White syndrome, cocaine, and anabolic steroids.

Among persons 30 years of age and older, an estimated 20% to 30% of sudden cardiac deaths are secondary to acute myocardial infarction[33] secondary to pump failure. Immedi-

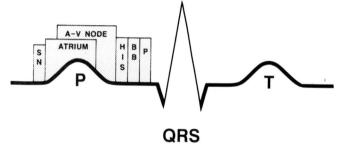

Figure **35-5**   Schematic drawing of cardiac activation related to the surface ECG. The timing of activation of the components of the conduction system is superimposed on the surface ECG. *SN,* Sinus node; *HIS,* common bundle of HIS; *BB,* bundle branches; *P,* Purkinje network. *(From Lounsberry P, Frye SJ:* Cardiac rhythm disorders: a nursing process approach, *ed 2, St. Louis, 1992, Mosby.)*

ate interventions include establishing an airway, supporting oxygenation, and providing circulation with chest compressions.[5,20] Airway management and oxygenation are discussed in greater detail in Chapter 34. Circulation for the pulseless patient is produced with chest compressions. Properly performed chest compressions can produce 30% of the patient's normal cardiac output, which is enough blood flow through the heart and brain to sustain tissue viability for a short time. Cerebral blood flow must be at least 50% of normal volume to maintain consciousness.

NORMAL

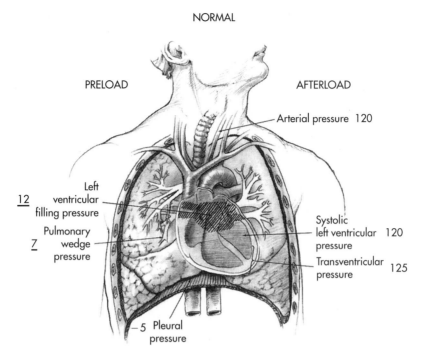

PRELOAD

AFTERLOAD

Arterial pressure 120

12 Left ventricular filling pressure

7 Pulmonary wedge pressure

Systolic left ventricular pressure 120

Transventricular pressure 125

–5 Pleural pressure

Figure **35-6**   The effects of normal pleural pressure on cardiac filling pressure. *(From Davis JH, Drucker WR et al: Clinical surgery, vol 1, St. Louis, 1987, Mosby.)*

Chest compressions are best accomplished with the victim on a firm surface to allow even compression of the thoracic cavity. Compressions should be forceful enough to generate a carotid or femoral pulse. Mechanical chest compression devices should be an adjunct to manual chest compressions and used only by trained personnel in limited situations, for example, reducing rescuer fatigue in prolonged resuscitation efforts.[4] The most common mechanical compression device is the compressed gas–powered plunger mounted on a backboard. During the use of such devices, remember to place the plunger in the correct location over the sternum to provide maximum cardiac output and minimize adverse events, for example, fractured ribs. Another mechanical device reported in the literature is a *CPR vest.* However, use of this device is still considered investigational.

Open thoracotomy and cardiac massage may be required in cases of penetrating wounds to the heart, penetrating abdominal trauma with deterioration and arrest, pericardial tamponade, tension pneumothorax, or crushing chest injuries. This technique may also be used for patients with chronic lung disease who have a barrel chest when other more conservative measures for chest compression have failed. Studies have demonstrated that direct cardiac chest massage provides better hemodynamics than closed chest compressions; however, this procedure must be performed within 15 minutes of the arrest to be effective.

Defibrillation. Advanced life support measures implemented in the ED augment basic life support measures with administration of drugs, fluids, and defibrillation.[4,20] Restor-

ing normal circulation for the patient who has experienced sudden cardiac arrest or cardiopulmonary arrest requires vigilance to restore and/or stabilize the cardiac rhythm. If the patient has ventricular fibrillation (VF) or pulseless ventricular tachycardia (VT), the intervention of choice is immediate defibrillation. For defibrillation to be effective, an electric current sufficient to depolarize a critical portion of the left ventricle must pass through the heart. When treating VF and pulseless VT in adults, up to three countershocks should be rapidly delivered, the first at 200 J, the second at 200 to 300 J, and the third at 360 J. Check pulse and ECG rhythm between shocks to determine if defibrillation has been effective.

When preparing to defibrillate, make sure the machine has a charged battery or is plugged into an electrical outlet. Turn the machine on and select "defib" or "unsynchronized" mode. Select energy level and prepare defibrillation paddle-electrodes by applying conducting gel or by placing defibrillation pregelled patches on the patient's chest. Saline-soaked gauze pads may be used if other conductive media are not available, but these are not ideal conductors. Most commonly, anterolateral paddle placement is used; however, anteroposterior paddle placement may also be used (Figure 35-7). To defibrillate, apply firm pressure, ensure the area around the patient is clear of personnel and electrical equipment, then discharge the paddles by depressing discharge buttons simultaneously.

An alternative to manually defibrillating the patient is automated external defibrillation (AED).[4,13,20] The AED device uses two large adhesive patches placed on the patient's chest in the anterolateral positions. These patches serve as elec-

Table **35-2**	**Differential Diagnosis of Cardiopulmonary Arrest***			
Causes	Specific cause	Signs and symptoms	Therapeutic intervention	Notes
Metabolic	Hypoglycemia	Physical signs of insulin or oral hypoglycemic agent usage; tachydysrhythmias; seizures; aspiration	Dextrose, 50%	Consider hypoglycemia a strong possibility in patients who have a history of diabetes
	Hyperkalemia	ECG Prolonged QT interval; peaked T waves; loss of P waves; wide QRS complexes	Calcium chloride; sodium bicarbonate	Often seen in hemodialysis and renal failure patients; also seen in patients taking spironolactone (Aldactone)
Drug-induced	Tricyclic antidepressants amitriptyline (Elavil), amitriptyline and perphenazine (Etrafon, Triavil), imipramine (Tofranil), doxepin (Sinequan), protriptyline (Vivactil)	Tachydysrhythmias	Sodium bicarbonate (to keep pH at 7.50); physostigmine (however, efficacy has been questioned)	Causes direct cardiac toxicity; often delayed toxicity in adults
	Narcotics	Bradydysrhythmias; heart blocks	Naloxone (Narcan)	There is a question of direct cardiac toxicity
	Propranolol	Cardiac Heart blocks; bradydysrhythmias; PVCs Respiratory Bronchospasm Metabolic Hypoglycemia	Isoproterenol (Isuprel) Atropine Aminophylline Dextrose, 50%	PVCs may be caused by slow rate
Pulmonary (any disease causing severe hypoxia)	Asthma	Severe bronchospasm causing hypoxia and respiratory acidosis ECG Tachydysrhythmias (especially ventricular fibrillation)	Endotracheal intubation and ventilatory support	Abuse of sympathomimetic inhalants
	Pulmonary embolus	Pleuritic chest pain; shortness of breath in high-risk patients (postoperative, those taking birth control pills); syncope (recent study shows 60% have syncope as part of initial complaint); tachydysrhythmias	Good ventilatory support; consider thrombolytic agents	Pathophysiology; acute hypoxia and cor pulmonale leading to tachydysrhythmias
	Tension pneumothorax	Distended neck veins; tracheal deviation; asymmetric chest expansion ECG Often electrical mechanical dissociation	Needle thoracotomy; chest tube	Often seen in patients with blunt chest trauma; often occurs during CPR because of chest compressions (especially in patients with COPD)

Table **35-2** Differential Diagnosis of Cardiopulmonary Arrest*—cont'd				
Causes	Specific cause	Signs and symptoms	Therapeutic intervention	Notes
Neurogenic	Increased intracranial pressure from any cause (e.g., subarachnoid hemorrhage; subdural hematoma)	Central neurogenic breathing; dilated pupil(s); decerebrate/decorticate posturing ECG Wide range of dysrhythmias, especially heart blocks	Central neurogenic hyperventilation (causes respiratory alkalosis, which results in cerebral vasoconstriction); steroids; diuretic agents; surgery	Damage to brain stem and autonomic centers
Hypovolemic	Anything that causes volume loss such as gastrointestinal bleeding, severe trauma with organ damage, ruptured ectopic pregnancy, dissecting or leaking aneurysm	Tachycardia; decreasing blood pressure; skin cool, clammy, pale; obvious signs of external blood loss	IV fluids; pneumatic antishock garment (PASG); shock position; surgery	A major cause of cardiopulmonary arrest that may be unrecognized
Other cardiac causes	Pericardial tamponade	Distended neck veins; decreasing blood pressure; distant heart sounds, widening pulse pressure ECG Electromechanical dissociation of bradydysrhythmias	IV fluids: PASG; atropine; isoproterenol; pericardiocentesis; thoracotomy	Look for it, especially in patients with blunt chest trauma or prolonged CPR efforts

*Many causes of cardiopulmonary arrest exist other than primary cardiac abnormalities. It is important for the nurse or rescuer to be familiar with these causes and to be alert to their signs and symptoms, as identification of these may modify the type of therapeutic intervention given. This table lists some of the conditions that may lead to cardiopulmonary arrest but are not primary cardiac abnormalities. All therapeutic interventions listed are in addition to basic and advanced cardiac life support measures.
SPECIAL NOTE FOR PREHOSPITAL CARE: Consider early transport for young patients in cardiac arrest, since definitive therapeutic intervention will most likely include procedures not performed in the field.

Table **35-3** Sympathetic Nervous System Receptors		
Sympathetic receptor	Location	Clinical response
α	Vascular smooth muscle	Vasoconstriction
β-1	Myocardium	Increased heart rate, contraction, automaticity, and conduction
β-2	Peripheral vasculature and lungs	Vasodilation of peripheral vasculature and bronchodilation
Dopaminergic	Renal, mesenteric, cerebral, and coronary arteries	Vasodilation

trodes to monitor the rhythm and to deliver the countershock. Some AED devices are considered fully automated because they analyze the ECG rhythm, determine rhythm lethality (e.g., VF, VT), charge, and deliver countershock as appropriate. Other AEDs are considered semiautomated or shock-advisory defibrillators. These devices monitor the rhythm, but require the nurse or physician to interpret the rhythm, charge the defibrillator, and discharge the countershock. Both types provide "hands-off" defibrillation. All personnel should be clear of the patient when the countershock is delivered; however, a bag-valve-mask can be safely used during defibrillation, as long as the rescuer touches only the bag. Compressions are stopped while the patient is defibrillated. Some AEDs have a minimum energy level of 200 J. This level of energy is contraindicated in patients who weigh <90 lb. Other AEDs allow the user to program the energy level appropriate for the size of the patient. When transporting a patient, the AED should be in the semiautomatic mode so that inappropriate discharge of energy does not occur if the AED interprets a motion artifact as VF or VT.

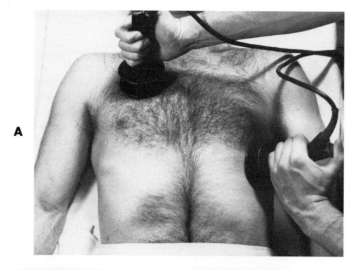

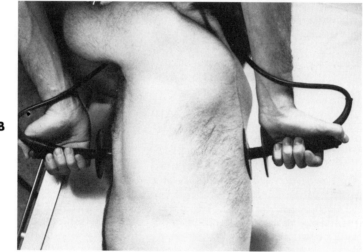

Figure **35-7** Defibrillation. **A,** Anterolateral paddle placement. **B,** Anteroposterior paddle placement. *(Photos by Richard Lazar.)*

Internal defibrillation during open cardiac massage requires internal paddles. Follow the same set-up procedure as external defibrillation. Apply sterile saline solution to sterile gauze sponges placed over the internal defibrillation paddles. The energy level for defibrillation is usually 10 to 50 J for adults.

Successful defibrillation depends on the metabolic state of the heart and decreasing resistance (i.e., thoracic impedance) to the countershock. Improved effectiveness of defibrillation can be accomplished with appropriately sized defibrillator paddle-electrodes, appropriate placement of defibrillator paddles, good interface between the defibrillator paddle and the patient's chest wall, and the electrode-chest contact pressure (Box 35-1).

Cardioversion. Synchronized cardioversion is used when the patient become hemodynamically unstable or pharmacologic intervention has been unsuccessful in management of sustained ventricular tachycardia, paroxysmal supraventric-

---

Box **35-1** **Improving Effectiveness of Defibrillation**
Defibrillator paddle-electrode of adequate size (i.e., 13 cm for adults)
Good interface of defibrillator paddle-electrode with chest wall, e.g., using electrode paste or gel, saline-soaked gauze pads
Defibrillator paddle-electrode placement
Anteroposterior: One paddle positioned anteriorly over precordium just left of lower sternal border with posterior paddle positioned behind the heart
Anterolateral: One paddle-electrode placed right of upper sternum just below the right clavicle; second paddle-electrode left of nipple in midaxillary line
Electrode-paddle to chest contact pressure minimum 11 kg (25 lb) per paddle

ular tachycardia, and atrial fibrillation or atrial flutter. In synchronized cardioversion, energy is delivered to the heart during the absolute refractory period, which occurs a fraction of a second after the QRS (i.e., ventricular depolarization). Synchronized cardioversion decreases potential energy delivery during the vulnerable period of repolarization, that is, the T wave of the ECG (Figure 35-8).

The procedure for cardioversion is the same as defibrillation with two exceptions. The machine must be set on synchronous mode and sedation may be given for the conscious patient. Sedatives such as diazepam (Valium) and/or midazolam (Versed) are administered slowly IV push in small incremental doses. Explain the procedure to the patient and obtain informed consent when possible. Check serum potassium; hypokalemia predisposes the heart to ventricular fibrillation. If the procedure is elective, ask the patient to empty his or her bladder and remove dentures prior to the procedure. A baseline 12-lead ECG is obtained prior to the procedure. After cardioversion, monitor vital signs, level of consciousness, and cardiac rhythm frequently until the patient is hemodynamically stable and returns to preintervention level of consciousness. Complications of cardioversion include asystole, junctional rhythms, premature ventricular contractions, ventricular tachycardia, ventricular fibrillation, embolization, and return to atrial fibrillation or atrial flutter.

Another method to cardiovert a patient's rhythm is through stimulation of the vagus nerve by a Valsalva maneuver, retching or emesis, or carotid sinus massage. Ocular pressure and application of ice water to the patient's face are no longer recommended for vagal stimulation.

Carotid sinus massage is accomplished by placing pressure on the carotid bodies, stimulating baroreceptors thereby stimulating the parasympathetic branch of the autonomic nervous system. Stimulation decreases blood pressure and heart rate. The patient should be supine with oxygen supplied at 4 to 6 L/min via nasal cannula. A patent IV line and ECG monitor should be present prior to the procedure. The physician auscultates the carotid arteries for bruits. Bruits are produced by turbulent flow through the carotid arteries and suggest presence of atherosclerotic plaque, which could break off if manipulated and cause a stroke. If a bruit is auscultated, carotid massage is not performed on that artery.

Start the carotid massage with the right carotid sinus. In more than 75% of the population, preferential massage of the right carotid body affects the SA node, whereas left carotid body massage affects the AV node. Even when the SA node is completely shut down, the AV node can provide pacemaker activity. If the left side is massaged first, complete block of the AV node may occur and lead to slow ventricular rate. Pressure is applied gently to the carotid artery just below the mandible in small, circular motions, rotating the fingers backward and medially. Carotid massage should not exceed 5 to 10 seconds and should be discontinued sooner if the rhythm changes. Even when properly performed, carotid massage may cause asystole for 15 to 30 seconds, followed by a few idioventricular complexes before a new pacemaker site becomes active. Emergency equipment and medications should always be available whenever carotid massage is performed. If carotid massage is successful, monitor the patient continuously for several hours after the procedure. Complications of carotid massage include further dysrhythmias (e.g., ventricular tachycardia, ventricular fibrillation, asystole), cerebral occlusion that leads to stroke, cerebral anoxia, and seizures.

Fluids. Use of intravenous fluids in sudden cardiac arrest or cardiopulmonary arrest must be guided by suspected etiology of arrest and patient response to fluids. Expansion of circulating volume is needed when there has been unexpected loss of blood volume (e.g., ruptured abdominal aortic aneurysm, trauma). Volume expansion is accomplished with crystalloids (e.g., normal saline, lactated Ringer's solution) or colloids (e.g., albumin). Fluid therapy is also beneficial in circumstances in which the patient has decreased cardiac output (e.g., secondary to an acute myocardial infarction (MI)).

Because of adverse effects on cerebral tissue, dextrose solutions are not recommended during CPR. Recommended fluids in cardiac arrest are normal saline or lactated Ringer's solution. Dextrose solutions are reserved for patients with actual or suspected hypoglycemia. All emergency drugs routinely administered for cardiac arrest are stable in 0.9% normal saline solution.

Drug therapy. Emergency drug therapy is dependent on ECG rhythm and hemodynamic stability.[20,22,47] Table 35-4

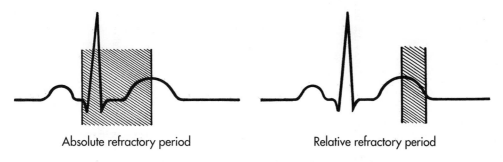

Absolute refractory period   Relative refractory period

Figure **35-8**   Relative and absolute refractory periods on the ECG.

Table 35-4   Drugs Commonly Used in Cardiopulmonary Resuscitation[31,32,38,46]

Drug	Category	Actions	Indications	Dose	Comments
Adenosine (Adenocard)	Unclassified antidysrhythmic	Slows conduction through the AV node; can interrupt reentry pathways through AV node to decrease heart rate	Paroxysmal supraventricular tachycardia (PSVT)	**PSVT:** 6 mg, rapid IV push over 1 to 3 sec; may give additional 12 mg rapid IV push if first dose not effective; may repeat 12 mg after 1 to 2 min Helpful to rapidly bolus 20 ml normal saline after giving adenosine to clear IV tubing completely	May cause brief heart block and/or transient asystole; may cause other dysrhythmias (e.g., PVC, PAC, sinus bradycardia, sinus tachycardia) during conversion from PSVT although symptoms usually brief due to short drug half-life (i.e., <10 sec) Contraindications include second- or third-degree AV block, or sick sinus syndrome
Atropine	Parasympatholytic; anticholinergic	Increases rate of SA node; increases conduction through AV node; decreases vagal tone	Hemodynamically significant bradycardia; asystole; AV blocks	**Bradycardia and AV blocks:** 0.5-1.0 mg (IV push) or intratracheally every 5 min to maximum dose of 0.04 mg/kg **Asystole:** 1.0 mg IV push or intratracheally; every 3-5 min to total dose of 0.04 mg/kg	May cause paradoxic slowing of heart rate when given slowly in doses less than 0.5 mg. May be ineffective in high-degree AV blocks
Bretylium (Bretylol)	Category III antidysrhythmic	Elevates threshold; suppresses reentry dysrhythmias; positive inotrope; transiently positive dromotrope	VF, VT, PVCs refractory to lidocaine	5 mg/kg IV push; may repeat twice at 10 mg/kg **VT:** 500 mg in 50 ml IV solution 5-10 mg/kg over 10 min; repeat every 1-2 hr when required Maximum dose: 30 mg/kg **IV infusion:** 1 g/250 ml D₅W (4 mg/ml) at 1-4 mg/min (15-60 micro-gtts/min)	May cause hypertension, syncope, bradycardia, vertigo, dizziness, nausea, and vomiting; patient should be supine; response not as rapid with VT as VF
Epinephrine (Adrenalin)	Sympathomimetic	α- And β-adrenergic effects; increases mean arterial pressure; decreases fibrillatory threshold; stimulates heart in asystole and idioventricular rhythms; increases cerebral and myocardial blood flow	Allergic reaction; cardiac arrest; bronchoconstriction or bronchospasm	Available as 1:10,000 solution (1 mg in 10 ml) **Cardiac arrest:** 1.0 mg IV push or intratracheally; repeat every 5 min when needed Intermediate/escalating doses: 2-5 mg IV push every 3 min High doses: 0.01 mg/kg IV push every 3-5 min	May cause tachycardia, palpitations, PVCs, angina, pallor
Isoproterenol (Isuprel)	Sympathomimetic	Nonspecific β-adrenergic stimulation	Hemodynamically significant bradycardia refractory to atropine	**Bradycardia:** 1 mg in 250 ml D₅W (4 μg/ml); 2-20 μg/min IV (30-300 micro-gtts/min); titrate to achieve heart rate of >60 beats/min	Causes increased workload for heart; use with extreme caution: exacerbates ischemia and extends infarct

Lidocaine (Xylocaine)	Category IB antidysrhythmic	Decreases automaticity; suppresses ventricular ectopy; depresses conduction through reentry pathways; elevates VF threshold	**VF & VT with collapse:** 1.5 mg/kg IV push or intratracheally; repeat in 3-5 min; not to exceed 3 mg/kg **PVCs & VT:** 1 mg/kg IV push or intratracheally; repeat at 0.5 mg/kg every 8-10 min; not to exceed 3 mg/kg **IV infusion:** 1 g in 250 ml D$_5$W (4 mg/ml) at 2-4 mg/min (30-60 micro-gtts/min) **Preintubation:** 1.5 mg/kg IV push, wait 90 sec then intubate	May cause central nervous system depression, drowsiness, dizziness, confusion, anxiety Contraindications: bradycardia-related PVCs, bradycardia, idioventricular rhythm; if given too rapidly, may cause seizures
Procainamide (Pronestyl)	Category IA antidysrhythmic	Suppresses PVCs; suppresses reentry dysrhythmias; may elevate VF threshold; negative chronotrope and dromotrope; mild negative inotrope; potent peripheral vasodilator	**IV push:** 100 mg IV (20 mg/min) repeat every 5 min; not to exceed 17 mg/kg **IV infusion:** 1 g in 250 ml D$_5$W (4 mg/ml) at 1 to 4 mg/min (15-60 micro-gtts/min)	May cause hypotension, bradycardia, widened QRS Contraindications: third-degree AV block, digoxin toxicity
Sodium bicarbonate	Alkalotic agent	Buffers or neutralizes metabolic acidosis	1 mEq/kg IV push; repeat 0.5 mEq/kg every 10 to 15 min when required	May inactivate catecholamines when given in the same IV line; use arterial blood gases to guide administration
Verapamil (Calan, Isoptin)	Category IV antidysrhythmic	Blocks entry of Ca^{2+} into cells; negative dromotrope and depresses atrial automaticity; negative chronotrope; negative inotrope; vasodilator	**IV push:** 0.075 to 0.15 mg/kg IV (slow IV push) Elderly patients: give 2 mg over period of 3 to 4 min Maximum dose = 10 mg	May cause hypotension

provides an overview of commonly used emergency medications. Epinephrine is the first-line drug in management of cardiac arrest, specifically for asystole, pulseless electrical activity (PEA), VF, and pulseless VT. Patients with VF and pulseless VT should be defibrillated before receiving epinephrine.

Patients with ventricular dysrhythmias associated with cardiac-cardiopulmonary arrest benefit from lidocaine (Xylocaine) administration. Once the ventricular dysrhythmia is controlled, an infusion of lidocaine is necessary to sustain therapeutic drug levels. Lidocaine should not be given to patients with third-degree atrioventricular (AV) block and with an escape rhythm or patients with bradycardia and PVCs.[26] Ectopic beats may contribute to the patient's cardiac output, so lidocaine could effectively reduce output and cause further decompensation or asystole. Other drugs used to manage ventricular dysrhythmias include procainamide (Pronestyl) and bretylium (Bretylol). Procainamide is also used for supraventricular dysrhythmias. Both bretylium and procainamide require IV infusions to maintain therapeutic drug levels.

Bradycardia dysrhythmias are usually managed with atropine, which blocks stimulation of the vagus nerve. Atropine may not be effective for high degree AV block dysrhythmias. Atropine can also be used for asystole and PEA. Isoproterenol (Isuprel) is a β-adrenergic agonist and may be used to increase cardiac output in bradydysrhythmias in some cases. Routine use of isoproterenol is not recommended because of its effects on ventricular irritability.

Supraventricular rhythms can impair effective cardiac output (because of decreased filling time) and hemodynamic stability. Adenosine (Adenocard) is an extremely rapid-acting agent (i.e., half-life ≤6 seconds) for reentry dysrhythmias. The drug must be given rapidly and followed with a 20-ml saline bolus to maximize effects. Side effects include transient bradycardia, transient asystole, ventricular ectopy, flushing, dyspnea, hypotension, and chest pain. Symptoms usually terminate spontaneously without further intervention. Verapamil (Calan) and diltiazem (Cardizem) are calcium channel–blocking agents used for controlling ventricular response rate in patients with supraventricular tachycardias (e.g., atrial fibrillation, atrial flutter, PSVT, atrial tachycardia). Monitor for bradycardia and hypotension when administering the drugs. Drugs should be used only for narrow complex SVT, because of the potential to induce and/or worsen reentry ventricular dysrhythmias.

Other miscellaneous drugs that may be used during cardiac arrest include sodium bicarbonate, calcium, and magnesium sulfate. Sodium bicarbonate is reserved for specific clinical situations including hyperkalemia, preexisting bicarbonate-responsive acidosis, and tricyclic antidepressant overdose. Magnesium is considered useful in the treatment of torsades de point, suspected hypomagnesemia, and refractory VF. Calcium, an ion essential to myocardial contraction and impulse formation, is recommended for hyperkalemia, hypocalcemia, and calcium channel–blocker toxicity.

During cardiopulmonary arrest, hemodynamic status is unstable and requires intervention to stabilize not only the patient's cardiac rhythm but also the cardiovascular system. Table 35-5 reviews the vasoactive drugs more commonly used during cardiac arrest. Some cardiovascular drugs can be given via endotracheal tube when IV access cannot be established (Table 35-6).

Acute Myocardial Infarction

Approximately 1.5 million persons experience acute myocardial infarction (AMI) annually in the United States; 40% die before reaching the hospital.[27] The majority of patients die in the first 2 hours after the onset of infarction. Mortality from infarction can be reduced significantly if the patient receives proper medical care in the early phases of infarction.[3]

The underlying disease process for AMI is atherosclerosis. An estimated 5.5 million people over 18 years of age in the United States have atherosclerosis. Pathogenesis of atherosclerosis includes accumulation of lipids on intimal lining of the arteries, calcific sclerosis of the medial layer of the arteries, and thickening of the walls of the arteries.[46] Generally, atherosclerosis affects the aorta as well as the coronary, cerebral, femoral, and other large or middle-sized arteries. Risk factors for atherosclerosis include smoking, hyperlipidemia, hypertension, diabetes mellitus, stress, lack of exercise, aging, diet high in fat and cholesterol, gender, and family history. Multiple existing risk factors increase a person's chance of having an AMI.

The major cause of the final event leading to AMI is thrombosis formation in a narrowed coronary artery from ruptured or fissured atherosclerotic plaque.[16] Subsequent vessel occlusion and thrombosis cause myocardial hypoxia and necrosis. Myocardial hypoxia may also be caused by coronary artery spasm and dissecting aortic aneurysm. Complete necrosis takes 4 to 6 hours to complete. The area surrounding the zone of necrosis is ischemic.[11] Damage to the myocardium predisposes the patient to pump failure and various dysrhythmias secondary to conduction defects and irritability of the myocardial tissue. Location and size of the infarct depend on which coronary artery is affected and where the occlusion occurred (Table 35-7). Most AMIs are caused by blockage of the left anterior descending coronary artery, causing involvement of the anterior wall of the myocardium.

When the coronary artery(s) becomes narrowed or occluded, myocardium becomes hypoxic, often resulting in classic retrosternal chest discomfort or angina pectoris. Pain is described as crushing, burning, sharp, heavy, or a variety of other descriptors. The pain lasts several minutes to several weeks and may vary in location. Local hypoxia, lactate buildup, and sensory response of the hypoxic myocardium contribute to pain. Pain may localize in the substernal area,

Table 35-5   Commonly Used Parenteral Vasoactive Drugs for Cardiovascular Emergencies[32,46]

Drug	Category	Actions	Indications	Dose	Comments
Esmolol (Brevibloc)	β-Adrenergic blocker	Depresses AV conduction and myocardial automaticity, especially the SA node; prolongs refractory period	SVT (e.g., PAT, atrial fibrillation-flutter, sinus tachycardia)	**IV push:** Initial loading dose 500 μg/kg over 1 min, followed by 50 μg/kg over 4 min. May repeat initial loading dose followed by 4 min. Infusion increased at increments of 50 μg/kg/min. (*Do not give over 200 μg/kg/min) **IV infusion:** Follow loading dose with infusion of 100 μg/kg/min	May cause significant bradycardia, hypotension, bronchospasm, heart failure Contraindications: heart block, CHF, severe asthma Immediate onset of action Duration of action approximately 30 min after infusion terminated
Calcium chloride	Electrolyte replacement	Improves vascular tone and myocardial contractility	Rapid electrolyte replacement In seriously hypotensive patients who respond poorly to fluid and vasopressors when hypocalcemia suspected	**IV push:** For Ca^{2+} replacement: 500 mg to 1 g (i.e., 7 to 14 mEq) For hyperkalemic ECG changes: 100 mg to 1 g For hypocalcemic tetany: 300 mg to 1.2 g For hypotension associated with Ca channel blockers: 500 mg to 2 g Administer slowly at rate not to exceed 0.7-1.4 mEq/min **IV infusion:** Administer diluted solution over 30-60 min (i.e., dilute calcium chloride in 50-100 ml D$_5$W, LR, or 0.9% NS)	May cause hypotension, bradycardia, dysrhythmias Contraindications: hypercalcemia, ventricular fibrillation
Diazoxide (Hyperstat)	Antihypertensive vasodilator	Direct relaxation of smooth muscle Inhibits release of pancreatic insulin	Significant hypertension	**IV push:** 1-3 mg/kg (e.g., approx. 50-150 mg) May repeat every 5-15 min as needed Maintenance dose = 50-150 mg every 4-24 hr	Inject drug rapidly—slow administration reduces hypotensive effects Onset of action <1 min, with peak in 2-5 min May cause hypotension CHF, dysrhythmias, myocardial and cerebral ischemia, and hyperglycemia

Continued

Table **35-5** **Commonly Used Parenteral Vasoactive Drugs for Cardiovascular Emergencies—cont'd**

Drug	Category	Actions	Indications	Dose	Comments
Diltiazem (Cardizem)	Calcium channel blocker	SA node automaticity decreased; AV conduction prolonged; increased refractoriness of AV node; vasodilation including coronary arteries	SVT (e.g., atrial fibrillation-flutter, PSVT)	**IV push:** 0.25 mg/kg administered over 2 min. May give additional dose in 15 min of 0.35 mg/kg if initial dose inadequate to control HR **Infusion:** 5-15 mg/hr	May cause hypotension, bradycardia, AV heart block Immediate onset when given IV, with peak effect in 15 min. Contraindications: heart block, accessory conduction pathways, or preexcitation syndromes
Dobutamine (Dobutrex)	Sympathomimetic β-1 adrenergic receptor agonist	Positive inotropic effects (e.g., increases force of myocardial contraction); increases heart rate at higher doses	To optimize cardiac output; may be used as concurrent therapy with afterload-reducing agents to increase cardiac output	**IV infusion:** Initially 2.5 μg/kg/min; continue titration to maintain effective cardiac output Maintenance dose usually 2.5-10 μg/kg/min Maximum dose = 40 μg/kg/min	May cause tachycardia, dysrhythmias (e.g., ventricular) Consider dose reduction if heart rate >10% above baseline
Dopamine (Intropin, Dopastat)	Sympathomimetic, β-1 and α-adrenergic agent; also dopaminergic stimulator	At low doses: vasodilates renal, mesenteric, and cerebral blood flow At intermediate doses: increases myocardial contractility and peripheral vasodilation At high doses: increases peripheral/renal vascular resistance and myocardial contractility	Low doses to increase urinary output Intermediate doses to increase cardiac output High doses to increase BP in shock with normovolemia	**IV infusion:** Low dose: 0.5-2 μg/kg/min Intermediate dose: 2-10 μg/kg/min High dose: >10 μg/kg/min Maximum dose = 20 μg/kg/min	May cause dysrhythmias Extravasation may cause tissue sloughing and necrosis
Enalapril (Vasotec)	Angiotensin converting enzyme (ACE) inhibitor	Reduces vascular tone	Significant hypertension	**IV push:** Initial dose 0.625 mg IVP; may repeat in 1 hr Maintenance dose = 1.25 mg every 6 hr IVP	May cause hypotension, pulmonary edema
Labetalol (Normodyne)	Selective α-adrenergic blocker and nonselective β-adrenergic blocker	Blocks sympathetic stimulation causing vasodilation	Hypertension	**IV push:** 20 mg (0.25 mg/kg) administered over 2 min. Additional doses of 40-80 mg can be given at 10 min intervals up to maximum 300 mg total.	Rapid injection may cause hypotension, heart block, cardiac/respiratory arrest Immediate onset when given IV Observe for hypermagnesemia: flushing, hypotension, bradycardia, confusion, weakness, depressed deep tendon reflexes, respiratory depression

Drug	Classification	Action	Indications	Dosage	Special Considerations
Nitroglycerin (Tridil)	Vasodilator	Relaxes vascular smooth muscle, promotes venous and coronary artery vasodilation; reduces venous return	Angina, hypertension	**IV infusion:** 5-10 µg/min Increase infusion by 5-10 µg/min every 5-10 min Maximum dose: 200 µg/min	May cause hypotension, headache, dizziness Nitroglycerin absorbed by many soft plastics; therefore dilute in glass bottle and consider using nonabsorbing, non-PVC tubing. If regular IV tubing used, flush line with 5-10 ml NTG solution.
Nitroprusside (Nipride)	Vasodilator	Relaxes vascular smooth muscle—lowering arterial and venous blood pressure; decreases afterload so CO decreases	Significant hypertension	**IV infusion:** Begin with 0.3-0.5 µg/kg/min Increase infusion by 1 to 2 µg/kg/min to attain desired hemodynamic effects Maximum infusion rate = 10 µg/kg/min	May cause hypotension, angina, increased ICP, seizures Protect from light by using light-resistant covering (e.g., aluminum foil, opaque plastic) Onset of action immediate, with peak action of 1-2 min
Norepinephrine bitartrate (Levophed)	Vasopressor	Peripheral venous-arterial vasoconstriction; cardiac stimulation	Short-term use for hypotension-shock	**IV infusion:** Begin with 2 µg/min and titrate to desired BP Usual range = 2-12 µg/min	May cause ventricular tachycardia-fibrillation (i.e., secondary to increased myocardial O_2 consumption) Extravasation may cause tissue sloughing and necrosis
Phenylephrine (Neo-synephrine)	Vasopressor	Potent postsynaptic α-adrenergic agonist	Short-term use for hypotension-shock	**IV push:** 0.1-0.5 mg over 1 min **IV infusion:** Dilute to yield solution of 0.1 ml and titrate every 10-15 min to achieve and to maintain BP >90 mm Hg	May cause hypertension, dysrhythmias, reflex bradycardia, cerebral hemorrhage Extravasation may cause tissue sloughing and necrosis
Propranolol (Inderal)	Nonselective β-adrenergic blocker and Class II antidysrhythmic	Blocks sympathetic stimulation of β-1 adrenergic receptors	Control of hypertension and suppression of rapid rate cardiac dysrhythmias	**IV push:** 0.5 to 3 mg Give slowly (1 mg/min); may repeat dose after 2 min	May cause bronchospasm, hypotension, heart block, angina

Table **35-6** **Alternate Routes for Drug Administration in Cardiovascular Emergencies**[26,29,30,31,37,43]

Route	Nursing management
Endotracheal (ET)	

When IV access not available, can administer selected emergency drugs:
    Epinephrine
    Atropine
    Lidocaine
    Naloxone
	Dilute drug in sterile saline or sterile water (i.e., 10 ml for adults and 1 to 2 ml for children)
	Administer medications as far down ET tube as possible; consider inserting intracatheter in ET tube and advancing to give medication

Consider dose 2.0 to 2.5 times recommended IV dose	Administer drug quickly down ET tube, follow with three to four rapid insufflations of ambu-bag to aerosolize medication in tracheobronchial tree
Intraosseous (IO)	
Used most often in children ≤6 years old Intraosseous needle placed in proximal tibia Can be placed in any portion of the tibia excluding the epiphyseal plates (e.g., distal tibia, midanterior distal one third of the femur, iliac crest, humerus); the sternum can be used as a site in patients ≥3 years of age	Use sterile technique to insert an intraosseous needle; alternative methods include using #16 or #18 gauge hypodermic, spinal, or bone marrow needle Confirm placement by aspiration of bone marrow, and freely flowing IV without evidence of infiltration Secure firmly with sterile dressing and tape to prevent dislodgement Monitor for extravasation and patency Flush with dilute saline or heparin to maintain patency Dilute hypertonic-alkaline solutions before administration

or radiate to the jaw and down the left arm. Associated symptoms include nausea, vomiting, diaphoresis, and hiccups if the phrenic nerve is stimulated.

Blood pressure decreases with AMI because poor pump action of the heart decreases cardiac output. Sodium and water retention may occur due to decreased cardiac output and increased venous pressure. When AMI occurs, ventricular failure occurs. With severe ventricular failure, stroke volume decreases and ventricular diastolic pressure increases, while the sympathetic response decreases blood flow to the periphery. Decreased blood flow and pressure to the kidneys leads to slow glomerular filtration rate (GFR). Decreased GFR stimulates renal cells to produce renin so angiotensin levels rise and aldosterone is secreted. Increased aldosterone and decreased GFR cause sodium and water retention and formation of interstitial edema.

Patient assessment. Prompt assessment of the patient with possible AMI is crucial because the incidence of ventricular fibrillation is 15 times greater during the first hour after onset of symptoms.[25] On average, the person experiencing AMI delays 3 hours before seeking medical care. Most patients are resting or engaged in only moderate activity when symptoms begin. Chest pain indicative of AMI is usually severe, lasts longer than 30 minutes, and is not relieved with rest or vasodilators such as nitroglycerin. Ironically, up to 20% of patients with AMI do not experience chest pain. Patients with diabetes mellitus are more prone to neuropathy and may not experience pain. Among patients older than 85 years, the classic symptom of AMI is shortness of breath.[2]

Heart transplant patients do not experience chest pain because pain receptors are disconnected during transplant.

Obtaining a concise, brief history of chest pain is crucial; the PQRST mnemonic is particularly useful for these patients[33] (Table 35-8). Patients who have chest pain must have a differential diagnosis made between angina pectoris and AMI. There are two types of angina—stable and unstable (Table 35-9). Stable angina, known as typical angina, occurs as a predictable event after activities such as exercise or body strain. Two categories of unstable angina are typical unstable angina and Prinzmetal's angina. Attacks of typical unstable angina, also called preinfarction angina, are prolonged, occur more frequently, and worsen with each episode.[24] Typical unstable angina is associated with higher incidence of left main and proximal left anterior descending coronary artery disease.[36] Half the patients with typical unstable angina have total or near-total occlusion (i.e., 70% to 100% stenosis) of a coronary artery. Prinzmetal's angina, or variant angina, occurs when the patient is at rest, usually at the same time each day. Prognosis with Prinzmetal's angina is poor, with 50% mortality during the first year.

In addition to assessing pain, assess for associated symptoms and pertinent medical history.[2] Associated symptoms include diaphoresis, nausea, vomiting, indigestion, dyspnea, palpitations, dizziness, or light-headedness. Evaluate risk factors for cardiac disease, for example, smoking, hypertension, hyperlipidemia, diabetes, and related medical history, that is, previous angina, previous AMI or cardiac surgery,

Table 35-7 Coronary Arteries in MI

Right coronary artery	Left coronary artery
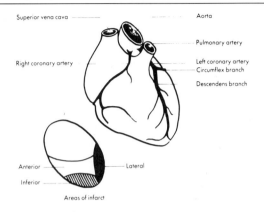	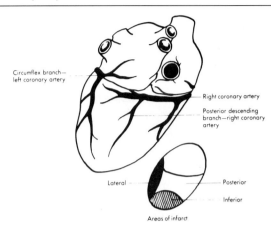

Supplies
    Right atrium
    Right ventricle
    Posterior surface left ventricle
    50%-60% sinoatrial node
    Bundle of His
Block causes
    Infarction posterior wall left ventricle
    Infarction posterior wall interventricular septum
    Anticipate second-degree heart block, Mobitz type 1 block,
        and Wenckebach block in inferior MI

Left circumflex branch

Supplies
    Left atrium
    Free wall left ventricle
    40%-50% sinoatrial node
    8%-10% arteriovenous node
    Bundle of His
    Right bundle
Block causes
    Lateral wall infarction
    Posterior wall infarction (near base)

Left anterior descending branch

Supplies: interventricular septum
Block causes
    Infarction anterior wall left ventricle
    Affects papillary muscle, which attaches to mitral valve
    Infarction anterior wall septum
    Anticipate second-degree heart block and Mobitz type 2 block
        in anterior MI

---

peripheral vascular disease, and immediate family history of AMI. Medication history may include antianginals, antidysrhythmics, antihypertensives, anticoagulants, and digitalis preparations. Such drugs as H_2 blockers, antacids, sucralfate, and nonsteroidal antiinflammatory drugs (NSAIDs) may assist in differentiating gastrointestinal problems and/or musculoskeletal discomfort.

In addition to cardiac disease, other etiologies may be associated with chest pain (Table 35-10). Hyperventilation, a common condition in the ED, may occur as a result of anxiety disorder, or may be a response to disease processes such as AMI, salicylate overdose, or intracerebral hemorrhage. Treat these patients with extreme caution and assess carefully for signs and symptoms of an underlying disorder.

A patient with hyperventilation is a difficult diagnostic problem. Hyperventilation may be a response to an organic process in which having the patient breathe in a paper bag may be detrimental. Hyperventilation is a sign of many illnesses and conditions, including anxiety, pregnancy, fever, liver disease, trauma, hypovolemia, pulmonary embolus, stress, ketoacidosis, high altitude, thyrotoxicosis, pulmonary hypertension, pulmonary edema, anemia, stroke, central nervous system lesion, and fibrotic lung disease. Hyperventilation causes partial arterial carbon dioxide pressure to drop and cerebral vasculature to constrict, resulting in respiratory alkalosis and tetany. Signs and symptoms include anxiety, panic, shortness of breath, paresthesia of the fingers, toes, and periorbital area, carpopedal spasms, confusion, syncope, and, occasionally, chest pain.

Therapeutic intervention includes calming and reassuring the patient. Have the patient talk; it is difficult to hyperventilate when speaking. As a last therapeutic intervention, have the patient breathe in a paper bag to facilitate carbon dioxide rebreathing.

Table **35-8**	**PQRST Mnemonic for Chest Pain Assessment**	
Factor		Description questions
P	Provokes, palliates, precipitating factors	What provoked the pain?
		What makes the pain better?
		What makes the pain worse?
		Have you had this type of pain before?
		What were you doing when the pain occurred?
Q	Quality	What does the pain feel like?
		Is it burning? Crushing? Tearing? Sharp?
R	Region, radiation	Show me where the pain is.
		How large an area is involved?
		Does the pain radiate? If so, where?
S	Severity, associated symptoms	How severe is the pain?
		If you were to rate the pain on a scale from 0 to 10 with 10 being the most severe pain you can imagine, how would you rate your pain?
		What else did you feel besides the pain?
T	Time, temporal relations	When did the pain start?
		How long did it last?
		Does it come and go?
		Were you awakened by the pain?
		Is the pain always present?

Chest pain may also be caused by abdominal illnesses such as hiatal hernia, gastric or peptic ulcer, pancreatitis, esophageal spasms, Mallory-Weiss syndrome, or Boerhaave's syndrome. Other problems that cause chest pain are musculoskeletal disorders involving trauma, degenerative disk disease, xiphoidalgia, costochondritis, Mondor's disease, and postherpetic syndrome.

Physical findings associated with AMI are usually consistent with a patient who is acutely ill. Because of hemodynamic effects of AMI, the patient may have a variety of heart rates and heart dysrhythmias. The patient may be hypertensive secondary to the low cardiac output and sympathetic stimulation or hypotensive from pump failure. The first heart sound may be decreased because of decreased myocardial contractility, whereas the second heart sound may be increased because of the increased pulmonary artery pressure. An S_3 sound (i.e., gallop) may be present as the result of ventricular dilation and increased ventricular fluid pressure. The presence of a new systolic murmur indicates ischemic mitral regurgitation or ventricular septal defect.

A transient pericardial friction rub may be heard as the result of the inflammatory response to the necrosis. There also may be an alternating pulse rate caused by left-sided heart failure. Increased pressure from congestion causes backflow of blood into the jugular veins and jugular vein distention when the patient is sitting at a 45-degree angle. There may also be a prominent V wave with rapid Y wave descent. The patient may also have an elevated temperature caused by inflammation and necrosis of myocardial tissue.

The patient is often diaphoretic and anxious. Diaphoresis is related to the autonomic nervous system response and anxiety may be due to pain and fever. Cyanosis may be caused by decreased oxyhemoglobin concentration and decreased blood supply to the peripheral vascular system.

ECG. Changes in the ECG provide information about the site of coronary artery occlusion, myocardial ischemia, and the presence of tissue necrosis. Lead placement of an ECG determines which area of the heart the ECG signal is representing (Figure 35-9 and 35-10). Changes in the ECG occur

Table **35-9** **Differential Diagnosis of Angina**		
Characteristic	Stable angina	Unstable (preinfarction) angina
Location of pain	Substernal; may radiate to jaws, neck, and down arms and back	Substernal; may radiate to jaws, neck, and down arms and back
Duration of pain	1-5 min	5 min; occurring more frequently
Characteristic of pain	Aching, squeezing, choking, heavy burning	Same as stable angina, but more intense
Other symptoms	Usually none	Diaphoresis; weakness
Pain worsened by	Exercise; activity; eating; cold weather; reclining	Exercise; activity; eating; cold weather; reclining
Pain relieved by	Rest; nitroglycerin; isosorbide	Nitroglycerin, isosorbide may give only partial relief
ECG findings	Transient ST depression; disappears with pain relief	ST segment depression; often T wave inversion; ECG may be normal

Table 35-10 **Etiologic Factors Considered in Differential Diagnosis of Chest Pain**[11,24,33,46]

Etiology	P Precipitating-palliating	Q Quality	R Radiating-region	S Severity-symptoms	T Time-temporal
Ischemia/angina	Precipitating factors: effort-related activity, large meals, emotional stress Palliation: ceases with activity abatement, relief with nitroglycerin and/or rest	Tightness, burning, deep, constrictive	Retrosternal, area affected the size of the palm of the hand Pain may radiate to left shoulder, left hand—especially the fourth and fifth finger, epigastrium, trachea, larynx Never involves region above level of the eye	Profuse diaphoresis, weakness, shortness of breath, nausea, vomiting	Gradual onset of pain builds to maximum pain intensity; usually anginal pain lasts 1-5 min
Myocardial infarction	Precipitating factors: effort-related activity, large meals, emotional stress	Severe chest pain	Chest pain; may radiate to back, jaw, or left arm	Palpitations, dyspnea, diaphoresis, nausea, vomiting, dizziness, weakness, sense of impending doom	Usually pain lasts 30 min or more
Acute pericarditis	Precipitating factors: may occur after AMI	Pain may be dull to severe with crushing type pain	Anterior chest pain with radiation to neck, arms, or shoulders; pain may be intensified by deep inspiration	Fever (i.e., between 101-102° F or 38.3-38.9° C); pericardial friction rub	
Dissecting aortic aneurysm	Sudden onset	Severe, ripping, tearing pain	Anterior and posterior chest	Dyspnea, tachypnea, CHF (i.e., secondary to aortic regurgitation caused by dissection); may also be CVA, syncope, paraplegia, and pulse loss associated with dissecting aneurysm	Sudden onset
Esophageal disorders	Precipitating factors: often triggered by exercise	Similar to AMI	Similar to AMI	Similar to AMI	Similar to AMI
Cocaine-induced	Precipitating factors: cocaine use Palliation: relieved with nitroglycerin	Heaviness, pressure of the chest	Substernal location, with radiation to both arms	Palpitations, diaphoresis, nausea, dizziness, syncope, dyspnea	Occurs 1 to 6 hours after cocaine use
Postoperative coronary artery bypass graft (CABG) caused by harvest of internal mammary artery (IMA)	Precipitating factors: use of IMA for graft of CABG patient	Mild to severe chest pain, burning, prickling, and dull sensations	Anterior chest, may radiate over entire chest wall, particularly over site of graft; may radiate to neck or axilla	Numbness, tenderness on palpation of sternum, hyperesthesia along incision line, delayed healing of the sternum	Persistent pain; shooting pain may last several seconds and occur several times per day

Continued

Table **35-10**   **Etiologic Factors Considered in Differential Diagnosis of Chest Pain—cont'd**

Etiology	P Precipitating-palliating	Q Quality	R Radiating-region	S Severity-symptoms	T Time-temporal
Mitral valve prolapse	Palliation: relief in recumbent position, no relief with nitroglycerin	Dull, aching	Nonretrosternal chest pain	Systolic murmur, unexplained dyspnea, weakness, mid-systolic (apical) click	
5-Fluorouracil therapy	Precipitating factors: following infusion of 5-FU Palliation: relief with nitroglycerin	Mild to severe pain	Central chest pain; radiates to left shoulder and left arm	Nausea, vomiting, tachycardia, hypertension	Occurs several hours after IV bolus or infusion of 5-FU; no chest pain between treatments
Tachydysrhythmias	Precipitating factors: anxiety, digitalis, toxicity, exercise, organic heart disease Palliation: terminated by anti-arrhythmics, direct current shock, vagal maneuvers	Sharp, stabbing chest pain; may have palpitations, "skipped beats"	Precordial chest pain	Weakness, fatigue, lethargy, palpitations, dizziness, vertigo	Paroxysmal in onset; lasts briefly to hours
Monosodium glutamate	Occurs with ingestion of food high in monosodium glutamate	Burning chest pain	Retrosternal chest pain	Facial pain, nausea, vomiting	Occurs shortly after meals or up to several hours after meal
Musculoskeletal	Precipitating factors: pain with inspiration or with musculo-skeletal movement	Generalized aching, stiffness with point tenderness, swelling	Tenderness of anterior chest wall	Persistent chest pain; no relief with rest	Duration of pain longer lasting than pain associated with angina

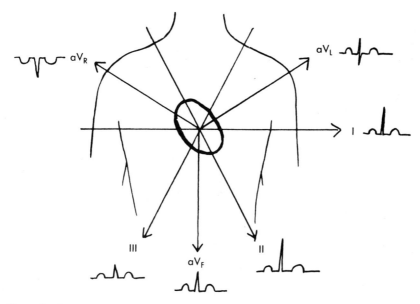

Figure **35-9**   Six-limb lead (leads I, II, III, aV$_R$, aV$_L$, and aV$_F$) normally appear as shown.

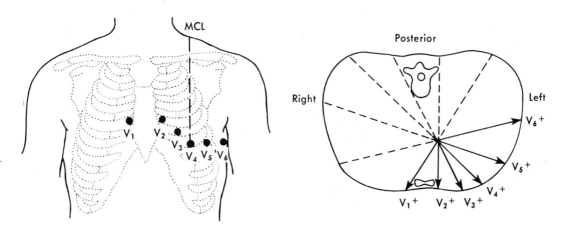

Figure **35-10**   Precordial or chest (V$_{1-6}$) leads.

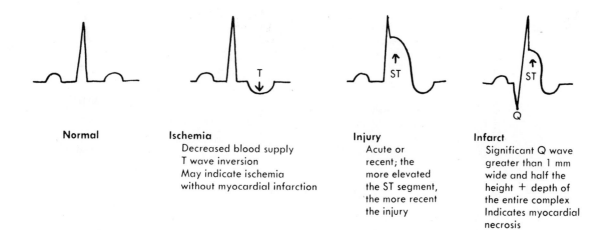

Normal

Ischemia
Decreased blood supply
T wave inversion
May indicate ischemia
without myocardial infarction

Injury
Acute or
recent; the
more elevated
the ST segment,
the more recent
the injury

Infarct
Significant Q wave
greater than 1 mm
wide and half the
height + depth of
the entire complex
Indicates myocardial
necrosis

Figure **35-11**   ECG changes.

due to changes in electrical current flow when there is myocardial damage and/or ischemia (Figure 35-11). When current flows toward a lead (arrowhead, positive electrode), an upward ECG deflection occurs. When current flows away from a lead (arrowhead, positive electrode), downward deflection occurs. When current flows perpendicular to a lead (arrowhead), biphasic ECG deflection occurs. Figures 35-12 through 35-15 illustrate ECG changes with myocardial infarction. Serial ECGs are used in conjunction with the patient assessment,

history, and other diagnostic measures to confirm the diagnosis of AMI. A single ECG cannot be used exclusively. ECG findings are sensitive only 50% of the time and ECG changes may occur with other conditions. Patients with stable angina may have ST segment depression, and ST segment elevation can occur with unstable angina and Prinzmetal's angina. Pericarditis may cause ST segment elevation in many leads, hemorrhagic stroke is associated with T wave inversion, and ventricular aneurysms may be associated with ST elevation.

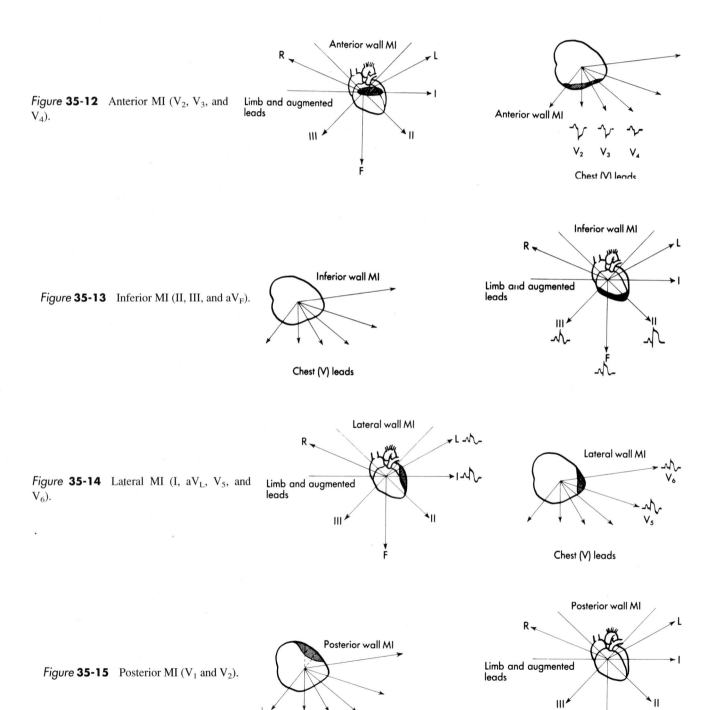

Figure **35-12**   Anterior MI (V_2, V_3, and V_4).

Figure **35-13**   Inferior MI (II, III, and aV_F).

Figure **35-14**   Lateral MI (I, aV_L, V_5, and V_6).

Figure **35-15**   Posterior MI (V_1 and V_2).

Elevation of the segment between the end of the S wave and the beginning of the T wave (ST segment) is indicative of myocardial injury and occurs minutes after occlusion of a coronary artery. The ST segment may remain elevated for 24 hours. T wave inversion occurs 6 to 24 hours after occlusion, may persist months to years, and is due to ischemia. Pathologic Q waves, measuring more than 0.04 seconds in width and at least 25% or more of overall QRS height, occur within 24 hours and indicate irreversible myocardial cell death. ST segment depression may also be associated with AMI. Reciprocal changes (i.e., ST segment depression and peaked T wave) may be seen in ECG leads that view the regions opposite to the damaged area.[11] In the Multicenter Chest Pain Study,[42] ECG changes achieved an overall 79% sensitivity and 44% specificity in detecting an AMI (Box 35-2).

A Q wave has been associated with a transmural AMI; however, studies now demonstrate both Q wave and non–Q wave infarcts can be transmural or subendocardial. In general, Q wave infarctions are associated with a larger region of myocardial necrosis, higher enzyme levels, fresh coronary thrombosis, frequent vomiting, congestive heart failure, conduction defects, dysrhythmias, and less collateral circulation.[11] When ST segment depression occurs in the in-

ferior (II, III, aV_F), lateral (I, aV_L, V_5, V_6), or anterior (V_1 through V_6) leads and cardiac enzymes are elevated, diagnosis of non–Q wave infarct is supported. ST elevation is most frequently associated with Q wave infarctions and almost 50% of non–Q wave infarctions.

All patients with suspected inferior and/or lateral AMI should be evaluated for right ventricular infarction. Right ventricular infarct is present in up to 40% of patients with inferior MIs due to occlusion of the right coronary artery. Changes noted on the ECG may include isolated ST segment elevation in V_1 or ST elevation in V_1 to V_4. A more reliable method of determining right ventricular infarct is use of right ventricular leads (V_{3R} to V_{6R}). Figure 35-16 and Box 35-3 illustrate right ventricular lead placement. Use of lead V_{4R} has 92% sensitivity for right coronary artery occlusion.[11]

ECG changes in posterior infarct include ST depression in V_1 to V_4, which represents reciprocal changes of the anterior wall, the portion of the heart opposite the posterior portion. Other changes include R waves > 0.04 seconds in V_1 and V_2 and R wave to S wave ratio ≥1 in V_1 and V_2. Further evaluation may include posterior ECG leads (V_7 to V_9) (see Box 35-3).

Continuous ECG monitoring in one or more leads is essential for the AMI patient. Dual lead and/or continuous ST seg-

---

Box 35-2   Criteria for Significant ECG Changes

Probable new transmural AMI

 ≥1 mm ST segment elevation in ≥two leads

OR

 abnormal Q waves in ≥two leads

New strain or ischemia

 ≥1 mm ST segment depression in ≥two leads

New ST or T wave changes of ischemia or strain

 ST depression <1 mm and T wave inversions (can represent ischemia or strain)

Box 35-3   Lead Placement for Right Ventricular and Posterior Leads

Right ventricular leads

V_{3R} = Between V_1 and V_{4R}
V_{4R} = Fifth intercostal space right midclavicular line
V_{5R} = Fifth intercostal space right anterior axillary line
V_{6R} = Fifth intercostal space right midaxillary line

Posterior leads

V_7 = Fifth intercostal space posterior axillary line
V_8 = Fifth intercostal space between V_7 and V_9
V_9 = Fifth intercostal space next to vertebral column

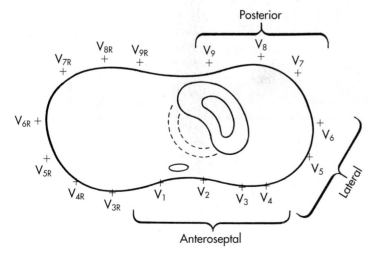

Figure **35-16** Right ventricular and posterior wall ECG lead placement. *(Modified from Hearns PA: Differentiating ischemia, injury, infarction: expanding the 12-lead electrocardiogram, Dimen Crit Care Nurs 13[4]:176, 1994.)*

ment monitoring is available to detect changes in the ECG and identify dysrhythmias. The best lead to use for diagnosing wide complex QRS rhythms is MCl₁ or MCl₆[19] (Figure 35-17). This combination of a limb lead and precordial lead is valuable in detecting both ST segment changes associated with further blockage of coronary arteries and for dysrhythmia detection. If bedside monitoring permits, the combination of leads V₁, I, and aV_F allows quick evaluation of ECG axis. Figure 35-18 provides an overview of axis based on leads I and

aV_F. Evaluation of axis during wide-complex QRS rhythms or dysrhythmias assists in differentiating supraventricular from ventricular dysrhythmias.[18] In one study, three lead combinations were 100% sensitive for ischemic changes in the major coronary vessels. Leads III, V₂, and V₅ reflect the coronary artery and left circumflex artery. Leads III, V₃, and V₅ reflect left anterior descending artery.[7] As technology evolves, multi-lead ECG monitoring and continuous ST segment monitoring may become increasingly common in the ED.

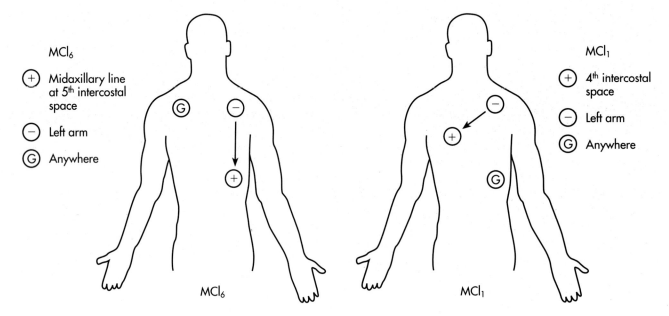

Figure **35-17** Monitoring on 3-lead ECG monitor. Leads MCl₆ and MCl₁ are the best leads for monitoring dysrhythmias.

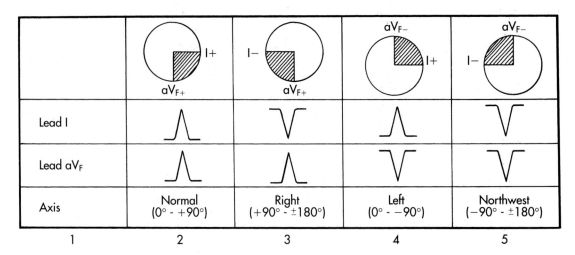

Figure **35-18** Determination of QRS axis. *(1)* Note predominant QRS polarity in leads I and aV_F. *(2)* If QRS during tachycardia is primarily positive in I and aV_F, axis falls within normal quadrant from 0 degrees to 90 degrees. *(3)* If complex is primarily negative in I and positive in aV_F, right axis deviation is present. *(4)* If complex is predominantly positive in I and negative in aV_F, left axis deviation is present. *(5)* If QRS is primarily negative in both I and aV_F, markedly abnormal "northwest" axis is present that is diagnostic of ventricular tachycardia. *(Modified from Drew BJ: Bedside electrocardiographic monitoring,* Heart Lung *20[6]:610, 1991.)*

Cardiac enzymes. In addition to ECG monitoring, cardiac enzymes are measured as part of the diagnostic workup for AMI. Primary cardiac enzymes evaluated in determining the presence of AMI are creatine kinase (CK) and the MB fraction of the CK. These enzymes are released from the necrotic myocardium.

Lactate dehydrogenase (LDH) is another enzyme that is elevated following AMI. Table 35-11 describes these and other enzymes released with myocardial tissue necrosis.

Other biochemical markers are myoglobin and troponin. Myoglobin is a nonspecific protein associated with muscle oxygen transport. Myoglobin levels elevate sooner (i.e., <1 hour) than CK after myocardial injury and peak in 2 to 4 hours. Myoglobin is found in the heart and the skeletal muscle, so it is used to rule out AMI.[34] Troponin is also a protein found in the myofibrils of muscle.[1] Two subforms, troponin T and troponin I, are very specific for the cardiac muscle. Troponin is detectable 4 to 6 hours following AMI, peaks at 10 to 24 hours, and remains elevated 5 to 7 days.

Further evaluation of the patient with AMI includes a chest radiograph to rule out other causes of chest pain such as pneumonia, pneumothorax, trauma, and malignancy. A chest radiograph is also valuable in determining the presence of cardiomegaly and pulmonary congestion. In some situations, an echocardiogram may be used to evaluate myocardial wall motion, valve abnormalities, and septal wall defect. Although not diagnostic of AMI, an echocardiogram is useful in determining the extent of damage to the myocardium. Extensive myocardial damage puts the patient at risk for complications such as heart failure and cardiogenic shock.

Patient management. While obtaining the history and assessing the patient's status, the emergency nurse should convey a calm and reassuring manner. Any patient with AMI or suspected AMI should have low flow oxygen (2 to 6 L/min) and the head of the bed elevated. Maintain oxygen saturation at ≥95%. If oxygenation cannot be maintained or the patient is acidotic, intubation and mechanical ventilation are indicated.[2]

After oxygen therapy is initiated, establish IV access for medications and fluid therapy. Insert at least two large-bore (i.e., 18-gauge or large-bore) catheters and infuse normal saline (NS) as needed. If thrombolytic therapy is possible, consider insertion of double-lumen catheters. Ongoing assessment includes frequent determination of blood pressure, continuous ECG monitoring, and continuous pulse oximetry monitoring. Assessment of pain intensity, location, radiation of pain, and applicable descriptors establishes baseline. Assessment parameters should be reassessed after any intervention for chest pain. Nitroglycerin is the initial drug of choice for treatment of chest pain related to angina pectoris and AMI. Nitroglycerin can be administered sublingually in 0.4 or 0.3 mg tablets or in a spray. One tablet or spray is administered every 5 minutes up to three doses. Nitroglycerin dilates coronary arteries, reduces afterload by dilating peripheral venous circulation, and reduces preload, that is, decreases venous return to the heart. Nitroglycerin is not usually given unless the systolic blood pressure (SBP) is at least 100 mm Hg because of potential decreased blood pressure that may occur with nitroglycerin. If sublingual nitroglycerin is not effective, IV nitroglycerin (Tridil) can be used. Initiate nitroglycerin infusion at 10 to 20 μg/min and titrate in increments of 5 to 10 μg/min up to 50 to 180 μg/min.

If nitroglycerin fails to relieve chest pain, the next drug of choice is morphine sulfate. This narcotic analgesic relieves chest pain and anxiety, which decreases myocardial oxygen consumption. If SBP is >100 mm Hg, administer morphine 2 to 4 mg IV every 5 to 10 minutes until pain is relieved. Monitor respiratory status and hemodynamic response carefully following morphine administration. If the patient is allergic to morphine, meperidine (Demerol) may be used. Approximately 75 to 100 mg of meperidine is equivalent to 10 mg of morphine and can be given in small incremental doses.

Once the patient is initially stabilized, aspirin should be given orally unless contraindicated (e.g., allergy, active GI bleeding). If the patient is unable to tolerate oral aspirin, one rectal suppository can be given. Recommended dosage ranges from 65 to 325 mg.

Thrombolytic therapy. Thrombolytic therapy for the patient with AMI is a crucial component of overall therapy to reduce patient mortality and morbidity.[8,9,28,48] Patients benefit from therapy if the thrombolytic agent is initiated within 12 hours of the onset of chest pain. The goal of thrombolytic

Table **35-11** **Serum Enzymes and Biochemical Markers for AMI**[40]			
Diagnostic test	Elevation (after AMI)	Peak	Return to normal
Creatine kinase (CK)	2 to 5 hours	24 to 48 hours	2 to 3 days
Creatine kinase-MB (CK-MB)	2 to 5 hours	24 to 48 hours	2 to 3 days
CK-MB subforms: MB1 and MB2	<1 hour	4 to 8 hours	
Lactic dehydrogenase (LDH)	8 to 12 hours	72 to 144 hours	10+ days
*LDH1/LDH2 ratio >0.76 is significantly associated with AMI			
Myoglobin	<1 hour	2 to 4 hours	
Troponin	4 to 6 hours	10 to 24 hours	5 to 7 days

therapy is to lyse coronary thrombi, restore blood flow to a hypoperfused myocardium, and abort or prevent complete evolution of the infarction process. When treatment begins within 3 hours of new symptoms, the incidence of successful reperfusion is 60% to 70% for all thrombolytic agents.

Thrombolytic therapy targets elements of the clotting process to cause **fibrinolysis,** the process of clot degradation. Lysis of the clot begins with activation of plasminogen, which converts to plasmin. Plasmin degrades or breaks down fibrin in the clot, circulating fibrinogen, factor V, and factor VIII. Thrombolytic agents are an exogenous source of plasminogen. Four thrombolytic agents are currently available— urokinase (Abbokinase), streptokinase (Streptase), tissue plasminogen activator (Alteplase), and anisoylated plasminogen streptokinase activator complex (APSAC, Eminase). Urokinase is usually administered via the intracoronary artery on the cardiac cath lab. Selection of the thrombolytic agent is based on the patient's history, physician preference, availability, funding, and mechanism of action. Various agents are compared in Table 35-12.

Thrombolytic agents have a significant potential for bleeding complications. Absolute contraindications for thrombolytic therapy include recent internal bleeding (<1 month ago), known bleeding diathesis, history of CVA, recent surgery (e.g., intracranial, intraspinal, or intraocular), intracranial AV malformations, uncontrolled hypertension (SBP >180 mm Hg, diastolic blood pressure [DBP] >110 mm Hg), recent trauma (in past 10 days), and CPR. Relative contraindications include minor trauma, diabetic retinopathy, pregnancy, concurrent anticoagulation, severe trauma (e.g., in past 6 months), any previous CNS event, and unsuccessful central venous puncture. If the patient will receive streptokinase or APSAC, the patient should be screened for recent history of a streptococcal infection (i.e., <6 months

Table **35-12** **Comparison of Thrombolytic Agents**			
Agent	**Action**	**Dose**	**Comments**
Streptokinase (Streptase, Kabikinase)	Exogenous plasminogen activator; not clot specific	**IV:** 1.5 million units IV over 1 hr **Intracoronary:** 10,000 to 30,000 units; followed by maintenance infusion of 2000 to 4000 units/min until thrombolysis occurs (e.g., 150,000 to 500,000 units total)	Half-life in plasma is 18 min; prolonged effect on coagulation because of fibrinogen depletion that persists 18 to 24 hr; antibodies to the drug present in persons who have been exposed to *Streptococcus* infection can cause allergic reaction (rash, fever, and chills); patients should not be retreated with streptokinase for 2 wk to 1 yr after initial administration because of secondary resistance
Urokinase (Abbokinase)	Proteolytic enzyme; directly activates plasminogen to plasmin; not clot specific	**Intracoronary:** 6000 units/min up to 2 hr **IV:** 2 to 3 million units IV bolus over 45 to 90 min	Half-life in plasma 10 to 16 min
Recombinant tissue plasminogen activator (rt-PA) (Activase)	Proteolytic enzyme; direct activator of plasminogen; high degree of clot specificity	**Standard IV dose:** 10 mg IV bolus followed by continuous infusion of 50 mg IV over 1 hr, then 20 mg/hr over 2 hr (total dose = 100 mg). **Front loaded dose:** 15 mg IV bolus, followed by 0.75 mg/kg (up to 50 mg) over 30 min; then 0.50 mg/kg (up to 35 mg) over remaining 60 min	Half-life in plasma 5 to 7 min; may cause sudden hypotension; in-line IV filters can remove as much as 47% of the drug; dose adjusted for patients who weigh <65 kg
Anisoylated plasminogen streptokinase activator complex (APSAC) (Eminase)	Inactivated derivative of thrombolytic enzyme synthesized from streptokinase and lysoplasminogen; promotes thrombolysis after activation within the body	**IV:** 30 units over 2 to 5 min; dilute only with 5 ml sterile water	Do not give to patients allergic to streptokinase; may not be as effective when administered more than 5 days after previous dose, after streptokinase therapy, or after streptococcal infection; discard if not used within 30 min of mixing

ago) or prior treatment with streptokinase or APSAC. Additional lab data such as a complete blood cell count, prothrombin time, partial thromboplastin time, fibrinogen, and platelet count can assist with determining potential bleeding problems and serve as baseline data.

Additional nursing management for the patient receiving thrombolytic therapy focuses on assessing for potential complications, monitoring for reperfusion, and minimizing tissue trauma. The major complication for the patient receiving thrombolytic therapy is bleeding and hemorrhage. Bleeding occurs most often at cut-down sites, arterial puncture sites, and injection sites. Systemic bleeding, that is, GI, urinary, vaginal, cerebral, or retroperitoneal, and neurologic impairment (e.g., CVA) may also occur. Monitor for hypotension, decreased hemoglobin and hematocrit, and tachycardia. The other major complication that occurs is an allergic reaction, particularly with use of streptokinase or APSAC. Monitor for respiratory distress, rash, or urticaria. Minimize tissue trauma by keeping the patient on bed rest, limiting arterial and venous punctures, and limiting use of noninvasive blood pressure cuffs. Reperfusion cannot be absolutely determined without benefit of cardiac angiography; however, markers of reperfusion that can be assessed by the emergency nurse include resolution of chest pain, normalizing of ST changes, and occurrence of reperfusion dysrhythmias such as accelerated idioventricular rhythms.

A heparin infusion is often used in conjunction with thrombolytic agents to prevent formation of a new clot and reocclusion of the coronary vessel. Intravenous heparin is initiated with a 5000 unit IV bolus followed with infusion at 1000 units/hr and titrated to maintain the patient's partial thromboplastin time (PTT) at 1½ to 2 times the control levels. Weight-based heparin therapy is also used.

Recent studies have recommended additional pharmacologic agents to provide further protection for the AMI patient from mortality and morbidity.[2] β-Blocker therapy is recommended if there are no specific contraindications such as asthma, chronic obstructive pulmonary disease (COPD), AV block, hypotension, congestive heart failure (CHF), and allergy. β-Blockers have proven especially useful in AMI patient with recurrent symptoms of ischemia, hypertension, sinus tachycardia, and in patients >65 years of age. Additional therapy that may be initiated in the ED includes angiotensin converting enzyme (ACE) inhibitor agents. ACE inhibitor use has been associated with reduced mortality. Known contraindications to ACE inhibitor therapy include allergies, Killip class III and IV, history of renal failure, or bilateral renal artery stenosis.

Dysrhythmias

Blood flow deprivation to the myocardium as a result of AMI can affect the heart's electrical conduction system, causing various dysrhythmias. Table 35-13 summarizes dysrhythmias and categories of antidysrhythmics according to modified Vaughn-Williams classification schema. By under-

standing the drug classifications, the emergency nurse can anticipate expected action of the drug and nursing implications for drug administration and patient assessment.

Premature ventricular contractions (PVCs) are the most common dysrhythmia associated with cardiac ischemia and AMI, occurring in approximately 85% of patients with AMI. After the initiation of oxygen therapy, lidocaine is the drug of choice for symptomatic PVCs. Lidocaine may be used prophylactically for AMI patients, even without PVCs, due to the high incidence of ventricular tachycardia and ventricular fibrillation that occurs without warning dysrhythmias. Some studies suggest that prophylactic use of lidocaine in patients with AMI may increase mortality; therefore lidocaine use must be considered with respect to the potential adverse effects. PVCs may also be caused by hypoxemia, acidosis, alkalosis, electrolyte imbalances, digoxin toxicity, and bradycardia. The underlying mechanism responsible for the patient's PVCs should be evaluated and treated.

Bradycardia is defined as a heart rate less than 60 beats/min and occurs in approximately 65% of AMI patients, particularly those with inferior wall infarction. Bradycardic dysrhythmias include atrioventricular (AV) blocks. Four different types may occur, depending on the area and degree of damage to the conduction system. These AV blocks are referred to as first-degree, second-degree Mobitz I (Wenckebach), second-degree Mobitz II, and third-degree or complete heart block. Blocks in conduction may be caused by myocardial infarction, infection, degenerative changes in the conduction system, rheumatic heart disease, and medications such as β-blockers, calcium

---

Box **35-4**   ***Systematic Evaluation of Cardiac Rhythms***

Rate

Bradycardia: <60 beats/min
Normal rate: 60 to 100 beats/min
Tachycardia: >100 beats/min

Rhythm

Is the rhythm regular or irregular?

P waves

Are P waves present? Does one P wave appear before each QRS? Is P wave deflection normal?

QRS complex

Normal is 0.06 to 0.12 second. Are the QRS complexes normal shape and configuration?

P/QRS relationship

Does QRS complex follow every P wave?

PR interval

Normal is 0.12 to 0.2 second. Is the interval prolonged? Shortened?

Table 35-13   Antidysrhythmic Agents Classified by Modified Vaughan-Williams Classification Schema[32,38,46,47]

Class	Pharmacologic action	Electrophysiologic effects	Indications	Drugs	Comments
I	Sodium channel blockade (stabilizes cell membrane)	Decreases conduction velocity; prolongs PR and QRS intervals	Ventricular dysrhythmias	Moricizine (Ethmozine)	Risk of prodysrhythmia potential
IA		Blocks and delays repolarization, lengthening action potential duration and effective refractory period	Atrial and ventricular dysrhythmias	Quinidine sulfate (Quinidex) Procainamide (Pronestyl) Disopyramide (Norpace)	Observe for heart block, hypotension, prolonged PR/QRS/QT intervals
IB		Shortens action potential duration	Ventricular dysrhythmias	Lidocaine (Xylocaine) Tocainide (Tonocard) Mexilitene (Mexitil)	Potential toxicity: dizziness, vertigo, confusion, seizures
IC		Slows conduction of electrical impulses in atria, AV node, and ventricular/His—Purkinje fibers	Ventricular dysrhythmias	Flecainide (Tambocar) Encainide (Enkaid) Propafenone (Rhythmol)	Risk of prodysrhythmia potential
II	β-Adrenergic blockade	Inhibition of sympathetic stimulation—reducing heart rate and decreasing myocardial irritability, shortens action potential	Supraventricular and ventricular dysrhythmias	Propranolol (Inderal) Esmolol (Brevibloc) Acebutolol (Sectral)	Observe for hypotension, bradycardia, heart block
III	Potassium channel blockade	Delayed repolarization and prolongation of action potential and delayed repolarization, thus decreasing myocardial irritability	Ventricular tachycardia and ventricular fibrillation	Bretylium (Bretylol) Amiodarone (Cordarone)	Observe for exacerbation of dysrhythmias, hypotension; pulmonary fibrosis may occur with amiodarone use
IV	Calcium channel blockade	Slows conduction of electrical impulses and decreases rate of impulse initiation	SVT and atrial dysrhythmias	Verapamil (Calan) Diltiazem (Cardizem) Nifedipine (Procardia)	Observe for hypotension, bradycardia, heart block
Unclassified	Potassium channel opener	Slows conduction through AV node and increases refractory period in AV node	SVT	Adenosine (Adenocard)	Has very rapid effect, short half-life

channel–blockers, and cardiac glycosides. Management of symptomatic bradycardias and heart blocks includes drugs such as atropine and isoproterenol. An external pacemaker or transvensous pacemaker may also be used. Second-degree Mobitz I heart block, associated with a conduction defect through the AV node, is usually benign and transient. This rhythm is commonly associated with inferior infarction because the right coronary artery supplies this area and the AV node. Second-degree Mobitz II AV block occurs when conduction through the bundle branches is impaired, usually because of blockage of the left coronary artery, which supplies the anterior wall and the bundle branches. This form of second-degree block is more likely than the other form to progress to a third-degree block.

Other dysrhythmias that commonly occur are supraventricular tachycardias, which may be indicative of myocardial ischemia or an anterior wall infarct. Often associated with chest pain, tachycardias are dangerous because they increase myocardial oxygen consumption and may extend the size of the infarct. Treatment depends on clinical findings. For hemodynamically unstable patients, therapy may include pharmacologic agents such as adenosine, verapamil, and procainamide, as well as vagal maneuvers or synchronized cardioversion.

Evaluation of dysrhythmias requires a systematic approach (Box 35-4). An overview of each rhythm is presented including rhythm strip in lead II, significance of the rhythm, and therapeutic interventions for adults.

Dysrhythmias originating in the sinus node

Normal sinus rhythm

Rate	60 to 100 beats/min
Rhythm	Regular
P waves	Present
QRS complex	Present; normal duration
P/QRS relationship	P wave preceding each QRS complex
PR interval	Normal

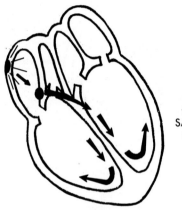

Impulse travels from SA to AV node through His bundle to Purkinje fibers

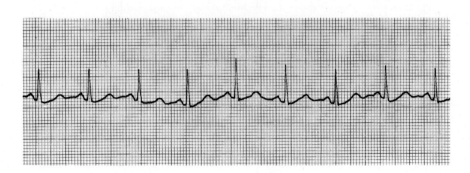

Significance: The sinoatrial (SA) node is the normal pacemaker of the heart and is influenced by parasympathetic and sympathetic branches of the autonomic nervous system.

Intervention: None required.

Sinus tachycardia

Rate	>100 beats/min; seldom >160 beats/min
Rhythm	Regular
P waves	Normal; present; with rapid rates, P waves may be buried in previous T wave
QRS complex	Present; normal duration
P/QRS relationship	P wave precedes each QRS complex
PR interval	Normal

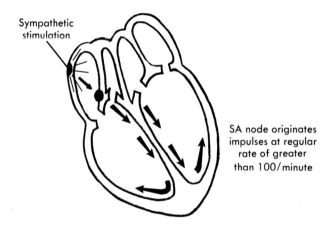

Sympathetic stimulation

SA node originates impulses at regular rate of greater than 100/minute

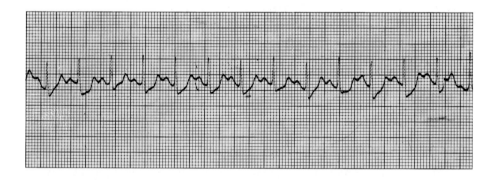

NOTE: If rate is exactly 150, consider possibility that rhythm is atrial flutter with a 2:1 conduction.

Significance: The normal pacemaker of the heart is firing at an increased rate because of anxiety, fever, pain, exercise, smoking, hyperthyroidism, heart failure, volume loss, specific drugs, or other reasons that cause increased tissue oxygen demands. Decreased vagal tone (parasympathetic stimulation) allows the sinus node to increase rate. Cardiac output may decrease with rates greater than 180 beats/min because of inadequate ventricular filling. Very rapid rates during AMI may lead to further ischemia and tissue damage.

Intervention: Treat the underlying cause. No specific drug is given for sinus tachycardia except in congestive heart failure; digitalis is usually the drug of choice.

Sinus bradycardia

Rate	<60 beats/min; seldom <30 beats/min
Rhythm	Regular or slightly irregular
P waves	Present; normal
QRS complex	Present; normal duration
P/QRS relationship	P wave precedes each QRS complex
PR interval	Normal

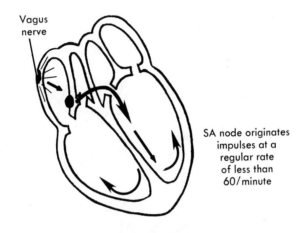

Vagus nerve

SA node originates impulses at a regular rate of less than 60/minute

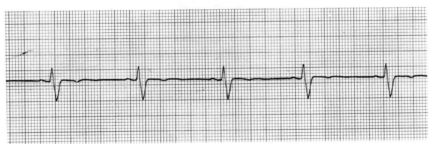

Significance: The normal pacemaker (SA node) is slowed by increased vagal tone (parasympathetic stimulation). Causes include rest, normal athletic heart, anoxia, hypothyroidism, increased intracranial pressure, acute myocardial infarction, vagal stimulation (such as vomiting, straining at stool, carotid sinus massage, or ocular pressure), and specific drugs.

Intervention: With heart rate less than 50 beats/min, cardiac output, coronary perfusion, and electrical stability may be reduced, causing PVCs. No treatment is needed if the patient is alert, has normal blood pressure, and no PVCs. Hypotension and PVCs should be treated. Symptomatic PVCs should be treated with oxygen and atropine, not lidocaine. Increasing the heart rate may eradicate the PVCs, whereas eliminating PVCs may decrease cardiac output.

Sinus arrhythmia

Rate	60 to 100 beats/min, but rate increases with inspiration and decreases with expiration
Rhythm	Regularly irregular
P waves	Present
QRS complex	Present; normal duration
P/QRS relationship	P wave precedes each QRS complex
PR interval	Normal

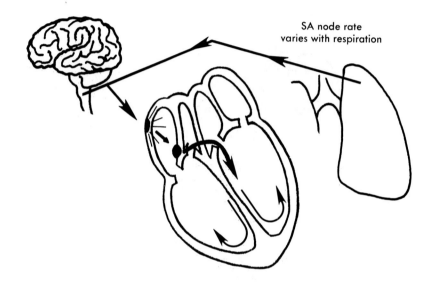

SA node rate
varies with respiration

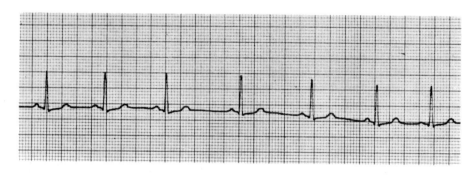

Significance: Normal finding in children and young adults with variation of vagal tone in response to respirations. As an abnormal finding, may occur in patients with mitral or aortic valve problems or as a response to increased intracranial pressure or specific drugs. To be considered a dysrhythmia, variation must exceed 0.12 seconds between the longest and shortest cycles.

Intervention: Observe the patient and document findings. If not related to respiratory problems, treat the underlying cause.

Dysrhythmias originating in the atria

Premature atrial contractions (extrasystoles)

Rate	Usually 60 to 100 beats/min
Rhythm	Usually regularly irregular; may be regular
P waves	Present, but premature P wave may appear different in configuration because it did not originate in the SA node
QRS complex	Present; normal duration
P/QRS relationship	P wave precedes each QRS complex
PR interval	Normal in regular beats, variable in premature atrial contractions (PACs)

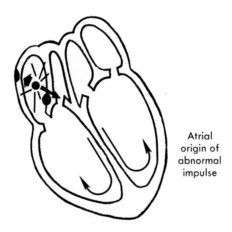

Atrial
origin of
abnormal
impulse

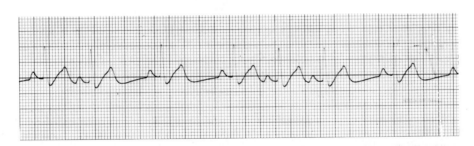

NOTE: Always describe underlying rhythm. For example, "Sinus tachycardia with approximately two PACs per minute."

Significance: PACs are the result of an irritable ectopic focus that may be caused by fatigue, alcohol, coffee, smoking, digoxin, congestive heart failure, or ischemia; sometimes the cause is unknown. PACs may be a prelude to atrial fibrillation, atrial flutter, or paroxysmal atrial tachycardia.

Intervention: Treatment is usually unnecessary. If the patient has symptoms, tranquilizers, quinidine, procainamide, verapamil, β-adrenergic blockers, and diltiazem may be tried. Encourage the patient to limit alcohol, coffee consumption, and smoking.

Supraventricular tachycardia

Rate	140 to 220 beats/min; atrial rate usually 160 to 240 beats/min
Rhythm	Atrial rhythm regular; ventricular rhythm usually regular, may be 2:1 AV block
P waves	Absent or abnormal; may be difficult to identify if P waves buried in preceding T wave; differ from normal sinus P waves
QRS complex	Normal or prolonged because of bundle branch block or aberrant conduction
P/QRS relationship	May be a block
PR interval	Normal or prolonged

Impulse travels from site above ventricles through HIS bundle to Purkinje fibers

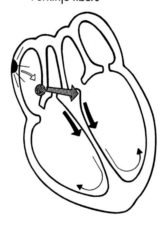

NOTE: Rhythm that is regular, greater than 150 beats/min, and associated with narrow QRS complex is considered supraventricular tachycardia. A part of the atria or AV junction, is serving as the pacemaker for the heart. Called paroxysmal supraventricular tachycardia when it begins and ends abruptly.

Significance: In elderly individuals and those with heart disease, rapid heart rates may precipitate myocardial ischemia, infarction, or pulmonary edema. May also be caused by digoxin overdose.

Intervention: Treatment should be initiated promptly when the patient has chest pain, hypotension, pulmonary edema, or signs of AMI. Determine whether the rhythm is paroxysmal supraventricular tachycardia or ventricular tachycardia. Vagal maneuvers, verapamil, adenosine, digoxin, overdrive pacing, and synchronized cardioversion are used to treat this rhythm.

Wandering atrial pacemaker

Rate	Usually 60 to 100 beats/min
Rhythm	Irregular
P waves	Present; configuration varies
QRS complex	Present; normal duration
P/QRS relationship	P wave preceding each QRS
PR interval	Normal, although may vary from beat to beat

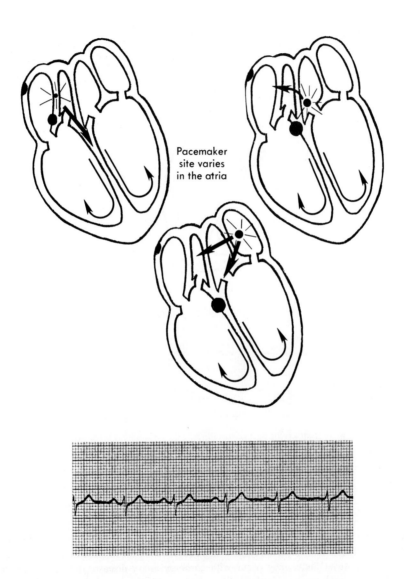

Pacemaker
site varies
in the atria

Significance: SA node is suppressed or other atrial foci become excited and take over pacemaker function of the heart. This dysrhythmia may be caused by specific drugs, inflammation, or chronic obstructive pulmonary disease.

Intervention: Treatment is usually unnecessary. Consider withholding digoxin until serum level confirmed. When necessary, treat the underlying cause.

Atrial flutter

Rate	Atrial rate of 240 to 360 beats/min
Rhythm	Regular or irregular
P waves	Saw-toothed pattern (F waves, or flutter waves)
QRS complex	Present; normal duration
P/QRS relationship	Ventricular response varies; because of rapid atrial rate, there may be regular or irregular ventricular response
PR interval	Not measurable

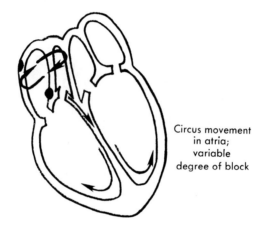

Circus movement
in atria;
variable
degree of block

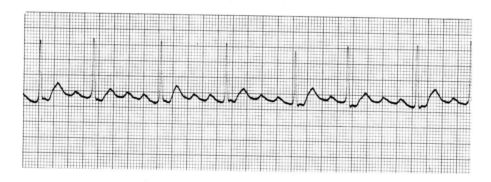

Significance: Irritable focus in the atria is responsible for this dysrhythmia. Usually a 2:1 AV block with ventricular rate approximately 150 beats/min. Ventricular response may be regular or irregular. New-onset atrial flutter is a dangerous dysrhythmia because ineffective atrial contractions may cause mural clots to form in the atria, which subsequently break loose and form pulmonary or cerebral emboli. Atrial flutter may occur with coronary artery disease, rheumatic heart disease, chronic obstructive pulmonary disease, shock, anoxia, electrolyte imbalance, hyperthyroidism, and in response to various drugs.

Intervention: Ventricular rate may be slowed with digitalis, verapamil, adenosine, diltiazem, or β-blocking agents. If pharmacologic therapy is unsuccessful, synchronized cardioversion is indicated. Verapamil and β-blockers may exacerbate bradycardia, congestive heart failure, or both.

Atrial fibrillation

Rate	Atrial rate 350 to 600 beats/min; ventricular rate 60 to 160 beats/min
Rhythm	Irregularly irregular
P waves	No P waves; F waves (fibrillatory) appear
QRS complex	Irregular rhythm; normal duration
P/QRS relationship	Indistinguishable P waves; irregular ventricular response
PR interval	Indistinguishable

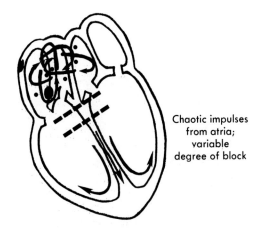

Chaotic impulses from atria; variable degree of block

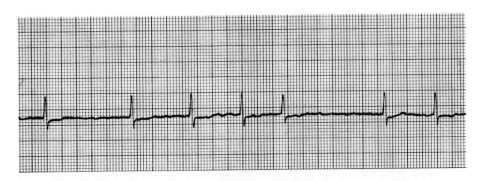

Significance: Multiple atrial pacemakers fire chaotically in rapid succession. Atria never firmly contract. Ventricles respond irregularly. Poor atrial emptying causes danger of mural clot formation and embolism. Cardiac output drops because there is no "atrial kick" (15% to 20% decrease in cardiac output). Patients who have chronic atrial fibrillation controlled with digitalis whose ventricular rate is less than 100 beats/min do not need treatment. Dysrhythmia frequently occurs in coronary artery disease, rheumatic heart disease, hyperthyroidism, and, most commonly, digitalis toxicity.

Intervention: Cardioversion is recommended for patients with ischemic heart disease. For asymptomatic patients, heart rate may be controlled with digitalis, calcium channel–blockers, or β-adrenergic blockers. Use of the latter two drugs in the undigitalized patient may not be effective and may cause congestive heart failure.

Dysrhythmias originating in the AV node
Nodal (junctional) rhythm

Rate	Usually 40 to 60 beats/min
Rhythm	Regular
P waves	May appear inverted before or after the QRS complex, or may be absent
QRS complex	Regular; normal duration
P/QRS relationship	Variable
PR interval	<0.12 second when the P wave precedes the QRS complex

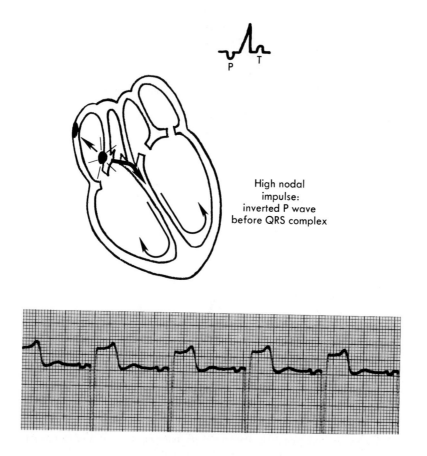

High nodal
impulse:
inverted P wave
before QRS complex

Significance: AV junction has assumed pacing function for the heart. There is retrograde depolarization of the atrium, which may or may not result in detectable P waves.

Intervention: If the patient has been receiving digitalis therapy, withhold digitalis and obtain serum digoxin level to check for toxicity. There is no specific therapy for this dysrhythmia. If the patient becomes symptomatic from decreased heart rate, atropine may be administered. If no response to the atropine, pacing is indicated.

Nodal (junctional) rhythm—cont'd

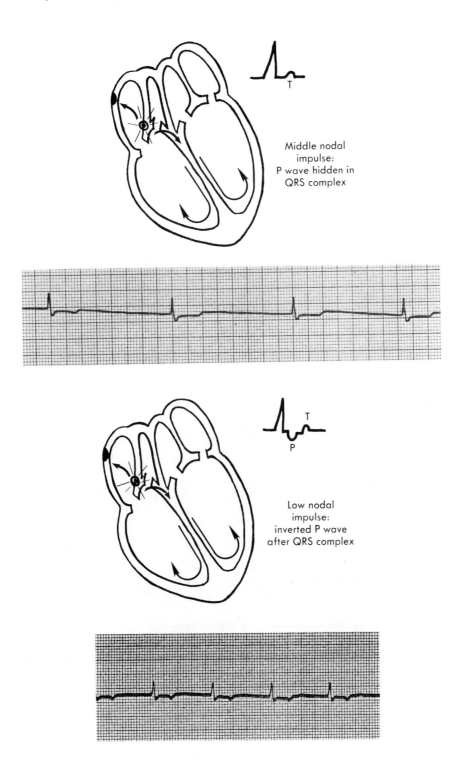

Middle nodal
impulse:
P wave hidden in
QRS complex

Low nodal
impulse:
inverted P wave
after QRS complex

Premature nodal contractions and premature junctional contractions

Rate	Usually normal or bradycardic
Rhythm	Irregularly irregular
P waves	May appear inverted or may be absent
QRS complexes	Regular; normal duration
P/QRS relationship	P waves may appear inverted, may be absent, and may occur before, during, and after the QRS complex
PR interval	<0.12 second when the P wave is seen in a premature beat

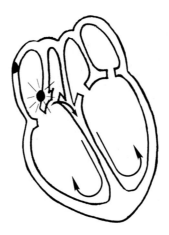

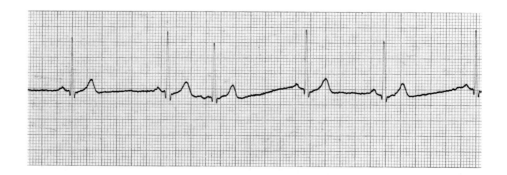

NOTE: See the description of premature atrial contractions.

Significance: AV junction serves episodically as pacemaker for the heart. Dysrhythmia is seen less frequently than premature atrial contractions or PVCs; may precede first-, second-, or third-degree heart block.

Intervention: Premature nodal contractions and premature junctional contractions are usually benign. If therapy is indicated, treatment is similar to that for premature atrial contractions.

Nodal tachycardia (junctional tachycardia)

Rate	100 to 800 beats/min
Rhythm	Regular
P waves	May appear inverted or may be absent
QRS complex	Regular; normal duration
P/QRS relationship	P waves may appear inverted before or after the QRS complex or may be absent
PR interval	<0.12 second when the P wave is present

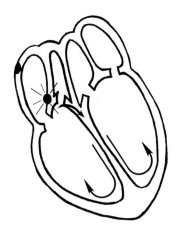

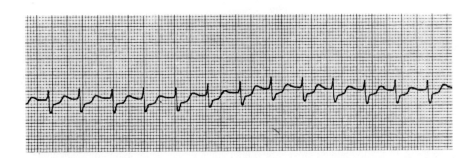

NOTE: Accelerated junctional rhythm is a junctional rhythm with increased sympathetic stimulation. Rate is 60 to 100 beats/min.

Significance: An irritable focus takes over as the heart's pacemaker. Nodal tachycardia may be caused by heart disease, electrolyte imbalance, chronic obstructive pulmonary disease, anoxia, or specific drugs.

Intervention: Dysrhythmia generally considered a variant of supraventricular tachycardia and is treated accordingly. In cases of nonparoxysmal episodes caused by digitalis intoxication, digitalis should be withheld and serum level checked. Serum potassium level should also be obtained.

First-degree AV block

Rate	Usually 60 to 100 beats/min
Rhythm	Usually regular
P waves	Present; normal configuration
QRS complex	Regular; normal duration
P/QRS relationship	P wave precedes each QRS complex
PR interval	>0.20 second

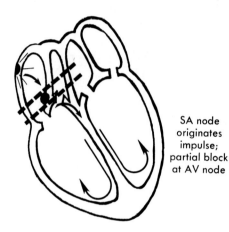

SA node
originates
impulse;
partial block
at AV node

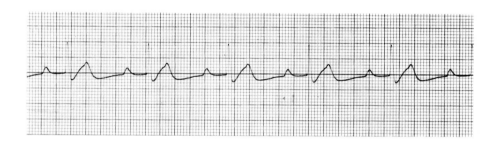

Significance: Conduction of impulse generated by the SA node is delayed through the atrioventricular node. Causes are varied and include anoxia, ischemia, atrioventricular node malfunction, edema after open-heart surgery, digitalis toxicity, myocarditis, thyrotoxicosis, rheumatic fever, clonidine, and tricyclic antidepressants.

Intervention: Usually no treatment is required. Observe the patient, noting level of consciousness and vital signs. If the patient becomes symptomatic (rarely), atropine is the drug of choice. If the patient is on a regimen of digitalis, withhold it and obtain serum digitalis and potassium levels.

Second-degree AV block (Mobitz I, Wenckebach)

Rate	Usually normal
Rhythm	Regularly irregular
P waves	One P wave preceding each QRS complex, except during regular dropped ventricular conduction at periodic intervals
QRS complex	Cyclic missed conduction; when QRS complex is present, duration normal
P/QRS relationship	P wave before each QRS complex, except during regular dropped ventricular conduction at periodic intervals
PR interval	Lengthens with each cycle until one QRS complex is dropped, then cycle is repeated

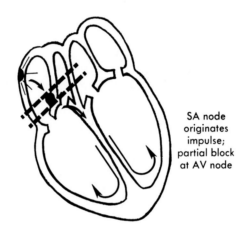

SA node
originates
impulse;
partial block
at AV node

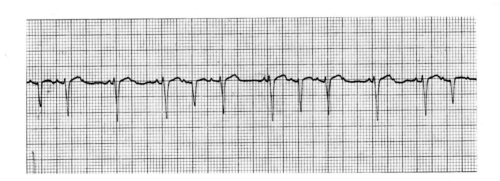

Significance: Each atrial impulse takes progressively longer to travel through the AV node until a beat is dropped, then the cycle begins again. Dysrhythmia is the less serious form of second-degree heart block; usually transient and reversible. In rare instances, dysrhythmia may progress to complete heart block. Commonly occurs after inferior wall infarct.

Intervention: Treatment needed when heart rate is <50 beats/min or if the patient becomes symptomatic. Therapy includes atropine, and temporary pacing.

Second-degree AV block (Mobitz II)

Rate	Atrial rate usually 60 to 100 beats/min; ventricular rate slower
Rhythm	Usually regularly irregular
P waves	Two or more P waves for every QRS complex; normal configuration; regular interval
QRS complex	Normal duration, when present
P/QRS relationship	One or more nonconducted impulses appearing as P waves not followed by QRS complexes
PR interval	Normal or delayed on the conducted beat but regular throughout the dysrhythmia

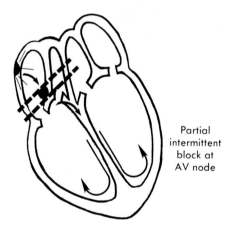

Partial
intermittent
block at
AV node

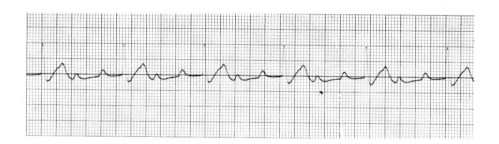

Significance: One or more atrial impulses are not conducted through the AV node to the ventricles. May occur in anterior myocardial infarction and progress rapidly to complete heart block. Other causes are anoxia, digitalis toxicity, and hyperkalemia.

Intervention: If the patient is asymptomatic, immediate treatment is not required. As with other heart block, atropine, and pacing measures are used. If the patient is taking digitalis, withhold medication and obtain serum level.

Third-degree AV block (complete heart block)

Rate	Atrial rate 60 to 100 beats/min; ventricular rate usually <60 beats/min
Rhythm	Usually normal for atria and ventricles when examined separately
P waves	Occur regularly
QRS complex	Slow; usually wide (>0.10 second)
P/QRS relationship	Completely independent of each other
PR interval	No PR interval because there is no consistent relationship between P wave and QRS complex

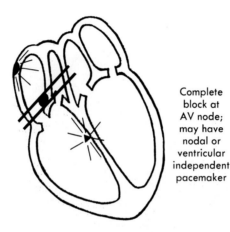

Complete block at AV node; may have nodal or ventricular independent pacemaker

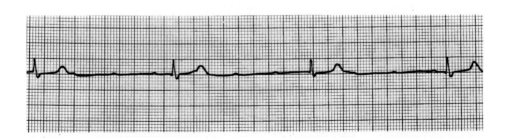

Significance: No SA impulses conducted through AV node. AV node or ventricle initiates impulse; the atria and ventricles beat independently. Bradycardia reduces myocardial perfusion and may lead to ventricular tachycardia or ventricular fibrillation.

Intervention: Pacemaker insertion is required. Transcutaneous pacing may be used until a transvenous pacer can be inserted. Atropine may be used until the pacing unit is available. Be prepared to perform CPR and advanced life support. Do not give lidocaine to a patient with complete heart block, even when wide, bizarre QRS complexes are present.

Dysrhythmias originating in the ventricles

Premature ventricular contractions (premature ectopic beats, extrasystoles, premature ventricular beats, ventricular premature beats)

Rate	Usually 60 to 100 beats/min
Rhythm	Irregular
P waves	Present with each sinus beat; do not precede premature ventricular contractions (PVCs)
QRS complex	Sinus-initiated QRS complex normal; QRS complex of PVC wide and bizarre: >0.10 second; full compensatory pause
P/QRS relationship	P wave before each QRS complex in normal sinus beats; no P wave preceding PVC; compensatory pause following PVC
PR interval	Normal in sinus beat; none in PVC

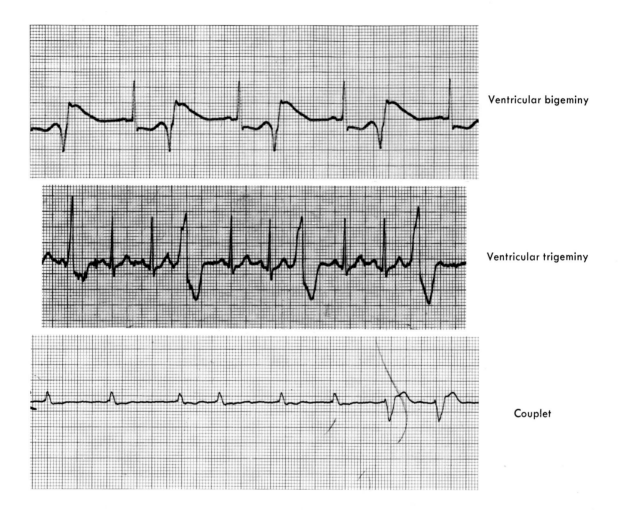

Ventricular bigeminy

Ventricular trigeminy

Couplet

Significance: PVCs indicate ventricular irritability. Impulse is initiated by ventricular pacemaker cell. PVCs may occur as a result of hypoxia, hypovolemia, ischemia, infarction, hypocalcemia, hyperkalemia, acidosis, or from alcohol, tobacco, coffee, or other stimulants. PVCs may originate from the same focus (unifocal) or from various foci (multifocal). Multifocal PVCs have various morphologies. PVCs may occur in repetitious patterns, every other beat (bigeminy), every third beat (trigeminy), in pairs (couplet), three contractions together (triplet). Four or more consecutive PVCs is referred to as a short run of ventricular tachycardia.

Intervention: Administer oxygen. If possible, treat the underlying cause. If treating the cause is not possible, pharmacologic therapy is indicated. First try lidocaine as a bolus. If this treatment is not successful, procainamide and bretylium may be used. After ectopy is resolved, IV drip of effective antidysrhythmic drug should be instituted. When the PVCs are related to a slow heart rate, atropine is the drug of choice.

Ventricular tachycardia

Rate	150 to 250 beats/min
Rhythm	May be slightly irregular
P waves	Not seen
QRS complex	Wide and bizarre; width is >0.12 second
P/QRS relationship	None
PR interval	None

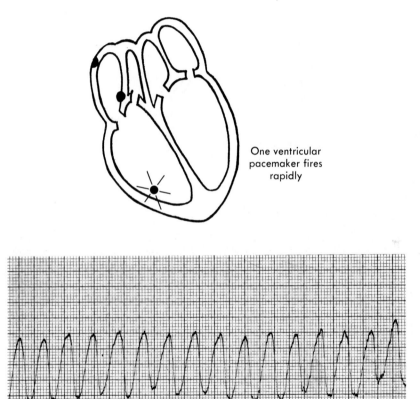

One ventricular
pacemaker fires
rapidly

Significance: Rhythm cannot be tolerated for long periods because cardiac output is significantly reduced. If the rhythm persists, will deteriorate into ventricular fibrillation and asystole.

Intervention: Pulseless ventricular tachycardia should be treated as ventricular fibrillation. If a pulse is present and the patient is stable, give an antidysrhythmic agent (lidocaine, procainamide, or bretylium). If the patient becomes unstable, cardioversion is the treatment of choice. Be prepared to begin CPR and initiate advanced life support measures.

Ventricular fibrillation

Rate	Rapid, disorganized
Rhythm	Irregular
P waves	Not seen
QRS complex	Absent; fibrillatory waves of varying size, shape, and duration occur
P/QRS relationship	None
PR interval	None

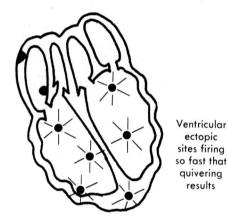

Ventricular ectopic sites firing so fast that quivering results

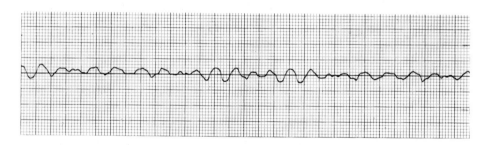

Significance: Dysrhythmia is the most common cause of sudden cardiac death. Ventricular fibrillation produces no cardiac output; cerebral death results when dysrhythmia persists more than 4 to 6 minutes. Ventricular fibrillation may be preceded by ventricular tachycardia.

Intervention: Begin CPR until a defibrillator is available. Check the rhythm, differentiating between asystole and fine ventricular fibrillation. Defibrillate, start with 200 J, continue with 200 to 300 J, and increase as high as 360 J if no response. If no pulse is present, continue CPR while establishing IV access, intubating the patient, or both. Next, administer epinephrine, defibrillate up to 360 J, administer lidocaine, defibrillate at 360 J, administer bretylium, and defibrillate again. At this stage, administration of antidysrhythmics is alternated with countershocks. Remember to check pulse and rhythm between each countershock. If ventricular fibrillation reoccurs after conversion, begin defibrillation at whatever energy level was previously successful.

Idioventricular rhythm

Rate	Usually <40 beats/min
Rhythm	Regular or irregular
P waves	None
QRS complex	Wide and bizarre (>0.10 second)
P/QRS relationship	None
PR interval	None

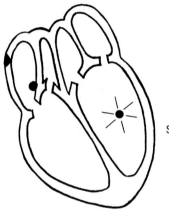

Slow impulses
from ectopic
site in
ventricle

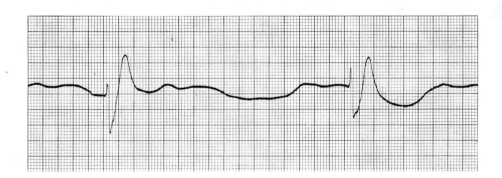

Significance: Rhythm is escape rhythm of ventricular origin. Effective cardiac contractions and pulses may or may not be present. May be caused by complete heart block, AMI, cardiac tamponade, or exsanguinating hemorrhage. Outcome is usually poor.

Intervention: Administer atropine; consider pacing. Treat the underlying cause.

Pulseless Electrical Activity (PEA)

Rate	Varies
Rhythm	No characteristic pattern
P waves	None
QRS complex	Relatively normal or wide and bizarre
P/QRS relationship	None
PR interval	None

NOTE: By definition a patient is having pulseless electrical activity (PEA) when current rhythm should be perfusing but the patient has no pulse. Idioventricular rhythm at rate of 20 beats/min without a pulse is *not* PEA, but normal sinus rhythm at 72 beats/min in a patient who is unconscious, pulseless, and apneic is PEA.

Significance: Electrical complexes are present without mechanical contraction of the heart. The most common causes of this dysrhythmia are hypoxemia, hypovolemia, tension pneumothorax, acidosis, cardiac tamponade, and pulmonary embolism.

Intervention: Perform CPR and treat the underlying cause. Intubate, establish IV access, and give epinephrine every 3 to 5 minutes. If the electrical rate is less than 60 beats/min, atropine is given.

Asystole (ventricular standstill)

Rate	None
Rhythm	None
P waves	May or may not appear
QRS complex	Absent or rare with bizarre configuration
P/QRS relationship	None
PR interval	None

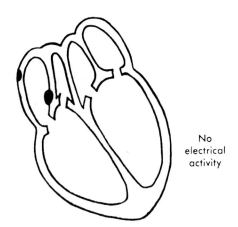

No
electrical
activity

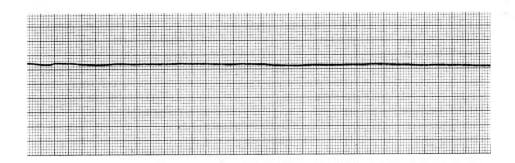

Significance: Mortality greater than 95%. Asystole often implies the patient's heart has been in arrest for a prolonged period. Confirm presence of asystole in two limb leads.

Intervention: Begin CPR. Differentiate between asystole and ventricular fibrillation. Intubate and establish IV access. Administer epinephrine; repeat every 3 to 5 minutes as needed. Next, give atropine (repeat once in 3 to 5 minutes) and use external pacemaker.

Pacemakers. Temporary pacing is used when a patient's condition deteriorates secondary to a bradycardic or tachycardic dysrhythmia unresponsive to other therapy. Indications for pacing include severe bradycardia, high-degree AV blocks, atrial tachycardia, atrial flutter, and recurrent ventricular tachycardia.

Three methods can be used for pacing, transthoracic, transvenous, and external (transcutaneous) methods. The transthoracic approach is not used in the ED because of associated risks, time required to complete the procedure, and interference with chest compressions. The transvenous method involves inserting a catheter electrode percutaneously into the right atrium or ventricle via the subclavian, internal jugular, brachial, or femoral vein. The procedure is guided by the changes in the ECG and/or fluoroscopy. Atrial pacing is used to suppress atrial tachycardia; ventricular pacing is used to suppress ventricular ectopy by overdrive pacing.

Transcutaneous or external pacing is used more often in the ED. A negative electrode is placed posteriorly at midthoracic level of the spine with a positive electrode placed anteriorly at chest lead V_3 position. This position provides a lower pacing threshold and is away from large skeletal muscles, thus decreasing muscle stimulation. Electrode placement should not interfere with defibrillation. The rate of pacing impulses may be "fixed" (asynchronous, competitive, or nondemand) or set to fire on demand. A fixed rate delivers electrical current at regular intervals and is usually used when patients have bradycardia causing hemodynamic instability, for example, complete heart block. The demand pacing mode senses the patient's own QRS complexes and generates an impulse only if the patient does not have an intrinsic QRS generated during a set time frame. Fixed-rate pacing is rarely used because of potential competition with the patient's own rhythm and/or ventricular fibrillation if the pacer discharges on the T wave (i.e., relative refractory period) of the patient's own cardiac cycle.

Successful pacing depends on the condition of the myocardium. Patients with severe bradycardia, heart block, or idioventricular rhythm who can generate a pulse with each QRS complex usually respond to cardiac pacing and have a better outcome. Patients in asystole are less likely to respond to pacing.

Factors that indicate successful pacemaker capture, that is, successful electrical stimulation followed by mechanical response, include combined pacing spike and QRS complex 0.14 seconds in duration and resolution of the dysrhythmia being treated. Mechanical capture occurs when the heart responds to pacing with effective contractions. Mechanical capture is evaluated by the presence of a pulse consistent with paced beats. Both types of capture must be present for effective pacing. Assess the patient's hemodynamic and neurologic response by palpating the carotid or femoral pulse, obtaining vital signs, and evaluating the level of consciousness.

Two major reasons for lack of capture are acidosis and hypoxemia. Evaluate the patient's oxygen saturation and acid-base levels to determine appropriate interventions for such disorders. Another reason for lack of capture is related to the external pacing device and pacing electrodes. Check all connections. Consider repositioning the posterior electrode to the fifth intercostal space, midaxillary line (i.e., V_6 chest lead position). Replace dry pacing electrodes. Make sure contact between external pacing electrodes and skin surface is adequate. Skin should be clean and dry before electrode application; benzoin may be used to improve adherence to the skin.

Implanted cardioverter defibrillator (ICD) therapy. The ICD is a device that may be used as a treatment modality to reduce the incidence of sudden death from AMI. Approved in 1985, ICD monitors the patient's cardiac rhythm and provides pacing and/or defibrillation to the patient depending on programming.[12,15] Newer models can deliver multiple or tiered therapies, antitachycardia pacing (i.e., fast pacing), single-chamber ventricular demand pacing for bradycardia (i.e., slow pacing), cardioversion, or defibrillation shocks.

ICD generators are implanted under skin and subcutaneous tissue. Depending on the type of ICD device, the ICD generator may be implanted in the abdomen or upper chest. Older ICD devices require a surgical approach for applying electrodes to the epicardial surface of the heart. Newer devices allow subcutaneous or submuscular insertion of the ICD patch along the left anterior axillary line, left midaxillary area, or left posterior area. The lead is then tunneled along the left anterior chest wall and connected to the ICD generator.

If the patient requires defibrillation, external defibrillation may still be performed. Defibrillator paddles should not be placed over the ICD generator. If defibrillation attempts are unsuccessful, consider anterior-posterior placement of paddles to improve conduction of electrical current around the ICD electrodes on the chest wall. Anyone in physical contact with the patient when the ICD device fires may experience a harmless, slight tingling sensation. If the ICD device is firing inappropriately, the physician may deactivate the device by placing a magnet over the ICD generator.

Congestive Heart Failure

Congestive heart failure (CHF) occurs when the heart fails to function adequately as a pump. This inadequacy results in venous congestion, decreased stroke volume, decreased cardiac output, and increased peripheral systemic pressure. Onset may be gradual or sudden. The primary precipitating event of heart failure is some type of myocardial damage that activates many compensatory mechanisms.[14] Over time, compensatory mechanisms are exhausted and cause adverse events. Heart failure rarely occurs at the same time as the AMI. Development is generally more insidious, over a period of time. Congestive heart failure may be seen alone or in conjunction with pulmonary edema. The onset of congestive heart failure is a symptom of an underlying problem such as

AMI, hypertension, fluid overload, intracranial injury, valvular heart disease, dysrhythmias, cardiomyopathy, hyperthyroidism, fever, and adult respiratory distress syndrome. CHF may also occur with oxygen toxicity syndrome, pneumothorax, uremic pneumonia, intracranial tumors, and drugs such as methotrexate, busulfan, hexamethonium, and nitrofurantoin.

Congestive heart failure is characterized by severe dyspnea, orthopnea, fatigue, weakness, abdominal discomfort secondary to ascites or hepatic engorgement, dependent edema, distended neck veins, bilateral rales, third heart sound (gallop), laterally displaced apical pulse, and hepatomegaly.[17] Assess patient and ensure adequate airway, breathing, and circulation, then check vital signs, monitor ECG rhythm, and oxygenation, auscultate lungs and heart, and observe for distended neck veins and peripheral edema.

Therapeutic interventions include maintaining the patient on bed rest in high Fowler's position; administering oxygen, digitalis and diuretics; maintaining an IV line at keep-open rate or use of a saline or heparin lock; monitoring intake and output; and weighing the patient daily. Additional therapy may include vasodilators to dilate arteries, decrease systemic vascular resistance (SVR), and increase cardiac output.

Acute Pericarditis

Acute pericarditis is inflammation of the pericardial sac caused by AMI, trauma, infection, or neoplasms. Among younger patients, infectious processes such as coxsackievirus, streptococci, staphylococci, tuberculosis, and *Haemophilus influenzae* can cause pericarditis. Early pericardial friction rub may occur with pericarditis in conjunction with AMI.[39] Friction rub occurs when an inflamed area over a transmural infarction causes the pericardial surface to lose its lubricating fluid. Pericarditis is most evident 2 to 3 days after an AMI.

Patients with pericarditis have severe chest pain that increases during inspiration and increased activity, fever, chills, and dyspnea. Tachycardia or other dysrhythmias may also be present. Pericardial friction rub increases in intensity when the patient leans forward. The patient has general malaise with ST segment elevations 1 to 3 mm in all ECG leads except aV_R and V_1. Therapeutic intervention includes oxygen by nasal cannula 4 to 6 L/min, sedation, analgesia, and bed rest. Antiinflammatory agents and steroids may also be indicated.

Aortic Aneurysm

An aneurysm is "irreversible dilatation of an artery secondary to a localized weakness of the arterial wall that may predispose the artery to thrombosis, distal embolization, or rupture."[10] Aneurysms can occur anywhere along the aorta; however, 80% occur in the abdominal aorta rather than the thoracic aorta.[21] Abdominal aortic aneurysms (AAA) are more common in people from 50 to 70 years of age. One postmortem study suggested 5% of men 65 to 74 years of age had AAA.

The primary etiology of AAA is atherosclerosis and related factors, that is, hyperlipidemia, smoking, diabetes, and hereditary factors. Other causes include arteritis, congenital abnormalities, trauma, infections, and syphilis. The atherosclerotic process contributes to weakening and eventual destruction of the medial wall of the artery. Over time hemodynamic forces of blood flow cause thickening of the wall and replacement of muscle fibers with fibrous tissue and calcium deposits. AAA enlarges over time and the wall tension of the aneurysm increases. Dilation of the aneurysm allows the development of a thrombus, which may be dislodged and cause thromboembolism distally in the patient's circulation, for example, lower extremities.

Three types of aneurysms are fusiform, saccular, and dissecting. Fusiform aneurysms are characterized by a segment of artery dilated around the entire circumference of the artery, whereas a saccular aneurysm dilates only a portion of the artery. A dissecting aneurysm actually results in a tear of the artery's intimal layer, which allows blood to flow between the intimal and medial layers (Figure 35-19). Dissecting aneurysms are further classified by the extent of the tear and location. Type I dissection occurs in the ascending aorta and extends beyond the aortic arch. Type 2 dissection occurs only in the ascending aorta. Type 3 dissection begins distal to the left subclavian artery.

As the aorta dissects, major vessels that branch off the aorta may be occluded. Occluded vessels include myocardial, cerebral, mesenteric, and renal vessels. Rupture of the dissection may cause pericardial tamponade or hemorrhage into the thoracic cavity, resulting in exsanguination, shock, and imminent death.

Patient assessment. Fifty percent of patients with AAA are asymptomatic. AAA may be discovered on physical exam suggested by widened midline pulsation proximal to the umbilicus. Patients who present to the ED with a leaking and/or rupturing AAA have a classic presentation characterized by

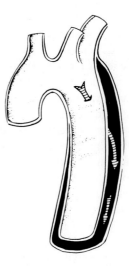

Figure **35-19** Dissecting aortic aneurysm.

extreme back pain accompanied by abdominal pain and tenderness with palpation.[21] Back pain may radiate to legs, groin, or lower back secondary to stretching of the anterior spinal ligament. Patients may also complain of excruciating substernal chest pain felt through to the posterior cavity. Rupture of the aneurysm compromises hemodynamic stability and blood flow distal to the aneurysm. Signs and symptoms include dyspnea, orthopnea, diaphoresis, pallor, apprehension, syncope, tachycardia, unilateral absence of major pulses, bilateral blood pressure differences, hypertension, pulsation at the sternoclavicular joint, murmur of aortic insufficiency, (i.e., in ascending aortic aneurysm), hemiplegia or paraplegia, and shock.

Patient management. The most common diagnostic test for AAA is the chest radiograph. Patients must be in an upright position to validate the widened mediastinum. Extremely large aneurysms may appear as soft masses, displace other organs, or cause abnormal gas patterns. Other diagnostic tests that may be used if the patient is hemodynamically stable include ultrasound and CT scan.

Therapeutic intervention includes placing the patient in a high Fowler's position, administering high-flow oxygen, and initiating two large-bore IV catheters with Ringer's lactate. Maintaining blood pressure control is critical. If hypertension is present such drugs as nitroprusside are used to decrease blood pressure. If patient has hypovolemic shock, intervention focuses on maintaining ABCs, fluid resuscitation, and preparing for emergency surgery.

Hypertensive Crisis

Hypertension can be defined as a systolic blood pressure of >140 mm Hg and/or diastolic pressure >90 mm Hg. When blood pressure becomes abruptly elevated to extreme levels, the patient has a life-threatening situation. An estimated 50 million Americans have hypertension. The actual incidence of hypertensive crisis is relatively rare, approximately 1% of the hypertensive population.

Hypertensive crisis is categorized by the degree of acute target end organ damage and the rapidity with which the blood pressure must be lowered.[44] Hypertensive crisis has been further categorized into hypertensive emergencies and hypertensive urgencies. Hypertensive emergencies are those clinical situations in which excessively high blood pressure must be lowered quickly, within minutes to hours, to prevent new or worsening organ damage. Hypertensive urgencies develop over days to weeks and generally demonstrate an elevated diastolic blood pressure without signs of end organ damage. Determination of end organ damage is made by clinical presentation.

Regardless of underlying mechanism of hypertension, elevated blood pressure increases systemic or peripheral vascular resistance and cardiac output. Increases perpetuate the cycle by stimulating release of catecholamines, which increases α-sympathetic activity and activates the reninangiotensin system. The net result is continued increases in blood pressure. Hypertensive crisis usually occurs in patients with a history of hypertension.[23] Other conditions that may cause or precipitate hypertensive crisis include cocaine, other sympathomimetic drugs such as amphetamines, phencyclidine, lysergic acid diethylamide (LSD), diet pills, and food-drug interactions such as MAO and tyramine interaction.

Patient assessment. Patients with hypertensive crisis usually have DBP of 120 mm Hg.[46] Primary symptoms are consistent with new or evolving end organ damage. Increase in the systemic-peripheral vascular resistance and sympathetic stimulation imposed by the significant hypertension increase the myocardial workload and myocardial oxygen consumption. Symptoms associated with cardiovascular manifestations include congestive heart failure, chest pain, angina, and AMI. Neurologic changes include headache, nausea, vomiting, dizziness, visual disturbances (e.g., blurred vision, temporary visual loss, decreased visual acuity, and photophobia), altered mental states (e.g., agitation, confusion, lethargy, coma), and seizures. Other neurologic symptoms include focal cranial nerve palsy, sensory deficits, motor deficits, aphasia, and hemiparesis.

Patient management. In addition to cardiac and vital sign monitoring, IV access should be established. An arterial line provides the most accurate blood pressure readings; however, a noninvasive blood pressure device can also be used for continuous BP monitoring. The goal of management is to lower SBP to 100 to 110 mm Hg.[23] Intravenous pharmacologic agents such as nitroprusside, labetalol, and propranolol are used so they can be titrated for safe, effective reduction of SBP. Assess the patient's response to these agents, that is, are the patient's presenting symptoms improved? Are there new symptoms?

SUMMARY

Cardiovascular attacks are frequent but challenging aspects of emergency nursing. Box 35-5 lists just a few nursing

Box **35-5**

NURSING DIAGNOSES FOR CARDIOVASCULAR EMERGENCIES

Altered tissue perfusion
Fluid volume excess
Fluid volume deficit
Decreased cardiac output
Impaired gas exchange
Ineffective breathing pattern
Inability to sustain spontaneous ventilation
Ineffective individual coping
Pain
Anxiety
Fear

diagnoses pertinent for patients with cardiovascular emergencies. Recent changes in management of these patients include new drugs, new doses for old drugs, and new diagnostic modalities. The emergency nurse is challenged to maintain an effective knowledge as new technologies emerge.

REFERENCES

1. Adams JE, Bodor GS, Davila-Roman VG et al: Cardiac troponin I: a marker with high specificity for cardiac injury, *Circulation* 88:101, 1993.
2. Albrich JM: Acute myocardial infarction: comprehensive guidelines for diagnosis, stabilization, and mortality reduction, *Emerg Med Rep* 15(6):51, 1994.
3. American College of Cardiology, American Heart Association Task Force: ACC/AHA guidelines for the early management of patients with acute myocardial infarction, *J Am Coll Cardiol* 16:249, 1990.
4. American Heart Association: *Advanced cardiac life support,* Dallas, 1987, The Association.
5. American Heart Association: *Basic cardiopulmonary life support,* Dallas 1988, The Association.
6. American Heart Association: *Heart facts,* Dallas, 1994, The Association.
7. Aragon D: Cardiac monitoring: follow these leads, *AJN* 94(12):56A, 1994.
8. Blank FSJ, Austin M, Bennett A et al: Decreasing "door to thrombolysis" time at one busy acute care hospital, *JEN* 21(3):202, 1995.
9. Burns D: Review of thrombolytic use in acute myocardial infarction, pulmonary embolism, and cerebral thrombosis, *Crit Care Nurs Q* 15(4):1, 1995.
10. Clochesy JM, Breu C, Cardin S et al: *Critical care nursing,* ed 2, Philadelphia, 1996, WB Saunders.
11. Colletti RC: Diagnosis of acute myocardial infarction in the emergency department, part 2, *JEN* 16(3):187, 1990.
12. Collins MA: When your patient has an implantable cardioverter defibrillator, *AJN* 94(3):34, 1994.
13. Cunningham CA: ICD and AED defibrillation, *Emerg* 18:23, 1995.
14. Cuny J, Enger EL: Medical management of chronic heart failure: direct-acting vasodilators and diuretic agents, *Crit Care Nurs Clin North Am* 5(4):575, 1992.
15. Davidson T, VanRiper S, Harper P et al: Implantable cardioverter defibrillators: a guide for clinicians, *Heart Lung* 23(3):205, 1994.
16. Dewood MA, Spores J, Notske R et al: Prevalence of total coronary occlusion during the early hours of transmural myocardial infarction, *N Engl J Med* 303:897, 1980.
17. Dracup K, Dunbar SB, Baker DW: Rethinking heart failure, *AJN* 95(7):23, 1995.
18. Drew BJ: Bedside electrocardiographic monitoring, *Heart Lung* 20(6):610, 1991.
19. Drew BJ, Tisdale LA: ST segment monitoring for coronary artery reocclusion following thrombolytic therapy and coronary angioplasty: identification of optimal bedside monitoring leads, *Am J Crit Care* 2(4):280, 1993.
20. Emergency Cardiac Care Committee and Subcommittees: American Heart Association guidelines for cardiopulmonary resuscitation and emergency cardiac care, *JAMA* 268(16):2172, 1992.
21. Fellows E: Abdominal aortic aneurysm: warning flags to watch for, *AJN* 95(5):27, 1995.
22. Foley JJ: Significant changes in advanced cardiac life support medication guidelines, *JEN* 19(6):516, 1993.
23. Foley JJ: Pharmacologic management of hypertensive crisis in the emergency department, *JEN* 20(2):134, 1994.
24. Futterman LG, Lemberg L: Angina, linked angina, chest pain: an enigma within a dilemma, *Am J Crit Care* 4(4):325, 1995.
25. Gibler WB, Lewis LM, Erb RE et al: Early detection of acute myocardial infarction for the early management of patients with acute myocardial infarction, *J Am Coll Cardiol* 16:249, 1990.
26. Grillo JA, Gonzalez ER: Changes in the pharmacotherapy of CPR, *Heart Lung* 22(6):548, 1993.
27. Gunby P: Cardiovascular disease remains nation's leading cause of death, *JAMA* 267:335, 1991.
28. Habib GB: Current status of thrombolysis in acute myocardial infarction: optimal selection and delivery of a thrombolytic drug, *Chest* 107:225, 1995.
29. Hazinski MF: Advances and controversies in cardiopulmonary resuscitation in the young, *J Cardiovasc Nurs* 6(3):74, 1992.
30. Iserson KV, Criss E: Intraosseous infusions: a usable technique, *Am J Emerg Med* 4:540, 1986.
31. Kayser SR: Pharmacological management of cardiac arrest: an updated perspective, *Prog Cardiovasc Nurs* 10(3):35, 1995.
32. Keen JH, Baird MS, Allen JH: *Mosby's critical care and emergency drug reference,* ed 2, St. Louis, 1996, Mosby.
33. Kernicki JG: Differentiating chest pain: advanced assessment techniques, *Dimen Crit Care Nurs* 12(2):66, 1993.
34. Lee HS, Cross SJ, Garthwaite P et al: Comparison of the value of novel rapid measurement of myoglobin, creatine kinase, and creatine kinase-MB with the electrocardiogram for the diagnosis of acute myocardial infarction, *Brit Heart J* 71:311, 1994.
35. Lounsbury P, Frye SJ: *Cardiac rhythm disorders: a nursing process approach,* ed 2, St. Louis, 1992, Mosby.
36. Matrisciano L: Unstable angina: an overview, *Crit Care Nurse,* 12(6):30, 1992.
37. Miccolo MA: Intraosseous infusion, *Crit Care Nurse* 10(10):35, 1990.
38. Morton PG: Update on new antiarrhythmic drugs, *Crit Care Nurs Clin North Am* 6(1):69, 1994.
39. Owen PM: *Sudden cardiac death: theory and practice,* Baltimore, 1991, Aspen.
40. Puleo PR, Meyer D, Wathen C et al: Use of rapid assay subforms of creatine kinase MB to diagnose or rule out acute myocardial infarction, *N Engl J Med* 331(9):561, 1994.
41. Rich BSE: Sudden death screening, *Med Clin North Am* 78(2):267, 1994.
42. Rouan GW, Lee TH et al: Clinical characteristics and outcome of acute myocardial infarction in patients with initially normal or non-specific electrocardiograms: a report from the Multicenter Chest Pain Study, *Am J Cardiol* 64(18):1087, 1989.
43. Soud T: Airway, breathing, circulation, and disability: what is different about kids? *JEN* 18(2):107, 1992.
44. Teplitz L: Hypertensive crisis: review and update, *Crit Care Nurse* 13(6):20, 1993.
45. Underhill SL, Woods SL, Froelicher ES et al: *Cardiovascular medications for cardiac nursing,* Philadelphia, 1990, Lippincott.
46. Underhill SL, Woods SL, Sivarajan ES et al: *Cardiac nursing,* ed 2, Philadelphia, 1994, Lippincott.
47. Weiner B: Hemodynamic effects of antidysrhythmic drugs, *J Cardiovas Nurs* 5(4):39, 1991.
48. Weiner B: Thrombolytic agents in critical care, *Crit Care Nurs Clin North Am* 5(2):355, 1993.
49. Woods SL, Sivarajan Froelicher ES, Halpenny CJ et al: *Cardiac nursing,* ed 3, Philadelphia, 1995, Lippincott.

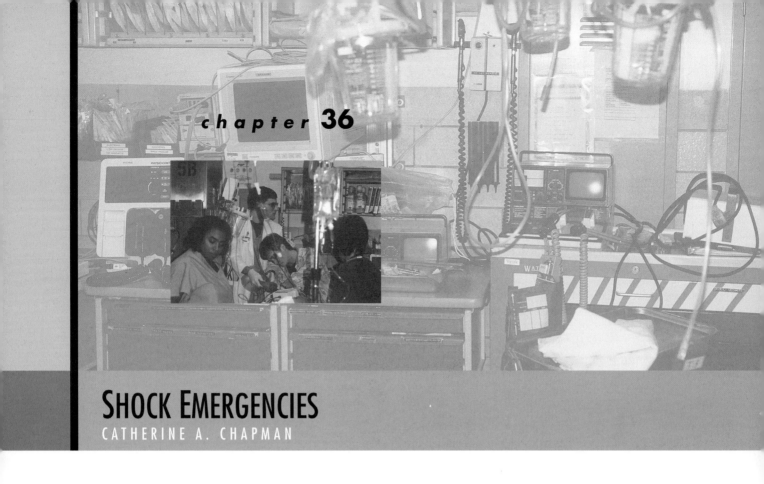

chapter 36

SHOCK EMERGENCIES

CATHERINE A. CHAPMAN

Shock has been superficially described as low blood pressure. The reality is much more complex. Low blood pressure may be the last thing to occur. Identifying the patient in shock requires astute assessment skills based on a strong clinical foundation. Shock is a potentially fatal condition that occurs when cells become hypoxic as a result of decreased perfusion. Clinically, shock is found in patients of all ages, as the result of blood loss, infection, myocardial infarction, and various other conditions that alter cellular perfusion. This chapter reviews the pathophysiology of shock, describes four categories of shock, and discusses patient assessment, evaluation, and treatment for each type of shock.

CATEGORIES OF SHOCK

Normal circulation and cellular perfusion is a product of adequate circulating volume, cardiac output, and peripheral vascular resistance. Changes or damage to any of these components alters cellular perfusion and oxygenation. Shock is categorized by which essential component is affected. Specific categories of shock are hypovolemic shock, cardiogenic shock, distributive shock, and obstructive shock. Box 36-1 lists categories of shock by causative agent.

Hypovolemic shock results from loss or redistribution of blood, plasma, or other body fluids, which ultimately leads to overall reduction in intravascular volume (preload). Hypovolemic shock is primarily an alteration in circulating volume. Volume loss can occur from traumatic injury, gastrointestinal bleeding, ruptured ectopic pregnancy, vaginal

bleeding, posterior nasal bleed, osmotic diuresis associated with diabetic ketoacidosis (DKA), nasogastric suctioning, or excessive vomiting and/or diarrhea. Redistribution of body fluids is most often caused by thermal injuries.

Cardiogenic shock occurs when loss of ventricular effectiveness (contractility) decreases cardiac output. Cardiac pump failure may result from myocardial infarction, myocardial contusion, cardiomyopathies, ruptured papillary muscle, dysrhythmias, or ruptured ventricular septum.

Distributive shock, or vasogenic shock, is caused by overall reduction in systemic vascular resistance (SVR) and vasodilation. Blood volume is normal; however, the circulating blood volume is decreased by massive vasodilation and decreased SVR. Distributive shock is categorized by etiology into neurogenic, septic, and anaphylactic shock.

Obstructive shock occurs when an obstruction decreases circulating volume by preventing the myocardium from mechanically emptying during systole or filling during diastole. Causes include pulmonary embolism, air embolism, tension pneumothorax, pericardial tamponade, intracardiac clot, vena cava obstruction, aortic stenosis, or aortic aneurysm. Obstructive shock decreases cardiac output.

PATHOPHYSIOLOGY

Shock is defined as an alteration in tissue perfusion that occurs at the cellular level. Conditions that result in hypoxia and/or poor cellular perfusion precipitate a complex clinical syndrome known as shock. In the presence of hypoxia and

Box 36-1   Causes of Shock

Hypovolemic shock	Massive external bleeding; hemothorax; hemoperitoneum; fractures; gastrointestinal bleeding; massive vomiting; massive diarrhea; massive diaphoresis; excessive diuretic use; burns; ascites
Cardiogenic shock	Myocardial infarction; cardiomyopathy; cardiac contusion; dysrhythmias; heart valve disease
Distributive shock	Sepsis; anaphylaxis; spinal cord injury; overdose; anoxia
Obstructive shock	Tension pneumothorax; pericardial tamponade; pulmonary embolus; intracardiac clot; vena cava clot; aortic aneurysm; aortic stenosis

Box 36-2   Cellular Effects of Shock

Decreased ATP production
Excess lactic acid production
Mitochondrial death
Cellular edema
Deterioration of the sodium-potassium pump
Hyperkalemia

Box 36-3   Shock Progression

Compensatory shock	Body responses initiated to increase cardiac output, tissue (cellular) and vital organ perfusion
Progressive shock	Body responses become inadequate to maintain perfusion and multisystem failure ensues
Irreversible shock	Pervasive cellular destruction; death is imminent

inadequate tissue perfusion, cells do not receive oxygen and nutrients or remove waste products. Cellular damage or death ensues when cellular oxygen demands exceed the tissue's oxygen supply.

Normal cell metabolism requires an aerobic environment to break down glucose and oxidize substrates. Enzyme-mediated chemical reactions transfer energy from this process into adenosine triphosphate (ATP). Oxidative energy synthesis of ATP is necessary for cell survival and is a fundamental characteristic of life. This process is also referred to as cellular respiration.

Cellular respiration occurs within organelles known as mitochondria, which are located in the cell's cytoplasm. Mitochondria are the site of ATP synthesis and energy production. Lysosomes in the cytoplasm store hydrolytic or digestive enzymes that mediate chemical reactions within the cell.

The production of cellular energy and synthesis of ATP is dependent on a continuous oxygen supply. Availability of oxygen is influenced by blood flow, oxygen saturation, and cardiac output. Oxygen consumption is the amount of oxygen removed by the tissues for metabolism. Oxygen debt refers to the difference between cellular demand for oxygen and cellular consumption of available oxygen. A continuous oxygen debt related to tissue hypoxia creates an anaerobic environment that adversely affects cellular metabolism.

In abnormal cell metabolism, the synthesis of ATP is altered, so pyruvic acid is reduced to lactic acid. Concurrently, the sodium-potassium pump deteriorates, so redistribution of ions and fluid occurs. Sodium and fluid move into the cell, displacing potassium extracellularly, causing hyperkalemia and cellular engorgement. Altered calcium ions within the mitochondria cause constriction of the mitochondria and eventually damage the mitochondrial membrane. Damage to the membrane exacerbates cellular engorgement

and leads to organelle death. Additionally, changes within the cell damage lysosomal membranes, leading to release of enzymes followed by further cell devastation. Lactic acid produced from the initial abnormal cellular metabolism precipitates metabolic acidosis. Box 36-2 summarizes adverse cellular effects of shock.

COMPENSATORY BODY RESPONSES

Regardless of the type of shock, the body mobilizes a series of responses to compensate for the evolving shock state. Compensatory responses are stimulated by decreasing tissue perfusion. Ideally, the outcome of these compensatory mechanisms is restoration of cardiac output and tissue perfusion. To accomplish this, blood is shunted from the kidneys, gastrointestinal tract, liver, and skin to vital organs, that is, the heart, lungs, and brain. Key compensatory responses include the baroreceptors, sympathetic nervous system, fluid shifts, and endocrine system. Without these compensatory mechanisms, shock progresses and ultimately death occurs. Box 36-3 summarizes the progression of the shock state.

Baroreceptors

Baroreceptors are a collection of specialized neural tissues located in the aortic arch and bifurcation of the common carotid arteries. Inhibition of baroreceptors by the vasomotor center of the brain in response to decreasing cardiac output results in sympathetic stimulation followed by peripheral vasoconstriction in an effort to maintain blood pressure.

Sympathetic Nervous System

Stimulation of the sympathetic nervous system by decreases in circulating volume and cardiac output results in release of epinephrine, norepinephrine, and other catecholamines that stimulate α- and β-receptors.

Stimulation of α-receptors is followed by arteriole and venous vasoconstriction. The chronotropic effect is tachycardia. β-Receptor stimulation has a positive inotropic effect, increasing myocardial contractility and improving coronary artery blood flow. The α-β adrenergic effects augment venous return, increasing ventricular filling or preload, heart rate, and myocardial contractility, which facilitates ventricular emptying and improves cardiac output and blood pressure.

Fluid Shifts

Normal distribution of body fluid is 75% intracellular and 25% extracellular. Of the extracellular fluid, one third is located intravascularly; the remainder is interstitial. Hydrostatic pressure and plasma colloid oncotic pressure (COP) are forces that maintain normal fluid distribution between the intravascular and interstitial compartments. Hydrostatic pressure pushes fluid from the arterial end of the capillary bed into the interstitial space. COP pulls fluid into the venous capillary bed because of plasma proteins such as albumin.

Alterations in circulating volume and/or cardiac output that reduce hydrostatic pressure cause less fluid to be distributed interstitially. However, the pressure gradient continues to push fluid into the intravascular space.

Endocrine Response

The endocrine system response to decreased circulating volume or decreased cardiac output is a product of the adrenal glands, the kidneys, the pituitary gland, and the lungs. Components are the renin-angiotensin-aldosterone system and antidiuretic hormone (ADH).

Renin-angiotensin-aldosterone system. Renal hypoperfusion and mediation of β-receptors by the sympathetic nervous system secondary to shock causes release of renin. Renin activates conversion of angiotensinogen to angiotensin I. Angiotensin is then converted by the lungs into angiotensin II, which causes release of aldosterone and produces vasoconstriction. Aldosterone promotes sodium reabsorption within the renal tubule. Water follows reabsorption of sodium so the net effect is water movement from the interstitial space into the intravascular space. Ideally, circulating volume and cardiac output increase. There is a corresponding decrease in urinary output as a result of this response.

Antidiuretic hormone. Antidiuretic hormone (ADH) is released by the posterior pituitary gland in response to increased plasma osmolarity, altered circulating volume, and in response to angiotensin. ADH causes sodium and water reabsorption from the distal renal tubules in an attempt to increase circulating volume and cardiac output. Urine output decreases and urine specific gravity increases as a result of this process.

PATIENT ASSESSMENT

Assessment, stabilization, and reassessment of the patient with actual or potential shock is critical for a positive patient outcome. Astute assessment and observation reveal subtle changes in clinical variables that indicate improvement or deterioration in the patient's status.

The initial approach to patient assessment is the *primary* assessment, which addresses airway, breathing, circulation, and level of consciousness.[2] Priority is given to controlling and maintaining the airway, effective breathing, and adequate oxygenation. Augmentation of circulating volume and cardiac output may also be required to support circulation. *Secondary* assessment follows the primary assessment and includes temperature, blood pressure, pulse, respiratory rate, history, and head-to-toe inspection, auscultation, and palpation of the patient. At this time, attention is directed to a focused assessment. The focused assessment is a detailed assessment of the patient's problem. It is guided by findings of the primary and secondary assessment. In most cases of shock, all systems require a focused assessment following the priority sequencing of the primary and secondary assessment.

History

History is an important part of the secondary assessment and may provide important information about the patient's clinical presentation, precipitating events, and preexisting health status. History may be determined by interviewing the patient, significant other(s), and/or prehospital personnel and can also be acquired during physical assessment. Box 36-4 highlights pertinent historical data.

Common Clinical Manifestations

Although shock occurs at the cellular level, manifestations of the shock state are evident at the systemic level.

Box 36-4   Pertinent Historical Data

Chief complaint	Vomiting, hematemesis
Pain, pressure (**PQRST**)	Diarrhea, melena
Provocation	Vaginal bleeding
Quality	Fever, chills
Radiation/region	Rash, urticaria
Severity (scale 0-10)	Polyuria, thirst
Time (time of onset)	Injury, location, mechanism,
Level of consciousness	force, protective device
Dizziness, syncope	Bleeding, site, estimated blood
Weakness, fatigue	loss
Difficulty breathing	Past medical-surgical history
Edema: location and type	Allergies

Clinical changes are noted in the respiratory and circulatory systems and in "nonessential" organs such as the kidneys and skin. Astute assessment depends on recognition of these common clinical manifestations of shock.

Respiratory. During shock, respiratory effectiveness is affected by hypoxia, decreasing level of consciousness, injury, and/or pulmonary congestion. Evaluation of respiratory rate, rhythm, and depth may reveal air hunger, accessory muscle use, and tachypnea. Breath sounds may be absent, unequal, or diminished. Wheezes, crackles, or coarse breath sounds indicating pulmonary congestion occur with cardiogenic shock.

Circulatory. Cardiac output is determined by preload, afterload, contractility, and heart rate. Preload is the volume in the right and left ventricles at the end of diastole. It is affected by circulating volume, right arterial pressure, and intrathoracic pressure. Preload affects myocardial stretch and the force of myocardial contractility. Afterload is the arterial pressure or resistance the ventricles must overcome with each contraction, that is, the amount of pressure necessary for the left ventricle to contract. Afterload is affected by aortic pressure, pulmonary arterial pressure, and systemic vascular resistance. An increase in afterload decreases stroke volume and subsequently decreases cardiac output. Contractility refers to the heart's contractile force.

Pulse rate increases when the sympathetic nervous system responds to decreased cardiac output in shock. A corresponding decrease in stroke volume results in weak, thready pulses. Evaluate peripheral pulses for presence, rate, equality, and quality.

A drop in systolic blood pressure occurs from decreased cardiac output and/or decreased venous return. In early shock, the diastolic blood pressure rises from sympathetic effect on peripheral vascular resistance, which causes vasoconstriction. Consequently, pulse pressure narrows in the presence of decreased systolic blood pressure. As shock progresses, sympathetic activity becomes less effective and diastolic blood pressure begins to fall.

A reduction in arterial distention caused by decreased cardiac output and a proportionate decrease in stroke volume causes flattened jugular veins when the patient is supine. However, the patient in obstructive shock and cardiogenic shock may have neck veins that appear full as a result of right-sided ventricular failure and/or increased pulmonary pressures. Assessment of neck veins may help determine the presence and cause of shock.

Auscultate heart sounds to evaluate rate, quality, the presence of abnormal sounds such as S_3 or S_4, and identify irregularities such as murmurs. Cardiac dysrhythmias develop frequently. Stimulation of the sympathetic nervous system causes tachycardia. Progression of shock and depletion of epinephrine stores leads to bradycardia, heart blocks, and ventricular dysrhythmia including ventricular fibrillation.

Level of consciousness (LOC) is a sensitive assessment measurement of shock and its progression. Decreased cerebral perfusion and hypoxia are initially manifested by restlessness, anxiety, and/or confusion. Continued progression of shock with significant cerebral hypoperfusion and hypoxia leads to an obtunded, unresponsive patient.

Nonessential organs. When tissue perfusion decreases, the body considers only three organs essential—the brain, heart, and lungs. All others, the kidneys, intestines, skin, are nonessential for self-preservation. Blood is shunted away from these nonessential organs in an attempt to maintain cardiac output and cerebral perfusion. Sympathetic nervous system activity and peripheral vasoconstriction shunt blood from the skin, causing cool skin, pallor, especially around the lips, cyanosis, and diaphoresis. Children develop mottled extremities. Capillary refill takes more than 2 seconds. Skin perfusion and capillary refill may be altered by hypothermia or preexisting peripheral vascular disease. Delayed capillary refill should be considered in light of other assessment findings for determining shock or impending shock.

Normal urinary output is 0.5 to 1 ml/kg/hr. In shock, urinary output falls, secondary to renal hypoperfusion and release of ADH. Urine specific gravity increases with reabsorption of water in the renal distal tubules. Reduction in hourly urine output with a rise in specific gravity may signify shock. BUN and creatinine increase as renal perfusion decreases.

Vasoconstriction leads to hypoperfusion of the gastrointestinal tract. Clinical manifestations include hypoactive or absent bowel sounds, leakage of pancreatic enzymes with an elevated serum amylase, and inability of the liver to metabolize substrates such as lactic acid. These effects worsen metabolic acidosis found in the patient in shock.

Initial Stabilization and Management

Stabilization is critical for a positive patient outcome. Adequate oxygenation and circulatory support to correct hypoxia and inadequate tissue perfusion are essential. An effective airway should be obtained and/or maintained along with support of effective breathing. Supplemental oxygen at 100% should be provided. Endotracheal intubation and mechanical ventilation should be anticipated. Management of circulation is directed toward augmentation of circulating volume and improving cardiac output through administration of crystalloids, colloids, and/or blood. Peripheral veins including the antecubital veins, external jugular veins, and saphenous veins should be cannulated with the largest gauge catheter possible. Central venous access can be obtained through the internal jugular veins and the subclavian veins. Warmed intravenous fluids are preferable in order to avoid hypothermia, which can inhibit resuscitative efforts to reverse metabolic acidosis. Options to enhance cardiac output and myocardial contractility include administration of inotropic medications such as dopamine or dobutamine; however, these should be used only after hypovolemia has been corrected.

Acid-base balance. In early shock, respiratory alkalosis occurs because of tachypnea, the body's attempt to increase oxygen levels. Unfortunately, carbon dioxide is blown off as respirations increase in the effort to take in more oxygen. Concurrently, continuing anaerobic metabolism increases serum lactic acid, which culminates in metabolic acidosis. At this time, respiratory rate drops and respiratory acidosis occurs. Management includes hyperventilation and administration of 100% oxygen. Administration of sodium bicarbonate is considered for metabolic acidosis documented by measurement of arterial blood gases and after hyperventilation and oxygenation.

Hemodynamic monitoring. Hemodynamic monitoring is now available in most EDs. Pulse oximetry and noninvasive blood pressure (NIBP) monitoring are as commonplace as the cardiac monitor. These monitoring avenues are an invaluable part of caring for the patient in shock. However, it is important to correlate these modalities with patient assessment.

Pulse oximetry is a noninvasive method of determining hypoxia through measurement of arterial hemoglobin saturation. Light is transmitted through tissue to a light detector attached to the patient's fingertip, nose, or ear. Variability of transmission is determined by pulsated arterial flow. The light absorption abilities of oxyhemoglobin and deoxyhemoglobin are calculated by the monitor to determine the percentage of arterial saturation.

Central venous pressure (CVP) is used to indirectly measure circulating volume, cardiac pump effectiveness, and vascular tone through measurement of pressures on the right side of the myocardium. Normal CVP measurements range from 4 to 10 cm H_2O pressure. A measurement less than 4 cm H_2O indicates decreased circulating volume. A measurement greater than 10 cm H_2O signifies excessive pressures on the right side of the myocardium—often the result of pulmonary edema, fluid overload, or obstruction such as pericardial tamponade or tension pneumothorax.

Arterial pressure may be measured invasively using an arterial line or indirectly using NIBP. Mean arterial pressure is between 70 and 90 mm Hg. A pressure less than 70 mm Hg indicates inadequate circulating volume with inadequate perfusion of the brain, kidneys, and coronary arteries. This may result from hypovolemia, pump failure, obstruction, and/or loss of systemic vascular resistance. Intraarterial lines may be inserted percutaneously or through a surgical incision.

HYPOVOLEMIC SHOCK

Hypovolemic shock is the type of shock seen most frequently by the emergency nurse. It is a direct result of reduction in intravascular volume. Decreased circulating volume can be caused by loss or redistribution of whole blood, plasma, or other body fluids. Redistribution or third-space sequestration occurs when fluid shifts from the intravascular compartment to the interstitial space. This can occur with changes in capillary permeability or capillary fluid pressures as in burn injuries. Actual volume loss is associated with traumatic injury, posterior nasal bleeds, intraabdominal hemorrhage, significant vaginal bleeding, gastrointestinal bleeding, or excessive vomiting and diarrhea. Diabetic ketoacidosis (DKA) causes extreme diuresis, which may reduce circulating volume.

Early identification and treatment are essential because the potential for good patient outcome declines with profound hypotension and progression to decompensated shock. Table 36-1 summarizes clinical manifestations associated with various levels of volume depletion. Age and preexisting health problems also affect the potential for a good patient outcome.

Inspection of the patient may reveal injury or other source of hemorrhage and fluid loss. In cases of trauma, impaled objects or penetrating injury may be present. Blunt injuries and/or deformities often result in sequestering of large amounts of blood because of occult bleeding. The presence of thermal injuries indicates the potential for substantial redistribution of fluid because of capillary injury. Clinical manifestations are related to the amount and rate of actual volume loss. Hypovolemia can occur suddenly or gradually as in some cases of gastrointestinal bleeding.

Initial complete blood count (CBC) analysis may be inaccurate, particularly in patients with sudden loss of large amounts of blood, because the serum to hematocrit/hemoglobin ratio does not change. Proportionate reductions in hematocrit and hemoglobin are usually demonstrated after fluid resuscitation.

Management of the patient in hypovolemic shock is directed toward controlling or preventing further loss of circulating volume and restoring intravascular volume. Control of external bleeding is accomplished with direct pressure to tamponade bleeding. Impaled objects are stabilized to pre-

Table **36-1**	**Classes of Shock**	
Class	Blood loss	Clinical manifestations
I	750 to 1500 ml	Tachycardia; narrowing pulse pressure; anxiety; restlessness; delayed capillary refill; mildly cool skin; slightly decreased urine output
II	1500 to 2000 ml	Tachypnea; tachycardia; hypotension; altered level of consciousness; pale, cool, moist skin; flat neck veins; decreasing urine output
III	2000 ml or more	Tachycardia progressing to pulselessness; shallow, agonal respirations; obtunded; unresponsive; anuria

vent further movement and bleeding. Volume replacement is initiated with large-bore intravenous access and fluid replacement. Crystalloids are administered at a 3:1 ratio for calculated fluid replacement, whereas blood products are administered at a 1:1 replacement ratio.

Blood is administered in cases of major trauma when there is no improvement in clinical status after 3 to 4 L of crystalloids. Type-specific blood is always preferable; however, O-negative blood can be given in extremely critical situations when there is no time to wait for type-specific blood. Autotransfusion can be done with intrapleural and mediastinal blood from a clean wound, usually with blood loss greater than 200 ml. Adequate renal and liver function is necessary given the potential red blood cell hemolysis. Crystalloids and blood products should be warmed before infusion to avoid hypothermia.

Fluid replacement and blood transfusions for hypovolemic shock can save the patient's life, but they can also complicate the patient's clinical course. Resuscitation can cause hypothermia, hyperkalemia, hypocalcemia, acidosis, alkalosis, clotting problems, and intravascular debris. These complications are summarized in Table 36-2. Patients who receive transfusions that replace more than 50% of their blood volume during a 3-hour period should be closely monitored for these adverse effects of resuscitation.

CARDIOGENIC SHOCK

Cardiogenic shock occurs when the heart fails as a pump, causing a significant reduction in ventricular effectiveness. Cardiac output decreases and tissue perfusion diminishes while left ventricular end-diastolic pressure increases. Injury to the myocardium impairs contractility, which decreases ventricular emptying. Cardiogenic shock carries a high mortality rate; most patients die within 24 hours, others may live only a few days. Cardiogenic shock is caused by myocardial infarction with damage to greater than 40% of the left ventricle, severe myocardial contusion, valvular heart disease, cardiomyopathies, ruptured papillary muscle, ruptured ventricular septum, and dysrhythmias such as third-degree heart block.

When pump failure occurs, the myocardium cannot forcibly eject blood. Stroke volume decreases because of decreased contractility, decreasing cardiac output and blood pressure. Subsequent alteration in tissue perfusion precipitates myocardial ischemia and extends the region of injury, which further compromises cardiac contractility. Myocardial contractility is also affected by hypoxemia, metabolic acidosis, ventricular diastolic volume, and sympathetic nervous system stimulation. Poor myocardial contractility causes inadequate emptying of the left ventricle.

Incomplete emptying of the left ventricle during diastole elevates pressures in the left ventricle, left atrium, and pulmonary vessels. There is a corresponding increase in pulmonary pressures as pulmonary capillaries leak fluid into the alveolar spaces, causing pulmonary edema. Elevated

Table **36-2**	**Adverse Effects of Fluid and/or Blood Replacement**
Problem	Description
Hypothermia	Transfusion of banked blood without warming can make the patient hypothermic. Hypothermia shifts the oxyhemoglobin dissociation curve to the left, i.e., oxygen is not available for the cells.
Hyperkalemia	Lysis of red blood cells releases potassium from the intracellular space so the patient becomes hyperkalemic. Monitor the patient's serum potassium and observe for cardiac rhythm problems.
Hypocalcemia	Banked blood contains citrate, which binds with free calcium. Calcium chloride is given after 10 units of blood.
Acidosis	The pH of banked blood is 7.1. With large amounts of banked blood, acidosis can occur. Monitor arterial blood gases and watch for dysrhythmias.
Alkalosis	With large amounts of banked blood, alkalosis can develop because the citrate is converted by the liver into bicarbonate. Monitor arterial blood gases.
Clotting problems	Clotting factors are lost in most banked blood. Coagulation times may be prolonged and clotting problems occur with massive blood transfusions. Usually, 1 unit of fresh-frozen plasma is given after 10 units of blood.
Intravascular debris	Banked blood contains debris as a result of processing. It is not known if this debris is harmful; therefore blood is always given through a filter.

pulmonary pressures increase right ventricular and atrial pressures, which contribute to right-sided heart failure.

Increased myocardial performance as a compensatory response to the shock translates to increased myocardial oxygen demand and increased myocardial ischemia, which further compromises cardiac output and eventually progresses to cardiovascular collapse.

Clinical manifestations of cardiogenic shock resemble those seen in myocardial infarction. The patient complains of chest pain or pressure as a result of myocardial ischemia, myocardial infarct, and/or dyspnea. There are electrocardiogram changes, dysrhythmias, and an elevation in cardiac enzymes. Elevated pulmonary and myocardial pressures cause distended neck veins. Decreasing cardiac output and hypotension contribute to absent or weak, thready peripheral pulses. Auscultation reveals muffled heart sounds with rhythm irregularities. Tachypnea occurs to compensate for pulmonary edema. Diffuse crackles and wheezes are usually present. Skin is pale, cool, and clammy. Central cyanosis is often present.

Management of cardiogenic shock begins with administering high-flow oxygen and establishing intravenous access. Subsequent management is predominately pharmacologic. Vasodilating agents such as nitroglycerin are given to reduce pain, increase coronary perfusion, and reduce preload and afterload. These agents also decrease left ventricular filling pressures and increase cardiac output. Sodium nitroprusside may be given to decrease afterload. Morphine sulfate reduces pain and anxiety, eases respiratory efforts, and decreases afterload. Inotropic medications such as dopamine and dobutamine increase contractility and improve systolic pressure.

The intraaortic balloon pump, a diastolic assist device that improves cardiac output, coronary artery perfusion, and oxygen delivery without increasing myocardial oxygen consumption, may also be used. Pulmonary arterial catheters are used to measure pulmonary artery wedge pressure (PAWP), a precise indication of left ventricular function and cardiac competence. These PAWP measurements guide fluid administration in cardiogenic shock.

DISTRIBUTIVE SHOCK

Distributive shock, also referred to as vasogenic shock, results from an alteration in systemic vasculature that causes maldistribution of intravascular volume to the circulatory network and interstitial spaces. Distributive shock is characterized by extreme vasodilation in the presence of normal blood volume and cardiac function. Three categories of distributive shock based on etiology are neurogenic, septic, and anaphylactic shock.

Neurogenic Shock

Neurogenic shock is most often associated with acute spinal cord disruption from trauma or spinal anesthesia. Other causes of neurogenic shock are brain injury, hypoxia, depressant drug actions, and hypoglycemia associated with insulin shock. In neurogenic shock, outflow from the vasomotor center in the medulla is inhibited or depressed, causing loss of sympathetic vasomotor regulation. Uncontested parasympathetic responses cause vasodilation and loss of sympathetic tone. Inhibition of sympathetic innervation impedes release of norepinephrine and interferes with the body's ability to vasoconstrict. Consequently, venous return and cardiac output decrease. Neurogenic shock is relatively uncommon. It is a transient shock state that usually requires only supportive treatment.

The combination of hypotension and loss of sympathetic innervation contributes to two manifestations unique to neurogenic shock: bradycardia and warm, dry, flushed skin. With cord disruption, skin above the disruption is pale, cool, and moist. The patient also manifests hypotension, tachypnea, and loss of sensation, mobility, and/or reflexes below the level of cord disruption. Rectal and bladder sphincter control are absent. Priapism is seen in male patients. Patients become poikilothermic, assuming the temperature of the surrounding environment.

Management is primarily supportive, maintenance and support of airway, breathing, and circulation with simultaneous spinal immobilization. Realignment and definitive spinal stabilization with halo ring device or insertion of tongs should be performed once the patient is stabilized. Measures to warm the patient should be instituted to maintain a normothermic core temperature. Vasopressors for hypotension and atropine for symptomatic bradycardia may be needed for supportive management.

Septic Shock

The most common cause of septic shock is untreated infection. Sepsis occurs in 1 of every 100 hospitalized patients—40% will develop septic shock.[1] The mortality rate for septic shock ranges from 40% to 90%. Survival depends on promptness of treatment. Septic shock is the most common form of distributive shock.

The systemic response in septic shock is caused by endotoxins of the infecting organisms, immunosuppression, or inability of the immune system to respond to the bacterial assault of an overwhelming infection. The most common causative organisms are gram-negative bacilli. Gram-positive bacteria, yeast, fungi, and viruses have also been implicated in septic shock. Endotoxins released by the invading organisms prompt release of hydrolytic enzymes from weakened cell lysosomes, which causes cellular destruction of bacteria and normal cells. The immune system responds by releasing histamine, prostaglandins, and chemical mediators, precipitating profound vasodilation, increased capillary permeability, and redistribution of fluid into the interstitial spaces. The resulting inadequate tissue perfusion, third-space sequestration of fluid, and altered cellular metabolism affect multiple organs.

Clinical manifestations of septic shock occur in two phases. The initial phase is the *hyperdynamic* or warm phase. The patient is febrile with a high cardiac output and decreased systemic vascular resistance. Skin appears flushed and petechiae may be present. The patient is tachycardic and tachypneic. This stage is followed by the *hypodynamic* or cold phase, characterized by decreased cardiac output and profound vasoconstriction. Skin is pale, cool, and moist with mottling progressing above the knees. Temperature is subnormal and respirations are rapid and shallow, progressing to Cheyne-Stokes respirations.

Management of the overwhelming infection follows support of airway, breathing, and circulation with high-flow oxygen and intravenous fluids. It is important to identify and remove potential sources of infection. Wounds and necrotic tissue should be debrided, existing invasive devices such as indwelling catheters should be removed. Cultures should be obtained from potential sites prior to administration of antibiotics. Antipyretics should be administered for temperatures >101°F. Inotropic medications are used to augment cardiac output and blood pressure.

Anaphylactic Shock

Anaphylaxis is an acute allergic reaction following exposure to a foreign protein to which the patient has been previously sensitized. Anaphylactic shock is a profound hypersensitivity reaction with a systemic antigen-antibody response. Clinical manifestations are usually acute and sudden; however, symptoms may occasionally be mild, evolving into respiratory distress and hypotension after several hours. Antigens commonly implicated in anaphylactic shock include medications such as antibiotics, iodine contrast dyes, foods such as shellfish or nuts, food additives such as MSG, and insect stings. Antibodies are formed upon initial exposure to a foreign protein. The antigen triggers release of vasoactive mediators that act on the vascular and pulmonary systems. The effect of these mediators is smooth muscle contraction, vasodilation, increased capillary permeability, and bronchoconstriction. Redistribution of fluid interstitially in combination with vasodilation decreases intravascular volume and causes urticaria and angioedema. Fluid leakage into the alveoli leads to pulmonary congestion.

Acute onset of angioedema of the upper airway and bronchospasm may progress rapidly to airway obstruction and respiratory arrest. Initial respiratory symptoms include respiratory difficulty, stridor, bronchospasm, and wheezing. Patients initially have warm, dry skin that becomes cool and pale. Chest tightness, dysrhythmias, and cardiac irritability may also be noted.

Management is directed toward maintaining a patent airway, effective breathing, and circulatory support. High-flow oxygen and intravenous access are followed by intravenous administration of epinephrine 0.1 to 0.5 ml of 1:10,000 solution, repeated in 5 to 15 minutes for profound vasoconstriction. Antihistamines such as diphenhydramine (Benadryl) and cimetidine (Tagamet) are given. Bronchodilators such as albuterol and/or aminophylline may be given for bronchoconstriction and bronchospasm. Cricothyrotomy may be required for severe airway compromise.

OBSTRUCTIVE SHOCK

Obstructive shock occurs from mechanical obstruction or compression of the great veins, pulmonary arteries, aorta, or the myocardium itself that prevents adequate circulating volume. Inadequate cardiac output and tissue hypoperfusion occur when the obstruction prevents adequate emptying of the myocardium during systole or filling during diastole. Pulmonary embolus prevents right ventricular emptying when a large portion of the pulmonary arterial cross-sectional area is obstructed. Incomplete right ventricular emptying causes decreased cardiac output, right ventricular failure, and increased right atrial pressure. Air embolus obstructs flow from the right atrium to the pulmonary outflow

tract, preventing emptying of the right ventricle during systole. Pericardial tamponade prevents filling during diastole because the atria and ventricles are unable to fill. Compression on the heart decreases stroke volume. Tension pneumothorax displaces the inferior vena cava, obstructing venous return to the right atrium, thereby reducing stroke volume. Other causes of obstructive shock include aortic aneurysm, intracardiac clot, and aortic stenosis.

Clinical manifestations vary depending on the cause of obstruction. Common manifestations include pain in the chest or back, dyspnea, tachypnea, tachycardia, profound hypotension, cyanosis, and diaphoresis. Management is directed toward removal of the obstruction and support of airway, breathing, and circulation.

COMPLICATIONS ASSOCIATED WITH SHOCK

Shock places the patient at risk for complications with long-term implications, including disability and even death. Specific complications include adult respiratory distress syndrome (ARDS), disseminated intravascular coagulation (DIC), acute renal failure, and multiorgan failure (MOF). Management of these clinical syndromes is discussed in greater detail in Chapter 34, Chapter 44, and Chapter 39, respectively.

Adult respiratory distress syndrome (ARDS) is acute pulmonary congestion and atelectasis with hyaline membrane formation associated with aggressive blood transfusions and/or fluid resuscitation, sepsis, trauma, pulmonary embolus, and other conditions. Hyaline membrane formation and atelectasis decrease lung compliance, reduce pulmonary surfactant, and increase lung capillary permeability. This is followed by significant interstitial and alveolar edema with mucus formation along the alveoli and acute pulmonary congestion. Ineffective oxygenation of tissues and ventilation-perfusion abnormalities worsen as hypoxemia occurs. Management is directed toward early identification of pulmonary congestion through frequent assessment of lung sounds. Endotracheal intubation and mechanical ventilation with positive end-expiratory pressure (PEEP) is used to manage ventilation-perfusion abnormalities and expand alveoli.

Disseminated intravascular coagulation (DIC) is widespread microvascular coagulation followed by depletion of clotting factors. Microthrombi form and are distributed to the microvasculature of various organs, producing infarction, tissue ischemia, and hemorrhagic necrosis when secondary fibrinolysis fails to lyse the fibrin quickly. Secondary fibrinolysis reduces clotting factors. Release of fibrin degradation products that act as anticoagulants is also impaired. These processes contribute to serious bleeding tendencies. The DIC syndrome may occur with aggressive transfusion with blood products or in association with ARDS. Patients should be observed for obvious or occult bleeding, hematuria, petechiae, and ecchymosis.

Acute renal failure (ARF) occurs from renal hypoperfusion, myocardial compromise, and/or fluid and electrolyte

Table **36-3**	Shock in the Pediatric, Elderly, or Pregnant Patient
Patient	Description
Pediatric	Increases cardiac output by increasing heart rate; fixed stroke volume; sustains arterial pressure despite significant volume loss; loses 25% of circulating volume before signs of shock occur; early clinical manifestations are tachycardia, tachypnea, pallor, and cool, clammy skin; volume replaced with 20 ml/kg bolus of crystalloid
Elderly	Shock progression often rapid; normal physiologic changes of aging reduce compensatory mechanisms; predisposed to hypothermia
Pregnant	Hypervolemia of pregnancy means patient can remain normotensive with up to 1500 ml blood loss; compression of inferior vena cava by gravid uterus reduces circulating volume by 30%; place patient on left side, manually displace uterus, or elevate right hip with towel; risk for aspiration due to decreased gastric motility and decreased gastric emptying; treat suspected hypovolemia to prevent placental vasoconstriction associated with catecholamine release; potential for fetal distress exists despite maternal stability

depletion and is characterized by oliguria, elevated BUN and creatinine levels, hyperkalemia, hyponatremia, azotemia, and acidosis. Oliguria occurs in response to extracellular volume depletion and myocardial compromise. Compensatory responses stimulate sodium and water reabsorption, cause a drop in glomerular filtration rate, and eventually lead to renal tubular dysfunction. This syndrome is often associated with DIC in the shock patient.

SPECIAL POPULATIONS

It is important for the emergency nurse to recognize that pediatric patients, elderly patients, and pregnant patients respond differently to volume depletion and other causes of shock. These varied responses are due to physiologic differences in these patients. Table 36-3 highlights some of these differences. Emergent conditions in these pop-

Box **36-5**

NURSING DIAGNOSES RELATED TO SHOCK
Altered tissue perfusion
Decreased cardiac output
Fluid volume deficit
Impaired gas exchange

ulations are covered in greater detail in other chapters of this text.

SUMMARY

Shock is a progressive, pervasive process caused by inadequate tissue perfusion and oxygenation. Regardless of etiology, the cellular effects of shock are the same. Nursing assessment, early recognition, and appropriate management are essential to prevent or reverse the shock process and ensure a positive patient outcome. Box 36-5 outlines the most critical nursing diagnoses for the patient in shock.

REFERENCES

1. Emergency Nurses Association: *Trauma nursing core course: instructors manual,* ed 4, Chicago, 1991, The Association.
2. Emergency Nurses Association: *Emergency nursing core curriculum,* ed 4, Philadelphia, 1994, WB Saunders.

SUGGESTED READING

Berkow R, Fletcher A: *The Merck manual,* ed 15, Rahway, NJ, 1988, Merck.

Emergency Nurses Association: *Emergency nursing pediatric course—instructors manual,* Chicago, 1993, The Association.

Garb S: *Laboratory tests in common use,* ed 5, New York, 1971, Springer.

Kitt S, Selfridge-Thomas J, Proehl J et al: *Emergency nursing: a physiologic and clinical perspective,* ed 2, Philadelphia, 1995, WB Saunders.

Kokiko J: Septic shock: a review and update for the emergency department clinician, *J Emerg Nurs* 19:102, 1993.

Littleton MT: Pathophysiology and assessment of sepsis and septic shock, *Crit Care Nurs Q* 11:30, 1988.

Selfridge-Thomas J: *Manual of emergency nursing,* Philadelphia, 1995, WB Saunders.

Sheehy S: *Manual of emergency care,* ed 4, St. Louis, 1995, Mosby.

Unruth S: Shock emergencies. In Emergency Nurses Association: *CEN review video series,* Chicago, 1991, The Association.

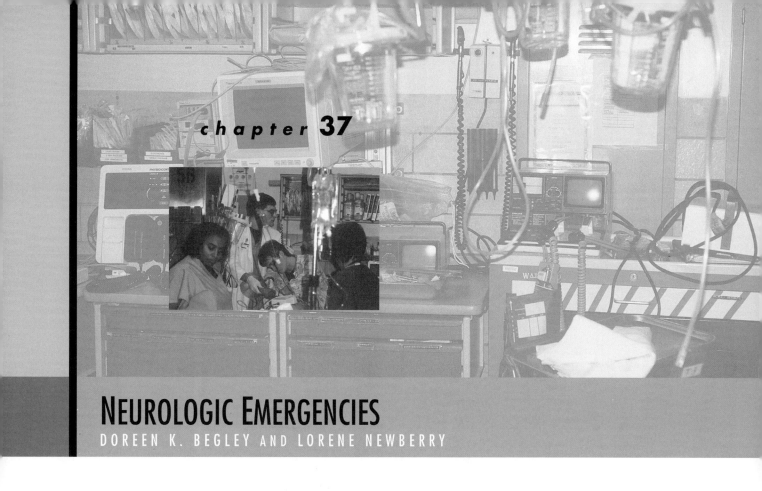

chapter 37

NEUROLOGIC EMERGENCIES

DOREEN K. BEGLEY AND LORENE NEWBERRY

The emergency nurse encounters a variety of neurologic emergencies related to illness or injury, including stroke, head injury, spinal cord injury, headache, and meningitis. Regardless of etiology, a neurologic emergency is one that causes severe temporary or permanent disability or is an immediate threat to the patient's life. This chapter focuses on assessment and treatment of neurologic conditions caused by disease or pathologic abnormality. Patient assessment and anatomy and physiology are also reviewed. Neurologic emergencies secondary to injury, that is, head injury and spinal cord injury, are covered in Chapters 23 and 24, respectively.

ANATOMY AND PHYSIOLOGY

The nervous system coordinates, interprets, and controls interactions between the individual and the surrounding environment. Major divisions, the central nervous system (CNS) and the peripheral nervous system, regulate most other body systems.

Central Nervous System

The central nervous system consists of the brain and the spinal cord. Functional units of the CNS are neurons, cells that relay signals between the body and the brain. Figure 37-1 illustrates a generic neuron and identifies essential neuronal structures. More than 100 billion neurons relay signals that control the body's various systems.[1] Signal relay between neurons is controlled by neurotransmitters located at the synapse, or junction, between two neurons. Examples of neurotransmitters include acetylcholine, dopamine, norepinephrine, epinephrine, histamine, insulin, glucagon, and angiotensin II. Signal movement along the neuron itself is an electrical phenomenon enhanced by the presence of myelin.

Brain. The adult brain weighs approximately 3 lb or 2% of total body weight. Brain tissue is the most energy-consuming tissue in the body, receiving approximately 20% of the cardiac output and using approximately 20% of the body's oxygen supply. Structurally the brain consists of external gray matter and internal white matter. The brain has three distinct parts—the cerebrum, brainstem, and cerebellum (Figure 37-2). The cerebrum, divided into two hemispheres, represents almost 90% of the brain's weight. Bands of connective tissue, called the corpus callosum, relay information between the two hemispheres. Each hemisphere consists of lobes named for the adjacent portion of the skull, that is, frontal, temporal, parietal, and occipital. The brainstem is continuous with the spinal cord and serves as an important relay and reflex center for the CNS. Nuclei for the cranial nerves found in the brainstem control respiration, the cardiovascular system, gastrointestinal functions, equilibrium, and eye movement.[1] The cerebellum controls activities below the level of consciousness, for example, posture and equilibrium. Within the brain, a series of interconnected cavities called ventricles produce cerebrospinal fluid.

In addition to the cranium, three connective tissue layers, called meninges, surround and protect the brain. Figure 37-3

525

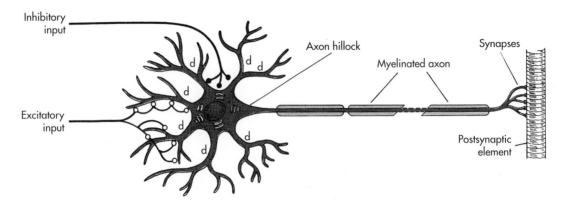

Figure **37-1** Schematic diagram of an idealized neuron and its major components; *d*, dendrites. *(From Berne RM, Levy MN:* Physiology, *ed 3, St. Louis, 1993, Mosby.)*

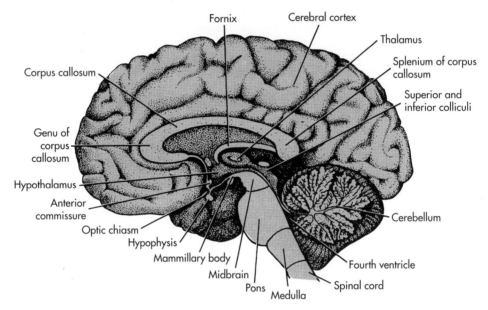

Figure **37-2** Midsagittal section of the brain. Note the relationships among the cerebral cortex, cerebellum, thalamus, and brainstem as well as the location of various commissures. *(From Berne RM, Levy MN:* Physiology, *ed 3, St. Louis, 1993, Mosby.)*

illustrates the dura mater, arachnoid, and pia mater and their relationship to the brain. The dura forms a tent over the brain and separates the cerebrum from the cerebellum. (This is the basis for the term *supratentorial.*) The subarachnoid contains sinuses that collect venous blood from the brain and return blood to the internal jugular veins. The pia mater extends below the spinal cord to form the filum terminale.

Cranial nerves. Twelve pairs of cranial nerves arise directly from the brainstem. Each nerve is identified with a Roman numeral and name. Cranial nerves may be sensory, motor, or both. Cranial nerve functions are not consciously controlled; therefore assessment of cranial nerves provides an accurate picture of brainstem activity and neurologic function. Table 37-1 lists cranial nerves and their function.

Cerebral blood flow. Two pairs of arteries anastomose to form the circle of Willis, which provides collateral circulation to the brain. The internal carotid arteries supply the anterior brain and vertebral arteries supply the posterior brain. Figure 37-4 illustrates arterial blood supply to the brain. Venous blood drains from the brain through sinuses in the dura mater into the internal jugular veins.

The brain occupies 80% of the cranium. Vascular volume and cerebrospinal fluid (CSF) represent the remaining 20%. Cranial rigidity limits the brain's ability to tolerate increases in any component. If one component increases, the other components must decrease to prevent pressure on the brain. This tenet of cerebral function is called the Monro Kelly hypothesis. Cerebral blood flow changes with cerebral perfu-

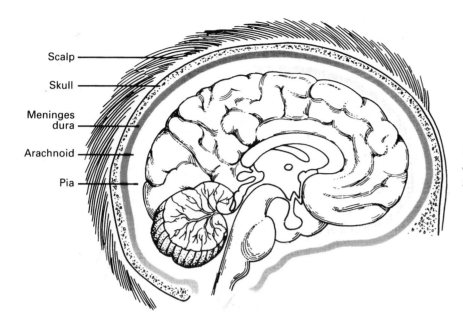

Scalp
Skull
Meninges
dura
Arachnoid
Pia

Figure **37-3** Cross section of the head. *(From Sheehy SB, Lombardi JE:* Manual of emergency care, *ed 4, St. Louis, 1995, Mosby.)*

Table **37-1**	**Cranial Nerves and Their Functions**	
Number	**Name**	**Function**
I	Olfactory	Smell
II	Optic	Vision
III	Oculomotor	Elevate upper lid, pupillary constriction, most extraocular movements
IV	Trochlear	Downward, inward movement of the eye
V	Trigeminal	Chewing, clinching the jaw, lateral jaw movement, corneal reflexes, face sensation
VI	Abducens	Lateral eye deviation
VII	Facial	Facial motor, taste, lacrimation, and salivation
VIII	Acoustic	Equilibrium, hearing
IX	Glossopharyngeal	Swallowing, gag reflex, taste on posterior tongue
X	Vagus	Swallowing, gag reflex, abdominal viscera, phonation
XI	Spinal accessory	Head and shoulder movement
XII	Hypoglossal	Tongue movement

sion pressure (CPP) and size of the cerebrovascular bed. CPP is a product of mean arterial pressure (MAP) minus intracranial pressure (ICP) (CPP = MAP − ICP). Normal CPP is 60 mm Hg, normal ICP is 10 to 15 mm Hg.

Cerebrospinal fluid. Cerebrospinal fluid is produced in the ventricles by the choroid plexus at a rate of 7 to 10 ml/hr. CSF protects the brain and spinal cord by forming a shock-absorbing cushion, providing nutrition via glucose transport, and removing metabolic waste products. CSF also compensates for changes in pressure and volume within the cranium. Table 37-2 summarizes normal CSF characteristics.

Spinal cord. The spinal cord lies in the spinal canal of the vertebral bodies and is covered by meningeal layers. The adult spinal cord is approximately 16 to 18 inches long and extends from the brainstem to the intervertebral disk between L-1 and L-2. Sensory and motor neurons in the spinal cord conduct impulses to and from the brain. Unlike the brain, the spinal cord has white matter on the exterior and gray matter on the interior. Figure 37-5 illustrates the spinal cord in cross-section. Reflex arcs into the spinal cord operate without voluntary or conscious control. Table 37-3 lists these reflexes.

Peripheral Nervous System

The peripheral nervous system consists of 31 spinal nerves and the autonomic nervous system. Spinal nerves innervate skeletal muscle and a segment of skin called a dermatome. Figure 37-6 shows these dermatomes with distinct borders; however, there is significant overlap between adjacent segments. In certain areas, spinal nerves form a network called a plexus; for example, the brachial plexus innervates the upper extremity.

Autonomic nervous system. The autonomic nervous system (ANS) controls the body's visceral functions. There is no sensory component; functions are entirely motor. Activity is regulated by the cerebral cortex, hypothalamus, and the brainstem. Two major divisions, the sympathetic and parasympathetic nervous systems, respond to stressors such as fear or blood loss to provide extra energy or conserve existing energy stores. The *sympathetic nervous system* provides the body energy, that is, the fight-or-flight response.

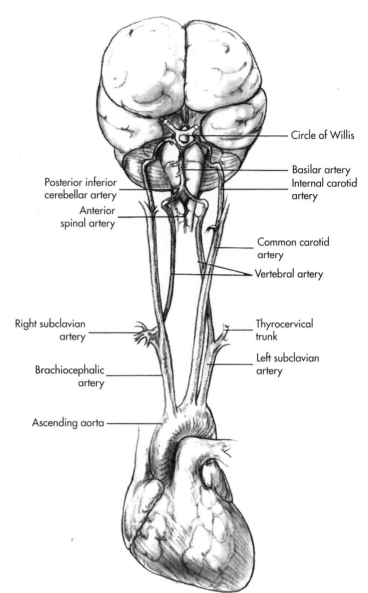

Figure **37-4** Origin and course of arterial supply to the brain. *(From Davis JH, Drucker WR et al:* Clinical surgery, *vol 1, St. Louis, 1987, Mosby.)*

Table 37-2   **Normal Cerebrospinal Fluid**

Quality	Value-description
Appearance	Clear, colorless, odorless
Cell count	WBC count 5/mm^3
	RBC count 0/mm^3
Pressure	80-180 mm H_2O
Glucose	60-80 mg/100 ml (2/3 serum glucose value)
Protein	15-45 mg/100 ml (lumbar)
pH	7.35-7.40
Sodium	140-142 mEq/L
Chloride	120-130 mEq/L
Volume	125-150 ml

Table 37-3   **Spinal Reflexes**

Reflex	Segmental level
Biceps	C5-6
Brachioradialis	C5-6
Triceps	C7-8
Knee	L2-4
Ankle	S1-2
Superficial abdominal (Above the umbilicus)	T8-10
Superficial abdominal (Below the umbilicus)	T10-12
Cremasteric	L1-2
Plantar	L4-5, S1-2

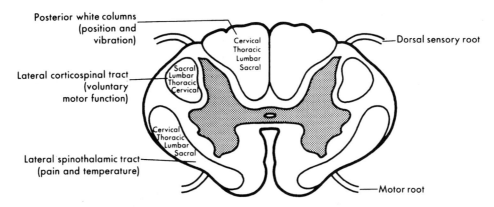

Figure **37-5** Cross section of the cervical spinal cord. *(From Rund DA, Barkin RM, Rosen P: Essentials of emergency medicine, ed 2, St. Louis, 1996, Mosby.)*

Table 37-4	Autonomic Nervous System Functions	
Sympathetic nervous system	**Parasympathetic nervous system**
Pupil dilation	Pupil constriction
Increased heart rate	Decreased heart rate
Increased conduction velocity	Decreased conduction velocity
Increased contractility	Decreased contractility
Coronary vasodilation	
Skeletal muscle vasodilation	Minimal peripheral vascular effects
Abdominal and cutaneous vasoconstriction	
Bronchodilation	Bronchoconstriction
Increased glucose release from liver	Slight glycogen synthesis
Decreased peristalsis	Increased peristalsis
Decreased gastric tone	Increased gastric tone
Increased basal metabolic rate (BMR)	No change in BMR
Increased coagulation	No effect on coagulation
Diaphoresis	Sweating of palms only
Piloerection	No effect

Box 37-1	Glasgow Coma Scale	
Eye Opening	
Spontaneous	4
To verbal command	3
To pain	2
No response	1
Best Motor Response	
Obeys commands	6
Localizes pain	5
Withdraws from pain	4
Abnormal flexion	3
Abnormal extension	2
No response	1
Best Verbal Response	
Oriented	5
Confused	4
Inappropriate words	3
Incomprehensible sounds	2
No response	1
Total	3-15

Receptors are scattered throughout the body, including the skin. Parasympathetic nervous system receptors distributed primarily in the head, chest, abdomen, and pelvis conserve the body's energy. Table 37-4 compares activities of these opposing systems.

PATIENT ASSESSMENT

The most reliable indicator of neurologic function is the patient's level of consciousness (LOC). Follow initial assessment with continuous evaluation to detect changes. Question the patient's family and significant other about changes in behavior, mood, or physical ability. Evaluate for signs of increasing ICP, that is, headache, nausea, vomiting, altered LOC. Assess cranial nerve function and pupil size, equality, reactivity, and accommodation. The pupil dilates when increased ICP causes pressure on cranial nerve III; however, this is a late indicator of increasing ICP. Serial assessment is essential to identify subtle changes indicating impending herniation. A universal tool such as the Glasgow Coma Scale is recommended (Box 37-1). Evaluating motor strength involves comparison of the patient's dominant hand with the evaluator's dominant hand. Sensory evaluation should include differentiation of dull and sharp objects. Assessment should also include identification of existing deficits such as muscle weakness, pupil abnormality, and gait disturbances.

Stabilization of the patient with a neurologic emergency begins with the airway, breathing, and circulation (ABCs). Specific interventions depend on patient complaint and acuity. The patient with a severe migraine headache has differ-

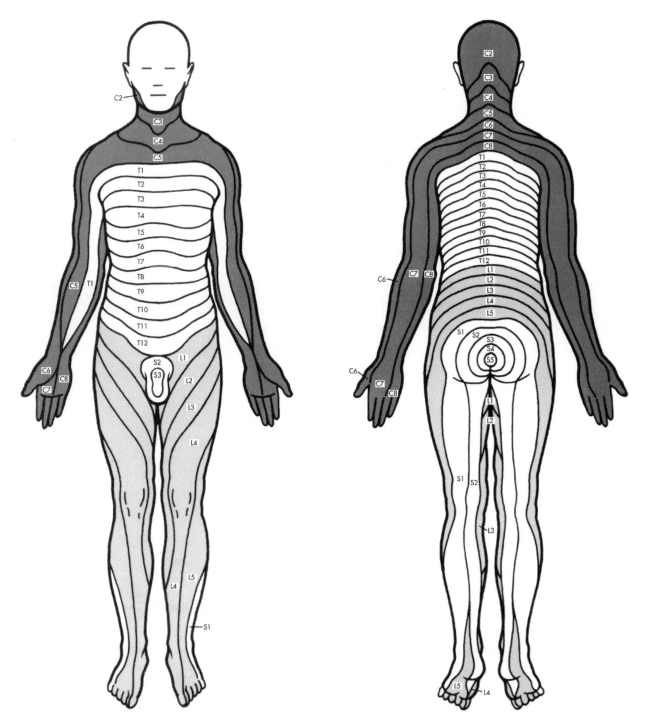

Figure **37-6** Sensory dermatomes. *(From Rund DA, Barkin RM, Rosen P:* Essentials of emergency medicine, *ed 2, St. Louis, 1996, Mosby.)*

ent priorities than a comatose patient. A patient with severe migraine requires pain management, whereas the comatose patient needs support of the ABCs, management of increased ICP, and monitoring for impending herniation. Herniation occurs when increased ICP forces the brain downward through the foramen magnum. Compression of the brainstem impairs respiratory and cardiovascular function, ultimately causing death. Figure 37-7 illustrates this process. Controlling increased ICP includes use of medications such as osmotic diuretics, sedatives, and analgesics. Elevating the patient's head facilitates venous drainage and decreased ICP; however, cervical spine injury should be ruled out prior to elevation. Decreasing stimulation such as noise and some procedures also affects ICP.

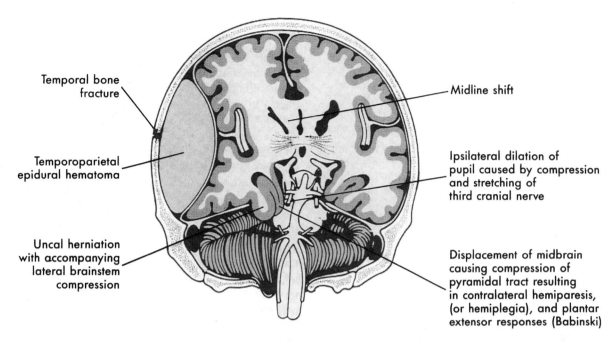

Temporal bone
fracture

Temporoparietal
epidural hematoma

Uncal herniation
with accompanying
lateral brainstem
compression

Midline shift

Ipsilateral dilation of
pupil caused by compression
and stretching of
third cranial nerve

Displacement of midbrain
causing compression of
pyramidal tract resulting
in contralateral hemiparesis,
(or hemiplegia), and plantar
extensor responses (Babinski)

Figure **37-7** Cross section showing herniation of lower portion of temporal lobe (uncas) through tentorium caused by temporoparietal epidural hematoma. Herniation may occur also in cerebellum. Note mass effect and midline shift. *(From Meeker MH, Rothrock JC:* Alexander's care of the patient in surgery, *ed 10, St. Louis, 1995, Mosby. Redrawn from Kintzel KC, editor:* Advanced concepts in clinical nursing, *ed 2, Philadelphia, 1977, JB Lippincott.)*

SPECIFIC NEUROLOGIC EMERGENCIES

Specific neurologic emergencies represent a threat to the patient's life, integrity of specific functions, that is, vision, or the quality of the patient's life. Specific emergencies include headache, seizures, stroke, meningitis, Guillain-Barré syndrome, and myasthenia gravis. A brief review from the emergency nurse's perspective is presented.

Headache

Headache is one of the most common complaints seen in the ED. Headache not caused by trauma accounts for 1% to 2% of ED visits.[4] However, headache is a symptom of an underlying disorder rather than a diagnosis. The headache may be minor or represent a life-threatening situation such as subarachnoid hemorrhage; therefore careful assessment is essential. Box 37-2 highlights key assessment questions for these patients.

Headaches may be caused by an extracranial or intracranial condition. Extracranial causes include acidosis, dehydration, hypoglycemia, uremia, and hepatic disorders. Ophthalmic causes of headache include glaucoma, refractory errors, inflammation, or allergic reactions (see Chapter 48). Poisoning and toxicologic emergencies also cause headache (see Chapter 45). Other extracranial causes include ear infection, upper respiratory infection, sinus congestion, facial trauma, temporomandibular joint syndrome, toothache, anemia, polycythemia, electrolyte imbalance, and systemic in-

Box 37-2	**Key Assessment Questions Related to Headache**

Is this the patient's first headache?
When did this headache start?
Has the patient been injured recently?
Have there been any personality changes?
Has the patient experienced any memory loss?
Has the patient had a recent infection?
Does the patient have any problems with vision?
Has the patient had any recent neurologic problems?
Does the patient have hypertension? For how long?
Does the patient have any emotional problems?
What medication is the patient currently taking?
Has the patient ever had a seizure?

fection. Identification and treatment of extracranial causes should relieve the headache.

Specific headaches related to intracranial conditions include migraine headache, tension headache, and temporal arteritis. Traumatic headaches may occur as an emergency or nonemergency. Nonemergency conditions include postconcussion or contusion headaches. Emergent conditions that cause severe headache include intracranial injury (see Chapter 23).

Migraine headache. Twenty-three million Americans suffer migraine headaches.[5] A diagnosis of migraine headache is based on the patient's history and presenting symptoms. Headache is never the only symptom. Before the diagnosis is reached, other causes should be ruled out. Migraine symptoms include nausea, vomiting, and visual disturbances. Approximately 12% of the U.S. population have migraine headaches, and almost 70% of those with migraines have a positive family history.[5]

Migraine headaches are classified as vascular or nonvascular. Muscular contraction or tension headache is an example of a nonvascular migraine headache. Skeletal muscle contraction in the head or neck produces steady, pulsatile pain and limited motion of the head, neck, and jaw. Pressure over contracted muscles worsens the pain. Pain also worsens with vasoconstrictive drugs such as ergotamines. Treatment is mild analgesia with identification and treatment of the underlying cause.

Vascular headaches occur suddenly and are described as intense, sharp, and piercing or pounding and throbbing. Table 37-5 describes specific vascular migraine headaches. Vascular migraine headaches have three distinct phases. During the prodromal phase, the patient may experience an aura. Fifteen percent of migraine patients experience an aura.[5] Author Lewis Carroll saw the distorted figures in *Alice in Wonderland* as part of a migraine attack. Most auras are visual; however, any sign or symptom of brain dysfunction can be a feature of an aura. During the second phase, inflammation and cerebral vasodilation cause the characteristic headache. The third phase, or the recovery phase, is characterized by extreme temporal and cranial tenderness. Migraines can be caused by changes in sleep patterns, physical exertion, sudden changes in barometric pressure, increased stress, dieting, heat, lights, cyclic estrogen levels, and certain foods, such as alcohol, caffeine, monosodium glutamate, ripened cheeses, and coffee.

Pharmacologic therapy used during a migraine attack includes analgesics, antiinflammatory agents, β-adrenergic blockers, serotonin antagonists, vasoconstrictors, and antidepressants. Diuretics, antihistamines, anticonvulsants, and short courses of steroids may be used. Female patients with migraines should avoid oral contraceptives. Other interventions include biofeedback, relaxation training, assertiveness training, family counseling, dietary counseling, allergy testing, and education.

Temporal arteritis. Temporal arteritis, inflammation of branches of the carotid artery, usually occurs in patients over 50 years of age. Women are affected four times more often than men. Headache is the most frequent and severe symptom. Pain is severe and stabbing in one or both temporal regions with decreased visual acuity. The patient may have difficulty sleeping and opening or closing the mouth because of pain. Weight loss, night sweats, aching joints, fever, and red nodules over the temporal region also occur. Untreated, this condition can result in blindness. Definitive diagnosis is biopsy of the temporal artery. ED management includes steroids and pain management with antiinflammatory drugs or stronger agents as necessary.[5]

Table **37-5**	**Types of Vascular Migraine Headaches**
Type	Description
Classic migraine	Aura that lasts 15-20 min; clears more quickly than it develops; severe pain, usually unilateral, can be bilateral; lasts 30 min to several days; photophobia, sound sensitivity, nausea, vomiting, and anorexia; worsened by walking, straining, or sudden changes in body position; occurs during increased stress and pregnancy *Treatment* includes ergotamines, sumatriptan (Imitrex)
Common migraine	Euphoria, hunger, depression, irritability, intense yawning, generalized edema, and photophobia present; usually does not occur in pregnancy *Treatment* includes ergotamines, sumatriptan
Cluster headache	Ten times more common in men; closely grouped attacks over several weeks followed by remission of months or years; may have 12 or more headaches per day; more frequent in spring and fall; excruciating, unilateral pain, usually behind eye or in temporal region; may travel to ear, nose, and cheek; facial flushing, nasal congestion, lacrimation, rhinorrhea, and salivation may be present; may wake patient from deep sleep or occur during periods of rest after exhaustion *Treatment* includes oxygen, ergotamines, sumatriptan, prednisone, and in some cases, lithium
Opthalmoplegic migraine	Begin during infancy or early childhood; headache and paralysis of cranial nerve III; if untreated, prominent visual field defects or blindness may occur *Treatment* includes ergotamines, sumatriptan, and steroids
Hemiplegic migraine	Visual field defects, numbness of mouth and/or extremities, and various paresthesias; unilateral extremity weakness or paralysis; family history positive for migraine *Treatment* includes rest, sedation, analgesia, and increasing CO_2 levels; ergotamines contraindicated
Facial migraine	Unilateral episodic facial pain; associated with cluster headache or common migraine
Migraine equivalent	All features of migraine present except headache; symptoms include vomiting, abdominal migraines, menstrual syndromes, precordial migraines, and periodic diarrhea, fever, mood changes, and sleep or trancelike states

Seizures

Approximately 1% to 2% of the U.S. population have a seizure disorder.[5] Seizure is a symptom of an underlying problem rather than an independent diagnosis. Defined as an abnormal period of electrical activity in the brain, seizures are classified as partial, generalized, or unclassified. Unclassified seizures are seizures that do not fall into other categories.

Initial treatment focuses on protection of the patient's ABCs and prevention of injury during the seizure. Oxygen therapy should be initiated and intravenous access obtained. Glucose level should be checked immediately since hypoglycemia may cause seizures. Additional treatment depends on the type of seizure and the underlying cause. Intravenous midazolam (Versed), diazepam (Valium), and lorazepam (Ativan) in conjunction with intravenous phenobarbital and phenytoin (Dilantin) are used to control seizure activity. Dextrose 50% and naloxone are administered as indicated.

Partial seizures. Partial, or focal, seizures are limited to one specific body part and may be further classified as simple or complex. The patient's mental status is not affected in a simple partial seizure, whereas there is loss of consciousness in a complex partial seizure. A partial seizure may consist of focal motor activity, somatic sensory symptoms, or disturbances in the patient's vision, hearing, smell, or taste. Focal motor activity may occur in a specific area or begin in one area and progress to surrounding areas in an organized manner (Jacksonian seizure). Somatic sensory symptoms include tingling or numbness.

Temporal lobe seizures are often preceded by an aura, such as foul smell, metallic or bitter taste, buzzing, ringing, or hissing sounds, or vague visceral feelings in the chest and abdomen. Feelings of familiarity in an unfamiliar setting (deja vu) or unfamiliarity in a familiar setting (jamais vu) have been reported. The most characteristic symptom of temporal lobe seizure is semipurposeful patterns of movement (automatism) such as lip-smacking, chewing, patting hands, or facial grimacing.

Partial seizures can occur with secondary generalized seizures. Seizure activity originates locally and progresses until the entire body is involved. There is an associated loss of consciousness.

Generalized seizures. There are two major types of generalized seizures—absence (petit mal) and tonic-clonic (grand mal) seizures. Absence seizures usually occur in children 4 to 12 years of age. Episodes are characterized by abrupt cessation of activity with momentary loss of consciousness, duration of less than 15 seconds, and may be accompanied by automatism.

Tonic-clonic seizures begin with sudden loss of consciousness and major tonic contractions of large muscle groups. Arms and legs extend stiffly as the person falls to the ground. A shrill cry may precede the event. During the tonic phase, the person is apneic, pupils are dilated and unresponsive, and bowel and bladder incontinence occur. The individual may also bite his or her tongue. During the clonic phase, strenuous, rhythmic muscle contractions occur. Hyperventilation, profuse sweating, tachycardia, and excessive salivation with frothing are usually present. A postictal phase follows as muscles relax. Deep breathing and a depressed level of consciousness are present. The person awakens confused with complaints of headache, muscle aching, and fatigue. There is generalized amnesia concerning the event and the person may sleep for hours afterward.

Status epilepticus. Status epilepticus is a series of consecutive seizures or one seizure that does not respond to conventional therapy. Uncontrolled seizure activity increases the patient's temperature, blood pressure, and pulse, interferes with cerebral blood flow, and increases the risk for hypoxic brain damage. Control of seizure activity is critical. Therapeutic interventions begin with the ABCs. Endotracheal intubation is used to maintain the airway and oxygenate the patient. Protect the patient from injury with restraints and other seizure precautions. Naloxone, dextrose 50%, and thiamine may be given. Sedation and anticonvulsant medications are given until seizure activity is controlled. If these medications fail, general anesthesia is considered.

Stroke

Decreased cerebral blood flow or cerebral perfusion pressure deprives the brain of oxygen and glucose. This leads to cellular ischemia and, ultimately, cerebral infarction. Strokes may be ischemic or hemorrhagic. Eighty percent to 85% of all strokes are ischemic.[5] Ischemic strokes are caused by occlusion of cerebral vessels by a thrombus or embolus. Hemorrhagic strokes occur with ruptured aneurysms, leaking venous malformations, or subarachnoid hemorrhage. Factors that increase the patient's risk of stroke are hypertension, diabetes mellitus, atherosclerosis, cardiac valve disease, and smoking. Approximately 500,000 Americans suffer a stroke each year, with a 20% mortality rate the first year.[5]

Approximately half of all strokes are caused by cerebral thrombosis. Thrombotic strokes occur as atherosclerotic plaque accumulates within the vessel. Carotid stenosis is a major cause of thrombotic stroke. Symptoms occur slowly as cerebral blood flow gradually decreases. Neurologic deficits depend on the area of the brain affected. Embolic strokes occur when a free-floating substance travels to the brain and occludes a vessel. Substances tend to fragment as they float, so multiple areas of the brain are affected. Multifocal neurologic deficits occur. Free-floating substances include blood clots, tumor particles, fat, air, or vegetation from a diseased heart valve. Patients with atrial fibrillation are at risk for embolic stroke because of formation of clots on the mitral valve.

Cerebral infarction, or stroke, may occur anywhere in the brain. Symptoms and lethality are determined by the location and size of the infarction. Surrounding the area of infarction is an area of ischemia called the penumbra.[3] Recog-

Table **37-6**	**Stroke Classification**
Type	Description
Transient ischemic attack (TIA)	Temporary disturbance of blood supply causes transient neurologic deficit; symptoms present less than 24 hrs; no permanent neurologic deficit
Reversible ischemic neurologic deficit	Neurologic deficits last a few days or weeks; minimal permanent neurologic deficits
Stroke in evolution	Progressive neurologic deterioration occurs; residual neurologic deficit present
Completed stroke	Patient appears stable with neurologic deficit permanent and unchanging

Table **37-7**	**Selected Agents for Treatment of Stroke**
Category	Agents*
Thrombolytic Agents	rt-PA, recombinant prurokinase
Anti-thrombotic agents	Fraxiparine
Antioxidants	PNA
NMDA receptor antagonists	Cerestat, ACPC, ACEA, GV150526
Opiate Antagonists	Cervene
GABA-A Agonists	Chlomethiazole
Defibrinogenating agents	Ancrod
Other neuroprotective agents	Enlimomab, Citicoline, Lubeluzole, Calpain inhibitors, Kinase inhibitors

*Includes agents currently in use and those under investigation.
Data from National Stroke Association: *The stroke/brain attack reporter's handbook*, Englewood, Colo, 1997, The Association.

nition and treatment of stroke focus on preservation and reperfusion of this ischemic area to prevent further cellular destruction. Duration of symptoms is a crucial factor in treatment. Table 37-6 describes four types of strokes by duration of symptoms.

Treatment of stroke patients begins with the ABCs. Significant respiratory impairment occurs when the stroke affects the respiratory center. The unconscious patient or one who is unable to manage oral secretions is also at risk for respiratory compromise. Endotracheal intubation may be required to ensure a patient's airway. If the patient is hypertensive ($\geq$220 mm Hg systolic, or $\geq$120 mm Hg diastolic), antihypertensive agents should be used. However, precipitous reduction of blood pressure is not recommended. Sudden rapid decrease in blood pressure can impair cerebral perfusion, reducing perfusion to the penumbra, thereby converting an area of ischemia to an area of infarction.[5]

Identification of stroke type is critical to successful treatment. Computed tomography (CT) scans are used to determine if the stroke is hemorrhagic or ischemic. This is essential since treatment for ischemic stroke, that is, anticoagulant therapy, is contraindicated in hemorrhagic stroke. In a few centers, thrombolytic agents are used to treat thromboembolic strokes. Hemorrhagic stroke usually requires surgical intervention to control hemorrhage and manage increased ICP.

A number of neuroprotective agents have been approved for use in cases of ischemic stroke. These agents preserve cerebral function by increasing perfusion of the penumbra.[2] Mechanism of action varies with type of agent. Table 37-7 reviews medications currently being studied. Some agents remove oxygen radicals, whereas others increase movement of calcium across the cell membrane. Agents are usually time-limited, that is, must be given within 6 to 12 hours of symptom onset. As more research occurs in this area, addi-

tional agents with a bigger window of opportunity for administration are anticipated.

Meningitis

Meningitis is inflammation of the meningeal layers surrounding the brain and spinal cord; it is a neurologic emergency and an infectious disease emergency. Infection may be viral, bacterial, or fungal. Viral meningitis is usually less acute with gradual onset of symptoms. Bacterial meningitis has acute onset of symptoms and is fatal in 50% of the patients. Common bacterial agents include *Streptococcus pneumoniae, Neisseria meningitides, Haemophilus influenzae,* group B streptococci, and *Listeria monocytogenes.*

Classic symptoms of meningitis are fever, headache, photophobia, nuchal rigidity, lethargy, seizures, vomiting, and chills. The patient may arrive at the ED with mild headache and severe confusion, or comatose with shock. Patients with meningococcemia may have purpura, petechiae, splinter hemorrhages, and pustular lesions.

Diagnosis is confirmed with lumbar puncture (LP) and CSF cultures. If a brain abscess is suspected, LP is contraindicated due to the potential for herniation. A CT scan may be obtained before the LP. Treatment includes support of the patient's ABCs, immediate administration of appropriate antibiotics, antipyretics, and anticonvulsants as indicated. Serial neurologic assessment is critical to identify changes in level of consciousness. The patient with bacterial meningitis should be isolated. Prophylactic antibiotics are given for intimate contact or documented exposure such as needle stick.

Guillain-Barré Syndrome

Guillain-Barré syndrome is an acute paralytic disease caused by decreased myelin at the nerve roots and in peripheral nerves. Individuals in their 20s and 30s are affected most often. Symptoms usually follow an acute febrile episode.[5] Signs and symptoms are tingling sensation in the extremities lasting for hours to weeks, severely decreased deep tendon reflexes, and a symmetrical paralysis that begins in the lower extremities and ascends. Paralysis eventually affects the diaphragm and intercostal muscles, causing respiratory paralysis and death. Emergency management focuses on support of the ABCs. Endotracheal intubation and ventilator support are often required. Provide general supportive care until the disease has run its course. Patients who survive this disease usually require a long program of rehabilitation.

Myasthenia Gravis

Myasthenia gravis, a defect in neuromuscular transmission, occurs more frequently in women and can occur at any age, but is predominant in adults age 20 to 30 years (an estimated 5 to 10 cases per 100,000 population).[5] In a crisis state, onset may be sudden, causing respiratory paralysis and arrest. Patients experience increasing fatigue; delayed muscle strength recovery; weak eye, facial, and jaw muscles; weak pharyngeal muscles; diplopia; dysphagia; and inability to swallow. Therapeutic intervention is support of ABCs, with possible endotracheal intubation and ventilator management. Pharmacologic therapy is neostigmine (Prostigmin), 1 mg IV, for crisis states, barbiturates, opiates, quinidine, quinine, corticotropin, corticosteroids, aminoglycosides, antibiotics, and muscle relaxants. Differentiation of "myasthenic crisis" from "cholinergic crisis" may be accomplished with administration of edrophonium, an anticholinesterase inhibitor. If the patient's condition worsens after edrophonium, cholinergic crisis should be suspected.[5]

SUMMARY

Neurologic emergencies represent a significant challenge for the emergency nurse. Life-threatening neurologic emergencies require rapid, organized assessment with simultaneous intervention. Patients with neurologic problems that are not life-threatening may fear loss of function or cognitive ability, or pain. Patients require supportive, therapeutic care

Box **37-3**

> **NURSING DIAGNOSES FOR NEUROLOGIC EMERGENCIES**
>
> Altered tissue perfusion
> Ineffective breathing pattern
> Pain
> Fear
> Anxiety
> Impaired verbal communication

to minimize discomfort and facilitate recovery. Box 37-3 summarizes nursing diagnoses for patients with neurologic emergencies.

Management of neurologic emergencies is undergoing rapid change. Old treatments such as hyperventilation to decrease ICP are being questioned. Research in management of stroke and preservation of cerebral function in other neurologic problems, for example, head injury, is rapidly changing. Changes represent an opportunity for improved patient outcomes with decreased mortality and morbidity. Diligence by the emergency nurse is essential to maintain a current knowledge base in the face of this rapidly changing information.

REFERENCES

1. Guyton AC, Hall JE: *Textbook of medical physiology,* ed 9, Philadelphia, 1996, WB Saunders.
2. Hilton G: Experimental neuroprotective agents: nursing challenge, *Dimen Crit Care Nurs* 14(4):181,
3. National Stroke Association: *Stroke/brain attack,* Englewood, Colo, 1994, The Association.
4. Rakel RE: *Conn's current therapy,* Philadelphia, 1997, WB Saunders.
5. Tintinalli JE, Ruiz E, Krome RL: *Emergency medicine: a comprehensive study guide,* ed 4, New York, 1996, McGraw-Hill.

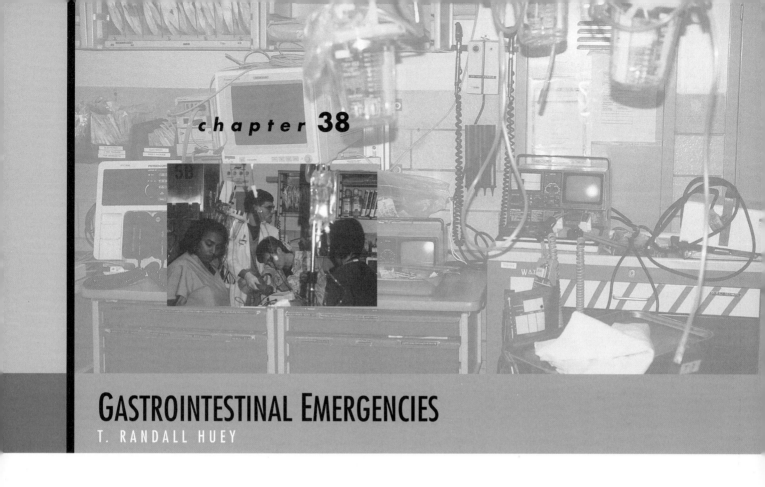

chapter 38

GASTROINTESTINAL EMERGENCIES
T. RANDALL HUEY

Gastrointestinal (GI) emergencies are a common reason for emergency department (ED) visits. GI emergencies vary from minor problems to more serious, potentially life-threatening problems. Cardinal symptoms that alert the emergency nurse to a problem in the GI system include heartburn, nausea, vomiting, constipation, diarrhea, belching, bloating, chest pain, abdominal pain, and bleeding.[13] A brief review of anatomy and physiology is followed by discussion of specific GI conditions, that is, gastroenteritis, gastrointestinal bleeding, appendicitis, cholecystitis, pancreatitis, and bowel obstruction.

ANATOMY AND PHYSIOLOGY

Normal GI function utilizes ingested nutrients and fluids, then eliminates waste products formed from metabolic activities. Major organs and structures of the GI system are the esophagus, stomach, intestines, liver, pancreas, gallbladder, and peritoneum (Figure 38-1).

Esophagus

The esophagus is a straight, collapsible tube approximately 25 cm long and up to 3 cm in diameter that extends from pharynx to stomach. Distinct esophageal layers are the mucous membrane, submucosa, and muscular layer. Secretions from mucous glands scattered throughout the submucosa keep the inner lining moist and lubricated. Striated muscle in the upper esophagus is gradually replaced by smooth muscle in the lower esophagus and GI tract. The up-

per esophageal sphincter is at the proximal end of the esophagus, and the lower esophageal sphincter (also known as the cardiac sphincter) is at the distal junction of the esophagus and stomach. The lower esophageal sphincter prevents regurgitation from the stomach into the esophagus. The major function of the esophagus is movement of food.

Stomach

Stomach functions include food storage, combining food with gastric juices, limited absorption, and moving food into the small intestine. The stomach is a J-shaped organ located below the diaphragm between the esophagus and small intestine. Identified regions of the stomach are pylorus, fundus, body, and antrum (Figure 38-2). The pyloric sphincter controls food movement from stomach to duodenum. Distinct layers of the stomach wall are outer serosa, muscular layer, submucosa, and mucosa. The mucosal layer contains multiple wrinkles called rugae that straighten as the stomach fills to accommodate more volume. Completely relaxed, the stomach holds up to 1.5 L.[7] Glands secrete gastric juices containing pepsin, hydrochloric acid, mucus, and intrinsic factor, which begin food breakdown. Acids in the stomach maintain the pH of gastric juices at 1.0.

Intestines

The small intestine is a tubular organ extending from the pyloric sphincter to the proximal large intestine. Secretions from the pancreas and liver complete digestion of nutrients

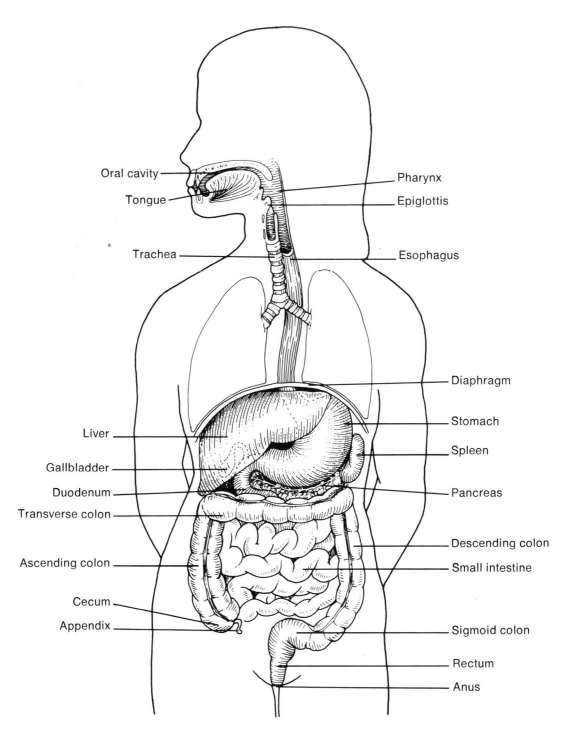

Figure **38-1** Anatomy of the gastrointestinal system. *(From Society of Gastroenterology Nurses and Associates [SGNA]: Gastroenterology nursing: a core curriculum, St. Louis, 1993, Mosby.)*

in chyme, the semiliquid mixture consisting of food and gastric secretions. The small intestine absorbs nutrients and other products of digestion and transports residue to the large intestine. The segments of the small intestine are the duodenum, jejunum, and ileum. The duodenum attaches to the stomach at the pyloric sphincter in the retroperitoneal space and represents the only fixed portion of the small

intestine. The duodenum is approximately 25 cm long and 5 cm in diameter. The jejunum and ileum are mobile and lie free in the peritoneal cavity.

The segments of the large intestine are the cecum, colon, rectum, and anal canal. The large intestine is approximately 1.5 m long, beginning in the lower right side of the abdomen where ileum joins cecum. The colon is divided into ascend-

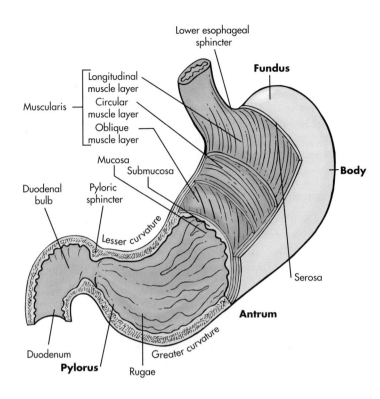

Figure **38-2** Parts of the stomach. *(From Lewis SM, Collier IC, Heitkemper MM:* Medical-surgical nursing: assessment and management of clinical problems, *ed 4, St. Louis, 1996, Mosby.)*

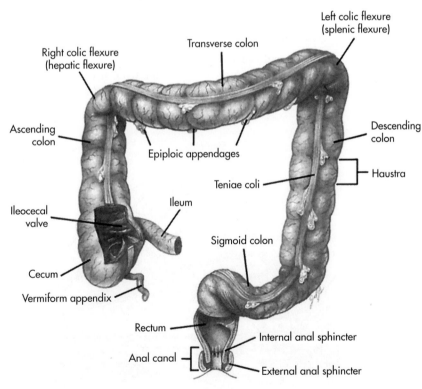

Figure **38-3** Large intestine showing the ascending colon, transverse colon, descending colon, and sigmoid colon. *(From Seeley RR, Stephens TD, Tate P:* Anatomy and physiology, *ed 3, New York, 1995, McGraw-Hill.)*

ing colon, transverse colon, descending colon, and sigmoid colon (Figure 38-3). Primary functions of the large intestine are absorption of water and electrolytes, formation of feces, and storage of feces. Approximately 1500 ml of chyme pass through the ileocecal valve each day.[7]

Liver

The liver is in the right upper quadrant of the abdomen and is divided into right and left lobes (Figure 38-4). Functional units of the liver are lobules, which contain sinusoids and Kupffer cells. Each lobule is supplied by a hepatic artery, sublobular vein, bile duct, and lymph channel (Figure 38-5). The liver is extremely vascular; approximately 1450 ml of blood flow through the liver each minute, accounting for 29% of resting cardiac output.[7] Sinusoids in lobules act as a reservoir for overflow of blood and fluids from the right ventricle.

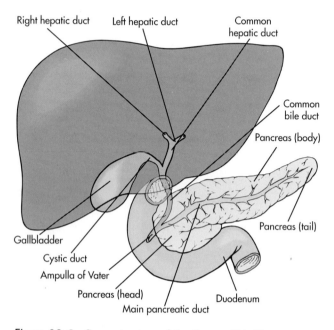

Figure **38-4** Gross structure of the liver, gallbladder, pancreas, and duct system. *(From Lewis SM, Collier IC, Heitkemper MM: Medical-surgical nursing: assessment and management of clinical problems, ed 4, St. Louis, 1996, Mosby.)*

Figure **38-5** Microscopic structure of liver lobule. *(Redrawn from Bloom W, Fawcett DW: A textbook of histology, ed 10, Philadelphia, 1975, WB Saunders. In Berne RM, Levy MN, editors:* Principles of physiology, *ed 3, St. Louis, 1993, Mosby.)*

A thick capsule of connective tissue known as Glisson's capsule covers the liver. The liver is involved in hundreds of metabolic functions including metabolism of nutrients, gluconeogenesis, and drug metabolism. Table 38-1 summarizes functions related to nutrition and waste removal. Production of bile is a major function of the liver, which secretes 600 to 1200 ml of bile per day. Bile is essential for digestion, absorption, and excretion of bilirubin and excess cholesterol. Bilirubin is an end product of hemoglobin destruction. Figure 38-6 illustrates processes involved in bilirubin conjugation.

Pancreas

The pancreas, a lobulated organ behind the stomach, contains endocrine and exocrine cells. The organ is divided into the head, body, and a thin, narrow tail (Figure 38-7). Cells in the islets of Langerhans secrete insulin and regulate glucose levels. Exocrine cells called pancreatic acini secrete pancreatic juices for digestion of fats, carbohydrates, proteins, and nucleic acids. Pancreatic enzymes, that is, lipase and amylase, enter the intestines through the pancreatic duct at the same juncture as the bile duct from the liver and gallbladder. Pancreatic and bile ducts join at a short dilated tube called the ampulla of Vater. A band of smooth muscles called the sphincter of Oddi surrounds this area and controls the exit of pancreatic juices and bile.

Gallbladder

The gallbladder is a pear-shaped sac located in a depression on the inferior surface of the liver. It's main functions are collection, concentration, and storage of bile. Maximum

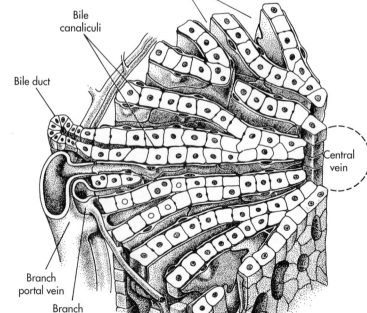

Table **38-1**	**Major Functions of the Liver**
Function	Description
Metabolic functions	
Carbohydrate metabolism	Glycogenesis (conversion of glucose to glycogen), glycogenolysis (process of breaking down glycogen to glucose), gluconeogenesis (formation of glucose from amino acids and fatty acids)
Protein metabolism	Synthesis of nonessential amino acids, synthesis of plasma proteins (except γ-globulin), synthesis of clotting factors, urea formation from NH_3 (NH_3 formed from deamination of amino acids and by action of bacteria on proteins in colon)
Fat metabolism	Synthesis of lipoproteins, breakdown of triglycerides into fatty acids and glycerol, formation of ketone bodies, synthesis of fatty acids from amino acids and glucose, synthesis and breakdown of cholesterol
Detoxification	Inactivation of drugs and harmful substances and excretion of their breakdown products
Steroid metabolism	Conjugation and excretion of gonadal and adrenal steroids
Bile synthesis	
Bile production	Formation of bile, containing bile salts, bile pigments (mainly bilirubin), and cholesterol
Bile excretion	Bile excretion by liver about 1 L/day
Storage	Glucose in form of glycogen; vitamins, including fat-soluble (A, D, E, K) and water-soluble (B_1, B_2, B_{12}, and folic acid); fatty acids; minerals (iron and copper); amino acids in form of albumin and β globulins
Mononuclear phagocyte system	
Kupffer cells	Breakdown of old RBCs, WBCs, bacteria, and other particles, breakdown of hemoglobin from old RBCs to bilirubin and biliverdin

From Lewis SM, Collier IC, Heitkemper MM: *Medical-surgical nursing: assessment and management of clinical problems,* ed 4, St. Louis, 1996, Mosby.
RBC, Red blood cell; *WBC,* white blood cell.

volume is 30 to 60 ml; however, input from the liver can reach 450 ml over 12 hours. Concentration of bile in the gallbladder can be 5 to 20 times that of bile in the liver.[7] Bile is 80% water, 10% bile acids, 4% to 5% phospholipid, and 1% cholesterol.[20]

Peritoneum

The peritoneum is a serous membrane covering liver, spleen, stomach, and intestines that acts as a semipermeable membrane, contains pain receptors, and provides proliferative cellular protection. Technically, all abdominal organs are behind the peritoneum and therefore are retroperitoneal; however, the liver, spleen, stomach, and intestines are suspended into the peritoneum and considered intraperitoneal organs. Omenta are folds of peritoneum that surround the stomach and adjacent organs. The greater omentum, which drapes the transverse colon and loops of small intestine, is extremely mobile, and spreads easily into areas of injury to seal off potential sources of infection. The lesser omentum covers parts of the stomach and proximal intestines and is not as movable as the greater omentum.

The peritoneum is permeable to fluid, electrolytes, urea, and toxins. Somatic afferent nerves sensitize the peritoneum to all types of stimuli. In acute abdominal conditions, the peritoneum can localize an irritable focus by producing sharp pain and tenderness, voluntary or involuntary abdominal muscle rigidity, and rebound tenderness.

PATIENT ASSESSMENT

Assessment of a patient with a GI emergency should initially focus on airway, breathing, and circulation (ABCs) with primary survey completed prior to focused assessment. After assessment and stabilization of ABCs, chief complaint, social or medical history, reason for seeking treatment, and treatment prior to arrival should be elicited from the patient, family members, significant other, friends, or EMS personnel.[8] Historical assessment should include questions related to gynecologic and genitourinary symptoms, since many gynecologic or GU conditions cause abdominal pain, nausea, and vomiting. Information related to food intake and alcohol consumption should be obtained during assessment of patient history.

Evaluate the patient for abnormal skin color, abdominal wall abnormalities, pain, and alterations in bowel patterns. Abdominal pain is a common chief complaint in the ED, caused by an acute event or chronic process. Abdominal pain may be visceral, somatic, or referred.

Visceral pain, caused by stretching of hollow viscus, is described as cramping or a sensation of gas. Pain intensifies, then decreases, and is usually centered on the umbilicus or below the midline. Diffuse pain makes localization of pain difficult. Diaphoresis, nausea, vomiting, hypotension, tachycardia, and abdominal wall spasms may be present. Conditions associated with visceral pain are appendicitis, acute pancreatitis, cholecystitis, and intestinal obstruction.

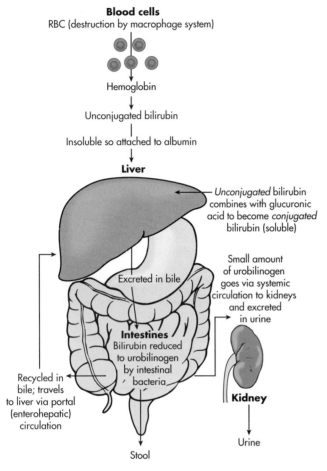

Blood cells
RBC (destruction by macrophage system)

Hemoglobin

Unconjugated bilirubin

Insoluble so attached to albumin

Liver

Unconjugated bilirubin combines with glucuronic acid to become *conjugated* bilirubin (soluble)

Excreted in bile

Small amount of urobilinogen goes via systemic circulation to kidneys and excreted in urine

Intestines
Bilirubin reduced to urobilinogen by intestinal bacteria

Recycled in bile; travels to liver via portal (enterohepatic) circulation

Kidney

Stool

Urine

Figure **38-6** Bilirubin metabolism and conjugation. *(From Lewis SM, Collier IC, Heitkemper MM: Medical-surgical nursing: assessment and management of clinical problems, ed 4, St. Louis, 1996, Mosby.)*

Somatic pain is produced by bacterial or chemical irritation of nerve fibers. Pain is sharp and usually localized to one area. A patient lies with legs flexed and knees pulled to the chest to prevent stimulation of the peritoneum and subsequent increase in pain. Associated findings include involuntary guarding and rebound tenderness.

Referred pain occurs at a distance from the original source of the pain and is thought to be caused by the development of nerve tracts during fetal growth and development. Biliary pain can be referred to the subscapular area, whereas peptic ulcer can cause back pain.

Assessment of abdominal pain must consider individual and cultural variations in expressions of pain. Each person reacts differently to pain. Elderly patients may not exhibit the same level of pain as younger patients and men may hide pain because expression of pain is not considered masculine in many cultures. Dramatic expression of pain may be expected in some cultures. Emergency nurses must remember that pain is a symptom—not a diagnosis. Interventions should focus on identification and treatment of the source of pain.

Table 38-2   PQRST Assessment of Abdominal Pain

Component	Description
Provocation	What makes pain better? Worse? Position? Vomiting?
Quality or character	What does pain feel like? Burning? Tight? Crushing? Tearing? Pressure? Cramping?
Radiation, location, referral	Where does pain radiate? Where is it most intense? Where does it start?
Severity	How severe is pain on a scale of 0 to 10?
Time	When did pain start? When did it end? How long did it last?

A systematic approach is recommended for assessment of abdominal pain. The PQRST mnemonic can be used to obtain appropriate historical information (Table 38-2). Identification of essential characteristics of pain such as location, description, and provocation, provides valuable clues to etiology of pain. Potential causes based on location of pain are listed in Table 38-3; Table 38-4 reviews pain descriptions associated with certain clinical conditions.

Abdominal assessment uses a sequence of inspection, auscultation, percussion, and palpation. Patient position should be noted, since patients assume positions of comfort. Observe facial expression for signs of discomfort. Note skin color, temperature, and moisture. Inspect abdominal wall for pulsations, movement, masses, symmetry, or surgical scars.

Auscultate bowel sounds in all four quadrants, determining frequency, quality, and pitch. Normal bowel sounds are irregular, high-pitched gurgling sounds occurring 5 to 35 times per minute. Decreased or absent bowel sounds suggest peritonitis or paralytic ileus whereas hyperactive bowel sounds associated with nausea, vomiting, and diarrhea suggest gastroenteritis. Frequent, high-pitched bowel sounds occur with bowel obstruction. Vascular sounds such as venous hums or bruits are abnormal findings.

Percussion should be performed in all four quadrants. Dull sounds occur over solid organs or tumors whereas tympanic sounds occur over air masses. Tympany is the normal sound heard when percussing the abdomen.

Palpation is the last step in abdominal assessment. Initially, palpate in an area away from areas of pain, noting areas of tenderness, guarding, or rigidity. Assess for abnormal masses and rebound tenderness.

Concurrent findings include fever and chills usually found with bacterial infection, appendicitis, or cholecystitis. Other signs associated with pain are nausea, vomiting, and anorexia. Intractable vomiting or feces in emesis suggest bowel obstruction. Blood in emesis occurs with gastritis or upper gastrointestinal bleeding. Assess bowel patterns for

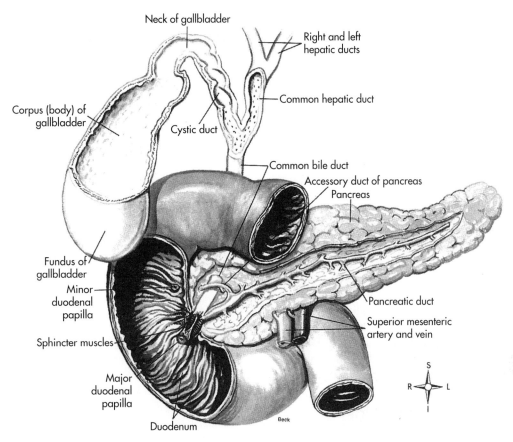

Figure **38-7** Associated structures of the gallbladder and exocrine pancreas. *(From Huether SE, McCance KL:* Understanding pathophysiology, *St. Louis, 1996, Mosby.)*

Table **38-3** **Potential Sources of Abdominal Pain by Location**

Location	Potential cause	
Right upper quadrant	Cholecystitis	Hepatomegaly
	Hepatic abscess	Pancreatic abscess
	Hepatitis	Duodenal ulcer perforation
Left upper quadrant	Pancreatitis	Left lung pneumonia
	Splenic rupture	Right renal pain
	Myocardial infarction	Pericarditis
	Gastritis	Right lung pneumonia
	Left renal pain	
Right lower quadrant	Appendicitis	Ovarian cyst
	Cholecystitis	Pelvic inflammatory disease
	Perforated ulcer	Endometriosis
	Intestinal obstruction	Right ureteral calculi
	Meckel's diverticulum	Incarcerated hernia
	Abdominal aortic aneurysm dissection or rupture	Gastric ulcer perforation
	Ruptured ectopic pregnancy	Colon perforation
	Twisted right ovary	
Left lower quadrant	Appendicitis	Pelvic inflammatory disease
	Intestinal obstruction	Endometriosis
	Diverticulum of the sigmoid colon	Left ureteral calculi
	Ruptured ectopic pregnancy	Left renal pain
	Twisted left ovary	Incarcerated hernia
	Ovarian cyst	Perforated descending colon
		Regional enteritis

Table 38-4	Description of Pain Associated With Certain Clinical Conditions
Pain description	**Associated clinical conditions**
Severe sharp pain	Infarction or rupture
Severe pain controlled by medication	Pancreatitis, peritonitis, small bowel obstruction, renal colic, biliary colic
Dull pain	Inflammation, low-grade infection
Intermittent pain	Gastroenteritis, small-bowel obstruction

abnormalities such as diarrhea or constipation, noting stool color and consistency. Diarrhea occurs with gastroenteritis; black, tarry stools suggest upper GI bleeding; and clay-colored stools are found with biliary tract obstruction. Fatty, foul-smelling, frothy stools occur with pancreatitis. Box 38-1 presents pertinent historical data related to assessment of diarrhea, Box 38-2 reviews causes of diarrhea, and Table 38-5 describes causes of infectious diarrhea.

SPECIFIC GASTROINTESTINAL EMERGENCIES

Specific GI emergencies may be caused by infection, structural abnormalities, or various pathologic processes. Heredity and lifestyle also play a role in the occurrence of GI emergencies. Excessive alcohol consumption can lead to GI bleeding, cirrhosis, or esophageal varices.

Gastrointestinal Bleeding

Bleeding can originate anywhere in the GI tract and occur at any age. The age group most often affected is individuals 50 to 80 years of age. Bleeding is functionally categorized by location as upper or lower GI bleeding. Figure 38-8 highlights various sites and causes of GI bleeding. Upper GI bleeding is more common in males, whereas lower GI bleeding is seen more often in females. Patients may have bright red blood from mouth or rectum or black, tarry stools. Bleeding stops spontaneously in 80% of hospitalized patients.[9]

Upper GI bleeding. Upper GI bleeding refers to blood loss between the upper esophagus and duodenum at the ligament of Treitz. Bleeding is categorized as variceal or nonvariceal. Gastroesophageal varices are enlarged, venous channels dilated by portal hypertension. As portal hypertension increases, varices continue to enlarge and eventually rupture, causing massive hemorrhage. The number one cause of portal hypertension in the United States is alcoholic cirrhosis, whereas schistosomiasis is the leading cause worldwide. Figure 38-9 highlights systemic manifestations of cirrhosis.

Nonvariceal bleeding is disruption of esophageal or gastroduodenal mucosa with ulceration or erosion into an un-

Box 38-1	Historical Information Relevant to Diarrhea

Character of stools
Amount
Consistency
Color
Odor
Mucus
Blood
Pus

Temporal characteristics
Acute
Chronic
Recurrent
Frequency
Time of day
Nocturnal
Duration
Urgency
Relationship to meals

Exogenous factors
Diet
Medications
Travel
Emotional stress
Exposure to others with same symptoms
Poisons/toxins
Operations
Irradiation
Institutionalization
Sexual habits
Daily activities

Associated symptoms
Fever
Anorexia
Nausea
Vomiting
Constipation
Flatulence
Abdominal pain
Tenesmus
Weight loss
Fluid intake and urine flow

Related past history
Known gastrointestinal disease
Acute cardiorespiratory disease
Acute central nervous system (CNS) disease
Endocrine
  Hyperthyroidism
  Hypoparathyroidism
  Diabetes mellitus
Adrenal insufficiency
Uremia

From Rosen P et al: *Emergency medicine*, vol 2, ed 3, St. Louis, 1992, Mosby.

| Box **38-2** | **Causes of Diarrhea** |

Decreased fluid absorption

Oral intake of poorly absorbable solutes (e.g., laxatives)

Maldigestion and malabsorption

Mucosal damage: tropical sprue, Crohn's disease, radiation injury, ulcerative colitis, ischemic bowel disease

Pancreatic insufficiency

Intestinal enzyme deficiencies (e.g., lactase)

Bile salt deficiency

Decreased surface area (e.g., intestinal resection)

Increased fluid secretion

Infectious: bacterial endotoxins (e.g., cholera, *Escherichia coli, Shigella, Salmonella, Staphylococcus, Clostridium difficile,* viral agents [rotavirus], and parasitic agents *[Giardia lamblia]*)

Drugs: laxatives, antibiotics

Hormonal: vasoactive intestinal polypeptide secretion from adenoma of the pancreas; gastrin secretion caused by Zollinger-Ellison syndrome; calcitonin secretion from carcinoma of the thyroid

Tumor: villous adenoma

Motility disturbances

Irritable bowel syndrome

Diabetic enteropathy

Visceral scleroderma

Carcinoid syndrome

Vagotomy

From Lewis SM, Collier IC, Heitkemper MM: *Medical-surgical nursing: assessment and management of clinical problems,* ed 4, St. Louis, 1996, Mosby.

derlying vein or artery. Ulcerations or erosions occur when hyperacidity, pepsin, or aspirin inhibit mucosal prostaglandins and overwhelm protective factors of the esophagus (i.e., esophageal motility, salivary secretions, and the lower esophageal sphincter) and gastric mucosa (i.e., mucus, rapid epithelial renewal, and tissue mediators). Common causes are drug-induced erosions and peptic ulcer disease, an infectious process caused by *Helicobacter pylori.*[12] Retching and vomiting seen with bulimia can also lead to upper GI bleeding.

Clinical signs and symptoms are variable. Presenting symptoms may include pallor, dizziness, weakness, and lethargy. Abdominal pain, nausea, vomiting, hematochezia, or melena can be present. Signs of hypovolemia such as tachycardia, orthostatic hypotension, and syncope may also occur. Mental confusion, jaundice, or ascites occur most often with variceal bleeding.

Management begins with maintenance of airway, breathing, and circulation (ABCs). Administer high-flow oxygen via nonrebreather mask for patients with hemodynamic compromise or decreased oxygen saturation. Fluid replacement begins with normal saline or Ringer's lactate solution followed by blood product (PRBCs or whole blood) replacement if the patient's condition does not improve. Cardiac monitor and continuous pulse oximetry are recommended for patients with significant blood loss or bright red bleeding. Elderly patients can have myocardial infarction secondary to ischemia caused by hypovolemia. Monitor vital signs and level of consciousness for signs of hemodynamic compromise. A nasogastric tube is inserted for gastric lavage with saline solution to remove blood clots. Lavage also clears the GI tract and facilitates endoscopy. Insert a urinary catheter to monitor output and fluid status.

Baseline laboratory values include complete blood count (CBC), type and cross-match (for a minimum of 2 units), electrolytes, blood urea nitrogen (BUN), creatinine, and serum glucose. Normal creatinine with increased BUN suggests bleeding with breakdown of blood in the gut, dehydration, or diuretic therapy. Liver function and coagulation studies are also recommended to rule out coagulopathies or liver disease. An upright chest radiograph can provide valuable information if perforation is suspected; however, this is not feasible if significant hemodynamic compromise is present. An electrocardiogram should be obtained to identify dysrhythmias or ischemic changes related to blood loss.

Additional treatment modalities include medications, endoscopic control of bleeding, and surgical interventions. Medical therapy for nonvariceal bleeding includes administration of antacids and H_2 antagonists (Table 38-6). Gastroesophageal variceal bleeding is treated with IV vasopressin (20 units in 200 ml saline at 0.25 to 0.5 units per minute) or Sengstaken-Blakemore, Minnesota, or Linton balloon tube to tamponade bleeding. Peptic ulcer disease is treated endoscopically with thermal coagulation or injection therapy, whereas gastroesophageal varices are treated endoscopically with injection sclerotherapy or variceal band ligation. Endoscopic procedures may be done on a limited basis in EDs across the country. Surgical intervention may be necessary for variceal or nonvariceal bleeding.[12,19] Complications related to upper GI bleeding include aspiration, pneumonia, respiratory failure, and hypovolemic shock.[14]

Lower GI bleeding. Lower GI bleeding is bleeding that occurs below the ligament of Treitz. Common causes are hemorrhoids, diverticulitis, angiodysplasia, colonic polyps, colon cancer, or colitis.[16] Diverticulosis and angiodysplasia are common causes of lower GI bleeding in the elderly, whereas hemorrhoids, anal fissures, and inflammatory bowel disease occur most often in younger patients.[3] Diverticulosis refers to pouchlike herniations on the colon (Figure 38-10). Figure 38-11 depicts internal and external hemorrhoidal veins, where hemorrhoids often erupt. Eighty-five percent of patients with lower GI bleeding experience acute

Table **38-5** **Causes of Acute Infectious Diarrhea**

	Onset	Duration	Symptoms and signs
Viral			
Rotavirus, Norwalk	18-24 hr	24-48 hr	Explosive, watery diarrhea; nausea; vomiting; abdominal cramps
Bacterial			
Escherichia coli	4-24 hr	3-4 days	Four or five loose stools per day, nausea, malaise, low-grade fever
Shigella	24 hr	7 days	Watery stools containing blood and mucus, fever, tenesmus, urgency
Salmonella	6-48 hr	2-5 days	Watery diarrhea, fever, nausea
Campylobacter species	24 hr	<7 days	Profuse, watery diarrhea; malaise; nausea; abdominal cramps; low-grade fever
Clostridium perfringens	8-12 hr	24 hr	Watery diarrhea, abdominal cramps, vomiting
Clostridium difficile toxin	4-9 days after start of antibiotics	1-3 wk	Associated with antibiotic treatment; symptoms range from mild, watery diarrhea to severe abdominal pain, fever, leukocytosis, hypoalbuminemia, leukocytes in stool
Parasitic			
Giardia lamblia	1-3 wk	Few days to 3 months	Sudden onset; foul, explosive, watery diarrhea; flatulence; epigastric pain and cramping; nausea
Entamoeba histolytica	4 days	Weeks to months	Frequent soft stools with blood and mucus (in severe cases, watery stools), flatulence, distention, cramping, fever, leukocytes in stool

From Lewis SM, Collier IC, Heitkemper MM: *Medical-surgical nursing: assessment and management of clinical problems,* ed 4, St. Louis, 1996, Mosby.

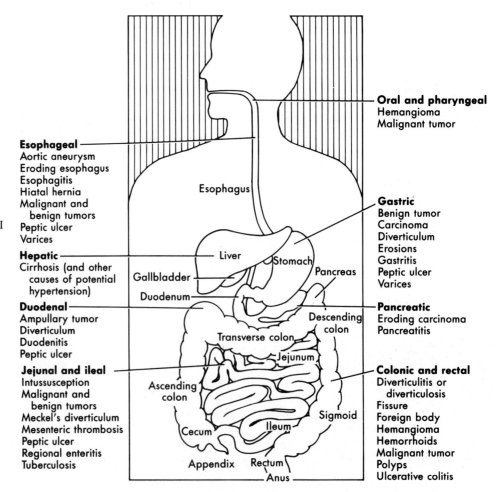

Figure **38-8** Sites and causes of GI bleeding. *(From SGNA: Gastroenterology nursing: a core curriculum, St. Louis, 1993, Mosby.)*

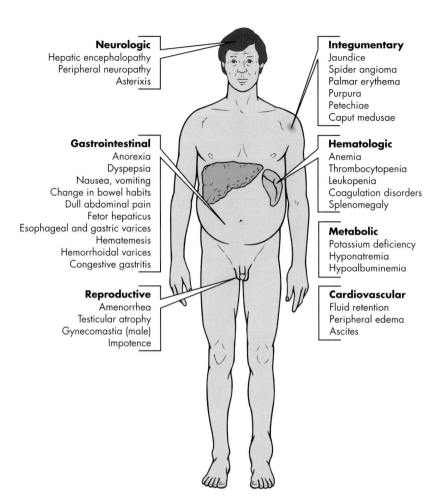

Neurologic
Hepatic encephalopathy
Peripheral neuropathy
Asterixis

Integumentary
Jaundice
Spider angioma
Palmar erythema
Purpura
Petechiae
Caput medusae

Gastrointestinal
Anorexia
Dyspepsia
Nausea, vomiting
Change in bowel habits
Dull abdominal pain
Fetor hepaticus
Esophageal and gastric varices
Hematemesis
Hemorrhoidal varices
Congestive gastritis

Hematologic
Anemia
Thrombocytopenia
Leukopenia
Coagulation disorders
Splenomegaly

Metabolic
Potassium deficiency
Hyponatremia
Hypoalbuminemia

Reproductive
Amenorrhea
Testicular atrophy
Gynecomastia (male)
Impotence

Cardiovascular
Fluid retention
Peripheral edema
Ascites

Figure **38-9** Systemic clinical manifestations of liver cirrhosis. *(From Lewis SM, Collier IC, Heitkemper MM: Medical-surgical nursing: assessment and management of clinical problems, ed 4, St. Louis, 1996, Mosby.)*

Table **38-6** **Drug Therapy for Gastrointestinal Bleeding**

Drug	Source of GI bleeding	Mechanism of action
Antacids	Duodenal ulcer, gastric ulcer, acute gastritis (corrosive, erosive, and hemorrhagic)	Neutralizes acid and maintains gastric pH above 5.5, elevated pH inhibits activation of pepsinogen
Histamine H₂-receptor antagonists Cimetidine (Tagamet), ranitidine (Zantac), famotidine (Pepcid), nizatidine (Axid)	Duodenal ulcer, gastric ulcer, esophagitis, acute gastritis (especially hemorrhagic)	Inhibits action of histamine at H₂ receptors of parietal cells and decreases acid secretion
Vasopressin	Acute gastritis (corrosive, erosive, and hemorrhagic)	Causes vasoconstriction and increases smooth muscle activity of the GI tract, reduces pressure in the portal circulation, and arrests bleeding

From Lewis SM, Collier IC, Heitkemper MM: *Medical-surgical nursing: assessment and management of clinical problems,* ed 4, St. Louis, 1996, Mosby.

bleeds that are self-limited and do not cause significant changes in hemodynamic status. Most patients with mild lower GI bleeding who are hemodynamically stable may be evaluated on an outpatient basis. Treatment includes identifying the source of bleeding with anoscopy, flexible sigmoid-oscopy, or air-contrast barium enema. Patients with severe symptomatic lower GI bleeding require hospital admission for resuscitation, diagnosis, and treatment. Colonoscopy may be performed to determine the source of bleeding after the patient is stabilized.[18]

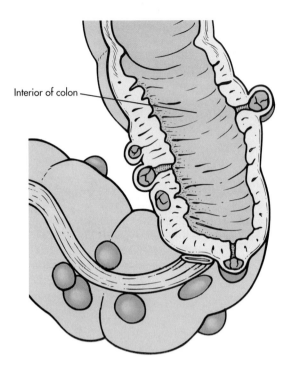

Figure **38-10** Diverticula are outpouchings of the colon. When they become inflamed, the condition is diverticulitis. The inflammatory process can spread to the surrounding area in the intestine. *(From Lewis SM, Collier IC, Heitkemper MM: Medical-surgical nursing: assessment and management of clinical problems, ed 4, St. Louis, 1996, Mosby.)*

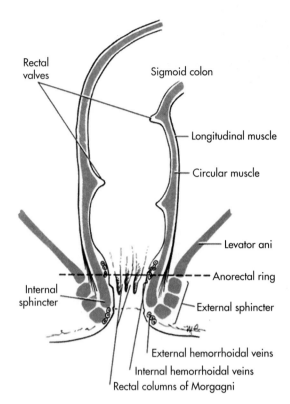

Figure **38-11** Anatomy of rectum and anus showing internal and external hemorrhoidal veins. *(From Price SA, Wilson LM: Pathophysiology: clinical concepts of disease processes, ed 5, St. Louis, 1997, Mosby.)*

The cardinal sign of lower GI bleeding is hematochezia. Patients may have maroon stools or occult blood in the stool. Cramplike abdominal pain may be present. Explosive diarrhea with foul odor is frequently present. Painless bleeding does occur. Pallor, diaphoresis, and decreased capillary refill are present with significant bleeding. Orthostatic changes in pulse and/or blood pressure occur in many patients. Pedal edema occurs in patients with chronic bleeding because of protein depletion.

Baseline laboratory studies include CBC, platelet count, and coagulation studies. The first priority is management of the ABCs followed by intravenous fluid resuscitation with normal saline or Ringer's lactate via large-bore intravenous catheter. Administration of PRBCs may be necessary in cases of significant blood loss. Determining the source of bleeding is a priority. Colonoscopy, bleeding scans, or angiography may be performed with surgical intervention required in some cases.[3]

Appendicitis

Obstruction of the entrance to the appendix decreases blood supply and leads to bacterial invasion. Untreated, inflammation progresses so that the appendix becomes nonviable and gangrenous, and eventually ruptures into the peritoneal space. Appendicitis affects both sexes and all ages, but is most common in males 10 to 30 years of age, and rarely occurs in infants less than 2 years of age.[17] Appendicitis is the most common problem requiring surgery in children.[10] Approximately 6% of the population develop appendicitis in their lifetime; one in 2200 pregnant women develops appendicitis.[20]

Patients may have abdominal pain and/or abdominal cramping, nausea, vomiting, tachycardia, malaise, and anorexia. Chills and fever also occur. Abdominal pain may be initially diffuse and periumbilical, and later become intense and localized to the lower right quadrant. Classic pain associated with appendicitis is located just inside the iliac crest at McBurney's point. Elderly patients may be afebrile without this classic pain.[1] Pressure on the lower left abdomen intensifies pain in the right lower quadrant (Rovsing's sign).[2] Pain may not always occur in this classic location because of normal variations in the location of the appendix (Figure 38-12). The position of comfort for most patients is supine with hips and knees flexed.

If the appendix ruptures, peritoneal signs increase and involuntary guarding develops. Increased fever and rebound tenderness occur when the appendix abscesses or ruptures. Diagnosis is made by clinical signs and symptoms in concert with physical examination. Diagnostic data include elevation of white blood cell count greater than 10,000 cells/mm^3

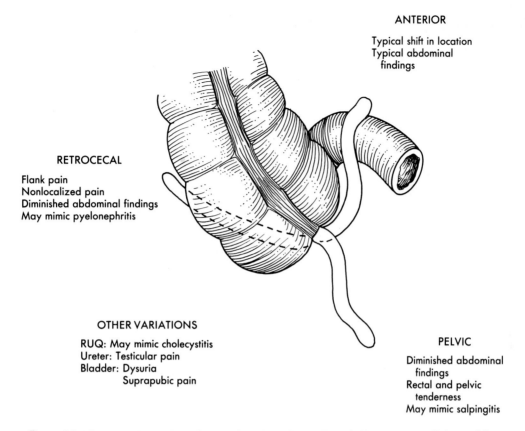

ANTERIOR

Typical shift in location
Typical abdominal
findings

RETROCECAL

Flank pain
Nonlocalized pain
Diminished abdominal findings
May mimic pyelonephritis

OTHER VARIATIONS

RUQ: May mimic cholecystitis
Ureter: Testicular pain
Bladder: Dysuria
     Suprapubic pain

PELVIC

Diminished abdominal
     findings
Rectal and pelvic
     tenderness
May mimic salpingitis

Figure **38-12**   Variable position of appendix. *(From Rosen P et al: Emergency medicine, vol 2, ed 3, St. Louis, 1992, Mosby.)*

with increased neutrophils, specifically bands.[17] WBC count is rarely greater than 20,000 cells/mm³. Ultrasound may occasionally demonstrate an enlarged appendix or collection of periappendicial fluid, with 75% to 90% sensitivity and 86% to 100% specificity.[1,20] Urinalysis should be performed to rule out genitourinary problems.

Definitive therapy for appendicitis is surgical intervention; laparoscopic surgery is the preferred method. Instruct the patient not to eat or drink, obtain IV access, and administer prophylactic broad-spectrum antibiotic. Narcotic pain medication is usually withheld until diagnosis is made. Complications such as perforation, peritonitis, and abscess formation can occur when treatment is delayed.

Cholecystitis

Inflammation of the gallbladder causes distention as the cystic duct becomes obstructed. Bacterial invasion, usually by *E. coli,* streptococcus, or salmonella, also causes cholecystitis. Gallstones may exacerbate cholecystitis; however, 5% of patients do not have gallstones.[6] Conversely, cholecystitis occurs in 16 to 20 million Americans with a million new cases each year.[20] Cholecystitis usually affects obese, fair-skinned women of increasing age and parity.

Symptoms include sudden onset abdominal pain, usually after ingestion of fried or fatty foods. Pain may radiate from epigastrium to the right upper quadrant or may be referred to the right supraclavicular area. Patients usually describe pain as colicky. Local and rebound tenderness may also be present. Marked tenderness and inspiratory limitation on deep palpation under the right subcostal margin (Murphy's sign) may also be present.[11] Low-grade fever (38° C or 100.4° F), tachycardia, nausea, vomiting, and flatulence are common findings. If the common bile duct is obstructed, the patient may appear slightly jaundiced. Table 38-7 highlights clinical signs associated with obstructed bile flow.

Diagnostic tests include urinalysis, CBC, serum electrolytes, BUN, creatinine, serum glucose, and serum bilirubin levels; however, these results are often normal.[20] Ultrasound is extremely useful in the emergency setting for detection of a thickened gallbladder wall, gallstones, and pericholecystic fluid.[6]

Treatment of cholecystitis includes administration of IV crystalloid solution and antiemetics for nausea and vomiting. A nasogastric tube may be necessary for gastric decompression. Monitor vital signs and intake and output. Broad-spectrum antibiotics are indicated for potential microbial infection. Narcotic analgesics are recommended for pain control. Definitive treatment for cholecystitis is surgery with traditional laparotomy or laparoscopic cholecystectomy.[6]

Table **38-7**	**Clinical Manifestations Caused by Obstructed Bile Flow**
Clinical manifestation	Etiology
Obstructive jaundice	No bile flow into duodenum
Dark amber urine, which foams when shaken	Soluble bilirubin in urine
No urobilinogen in urine	No bilirubin reaching small intestine to be converted to urobilinogen
Clay-colored stools	Same as above
Pruritus	Deposition of bile salts in skin tissues
Intolerance for fatty foods (nausea, sensation of fullness, anorexia)	No bile in small intestine for fat digestion
Bleeding tendencies	Lack of or decreased absorption of vitamin K, resulting in decreased production of prothrombin
Steatorrhea	No bile salts in duodenum, preventing fat emulsion and digestion

From Lewis SM, Collier IC, Heitkemper MM: *Medical-surgical nursing: assessment and management of clinical problems,* ed 4, St. Louis, 1996, Mosby.

Table **38-8**	**Diagnostic Studies for Acute Pancreatitis**	
Laboratory test	Abnormal finding	Etiology
Primary tests		
Serum amylase	Increased (>200 U/L [3.34 μkat/L])	Pancreatic cell injury
Serum lipase	Elevated	Pancreatic cell injury
Urinary amylase	Elevated	Pancreatic cell injury
Secondary tests		
Blood glucose	Hyperglycemia	Impairment of carbohydrate metabolism due to β-cell damage and release of glucagon
Serum calcium	Hypocalcemia	Saponification of calcium by fatty acids in areas of fat necrosis
Serum triglycerides	Hyperlipidemia	Release of free fatty acids by lipase

From Lewis SM, Collier IC, Heitkemper MM: *Medical-surgical nursing: assessment and management of clinical problems,* ed 4, St. Louis, 1996, Mosby.

Acute Pancreatitis

Acute pancreatitis results from inflammation of the pancreas; however, the exact mechanism is not clear. Theories include bile or duodenal reflux, bacterial infection, pancreatic enzyme activation with autolysis, and ductal hypertension. Etiology can be traced to biliary disease or alcohol consumption. Seventy percent to 80% of pancreatitis cases are due to biliary disease,[4,6] probably obstruction of the common bile duct resulting in ductal hypertension and pancreatic enzyme activation. Alcohol abuse causes toxic metabolites that injure the pancreas, leading to inflammation. Other causes include chronic hypercalcemia, surgery, abdominal trauma, infections (mumps, cytomegalovirus infection), drugs, toxins (organophosphate insecticides, scorpion venom), or endoscopic retrograde cholangiopancreatography (ERCP).[5] Regardless of mechanism, pancreatitis is characterized by acinar cell damage that leads to necrosis, edema, and inflammation. Acute pancreatitis affects 1.5 persons per 100,000 population, but varies with the population.[6]

A clinical hallmark in 95% of patients with pancreatitis is abdominal pain originating in the epigastric region and radiating to the back.[15] Abdominal tenderness, rebound, and guarding are usually present. Nausea, vomiting, and abdominal distention may be present. Patients may be febrile, with tachycardia, tachypnea, and hypotension. Decreased gastric motility causes hypoactive or absent bowel sounds.

Certain laboratory values aid in diagnosis of acute pancreatitis (Table 38-8). Elevated serum amylase and lipase levels are pathognomonic for pancreatitis. Leukocytosis, decreased hematocrit, hyperglycemia, and glucosuria may also be present. Continuing decreases in hematocrit suggest hemorrhagic pancreatitis.[20] Serum calcium is decreased, whereas serum glutamic oxaloacetic transaminase (SGOT) is elevated. Persistent hypocalcemia is associated with poor prognosis.[20]

Radiographic studies are useful in diagnosing acute pancreatitis. A chest radiograph may reveal pleural effusions or pulmonary infiltrates and ileus may be detected on abdominal radiographs. Abdominal ultrasound can identify gallstones as an underlying cause. Abdominal CT scan may also contribute to the diagnosis of acute pancreatitis by identification of pancreatic edema or fluid around the pancreas.[20]

Management includes maintaining strict NPO status. Obtain IV access for fluid and electrolyte replacement with balanced salt solution to ensure renal perfusion. Antiemetics are administered for nausea, vomiting, and to minimize further fluid loss. Pain control is a high priority for the patient with pancreatitis. Meperidine is less likely than morphine to increase pressure in the sphincter of Oddi, a suspected source of pain.[5] Table 38-9 highlights drugs used for management of acute pancreatitis. Nasogastric suction helps al-

Table 38-9 Drugs Used in Treatment of Acute Pancreatitis

Drug	Mechanisms of action
Meperidine (Demerol)	Relief of pain
Nitroglycerin or papaverine	Relaxation of smooth muscles and relief of pain
Antispasmodics (e.g., dicyclomine [Bentyl], propantheline bromide [Pro-Banthine])	Decrease of vagal stimulation, motility, pancreatic outflow (inhibition of volume and concentration of bicarbonate and enzymatic secretion); contraindicated in paralytic ileus
Carbonic anhydrase inhibitor (acetazolamide [Diamox])	Reduction in volume and bicarbonate concentration of pancreatic secretion
Antacids	Neutralization of gastric secretions; decrease in hydrochloric acid stimulation of secretin, which stimulates production and secretion of pancreatic secretions
Histamine H_2-receptor antagonists (cimetidine [Tagamet], ranitidine [Zantac])	Decrease in hydrochloric acid by inhibiting histamine (hydrochloric acid stimulates pancreatic activity)
Calcium gluconate	Treatment of hypocalcemia to prevent or treat tetany
Adrenocortical steroids	Use only for seriously ill patients with hypotension or shock
Aprotinin (Trasylol)	Antitryptic and antikallikreinic actions
Glucagon	Reduction in pancreatic inflammation and decrease in serum amylase, suppression of pancreatic secretions
Somatostatin	Inhibition of pancreatic secretions

Modified from Lewis SM, Collier IC, Heitkemper MM: *Medical-surgical nursing: assessment and management of clinical problems*, ed 4, St. Louis, 1996, Mosby.

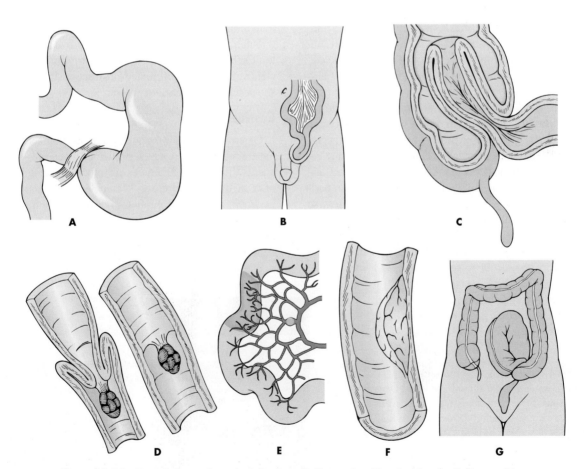

Figure **38-13** Bowel obstructions. **A,** Adhesions. **B,** Strangulated inguinal hernia. **C,** Ileocecal intussusception. **D,** Intussusception from polyps. **E,** Mesenteric occlusion. **F,** Neoplasm. **G,** Volvulus of the sigmoid colon. *(From Lewis SM, Collier IC, Heitkemper MM: Medical-surgical nursing: assessment and management of clinical problems, ed 4, St. Louis, 1996, Mosby.)*

leviate nausea, vomiting, and abdominal distention. Ongoing monitoring of respiratory, cardiovascular, and renal functions is recommended. Prophylactic administration of antibiotics should be considered.

Severe life-threatening complications with acute pancreatitis are pleural effusions and adult respiratory distress syndrome (ARDS). Significant hypovolemia can lead to hypovolemic shock and ischemia of lungs, heart, and kidneys. Electrolyte imbalances such as hyperglycemia and hypocalcemia also occur. Septic complications include formation of pancreatic abscess.[15]

Bowel Obstruction

Bowel obstruction occurs in either sex, at any age, from a variety of causes.[5] The most common cause is adhesions from previous abdominal surgery, followed by incarcerated inguinal hernia.[20] Other causes include foreign bodies, volvulus, intussusception, strictures, tumors, congenital adhesive bands, fecal impaction, gallstones, and hematomas (Figure 38-13).

Bowel obstructions are classified as mechanical or nonmechanical. Mechanical obstruction results from a disorder outside the intestines or blockage inside the lumen of the intestines (Figure 38-14). Intussusception, telescoping of the bowel within itself by peristalsis, is an example of a mechanical obstruction (Figure 38-15). Nonmechanical obstruction results when muscle activity of the intestine decreases and movement of contents slows, for example, paralytic ileus (Figure 38-16).

When obstruction occurs, bowel contents accumulate above the obstruction. Distention occurs when intestines can no longer absorb contents or move contents down the intestinal tract. Peristalsis increases so more secretions are released, which worsens distention, causes bowel edema, and increases capillary permeability. Plasma leaks into the peritoneal cavity with fluid trapped in the intestinal lumen, so absorption of fluid and electrolytes decreases.

Clinical signs vary with the location of the obstruction. Table 38-10 compares clinical manifestations of obstructions in the large and small intestines. Symptoms include colicky, crampy, intermittent, and wavelike abdominal pain. At times pain may be severe. Abdominal distention may also be present. Patients may have diffuse abdominal tenderness, rigidity, and constipation. Hyperactive bowel sounds (borborygmi) or absent bowel sounds may be noted. The patient may also be febrile, tachycardic, and hypotensive with nausea and vomiting. Emesis usually has an odor of feces.

Laboratory studies include CBC, BUN, serum glucose, electrolytes, serum creatinine, and arterial blood gas measurements. A white cell count greater than 20,000/μL suggests bowel gangrene, whereas elevations greater than 40,000/μL occur with mesenteric vascular occlusion.[20] Abdominal radiographs show dilated, fluid-filled loops of bowel. Table 38-11 highlights radiographic differences with specific obstructions. Management includes IV access for fluid and electrolyte replacement using crystalloid solution to maintain hemodynamic values and renal perfusion. Intake, output, and patient response to therapy should be monitored to prevent fluid overload. Bowel sounds should be evaluated frequently to identify changes. Nasogastric tube is inserted to decompress the stomach and reduce vomiting. Evaluate pain for worsening of the condition. Prophylactic administration of antibiotics is recommended. Surgical intervention may be required for some patients. Life-threatening complications of bowel obstruction include peritonitis, bowel strangulation and/or perforation, renal insufficiency, and death. Untreated obstruction that progresses to shock has a 70% mortality rate.[20]

Gastroenteritis

Gastroenteritis is inflammation of the stomach and intestinal lining caused by viral, protozoal, bacterial, or parasitic agents (Table 38-12). Bacterial infection accounts for 20% of acute diarrheal disease.[20] Table 38-13 highlights bacterial gastroenteritis, a common source of epidemics. Gastroenteritis may be caused by an imbalance of normal flora (*E. coli*) resulting from the ingestion of contaminated food. Patients have nausea, vomiting, diarrhea, and abdominal cramps.

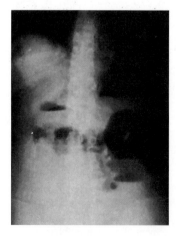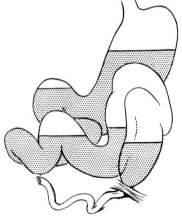

Figure **38-14** Mechanical bowel obstruction. Localized air-fluid levels seen on upright film of abdomen. Diagram shows dilated proximal bowel and stomach air-fluid levels, and adhesive band causing obstruction. *(From Liechty RD, Soper RT: Fundamentals of surgery, ed 6, St. Louis, 1989, Mosby.)*

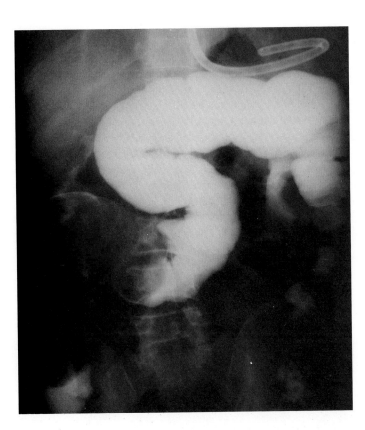

Figure **38-15** Intussusception with thin layer of barium around invaginating intestine. *(From Rosen P et al:* Emergency medicine, *ed 3, St. Louis, 1992, Mosby.)*

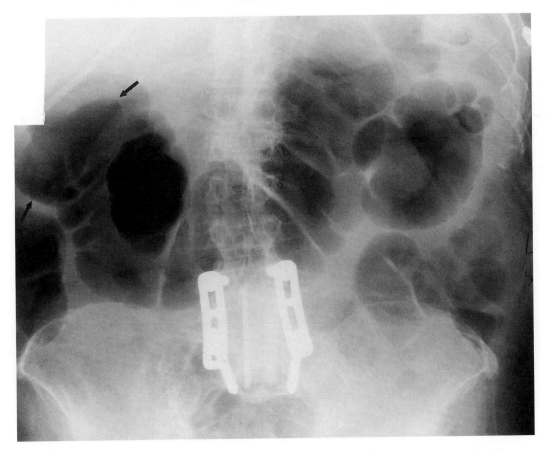

Figure **38-16** Ileus on abdominal radiograph. Note dilated loops of bowel. *(From Dettenmeier PA:* Radiographic assessment for nurses, *St. Louis, 1995, Mosby.)*

Table 38-10	Clinical Manifestations of Small and Large Intestinal Obstructions	
Clinical manifestation	Small intestine	Large intestine
Onset	Rapid	Gradual
Vomiting	Frequent and copious	Rare
Pain	Colicky, cramplike, intermittent	Low-grade, crampy abdominal pain
Bowel movement	Feces for a short time	Absolute constipation
Abdominal distention	Minimally increased	Greatly increased

From Lewis SM, Collier IC, Heitkemper MM: *Medical-surgical nursing: assessment and management of clinical problems,* ed 4, St. Louis, 1996, Mosby.

Hyperactive bowel sounds, fever, and headaches are also present. Anal excoriation occurs with frequent episodes of diarrhea. Diarrhea accounts for 5 to 10 million deaths annually in Asia, Africa, and Latin America.[20]

Laboratory data include CBC, electrolytes measurement, and stool culture. Obtain IV access for replacement of fluid and electrolytes. Administer antiemetics and analgesics as needed. Antibiotics are determined by patient history and presenting symptoms. Successful treatment is based on identifying the causative agent and resting the intestinal tract. Oral hydration with clear liquids is possible in most patients. Suggested fluids include cola, ginger ale, apple juice, tea, broth, and Gatorade. Fluid replacement in children is critical to prevent dehydration. Rice, applesauce, bananas, and toast can be started as soon as diarrhea subsides. Feeding should begin as soon as possible in children and adults.

SUMMARY

GI emergencies can be minor or life threatening. Most GI emergencies present with similar clinical manifestations, so triage history and physical assessment play an important role in management of these patients. Ability to differentiate

Table 38-11	Radiographic and Clinical Evidence of Specific Bowel Obstructions	
Type	Radiographic findings	Clinical signs and symptoms
Bowel obstructions (general)	Air-fluid levels may appear as "string of beads" and thus serve as important diagnostic clue to mechanical obstructions. More than two air-fluid levels reflect mechanical obstruction, adynamic ileus, or both. Fluid-filled loops form proximal to impediment and are indicative of bowel obstruction. Routine films or contrast studies show air-fluid levels, distortion, abscess formation, narrow lumens, mucosal destruction, distension, and deformities at site of torsion.	Pain, distension, vomiting, obstipation, and constipation
Strangulation obstruction	"Coffee bean" sign appears on radiograph (dilated bowel loop bent on itself, assuming shape of coffee bean). Gas- and fluid-filled loops may have unchanging locations on multiple projection films. Pseudotumor (closed-loop obstruction filled with water that looks like tumor) may be present.	Abdominal tenderness, hyperactive bowel sounds, leukocytosis, rebound tenderness, fever
Gallstones	Air in gallbladder tree, distension of small bowel, and visualization of stone.	
Hernia		Extraabdominal or intraabdominal hernia may be present: in men, most commonly inguinal; in women, right-sided femoral hernias
Volvulus		Torsion of mesenteric axis creating digestive disturbances
Intussusception	"Coiled spring" appearance seen on contrast radiograph	

Table **38-12**	**Etiology of Gastroenteritis**
Type	Example
Bacteria	*Salmonella, E. coli, C. difficile, Campylobacter fetus jejuni*
Virus	Rotavirus, parvovirus, enterovirus
Protozoa	*G. lamblia,* cryptosporidium

Box **38-3**

NURSING DIAGNOSES FOR GI EMERGENCIES

Pain
Fluid volume deficit
Knowledge deficit
Risk for infection
Anxiety
Impaired gas exchange

Table **38-13**	**Epidemiologic Aspects of Invasive Bacterial Gastroenteritis**			
	Source	Incubation period	Features	Duration
Shigella	Person to person, fecal-oral	24 to 48 hours	Confined populations; poor personal hygiene and sanitation	4 to 7 days
Salmonella	Poultry, eggs, water, and domestic pets	8 to 24 hours	Family and cafeteria-type outbreaks common	2 to 5 days
Campylobacter fetus	Poultry, wild birds, water	2 to 5 days	High relapse rate; summer months; cases sporadic	5 to 14 days
Yersinia enterocolitica	Food or drink and person to person	12 to 48 hours (?)	Appendicitis; mesenteric adenitis-like syndromes; winter months	10 to 14 days
Vibrio parahaemolyticus	Seafood, especially shellfish	8 to 24 hours	High attack rates; summer months	24 to 48 hours

From Rosen P et al: *Emergency medicine,* ed 2, vol 2, St. Louis, 1988, Mosby.

conditions that require immediate attention is a requisite skill for the emergency nurse. Box 38-3 highlights selected nursing diagnoses for GI emergencies.

REFERENCES

1. Birnbaumer DM: Abdominal emergencies in later life, *Emerg Med* 25(5):75, 1993.
2. Cummings SP, Cummings PH: Abdominal emergencies. In Klein AR, Lee G, Manton A et al, editors: *Emergency nursing core curriculum,* ed 4, Philadelphia, 1994, WB Saunders.
3. DeMarkles MP, Murphy JR: Acute lower gastrointestinal bleeding, *Med Clin North Am* 77(5):1085, 1993.
4. Grendell JH: Acute pancreatitis. In Grendell JH, McQuaid KR, Freidman SL, editors: *Current diagnosis and treatment in gastroenterology,* Stamford, Conn, 1996, Appleton & Lange.
5. Grendell JH: Miscellaneous disorders of the stomach and small intestine. In Grendell JH, McQuaid KR, Freidman SL, editors: *Current diagnosis and treatment in gastroenterology,* Stamford, Conn, 1996, Appleton & Lange.
6. Guss D: Disorders of the liver, biliary tract, and pancreas. In Rosen P Barkin RM et al, editors: *Emergency medicine: concepts and clinical practice,* ed 3, St. Louis, 1992, Mosby.
7. Guyton AC, Hall J: *Textbook of medical physiology,* ed 9, Philadelphia, 1996, WB Saunders.
8. Heiser R: Abdominal conditions. In Kidd PS, Sturt P, editors: *Mosby's emergency nursing reference,* St. Louis, 1996, Mosby.
9. Henneman PL: Gastrointestinal bleeding. In Rosen P et al, editors: *Emergency medicine: concepts and clinical practice,* ed 3, St. Louis, 1992, Mosby.
10. Hockberger RS, Henneman PL, Boniface K: Disorders of the small intestine. In Rosen P et al, editors: *Emergency medicine: concepts and clinical practice,* ed 3, St. Louis, 1992, Mosby.
11. Jacobson IM: Gallstones. In Grendell JH et al, editors: *Current diagnosis and treatment in gastroenterology,* Stamford, Conn, 1996, Appleton & Lange.
12. Jutabha R, Jensen DM: Acute upper gastrointestinal bleeding. In Grendell JH et al, editors: *Current diagnosis and treatment in gastroenterology,* Stamford, Conn, 1996, Appleton & Lange.
13. Kearney DJ, McQuaid KR: Approach to the patient with gastrointestinal disorders. In Grendell JH et al, editors: *Current diagnosis and treatment in gastroenterology,* Stamford, Conn, 1996, Appleton & Lange.
14. Kerber K: The adult with bleeding esophageal varices, *Crit Care Nurs Clin North Am* 5(1):153, 1993.
15. Krumberger JM: Acute pancreatitis, *Crit Care Nurs Clin North Am* 5(1):185, 1993.
16. Manten HD, Green JA: Acute lower gastrointestinal bleeding: a guide to initial management, *Postgrad Med* 97(4):154, 1995.
17. McQuaid KR: Alimentary tract. In Tierney LM, McPhee SJ, Papadakis MA, editors: *Current medical diagnosis and treatment 1995,* Norwalk, Conn, 1995, Appleton & Lange.
18. Savides TJ, Jensen DM: Acute lower gastrointestinal bleeding. In Grendell JH et al, editors: *Current diagnosis and treatment in gastroenterology,* Stamford, Conn, 1996, Appleton & Lange.
19. Stein C, Korula J: Variceal bleeding: what are the treatment options? *Postgrad Med* 98(6):143, 1995.
20. Tintinelli JE, Ruiz E, Krome RL: *Emergency medicine—a comprehensive study guide,* ed 4, New York, 1996, McGraw-Hill.

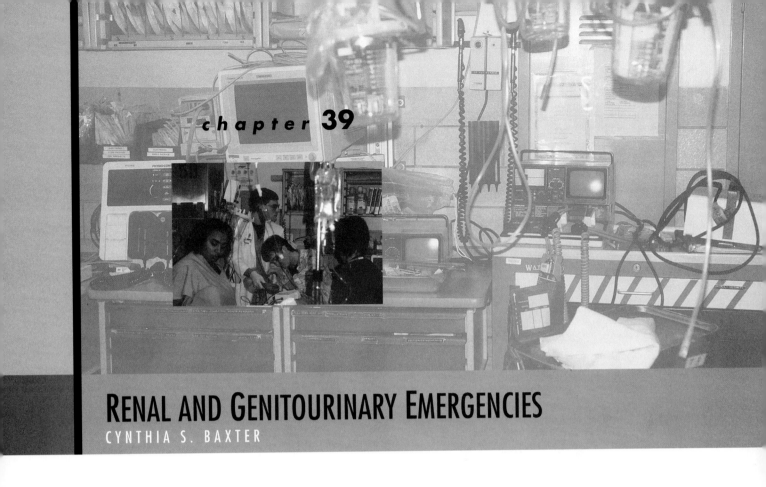

chapter 39

RENAL AND GENITOURINARY EMERGENCIES

CYNTHIA S. BAXTER

Genitourinary (GU) problems are a common complaint in the emergency department (ED). Urinary tract infections (UTIs) are the third most common infection in ambulatory patients—up to 3% of all females experience one or more infections per year.[2] Renal calculi affect up to 6% of the American population and account for seven of 1000 hospitalizations.[6] Sexually transmitted diseases (STDs) are increasing in the United States, especially among low income, urban, minority adolescents.[4] Incidence of end-stage renal disease (ESRD) is rising in all industrialized nations, but the etiology is not clear. ESRD affects blacks three times more often than whites, and is most prevalent in those with diabetes or hypertension, occurring six times more often in patients with hypertension. In persons 65 years of age or older, incidence of renal failure increases sixfold; however, 66% of all diabetes-induced renal failure occurs before age 64. Males account for 65% of the ESRD population.[3] Acute tubular necrosis (ATN), the most common type of acute renal failure, accounts for 5% of all hospital admissions.[5] Patients with compromised renal function often arrive at the ED with life-threatening fluid and electrolyte imbalances.

Genitourinary emergencies can also occur as a result of trauma (Chapter 27). Specific GU emergencies discussed are acute azotemia, urinary tract infections, urinary calculi, testicular torsion, priapism, and STDs. Refer to Chapter 46 for additional discussion of STDs in women.

ANATOMY AND PHYSIOLOGY

The genitourinary tract consists of the kidneys, ureters, urinary bladder, urethra, and external genitalia. Urine is produced by the kidneys as a way to regulate fluid volume and electrolyte balance. Ureters transport urine to the bladder for temporary storage. Urine is drained from the bladder to the outside by the urethra. Figure 39-1 shows structures of the GU system. External structures of the male GU system have reproductive functions.

The kidneys are located on the posterior abdominal wall behind the peritoneum on either side of the vertebral column. Figure 39-2 shows the kidney in cross section. On the medial aspect of each kidney is the hilum, where the renal artery and nerve enter and renal vein and ureter exit. The hilum opens into the renal pelvis, an enlargement of the urinary channel. Renal calyces, shaped like the cup of a flower, open into the renal pelvis. Each kidney contains two or three major calyces and 20 minor calyces that open into major calyces. The kidney has an outer cortex and inner layer or medulla. Cone or triangular-shaped structures called medullary pyramids located in the renal medulla open into a minor calyx. The cortex surrounds the medulla and extends between pyramids in columns to the renal pelvis. Blood flow to the kidney is supplied by the renal artery, which branches off the abdominal aorta and enters the kidney through the renal sinus. Blood leaves the kidney through the renal vein, which empties into the abdominal inferior vena cava.

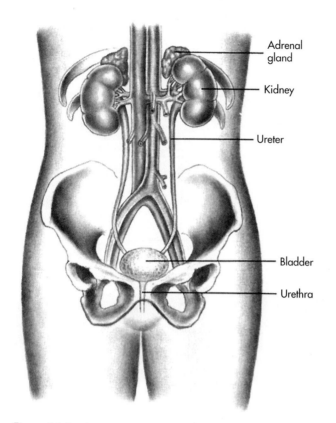

Figure **39-1** Components of the urinary system. *(From Thompson JM et al:* Mosby's clinical nursing, *ed 4, St. Louis, 1997, Mosby.)*

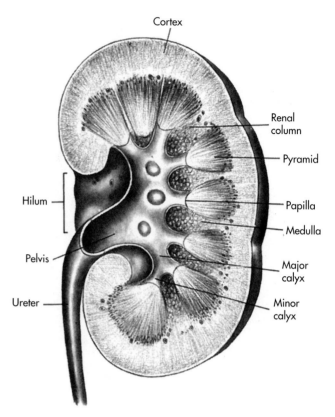

Figure **39-2** Cross section of kidney. *(From Thompson JM et al:* Mosby's clinical nursing, *ed 4, St. Louis, 1997, Mosby.)*

The nephron, the functional unit of the kidney, is composed of the renal corpuscle, proximal convoluted tubule, Henle's loop, distal convoluted tubule, and collecting ducts (Figure 39-3). Each kidney contains an estimated 1 million nephrons that are individually capable of producing urine. These nephrons cannot be reproduced once destroyed. The renal corpuscle contains the glomerulus, a web of tightly convoluted capillaries, and Bowman's capsule, which surrounds and supports these structures. Blood flows through the afferent arteriole into the glomerulus and out the efferent arteriole. Renal blood flow accounts for 21% of cardiac output or 1200 ml/min.[1] Specialized cells called juxtaglomerular cells are located at the entrance to the glomerulus of the afferent arteriole in 15% of nephrons. Juxtaglomerular cells form a cuff and combine with the macula densa, a portion of the distal convoluted tubule that lies adjacent to the renal corpuscle between afferent and efferent arterioles. The juxtaglomerular cells and the macula densa form the juxtaglomerular apparatus, which senses changes in pressure and sodium concentration and plays a role in the renin-angiotensin-aldosterone (RAA) system. Juxtaglomerular nephrons have a greater capacity to concentrate urine because they have longer Henle's loops, which extend into the medulla.

Filtration of plasma in the renal corpuscle is the first step in urine production and helps the kidney to rid the body of wastes and retain water and essential solutes. Pressure gen-

erated as blood courses through the tight web of capillaries in the glomerulus, along with oncotic pressure within the blood, is greater than pressure created by Bowman's capsule, so plasma or filtrate and small solutes cross the semipermeable epithelial capillary lining. Injury to the glomerulus, such as ischemia or inflammation, increases permeability of the capillary membrane and allows larger molecules (RBCs, epithelial casts, protein, or WBCs) to cross. Decreased oncotic pressure, often due to decreased serum albumin levels, or decreased pressure within the glomerulus produced by systemic hypotension decreases glomerular filtration rate (GFR) and eventually urine output. GFR in the average adult is 125 ml/min or 180 L/day.

Tubules, Henle's loop, and collecting ducts excrete waste products (urea, nitrogen, creatinine, drug metabolites, etc.), reabsorb water and solutes (K, Na, Cl, H, glucose, and amino acids) from filtrate, and secrete excess solutes into filtrate the body doesn't need. Osmosis, diffusion, and active transport occur between the nephron and surrounding capillaries. Hormonal control regulates reabsorption and secretion in the nephron.

The RAA system (Figure 39-4) and antidiuretic hormone (ADH) are feedback loop systems within the body that maintain homeostasis. Serum osmolarity increases and causes stimulation of the hypothalamus, which releases ADH. Nephron permeability increases, so additional water

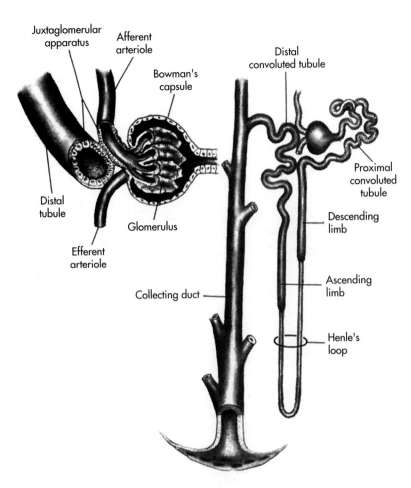

Figure **39-3** Components of nephron. *(From Thompson JM et al:* Mosby's clinical nursing, *ed 4, St. Louis, 1997, Mosby.)*

is absorbed, serum osmolarity returns to normal, and ADH release stops. Pressure changes in the glomerulus are overcome by vasodilation and constriction of the afferent arteriole by a process called autoregulation, which keeps pressure in the glomerulus within a wide range of systolic blood pressures. When range is exceeded, autoregulation fails and epithelial damage occurs with eventual scarring and sclerosis followed by decreased permeability, glomerular filtration rate, and urine output. Inadequate nephron perfusion stimulates the juxtaglomerular apparatus to secrete renin that converts angiotensin to angiotensin I, which stimulates aldosterone release from the adrenal cortex and reabsorption of sodium and water by the nephron. Angiotensin I converted to angiotensin II by an enzyme in the lung causes peripheral vasoconstriction. Perfusion increases to the nephron and the cycle is altered.

Without a functioning kidney and adequate urine production, homeostasis is severely impaired. Fluid and electrolyte imbalance, accumulation of urea and creatinine, decreased excretion of drug metabolites, and inadequate reabsorption of amino acids and glucose occur. The kidneys also help convert vitamin D into the active form (1, 25-vitamin D_3) to ensure calcium absorption from intestines and secrete erythropoietin for stimulation of RBC production in bone marrow.

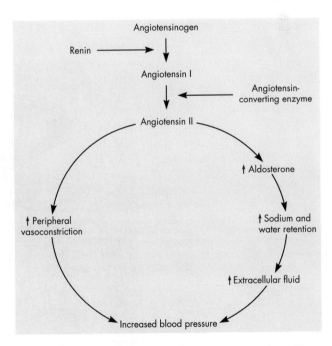

Figure **39-4** Renin-angiotensin-aldosterone mechanism. *(From Lewis SM, Collier IC, Heitkemper MM:* Medical-surgical nursing: assessment and management of clinical problems, *ed 4, St. Louis, 1996, Mosby.)*

Consequently, altered renal function decreases bone mineralization and the oxygen-carrying capacity of the blood.

The renal pelvis narrows to enter the ureter where urine is moved to the bladder by peristaltic contractions. The muscular bladder stores urine until release to the urethra by the micturition reflex.

External genitalia are also part of the GU system. Female genitalia consist of the vestibule, the space into which the urethra and vagina open, and surrounding labia minora and majora (Figure 39-5). Anatomic position and short length of the female urethra are responsible for the high frequency of urinary tract infection in females.

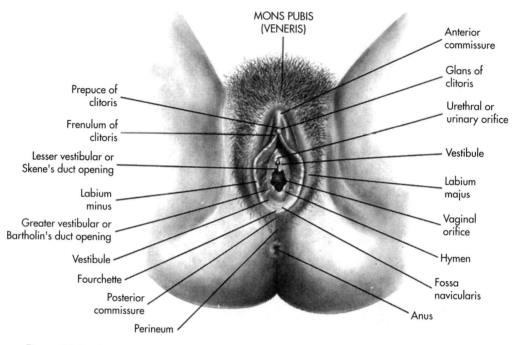

Figure **39-5**   External female genitalia. *(From Lowdermilk DL:* Maternity and women's health care, *ed 6, St. Louis, 1997, Mosby.)*

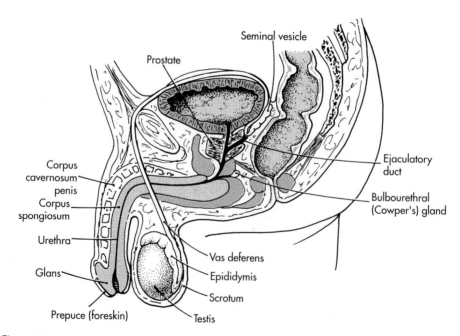

Figure **39-6**   External and internal male genitalia. *(From Price SA, Wilson LM:* Pathophysiology: clinical concepts of disease processes, *ed 5, St. Louis, 1997, Mosby.)*

Male external genitalia include penis, scrotum, and scrotal contents (Figure 39-6). Scrotal contents include the testes, tubules that carry developing sperm cells and secrete testosterone, and the epididymis, which lies along the posterior testes and is the final maturation area for sperm. The prostate is glandular and muscle tissue that surrounds the urethra at the base of the bladder. Enlargement of the prostate can cause outlet obstruction and urinary retention. The penis consists of three columns of erectile tissue that become engorged with blood, producing erection (Figure 39-7). Two columns of corpora cavernosa form the dorsum and sides of the penis and the corpus spongiosum forms the base and glans. Clinical manifestations of GU disease frequently involve external genitalia.

PATIENT ASSESSMENT

Assessment of the GU system should determine history of hypertension, diabetes, previous infections, prostatitis, urethritis, bladder or urethral damage during delivery, history of calculi, and recurrent urinary tract infections. A detailed drug list, including prescription, over-the-counter (OTC), and illegal drug use along with exposure to occupational chemicals or toxins, may identify contact with nephrotoxic substances. The sexual history should include discussion of risk factors for GU symptoms including contraceptive jellies or creams, multiple partners, abnormal penile or vaginal discharges, unsafe sexual practices, and history of STDs. GU complaints often arise from changes in urinary patterns, for example, frequency, dysuria, urgency, dribbling, or incontinence.

Hematuria or urine discoloration may be the primary complaint or occur with other symptoms. A detailed medication and diet history may uncover other causes for the discoloration of urine. Box 39-1 highlights possible causes of red or dark red urine. Hematuria can be confirmed by urinalysis (UA); however, microscopic hematuria on a single test is common. Early stream hematuria suggests bleeding from the urethra, hematuria throughout the stream indicates upper GU tract bleeding, and bleeding at the end suggests bladder neck or urethral bleeding. Complete urinalysis and urine cytology may indicate the need for further diagnostic testing for urologic cancer, renal disease, infection, or calculi as the source of hematuria. Box 39-2 highlights drugs and chemicals that cause hematuria.

Pain should be assessed using the PQRST mnemonic—provocation, quality, region or radiation, severity, and timing. The most severe pain associated with the GU system is renal colic caused by calculi. Increased pressure and dilation of the kidney and urinary collecting system cause sudden, unbearable pain. The patient is pale and restless with flank

Box **39-1**	**Nonhematuric Causes of Red or Dark Red Urine**
Food	**Drugs**
Beets	Cascara
Rhubarb	Desferol
Blackberries	Adriamycin
	Phenothiazides
	Phenytoin (Dilantin)
	Rifampin

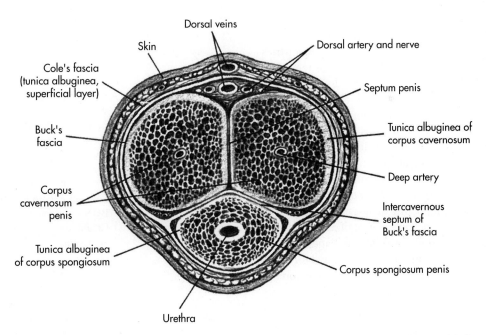

Figure **39-7** Cross section of penis. *(From Thompson JM et al: Mosby's clinical nursing, ed 4, St. Louis, 1997, Mosby.)*

Box **39-2**	**Drugs and Chemicals That Cause Hematuria**

Antibiotics

Amphotericin
Ampicillin
Colistimethate
Kanamycin
Methicillin
Penicillin
Polymyxin
Sulfonamides

Anticoagulants

Heparin
Warfarin

Drugs

Amitriptyline
Aspirin (acetylsalicylic acid)
Benztropine (Cogentin)
Cantharides
Chlorothiazide
Chlorpromazine
Colchicine

Corticosteroids
Cyclophosphamide
Indomethacin
Methenamine
Phenacetin
Phenylbutazone
Probenecid
Trifluoperazine (Stelazine)

Metals

Arsenic
Copper sulfate
Gold
Lead
Phosphorus

Organic solvents

Carbon tetrachloride
Phenol
Propylene glycol
Turpentine

From Kendall AR, Karafin L: *Urology,* New York, 1973, Harper & Row.

pain radiating to the abdomen and groin. If the stone lodges in the bladder, urinary frequency and urgency develop. Pain may cause tachypnea and tachycardia with elevated blood pressure. Relief of renal colic requires substantial amounts of narcotics, so drug seekers may feign renal colic pain and give a history of allergy to intravenous pyelography (IVP) dye.

Oliguria, defined as urine output <400 ml in 24 hours, or anuria, <75 ml in 24 hours, may be presenting symptoms. The cause is usually obstruction; however, blood chemistries should be evaluated for azotemia, which indicates renal failure from prolonged obstruction leading to hydronephrosis or other causes. If the patient has a urinary catheter, patency must be assessed. A physical examination can identify urinary retention by palpating the firm mass above the symphysis pubis, with an urge to void on palpation. A history should be obtained to identify drugs that contribute to retention, including OTC nasal decongestants containing anticholinergic ingredients. A neurologic examination should be performed to rule out spinal cord injury or disease that can interfere with the micturition reflex. The prostate is examined for enlargement as the cause of obstruction. After the patient has attempted to void, a urethral catheter may be inserted for residual volume. If the catheter cannot be inserted without force, a suprapubic bladder tap or assistance from a urologist may be necessary. With residual volume over 500 ml, the catheter may be left in place to allow the bladder to regain muscle tone. If residual volume is minimal, further diagnostic evaluation is aimed at identifying the cause.

SPECIFIC CONDITIONS
Acute Azotemia

Azotemia, or uremia, refers to accumulation of nitrogen waste products in the blood. Acute azotemia generally refers to the patient with acute renal failure (ARF), usually over a period of days; however, chronic renal failure patients can experience acute episodes because of noncompliance or other medical conditions. Causes of ARF, specific pathophysiology, general treatment, and diagnostic markers are listed in Box 39-3. Table 39-1 highlights clinical manifesta-

Table **39-1**	**Clinical Manifestations of Acute Uremia**
Body system	**Clinical manifestations**
Urinary	↓ Urinary output
	Proteinuria
	Casts
	↓ Specific gravity
	↓ Osmolality
	↑ Urinary sodium
Cardiovascular	Volume overload
	Congestive heart failure
	Hypotension (early)
	Hypertension (after development of fluid overload)
	Pericarditis
	Pericardial effusion
	Dysrhythmias
Respiratory	Pulmonary edema
	Kussmaul's respirations
	Pleural effusions
Gastrointestinal	Nausea and vomiting
	Anorexia
	Stomatitis
	Bleeding
	Diarrhea
	Constipation
Hematologic	Anemia (development within 48 hr)
	Leukocytosis
	Defect in platelet functioning
Neurologic	Lethargy
	Convulsions
	Asterixis
	Memory impairment
Others	↑ Susceptibility to infection
	↑ BUN
	↑ Creatinine
	↑ Potassium
	↓ pH
	↓ Bicarbonate
	↓ Calcium
	↑ Phosphate

From Lewis SM, Collier IC, Heitkemper MM: *Medical-surgical nursing: assessment and management of clinical problems,* ed 4, St. Louis, 1996, Mosby.
BUN, Blood urea nitrogen.

Box **39-3** **Common Causes of Acute Renal Failure**

Prerenal

Hypovolemia caused by:
  Hemorrhage
  Burns
  Dehydration
  Prolonged diarrhea or vomiting
Decreased cardiac output caused by:
  Myocardial infarction
  Cardiac dysrhythmias
  Congestive heart failure
  Cardiogenic shock
  Pericardial tamponade
  Surgery (e.g., open heart)
Decreased peripheral vascular resistance
  caused by:
  Septic shock
  Anaphylaxis
Renal vascular obstruction caused by:
  Thrombosis of renal arteries
  Bilateral renal vein thrombosis
  Embolism

Intrarenal

Nephrotoxic injury from the following:
  Drugs (aminoglycosides [gentamicin, tobramycin,
    amikacin], amphotericin B, cisplatin)
  Radiographic contrast agents
  Hemolytic blood transfusion reaction (hemoglobin
    blocks tubules)
  Severe crushing injury (myoglobin released from
    muscles blocks tubules)
  Chemicals (ethylene glycol, mercuric chloride, carbon
    tetrachloride, lead, arsenic)
Acute glomerulonephritis
Acute pyelonephritis
Toxemia of pregnancy
Malignant hypertension
Systemic lupus erythematosus
Interstitial nephritis
  Allergic (antibiotics [sulfonamides, rifampin], non-
    steroidal antiinflammatory drugs, ACE inhibitors)
  Infection (bacterial [e.g., acute pyelonephritis], viral
    [e.g., CMV], fungal [e.g., candidiasis])

Postrenal

Calculi formation
Benign prostatic hyperplasia
Prostate cancer
Bladder cancer
Trauma (to back, pelvis, or
  perineum)
Strictures
Spinal cord disease

ACE, Angiotensin-converting enzyme; CMV, cytomegalovirus.
From Lewis SM, Collier IC, Heitkemper MM: *Medical-surgical nursing: assessment and management of clinical problems,* ed 4, St. Louis, 1996, Mosby.

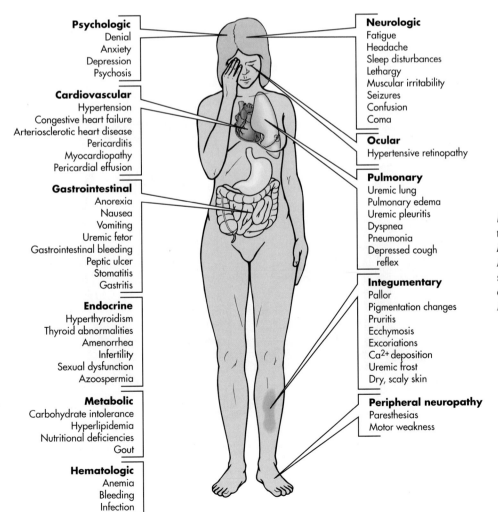

Psychologic
Denial
Anxiety
Depression
Psychosis

Cardiovascular
Hypertension
Congestive heart failure
Arteriosclerotic heart disease
Pericarditis
Myocardiopathy
Pericardial effusion

Gastrointestinal
Anorexia
Nausea
Vomiting
Uremic fetor
Gastrointestinal bleeding
Peptic ulcer
Stomatitis
Gastritis

Endocrine
Hyperthyroidism
Thyroid abnormalities
Amenorrhea
Infertility
Sexual dysfunction
Azoospermia

Metabolic
Carbohydrate intolerance
Hyperlipidemia
Nutritional deficiencies
Gout

Hematologic
Anemia
Bleeding
Infection

Neurologic
Fatigue
Headache
Sleep disturbances
Lethargy
Muscular irritability
Seizures
Confusion
Coma

Ocular
Hypertensive retinopathy

Pulmonary
Uremic lung
Pulmonary edema
Uremic pleuritis
Dyspnea
Pneumonia
Depressed cough
  reflex

Integumentary
Pallor
Pigmentation changes
Pruritis
Ecchymosis
Excoriations
Ca^{2+} deposition
Uremic frost
Dry, scaly skin

Peripheral neuropathy
Paresthesias
Motor weakness

Figure **39-8** Clinical manifestations of chronic uremia. *(From Lewis SM, Collier IC, Heitkemper MM: Medical-surgical nursing: assessment and management of clinical problems, ed 4, St. Louis, 1996, Mosby.)*

tions of acute uremia, and Figure 39-8 describes clinical manifestations of chronic uremia.

Symptoms include short-term weight gain or loss, nausea and vomiting, hematemesis, melena, dysrhythmias, dyspnea, stupor, or coma. Compromise of airway, breathing, circulation, and neurologic function require intervention. Fever may be associated with infectious or inflammatory events. Reducing measures should be instituted to prevent continued rise of nitrogenous waste products by catabolic effect of fever.

Hyperkalemia, hyponatremia, hypocalcemia, hyperphosphatemia, and volume overload are the most common fluid and electrolyte imbalances due to the loss of kidney's ability to excrete K^+ and PO_4^{3-}, conserve Na^+, and eliminate excess volume. Calcium is inversely related to PO_4^{3-} and is low secondary to a rise in PO_4^{3-}, along with the inability of the kidney to convert vitamin D to the active form for calcium absorption from the gut. ECG may reveal tall peaked T waves, widened QRS, and prolonged PR interval secondary to hyperkalemia. Administration of IV calcium may be needed to antagonize the membrane and improve cardiac conductivity until removal of excess K^+ by emergency dialysis can be initiated. Intravenous calcium works within min-

utes, but duration is short, as evidenced by return of ECG changes. Administration of IV $NaHCO_3$, glucose, and insulin redistributes extracellular K^+ into the intracellular fluid, works within 15 to 30 minutes, and lasts approximately 4 hours. Potassium can be removed by cation exchange resin (Kayexolate) but the onset of action is 60 minutes when given rectally and 120 minutes for oral administration.

Urine output may be increased or decreased. If ARF is nonoliguric, large volumes of fluid can be lost, so the patient may be dehydrated and hypotensive. Volume replacement with normal saline or volume expanders is guided by monitoring jugular vein distention and vital signs or by invasive lines such as central venous pressure (CVP) and Swan-Ganz catheters to avoid further ischemic injury to renal tissue. If ARF presents with oliguria, the patient may be volume overloaded and hypertensive so minimal fluid is given until the volume can be removed by diuretics or hemodialysis. Metabolic acidosis occurs because renal tubules can no longer regulate the concentration of H^+ ions. Intravenous $NaHCO_3$ may be used unless contraindicated by volume status.

Indications for emergency dialysis include stupor or coma (caused by rising nitrogen waste products in blood and

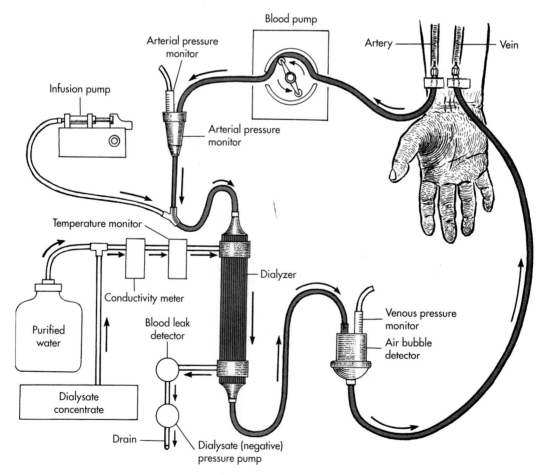

Figure **39-9**   Components of a hemodialysis system. (*From Thelan LA, Davie JK, Urden LD:* Textbook of critical care, *St. Louis, 1990, Mosby.*)

metabolic changes), volume overload and pulmonary edema, dangerous hyperkalemia, and acidosis. Emergency hemodialysis requires vascular access (usually a temporary femoral or subclavian dual lumen catheter or an internal shunt), an artificial kidney (dialyzer) to act as a semipermeable membrane, dialysate low in ions that the body needs to excrete and high in those to be reabsorbed, and a blood pump to move blood through the dialyzer (Figure 39-9).

After initial stabilization, history and diagnostic testing focus on identifying the cause of ARF and may include serial blood chemistries, UA with Na^+ and K^+ concentrations, chest radiograph, renal ultrasounds and Doppler studies, or CT scan. Imaging procedures are usually done without contrast media because of the toxic effects of media on renal tubules.

Dialysis Access Complications

Major etiologies of chronic renal failure (CRF) are vascular changes caused by diabetes, hypertension, or progressive glomerulonephritis. Renal replacement therapy may be provided by peritoneal dialysis or hemodialysis. Peritoneal dialysis involves instilling 1 to 2 L of dialysate fluid containing varying amounts of glucose, magnesium, calcium, chloride, and lactate into the abdomen. The peritoneal membrane acts as a semipermeable pathway for exchange of solutes and water between the vascular peritoneal space and dialysate by osmosis and diffusion (Figure 39-10). Access to the peritoneal cavity is achieved through a plastic catheter held in place by a dacron cuff (Figure 39-11). Peritonitis and exit site infections may bring the patient to the ED with complaints of abdominal pain, nausea and vomiting, fever, and cloudy dialysate fluid. Antibiotics may be given IV and added to dialysate. If this is unsuccessful, the catheter should be removed and hemodialysis initiated until the peritonitis clears. Unless scarring impairs the permeability of the peritoneal membrane, the catheter can be surgically replaced and peritoneal dialysis reinitiated.

Clotted vascular access frequently brings patients with CRF to the ED. Arteriovenous fistulas are surgical connections of a native artery and vein in an extremity or insertion of Gortex graft material to form the connection (Figure 39-12). Available sites suitable for vascular access become exhausted, so permanent subclavian dual lumen catheters are placed for hemodialysis. Clotted vascular access should be emergently declotted with the use of locally instilled or infused thrombolytics or surgery. Grafts, fistulas, and insertion sites also become infected and may progress to septicemia. Local symptoms include redness, drainage, or edema. Blood cultures and CBC should be obtained to rule out systemic infection. Access removal may be necessary, so temporary subclavian or femoral access that is replaced every 2 or 3 days can be used until blood is free of infection.

Urinary Tract Infections

Common symptoms of GU tract infection include pyuria, hematuria, chills and fever, leucocytosis, nausea and vomiting, and signs of bladder irritability such as frequency,

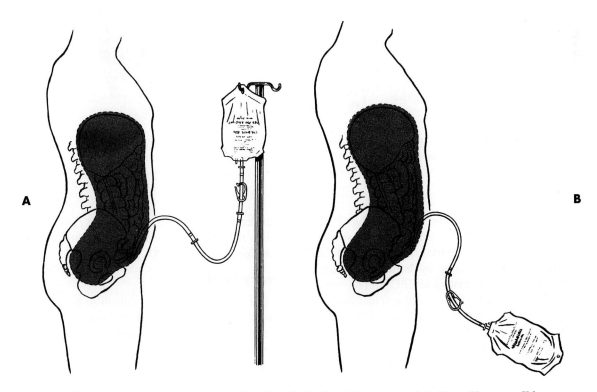

Figure **39-10**   Peritoneal dialysis. **A,** Inflow. **B,** Outflow (drains to gravity). *(From Thompson JM et al: Mosby's clinical nursing, ed 4, St. Louis, 1997, Mosby.)*

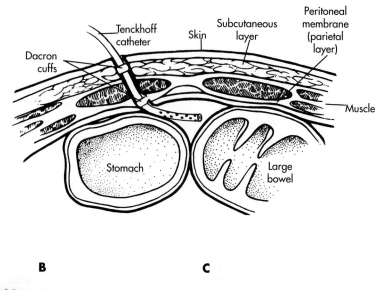

Figure **39-11** Peritoneal catheter. *(From Thompson JM et al:* Mosby's clinical nursing, *ed 4, St. Louis, 1997, Mosby.)*

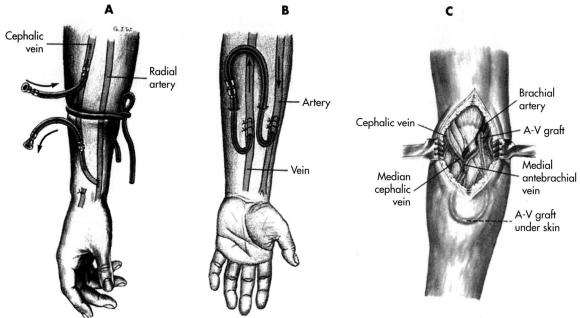

Figure **39-12** Circulatory access for hemodialysis. **A,** External (temporary) arteriovenous cannula (shunt). **B,** Internal (permanent) arteriovenous fistula. **C,** Internal (permanent) arteriovenous graft. *(From Thompson JM et al:* Mosby's clinical nursing, *ed 4, St. Louis, 1997, Mosby.)*

dysuria, and urgency. With renal involvement, dull flank pain and costovertebral angle (CVA) tenderness may also be present. Figure 39-13 illustrates infectious processes of the urinary system. Diagnosis is made by history, presenting signs, UA, urine culture-sensitivity, and CBC with differential. KUB (kidneys-ureters-bladder) radiograph may show a hazy outline of the kidney secondary to edema. BUN, creatinine, and electrolytes values are obtained to rule out alteration in renal function. Persistent microscopic or gross hematuria, symptoms of obstruction, or presence of urea-splitting bacteria associated with staghorn renal calculi require work up with renal ultrasound, cystogram, or IVP. Infection with *Chlamydia trachomatis* or *Neisseria gonorrhoeae* should be

considered with urethral infection and pyuria that has negative culture. Table 39-2 compares common GU tract infections that present to the ED.

Urinary Calculi

A primary risk factor for calculi is hypercalciuria; however, there is also an association with UTI, gout, excessive ingestion of certain foods, family history, dehydration, and pregnancy (Box 39-4). Seventy-five percent of stones are composed of calcium combined with oxalate or phosphate, the remaining 25% are composed of struvite, cystine, or uric acid (Table 39-3). Calculi are asymptomatic until movement causes intermittent backache, urge to void, dysuria, renal

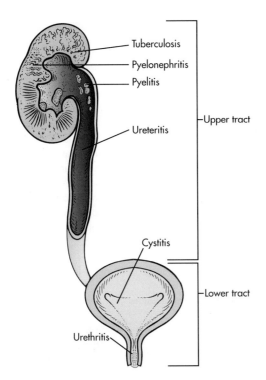

Figure **39-13** Sites of infectious processes in the urinary tract. *(From Lewis SM, Collier IC, Heitkemper MM: Medical-surgical nursing: assessment and management of clinical problems, ed 4, St. Louis, 1996, Mosby.)*

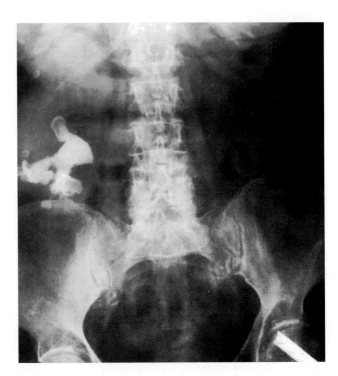

Figure **39-14** Radiograph of a staghorn calculus. *(Courtesy Harborview Medical Center, University of Washington, Seattle.)*

colic, and hematuria. Bacteremia and proteinuria may also be present. Diagnostic studies include CBC, BUN, creatinine, electrolytes, uric acid, UA with culture and sensitivity (C and S), KUB, and IVP. Figure 39-14 shows staghorn calculus on a KUB radiograph. Ninety percent of stones exit spontaneously; however, if unpassed, they may be removed by laparoscopy, lithotripsy, or surgical removal. Figure 39-15 illustrates shock wave lithotripsy. Nursing interventions include input and output measurement, straining all urine, sending solid material for lab analysis, and increased fluids. Complications include ischemia at obstructive site, altered elimination, and UTI. Criteria for admission include need for frequent pain medicine, large-diameter stones, solitary kidney, ileus, bladder stones, and infection. If discharged, information should be provided to return in case of increasing pain, excessive vomiting, or fever and chills. Dietary restrictions should also be included (see Box 39-4).

Testicular Torsion

Testicular torsion causes vascular compromise of the testes within 6 to 12 hours and can lead to infarction with resultant atrophy and loss of spermiogenesis. Most cases occur in adolescent males, 50% during sleep, and are associated with congenital abnormality of the tunica vaginalis, the canal from which the testes descend. Clinical manifestations include upwardly retracted testes with redness and

Text continued on p. 572

Box 39-4 Risk Factors in the Development of Urinary Tract Calculi

Metabolic

Abnormalities that result in increased urine levels of calcium, oxaluric acid, uric acid, or citic acid

Climate

Warm climates that cause increased fluid loss, low urine volume, and increased solute concentration in urine

Diet

Large intake of dietary proteins that increases uric acid excretion

Excessive amounts of tea or fruit juices that elevate urinary oxalate level

Large intake of calcium and oxalate

Low fluid intake that increases urinary concentration

Genetic factors

Family history of stone formation, cystinuria, gout, or renal acidosis

Lifestyle

Sedentary occupation, immobility

From Lewis SM, Collier IC, Heitkemper MM: *Medical-surgical nursing: assessment and management of clinical problems,* ed 4, St. Louis, 1996, Mosby.

Table **39-2**   **Common Genitourinary Infections**

Type	Description	Additional signs and symptoms	Interventions	Complications and comments
Pyelonephritis	Involves renal parenchyma and pelvis Usually unilateral Kidneys enlarged by edema More prevalent in women and diabetics Most commonly caused by ascending *Escherichia coli* infection from lower GU tract		Antibiotics specific to C and S Antipyretics and anti-emetics Adequate hydration Monitor intake and output Bed rest	Complications uncommon but may include septicemia Follow-up urine C and S to ensure effective antibiotic therapy Recurrence may require continuous antibiotic prophylactic suppression
Urethritis	More common in women *E. coli* most common organism Behavioral factors associated include sexual intercourse, diaphragm and/or spermicide use, not voiding within 10-15 minutes after intercourse		Short-term antibiotics May need continuous antibiotic, prophylactic suppression, or post-coital antibiotic	Behaviors associated with UTIs Direction of wiping after defecation Tampon use Bubble bath Douche Tight clothing Carbonated beverages, coffee, alcohol Resisting urge to void Decreasing PO fluids Synthetic underwear
Epididymitis	Bacterial infection in older men Usually preceded by STD or urethritis in young men	*P* lifting, sexual excitement, trauma *Q* Dull ache, sharp *R* Scrotum, lower abdomen *S* Increased with sex, decreased with elevation and support *T* Gradual onset Scrotum red, swollen, and warm	Antibiotics Posttreatment culture Bed rest Scrotal support Avoid heavy lifting and straining	Teach safe sex and condom use, complete antibiotic regimen
Prostatitis	Expressed prostate secretions have more WBCs than urine	May have bladder outlet obstruction Low back pain Tender, boggy, hot prostate on manual exam	Antibiotics, UA C and S and expressed prostate fluid C and S	
Nonspecific urethritis	Causative agents: *E. coli, Staphylococcus, Klebsiella, Pseudomonas*	White discharge Urethral itching Perineal, suprapubic, or testicular pain	Antibiotics as result of discharge C and S	

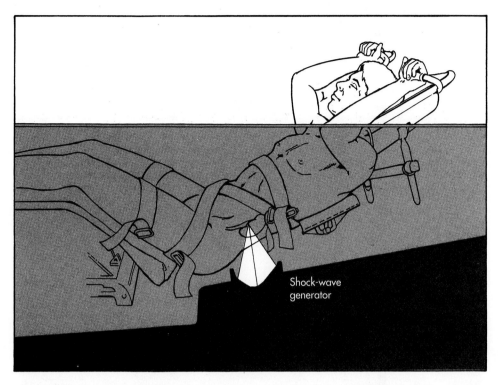

Figure **39-15** Patient positioned for shock-wave lithotripsy. Area of flank is exposed for efficient shock-wave conduction. *(From Brundage DJ:* Renal disorders, *St. Louis, 1992, Mosby.)*

Table **39-3**	**Types of Urinary Tract Calculi**			
Urinary stone	Incidence (%)	Characteristics	Predisposing factors	Therapeutic measures
Calcium oxalate*	35-40	Small, often possible to get trapped in ureter; more frequent in men than in women	Idiopathic hypercalciuria, hyperoxaluria, independent of urinary pH, family history	Increase hydration; reduce dietary oxalate; give thiazide diuretics, phosphate therapy; give cholestyramine to bind oxalate; give calcium lactate to precipitate oxalate in gastrointestinal tract
Calcium phosphate	8-10	Mixed stones (typically), with struvite or oxalate stones	Alkaline urine, primary hyperparathyroidism	Treat underlying causes and other stones
Struvite (MgNH$_4$PO$_4$)	10-15	Three to four times as common in women than men, always in association with urinary tract infections, large staghorn type (usually)	Urinary tract infections (usually *Proteus* organisms)	Administer antimicrobial agents, acetohydroxamic acid; use surgical intervention to remove stone; take measures to acidify urine
Uric acid	5-8	Predominant in men, high incidence in Jewish men	Gout, acid urine, inherited condition	Reduce urinary concentration of uric acid; alkalinize urine, administer allopurinol
Cystine	1-2	Genetic autosomal recessive defect, defective absorption of cystine in gastrointestinal tract and kidney, excess concentrations causing stone formation	Acid urine	Increase hydration; give α-penicillamine to prevent cystine crystallization; give sodium bicarbonate to maintain alkaline urine.

From Lewis SM, Collier IC, Heitkemper MM: *Medical-surgical nursing: assessment and management of clinical problems,* ed 4, St. Louis, 1996, Mosby.
*Calcium stones can exist as calcium oxalate, calcium phosphate, or a mixture of both. Calcium stones account for the majority of all stones.

Table 39-4   Common Sexually Transmitted Diseases

Virus	Epidemiology	Clinical presentation	Diagnosis	Treatment
Herpes simplex	Most common cause of nongonococcal proctitis in sexually active homosexual men Incubation 1-12 days for first episode Recurrence in 60% of cases, usually less severe HSV1 can occur genitally but HSV2 is more common, both can occur orally	Pain, itching, dysuria, vaginal or urethral purulent discharge Classic small painful vesicles on erythematous base that may ulcer Crusting of vesicles indicates healing Lymph enlargement occurs with primary infection 33% develop meningitis	Culture lesions Serum test for virus	Acyclovir topically, orally, or IV to decrease time of viral shedding, local symptoms, and healing time 400 mg TID or 200 mg 5 times a day for 7-10 days 6-8 recurrences/year need suppressive therapy 200 mg TID or 400 mg TID to decrease recurrence
Cytomegaly	Viral member of herpes family Primary infection followed by latency and may recur with immunosuppression Transmitted via secretions of the oropharynx, vagina, cervix, urine, breast milk, semen, and blood High prevalence in HIV-positive patients	Fever, fatigue, arthralgia, myalgia, headache, hepatitis Immunosuppressed patients may have life-threatening illness	Serum test for virus	Gancyclovir—may have increased benefit with retinitis and GI CMV
Gonorrhea	Gram-negative diplococcus bacteria Asymptomatic carriage in pharynx, urethra, rectum, and cervix common 3-5 day incubation	Urethritis in men with dysuria and mucoid drainage Endocervicitis usual form of infection in women with dysuria, frequency, abnormal discharge Anorectal infection from pruritus to proctitis Pharyngitis may occur Yellow mucopurulent drainage	Gram stain exudate on Thayer-Martin medium (prewarmed) in ED (or transported directly to lab) Resistant strains increasing in incidence	Ceftriaxone drug of choice 125-150 mg IM

Chlamydial	Intracellular parasitic infection with *C. trachomatis* 5-10+ days incubation period	Pelvic inflammatory disease in women Epididymitis in men Urethritis with mucopurulent drainage	Cytology of discharge	Doxycycline 100 mg BID for 7 days Erythromycin 500 mg QID for 7 days Azithromycin 1 g for one dose
Condyloma acuminatum (venereal warts)	Incubation 3-6 months	No discharge Pink-gray soft lesions, singular or grouped Lesions are tall and may bleed		Topical 10%-25% podophyllin in tincture of benzoin OR 50% trichloroacetic acid or liquid nitrogen (treatment of choice for pregnancy)
Trichomonas vaginalis	Incubation period of 1 week	Copious, thin, frothy, greenish, gray, foul-smelling discharge Severe pruritus Edema and redness of vagina Worse following menstrual bleeding	Culture and sensitivity	Metronidazole
Gardnella vaginalis	Incubation period 5-10 days	Fishy odor Gray, white, frothy discharge in lesser amounts than with *T. vaginalis* Mild itching	Culture and sensitivity	Metronidazole or ampicillin
Syphilis	Spirochete infection with *Treponema pallidum* Transmitted via sexual contact with moist skin lesions 3-6 weeks incubation for the primary stage (chancre) 6-8 weeks later secondary stage with disseminated bacteremia Tertiary stage if untreated with endocarditis and granuloma formation	Papule that progresses to indurated ulcer that is painless and associated with lymphadenopathy	VDRL serology Lesion culture	PCN 2.4 million units IM Doxycycline 100 mg BID for 14 days Erythromycin 500 mg PO QID for 14 days
Chancroid	Caused by *Haemophilus ducreyi* 3-14 days incubation	Acute painful ulcers that are nonindurated with nonspecific edges Inguinal tender lymphadenopathy Dysuria	Culture and gram stain of lesion	Ceftriaxone 250 mg IM for one dose Azithromycin 1 g PO for one dose Erythromycin 500 mg PO QID for 7 days Ciprofloxacin 500 mg PO BID for 3 days

A   **B**   **C**

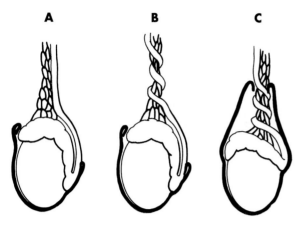

Figure **39-16** Testicular torsion. **A,** Normal tunica vaginalis insertion. **B,** Extravaginal torsion. **C,** Intravaginal torsion with abnormally high vaginal insertion. *(From Price SA, Wilson LM: Pathophysiology: clinical concepts of disease processes, ed 5, St. Louis, 1997, Mosby.)*

edema to the site of the torsion, abdominal pain, and nausea and vomiting. Figure 39-16 compares normal testicular structures with testicular torsion. Intervention with manual detorsion under local anesthesia or surgery must be performed within 48 hours or orchiectomy may be necessary. Testicular torsion is differentiated from epididymitis by absence of pyuria and age of occurrence; epididymitis is rare in puberty.

Priapism

Priapism is persistent, painful erection not associated with sexual desire. Engorgement is limited to the corpora cavernosa; the corpus spongiosum and glans are not involved. Obstruction of venous drainage causes the build up of viscous deoxygenated blood, interstitial edema, and eventual fibrosis. Pain severity increases with duration. With urinary obstruction and bladder distention, pain can last as long as 24 hours. Etiologies include sickle cell crisis, spinal cord injury, multiple sclerosis, psychotropic drugs, or prolonged sexual activity. Priapism from use of papaverine for impotence is being seen more frequently.

Pharmacologic management of priapism includes subcutaneous terbutaline.[7] Acute detumescence is accomplished surgically with a large-bore needle, after regional nerve block with an adrenergic agent such as Neosynephrine. Surgical stinting may be necessary by tissue removal to relieve obstruction or by anastomosis of veins between glans and cavernosa. CBC with increased reticulocyte count may identify sickling cells as the underlying cause, so supplemental oxygen along with transfusion may be effective. Fifty percent of cases require a urinary catheter for bladder obstruction and distention. Development of fibrosis and scarring in cavernous spaces is related to the duration of priapism and decompression and can cause impotence.

Box **39-5**

NURSING DIAGNOSES RELATED TO GU EMERGENCIES

Altered tissue perfusion
Fluid volume deficit
Fluid volume excess
Electrolyte imbalance
Pain
Risk for infection
Altered urinary elimination
Knowledge deficit
Anxiety

Sexually Transmitted Diseases

Sexually transmitted diseases are spread through intimate sexual contact and can present with a variety of symptoms. History should be elicited to include location, color, smell, character, and quantity of discharge. Pain usually presents as pruritus and burning at the urethra, vagina, perineum, or pharynx, which can be mild to severe with associated lesions. Sexual activity, past medical history, and the date of last menstrual period should be obtained. A pelvic examination may be performed with warm water employed as the only lubricant. A rectal examination and sigmoidoscopy may also be indicated. Diagnostic studies include C and S of lesions or drainage, VDRL, wet mount (saline and KOH), UA with C and S, and cytology smear. Along with antibiotics, discharge teaching should include abstinence until treatment is completed and lesions are healed, need for partner treatment, use of condoms, 7- to 10-day follow up, and consideration of HIV testing. Complications of untreated STDs include endocarditis, arthralgias, meningitis, salpingitis, chronic pelvic inflammatory disease (PID), severe proctitis, and sterility. Table 39-4 compares common STDs excluding acquired immunodeficiency syndrome (AIDS), which is reviewed further in Chapter 42.

SUMMARY

GU emergencies require evaluation of renal function to rule out renal involvement. The GU system functions to maintain homeostasis, so disruption of renal function interrupts almost all organ systems, as evidenced by the priority nursing diagnoses listed in Box 39-5. Emerging strains of resistant bacteria are challenging health care professions in treatment and prevention. Public education regarding safe sexual practice should be included in all discharge teaching for STDs. The emergency nurse has many opportunities to play an important role in the detection and prevention of GU diseases.

REFERENCES

1. Guyton AC, Hall J: *Textbook of medical physiology,* ed 9, Philadelphia, 1996, WB Saunders.
2. Leiner S: Recurrent urinary tract infections in otherwise healthy adult women, *Nurse Pract: Am J Prim Health Care* 20(2):48, 1995.
3. Schrier RW: *Manual of nephrology,* ed 4, Boston, 1994, Little, Brown.
4. Smith M, Singer C: Sexually transmitted viruses other than HIV and papillomavirus, *Urol Clin North Am* 19(1):47, 1992.
5. Stark JL: Acute tubular necrosis: differences between oliguria and anuria, *Crit Care Nurs Q* 14(4):22, 1992.
6. Stine R, Chudnofsky C: *A practical approach to emergency medicine,* ed 2, Boston, 1994, Little, Brown.
7. Tintinalli JE, Ruiz E, Krome RL: *Emergency medicine: a comprehensive review,* ed 4, New York, 1996, McGraw-Hill.

SUGGESTED READING

Bellinger M: Spermatic cord torsion: a true emergency, *Emerg Med* 26(16):50, 1994.
Cooper C: What color is that urine specimen? *Am J Nurs* 93(8):37, 1993.
Danis D, Halm K: Sexually transmitted disease treatment guidelines revisited, *J Emerg Nurs* 20:239, 1994.
Daugirdas J, Ing T: *Handbook of dialysis,* ed 2, Boston, 1994, Little, Brown.
Drach G: *Campbell's urology,* ed 6, vol 3, Philadelphia, 1992, WB Saunders.

Emergency Nurses Association: *Emergency nursing core curriculum,* ed 4, Park Ridge, Ill, 1994.
Fihn SD: Urinary tract infection, *Consultant* 32(10):43, 1992.
The hematuria work-up: one step at a time, *Emerg Med* 22(20):18, 1990.
Kitt S, Selfridge-Thomas J et al: *Emergency nursing: a physiologic and clinical perspective,* ed 2, Philadelphia, 1995, WB Saunders.
Lewis SM, Collier IC, Heitkemper MM: *Medical-surgical nursing: assessment and management of clinical problems,* ed 4, St. Louis, 1996, Mosby.
Miller LR: Pyelonephritis, *Hosp Prac* 28(suppl 2):31, 1993.
Peterson NE: Treating acute oliguria or anuria, *Patient Care* 27(1):162, 1996.
Rutecki GW: The rules of three in oliguria: how to use this technique for evaluation, *Consultant* 33(1):43, 1993.
Ruth-Sand L: Renal calculi, *Am J Nurs* 95(11):50, 1995.
Schrier RW: *Renal and electrolyte disorders,* ed 5, Boston, 1997, Little, Brown.
Seeley RR, Stephens TD, Tate P: *Anatomy and physiology,* ed 3, St. Louis, 1995, McGraw-Hill.
Tanagho E, McAninch J: *Smith's general urology,* ed 14, Los Altos, Calif,1994, Lange Medical Publishers.
Thompson JM, McFarland GK, Hirsch JE et al: *Mosby's clinical nursing,* ed 4, St. Louis, 1997, Mosby.
Tonetti J, Tonetti F: Testicular torsion or acute epididymitis? Diagnosis and treatment, *J Emerg Nurs* 16(2):96, 1990.

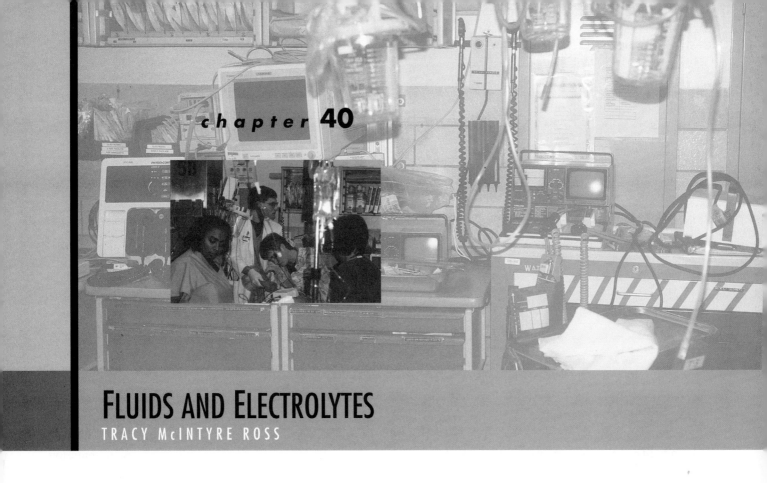

chapter 40

FLUIDS AND ELECTROLYTES

TRACY McINTYRE ROSS

Water is the most abundant fluid medium in the body, composing 60% of total body weight in the average adult, 80% in an infant, and as little as 40% in an elderly adult[6] (Figure 40-1). In a healthy physiologic state, this fluid medium has a constant balance of electrolytes controlled by a unique system of checks and balances. Effects of fluid and electrolyte disturbances are often a primary or secondary reason for many emergency department (ED) visits. Gastrointestinal, urologic, cardiac, respiratory, and endocrine diseases as well as many forms of traumatic injury cause fluid and electrolyte abnormalities.

This chapter describes the interrelation of water, water metabolism, and electrolyte composition. Fluid and electrolyte control mechanisms, signs and symptoms, etiology, and treatment of specific fluid and electrolyte abnormalities are also discussed.

PATHOPHYSIOLOGY

Water and electrolytes are interdependent. Pathophysiology of one affects function and value of the other. Normal fluid and electrolyte levels are the result of structural, physiologic, and environmental factors.

Water

Water has many important metabolic functions including transport of nutrients and other essential substances, removal of metabolic waste products, normal cell metabolism, and maintenance of normal body temperature. Individual fluid requirements are determined by age, weight, body fat, and environmental factors such as ambient temperature. Fat is virtually water free; therefore increases in body fat are associated with decreases in body water. The average adult ingests 1500 to 3000 ml of water per day through the gastrointestinal tract.[2] Water intake attributed to oxidation of hydrogen in food is approximately 150 to 250 ml/day, depending on individual metabolic rate.[4] Water output is dependent on factors such as ambient temperature and activity level. An average resting adult in an ambient temperature of 68° F loses approximately 1400 ml of water per day in urine, 100 ml in sweat, 100 ml in feces, and 700 ml in insensible water loss.[4] Conditions such as vomiting, diarrhea, denuding of the skin (i.e., burns), increased ambient temperature, or intense physical exercise significantly increase water loss.

Total body water (TBW) is distributed between the extracellular and intracellular compartments. Extracellular fluid (ECF) constitutes one third of TBW, or approximately 15 L. ECF consists of plasma, interstitial fluid, cerebrospinal fluid, intraocular fluid, fluids of the gastrointestinal tract, and fluids of potential spaces (i.e., pleural space, peritoneal space). Intracellular fluid (ICF) accounts for two thirds of TBW and represents the sum of the fluid content for all the cells in the body, approximately 25 L.

Two regulatory mechanisms influential in maintaining normal water volume and tonicity or osmotic pressure are thirst and renal function. Thirst, the primary regulator for intake of water, is defined as the "conscious desire for water."[4]

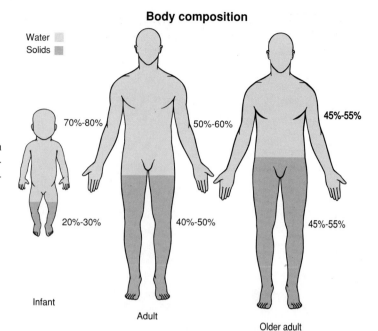

Body composition

Water

Solids

70%-80%   50%-60%   45%-55%

20%-30%   40%-50%   45%-55%

Infant

Adult

Older adult

Figure **40-1** Changes in body water content correlated with age. *(From Lewis SM, Collier IC, Heitkemper MM:* Medical-surgical nursing: assessment and management of clinical problems, *ed 4, St. Louis, 1996, Mosby.)*

Thirst ensures adequate replacement of fluid losses and is stimulated by ECF hypertonicity and decreased ICF volume. Conversely, thirst is depressed by ECF hypotonicity and increased ICF volume. Any factor that causes intracellular dehydration stimulates a small area in the hypothalamus called the thirst center and promotes water consumption. Figure 40-2 illustrates stimuli that affect the thirst mechanism. Since the thirst mechanism is triggered by increased osmolarity, thirst is not effective in hypotonic or hyponatremic dehydration where water and sodium loss are equal. Factors

that adversely affect the thirst mechanism include brain injury and psychosocial factors such as depression, confusion, and fear of incontinence.

Renal regulation of water balance is twofold, affecting both tonicity and body water. When the glomerular filtrate is hypertonic, osmoreceptors in the hypothalamus are stimulated, and antidiuretic hormone (ADH) is released by the pituitary gland. ADH makes renal collecting tubules more permeable to water, so water is reabsorbed into the body, diluting blood and concentrating urine (Figure 40-3). If plasma

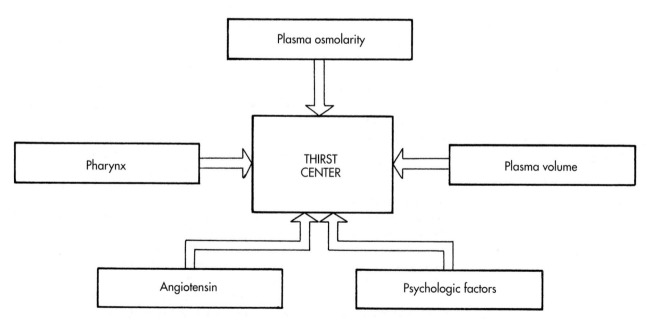

Plasma osmolarity

Pharynx   THIRST CENTER   Plasma volume

Angiotensin   Psychologic factors

Figure **40-2** Stimuli affecting the thirst mechanism. *(Modified from Groer MW:* Physiology and pathophysiology of the body fluids, *St. Louis, 1981, Mosby.)*

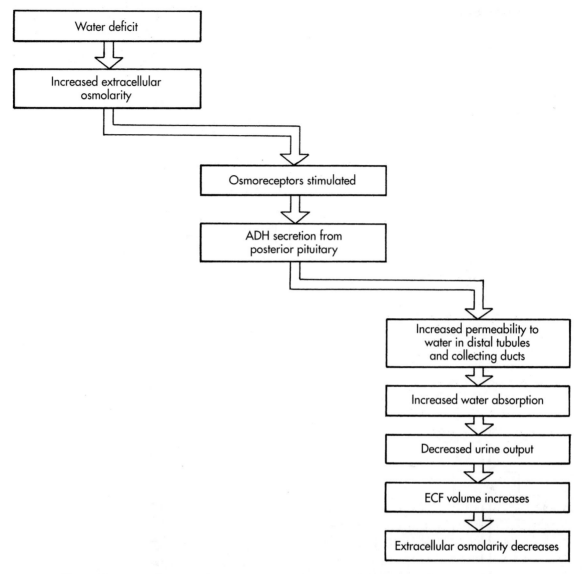

Figure **40-3** Osmoreceptor-ADH feedback mechanism for regulating osmolarity in response to water deficit.

or glomerular filtrate is hypotonic, ADH secretion is inhibited, and collecting tubules reabsorb less water. Blood becomes concentrated and the urine is diluted as more water exits the kidneys.

Volume of body water is also regulated by the kidney through the renin-angiotensin-aldosterone system (Figure 40-4). When ECF volume, specifically blood volume, is low, receptors in the kidneys secrete an enzyme called renin. Renin stimulates angiotensinogen (a normal plasma protein) to release angiotensin I, which is then converted to angiotensin II by another enzyme, primarily in the lungs. Angiotensin II stimulates the adrenal cortex to secrete aldosterone, which increases sodium reabsorption from glomerular filtrate in exchange for potassium and hydrogen ions. This exchange increases plasma tonicity, which leads to ADH secretion, water retention, and increased volume. With

excessive ECF volume (blood volume), aldosterone secretion is depressed, so tubular reabsorption of sodium and water decreases (Figure 40-5).

Electrolytes

An electrolyte is a substance capable of carrying an electrical charge. An electrolyte with a positive charge is called a *cation,* whereas an electrolyte with a negative charge is an *anion.* Electrolytes are found in varying concentrations in the ECF and ICF (Figure 40-6). For the purposes of this chapter, serum electrolyte measurements are equivalent to extracellular electrolyte values (Table 40-1). Direct measurement of intracellular electrolyte concentrations in the clinical setting is not yet feasible. ICF electrolyte concentrations must be inferred from serum electrolyte values.

Table **40-1**	**Normal Serum Electrolyte Values**
Anions	**Normal value**
Bicarbonate (HCO$_3^-$)	20-30 mEq/L (20-30 mmol/L)
Chloride (Cl$^-$)	96-106 mEq/L (96-106 mmol/L)
Phosphate (PO$_4^{3-}$)	2.8-4.5 mg/dl (0.90-1.45 mmol/L)
Protein	6-8 g/dl (60-80 g/L)
Cations	**Normal value**
Potassium (K$^+$)	3.5-5.5 mEq/L (3.5-5.5 mmol/L)
Magnesium (Mg^{2+})	1.5-2.5 mEq/L (0.75-1.25 mmol/L)
Sodium (Na$^+$)	135-145 mEq/L (135-145 mmol/L)
Calcium (Ca^{2+})	9-11 mg/dl
	4.5-5.5 mEq/L (2.25-2.75 mmol/L)

From Lewis SM, Collier IC, Heitkemper MM: *Medical-surgical nursing: assessment and management of clinical problems,* ed 4, St. Louis, 1996, Mosby.

All fluids outside the cells are collectively referred to as the ECF. Electrolytes in the ECF, from greatest to least concentration, are sodium, chloride, potassium, bicarbonate, and hydrogen. ECF also contains oxygen, carbon dioxide, proteins, and a few miscellaneous anions.

ICF represents fluid found in approximately seventy-five trillion cells in the body, about 25 L. Electrolytes in the ICF, from greatest to least concentration, are potassium, phosphate and sulphate combined, magnesium, and lastly sodium, hydrogen, and bicarbonate in equal concentrations. The ICF also contains a number of proteins.

The delicate balance of water and electrolytes between intracellular and extracellular compartments is an ongoing process of checks and balances easily disturbed by disease or injury. Regulatory processes and the role each electrolyte plays in the body are described in the following sections.

Sodium

Sodium, the principal cation in the ECF, is primarily responsible for osmotic pressure. Forty percent of the body's sodium is in the blood and ECF; the remainder is intracellular and in bone and connective tissue. Sodium is exchange-

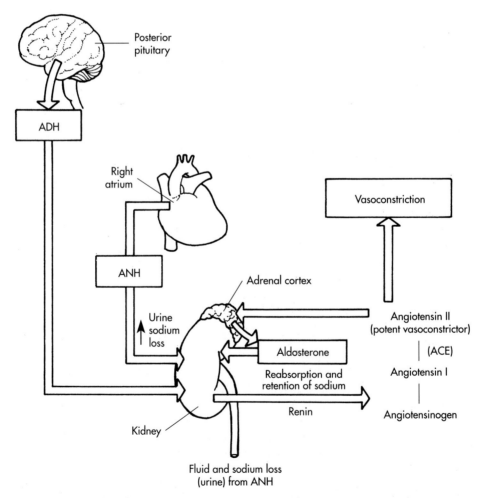

Figure **40-4** Renin-angiotensin-aldosterone system. *(From Huether SE, McCance KL:* Understanding pathophysiology, *St. Louis, 1996, Mosby.)*

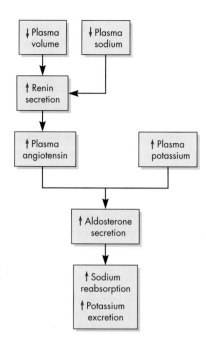

Figure **40-5** Influences of aldosterone secretion. *(From Lewis SM, Collier IC, Heitkemper MM:* Medical-surgical nursing: assessment and management of clinical problems, *ed 4, St. Louis, 1996, Mosby.)*

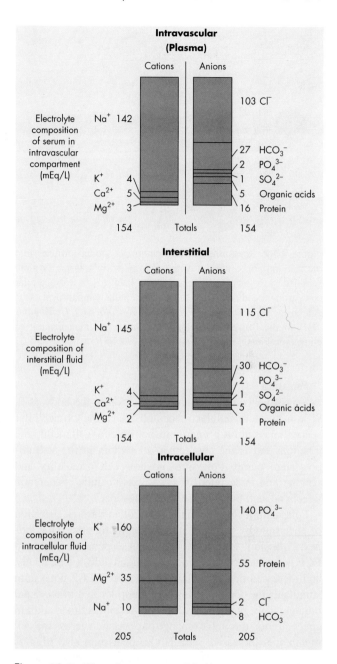

Figure **40-6** Electrolyte content of fluid compartments. *(From Lewis SM, Collier IC, Heitkemper MM:* Medical-surgical nursing: assessment and management of clinical problems, *ed 4, St. Louis, 1996, Mosby.)*

able across cell membranes to maintain sodium and water balance as well as normal arterial pressure. Sodium and chloride play an important role in maintaining body water; in movement of glucose, insulin, and amino acids across cell membranes; and in maintaining muscle strength, neural function, and urinary output. Sodium is essential for the sodium-potassium pump, which moves sodium and potassium across the cell membrane during repolarization (Figure 40-7).

Sodium levels are maintained through the renin-angiotensin-aldosterone system, sympathetic nervous system, and a less well-defined system mediated by atrial natriuretic factor. Decreased fluid volume decreases blood flow and arterial pressure, which stimulates baroreceptors in the kidneys (Figure 40-8). Baroreceptors stimulate the sympathetic nervous system, which leads to vasoconstriction of renal arterioles, decreased glomerular filtration rate, and retention of sodium and water. The opposite sequence of events occurs when fluid intake (or blood volume) rises above normal.

Atrial natriuretic factor, released from the atria in the heart in response to increased arterial pressure, produces natriuresis (excretion of abnormal amounts of sodium in the urine), diuresis, vasodilation, decreased thirst, and antagonistic effects on ADH release, renin, and aldosterone.[5] The resulting increase in sodium excretion eliminates excess volume.

Chloride

Chloride, the principal anion of blood and ECF, is secreted in various body fluids along with other electrolytes.

Sodium and chloride are excreted in sweat, bile, pancreatic fluids, and intestinal fluids. Gastric juice contains chloride and hydrogen. Like sodium, chloride plays a cooperative role in maintaining acid-base balance and takes part in exchange of oxygen and carbon dioxide in red blood cells. Serum chloride levels are passively regulated by serum sodium levels. When serum sodium increases, serum chloride also increases. However, chloride levels are inversely related to bicarbonate levels, since chloride is sacrificed in the kidneys to produce more bicarbonate.

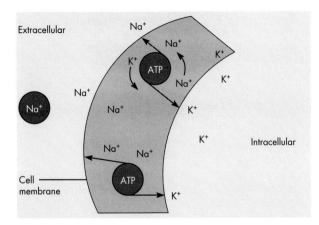

Figure **40-7** Sodium-potassium pump. As sodium diffuses into the cell and potassium out of the cell, an active transport system supplied with energy delivers sodium back to the extracellular compartment and potassium to the intracellular compartment. *ATP,* Adenosine triphosphate. *(From Lewis SM, Collier IC, Heitkemper MM: Medical-surgical nursing: assessment and management of clinical problems, ed 4, St. Louis, 1996, Mosby.)*

Potassium

Potassium is the most abundant cation in the body, with 98% in the intracellular space and 2% in the extracellular space. Potassium is primarily responsible for cell membrane potential and is the counterpart to sodium in the sodium-potassium pump. Potassium governs cell osmolality and volume and is secreted in sweat, gastric juice, pancreatic juice, bile, and fluids of the small intestine.

Potassium level is primarily controlled through secretion of potassium by the distal and collecting tubules in the kidney. Potassium secretion increases in response to increased ECF potassium concentration, increased aldosterone levels, and increased distal tubular flow. A rise in ECF potassium stimulates the sodium-potassium pump located in the renal tubules. This pump maintains a low intracellular sodium concentration through exchange of potassium across the cell membrane. Increased extracellular potassium also triggers aldosterone secretion by the adrenal cortex. Aldosterone increases the rate at which tubular cells secrete potassium and permeability of the renal tubular lumen for potassium. This is a negative feedback system regulated by the serum potassium level. Finally, increased distal tubular flow causes rapid secretion of potassium into the urine.

Alkalosis temporarily decreases serum potassium by driving potassium into the cells in exchange for hydrogen ions. Conversely, the major factor that decreases potassium secretion and increases serum potassium is acute acidosis. Acute acidosis increases hydrogen ion concentration in the ECF, so potassium moves out of the cell in exchange for excess hydrogen ions.

Calcium

Approximately 99% of the body's calcium is found in the bone, with 1% in the ICF and 0.1% in the ECF.[4] Bone acts as a large reservoir for calcium when ECF calcium levels fall. Calcium is transported in the blood in two forms. Half is bound to plasma proteins, usually albumin, and the rest exists as an ionized form that is free and metabolically active. A small amount of nonionized calcium forms complexes with anions such as phosphate, citrate, and sulfate. Most ionized calcium is found in the ECF. Because of the large amount of calcium bound to plasma proteins, assessment of total serum calcium without simultaneous measurement of serum proteins has limited value in determining hypo- or hypercalcemia.

Calcium has many important functions—in smooth and skeletal muscle contraction, in bone and brain metabolism, in blood clotting, and as a primary ingredient in lung surfactant. Calcium is essential for membrane polarization and depolarization, action potential generation, neurotransmission, and muscle contraction. Calcium channels in myocardial cells allow transmembrane calcium transport.

The most important regulatory factors for calcium homeostasis are parathyroid hormone (PTH), calcitonin, and vitamin D. When ECF calcium falls below normal levels, parathyroid glands release PTH, which acts directly on the bones to stimulate release of large amounts of calcium into ECF. With an elevated calcium ion concentration, PTH secretion decreases, so excess calcium is deposited into the bones.

Bones rely on proper intake and absorption of calcium to maintain calcium stores. Calcium absorption in the gastrointestinal tract and kidneys is regulated by PTH levels. In hypocalcemic states, PTH activates vitamin D_3, the form of vitamin D necessary to increase intestinal calcium reabsorption. PTH also directly stimulates the kidneys to increase renal tubular calcium reabsorption, which prevents loss of calcium in the urine.

Another factor that influences calcium reabsorption is the plasma concentration of phosphate. Serum calcium levels are inversely related to serum phosphate levels. Increases in plasma phosphate stimulate PTH, which increases calcium reabsorption by the renal tubules and reduces calcium loss in the urine.

The thyroid gland secretes a hormone called calcitonin in response to elevated calcium levels. The effect of calcitonin on plasma calcium levels is directly opposite that of PTH. Calcitonin decreases plasma calcium levels by increasing calcium deposits in the bone and decreasing formation of new osteoclasts, the cells responsible for breakdown and removal of bone. Calcitonin also has very minor effects on calcium absorption in the renal tubules and gastrointestinal tract.

Phosphate/phosphorus

Phosphorus, the major anion in the ICF, is essential for metabolism of carbohydrate, lipids, and protein. Phosphate also plays a role in various hormonal activities and acid-base balance. Phosphate has a close relationship with calcium in maintaining homeostasis. Clinical studies have shown that

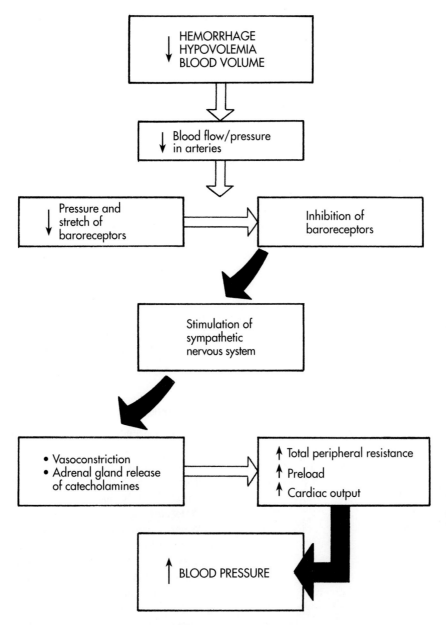

Figure **40-8**   Baroreceptor response.

changing the phosphate level in the ECF far below or far above normal levels does not cause immediate effects on the body.[4] However, even minute increases or decreases in calcium ions in ECF can cause significant physiologic effects.

Renal tubules maintain a normal phosphate level by an "overflow" mechanism. When the phosphate level in the glomerular filtrate falls below this set level, essentially all filtered phosphate is reabsorbed. When extra phosphate is present in the glomerular filtrate, excess phosphate is excreted in the urine.

PTH also plays a significant role in phosphate regulation. When PTH is present, bones dump phosphate salts and calcium into the ECF. PTH then stimulates the kidneys to dump more phosphate into the urine.

Magnesium

Magnesium is the second most important intracellular cation. More than half the body's magnesium is stored in bones, with the rest in cells, particularly muscle. Only a small fraction of the body's magnesium is found in the ECF. Magnesium is involved in numerous biochemical processes in the body, so normal concentrations must be carefully maintained. Although the exact mechanism is unclear, magnesium excretion is probably regulated by altering renal tubular reabsorption. With excess magnesium, renal tubules allow excretion of extra magnesium in the urine. In magnesium depletion, renal excretion dramatically decreases.

FLUID AND ELECTROLYTE ABNORMALITIES

Imbalances in fluid and electrolytes may be due to physiologic abnormalities, injury, or stress (Figure 40-9). Fluid and electrolyte levels are closely related. For example, sodium losses are almost always associated with water losses, just as sodium retention is associated with water excess.

Fluid and electrolyte therapy has three objectives: maintain daily requirements, restore previous losses, and prevent further losses. Oral electrolyte replacement is preferred. However, most patients who present to the ED with vomiting, diarrhea, and other fluid losses can no longer treat losses orally. Treatment of electrolyte abnormalities focuses on slowly restoring previous balance and carefully correcting the underlying cause. Electrolyte levels, hydration, and cardiovascular, renal, and neurologic function should be carefully monitored.

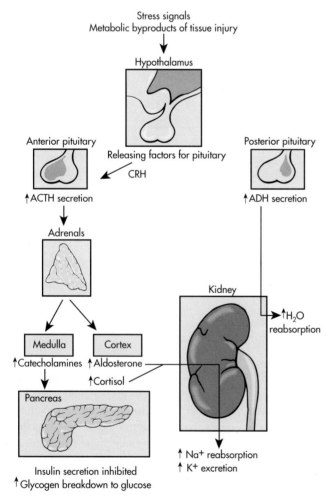

Figure **40-9** Effects of stress on fluid and electrolyte balance. *ACTH,* Adrenocorticotropic hormone; *ADH,* antidiuretic hormone; *CRH,* corticotropin-releasing hormone. *(From Lewis SM, Collier IC, Heitkemper MM: Medical-surgical nursing: assessment and management of clinical problems, ed 4, St. Louis, 1996, Mosby.)*

Box **40-1** Causes of ECF Volume Imbalances	
ECF volume deficit	**ECF volume excess**
Increased loss	*Increased retention*
Vomiting	Congestive heart failure
Diarrhea	Cushing's syndrome
Fistula drainage	Chronic liver disease with portal
GI tract suction	hypertension
Excessive sweating	Long-term use of corticosteroids
Fever	Renal failure
Third-space fluid shifts	
(e.g., burns, intestinal	
obstruction)	
Overuse of diuretics	
Hemorrhage	
Decreased intake	*Increased intake*
Nausea	Rare with adequate renal function
Anorexia	Excessive IV administration of
Inability to drink	fluids
Inability to obtain water	

From Lewis SM, Collier IC, Heitkemper MM: *Medical-surgical nursing: assessment and management of clinical problems,* ed 4, St. Louis, 1996, Mosby.
ECF, Extracellular fluid; *GI,* gastrointestinal; *IV,* intravenous.

Water Abnormalities

Water abnormalities may be due to underlying disease, iatrogenic causes, environmental factors, or psychologic abnormalities (Box 40-1). Determining the cause should occur concurrently with fluid replacement. Table 40-2 describes specific fluid imbalances.

Water depletion

Water depletion may be due to reduced water consumption, diarrhea, vomiting, excessive sweating, excessive respiration, renal disease, and ADH deficiency (i.e., diabetes insipidus). Water deficiency is almost always associated with loss of sodium. True water deficiency without concurrent sodium loss is rarely seen in the ED.

Signs and symptoms of water deficiency include thirst, loss of eyeball and skin turgor, dry mucous membranes, flushed skin, decreased urinary output, increased urine specific gravity, increased temperature, tachycardia, delirium, and coma. Most patients with water deficiency are also deficient in sodium and other electrolytes, so oral or parenteral fluid replacement must be determined on an individual basis. Frequently selected fluids to replenish water and sodium loss include normal saline (0.9%) and hypotonic half-normal saline (0.45%). Serial electrolyte and plasma osmolarity levels are required to determine appropriate fluid replacement. With true water depletion and normal serum sodium, 5% dextrose in water (D_5W) may be used. Table 40-3 describes various crystalloids used for fluid replacement.

Water excess

Water excess is characterized by weight gain, muscle twitching and cramps, pulmonary and peripheral edema, hy-

Table 40-2	Fluid Imbalances		
Imbalance	Clinical signs and symptoms	Therapy	Precursors
Dehydration	Thirst, anxiety, weight loss, poor skin turgor, slow vein filling, elevated temperature, tachycardia, dry mucous membranes, decreased level of consciousness, increased hematocrit, increased level of blood urea nitrogen, increased red blood cell concentration	Volume replacement	Any condition in which water output exceeds intake; vomiting, diarrhea
Edema	Weight gain exceeding 5%, rales, dyspnea, puffy eyelids, swollen ankles, bounding pulse	Salt-poor albumin, exchange resins, diuretics	Protein deficiency, venous obstruction, heart failure, obstructed lymphatic system, toxin ingestion, liver disease, renal disease
Third space syndrome	Hypotension, tachycardia, peripheral vasoconstriction, oliguria, no weight loss, increased hematocrit with no evidence of fluid loss	Plasma, salts, water replacement, diuretics, paracentesis, thoracentesis	Ascites, cellulitis, crush injuries, vascular occlusion, intestinal obstructions

perventilation, confusion, hallucination, coma, and convulsions. Water excess may be due to increased water ingestion, excessive intravenous therapy, renal disease, excess ADH, and inadequate water transport to the kidney (e.g., shock, congestive heart failure).

Treatment includes fluid restriction, with some patients limited to 1000 ml or less per day. In clinical emergencies, hypertonic saline may be used, followed by a diuretic such as furosemide to eliminate excess salt and water. If water excess is due to compulsive water consumption, psychiatric evaluation is recommended as soon as the patient's condition permits.

Electrolyte Abnormalities

Electrolyte abnormalities may be caused by an underlying disease or may be the result of starvation, therapeutic drugs, drug overdose, or other iatrogenic cause (Table 40-4). Electrolyte abnormalities are almost always associated with some degree of neuromuscular dysfunction (Table 40-5). Cardiac abnormalities are another common occurrence with many electrolyte abnormalities (Table 40-6).

Anion gap

The balance between positive and negative electrolytes is measured by calculating the anion gap (Box 40-2). This measurement is particularly useful in determining whether metabolic acidosis is due to acid excess or bicarbonate loss. Normal anion gap is 12 ± 4. Abnormalities in the anion gap may be due to a change in unmeasured anions or cations or an error in measurement of sodium, chloride, or bicarbonate.

A anion gap greater than 16 is associated with increased acids, as seen in diabetic ketoacidosis, alcoholic ketoacidosis, uremic acidosis, dehydration, salicylate intoxication,

Box 40-2	Anion Gap Calculation

$$\text{Anion gap} = Na^+ - (Cl^- + HCO_3^-)$$

and renal failure. A normal anion gap is seen in diarrhea, renal tubular acidosis, Addison's disease, and metabolic acidosis caused by diuretics. Albumin administration may cause a falsely elevated anion gap.[5] A decreased anion gap may be due to an error in electrolyte measurement.

Sodium abnormalities

Sodium and chloride travel together across most membranes, so sodium abnormalities are usually associated with chloride abnormalities. For the purpose of this discussion, abnormalities are described separately. Clinical manifestations of sodium abnormalities and various causes are presented in Table 40-7.

Hyponatremia

Hyponatremia is probably the most common electrolyte imbalance seen in the clinical arena. Hyponatremia is characterized by vague signs and symptoms, so diagnosis can rarely be made from clinical evaluation. Clinical manifestations are due to decreased osmolarity and cerebral edema and include anorexia, nausea, weakness, confusion, agitation, and disorientation. As serum sodium falls below 110 mEq/L, seizures, coma, or death may occur.

Mild hyponatremia does not require treatment. If the primary cause of hyponatremia is a fluid imbalance, normal saline is the treatment of choice. In severe symptomatic hyponatremia, hypertonic (3%) saline solution may be cautiously administered, usually 250 ml or less, with an infusion

Table **40-3**   **Composition and Use of Commonly Prescribed Crystalloid Solutions**

Solution	Tonicity	mOsm/L (mmol/L)	Glucose (g/L)	Indications and considerations
Dextrose in water				
5%	Isotonic	278	50	▪ Provides free water necessary for renal excretion of solutes ▪ Used to replace water losses and treat hypernatremia ▪ Provides 170 calories/L ▪ Does not provide any electrolytes
10%	Hypertonic	556	100	▪ Provides free water only, no electrolytes ▪ Provides 340 calories/L
Saline				
0.45%	Hypotonic	154	0	▪ Provides free water in addition to Na^+ and Cl^- ▪ Used to replace hypotonic fluid losses ▪ Used as maintenance solution although it does not replace daily losses of other electrolytes ▪ Provides no calories
0.9%	Isotonic	308	0	▪ Used to expand intravascular volume and replace extracellular fluid losses ▪ Only solution that may be administered with blood products ▪ Contains Na^+ and Cl^- in excess of plasma levels ▪ Does not provide free water, calories, other electrolytes ▪ May cause intravascular overload or hyperchloremic acidosis
3.0%	Hypertonic	1026	0	▪ Used to treat symptomatic hyponatremia ▪ Must be administered slowly and with extreme caution because it may cause dangerous intravascular volume overload and pulmonary edema
Dextrose in saline				
5% in 0.225%	Isotonic	355	50	▪ Provides Na^+, Cl^-, and free water ▪ Used to replace hypotonic losses and treat hypernatremia ▪ Provides 170 calories/L
5% in 0.45%	Hypertonic	432	50	▪ Same as 0.45% NaCl except provides 170 calories/L
5% in 0.9%	Hypertonic	586	50	▪ Same as 0.9% NaCl except provides 170 calories/L
Multiple electrolyte solutions **Ringer's solution**	Isotonic	309	0	▪ Similar in composition to plasma except that it has excess Cl^-, no Mg^{2+}, and no HCO_3^- ▪ Does not provide free water or calories ▪ Used to expand the intravascular volume and replace extracellular fluid losses
Lactated Ringer's (Hartmann's) solution	Isotonic	274	0	▪ Similar in composition to normal plasma except does not contain Mg^{2+} ▪ Used to treat losses from burns and lower gastrointestinal tract ▪ May be used to treat mild metabolic acidosis but should not be used to treat lactic acidosis ▪ Does not provide free water or calories

From Lewis SM, Collier IC, Heitkemper MM: *Medical-surgical nursing: assessment and management of clinical problems,* ed 4, St. Louis, 1996, Mosby.

pump.[3] The patient should be carefully monitored in the intensive care unit for fluid overload secondary to sodium replacement. Furosemide may be administered concurrently to reduce the likelihood of fluid overload. Any potassium deficits that occur as a result of treatment should be corrected.

Hypernatremia

Hypernatremia is a significant risk for infants, the elderly, and debilitated patients because of their inability to independently replace fluid losses. Clinical signs and symptoms are similar to those seen with hyponatremia but are secondary to hyperosmolarity and cellular dehydration. The patient is

Table 40-4 Iatrogenic Electrolyte Abnormalities

Cause	Effect on electrolytes
Diuretic therapy	Hyponatremia, hypochloremia, hyperkalemia, hypomagnesemia, elevated serum proteins, normal or elevated HCO_3^-
Starvation	Normal potassium or hyperkalemia, normal elevated H^+, decreased HCO_3^-, decreased protein, normal or decreased pH
Milk-alkali syndrome*	Hypokalemia, hypocalcemia, elevated HCO_3^-, hypercalcemia, elevated pH
Salicylate intoxication	Normal sodium or hypernatremia; hyperchloremia; normal potassium or hypokalemia; decreased HCO_3^-; early pH elevation, which later drops; early decrease in H^+, followed by increased H^+
Barbiturate intoxication	Hypochloremia, elevated H^+, elevated HCO_3^-, decreased pH, increased PCO_2

*Syndrome caused by ingestion of large amounts of nonabsorbable antacids such as calcium carbonate with or without milk.

thirsty and appears dehydrated. Early symptoms include anorexia, nausea, and vomiting. As serum sodium rises above 160 mEq/L, neurologic symptoms such as agitation, irritability, lethargy, coma, muscle twitching, and hyperreflexia may occur. Intracranial hemorrhages may result from shrunken brain tissue or engorged vasculature.

Treatment of sodium excess focuses on restoring normal fluid volume and osmolarity. Fluid replacement is the first step when hypovolemia is the cause of sodium excess. The patient initially requires administration of normal saline until the blood pressure stabilizes.[3] Treatment is followed by half-normal saline solution. Patients with pure water loss should receive oral hydration, intravenous D_5W, or hypotonic saline. Normovolemic patients with hypernatremia should receive D_5W and furosemide.[3] In all cases, slow correction of the imbalance is essential to avoid neurologic problems such as cerebral edema and seizures.

Chloride abnormalities

Chloride abnormalities rarely occur independently but usually occur in conjunction with sodium or potassium abnormalities.

Hypochloremia

Hypochloremia occurs in conjunction with hyponatremia and may also be seen with hyperkalemia caused by excretion of potassium chloride. Symptoms of chloride deficiency are basically the same as hyponatremia with the additional problems of profound muscle weakness, twitching, tetany, slow shallow respirations, and respiratory arrest. Treatment includes chloride and sodium replacement with careful monitoring of serum levels to determine effectiveness.

Table 40-5 Neuromuscular Manifestations of Electrolyte Abnormalities

	Hypokalemia	Hyperkalemia	Hypophosphatemia	Hypomagnesemia	Hypermagnesemia	Hypocalcemia	Hypercalcemia	Hyponatremia	Hypernatremia
Weakness	++	+	++	+	+	+	++	+	+
Paralysis	+	+	−	−	+	−	−	−	−
Myalgias	+	−	+	+	−	+	−	−	+
Fasciculations	+	+	+	+	−	+	−	+	−
Cramps	+	−	−	+	−	+	−	+	+
Restless legs	+	−	−	−	−	−	−	−	−
Tetany	−	−	−	+*	−	+	−	−	−
Myotonia	−	+†	−	−					
Areflexia	+	+	+	−					
Hyperreflexia	−	+	−	+		+	+	+	+
Choreoathetosis	−	−	−	+				−	−
Rhabdomyolysis	+	−	+	+‡				+‖	+

From Knochel JP: Neuromuscular manifestations of electrolyte disorders, *Am J Med* 72:521, 1982.
*Indefinite, may be due to associated hypocalcemia.
†Myotonia may occur in familial hyperkalemic periodic paralysis.
‡Experimental animals (dog, rat) only.
‖Biochemical evidence only (CPK increase, creatinuria).

Hyperchloremia

Hyperchloremia produces all the signs and symptoms seen with hypernatremia and also causes deep, labored breathing. Causes of hyperchloremia are the same factors that cause hypernatremia, with two exceptions: ammonium chloride ingestion and salicylate intoxication cause hyperchloremia but do not affect serum sodium. Treatment of hyperchloremia is essentially the same as for hypernatremia.

Potassium abnormalities

Potassium is subject to multiple influences within the body. Alkalosis, aldosterone, insulin, and β_2-agonists drive potassium into the cell, whereas acidosis and hyperosmolarity cause potassium to leave the cell. Table 40-8 highlights the causes and clinical manifestations of potassium abnormalities. Potassium abnormalities are almost always associated with electrocardiogram (ECG) changes, which may or may not correlate with severity (Figure 40-10).

Hypokalemia

Hypokalemia is characterized by muscle weakness, cramps, paralysis, hyporeflexia, paralytic ileus, paresthesia, latent tetany, cardiac dysrhythmias, and hyposthenuria (inability to form urine with a high specific gravity). Muscle weakness is usually more pronounced in the lower extremities and proximal muscle groups. Respiratory muscle weakness may lead to respiratory failure and arrest. Rhabdomyolysis may also occur. ECG changes such as flattened or inverted T waves and U waves do not correlate well with clinical severity (Figure 40-10). Ventricular ectopy is the most common dysrhythmia. Hypokalemia is due to decreased potassium intake or shifts of potassium from the ECF to the cells. Vomiting, diarrhea, intestinal obstruction, gastrointestinal suctioning, renal insufficiency, nephritis, diabetic ketoacidosis, diuretics, aldosteronism, Cushing's syndrome, and steroid therapy are all associated with hypokalemia.

Treatment is recommended when potassium is less than 3.5 mEq/L.[1] Potassium chloride is administered at 10 to 30 mEq/hr over 3 to 4 hours through a large-bore peripheral or central intravenous catheter.[1] An infusion pump is recommended when the entire amount of potassium in the IV bag exceeds 40 mEq. Potassium is extremely irritating to the veins, so the concentration infused through peripheral veins should not exceed 80 mEq/250 ml with the rate less than 40 mEq/hr. Additional potassium can be added to intravenous maintenance fluids at 10 to 40 mEq/L.[6] Frequent assessment of potassium levels and vital signs is necessary. Cardiac monitoring and serial evaluation of potassium levels are recommended to prevent inadvertent hyperkalemia secondary to potassium replacement. In less acute situations, oral potassium may be used, or potassium may be added to enteral feedings. Serum magnesium levels should be checked, since both electrolytes may be depleted with persistent hypokalemia.

Table **40-6**	**ECG Changes Associated with Electrolyte Abnormalities**
Electrolyte abnormality	ECG changes
Hypokalemia	Flattened or inverted T waves, depressed ST segment, U waves, ventricular ectopy
Hyperkalemia	Tall, peaked T waves; widened QRS complexes; prolonged PR interval; loss of P waves; sine wave or biphasic tracing; dysrhythmias including sinus bradycardia, sinus arrest, first degree heart block, nodal rhythm, idioventricular rhythm, ventricular fibrillation, and rarely asystole
Hypocalcemia	Prolonged QT interval
Hypercalcemia	Shortened QT interval
Hypomagnesemia	Torsades de pointes, ventricular tachycardia, ventricular fibrillation
Hypermagnesemia	Heart block, asystole

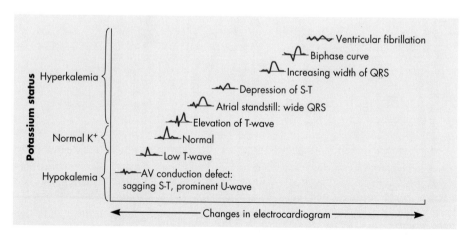

Figure **40-10** Electrocardiogram changes associated with alterations in potassium status. *(From Lewis SM, Collier IC, Heitkemper MM:* Medical-surgical nursing: assessment and management of clinical problems, *ed 4, St. Louis, 1996, Mosby.)*

Table **40-7**   **Sodium Imbalances: Causes and Clinical Manifestations**

Hyponatremia (Na$^+$ <135 mEq/L [mmol/L])	Hypernatremia (Na$^+$ >145 mEq/L [mmol/L])
CAUSES	

Sodium loss
GI losses: Diarrhea, vomiting, fistulas, NG suction
Renal losses: Diuretics, adrenal insufficiency, Na$^+$ wasting,
   renal disease
Skin losses: Burns, wound drainage
 	
Water gain
SIADH
Congestive heart failure
Excessive hypotonic IV fluids
Primary polydipsia
	Water loss
	Increased insensible water loss or perspiration
	   (high fever, heatstroke)
	Diabetes insipidus
	Osmotic diuresis
	
	Sodium gain
	IV hypertonic NaCl
	IV sodium bicarbonate
	IV excessive isotonic NaCl
	Primary aldosteronism
	Saltwater near drowning

CLINICAL MANIFESTATIONS	
Decreased ECF volume (sodium loss) Irritability, apprehension, confusion Postural hypotension Tachycardia Rapid, thready pulse Decreased CVP Decreased jugular venous filling Nausea, vomiting Dry mucous membranes Weight loss Tremors, seizures, coma	*Decreased ECF volume (water loss)* Intense thirst, dry, swollen tongue Restlessness, agitation, twitching Seizures, coma Weakness Postural hypotension, decreased CVP Weight loss
Normal or increased ECF volume (water gain) Headache, lassitude, apathy, weakness, confusion Nausea, vomiting Weight gain Increased blood pressure, increased CVP Muscle spasms, convulsions, coma	*Normal or increased ECF volume (sodium gain)* Intense thirst Restlessness, agitation, twitching Seizures, coma Flushed skin Weight gain Peripheral and pulmonary edema Increased blood pressures, increased CVP

From Lewis SM, Collier IC, Heitkemper MM: *Medical-surgical nursing: assessment and management of clinical problems,* ed 4, St. Louis, 1996, Mosby.

CVP, Central venous pressure; *ECF,* extracellular fluid; *GI,* gastrointestinal; *IV,* intravenous; *NG,* nasogastric; *SIADH,* syndrome of inappropriate antidiuretic hormone.

Hyperkalemia

Hyperkalemia is characterized by prominent cardiac changes (Table 40-8) and neuromuscular effects such as paresthesia and muscle weakness leading to flaccid paralysis. Various ECG changes correlate well with severity in hyperkalemia. Elevated T waves occur when serum potassium reaches 7 mEq/L, whereas prolonged PR interval and widened QRS complexes are evident when the level reaches 9 to 10 mEq/L. Dysrhythmias include sinus bradycardia, sinus arrest, first degree heart block, nodal rhythm, idioventricular rhythm, and ventricular fibrillation. Asystole may also occur. Hyperkalemia may be due to increased oral or intravenous intake, acute renal disease, potassium sparing diuretics, adrenal insufficiency, acidosis, anoxia, and hyponatremia.

Intravenous calcium chloride or calcium gluconate is the most rapid method for neutralizing neuromuscular effects of hyperkalemia. Serum potassium is rapidly reduced by administration of glucose (D$_{50}$W), insulin, and sodium bicarbonate, which drives potassium into the cell in exchange for sodium. However, this intervention provides only temporary reduction in serum potassium. Urinary potassium excretion is promoted with loop or osmotic diuretics. If these efforts fail, renal dialysis may be needed for significant hyperkalemia. Ion exchange resins such as sodium polystyrene sulfonate (Kayexalate, oral or rectal) may also be used in nonemergency situations. Continuous cardiac monitoring and serial potassium levels are essential for the patient with hyperkalemia.

Table **40-8**　Potassium Imbalances: Causes and Clinical Manifestations

Hypokalemia (K$^+$ <3.5 mEq/L [mmol/L])	Hyperkalemia (K$^+$ >5.5 mEq/L [mmol/L])	Hypokalemia (K$^+$ <3.5 mEq/L [mmol/L])	Hyperkalemia (K$^+$ >5.5 mEq/L [mmol/L])
Causes		**Cardiovascular—cont'd**	
Vomiting	Renal failure	Bradycardia, first- and	Complete heart block
Diarrhea	Early stage of burns	second-degree heart	Ectopic beats
Potent diuretics	Adrenal insufficiency	block, atrial	Ventricular fibrillation →
Aldosterone-producing tumor	Massive crushing injury	dysrhythmias	ventricular standstill
Potassium-free IV solutions	Excess IV administration of K$^+$	PVCs, especially for patients	
Recovery phase of diabetic	Metabolic acidosis	on digitalis	
acidosis		Postural hypotension	
Fistulas		**Gastrointestinal**	
Metabolic alkalosis		Anorexia, nausea	Nausea
Anorexia		Paralytic ileus	Vomiting
Starvation		Constipation	Cramping pain
Malnutrition			Diarrhea
Appearance		**Neuromuscular**	
Drowsiness	No specific findings	Hyporeflexia	Twitching
Behavior		Muscle	Seizures
Confusion	No alteration in mentation	weakness→paralysis	Paresthesias
Irritability	Irritability	Muscle cramps and	Paralysis when severe
Lethargy		paresthesias	
Depression		**Urinary findings**	
Cardiovascular		Urinary output ↑	Urine potassium ↑
ECG changes	ECG changes	Specific gravity ↓	
ST depression	Peaked T waves	May have decreased output	
T wave inversion or	PR interval prolongation	because of urinary retention	
flattening	Disappearance of P wave	**Serum values**	
U waves	Widening of QRS	Serum potassium ↓	Serum potassium ↑
		pH ↑	pH ↓

From Lewis SM, Collier IC, Heitkemper MM: *Medical-surgical nursing: assessment and management of clinical problems,* ed 4, St. Louis, 1996, Mosby.
ECG, Electrocardiogram; *IV,* intravenous; *PVC,* premature ventricular contractions.

Calcium abnormalities

Calcium abnormalities may be due to diet, medications, injury, or disease (Table 40-9). Bones provide a large reservoir of calcium; however, adequate dietary intake is necessary to maintain stores. Calcium abnormalities are often associated with phosphorus and magnesium abnormalities.

Hypocalcemia

Hypocalcemia makes the nervous system more excitable, which can lead to cardiac dysrhythmias, constipation, and lack of appetite. In skeletal muscle, excitability can lead to tetanic muscle contractions. Seizures are occasionally seen as a result of increased excitability of brain tissue. Clinical signs include a positive Trousseau's sign and a positive Chvostek's sign (Figure 40-11). Other manifestations include muscle twitching and cramping; facial grimacing; numbness and tingling of fingers, toes, nose, lips, and earlobes; hyperactive deep tendon reflexes; and abdominal pain. The ECG may show a prolonged QT interval, and the patient may appear anxious, irritable, and even psychotic.

More severe symptoms include laryngospasms, bronchospasms, seizures, and cardiac failure.

Calcium abnormalities occur with hypoparathyroidism, hypovitaminosis D, malabsorption syndrome, malnutrition, chronic nephrotic syndrome, chronic nephritis, Cushing's syndrome, and metastatic carcinoma of the bone. Overdose of calcium channel blockers can also cause hypocalcemia. Multiple blood transfusions, usually more than 10 units, are associated with hypocalcemia because of citrate in banked blood, which binds with calcium, making it inactive.

Before treatment for hypocalcemia is begun, hypomagnesemia should be excluded, since patients with low serum magnesium respond poorly to calcium replacement. Hypocalcemia is easily managed with intravenous calcium. One to two ampules of 10% calcium gluconate mixed in D$_5$W is administered over 10 to 20 minutes.[1] In severe deficits, a continuous infusion may be necessary after the initial bolus. Calcium levels, cardiac rhythm, and blood pressure should be carefully monitored during calcium administration.

Table 40-9   Calcium Imbalances: Causes and Clinical Manifestations

Hypocalcemia (<9 mg/dl [2.25 mmol/L])	Hypercalcemia (>11 mg/dl [2.75 mmol/L])	Hypocalcemia (<9 mg/dl [2.25 mmol/L])	Hypercalcemia (>11 mg/dl [2.75 mmol/L])
Causes		**Cardiovascular**	
Acute pancreatitis	Excess milk-product ingestion	Electrocardiogram changes	Electrocardiogram
Primary hypoparathyroidism	Hyperparathyroidism	Prolonged QT	Depressed T waves
Steatorrhea	Prolonged immobilization	Dysrhythmias	Shortened QT interval
Generalized peritonitis	Multiple myeloma		Hypertension
Chronic renal failure	Thyrotoxicosis		Cardiac arrest
Vitamin D deficiency	Vitamin D excess	**Gastrointestinal**	
Surgical removal of parathyroids		Colicky discomfort	Anorexia
Excess administration of citrated blood		Diarrhea	Nausea
Diuretic therapy			Constipation
Alcoholism			Paralytic ileus
Malabsorption		**Neuromuscular**	
Total parenteral nutrition		Hyperreflexia	Decreased muscle strength
Appearance		Muscle cramps	Depressed reflexes
Tonic and clonic convulsions	Lethargy	Numbness and tingling in extremities	
	Weight loss	Carpopedal spasms	
	Dehydration	Chvostek's sign	
		Trousseau's sign	
		Seizures	
Behavior		Tetany	
Personality changes	Decreased intellectual function	**Respiratory**	
Depression	Malaise	Laryngeal spasm	Hypoventilation
Irritability	Confusion	Respiratory arrest	
Easy fatigability	Psychosis	**Urinary findings**	
Anxiety	Coma	No specific findings	Increased urinary output
Confusion	Increased thirst		
	Impaired memory	**Serum values**	
	Fatigue	Overcorrection of acid pH (may precipitate symptomatic hypocalcemia)	
Musculoskeletal		↓Serum albumin (patient may not have symptoms despite decreased Ca^{2+})	
Bone pain	Bone pain		
Fractures	Fractures		
Rickets	Pseudogout		

From Lewis SM, Collier IC, Heitkemper MM: *Medical-surgical nursing: assessment and management of clinical problems,* ed 4, St. Louis, 1996, Mosby.

Hypercalcemia

Hypercalcemia is characterized by vague symptoms such as headache, irritability, fatigue, malaise, difficulty concentrating, anorexia, nausea, vomiting, and constipation. Neurologic effects are often the primary symptoms. Patients may be lethargic and confused and have a depressed level of consciousness. Deep tendon reflexes may be depressed, the QT interval may be prolonged, and the patient may have polyuria, polydipsia, or an ileus. Chronic hypercalcemia is associated with renal lithiasis, peptic ulcer, and pancreatitis.

Although rarely seen in the ED, serum calcium levels that exceed 14 to 15 mg/dl are considered a medical emergency.[1] Correction of hypercalcemia includes treating the underlying cause and increasing renal excretion of calcium with intravenous hydration and loop or osmotic diuretics. Other therapeutic options depend on the specific clinical situation and include glucocorticoid administration to decrease intestinal calcium absorption and increase urinary calcium excretion. Administration of calcitonin or phosphate inhibits bone reabsorption. In life-threatening emergencies, agents such as ethylenediaminetetraacetic acid (EDTA) are used to chelate ionized calcium.[1]

Phosphate abnormalities

Phosphate abnormalities are associated with a reciprocal calcium abnormality. Phosphate elevations occur with calcium losses, whereas phosphate depletion occurs with calcium excess. The patient with a phosphate abnormality should be carefully monitored for the effects of a calcium abnormality. Causes of phosphate abnormalities are listed in Box 40-3.

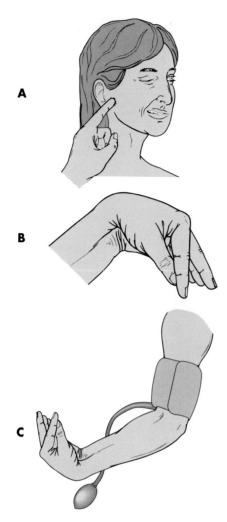

Figure **40-11** Tests for hypocalcemia. **A,** Chvostek's sign is a contraction of facial muscles in response to a light tap over the facial nerve in front of the ear. **B,** Trousseau's sign is a carpal spasm induced by **C,** inflating a blood pressure cuff above the systolic pressure for a few minutes. *(From Lewis SM, Collier IC, Heitkemper MM: Medical-surgical nursing: assessment and management of clinical problems, ed 4, St. Louis, 1996, Mosby.)*

Hypophosphatemia

Hypophosphatemia has a variable clinical presentation ranging from no symptoms to anorexia and muscle weakness, rhabdomyolysis, respiratory failure, hemolysis, and altered mental status. Causes include hyperparathyroidism, vitamin D deficiency, intestinal malabsorption, and renal tubular acidosis.

Treatment of severe hypophosphatemia begins with intravenous phosphate (20 mmol over 4 to 6 hours).[1] Potential complications of phosphate administration include hypocalcemia and hypotension, so patients with less severe deficiency are treated with enteric or oral phosphate preparations.

Hyperphosphatemia

Hyperphosphatemia is associated with a reciprocal fall in serum calcium and the resultant clinical effects of hypocal-

---

Box 40-3 **Causes of Phosphate Imbalances**

Hypophosphatemia	Hyperphosphatemia
Malabsorption syndrome	Renal failure
Nutritional recovery syndrome	Chemotherapeutic agents
Glucose administration	Enemas containing phosphorus (e.g., Fleet's)
Hyperalimentation	Excessive ingestion (e.g., milk, phosphate-containing laxatives)
Alcohol withdrawal	
Phosphate-binding antacids	
Diabetic ketoacidosis	Large vitamin D intake
Respiratory alkalosis	Hypoparathyroidism

From Lewis SM, Collier IC, Heitkemper MM: *Medical-surgical nursing: assessment and management of clinical problems,* ed 4, St. Louis, 1996, Mosby.

cemia. Hyperphosphotemia is also associated with and may even produce acute renal failure. The most serious effect of excess phosphate relates to precipitation of calcium phosphate crystals in soft tissues such as the cornea, lung, kidney, and blood vessels. Causes include hypoparathyroidism, chronic renal disease, Addison's disease, leukemia, sarcoidosis, osteolytic metastatic bone tumor, and milk-alkali syndrome.

Treatment includes limiting phosphate intake, using oral phosphate binding agents such as aluminum hydroxide, and increasing excretion. Intravenous hydration with saline is followed by diuretics to enhance excretion.

Magnesium abnormalities

Specific causes of magnesium abnormalities are identified in Box 40-4. Magnesium abnormalities are frequently associated with other electrolyte abnormalities. Clinically, hypo- and hypermagnesemia have the same effect on release of PTH and calcitonin as hypo- and hypercalcemia. Calcium and magnesium excretion are interdependent. A sudden calcium load causes excretion of both calcium and magnesium.

Box 40-4 **Causes of Magnesium Imbalances**

Hypomagnesemia	Hypermagnesemia
Diarrhea	Renal failure (especially if patient is given magnesium products)
Vomiting	
Chronic alcoholism	
Impaired gastrointestinal absorption	Excessive administration of magnesium for treatment of eclampsia
Malabsorption syndrome	
Prolonged malnutrition	Adrenal insufficiency
Large urine outputs	
Nasogastric suction	
Diabetic ketoacidosis	
Hyperaldosteronism	

From Lewis SM, Collier IC, Heitkemper MM: *Medical-surgical nursing: assessment and management of clinical problems,* ed 4, St. Louis, 1996, Mosby.

Box **40-5**

NURSING DIAGNOSES FOR FLUID AND ELECTROLYTE ABNORMALITIES

Fluid volume deficit
Fluid volume excess
Decreased cardiac output
Bowel incontinence
Constipation
Altered urinary elimination
Altered nutrition
Ineffective breathing pattern

Hypomagnesemia

Hypomagnesemia may result from malabsorption syndrome, ulcerative colitis, ileal bypass, cirrhosis, alcoholism, chronic renal disease, diabetic ketoacidosis, diuretic therapy, and malnutrition. Symptoms include nausea, vomiting, sedation, decreased deep tendon reflexes, and muscle weakness. With significant hypomagnesemia, hypotension, bradycardia, coma, respiratory paralysis, and cardiac arrest may occur.[5] Severe hypomagnesemia can also exist in the absence of clinical symptoms. When symptoms do occur, they are usually confined to the neuromuscular and cardiovascular systems. Generalized weakness, muscle fasciculations, and positive Trousseau's and Chvostek's signs may be seen (Figure 40-11). Dysrhythmias such as torsades de pointes, ventricular tachycardia, and ventricular fibrillation have been associated with hypomagnesemia.

Treatment depends on severity of symptoms. Magnesium sulfate, 2 to 3 g (10 to 15 ml of a 20% solution) is administered intravenously over 1 minute followed by a continuous infusion.[1] Vital signs, deep tendon reflexes, fluid intake, urinary output, and magnesium levels should be carefully monitored.

Hypermagnesemia

Hypermagnesemia may result from reduced excretion secondary to advanced renal failure and adrenocortical insufficiency, overdose of therapeutic magnesium, or routine doses of magnesium in the patient with renal compromise. Treatment of hypermagnesemia also depends on the severity of symptoms. Calcium chloride, 100 to 200 mg every 3 to 5 minutes until symptoms are reversed, is followed by a continuous infusion.[6] Saline diuresis and furosemide may also be used. In severe cases, hemodialysis may be required. Serial magnesium levels, vital signs, and deep tendon reflexes should be closely monitored.

SUMMARY

Whether caring for a trauma patient, chronically ill geriatric patient, or previously healthy person with acute simple gastroenteritis, the emergency nurse should anticipate electrolyte abnormalities. Recognition of abnormalities and potential adverse effects is essential for effective treatment and prevention of complications. Box 40-5 identifies nursing diagnoses appropriate for patients with fluid or electrolyte abnormalities.

REFERENCES

1. Andrews BT: Fluid and electrolyte disorders in neurological intensive care, *Neurosurg Intensive Care* 5:707, 1994.
2. Collins RD: *Illustrated manual of fluid and electrolyte disorders,* ed 2, Philadelphia, 1983, JB Lippincott.
3. Danis D: Metabolic and endocrine emergencies. In Sheehy SB, editor: *Emergency nursing: principles and practice,* ed 3, St. Louis, 1992, Mosby.
4. Guyton AC, Hall JE: *Textbook of medical physiology,* ed 9, Philadelphia, 1996, WB Saunders.
5. Kokko JP, Tannen RL: *Fluids and electrolytes,* ed 3, Philadelphia, 1996, WB Saunders.
6. O'Donnell ME: Assessing fluid and electrolyte balance in elders, *Am J Nurs* 96(11):41, 1995.

SUGGESTED READING

Bove LA: Restoring electrolyte balance: sodium and chloride, *RN,* p 25, Jan 1996.
Faber MD et al: Common fluid-electrolyte and acid-base problems in the intensive care unit: selected issues, *Semin Nephrol* 14:8, 1994.
Gilmour J, Penny S: Hydration and aging, *NZ Nurs J,* p 15, Nov 1991.
Perez A: Restoring electrolyte balance: hypokalemia, *RN,* p 33, Dec 1995.
Rutherford C: Fluid and electrolyte therapy: considerations for patient care, *J Intravenous Nurs* 12(3):173, 1989.

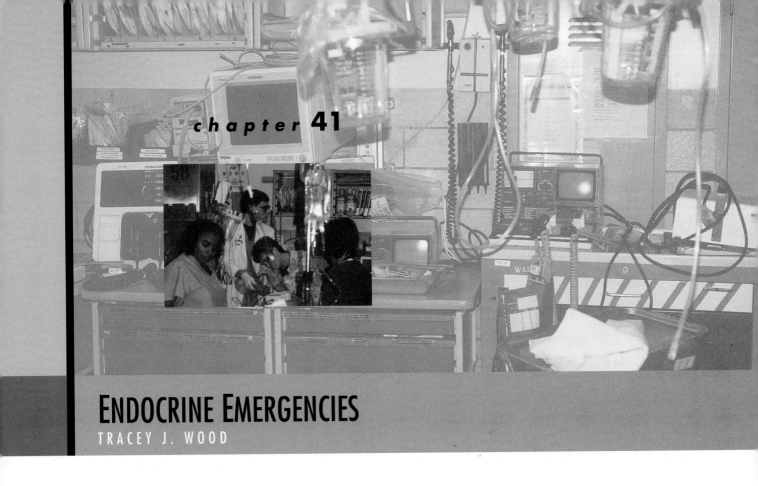

chapter 41

ENDOCRINE EMERGENCIES

TRACEY J. WOOD

The endocrine system is a regulatory system that uses hormones to control metabolic, renal, and neural functions. Endocrine disturbances lead to critical physiologic consequences if not promptly identified and treated. Most common endocrine emergencies involve diabetes and alcohol-related illnesses; however, thyroid and adrenal crises also have potentially serious outcomes. Specific endocrine emergencies described are alcoholic ketoacidosis (AKA), adrenal crisis, diabetic ketoacidosis (DKA), hyperosmolar hyperglycemic nonketotic coma (HHNC), hypoglycemia, thyroid storm, myxedema coma, and syndrome of inappropriate antidiuretic hormone (SIADH). A brief review of anatomy and physiology is provided to facilitate understanding of clinical material.

ANATOMY AND PHYSIOLOGY

The endocrine system consists of the hypothalamus, pituitary, thyroid, parathyroids, adrenals, testes, and ovaries (Figure 41-1). Each gland produces and stores one or more hormones, which have specific, unique functions. Table 41-1 identifies the hormones produced by the major endocrine glands, their target tissue, and their functions. Activities of the testes and ovaries are addressed in Chapters 39 and 46.

Hormone activity is the result of feedback loops, nerve stimulation, and intrinsic rhythms. Renal and liver function, as well as external factors such as pain, fear, and stress, also affect hormone release. Negative feedback loops are activated by circulating hormone levels above or below normal

level.[6] Excessive amounts of circulating hormones inhibit hormone release, whereas low levels lead to increased hormone release. Neural stimulation triggers increased glandular activity and release of hormones such as glucagon. Intrinsic rhythms vary from hours to weeks and provide another method of hormone control.

Hypothalamus

The hypothalamus creates part of the walls and floor of the third ventricle. Various centers in the anterior and posterior hypothalamus control most endocrine functions as well as many emotional behaviors. Table 41-2 reviews these control centers and target areas or processes. Nerve tracts from the hypothalamus join the posterior pituitary, which lies just below (Figure 41-2). Posterior pituitary hormones are actually synthesized in the hypothalamus and then transferred along axons for storage in the posterior pituitary. The hypothalamus regulates anterior pituitary action by inhibiting or releasing certain hormones.

Pituitary

The pituitary gland is approximately 1 cm in all directions and lies within the sella turcica of the middle cranial fossa (Figure 41-2). Two physiologically distinct areas are found in the pituitary. The anterior pituitary contains secretory cells, whereas the posterior pituitary consists of neural cells, which serve as a supporting structure for nerve fibers and nerve endings. Hormones secreted by the anterior pituitary

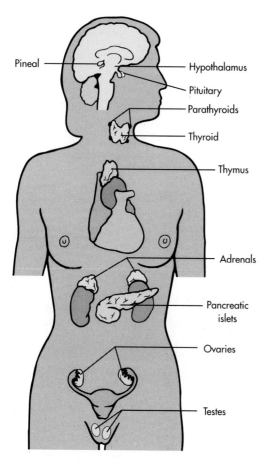

Figure **41-1** Location of the major endocrine glands. Parathyroid glands actually lie on the posterior surface of the thyroid. *(From Lewis SM, Collier IC, Heitkemper MM: Medical-surgical nursing: assessment and management of clinical problems, ed 4, St. Louis, 1996, Mosby.)*

include growth hormone, adrenocorticotropic hormone (ACTH), thyroid-stimulating hormone (TSH), prolactin, follicle-stimulating hormone, and luteinizing hormone. Hormones secreted by the posterior pituitary are antidiuretic hormone (ADH) and oxytocin.

Thyroid

The thyroid gland consists of two lobes connected by an isthmus (Figure 41-3). This butterfly-shaped gland in the anterior neck below the cricoid cartilage partially surrounds the trachea. Thyroid hormone release is regulated through a complex feedback system between the hypothalamus and anterior pituitary. This main metabolic regulator contains follicular cells that secrete thyroxine (T_4) and triiodothyronine (T_3) in response to stimulation by the pituitary. Calcitonin originating in parafollicular cells affects calcium metabolism.

Adrenals

The adrenal glands, located in the retroperitoneal area above the upper pole of each kidney, consist of an outer cor-

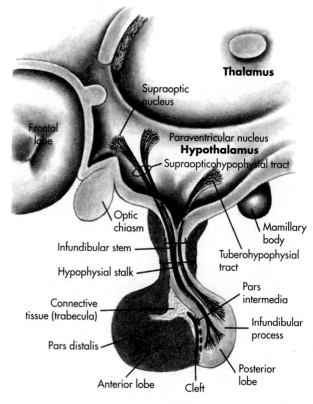

Figure **41-2** Anatomy of the hypothalamus and pituitary. *(From Thompson JM et al:* Mosby's clinical nursing, *ed 4, St. Louis, 1997, Mosby.)*

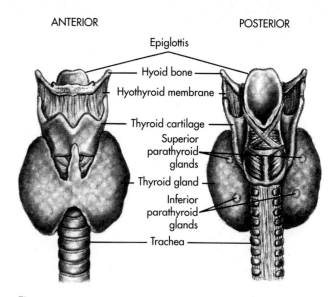

Figure **41-3** Thyroid gland. *(From Thompson JM et al:* Mosby's clinical nursing, *ed 4, St. Louis, 1997, Mosby.)*

tical layer and an inner medullary layer (Figure 41-4). The adrenal cortex produces the mineralocorticoids aldosterone, glucocorticoids, and androgens. Aldosterone is critical for maintaining internal fluid balance, whereas glucocorticoids are a major player in the body's ability to resist stress. The

Table 41-1 Major Endocrine Glands and Hormones

Hormones	Target tissue	Functions
Posterior pituitary (neurohypophysis)		
■ Oxytocin (Pitocin)*	Uterus, mammary glands	Stimulates milk secretion; uterine motility
■ Antidiuretic hormone (ADH) or vasopressin*	Renal tubules, vascular smooth muscle	Promotes reabsorption of water
Anterior pituitary (adenohypophysis)		
■ Growth hormone (GH) or somatotropin	All body cells	Promotes protein anabolism (growth, tissue repair), lipid mobilization, and catabolism
■ Thyroid-stimulating hormone (TSH) or thyrotropin	Thyroid gland	Stimulates synthesis and release of thyroid hormones, growth and function of thyroid (stimulation of thyroidal iodine uptake)
■ Adrenocorticotropic hormone (ACTH) or corticotropin	Adrenal cortex	Fosters growth of adrenal cortex; stimulates secretion of glucocorticoids
■ Prolactin or lactogen	Ovary and mammary glands in females	Stimulates milk production, protein synthesis, mammary gland development; unclear function in males
■ Gonadotropic hormones (e.g., follicle-stimulating [FSH] and luteinizing hormones [LH])	Reproductive organs	Stimulates sex hormone secretion, reproductive organ growth, reproductive processes
■ Melanocyte-stimulating hormone (MSH)	Melanocytes in skin	Increases melanin production in melanocytes to make skin darker in color
■ Prolactin	Ovary and mammary glands in females	Stimulates milk production in lactating women; increases response of follicles to LH and FSH; increase causes gynecomastia in men
Thyroid		
■ Thyroxine (T_4)	All body tissues	Precursor to T_3
■ Triiodothyronine (T_3)	All body tissues	Regulates metabolic rate of all cells and processes of cell growth and tissue differentiation
■ Calcitonin (CT)	Bone tissue	Regulates calcium and phosphorus blood levels, lowering of blood Ca^{++} levels
Parathyroids		
■ Parathyroid hormone (PTH) or parathormone	Bone, intestine, kidneys	Regulates calcium and phosphorus blood levels (bone demineralization, increased intestinal absorption)
Pancreas (islets of Langerhans)		
■ Insulin (from beta cells)	Liver, fat, and liver cells	Promotes utilization and storage of fuels (carbohydrates, protein, fats)
■ Glucagon (from alpha cells)	Liver	Promotes hepatic glucogenolysis and gluconeogenesis
■ Somatostatin (from delta cells)	Pancreas	Inhibits insulin and glucagon secretion
Adrenal medulla		
■ Epinephrine (adrenalin)	Sympathetic effectors	Enhances and prolongs effects of sympathetic division of ANS
■ Norepinephrine	Sympathetic effectors	Responds to stress; enhances and prolongs effects of sympathetic division of ANS
Adrenal cortex		
■ Corticosteroids (e.g., cortisol, hydrocortisone)	All body tissues	Promotes organic metabolism, response to stress
■ Androgens (e.g., testosterone, androsterone) or estrogen	Sex organs	Promotes masculinization in men, growth and sexual activity in women
■ Mineralocorticoids (e.g., aldosterone)	Kidney	Regulates sodium and potassium balance and thus water balance

ANS, Autonomic nervous system.
*These hormones are synthesized in the hypothalamus; the posterior pituitary stores and secretes them.

Continued

Table 41-1   Major Endocrine Glands and Hormones—cont'd

Hormones	Target tissue	Functions
Gonads		
Women: ovaries		
■ Estrogen	Reproductive system, breasts	Stimulates development of secondary sex characteristics, preparation of uterus for fertilization and fetal development; stimulates bone growth
■ Progesterone	Reproductive system	Maintains lining of uterus necessary for successful pregnancy
Men: testes		
■ Testosterone	Reproductive system	Stimulates development of secondary sex characteristics; stimulates epiphyseal closure

From Lewis SM, Collier IC, Heitkemper MM: *Medical-surgical nursing: assessment and management of clinical problems,* ed 4, St. Louis, 1996, Mosby.

Table 41-2   Control Centers of the Hypothalamus

Posterior hypothalamus		Anterior hypothalamus	
Control center	Effect	Control center	Effect
Posterior hypothalamus	Increased BP; pupillary dilation; shivering	Paraventricular nucleus	Oxytocin release; water conservation
Dorsomedial nucleus	GI stimulation	Medical preoptic area	Bladder contraction; decreased heart rate; decreased BP
Perifornical nucleus	Hunger; increased BP; rage	Supraoptic nucleus	Vasopressin release
Ventromedial nucleus	Satiety; neuroendocrine control	Posterior preoptic and anterior hypothalamic area	Temperature regulation; panting, sweating, thyrotropin inhibition
Mamillary body	Feeding reflexes		
Arcuate nucleus and periventricular zone	Neuroendocrine control		
Lateral hypothalamic area	Thirst; hunger		

From Guyton AC, Hall JE: *Textbook of medical physiology,* ed 9, Philadelphia, 1996, WB Saunders.
BP, Blood pressure; *GI,* gastrointestinal.

Table 41-3   Catecholamine Functions

Class and function	α-Adrenergic	β-Adrenergic	Dopaminergic
Agonist	Norepinephrine	Epinephrine	Dopamine
Antagonist	Phentolamine	Propranolol	Haloperidol
Actions			
Heart		Inotropic and chronotropic	Inotropic
Smooth muscle	Contracts	Relaxes	Mixed
Metabolic		Lipolysis	
		Glycogenolysis	
		Gluconeogenesis	
Molecular	Decreases cAMP	Increases cAMP	Increases cAMP

From Korenman et al: *Practical diagnosis/endocrine disease,* Boston, 1978, Houghton-Mifflin.
cAMP, cyclic adenosine monophosphate.

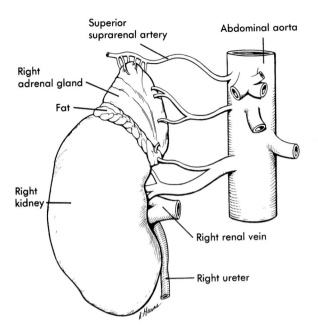

Figure **41-4**   Adrenal gland. *(From Seeley RS, Stephens TD, Tate P: Anatomy and physiology, ed 2, St. Louis, 1992, Mosby. Used with permission of the McGraw-Hill Companies.)*

adrenal medulla releases the catecholamines epinephrine and norepinephrine in response to sympathetic stimulation. Epinephrine is 5 to 10 times more potent than norepinephrine; however, norepinephrine has a longer duration of action. Table 41-3 summarizes the major functions of these catecholamines.

Pancreas

The pancreas is situated behind the stomach in the retroperitoneal space. The body of the pancreas extends horizontally across the abdominal wall with the head in the curve of the abdomen and the tail touching the spleen (Figure 41-5). Exocrine and endocrine cells are found in the pancreas. Acini are exocrine cells that release amylase, lipase, and other enzymes that aid in digestion. Three types of endocrine cells within the islet of Langerhans produce hormones that regulate serum glucose levels. Alpha cells secrete glucagon, beta cells produce insulin, and delta cells secrete somatostatin, which inhibits glucagon and insulin release.[14] Table 41-4 describes the physiologic actions of insulin.

PATIENT ASSESSMENT

Arrival of an unresponsive patient in the emergency department (ED) creates a flurry of activity that begins with as-

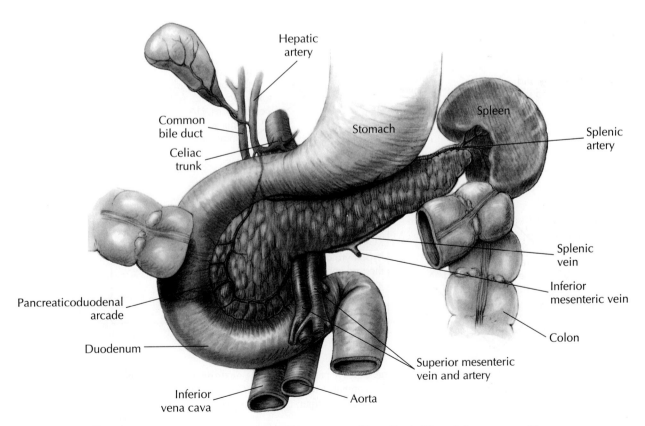

Figure **41-5**   The pancreas and surrounding structures. *(From Davis JH et al: Surgery: a problem-solving approach, ed 2, vol 2, St. Louis, 1995, Mosby.)*

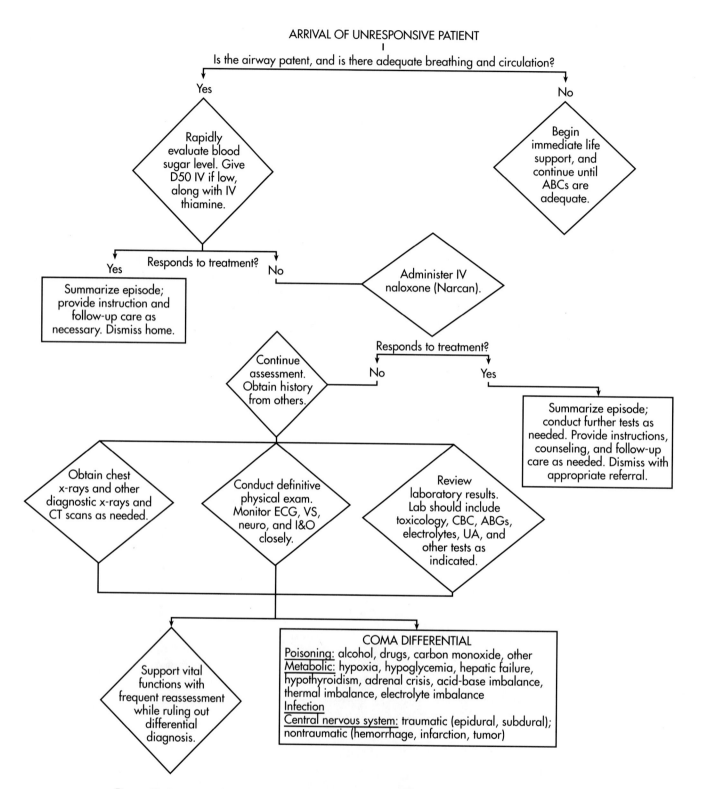

Figure **41-6** Management of the unresponsive patient. *D50,* 50% dextrose; *IV,* intravenous; *ABCs,* airway, breathing, and circulation; *CT,* computed tomography; *ECG,* electrocardiogram; *VS,* vital signs; *neuro,* neurologic status; *I&O,* intake and output; *CBC,* complete blood count; *ABGs,* arterial blood gases; *UA,* urinalysis.

sessment and stabilization of the airway, breathing, and circulation (ABCs) followed by assessment, treatment, and reassessment of patient condition (Figure 41-6). Once a differential diagnosis is reached, individualization of care can begin. An important aspect of care common to all endocrine emergencies is identification of the stressor or precipitating event. Identification may come through patient history, family interviews, laboratory findings, radiographic analysis, and other diagnostic procedures.

SELECTED ENDOCRINE EMERGENCIES

Endocrine emergencies represent a significant threat to the patient's life. Numerous endocrine problems exists; however, most do not present as a problem for the emergency nurse. Conditions covered in this chapter include those situations most likely to be encountered by the emergency nurse.

Alcoholic Ketoacidosis

An estimated 13 million American adults are alcoholics, with women accounting for approximately 50% of the total alcoholic population.[17] Emergencies related to alcohol include acute intoxication and withdrawal; injuries related to domestic violence, motor vehicle collisions, homicides, suicides, and other accidents; gastrointestinal bleeding, pancreatitis, liver failure, and diverse acute and chronic conditions; and various psychiatric crises. Increased amounts of adipose tissue place women at higher risk for AKA because estrogen appears to increase fatty acid production in adipose tissue. AKA typically occurs after an alcoholic patient consumes a significant amount of alcohol and tends to recur in patients previously diagnosed with AKA.[18]

Major aggravating factors for development of AKA are insulin deficiency, decreased glycogen stores, and volume depletion. Liver and pancreatic damage secondary to chronic alcohol consumption decreases glycogen stores and insulin levels. Glycogen stores are further diminished by starvation or inadequate nutritional stores. Inadequate glycogen leads to utilization of fat and muscle tissue for energy. Subsequent increased fatty acid production enhances an existing acidotic state. Decreased insulin availability decreases glucose utilization, which also leads to increased fatty acid levels and acidosis. Actual alcohol metabolism decreases gluconeogenesis and compounds the altered metabolic state. Profound dehydration increases circulating levels of epinephrine, cortisol, and growth hormones, which alter glucose utilization, so the ketoacidotic cycle continues.

Patients complain of abdominal pain, nausea, and vomiting. Tachycardia, tachypnea, and altered mental status are usually present, with altered mental status often attributed more to intoxication than to ketoacidosis. The skin may be cool and dry, and the patient may have a strong odor of ketones on the breath. Initial laboratory studies show decreased pH, normal to slightly decreased potassium, hypoglycemia, elevated liver function tests and amylase, and elevated blood alcohol.

Management in the ED focuses on correction of volume and glycogen depletion to restore metabolic functions. Moderate fluid replacement, usually with 5% dextrose in normal saline at 125 to 250 ml/hr, increases the serum bicarbonate level, so sodium bicarbonate administration may not be necessary except in severe cases. Glucose administration triggers increased insulin production, which interrupts ketogenesis. Consequently, intravenous fluids with dextrose often produce quicker results than saline alone unless the patient is hyperglycemic. Diabetic ketoacidosis should be ruled out when hyperglycemia is present. Potassium supplements may be necessary if fluid therapy and shifting glucose molecules lead to hypokalemia. Magnesium replacement helps correct calcium and potassium disturbances and also forestalls acute alcohol withdrawal. Table 41-5 identifies drugs used in treatment of alcohol withdrawal. The patient with AKA needs close monitoring and supportive care. Frequent assessment of vital signs, intake and output, neurologic status, and electrolyte values is necessary to monitor effectiveness of therapy and to ensure an uncomplicated return to the patient's normal metabolic state.

Adrenal Crisis

Adrenal crisis is a rare occurrence with life-threatening potential that develops after acute stressors deplete adrenal glucocorticoids and mineralocorticoids. Long-term steroid therapy patients may experience adrenal crisis after abrupt

Table 41-4	**Action of Insulin**		
	Liver	Adipose tissue	Muscle
Anticatabolic effects	Decreased glycogenolysis Decreased gluconeogenesis Decreased ketogenesis	Decreased lipolysis	Decreased protein catabolism Decreased amino acid output Decreased amino acid oxidation
Anabolic effects	Increased glycogen synthesis Increased fatty acid synthesis	Increased glycerol synthesis Increased fatty acid synthesis	Increased amino acid uptake Increased protein synthesis Increased glycogen synthesis

From Ellenberg M, Rifkin H, editors: *Diabetes mellitus: theory and practice*, ed 3, New York, 1983, Medical Examination Publishing. By permission of Appleton & Lange.

Table **41-5**	**Medications for Alcohol Withdrawal**		
Medications	Indication	Dose and route	Considerations
Atenolol (Tenormin)	Minor withdrawal	50-100 mg PO	Provides symptomatic relief; contraindicated in congestive heart failure, diabetes, bronchospasm
Chlordiazepoxide (Librium)	Minor withdrawal; anticonvulsant	25-100 mg PO	Titrate dose to achieve sedation
Clonidine (Catapres)	Minor withdrawal	0.1-0.4 mg PO	Provides symptomatic relief
Diazepam (Valium)	Delirium tremens; anticonvulsant	5-10 mg IV; may be given PO for minor symptoms	Titrate dose to achieve sedation; may need repeat doses; large doses may be necessary; watch for respiratory depression; IV rate is 5 mg/min
Lorazepam (Ativan)	Delirium tremens; minor withdrawal	1-5 mg PO, IV, or IM	Recommended for elderly patients or patients with liver disease
Phenytoin (Dilantin)	Anticonvulsant	100-300 mg PO; 500-100 mg IV loading dose	Not usually needed for simple alcohol-related seizures; IV rate < 50 mg/min; do not mix with other drugs or dextrose solutions; with IV use, monitor heart rate and rhythm, blood pressure, and central nervous system

discontinuation of medications. Prolonged steroid use suppresses adrenal activity, so the system cannot compensate sufficiently with abrupt removal of steroids. Other stressors include trauma, infection, hemorrhage, surgery, hypothermia, and metastatic disease of the adrenal glands.[12] Stress demands increased cortisol output from the adrenal system, so inability to meet increased demands begins the sequence of events that leads to crisis.

When the adrenal system fails, the resulting decrease in cortisol and aldosterone levels leads to massive sodium and water loss from the kidneys and gastrointestinal tract. Water loss results in hypotension and hypovolemia, which can progress to hypovolemic shock, coma, and death. While sodium decreases, serum potassium increases, which leads to hyperkalemia and potentially fatal dysrhythmias.

Gluconeogenesis, the normal hepatic response to stress, fails without sufficient levels of cortisol; therefore hypoglycemia often occurs in concert with adrenal crisis. Decreased cortisol levels also alter activities of the adrenal medulla, which normally responds to stress through release of catecholamines to increase heart rate and serum glucose. Without a catecholamine response, the severity of hypoglycemia and hypotension is magnified (Figure 41-7).

The patient in acute adrenal crisis presents with multiple symptoms including weakness, fatigue, nausea, vomiting, abdominal pain, and palpitations. The patient may describe salt craving. An accurate history of prior illnesses (e.g., asthma with *steroid* therapy), recent medication changes, recent surgery, or injury helps determine precipitating factors.

Objective assessment findings include poor skin turgor and dry mucous membranes, signs of hypovolemic shock (hypotension, tachycardia, and tachypnea), electrocardiogram changes (elevated T waves with progression to widened QRS complexes), fever related to predisposing infection, and confusion and/or lethargy.[7]

Hyponatremia, hyperkalemia, hypoglycemia, and hypercalcemia are usually present. Decreased volume also increases blood urea nitrogen (BUN). ACTH challenge does help with diagnosis but is not useful in the emergency setting. Challenge consists of obtaining the baseline serum cortisol level, administering synthetic ACTH, and repeating the serum cortisol level 6 to 8 hours later. If the adrenal glands are functioning appropriately, the repeat cortisol level should be at least twice the baseline level.[16]

Maintenance of ABCs, replacement of glucocorticoids, and correction of electrolyte and fluid disturbances are cornerstones of care. Oxygen should be administered to alleviate increased oxygen demands caused by tachycardia. Hydrocortisone is given as the primary glucocorticoid replacement to stimulate gluconeogenesis, inhibit inflammatory response, and allow the body to increase the response to stress. Mineralocorticoids (dexamethasone, prednisone) should be used as secondary replacers because of the potential for excessive sodium retention.

Rapid intravenous fluid replacement assists in correcting volume deficit. Intravenous insulin and 50% dextrose (D50) drive potassium from vascular space into the cell, so serum potassium levels decrease. Kayexalate administration may also facilitate serum potassium reduction. Close cardiac monitoring is essential. Frequent reassessment of electrolyte levels is necessary to evaluate care and prevent complications. Observation of neurologic function, intake and output, and vital signs provides information on patient response to treatment.

The patient with acute adrenal insufficiency is critically ill, so care must focus on fluid replacement, electrolyte correction, and rejuvenation of the adrenal system. Maintaining ABCs and providing the patient and family with necessary support and information lead to a positive outcome.

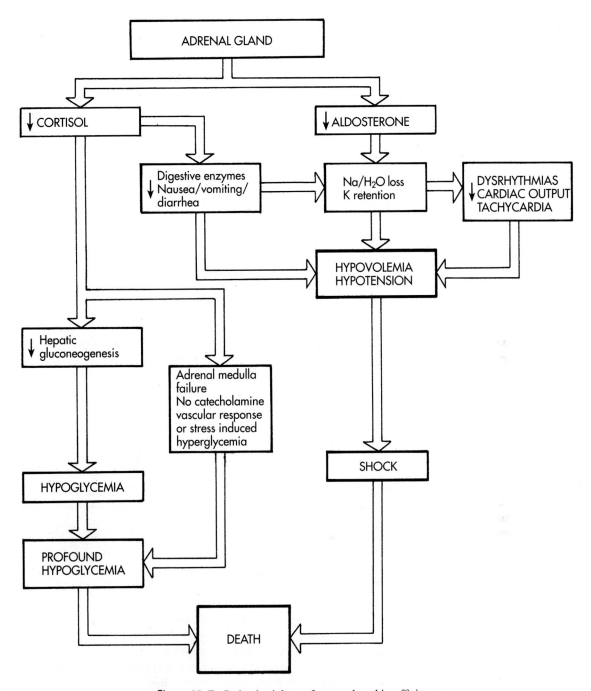

Figure **41-7** Pathophysiology of acute adrenal insufficiency.

Diabetic Ketoacidosis

DKA develops when a patient experiences relative or absolute depletion of circulating insulin. Occurring primarily in type I diabetes, DKA is responsible for 10% of all diabetic-related hospital admissions. DKA may occur in patients with new-onset diabetes, so acute presentation can lead to initial diagnosis of diabetes. Stressors such as infection, illness, pregnancy, or situational stressors can lead to gluconeogenesis, which creates a relative insulin deficiency. Poor dietary management may also lead to excess circulating glucose,

which overwhelms an already stressed system. Absolute deficiency may occur in the noncompliant patient who experiences stress and fails to follow the prescribed insulin regimen or in the diabetic patient who becomes ill and fails to take insulin. The latter example demonstrates why diabetic education is so critical.

After prolonged insulin deficiency, the patient can present with four acute problems: hyperglycemia, dehydration, electrolyte depletion, and metabolic acidosis. Stress causes release of regulatory hormones, which leads to onset of gluco-

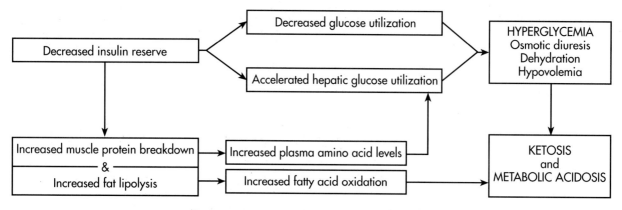

Figure **41-8** Pathophysiology of diabetic ketoacidosis.

neogenesis (Figure 41-8). Gluconeogenesis progresses to severe hyperglycemia, which leads to onset of osmotic diuresis. Excessive loss of water, sodium, and potassium can lead to hypovolemia. Profound hyperglycemia overwhelms available insulin, so the body is unable to metabolize glucose. Fats and muscle proteins are metabolized for energy. Ensuing lipolysis leads to buildup of fatty acids, which overwhelms the body's natural buffering system, leading to ketoacidosis.

DKA develops over a relatively short time period, usually 2 to 3 days, and is seen most often in young adults. The patient describes a steady progression of symptoms including polydipsia, polyuria, fatigue, and weakness. Patients with new-onset diabetes may report recent weight loss. As ketoacidosis worsens, nausea, vomiting, decreased appetite, and abdominal discomfort occur. The patient appears in moderate to severe distress with possible altered level of consciousness, confusion about recent events, or slow response to questions. Rapid, deep Kussmaul's respirations are present, with fruity odor on the breath. This acetone smell indicates worsening ketoacidosis. The skin is usually hot and dry, skin turgor is diminished, and mucous membranes are dry. The cardiac monitor displays tachycardia with dysrhythmias related to electrolyte disturbances (Table 41-6).

Laboratory studies should be obtained early. Fluid therapy should begin on arrival. Serum glucose greater than 300 mg/dl and normal or elevated potassium levels are usually present. Creatinine and BUN levels are also elevated as a result of dehydration. Serum osmolality is greater than 310 mosm/kg, and serum acetone titrations are positive. Serum acetone levels may be helpful in diagnosis but should not be used to monitor patient condition, since the acetoacetate level may actually rise once the patient begins to improve.[10] Urinalysis reveals elevated ketones and glucose. Blood gas results show normal PaO_2, respiratory alkalosis, and metabolic acidosis.

Treatment focuses on correction of hyperglycemia, dehydration, electrolyte imbalances, and metabolic acidosis.

Table 41-6	Clinical Manifestations of Diabetic Ketoacidosis
System	**Clinical manifestations**
Neurologic	Lethargy, confusion, coma, hyperthermia
Pulmonary	Kussmaul's respirations, fruity acetone breath
Cardiovascular	Tachycardia, hypotension, dysrhythmias
Integumentary	Flushed skin, dry membranes, poor skin turgor
Renal	Polyuria, ketonuria, glucosuria
Gastrointestinal	Nausea, vomiting, abdominal cramps, ileus

Close monitoring with frequent reassessment is essential to prevent complications. Oxygen therapy should be initiated for any signs of compromise or altered mental status.

Intravenous fluid replacement should start immediately with 1 to 2 L of normal saline over the first 1 to 2 hours of treatment. The patient may require 8 to 10 L of fluid to replace lost volume. Once serum glucose reaches 250 to 300 mg/dl, fluids should be converted to 5% dextrose in normal saline to provide fuel until the patient is able to eat. Close observation of intake and output should be stressed. Rapid fluid infusion creates potential for complications. Foley catheter placement ensures accurate output assessment and may help identify the onset of complications.

Insulin drip (normal saline with regular insulin) should be initiated as soon as serum glucose is known. Short duration of action for regular insulin allows better control of serum glucose. Insulin drip rates are generally low (5 to 10 U/hr), with sliding-scale parameters to cover frequent glucose monitoring. Serum glucose is reduced gradually, usually 75 to 100 mg/dl/hr. Intravenous tubing should be flushed with 50 to 60 ml of insulin solution prior to administration, since tubing absorbs part of the insulin.

Acidosis is treated with sodium bicarbonate if pH is less than 7.0 to 7.1. Bicarbonate given with higher pH causes rebound alkalosis, which can worsen hypokalemia. With higher pH levels, acidosis generally corrects with insulin therapy. By decreasing hyperglycemia, insulin helps decrease circulating amino and fatty acids, which cause ketoacidosis.

Fluid replacement dilutes serum potassium, so potassium replacement should begin after the initial liter of intravenous fluids. Serum potassium also decreases in response to the insulin as insulin forces potassium out of the vascular area into the cells. Cardiac dysrhythmias can develop with significant hypokalemia.

Management in the ED should be aggressive. Controlling nausea and vomiting not only improves patient comfort but also prevents worsening dehydration. The patient may require analgesia to relieve abdominal pain, headaches, or other somatic complaints. Providing a quiet, calm environment may also improve patient comfort. Stress reduction plays an important part in patient recovery. Thorough explanation of treatment, medications, and plan of care can alleviate stress related to hospitalization.

Infection can precipitate DKA. Blood cultures and urine culture should be obtained if infection is suspected. Once cultures are obtained, antibiotic therapy should begin. Radiographs may also be ordered to determine the primary site of infection.

Potential complications in treatment include hypoglycemia, hypokalemia, dysrhythmias, and cerebral edema. Monitor laboratory values, vital signs, intake and output, and neurologic status carefully. If serum glucose falls rapidly, the resulting fluid shift can lead to cerebral edema, which is associated with higher mortality rate. Cerebral edema is a greater threat for children than adults. If the patient exhibits signs of hypoglycemia, the insulin drip should be discontinued, and the physician should be notified.

Hyperosmolar Hyperglycemic Nonketotic Coma

HHNC threatens non–insulin-dependent (type II) diabetic patients with mortality rates as high as 50% to 70%.[10] Undiagnosed type II diabetics, alcoholics, and dialysis patients face the greatest risk. Type II diabetic patients are typically over 50 years old and may have other contributing health problems that account for high mortality rates. When stressed with illness, surgery, or injury, the body responds with increased glucose levels. Type II diabetics produce enough insulin to avoid ketoacidosis but not enough to prevent profound hyperglycemia, dehydration, and hyperosmolality, which are the hallmark conditions of HHNC (Table 41-7).

Increased serum glucose acts as an osmotic diuretic, leading to severe dehydration. Patients are unable to replace lost fluids, so their condition progressively worsens. Severe dehydration may also predispose patients to thrombus formation, which can lead to disseminated intravascular coagulation. Lack of sufficient circulating insulin causes the body to metabolize fat and muscle tissues, which increases amino

Table **41-7**	**Clinical Manifestations of Hyperosmolar Hyperglycemic Nonketotic Coma**
System	**Clinical manifestations**
Neurologic	Confusion, lethargy, seizures, coma
Pulmonary	Shallow or normal respirations
Cardiovascular	Tachycardia, elevated T waves, dysrhythmias
Renal	Polyuria, glucosuria
Gastrointestinal	Mild abdominal discomfort, nausea, vomiting

acid levels. The resulting hepatic gluconeogenesis compounds existing hyperglycemia.

Onset of symptoms is much longer than with DKA, developing over days or even weeks. Subtlety of symptoms may account for delay in seeking treatment. The patient may notice vague abdominal pain, decreased appetite, polydipsia, and polyuria. As the disease progresses, headaches, blurred vision, and confusion develop. Changes in level of consciousness, seizures, or coma also occurs. Tachycardia, dysrhythmias, and hypotension may also be present. Respirations may be increased but do not have the fruity smell associated with DKA (Figure 41-9).

Laboratory analysis includes complete blood count (CBC), electrolytes, urinalysis, and arterial blood gases. Blood gas analysis indicates normal PaO_2 unless respiratory infection is the stressor. Slightly decreased to normal serum pH may be present. Urinalysis shows positive glucosuria without ketonuria. Elevated white blood cell (WBC) count is present with infection. Serum glucose is usually greater than 600 mg/dl and is often greater than 1000 mg/dl. Serum sodium and potassium may be normal or elevated depending on the level of dehydration.

Correction of hyperglycemia, dehydration, and electrolyte imbalances is the focus for treatment. If the patient exhibits respiratory compromise or altered level of consciousness, oxygen therapy should be initiated immediately. Rapid intravenous fluid replacement is initiated with half-normal or normal saline in adults or normal saline in children and the elderly. Dehydration in HHNC can require 12 L or more of intravenous fluid. Continual assessment and reassessment are the key to preventing complications associated with fluid therapy. Most patients with type II diabetes are over 50 years old, so circulatory overload is a risk with rapid fluid therapy. Foley catheter placement assists with intake and output monitoring. Intravenous potassium supplements help prevent hypokalemia from hemodilution and insulin therapy. Cardiac monitoring allows observation for potential cardiac complications related to the potassium deficits.

Once the serum glucose level is known, an insulin drip may be started but is not always necessary. Serum glucose

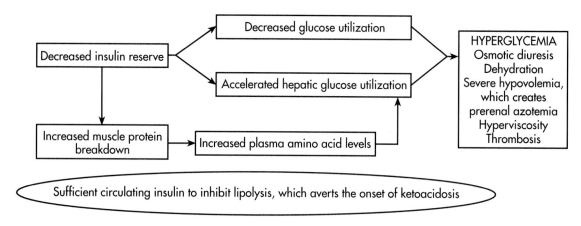

Figure **41-9** Pathophysiology of hyperosmolar hyperglycemic nonketotic coma.

Table **41-8** **Comparison of Hyperglycemic Hyperosmolar Nonketotic Coma (HHNC) and Diabetic Ketoacidosis (DKA)**

Clinical picture	HHNC	DKA
General	More dehydrated, not acidotic	More acidotic and less dehydrated
	Frequently comatose	Rarely comatose
	No hyperventilation	Hyperventilation
Age frequency	Usually elderly	Younger patients
Type of diabetes mellitus	Type II or non–insulin-dependent	Type I or insulin-dependent
Previous history of diabetes mellitus	In only 50%	Almost always
Prodromes	Several days' duration	Less than 1 day
Neurologic symptoms and signs	Very common	Rare
Underlying renal or cardiovascular disease	About 85%	About 15%
Laboratory findings		
Blood sugar	Over 800 mg/dl	Usually less than 800 mg/dl
Plasma ketones	Less than large in undiluted specimen	Positive in several dilutions
Serum sodium	Normal, elevated, low	Usually low
Serum potassium	Normal or elevated	Elevated, normal, or low
Serum bicarbonate	Over 16 mEq	Less than 10 mEq
Anion gap	10-12 mEq	Over 12 mEq
Blood pH	Normal	Less than 7.35
Serum osmolality	Over 350 mOsm/L	Less than 330 mOsm/L
Serum BUN	Higher than DKA (↑↑↑ to ↑↑↑↑)	Not as high as in HHNC (↑↑)
Free fatty acids	Less than 1000 mEq/L	Over 1500 mEq/L
Complications		
Thrombosis	Frequent	Very rare
Mortality	20%-50%	1%-10%
Diabetes treatment after recovery	Diet alone or oral agents (sometimes)	Always insulin

From Kozak G, editor: *Clinical diabetes mellitus,* Philadelphia, 1982, WB Saunders.

should be lowered gradually, since reductions greater than 100 mg/dl/hr may predispose the patient to cerebral edema because of associated fluid shifts. Once serum osmolality begins to normalize or serum glucose reaches 200 to 300 mg/dl, intravenous fluids may be converted to 5% dextrose in normal or half-normal saline to provide energy until oral intake improves.

Differentiation between HHNC and DKA may be initially difficult; however, this should not alter the basic course of treatment. Intravenous fluid therapy should begin immediately. Nursing actions are similar in both instances and include close observation of vital systems to prevent complications of therapy. Table 41-8 compares the clinical pictures of HHNC and DKA.

Hypoglycemia

Of three specific diabetic emergencies, hypoglycemia progresses the quickest. Prompt nursing assessment and action are imperative to avoid fatal consequences (Box 41-1). Type I diabetics are more susceptible because of insulin's quick onset of action. Hypoglycemia should be considered a causative agent in all unresponsive patients until established otherwise. Factors that contribute to hypoglycemia include lack of dietary intake, increased physical stress, liver disease, changes in type of insulin or oral agents, pregnancy, alcohol ingestion, and certain drugs (nonsteroidal antiinflammatory drugs, phenytoin, thyroid hormone, propranolol).

Serum glucose less than 70 mg/dl indicates hypoglycemia; however, this number may be higher depending on the patient's "normal" glucose level. The axiom "Treat the patient, not the monitor" is applied here. Treat the patient's symptoms, not just the serum glucose.

Rapid decline in glucose deprives the body of normal compensatory responses, that is, glucagon and epinephrine. Normally, the body senses declining serum glucose, so glucagon and epinephrine are released to increase release of glycogen stored in the liver. Glycogen functions as an alternate energy source; however, in acute hypoglycemia, glycogen stores cannot be broken down quickly enough to overcome insulin. Epinephrine release decreases utilization of existing glucose.

Mild symptoms of palpitations, tachycardia, shakiness, perspiration, and hunger are attributed to epinephrine. The known diabetic patient can usually recognize these symptoms and self-treat. β-Blocker therapy masks the sympathetic response, so these patients may not recognize onset of hypoglycemia.

Moderate symptoms include altered levels of consciousness, slurred speech, headache, and decreased reaction time. As neuroglycopenia worsens, confusion with decreased ability to make decisions results. The patient may or may not be able to self-treat or seek treatment at this point. Without treatment, moderate hypoglycemia can lead to disorientation, seizures, and eventually coma (Table 41-9). Family education is critical. Often, the family must initiate treatment after recognizing changes in the patient's behavior. Patients on insulin pumps may be especially vulnerable.

Treatment of the conscious patient consists of oral intake of 10 to 15 g of carbohydrates followed by a more complex carbohydrate snack or small meal (Box 41-2). In the lethargic or unconscious patient, rapid administration of intravenous glucose (1.5 ampules of D50) remains the treatment of choice. If intravenous access cannot be obtained, intramuscular glucagon should be administered. Glucagon, 1 mg IM, stimulates the liver to release glycogen, which is converted to glucose. If the patient has an insulin pump, the pump must be stopped. If the patient has a seizure, protect the patient from injury by placing in the recovery or left lateral position to maintain the airway. In the hospital setting, priorities include ensuring patient safety and initiating oxygen therapy.

Laboratory studies obtained prior to glucose administration provide helpful information; however, administration of D50 should not be delayed to obtain laboratory samples. Severe neurologic deficits can result if the central nervous system is left without glucose. Once alert, the patient should be given a diet tray to provide complex carbohydrates as the D50 begins to wear off. After this meal and a glucose recheck, the patient is usually discharged unless the patient is on oral antihyperglycemic medications that have a longer half-life.

Thyroid Storm

Thyroid emergencies are rare but can have life-threatening outcomes. The thyroid gland regulates the body's metabolic

---

Table 41-9 Clinical Manifestations of Hypoglycemia

System	Clinical manifestations
Neurologic	Confusion, combativeness, seizures, coma
Pulmonary	Hyperventilation, shallow respirations
Cardiovascular	Palpitations, tachycardia
Integumentary	Cool, pale, clammy, diaphoretic
Gastrointestinal	Hunger, severe hypoglycemia

Box 41-1 Diabetic Emergency Initial Management

Secure airway.

Obtain intravenous access.

Institute cardiac monitoring with central monitoring as needed.

Obtain laboratory samples if possible; initiate intravenous fluids.

Administer D50 if patient is unconscious, and consider thiamine and naloxone administration if alcohol and/or drug involvement is suspected.

Place Foley catheter; send for urinalysis and urine culture and sensitivity; monitor intake and output closely.

Obtain arterial blood gases to monitor oxygen therapy and assess acid-base balance.

Frequently reassess with close monitoring to ensure patient safety and condition improvement.

Box 41-2 Quick Glucose Sources

The following foods provide a quick glucose source (approximately 10-15 g of carbohydrates):

4-6 oz of orange juice, apple juice, or ginger ale

5-6 Lifesaver candies

½-¾ cup of nondiet soda

6 oz of milk

2-3 glucose tablets

rate, so hyperactivity or hypoactivity results in multisystem symptoms. Thyroid storm commonly occurs as a complication of Graves' disease (thyroid hyperactivity) and is seen primarily in women 30 to 40 years old.

The hypothalamic-pituitary-thyroid counterregulatory system is responsible for normal thyroid function. Thyroid crisis occurs when any part of the circuit malfunctions. Thyroid gland activity depends on the hypothalamus secreting thyrotropin-releasing hormone (TRH), which is responsible for release of thyrotropin or TSH by the anterior pituitary, which causes T_3 and T_4 release. Circulating T_4 also converts to T_3 (Figure 41-10). The amount of TSH depends on the amount of TRH, which can be influenced by physical stressors such as surgery, infection, and extremely cold temperatures. Circulating levels of T_3 and T_4 also affect the amount of TRH released.

Hyperthyroidism can be divided into three categories. True hyperthyroidism is characterized by an overactive thyroid gland and excessive production of thyroid hormones. In Graves' disease, thyroid-stimulating immunoglobulins increase thyroid activity. Tumors and thyroid nodules also increase thyroid activity. A type of thyrotoxicosis occurs with an increased amount of circulating hormones without concurrent overactivity from the thyroid, as in thyroiditis or ingestion of thyroid hormones (intentionally or unintentionally). Certain drugs, especially iodine and iodine-containing agents such as amiodarone and lithium, induce hyperthyroidism.

Thyroid storm occurs with rapid elevation in thyroid hormone levels. Actual levels may be less important than rapidity of elevation.[15] The end result is a hypermetabolic state characterized by hyperthermia, agitation, tachydysrhythmias, and other symptoms that stress the body. Elevated hormone levels may occur in response to hospitalization, surgery, infection, emotional stressors, trauma, childbirth, sudden discontinuation of antithyroid medications, and overmanipulation of the thyroid.

Gathering a concise history regarding past and recent illnesses and current medications is important. The patient may have recently discontinued a medication or experienced a recent change in therapy. The patient usually has a history of Graves' disease. Patients often report recent weight loss despite increased appetite and increased caloric intake. Complaints of abdominal pain are common. Pregnant women may present with hyperemesis gravidarum.[13]

The patient is restless with shortened attention span and may switch topics of conversation frequently. Tremors and manic behaviors are also common. In late stages, the patient may have altered mental status, which progresses to coma. Hyperthermia may be extreme, with temperatures reaching 105° to 106° F. Tachycardia with rates as high as 200 to 300 beats/min increases the patient's risk for cardiac failure and arrest.[15] Rales secondary to cardiac failure may be heard. The skin often progresses from warm and diaphoretic to hot and dry as dehydration worsens. Nausea, vomiting, and diarrhea are caused by increased gastric motility. Hepatic tenderness and jaundice may occur. Hair may thin and goiter, an enlarged thyroid gland, develops as the condition progresses. Eyes become protuberant, periorbital edema develops, and the patient may have a staring gaze with heavy eyelids. Table 41-10 summarizes the clinical manifestations of thyroid storm.

Thyroid hormone levels may help differentiate the causative factor, but long turnaround times offer little help in the emergency setting. Even elevated levels do not necessarily discriminate between thyroid storm and thyrotoxicosis.

Immediate goals for management of thyroid storm include oxygen therapy, heart rate reduction, thyroid loop interruption, temperature reduction, and fluid administration.[4] Rapid, aggressive therapy is essential to reduce hormone levels and preserve hemodynamic integrity. Interventions include fluid replacement, management of hormone effects, supportive care, and identification of precipitants. Providing supplemental oxygen assists with increased multisystem oxygen demands.

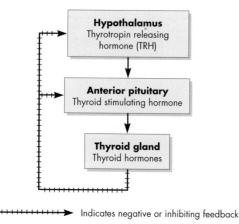

Figure **41-10** Thyroid regulation. (*From Lewis SM, Collier IC, Heitkemper MM:* Medical-surgical nursing: assessment and management of clinical problems, *ed 4, St. Louis, 1996, Mosby.*)

Table **41-10**	**Clinical Manifestations of Thyroid Storm**
System	Clinical manifestations
Neurologic	Nervousness, restlessness, tremors, confusion
Pulmonary	Tachycardia, dysrhythmias, hypertension
Respiratory	Shortness of breath, dyspnea, rales, congestive heart failure
Gastrointestinal	Hyperactive bowel, abdominal pain, decreased appetite, weight loss, diarrhea, jaundice
Ocular	Exophthalmus, lid lag, staring gaze
Integumentary	Hyperthermia, flushed, diaphoresis, poor turgor

High priority must be given to eliminating the hypermetabolic state. Propylthiouracil and methimazole may be used to block further synthesis of thyroid hormones. Most clinicians prefer propylthiouracil because of inhibition of peripheral conversion of T_4 to T_3. Medications may be given orally or through a gastric tube. Onset of action is quite rapid, usually within 1 hour. Methimazole may be given rectally.[13] Another medication option includes iodide to prevent thyroid release of stored hormones. Iodides should be given 1 hour after antithyroid medications. If given sooner, iodide may actually be used to create new hormones. Iodides may be given orally (Lugol's solution) or by slow intravenous infusion. Blocking conversion of T_4 to T_3 improves the patient's condition. Lithium can be given to prevent T_4 release. Patients with Graves' disease and thyroid crisis metabolize and utilize cortisol faster than normal, so administration of glucocorticoids has been shown to increase survival rates. Glucocorticoids prevent adrenal compromise and inhibit T_4 conversion to T_3.

Heart rate reduction requires immediate attention, usually by administration of intravenous propranolol, which not only helps tachycardia but also prevents further conversion of T_4 to T_3. Large doses of propranolol (160 to 480 mg/day) may be required, especially in younger patients and those in severe crisis.[15] If β-blockers fail, reserpine may be tried. Digoxin may be used to decrease heart rate. Small amounts of diuretics may be required to help prevent or minimize fluid overload. Intake and output should be closely monitored to ensure fluid balance and assess response to therapy. If the causative agent is overload of thyroid medications, these can be removed through lavage or peritoneal dialysis.

Increased body temperature raises metabolic demands, which increases the percentage of free T_4. Acetaminophen is preferred over salicylates, which displace thyroid hormones from binding sites and worsen the situation. Cooling blankets may be necessary. Cool cloths to the axilla and groin are also helpful. Fluid replacement therapy replenishes fluids lost through hyperthermia, vomiting, and diarrhea. Administration of antiemetic and antidiarrheal agents helps the patient conserve fluids. The fluid of choice is determined by the patient's hemodynamic status and electrolyte levels.

Once the patient stabilizes, close evaluation and assessment are necessary to identify the aggravating agent or illness. Laboratory analysis includes cultures, toxicology screens, thyroid functions, electrolyte levels, and CBC. Radiographs may be ordered to rule out infectious sources, and head and neck computed tomography scans may be ordered to identify existing neoplasms or structural abnormalities. Antibiotic therapy may be started when infection is suspected as a causal agent.

Myxedema Coma

Myxedema coma affects women more than men, with crisis occurring most often in women 40 to 60 years old. Survival rates increase when patients receive prompt hormone replacement with intensive supportive care; however, mortality approaches 50%.

Untreated hypothyroidism progresses over months to years before culminating in myxedema coma. Primary hypothyroidism from thyroid malfunction accounts for 95% of cases.[1] Dysfunction may be related to autoimmune thyroiditis, ablation therapy (treatment for hyperthyroidism), iodine deficiency, tumor activity, or drug therapy. Medications such as lithium, amiodarone, and certain anticonvulsants can create hypothyroid conditions. Secondary hypothyroidism stems from pituitary dysfunction. Alterations in pituitary function decrease TSH release, which lowers thyroid hormone secretion. Tertiary hypothyroidism occurs when the hypothalamus secretes inadequate amounts of TRH or TRH fails to reach the pituitary gland.

With hypoactive thyroid, the entire system slows down. Fever, tachycardia, and diaphoresis are absent, so the crisis state may not be noticed initially. The patient may complain of pronounced fatigue, decreased activity tolerance, episodes of shortness of breath, and weight gain. Tongue swelling or macroglossia may also occur. Patients may answer questions slowly and exhibit significant confusion. Altered mental status can progress to coma. "Myxedema madness" refers to associated psychiatric symptoms such as hallucinations, paranoia, depression, combativeness, and decreased concern for personal appearance.

The tongue may be thick and can obstruct the airway of a semiconscious or unconscious patient. Weak respiratory effort with decreased drive leads to alveolar hypoventilation and can predispose the patient to infections. Alveolar hypoventilation also leads to hypercarbia, which can cause altered mental status. Obesity-related sleep apnea can further compromise the respiratory system. Table 41-11 summarizes the clinical manifestations of myxedema.

Cardiac changes include bradycardia, decreased stroke volume, and decreased cardiac output. There may be widespread ST- and T-wave changes with prolonged QT inter-

Table **41-11**	**Clinical Manifestations of Myxedema Coma**
System	Clinical manifestations
Neurologic	Confusion, lethargy, coma
Pulmonary	Decreased stroke volume, decreased cardiac output, bradycardia, peripheral vasoconstriction, inverted T waves, prolonged QT interval
Respiratory	Macroglossia, obesity-related sleep apnea, pneumonia, hypoventilation, hypercarbia
Gastrointestinal	Hypoglycemia, constipation
Renal	Decreased renal blood flow, decreased sodium reabsorption, hyponatremia

vals. Peripheral vasoconstriction is the body's attempt to conserve heat, so skin is cool and pale.

Renal blood flow and glomerular filtration rates decrease, but sodium reabsorption also decreases. Patients cannot excrete the usual amount of fluid; however, urine osmolality does not reflect serum hypoosmolality. Generalized nonpitting edema may be observed. Occasionally, hypoglycemia develops as a result of increased insulin sensitivity and decreased oral intake. Systemic slowing affects the gastrointestinal tract, so constipation occurs. Oral medications in initial stages may not be adequately absorbed because of decreased gastric motility.

Diagnostic tests reveal decreased WBC count, decreased hemoglobin and hematocrit caused by low erythropoietin, and decreased thyroid levels. Creatinine kinase may be elevated, with elevations of MM bands.

Care focuses on thyroid hormone replacement after the ABCs have been stabilized. The patient may require mechanical ventilation to secure the airway to correct the increased carbon dioxide levels and improve oxygenation. Hormone replacement may take the form of intravenous levothyroxine (T_4). Large doses saturate empty sites and replenish peripheral circulating levels. T_4 avoids the adverse cardiac effects that might occur with a sudden increase in T_3. Some clinicians recommend a combination of T_4 and T_3 therapy.[3,8] T_3 does have a quicker onset of action, but controversy still exists related to increased mortality associated with sole T_3 use.[8,13] Once the patient can tolerate oral fluids, oral T_4 therapy may begin. Glucocorticoid administration may help prevent adrenal crisis in patients with compromised adrenal systems.

Slow warming is recommended; increased oxygen demands related to warming can add stress to an overstressed system. Passive warming with blankets or heated, humidified mist is recommended. Supportive care includes analgesic administration, Foley catheter placement, and a nasogastric tube to decrease abdominal pressure and distention.

Infection accounts for 35% of precipitating factors.[8] Medications such as sedatives and tranquilizers also contribute to hypothyroid crisis. Scans, radiographs, and further diagnostic tests are done once the patient stabilizes. Severe systemic slowing exhibited in myxedema coma should not be underestimated. Nursing care focuses on ABC stabilization, medication administration to correct thyroid hormone deficiencies, close observation to avoid complications, and initiation of patient education.

Syndrome of Inappropriate Antidiuretic Hormone

SIADH occurs when the pituitary gland releases excessive amounts of ADH because of failure of ADH's negative feedback system (Figure 41-11). Any disease process that alters the hypothalamic osmoreceptors or hypothalamic-pituitary-adrenal circuit may precipitate SIADH.[2] Diseases such as oat cell lung cancer, pancreatic cancer, and thyroid and pituitary

Syndrome of Inappropriate Antidiuretic Hormone (SIADH)

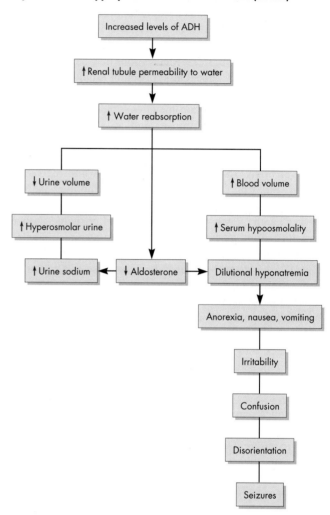

Figure **41-11** Pathophysiology of syndrome of inappropriate antidiuretic hormone (SIADH). *(From Lewis SM, Collier IC, Heitkemper MM: Medical-surgical nursing: assessment and management of clinical problems, ed 4, St. Louis, 1996, Mosby.)*

lesions place the patient at increased risk for SIADH.[9] Narcotics, tricyclic antidepressants, oral hypoglycemics, and certain anticonvulsants (carbamazepine) may precipitate SIADH. Other associated disorders include abscesses, pneumonia, tuberculosis, hypothyroid disorders, porphyria, and head injury. Box 41-3 summarizes causes of SIADH.

ADH is generated in the hypothalamus and stored in the pituitary gland. Water balance is controlled by ADH through increased distal renal tubular permeability to water, which decreases urine volume and returns water to the systemic circulation. Serum osmolality and circulating blood volume influence ADH release. Hypothalamic osmoreceptors sense increased serum concentration and stimulate release of ADH. Serum concentration decreases when the kidneys respond with increased water reabsorption. As circulating volume ex-

Box **41-3**   **Causes of Syndrome of Inappropriate Antidiuretic Hormone**

- Malignant neoplasms
    - Small-cell carcinoma of lung
    - Carcinoma of pancreas and duodenum
    - Lymphosarcoma, reticulum cell sarcoma, Hodgkin's disease
    - Thymoma
- Nonmalignant pulmonary diseases
    - Tuberculosis
    - Lung abscess
    - Pneumonia
    - Empyema
    - Chronic obstructive pulmonary disease
- Central nervous system disorders
    - Skull fracture
    - Subdural hematoma
    - Subarachnoid hemorrhage
    - Cerebral vascular thrombosis
    - Cerebral atrophy
    - Encephalitis
    - Meningitis
    - Guillain-Barré syndrome
    - Systemic lupus erythematosus
- Drugs
    - Chlorpropamide
    - Vincristine
    - Vinblastine
    - Cyclophosphamide
    - Carbamazepine
    - Oxytocin
    - General anesthesia
    - Narcotics
    - Tricyclic antidepressants
- Miscellaneous causes
    - Hypothyroidism
    - Positive pressure mechanical ventilation

From Moses A, Streeten D: Disorders of the neurohypophysis. In Isselbacher K et al, editors: *Harrison's principles of internal medicine*, ed 13, New York, 1994, Mosby. Used with permission of the McGraw-Hill Companies.

Box **41-4**

NURSING DIAGNOSES FOR ENDOCRINE EMERGENCIES

Fluid volume deficit
Fluid volume excess
Altered cardiopulmonary and cerebral tissue perfusion
Impaired gas exchange
Decreased cardiac output
Hyperthermia

pands, urinary output diminishes. The resulting hemodilution creates fluid overload with associated hyponatremia.

Baroreceptors in the left atrium sensitive to blood pressure changes respond to increased blood volume, so ADH release is inhibited, urinary output increases, and blood volume returns to normal. The reverse actions occur when baroreceptors sense decreased blood pressure. Distur-bances in this feedback loop may be responsible for ADH crisis.

Subjective complaints include weakness, nausea, vomiting, diarrhea, abdominal and muscle cramps, sudden weight gain, and confusion. The patient may also note decreased urinary output despite regular oral intake, but the greatest changes may be in neurologic function. The patient appears confused and disoriented, with seizures as hyponatremia worsens. Severe hyponatremia leads to fluid shifts, which result in cerebral edema.[5] Deep tendon reflexes decrease.

Laboratory tests reveal marked hyponatremia of less than 120 mEq/L and low serum osmolality. Blood urea nitrogen and creatinine are low to normal. Urine specific gravity demonstrates serum dilution below 1.002. Renal function tests are usually normal.

Fluid restriction is a hallmark for treatment of SIADH.[2] Restrictions often start at 800 to 1000 ml/day; however, restrictions as severe as 500 ml/day may be seen. The importance of accurate intake and output monitoring cannot be overemphasized. Fluid replacement therapy consists of hypertonic solutions such as 3% or 5% normal saline, which help move fluid out of edematous cerebral tissue. Intravenous therapy begins at 75 to 125 ml/hr. Close monitoring is necessary for early identification of circulatory overload. Small amounts of loop diuretics increase urinary output, which may prevent overload. Serial electrolyte evaluations help avoid complications in therapy and assist in monitoring therapy progress. Administration of demeclocycline, 600 to 1200 mg/day, interferes with ADH action. Lithium may also be given because of interference with ADH action and increased urinary output. However, these medications simply augment fluid restriction therapy. Ultimately, serum sodium and osmolality should improve. Once the patient stabilizes, identification and treatment of the precipitating event become a primary goal.

Uncorrected, SIADH can have serious consequences. Failure of the ADH regulatory feedback loop leads to vascular water overload with severe serum hyponatremia. Fluid restriction is the primary management tool, with close observation and timely management to ensure patient safety and prevention of complications.

SUMMARY

Endocrine emergencies affect all body systems because of the diversity of hormones and their effects. Support of hemodynamic functions and identification of precipitating events are essential for survival of these patients. Box 41-4 highlights priority nursing diagnoses for the patient with an endocrine emergency.

REFERENCES

1. Angelucci P: Caring for patients with hypothyroidism, *Nursing95* 25(5):60, 1995.
2. Bryce J: SIADH, *Nursing94* 24(4):33, 1994.
3. Burch H, Wartofsky L: Life-threatening thyrotoxicosis, *Endocrinol Metab Clin North Am* 22(2):263, 1993.
4. Corsetti A, Buhl B: Managing thyroid storm, *Am J Nurs* 94(11):39, 1994.
5. Emergency Nurses Association: *Emergency nursing core curriculum,* ed 4, Philadelphia, 1994, WB Saunders.
6. Guyton AC, Hall JE: *Textbook of medical physiology,* ed 9, Philadelphia, 1996, WB Saunders.
7. Handerhan B: Recognizing adrenal crisis, *Nursing92* 22(4):33, 1992.
8. Jordan R: Myxedema coma pathophysiology, therapy, and factors affecting prognosis, *Med Clin North Am* 19(1):185, 1995.
9. Lindaman S: SIADH: is your patient at risk? *Nursing92* 22(6):60, 1992.
10. Peragallo-Dittko V: Diabetes 2000 acute complications, *RN* 58(8):36, 1995.
11. Rosen P, et al: *Essentials of emergency medicine,* ed 3, St. Louis, 1992, Mosby.
12. Serrano S, et al: Addisonian crisis as the presenting feature of bilateral primary adrenal lymphoma, *Cancer* 71(12):4030, 1993.
13. Smallridge R: Metabolic and anatomic thyroid emergencies: a review, *Crit Care Med* 20(2):276, 1992.
14. Strowig S: Diabetes 2000 insulin therapy, *RN* 58(8):36, 1995.
15. Tietgens S, Leinung M: Thyroid storm, *Med Clin North Am* 79(1):169, 1995.
16. Tintinalli JE, Ruiz E, Krome RL: *Emergency medicine: a comprehensive study guide,* ed 4, New York, 1996, McGraw-Hill.
17. Wilson S: Can you spot an alcoholic patient? *RN* 57(1):46, 1994.
18. Wrenn K, et al: The syndrome of alcoholic ketoacidosis, *Am J Med* 91:119, 1991.

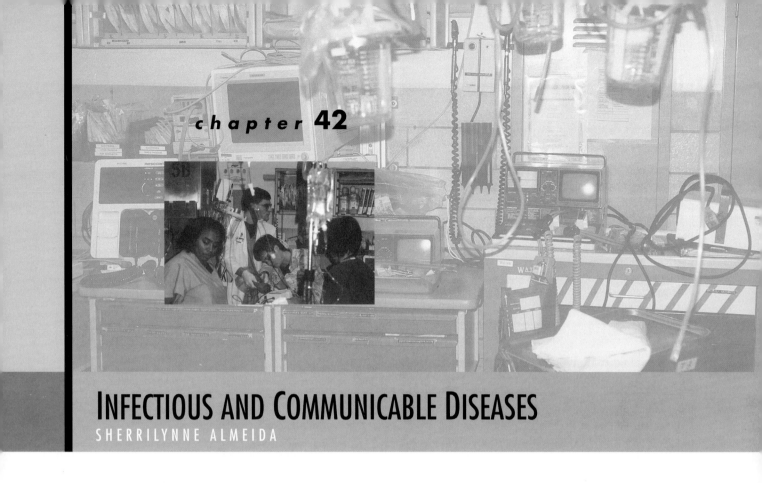

chapter 42

INFECTIOUS AND COMMUNICABLE DISEASES

SHERRILYNNE ALMEIDA

Infection is entry and development or multiplication of an infectious agent in the body. Three factors represent the chain of infection: agent, host, and mode of transmission.[13] The agent or microorganism can be a bacterium, virus, fungus, or parasite. The property of an infectious agent that determines the extent to which overt disease is produced or the power of an organism to produce disease is called *pathogenicity.* Some agents are highly pathogenic and almost always produce disease, whereas others multiply without invasion and rarely cause disease.

A susceptible host is one who lacks effective resistance to a pathogenic agent. Characteristics that influence susceptibility include age, sex, medical history, underlying pathology, lifestyle, nutrition, immunizations, medications, and specific insult to the body, such as trauma.

Transmission is the interaction between an infectious agent and a susceptible host. Major modes of transmission are direct, indirect, and airborne exposure. Direct transmission occurs when person-to-person contact occurs between an infected source and a susceptible host with a receptive portal through which human or animal infection can enter. Direct contact includes touching, biting, kissing, sexual intercourse, direct inoculation with contaminated blood (needle stick injury), or direct projection of droplet spray onto the conjunctiva of the eye, nose, or mouth during sneezing, coughing, spitting, or vomiting.[2] Indirect transmission occurs when susceptible hosts come in contact with a contaminated object. Any substance by which an infectious agent is transported and introduced into a susceptible host through a suitable portal of entry is vehicle-borne.

Vehicle-borne agents are contaminated, inanimate materials such as patient care equipment, soiled linen, surgical instruments, dressings, food, water, milk, and biologic products such as blood, serum, plasma, tissues, or organs. Vector-borne transmission occurs with injection of saliva during biting, regurgitation, or dermal exposure to feces or other material capable of penetrating nonintact skin. And finally, airborne transmission is defined as dissemination of microbial aerosols through a portal, usually the respiratory tract. Close contact with an infected source who is coughing or sneezing can transmit large infectious particles through the air. Factors that influence airborne transmission include ambient air flow, proximity, and spatial orientation to the person who is coughing or sneezing.

PREVENTION OF INFECTION

In the hospital environment, transmission of an infectious agent to a susceptible host occurs by direct and indirect contact.[1] Nosocomial infection, the most common form of hospital infection, is an infection acquired by a patient who had no infection at the time of arrival. Inappropriate or lack of hand washing is the most significant reason for development of nosocomial infections. In the absence of a true emergency, personnel should always wash their hands prior to patient contact.[7] Box 42-1 highlights critical times when hand washing should occur. Products containing antimicro-

---

Box 42-1 Hand-Washing Essentials

Before performing invasive procedures, i.e., intravenous catheter insertion, ureteral catheterization, tracheal suctioning

Before caring for susceptible patients, i.e., the immunosuppressed patient, newborns, and the elderly

Before and after touching wounds

When exposure to microbial contamination may occur, i.e., contact with mucous membranes, blood, body fluids, secretions, or excretions

After touching contaminated inanimate objects, e.g., suction equipment, urine collection devices

Between contact with patients

After removing protective gloves

Box 42-2 Universal Precautions

Do apply

Blood, semen, vaginal secretions, cerebrospinal fluid, synovial fluid, pleural fluid, peritoneal fluid, pericardial fluid, and amniotic fluid

Do not apply

Feces, nasal secretions, sputum, sweat, tears, urine, vomitus unless contaminated with blood

---

Box 42-3 Guidelines to Minimize Exposure to Blood-Borne Pathogens

Do not perform direct patient care or handle contaminated equipment without barrier protection when open skin lesions are present.

Use special caution if pregnant when working with patients or contaminated equipment, supplies, or materials.

Use disposable gloves when performing arterial or venous punctures, aspirating blood from existing arterial or venous catheters, handling blood or body fluid specimens, hanging or changing blood bags or transfusion tubing, emptying bedpans and urinals, and providing stoma care.

Remove damaged gloves. Wash hands, and then don new gloves.

Wash hands immediately if exposed to blood or body fluids, between patient contacts, after touching contaminated objects, and after removing gloves.

Wear impervious gowns, masks, and/or eye covering when extensive blood or body fluid exposure is possible, e.g., trauma resuscitation, emergency delivery, and gastric lavage.

Use artificial airways and resuscitation masks rather than mouth-to-mouth ventilations.

Do not recap, bend, or break needles. Do not place needles on the bed or drop on the floor. Discard needles in an appropriate sharps container.

Carry nondisposable sharp instruments in a puncture-resistant container.

Scrub reusable equipment to remove debris and blood (wear gloves).

Wipe contaminated surfaces with absorbent toweling to remove excess material, and then wash with an appropriate germicide. Clothing may be washed in the regular laundry.

Remove contaminated gloves before touching the telephone or other nonclinical surfaces.

---

bial agents such as foams and rinses can be used when water is not available.[9]

There will always be patients in the emergency department (ED) with infections or infectious diseases. Risk to the emergency nurse is probably no greater for these infections than risk to the community. Emergency nurses have a greater risk of exposure to blood-borne pathogens such as hepatitis B (HBV) and human immunodeficiency virus (HIV) because of frequent exposure to blood and the unknown status of the patient. The emergency nurse must use universal precautions, treating all blood and most body fluids as infectious. Blood is the single most important source of HIV, HBV, and other blood-borne pathogens; however, universal precautions also apply to other body fluids. Box 42-2 identifies precautions for various body fluids. Box 42-3 summarizes guidelines to minimize exposure to blood-borne pathogens.

SPECIFIC TYPES OF INFECTIOUS DISEASES

The emergency nurse may encounter a number of infectious and communicable diseases, depending on where the nurse works and how mobile the patient population is. This chapter focuses on infectious diseases that are most prevalent: hepatitis, acquired immunodeficiency syndrome (AIDS), and tuberculosis. Childhood illnesses such as measles, mumps, and chickenpox are discussed in Chapter 50.

Hepatitis

Hepatitis is an acute or chronic viral infection of the liver, which may be mild or life-threatening. Four types of hepatitis are currently recognized: hepatitis A, B, C, and D. Emergency nurses are more likely to develop hepatitis than HIV infection from an occupational injury. Universal precautions are the first line of protection against this and other infectious processes.

Hepatitis A

Hepatitis A virus (HAV) is a widely distributed pathogen known to cause epidemics. In developing countries, adults are usually immune and HAV epidemics uncommon. However, outbreaks are increasing because improved sanitation in many parts of the world is increasing susceptibility. In developed countries, disease transmission is frequent in day care centers, through household and sexual contact, and among travelers to countries where the disease is endemic.

Epidemics can evolve slowly or explosively from common-source epidemics. Outbreaks resulting from food contamination by food handlers, contaminated produce, and contaminated water continue to occur. In recent years, community-wide outbreaks have accounted for most disease transmission.

HAV is transmitted via the fecal-oral route. The infectious agent reaches peak levels 1 or 2 weeks before onset of symptoms and diminishes rapidly after liver dysfunction or symptoms appear. Liver dysfunction and symptoms are concurrent with appearance of circulating antibodies to HAV. Incubation period ranges from 15 to 50 days depending on the dose of the inoculum. Average incubation period is 28 to 30 days.

Studies of transmission in humans and epidemiologic evidence indicate maximum infectivity occurs during the latter half of the incubation period and continues a few days after onset of jaundice. Most cases are probably not infectious after the first week of jaundice, although prolonged viral excretion (up to 6 months) has been documented in infants born prematurely.[1]

The disease varies in clinical severity from mild illness lasting 1 to 2 weeks to a severe, disabling disease lasting several months (rare). In general, severity increases with age, but complete uncomplicated recovery without recurrence is the norm. Abrupt onset of fever, malaise, anorexia, nausea, and abdominal discomfort is followed within a few days by jaundice. Many infections are asymptomatic. Mild cases can occur without jaundice, especially in children. Diagnosis is made by identification of IgM antibodies against HAV (IgM anti-HAV) in the serum of the acutely or recently ill patient. Antibodies remain detectable 4 to 6 months after onset of symptoms. Epidemiologic evidence can provide support for diagnosis if laboratory analysis is not available.

An inactive hepatitis A vaccine, now available, has been shown to be safe, immunogenic, and efficacious. Protection against clinical HAV may begin in some persons 14 to 21 days after a single dose of vaccine; nearly all have protective antibodies by 30 days. Hepatitis A immunization is recommended for anyone who plans to travel repeatedly or reside for long periods in areas where HAV is highly endemic. Individuals employed in hospitals or day care centers should also be immunized.

For proven cases of hepatitis A, enteric precautions are necessary during the first 2 weeks of illness, but no more than 1 week after onset of jaundice. Passive immunization with intramuscular immune globulin, 0.02 ml/kg of body weight, should be given as soon as possible after exposure to all household and sexual contacts.[17] In a day care center, immune globulin should be given to all classroom contacts including staff. Immunizations are not recommended after 2 weeks of illness.

Hepatitis B

HBV is a widely distributed pathogen that produces acute and chronic infection. Chronically infected persons represent the major source of infection. Individuals have an increased risk of mortality and morbidity associated with chronic liver disease and primary hepatocellular carcinoma. HBV is a worldwide problem existing even in the most remote and isolated populations of the world. Prevalence of HBV infection varies widely. The disease is a highly endemic disease in most of the developing world but is minimally endemic in developed countries.[14] An estimated 300 million persons worldwide are chronically infected with HBV; over 250,000 persons die annually from HBV-associated acute and chronic liver disease.[14] Acute and chronic consequences of HBV infection are major health problems in the United States. Each year, an estimated 300,000 persons, primarily young adults, are infected with HBV. The reported incidence of acute HBV increased by 37% from 1979 to 1989. One quarter of patients with HBV develop jaundice, more than 10,000 patients require hospitalization, and an average of 250 die of fulminant disease. Approximately 4000 to 5000 persons die annually from chronic liver diseases.[5]

HBV is a major infectious occupational hazard for health care workers. Risk of infection is associated with exposure to blood or potentially infectious body fluids contaminated with blood.[8] Correcting for underreporting and subclinical infection, the Centers for Disease Control and Prevention (CDC) estimate that approximately 15,000 HBV infections are associated with health care workers each year. Fortunately, the number of cases of HBV reported in health care workers has dropped since 1985.

In the United States, most persons with HBV acquire the infection as adolescents or adults. Specific modes of transmission include sexual contact, parenteral drug use, occupational exposure, household contact with an individual who has an acute infection or is a carrier, specific blood products, or hemodialysis treatments. The virus is passed directly from those who are already infected or indirectly from their body fluids. The most common modes of HBV transmission are through the skin by way of cuts, scrapes, needle sticks or needle sharing; through the eyes, mouth, or nose by exposure to blood or other body fluids; sexual contact; and contact between an infected mother and her newborn child during birth and in early infancy.

The incubation period averages 60 to 80 days, with the norm 45 to 180 days; however, incubation period can range from 2 weeks to 6 to 9 months when hepatitis B surface antigen (HBsAg) appears. Extreme variation in the incubation period is related in part to the amount of virus in the inoculum, mode of transmission, alteration of viral pathogenicity by chemical or physical means, administration of a specific antibody, and unusual virus-host interactions.

All persons who are HbsAg and hepatitis B e antigen (HBeAg) positive are potentially infectious. Both antigens are detectable 1 to 3 weeks after exposure and 4 to 5 weeks prior to onset of jaundice. The infectivity of chronically infected individuals varies from highly infectious (HBeAg positive) to sparingly infectious (anti-HBe positive).

Diagnosis of HBV is based on clinical, serologic, and epidemiologic findings. Detection of HBV infection serologic markers, HBsAg, confirms hepatitis B infection. Infection may present with a variety of symptomatology: acute illness with jaundice followed by recovery, subclinical infection followed by recovery, acute illness that progresses to chronic active hepatitis, subclinical infection followed by chronic active hepatitis, and fulminant disease.[10] Viral hepatitis is the most common infectious etiology of jaundice. A short prodromal phase, varying from several days to more than a week, may precede the onset of jaundice. Typical symptoms include anorexia, weakness, and fatigue. Nausea, vomiting, and diarrhea may also occur. Many patients complain of right upper quadrant abdominal pain. The preicteric phase may be characterized by fever (usually <103° F), malaise, myalgia, and headache. Other symptoms are similar to serum sickness: arthritis, arthralgia, and urticaria or maculopapular rash.[10] The icteric phase begins with appearance of dark urine due to bilirubinuria, followed by light or gray stools and yellowish discoloration of the mucous membranes, sclerae, conjunctivae, and skin. Jaundice becomes apparent when total bilirubin levels exceed 2.0 to 3.0 mg/dl. Hepatic tenderness and hepatomegaly are also present.[10] Recovery begins with the disappearance of jaundice and other symptoms. HBsAg and HbeAg also disappear. The appearance of antibodies (anti-HBs and anti-HBc) indicates the infection is subsiding. Liver failure may occur in 1% to 3% of patients with acute hepatitis B. This disease is potentially fatal and is characterized by mental confusion, emotional instability, bleeding manifestations, and coma. Overall survival rate varies with age—7% in the elderly, 37% in patients under 16 years of age.

The Occupational Safety and Health Administration (OSHA) has stated the most effective method of infection control against hepatitis B is the hepatitis B vaccine. Over 90% of all people vaccinated develop immunity to HBV. Vaccines available in the United States contain no blood or blood products; they are made from yeast cells changed by genetic engineering. Current prevention strategy in the United States includes screening all pregnant women for the presence of HBsAg; hepatitis B immune globulin and hepatitis B vaccine for infants of HBsAg-positive mothers; hepatitis B vaccine for susceptible household contacts; routine hepatitis B immunization for all infants; catch-up immunization for children 1 to 10 years old in groups with high rates of chronic HBV infection; catch-up immunization for adolescents 11 to 12 years old; and intense efforts to immunize high-risk adolescents and adults. Health care workers are reminded that universal precautions should be employed when caring for all patients when there is potential for exposure to blood or body fluids.

Hepatitis C

Hepatitis C virus (HCV) is parenterally transmitted. This infection has been found in every part of the world where it has been sought. HCV is the most common posttransfusion hepatitis in the United States, accounting for approximately 90% of this disease, and is more common when paid blood donors are used. Overall, most hepatitis cases are not associated with blood transfusion; however, HCV accounts for 15% to 40% of community-acquired hepatitis cases. The prevalence of antibodies to HCV (anti-HCV) is highest in intravenous drug users and hemophilia patients (70% to 90%), moderate in hemodialysis patients (10% to 20%), low in heterosexuals with multiple sexual partners, homosexual men, health care workers, and family contacts of HCV-infected persons (1% to 5%), and lowest in volunteer blood donors (0.3% to 0.5%).[1]

HCV transmission occurs by percutaneous exposure to contaminated blood and plasma derivatives. As in HBV infection, contaminated needles and syringes are important vehicles of spread, especially among parenteral drug users and dialysis patients. Health care workers frequently contact blood, so there is an increased risk for infection. Household or sexual contact with persons who had hepatitis in the past has also been documented in some studies as risk factors for acquiring HCV. The importance of person-to-person contact and sexual activity in transmission of this disease has not been well defined. Transmission from mother to child appears to be uncommon; however, only small numbers of infants have been studied. More than 40% of HCV-infected patients have no obvious route or source of transmission.[4] Incubation period ranges from 2 weeks to 6 months, most commonly 6 to 9 weeks.

The period of communicability may range from one or more weeks before the onset of first symptoms and may persist indefinitely. Based on infectivity studies in chimpanzees, the titer of HCV in the blood appears to be relatively low. Peaks in virus concentration appear to correlate with peaks in serum alanine transaminase activity.

Onset is usually insidious, with severity ranging from inapparent cases to rare fulminating, fatal cases. Symptoms include anorexia, vague abdominal discomfort, nausea, and vomiting. Symptoms progress to jaundice less frequently than with hepatitis B. The disease is usually less severe in the acute stage, but chronicity is common, occurring more frequently than with hepatitis B in adults. Chronic infection may be symptomatic or asymptomatic. Chronic hepatitis C may progress to cirrhosis, and there also appears to be an association between HCV infection and hepatocellular carcinoma.

Diagnosis depends on the identification of anti-HCV. Some patients may not test positive for 6 to 9 months after onset of illness. Tests are not yet available to distinguish acute from chronic HCV infection or direct detection of antigen.

General control measures against blood-borne pathogens apply. The value of prophylactic immune globulin is not clear. Data suggest postexposure prophylaxis with immune globulin is not effective in preventing infection.

Hepatitis D

Prevalence of hepatitis D virus (HDV) varies widely, occurring epidemically and endemically in populations at high risk of acquiring HBV, including drug addicts, hemophiliacs, and others who have frequent contact with blood; in institutions for the developmentally disabled; and to a lesser extent in male homosexuals. Mode of transmission is thought to be similar to HBV, including exposure to blood and serous body fluids, needles, syringes, plasma derivatives, and sexual contact. Blood is potentially infectious during all phases of active HDV infection. Peak infectivity probably occurs before the onset of acute illness.

Onset is usually abrupt, with signs and symptoms resembling those of HBV infection. Symptoms may be severe and are always associated with a coexisting HBV. HDV infection may be self-limiting or may progress to chronic hepatitis. Diagnosis is made by detection of total antibody to HDV (anti-HDV).

General control measures against blood-borne pathogens apply. Prevention of HBV infection with hepatitis B vaccine prevents infection with HDV. Hepatitis B immune globulin, immune globulin, and hepatitis B vaccine do not protect HBV carriers from infection by HDV.

Acquired Immunodeficiency Syndrome

AIDS was first reported in 1981; however, isolated cases occurred in the United States and other areas of the world during the 1970s. By mid 1990, over 130,000 cases had been reported in the United States. Although the United States has recorded the largest number of cases, AIDS has been recorded in virtually all countries, among all races, ages, and social classes. Worldwide, the World Health Organization estimates close to 600,000 cases occurred by 1990. The CDC reported in 1994 that 79,647 persons over 13 years old had AIDS. In 1992, homosexual and bisexual men accounted for almost 61% of the total number of Americans with AIDS. Other populations with increased risk include heterosexual male and female intravenous drug users and heterosexual partners of HIV-infected individuals. Although the majority of the American patients with AIDS are homosexual and bisexual men, AIDS is now recognized as a pandemic global disease affecting men, women, and children.

Epidemiologic data indicate that transmission of this disease is limited to sexual, parenteral, and maternal-infant routes. Routes of transmission are analogous to those of HBV. There is no evidence supporting other routes of HIV transmission. Substantial evidence indicates transmission does not occur through casual contact, despite reports that HIV has been isolated in small amounts from saliva and tears.[6] From 15% to 30% of infants born to HIV-infected mothers are infected before, during, or shortly after birth. Treatment of pregnant women has resulted in a marked reduction of infant infections. Breast-feeding by HIV-infected women can transmit infection to the infant. Following direct exposure of health care workers to HIV-infected blood through injury with needles and other sharp objects, the rate of seroconversion is less than 0.5%—much lower than the risk of HBV infection (about 25%) after a similar exposure.[1]

The incubation period from HIV infection until the emergence of AIDS has proved to be much longer than originally predicted. Median incubation time for homosexual men based on several studies appears to be approximately 10 years. Incubation may differ in different populations and is influenced by numerous cofactors.

The period of communicability is unknown but is presumed to begin soon after onset of HIV infection and extend throughout life. Epidemiologic evidence suggests infectivity increases with increasing immune deficiency, clinical symptoms, and presence of other sexually transmitted diseases. Recent studies suggest infectiousness may be high during the initial period after infection.[1]

AIDS is a severe, life-threatening clinical condition. This syndrome represents the late clinical stage of infection with HIV and is most often the result of progressive damage to the immune and other organ systems. Within several weeks to months after infection with HIV, many individuals develop an acute self-limited mononucleosis-like illness lasting for 1 to 2 weeks. Infected individuals may then be free of clinical signs or symptoms for months to years. Onset of clinical illness is usually insidious with nonspecific symptoms such as lymphadenopathy, anorexia, chronic diarrhea, weight loss, fever, and fatigue. More than a dozen opportunistic infections are considered AIDS infections, including several cancers, pulmonary and extrapulmonary tuberculosis (TB), recurrent pneumonia, wasting syndrome, neurologic disease (HIV dementia or sensory neuropathy), and invasive cervical cancer. In HIV-infected people, a CD4+ cell count of less than 200/µl or a CD4 T-lymphocyte percentage of total lymphocytes of less than 14%, regardless of their clinical status, is regarded as an AIDS case.

The most commonly used screening test, ELISA, is highly sensitive and specific. When this test is reactive, an additional test such as the Western blot or indirect IFA should be obtained. Most individuals infected with HIV develop detectable antibodies within 1 to 3 months after infection.

For health care workers, universal precautions are the most available method to control transmission of the HIV virus. The health care worker must also be cognizant that multiple sexual partners and sharing drug paraphernalia increase the risk of infection with HIV.

Management of the patient with AIDS in the ED is based on treatment of the specific opportunistic infection that may be present. Care should be provided in a nonjudgmental manner to support the patient, family, and significant other. Universal precautions should be used, but the patient should not be made to feel ostracized.

Tuberculosis

TB is caused by *Mycobacterium tuberculosis* and usually infects the lungs (pulmonary TB) or respiratory system. TB can spread to other organs such as the kidneys, bones and joints, skin, intestines, peritoneum, eyes, lymph nodes, pericardium, and pleura. Extrapulmonary TB occurs frequently in persons infected with HIV. TB should be initially considered in anyone with respiratory symptoms including fatigue, weight loss, fever, cough, chest pain, hemoptysis, and hoarseness. A person's general immune status affects the risk of TB infection. Advanced age, corticosteroid medication, cancer chemotherapy, HIV infection, malnutrition, or chronic illness can reduce immunity and increase the risk for TB infection.

Prevalence of TB is not distributed evenly throughout the U.S. population. Some subgroups or individuals have a higher risk for TB because they are more likely than others in the general population to be exposed and infected or because their exposure is more likely to progress to active TB. Groups of persons with a higher prevalence of TB infection include intimate contacts with individuals with active TB, foreign-born persons from areas with a high prevalence of TB, medically underserved populations, homeless persons, current or former correctional facility inmates, alcoholics, parenteral drug users, and the elderly.

In 1993, 25,313 cases of TB (9.8 cases per 100,000 population) were reported to the CDC from the 50 states and the District of Columbia, a 5.1% decrease from 1992 (26,673 [10.5 cases per 100,000]). However, this represented a 14% increase from 1985, the year with the lowest number of TB cases since national reporting began in 1953. From January 1, 1993, through May 25, 1994, antibiotic-susceptible isolates for tuberculosis were reported for 10,941 (54%) of the 20,090 persons with culture-positive TB. Worldwide, an estimated one third of the population is infected with TB, with 8 million new cases each year. Nearly 3 million people die annually from tuberculosis, making it the leading worldwide cause of death due to an infectious agent.[3]

Transmission of TB is a recognized risk in health care facilities. The magnitude of risk varies considerably with the type of health care facility, prevalence of TB in the community, patient population served, health care worker's occupational group, area of the health care facility where the health care worker works, and effectiveness of TB infection control interventions.[12] Nosocomial transmission of TB has been associated with close contact with persons who have infectious TB and with performance of procedures such as bronchoscopy, endotracheal intubation, suctioning, open abscess irrigation, and autopsy. Sputum induction and aerosol treatments that induce coughing may also increase the potential for transmission. Several TB outbreaks among persons in health care facilities have been reported (CDC, unpublished data). Many outbreaks involve transmission of multidrug-resistant strains of TB to both patients and health care workers. Mortality associated with these outbreaks was high (range, 43% to 93%). Factors contributing to outbreaks include delayed diagnosis, recognition of drug resistance, and initiation of effective therapy.

In general, persons infected with TB have approximately 10% risk for developing active TB during their lifetime. Risk is greatest during the first 2 years after infection. TB is

carried in airborne particles or droplet nuclei generated when persons with pulmonary or laryngeal TB sneeze, cough, speak, or sing.[1] Infection occurs when a susceptible person inhales droplet nuclei containing TB. Droplet nuclei traverse the mouth or nasal passages, upper respiratory tract, and bronchi to reach the alveoli of the lungs.

The incubation period from infection to demonstrable primary lesion or significant tuberculin reaction is about 4 to 12 weeks. Subsequent risk of progressive pulmonary or extrapulmonary TB is greatest within the first year or two after infection. Latent infection may persist for life.

Degree of communicability depends on the number of bacilli in the droplets, virulence of the bacilli, adequacy of ventilation, exposure of bacilli to sun or ultraviolet light, and opportunities for aerosolization. Theoretically, as long as viable tubercle bacilli are discharged in the sputum, the person may be infectious. Diagnosis is confirmed by recovery of TB from a sputum sample, positive chest radiograph, and positive tuberculin skin test.

TB prevention and control programs should be established in all institutional settings where health care is provided. Therapeutic interventions include respiratory isolation to prevent spread, administration of antituberculin drugs, and supportive care. Controlled air flow rooms are recommended for isolation of these patients. Triage guidelines should include identification of potential TB patients (Box 42-4). Table 42-1 summarizes current therapy for tuberculosis.

Box 42-4 Triage Assessment for Possible Tuberculosis

Historical and social information

Homeless

Live in crowded, unsanitary conditions

Recently moved from or traveled to a high-risk country in Asia, Africa, Latin America

Previous history of tuberculosis with no treatment or poor compliance with treatment regimen

Resident of long-term care facility, nursing home, correctional institution, mental hospital, homeless shelter

Close contact with an infected person

Intravenous drug abuse or alcohol abuse

Health care worker

Objective clinical information

Weight loss, anorexia, malaise

Cough worsening over weeks or months

Productive cough with mucopurulent or blood-streaked sputum

Night sweats, chills, low-grade fevers

Malnourished

Coinfection with HIV

Preexisting medical conditions, i.e., diabetes mellitus, hematologic disorders, end-stage renal disease

Prolonged steroid or immunosuppressive therapy

Table 42-1 Drug Therapy Used in Tuberculosis

Drug	Mechanisms of action	Side effects	Comments
First-line drugs			
• Isoniazid (INH)	Interferes with DNA metabolism of tubercle bacillus	Peripheral neuritis, hepatotoxicity, hypersensitivity (skin rash, arthralgia, fever), optic neuritis, vitamin B_6 neuritis	Metabolism primarily by liver and excretion by kidneys, pyridoxine (vitamin B_6) administration during high-dose therapy as prophylactic measure, use as single prophylactic agent for active TB in individuals whose PPD converts to positive, ability to cross blood-brain barrier
• Rifampin	Has broad-spectrum effects, inhibits RNA polymerase of tubercle bacillus	Hepatitis, febrile reaction, GI disturbance, peripheral neuropathy, hypersensitivity	Most common use with isoniazid, low incidence of side effects, suppression of effect of birth control pills, possible orange urine
• Ethambutol (Myambutol)	Inhibits RNA synthesis and is bacteriostatic for the tubercle bacillus	Skin rash, GI disturbance, malaise, peripheral neuritis, optic neuritis	Side effects uncommon and reversible with discontinuation of drug, most common use as substitute drug when toxicity occurs with isoniazid or rifampin
• Streptomycin	Inhibits protein synthesis and is bactericidal	Ototoxicity (eighth cranial nerve), nephrotoxicity, hypersensitivity	Cautious use in older adults, those with renal disease, and pregnant women
Second-line drugs			
• Ethionamide	Inhibits protein synthesis	GI disturbance, hepatotoxicity, hypersensitivity	Valuable retreatment of resistant organisms Contraindication in pregnancy
• Capreomycin	Inhibits protein synthesis and is bactericidal	Ototoxicity, nephrotoxicity	Cautious use in older adults
• Kanamycin	Interferes with protein synthesis	Ototoxicity, nephrotoxicity	Use in selected cases for retreatment of resistant strains
• Pyrazinamide	Bactericidal effect (exact mechanism is unknown)	Fever, skin rash, hyperuricemia, jaundice (rare)	High rate of effectiveness when used with streptomycin or capreomycin
• Para-aminosalicylic acid (PAS)	Interferes with metabolism of tubercle bacillus	GI disturbance (frequent), hypersensitivity, hepatotoxicity	Interference with absorption of rifampin, infrequent use
• Cycloserine	Inhibits cell-wall synthesis	Personality changes, psychosis, rash	Contraindication in individuals with a history of psychosis, use in retreatment of resistant strains

From Lewis SM, Collier IC, Heitkemper MM: *Medical-surgical nursing: assessment and management of clinical problems*, ed 4, St. Louis, 1996, Mosby.
DNA, Deoxyribonucleic acid; *GI*, gastrointestinal; *PPD*, purified protein derivative; *RNA*, ribonucleic acid; *TB*, tuberculosis.

SUMMARY

Recognition of the potential for infectious disease is paramount in the care of any ED patient. Box 42-5 highlights potential nursing diagnoses for these patients. With the prevalence of life-threatening infectious diseases, one must assume that any patient may be a potential source of the infection and employ universal precautions whenever a potential for exposure exists. Careful attention to this matter reduces the spread of infection and contamination.

Box **42-5**

NURSING DIAGNOSES FOR INFECTIOUS DISEASES

Infection
Fluid volume deficit
Fluid volume excess
Altered nutrition requirements

REFERENCES

1. Bensenson A: *Control of communicable diseases in man,* ed 16, Washington, DC, 1995, The American Public Health Association.
2. Berg R, editor: *The APIC curriculum for infection control practice,* vol III, Dubuque, Iowa, 1988, Kendall/Hunt.
3. Bloom B, Murray C: Tuberculosis: commentary on a reemergent killer, *Science* 257:1055, 1064, 1992.
4. Bozzette B, et al: Familial cluster of hepatitis C virus type I, *J Infect Dis* 170:1042, 1994.
5. Centers for Disease Control and Prevention: Protection against viral hepatitis: recommendations of the Immunization Practices Advisory Committee (ACIP), *MMWR* 39:5, 1990.
6. Friedland G, et al: Lack of transmission of HTLV-III/LAV infection to household contacts of patients with AIDS or AIDS-related complex with oral candidiaseis, *N Engl J Med* 314:344, 1986.
7. Garner, Favero: CDC guidelines for handwashing and hospital environmental control, *Infect Control* 7(4):231, 1986.
8. Hadler S, et al: Occupational risk of hepatitis B infection in hospital workers, *Infect Control* 6:24, 1985.
9. Halpern J: Precautions to prevent transmission of human immunodeficiency virus infections in emergency settings, *J Emerg Nurs* 13(5):298, 1987.
10. Hollinger F: Features of viral hepatitis. In Fields BN et al, editors: *Virology,* New York, 1985, Raven.
11. Lett S: Measles and nosocomial measles control. Talk presented at APIC 17th Annual Education Conference, Washington, DC, June 7, 1990.
12. Madsen L: Tuberculosis today, *RN,* p 45, March 1990.
13. Mandell G, Douglas R, Bennett J, editors: Principles and practices of infectious diseases, ed 3, New York, 1990, Churchill Livingstone.
14. Margolis H, Alter M, Hadler S: Hepatitis B: evolving epidemiology and implications for control, *Semin Liver Dis* 11:84.

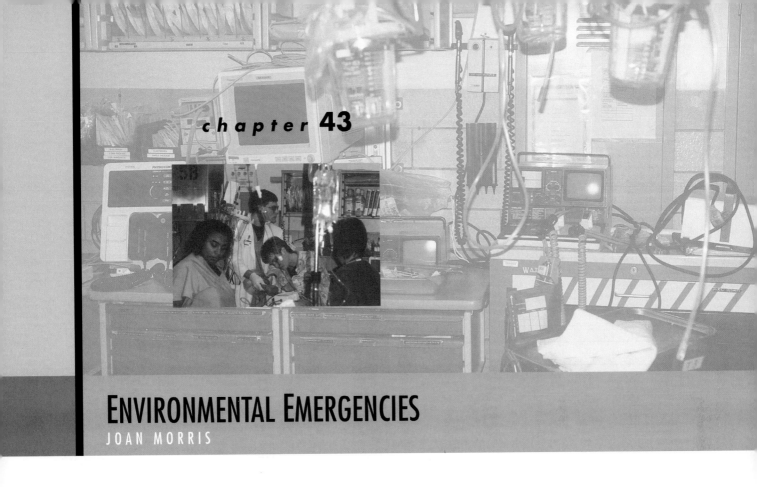

chapter **43**

ENVIRONMENTAL EMERGENCIES

JOAN MORRIS

Outdoor activities are extremely popular with individuals of all ages. Activities such as hiking, jogging, biking, swimming, and diving place the individual at risk for illness and injury secondary to the weather, the activity, and various animals. Environmental hazards may be encountered during voluntary participation in an outdoor activity or involuntary exposure caused by confusion, mental illness, alcohol, or drugs. Specific environmental emergencies discussed in this chapter are related to heat and cold stress, water immersion, bites, and stings.

HEAT-RELATED EMERGENCIES

Heat illness has occurred since the beginning of recorded history, and many cases occur annually in the United States. Only head injury, spinal cord injury, and heart failure are responsible for more deaths in athletes than heat illness. Regardless of physical condition, anyone can suffer ill effects from heat stress if the exposure is intense or prolonged. The effects of environmental heat stress can be mild or severe, depending on the degree of heat and length of exposure.

Ambient temperature is a product of environmental temperature and moisture in the air. For example, an environmental temperature of 90° F creates an ambient temperature of 93° F if the dew point is 65° F; however, ambient temperature increases to 111° F if the dew point is 83° F. Table 43-1 presents ambient temperature for various thermometer readings and dew point in degrees Fahrenheit.

Emergencies related to heat stress include heat edema, heat cramps, heat exhaustion, and heat stroke. Heat edema is the least acute situation, usually a minor inconvenience for most individuals. Heat stroke, however, is life-threatening.

Heat Edema

Heat edema occurs in nonacclimatized individuals during prolonged periods of standing or sitting. Characteristic swelling of the feet and ankles resolves in a few days. Treatment includes rest, elevation of the legs, and support hose. Heat edema is self-limiting and generally does not require further treatment.

Heat Cramps

Heat cramps are severe cramps of specific muscles, usually in the shoulders, thighs, and abdominal wall. Associated symptoms include weakness, nausea, tachycardia, pallor, profuse diaphoresis, and cool, moist skin. The core temperature may be normal or slightly elevated. Heat cramps develop suddenly when the victim is resting after exertion in a hot environment or one with high humidity. Salt depletion secondary to excessive perspiration in combination with excessive water consumption leads to heat cramps. Increased water intake does not replace sodium losses caused by perspiration. Instead, water dilutes serum sodium, causing hyponatremia, the key factor in the development of heat cramps.

Treatment includes removal from heat, rest, and electrolyte replacement with oral or parenteral fluids. Discharge

Table **43-1** **Heat Index Chart**

Dew point	Temperature (° F)															
	90	91	92	93	94	95	96	97	98	99	100	101	102	103	104	105
65	93	94	95	97	98	99	100	101	103	104	105	106	107	108	110	111
66	94	95	96	97	99	100	101	102	103	104	106	107	108	109	111	112
67	94	95	97	98	99	100	102	103	104	105	106	108	109	111	112	113
68	95	96	98	99	100	101	102	104	105	106	107	108	110	112	113	114
69	96	97	98	99	101	102	103	104	106	107	108	109	111	112	114	115
70	96	97	99	100	101	103	104	105	107	108	109	110	112	113	114	116
71	97	98	100	101	102	104	105	106	108	109	110	111	113	114	115	117
72	98	99	101	102	103	105	106	107	109	110	111	112	114	115	116	118
73	99	100	102	103	104	106	107	108	110	111	112	113	115	117	118	119
74	100	101	103	104	105	107	108	109	111	112	113	115	116	118	119	121
75	101	102	104	105	106	108	109	111	112	113	115	116	117	119	120	122
76	102	103	105	106	108	109	110	112	113	115	116	117	119	120	122	123
77	103	105	106	107	109	110	112	113	114	116	117	119	121	122	123	125
78	104	106	107	109	110	112	113	115	116	118	119	121	122	123	124	126
79	105	107	109	110	112	113	114	116	118	119	121	122	124	125	126	128
80	107	108	110	111	113	115	116	117	119	121	122	124	125	127	128	129
81	108	110	111	113	115	116	118	119	121	123	124	126	127	128	130	132
82	109	111	113	115	116	118	119	121	123	124	126	127	129	130	132	133
83	111	113	115	117	118	120	121	123	125	126	128	129	130	132	133	135

instructions should stress the importance of drinking commercially prepared electrolyte supplements (e.g., Gatorade, Powerade, All Sport) when working outdoors or participating in strenuous recreational activities during hot weather. Strenuous activity should be avoided for at least 12 hours after discharge.

Heat Exhaustion

Heat exhaustion is a clinical syndrome caused by prolonged heat exposure, usually over hours or days. Excessive perspiration and inadequate fluid and electrolyte replacement lead to fluid loss and dehydration. Heat exhaustion occurs most often in individuals working in hot environments. The elderly and the very young are also at risk because they cannot increase fluid intake sufficiently to compensate for increased fluid losses from sweating.

Heat exhaustion is characterized by syncope and collapse, extreme thirst, general malaise, muscle cramping, headache, nausea, vomiting, anxiety, and tachycardia. As-

sociated dehydration may cause orthostatic hypotension and mild to severe temperature elevation (98.6° to 105° F [37° to 40.6° C]). Diaphoresis may or may not be present. Untreated, heat exhaustion can progress to heat stroke.

Initial treatment begins with moving the patient to a cool, quiet environment and removing constricting clothing. When significant hyperthermia is present, moist cloths placed on the patient reduce temperature by evaporation. Fluid and electrolyte replacement should be initiated. Oral replacement with a balanced commercial salt preparation can be used if the patient is not nauseated. Intravenous 0.9% saline solution should be used if the patient is nauseated or vomiting. Salt tablets are not recommended because of potential gastric irritation and hypernatremia. Monitor the patient's temperature carefully. Hypotension may be corrected initially with a 300- to 500-ml bolus of 0.9% normal saline. Subsequent infusions should be correlated to clinical and laboratory findings. Patients with hypotension or a history of cardiac disease should be placed on a cardiac monitor, since heat exhaustion can rapidly evolve into heat stroke. Admission should be considered for any patient who does not improve significantly with 3 to 4 hours of emergency treatment.

Heat Stroke

Heat stroke is the least common but most severe presentation of heat illness. Mortality can be as high as 70%. With heat stroke, the core temperature exceeds 105° F (40.6° C). Heat stroke occurs when exposure to severe heat stress destroys the thermoregulatory system. The outcome of heat stroke is affected by environmental factors and the patient's ability to dissipate heat. Common predisposing factors associated with heat stroke are summarized in Box 43-1. Individuals with one or more risk factors are at much greater risk for hyperthermia when exacerbating environmental conditions are present.

The onset of heat stroke is usually sudden; however, the elderly and patients in predisposing environments can de-

---

Box 43-1   **Risk Factors Associated With Heat Stroke**

Age
Elderly
Infants

Environmental conditions
High environmental temperature
High relative humidity
Low wind

Preexisting illness
Cardiovascular disease
Previous stroke or other central nervous system lesion
Obesity
Diabetes
Cystic fibrosis
Skin disorders (e.g., large burn scars)

Prescription drugs
Anticholinergics
Phenothiazines
Butyrophenones
Tricyclic antidepressants
Antihistamines
Antispasmodics
Diuretics
Antiparkinsonian drugs
β-Blockers

Street drugs
Lysergic acid diethylamide (LSD)
Jimsonweed
Amphetamines
Phencyclidine (PCP)
Alcohol

---

velop heat exhaustion several hours before heat stroke develops. Heat stroke may present with changes in neurologic function such as anxiety, confusion, hallucinations, loss of muscle coordination, and combativeness. Direct thermal damage to the brain combined with decreased cerebral blood flow can lead to cerebral edema and hemorrhage. The brain, particularly the cerebellum, is extremely sensitive to thermal injury; therefore the range of neurologic symptoms is broad.

Management of heat stroke is directed at reducing core temperature as rapidly as possible and treating subsequent complications. Maintenance of airway, breathing, and circulation (ABCs) is crucial for patient recovery. Establish an airway, and administer supplemental oxygen by the method most appropriate for the patient's level of consciousness. Fluid volume is not depleted in most victims of hyperthermia; therefore, 1 to 2 L of isotonic saline solution during the first 4 hours is usually adequate. Ringer's lactate solution is not recommended, since the liver may not be able to metabolize lactate. Careful hemodynamic monitoring is indicated until normal vital signs are restored. Once the ABCs are secured, rapid, aggressive cooling is the primary intervention.

Prehospital treatment starts with removing the patient from the external source of heat and stripping all clothing. Spray the patient with tepid water while fanning the entire body to promote cooling by evaporation. Well-padded ice packs in vascular areas such as the groin, axilla, and neck are also useful. Once the patient is in the emergency department (ED), aggressive cooling measures can be used, such as ice water gastric and peritoneal lavage.

Cooling blankets may be used; however, cooling from wet skin is 25 times more effective than cooling from dry skin. Immersion in an ice water bath is contraindicated. In addition to being unpleasant for the patient and caregiver, access to the patient is limited. Ice water immersion can also cause shivering, which dramatically increases oxygen consumption and can increase body temperature. Intravenous chlorpromazine (Thorazine), 10 to 25 mg, may be used to prevent shivering during the cooling process. Massive peripheral vasoconstriction from ice water immersion can act as an insulator and prevent adequate cooling.

Cooling should be continued until the rectal temperature is 102° F (39° C) or less. The core temperature should be monitored frequently during the cooling phase to prevent inadvertent hypothermia. Aspirin and acetaminophen have not proved effective in reducing hyperthermia secondary to heat stroke. Corticosteroid therapy, usually with methylprednisolone, may be used to treat cerebral edema. Intracranial pressure monitoring may be helpful with some patients. Intravenous mannitol, 0.25 g/kg, is recommended in patients whose urinary output is less than 50 ml/hr.

High-output cardiac failure may develop with heat stroke; therefore patients should be placed on a cardiac monitor. Central venous pressure and pulmonary capillary wedge pressure monitoring may be considered in the critical phase to evaluate fluid status. Protecting the kidneys and liver from thermal and low-flow damage is critical. Myoglobinuria and poor renal perfusion put the kidneys at risk for renal failure; therefore urine should be carefully monitored for color, amount, pH, and hemoglobin.

COLD-RELATED EMERGENCIES

Approximately 700 fatalities occur annually from cold exposure.[2] Most deaths do not occur in the extreme northern areas. Most reported cold injuries occur in temperate regions, urban areas in poorly heated apartments, and among the homeless. Urban cold exposure is usually related to alcohol or a preexisting condition such as diabetes.

Injuries related to cold exposure are localized or generalized. Localized cold emergencies include chilblains, immersion foot, and frostbite, whereas hypothermia is a generalized cold emergency. Cold-related emergencies occur with prolonged exposure to cold ambient temperatures, from immersion in cold water, or as a result of factors such as alcohol. Ambient temperature is a product of air temperature and wind speed: the greater the wind speed, the lower the ambient temperature (Table 43-2). Heat loss occurs 32 times more quickly with immersion in cold water.

Chilblains

Chilblains, also known as pernio, are localized areas of itching and redness accompanied by recurrent edema on exposed or poorly insulated body parts such as the ears, fingers, and toes. Chilblains are usually seen in cool, damp climates with temperatures above freezing. Chilblain is probably a mild form of frostbite. Symptoms occur gradually. There is generally no pain; however, the patient may experience transient numbness and tingling. Initial pallor or redness of the nose, digits, or ears may evolve into plaques and small, superficial ulcerations over chronically exposed areas.

Prehospital treatment begins with removal to a warm area in conjunction with covering the affected area with a warm hand or placing the fingers under the axilla. Elevation of the affected area decreases edema, which increases circulation and allows gradual warming at room temperature. Never rub or massage injured tissue. Avoid direct heat application. Tissue damage is rarely seen with chilblains; however, the patient should be instructed to protect the area from injury and further environmental exposure and to watch for signs of secondary infection.

Immersion Foot

Immersion foot, or trench foot, refers to prolonged or constant contact between a wet foot and cold temperature, usually when the patient is wearing a watertight boot that does not allow normal evaporative "breathing." This condition is commonly seen in hunters and soldiers on outdoor maneuvers. Initially, feet appear cold, damp, numb, and edematous. However, the foot appears warm within 24 to 48 hours. Warming leads to intense burning and tingling pain secondary to vasodilatation and hyperemia. Prolonged and repeated exposure can lead to lymphangitis, cellulitis, thrombophlebitis, and liquification gangrene.

Therapeutic interventions include drying the feet and changing frequently into dry socks. Once in a controlled environment, rewarm injured areas gradually by exposing to air or soaking in warm water. Immersion foot is reversible with timely treatment. Patients are usually hospitalized for observation and prevention of complications.

Table **43-2**   **Windchill Index***

Wind speed (mph)	Air temperature (° F)														
	35	30	25	20	15	10	5	0	−5	−10	−15	−20	−25	−30	−35
4	35	30	25	20	15	10	5	0	−5	−10	−15	−20	−25	−30	−35
5	32	27	22	16	11	6	0	−5	−10	−15	−21	−26	−31	−36	−42
10	22	16	10	3	−3	−9	−15	−22	−27	−34	−40	−46	−52	−58	−64
15	16	9	2	−5	−11	−18	−25	−31	−38	−45	−51	−58	−65	−72	−78
20	12	4	−3	−10	−17	−24	−31	−39	−44	−51	−59	−66	−74	−81	−88
25	8	1	−7	−15	−22	−29	−36	−44	−51	−59	−66	−74	−81	−88	−96
30	6	−2	−10	−18	−25	−33	−42	−49	−56	−64	−71	−79	−86	−93	−101
35	4	−4	−12	−20	−27	−35	−43	−52	−58	−67	−74	−82	−89	−97	−105
40	3	−5	−13	−21	−29	−37	−45	−53	−60	−69	−76	−84	−92	−100	−107

*Shaded area indicates increasing danger from freezing of exposed flesh within 1 minute of exposure.

Frostbite

Frostbite is the most prevalent injury caused by extreme cold. Tissue freezes, so ice crystals form in the body's intracellular spaces.[5] The crystals enlarge and compress cells, causing membrane rupture, interruption of enzymatic activity, and altered metabolic processes. Histamine release increases capillary permeability, red cell aggregation, and microvascular occlusion. Once frostbite occurs, damage is irreversible. Further exposure to extreme cold or trauma worsens the injury and increases tissue damage. The patient with frostbite may also have hypothermia. Treatment of hypothermia takes priority over management of frostbite. Frostbite can be superficial or deep, depending on severity of the cold and length of exposure. Estimation of the extent of injury may not be possible until several days after exposure.

Superficial frostbite

Superficial frostbite involves skin and subcutaneous tissue and is similar to a superficial burn. Fingertips, ears, nose, toes, and cheeks are the areas most commonly affected. Symptoms include tingling, numbness, a burning sensation, and a white, waxy color. Frozen skin feels cold and stiff. Once the tissue thaws, the patient may feel a hot, stinging sensation. Affected areas become mottled; however, blisters develop within a few hours. Frostbite tissue is extremely sensitive to subsequent exposure to cold.

Injured tissue is friable, so recovery depends on *very gentle handling.* Do not rub the affected area. Apply warm soaks (104° to 110° F [40° to 43° C]), and elevate the extremity. Place the patient on bed rest for several days until the full extent of the injury has been evaluated and normal circulation has returned. The patient's room should be warm; however, heavy blankets should be avoided, since friction and weight on the affected area can lead to sloughing.

Deep frostbite

Deep frostbite occurs when the temperature of a limb is lowered. Deep frostbite usually involves muscles, bones, and tendons. The degree of frostbite depends on ambient temperature, windchill factor (Table 43-2), duration of exposure, whether the patient was wet while exposed or in direct contact with metal objects, and the type of clothing worn. Other factors that may contribute to the severity of frostbite are outlined in Box 43-2.

Deep frostbite appears white or yellow-white and is hard, cool, and insensitive to touch. The patient has a burning sensation followed by a feeling of warmth and then numbness. Blisters appear 1 to 7 days after injury. Edema of the entire extremity occurs and may persist for months (Figure 43-1). A gray-black mottling eventually progresses to gangrene (Figure 43-2).

Prehospital treatment includes transport with gentle handling and moderate elevation of the affected part. Rewarming is deferred until the patient reaches the ED. *Do not rub* the part with snow or ice. If the extremity has thawed, keep it immobile. Prevent heat loss by removing wet clothing, covering the patient with dry blankets, and removing the patient from the cold environment. If the patient is transported in a ground or air ambulance, warmed oxygen is recommended. Wool head coverings help prevent further heat loss.

Rapid rewarming under controlled conditions is the ideal treatment for maintaining tissue viability. Rewarming the patient with hypothermia and severe frostbite should occur with strict medical control. Once the patient reaches the ED, obtain a baseline core temperature (rectal or esophageal), and then immerse the affected area in warm water (104° to 110° F [40° to 43° C]). Thawing frozen tissue is *extremely* painful, so parenteral narcotics are needed in severe cases. Warm intravenous fluids prior to administration. Assess tetanus immunization status, and consider antibiotic therapy

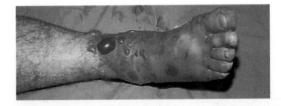

***Figure* 43-1** Edema and blister formation resulting from frostbite injury. *(From Auerbach P, editor:* Wilderness medicine: management of wilderness and environmental emergencies, *ed 3, St. Louis, 1995, Mosby.)*

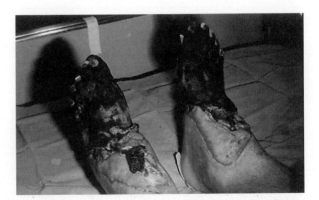

***Figure* 43-2** Gangrenous necrosis resulting from frostbite injury. *(From Auerbach P, editor:* Wilderness medicine: management of wilderness and environmental emergencies, *ed 3, St. Louis, 1995, Mosby.)*

Box **43-2** **Factors Affecting Severity of Frostbite**
Skin color (dark-skinned people are more prone to frostbite)
Lack of acclimatization
Previous history of frostbite injury
Poor peripheral vascular status
Anxiety
Exhaustion

for deep infections. If hypothermia is not present, administer warm oral liquids. Cover the patient with warm blankets, but avoid friction and pressure on the affected area. Protect the thawed part with a large, soft, bulky dressing. Elevate the affected area to minimize edema.

If severe vasoconstriction is present, escharotomy may be required. Final determination of the depth of the injury may not be possible for several weeks; therefore amputation is not considered in the ED.

Hypothermia

Hypothermia is defined as a core temperature below 95° F (35° C). Severe hypothermia is a core temperature less than 90° F (32.2° C). Death usually occurs when the core temperature falls below 78° F (25.6° C).

The body's metabolic responses depend on a normal temperature. As the core temperature drops, there is a progressive decrease in cellular activity and organ function. When the temperature drops by 18° F (10° C), the basal metabolic rate drops two to three times. The most obvious response is seen in the central nervous system (CNS). The patient becomes apathetic, weak, and easily fatigued, with impaired reasoning, coordination, and gait, and slow or slurred speech. Renal blood flow decreases, so glomerular filtration rate declines. Impaired water reabsorption leads to dehydration. Decreased respiratory rate and effort lead to carbon dioxide retention, hypoxia, and acidosis. Shivering consumes glucose stores, causing the patient to become hypoglycemic. Insulin levels fall, so available glucose decreases, which forces the body to metabolize fat for energy. Drug metabolism in the liver is sluggish, so medications may last longer.

The cardiovascular system is also dramatically affected. Cold heart muscle is irritable and prone to dysrhythmias. The characteristic Osborne or J wave may be seen on the electrocardiogram (Figure 43-3). The most common dysrhythmias are atrial and ventricular fibrillation. The cold patient is in great danger of ventricular fibrillation when the core temperature falls below 82° F (28° C). Ventricular fibrillation at these extremely cold temperatures does not respond to conventional treatment without prior rewarming. Only one attempt at defibrillation should be made and should be performed simultaneously with aggressive rewarming. Defibrillation should not be repeated until the patient is warmer than 85° F (29.5° C). Careful handling of hypothermic patients, especially when temperatures reach the vulnerable mid-80s range, is imperative because even turning may cause ventricular fibrillation.

The goal in mild hypothermia (84° to 94° F [29° to 34° C]) if the patient is still shivering, alert, and oriented is to prevent further heat loss and rewarm the patient as rapidly as possible. Patients with mild hypothermia usually respond well to passive rewarming techniques such as moving the patient to a warm environment, replacing wet clothing with dry material, and wrapping with warm blankets. Administer warmed, humidified oxygen, and give warmed, oral fluids that contain glucose or other sugars to provide more heat through calories. Passive rewarming raises the temperature 0.5° to 2.0° C/hr. Warmed oxygen and intravenous fluids raise the body

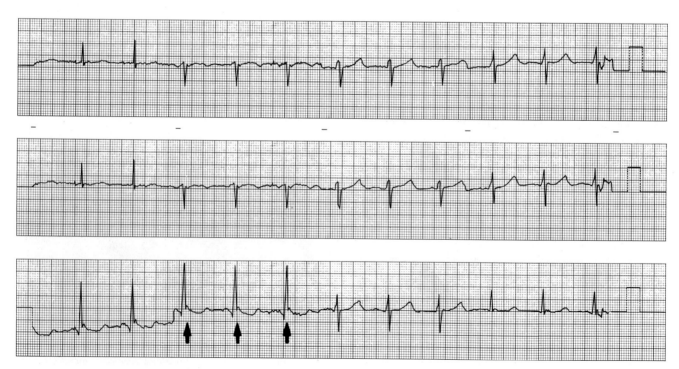

Figure **43-3**   Hypothermic J waves with QT prolongation. *(From Rosen P et al:* Emergency medicine: concepts and clinical practice, *ed 3, vol 1, St. Louis, 1992, Mosby.)*

temperature slightly. Gradual rewarming minimizes the risk of active rewarming shock.

In moderate hypothermia (78.8° to 89.4° F [26° to 31.9° C]), rewarm truncal areas at 0.5° C/hr using heating blankets such as the Bear Hugger, radiant heating lamps, and hot-water bottles. Monitor closely for marked vasodilation and subsequent hypotension.

In severe hypothermia (less than 78.8° F [26° C]), active internal (core) rewarming in conjunction with active external rewarming procedures is essential to prevent rewarming shock. Heated inhalation via endotracheal tube, warmed intravenous fluid, peritoneal lavage, gastrointestinal irrigation, extracorporeal rewarming cardiopulmonary bypass, and hemodialysis may all be used.

Successful rewarming depends on age, the patient's general condition before the hypothermic event, length of exposure, and careful handling. To prevent hyperthermia, discontinue active rewarming when the temperature reaches (89.6° to 93° F [32° to 34° C]). Rewarming shock can occur when the core temperature continues to drop after rewarming is initiated. The temperature drops as cold peripheral blood returns to the central circulation. Circulation of cold blood through the heart also increases ventricular irritability and leads to fibrillation. Rewarming may cause peripheral vasodilation, which leads to hypotension and cardiovascular collapse.

DROWNING AND NEAR DROWNING

Drowning claims approximately 9000 lives per year, with an additional 50,000 near drownings reported annually in the United States.[7] Drowning is the third leading cause of accidental death, with 40% of victims under age 5 years.[9] Toddlers and young children are at risk because of their naturally inquisitive nature and inadequate supervision. Near drowning is defined as survival from potential drowning. Rapid identification and initiation of resuscitation measures are vital for survival. Many victims of cold water immersion have a good chance of survival without neurologic sequelae when basic cardiac life support is initiated early.

Drowning stimulates various physiologic responses; however, death is caused by hypoxia secondary to asphyxiation. In any near drowning or drowning event, the victim is immersed in water for a prolonged time. Water is swallowed and aspirated into the lungs as the victim becomes unconscious. Dry drowning occurs secondary to intense laryngospasm; 10% of the victims do not aspirate water. Death is secondary to airway obstruction rather than pulmonary edema. Mortality is essentially the same for dry and wet drowning victims.

Freshwater and saltwater drowning victims present with similar clinical pictures—pulmonary edema. The difference is how pulmonary edema develops. With freshwater drowning, water is absorbed across the alveolar-capillary membrane because of hypotonicity relative to plasma. Hypervolemia occurs as more and more water moves into the capil-

laries. Red cells absorb excess water, so lysis may account for hemoglobinuria found in some freshwater near-drowning victims. Dilutional electrolyte problems, that is, decreased sodium and chloride, accompany even mild hypervolemia. Electrolyte abnormalities resolve when blood volume normalizes. Damage to the delicate alveolar membranes is a greater concern. Surfactant activity decreases, so lung compliance is impaired. Alveoli may rupture or become engorged, which leads to pulmonary edema. Decreased gas exchange, hypoxemia, and acidosis ultimately cause death.

Saltwater aspiration causes hypovolemia secondary to hypertonicity relative to plasma. Plasma is pulled across the alveolar-capillary membrane into the lungs, causing pulmonary edema, impaired gas exchange, and hypoxemia. The resulting hemoconcentration increases electrolyte concentration (e.g., sodium, potassium). Electrolyte abnormalities can be reversed with restoration of adequate circulating volume.

Secondary drowning can occur up to 72 hours after the event; therefore every near-drowning victim should be taken to the hospital for observation, regardless of how they appear at the scene. Inflammatory reactions in the lung injure the alveolar-capillary membrane and alter surfactant function. Approximately 10% to 15% of deaths associated with drowning are due to secondary drowning. Near-drowning victims should be observed for at least 24 hours.

Immersion in cold water may cause sudden death from cardiac dysrhythmias rather than drowning. Immersion syndrome occurs when cold water stimulates the vagus nerve, causing bradycardia or cardiac arrest. Alcohol is a significant factor in immersion syndrome because of altered judgment and impaired coordination. Sixty percent of all teenage drownings involve alcohol.

Presenting symptoms with near drowning vary with length of submersion, water temperature, quality of water, associated injuries, onset of cardiopulmonary resuscitation, and the patient's resuscitative response. Occasionally near-drowning victims may be asymptomatic; however, most present with mild dyspnea, a deathlike appearance with blue or gray coloring, apnea or tachypnea, hypotension, heart rate as slow as 4 to 5 beats/min or pulselessness, cold skin, dilated pupils known as fish eyes, hypothermia, and vomiting.

Field resuscitation of the near-drowning victim is crucial for survival. Immediate cardiopulmonary resuscitation (CPR) after removal from the water has been cited as a significant factor in survival. Regardless of advanced life support availability, increased survival results from excellent, prompt, field-initiated CPR. Initial resuscitation focuses on correcting hypoxia, acidosis, and hypotension. Box 43-3 highlights essential prehospital resuscitation. There is a high incidence of cervical spine injury in drowning victims, so cervical spine precautions are essential.

Once the victim reaches the medical facility, resuscitation includes stabilization of ABCs and continued warming. Box 43-4 summarizes factors affecting survival. Rewarming efforts should be aggressive if the core temperature is below 90° F (32° C). The heart is resistant to drug therapy and electroconversion when the core temperature is lower than 86° F (30° C); therefore early rewarming is essential to prevent ventricular fibrillation. Box 43-5 outlines essential steps for hospital resuscitation.

Complications associated with near drowning are the direct result of the hypoxic event. Primary complications are pulmonary, cerebral, and cardiovascular, including pulmonary edema, pneumonitis, adult respiratory distress syndrome, anoxic encephalopathy, and cardiopulmonary arrest. Later complications include cerebral edema, disseminated intravascular coagulation, acute tubular necrosis, and renal failure.

Box 43-3 Essential Guidelines for Near-Drowning Management

Determine duration of submersion.

Clear airway using cervical spine precautions, assess breathing, and provide rescue ventilations as soon as possible.

Assess circulation. If pulse is not palpated, begin chest compressions immediately. If advanced cardiac life support is available, proceed with gentle intubation.

Assess carefully for associated injuries when indicated by history and mechanism of injury.

Remove wet clothing, and gently wrap victim in dry blankets.

Do not attempt to warm victim if medical facility is less than 15 minutes away.

Initiate warming techniques, i.e., warm oxygen, warm IV fluids, or well-padded heat packs, if medical facility is more than 15 minutes away.

Transport the victim to a medical facility, even if victim recovers at the scene.

Box 43-4 Near-Drowning Survival

Factors that increase survival

Immediate, quality CPR
Colder water (<70° F)
Cleaner water
Shorter immersion time
Less struggle
No associated injuries

Factors that have no effect on survival

Sex
Race
Swimming ability
Eating a meal before the event
Type of water (saltwater or freshwater)
Use of the Heimlich maneuver during resuscitation attempts
Concurrent illnesses, i.e., cardiac or pulmonary disease

DIVING EMERGENCIES

Over the past few decades, self-contained underwater breathing apparatus (scuba) diving has enjoyed increased popularity. As equipment comfort and safety have improved, the recreational market has expanded significantly.[4] Nearly 200,000 Americans receive scuba instruction each year. There are thousands of commercial and military divers; however, most of the five million scuba divers in the United States are recreational divers. As the number of divers increase,[5] dive-related accidents increase. Most accidents occur because the human body is not designed for the marine environment. Cold water, lack of available oxygen, and inability to run away from hazards are intrinsic problems for which the diver must compensate. Diving accidents are increasing in all areas of the country, not just warm coastal resort areas. The most serious injuries discussed in this section are air embolism, nitrogen narcosis, and decompression sickness.

Divers are exposed to pressure changes related to water. Water is denser than air so that pressure changes are greater under water, even at relatively shallow depths (Table 43-3). Boyle's law states that gas volume is inversely related to pressure at a constant temperature. For the diver, this means volume decreases and pressure increases as the diver descends. This principle is the mechanism behind all types of

---

Box 43-5 Essential ED Resuscitation for Near Drowning

Obtain history of the event, treatment, and progress during transport.

Establish airway and provide ventilation as rapidly as possible.

Continue CPR, and begin active rewarming as indicated.

Perform endotracheal intubation as soon as possible, and provide high-flow oxygen with positive pressure ventilation.

Handle victim gently to prevent hypothermia-induced ventricular dysrhythmias.

Monitor core temperature continuously. Anticipate further decrease in core temperature with continued rewarming.

Intubate and provide assisted ventilation with positive end-expiratory pressure (PEEP) if there is evidence of pulmonary edema.

Insert a nasogastric tube to prevent gastric dilatation and possible aspiration.

Administer antibiotics for fever secondary to pneumonitis. (Prophylactic antibiotics are contraindicated for aspiration unless infection is present.)

Treat bronchospasm with a β-agonist such as albuterol by metered dose inhaler.

Anticipate profound neurologic depression. Treat with hyperventilation, intraventricular monitoring, diuretics, and possibly barbiturates. Treat hypoxic seizures with oxygen, ventilation, diazepam, and phenytoin. Corticosteroids have no proven benefit in treatment of anoxic brain injuries and should not be routinely utilized.

Table 43-3 Pressure-Volume Relationships According to Boyle's Law

	Depth (feet)	Gauge pressure (atmospheres)	Absolute pressure (atmospheres)	Gas volume (%)*	Bubble diameter (%)*
Air	0	0	1	100	100
Seawater	33	1	2	50	79
	66	2	3	33	69
	99	3	4	25	63
	132	4	5	20	58
	165	5	6	17	54

*Bubble diameter is probably a more important consideration than gas volume when considering the ability of recompression to restore circulation to a gas-embolized blood vessel.

barotrauma, the most common medical problem that occurs with divers. Table 43-4 illustrates this principle using the lung as an example. When a diver uses a scuba tank of pressurized air, lung volume remains constant at various depths. If the diver ascends but does not exhale, water pressure decreases and gas in the lungs expands, greatly increasing pressure in the lungs (Table 43-5).

Air Embolism

Air embolism is the most serious and dangerous of all diving emergencies, second only to drowning as cause of death among divers. As gas expands, lungs expand to the point of rupture, causing pneumothoraces. High-pressure air is forced into the circulatory system, producing air embolism. Air embolism is prevented by exhaling during controlled, slow ascent. Divers risk injury when they ascend too rapidly or when they hold their breath during ascent.

Air embolism appears within seconds to minutes of ascent, usually less than 10 minutes from time of alveolar rupture. Symptoms are neurologic and may include vertigo, limb paresthesias, unilateral paralysis, seizures, and loss of consciousness. Other signs and symptoms include chest tightness; shortness of breath; pink, frothy sputum; simple pneumothorax; and tension pneumothorax.

Death is an immediate threat to the diver with air embolism. If the patient is unconscious, intubate immediately. Ensure proper ventilation with positive pressure ventilation and 100% oxygen. Perform needle thoracentesis for tension pneumothorax. Place the patient in the left lateral position to avoid cerebral embolism. If air transport is necessary, cabin altitude should not exceed 100 feet. Definitive treatment is prompt recompression and controlled decompression in a hyperbaric chamber.

Complications of air embolism depend on the end point of the air bubbles. If bubbles enter the coronary arteries, the patient may have signs of myocardial infarction, whereas an embolism entering the cerebral circulation causes neurologic symptoms. Other complications include blocked vascular flow to the spinal cord causing spinal cord injury, altered blood coagulation leading to disseminated intravascu-

Table 43-4 Lung Volumes During Descent

Depth (feet)	Lung volume under pressure (cc)
Sea level	1000
33	500
100	200
233	123

Table 43-5 Lung Volumes During Ascent Without Exhalation

Depth (feet)	Air in each lung (cc)
233	1000
100	2000
33	4000
Sea level	8000

lar coagulation, and hemoconcentration. Table 43-6 highlights gas toxicities related to diving.

Nitrogen Narcosis

Solubility of any gas in a liquid is almost directly proportional to pressure of the liquid at a constant temperature (Henry's law). The composition of room air is 79% nitrogen. Nitrogen narcosis occurs when nitrogen becomes dissolved in solution because pressures are greater than normal. Symptoms begin to appear at depths of 99 feet or more and resolve with ascent (Table 43-5). Experienced divers usually have fewer problems than novices, although nitrogen narcosis is an inescapable problem for all divers.

Dissolved nitrogen produces neurodepressant effects similar to alcohol. Every 50 feet of descent is comparable to one martini. The "martini" rule is used to evaluate effects of dives to different depths. Initially, the diver may exhibit im-

Table **43-6**	**Gas Toxicities in Diving**	
Gas	Signs and symptoms	Therapeutic interventions
Oxygen (100%)	Twitching, nausea, dizziness, tunnel vision, restlessness, paresthesias, seizures, confusion, pulmonary edema, atelectasis, shock lung	Maintain airway, breathing, and circulation; intubation, controlled ventilation to reduce FiO_2, decompression, positive end-expiratory pressure
Carbon dioxide (8%-10%)	Dizziness, lethargy, heavy labored breathing, unconsciousness	Ascent to surface, ABCs, 100% oxygen
Carbon monoxide (from contaminated tank)	Dizziness, pink or red lips and mouth, euphoria	Ascent to surface, ABCs (CPR if necessary), 100% oxygen in hyperbaric chamber at 3 atmospheres for 1 hour

paired judgment, a feeling of alcohol intoxication, slowed motor response, loss of proprioception, and euphoria. Below 200 feet, nitrogen narcosis renders the diver unable to work; however, individual divers have varying tolerance levels for nitrogen narcosis. Loss of consciousness occurs at approximately 300 feet.

Nitrogen narcosis has no real metabolic significance. The risk lies with impairment of the diver's judgment. Jacques Cousteau aptly described this condition as "rapture of the deep." Divers become euphoric, silly, and unaware of the dangerous situation and the need to surface. Ascent to the surface causes symptoms to disappear completely, so no further therapy is required. Nitrogen narcosis can be avoided by limiting the depth of dives.

Decompression Sickness

Decompression sickness, also called the bends, dysbarism, caisson disease, and diver's paralysis, is the most common form of diving emergency. Symptoms occur following rapid ascent. Speed of safe ascent is defined for each dive, depending on the depth-time relationship of the dive using standard U.S. Navy air decompression tables. According to Henry's law, gradual ascent allows the ambient pressure of nitrogen to reach an equilibrium that permits nitrogen escape through respired air. Decompression sickness occurs during ascent and only when equilibrium cannot be established. Bubbles are squeezed into blood and tissues, obstructing flow and impairing tissue perfusion. Effects are seen in almost every organ of the body.

Typically, symptoms of decompression sickness begin within 30 minutes of ascent but may be delayed up to 36 hours. Most individuals exhibit symptoms within 6 hours. Factors that increase severity are described in Box 43-6. Nitrogen bubbles can develop in any tissue. The most significant mechanical effect is vascular occlusion in any tissue. For example, supersaturation of lymphatic tissue with nitrogen causes lymphedema, cellular distention, and membrane rupture. Biophysical effects are poor tissue perfusion and ischemia. Other symptoms characteristic of decompression sickness include cough, shortness of breath, and dysp-

Box **43-6**	**Factors that Increase Severity in Decompression Sickness**
Extremes in water temperature Increasing age Obesity Fatigue Poor physical condition Alcohol consumption Peripheral vascular disease Heavy work during diving	

nea (chokes); joint pain (bends); and neurologic symptoms including fatigue, diplopia, headaches, dizziness, unconsciousness, paresthesias, and seizures.

Initial treatment begins with high-flow oxygen to improve oxygenation and eliminate nitrogen. Fluid replacement is done with intravenous normal saline or Ringer's lactate. Narcotic analgesics should be avoided because of their respiratory depressant effect. Definitive treatment is immediate transfer to a recompression facility. When more information is required, 24-hour assistance is available through the National Divers Alert Network at Duke University, the local health department, or the nearest naval facility (Box 43-7).

Bends can occur at depths less than 33 feet, or 1 atmospheric pressure, if ascent is too rapid. Any joint pain within 24 to 48 hours of a dive should be treated as decompression sickness. Upper extremities are affected more often than lower extremities. A simple test for "joint bends" is inflation of a blood pressure cuff to 250 mm Hg or greater around the affected joint. Pain from the bends subsides as long as the cuff remains inflated.

Complications of decompression sickness are often related to failure to report symptoms, treat when the cause is unclear, or identify severe symptoms that result from a dive-related accident. Complications similar to air embolism may occur, such as spinal cord and cerebral lesions.

Box 43-7 References for Diving Accidents: Advice and Location of Dive Chambers

**U.S. Navy Experimental Diving Unit, Washington, DC
(202) 433-2790**

Operational 24 hours a day, 7 days a week. Ask to speak with a duty officer who provides the name, location, and telephone number of the nearest decompression chamber.

**National Divers Alert Network, Duke University
(919) 684-8111**

Alert person answering the phone that a dive-related emergency has occurred. Request the dive physician on duty. A physician familiar with dive-related emergencies will advise emergency care techniques and location of the nearest decompression chamber.

Remaining within a safe range of depth and time during repeated dives prevents decompression sickness. Gradual ascent with delays at certain depths allows nitrogen absorption and can be accomplished with decompression tables to calculate rate of nitrogen absorption. The depth and length of each dive should be limited. The diver should carry a scuba identification card for at least 48 hours after a dive.

Other Diving Problems

The squeeze

The squeeze occurs when air is trapped in hollow chambers such as the ears, sinuses, pulmonary tree, gastrointestinal tract, teeth, and added air space such as the face mask or diving suit. Severe, sharp pain occurs when external pressure in these spaces exceeds internal pressure. The squeeze occurs if the diver descends to depths without exhalation. Symptoms include pain, edema, capillary dilation, rupture, and bleeding. Treatment for all squeeze-related problems is gradual ascent to shallow depths to decrease pressure and maintenance of the ABCs.

Middle-ear squeeze is caused by a blocked eustachian tube or paranasal sinus with inability to equalize pressure in these spaces. Diving should be avoided when these chambers are congested from colds or allergies. When diving, gradual descents allow pressures in air-filled chambers to equalize.

A more serious but less common type of aural squeeze is inner-ear barotrauma. Structures of the inner ear may rupture with sudden pressure changes between the middle and inner ear. Permanent nerve damage and deafness can occur. Consultation with an otolaryngologist is recommended for the dive patient with tinnitus, vertigo, or deafness.

Barotrauma of ascent

Barotrauma of ascent is the reverse of the squeeze. Although air-filled chambers may equalize during descent, air trapped in these spaces expands as atmospheric pressure decreases during ascent. If air cannot escape, barotrauma oc-

curs. This condition is uncomfortable; however, no treatment is required, since the condition subsides with time as the pressure gradually equalizes.

Hyperpnea exhaustion syndrome

Diver fatigue is usually responsible for hyperpnea exhaustion syndrome. Symptoms include tachypnea, anxiety, feeling of impending doom, difficulty floating, and exhaustion. Treatment consists of returning to the surface and rest.

CARBON MONOXIDE POISONING

Carbon monoxide (CO) gas is odorless and colorless. Most severe cases of CO intoxication are associated with inhalation of smoke from house fires; however, engine exhaust, improperly vented stoves, and faulty stoves or heating systems are also significant causes of accidental poisoning. CO poisoning from engine exhaust is a common means of suicide. Poisoning occurs primarily during the winter, usually because of faulty heating systems. CO poisoning is the most frequent source of poisoning in the United States. Accidental and intentional CO poisoning accounts for 3500 to 4000 deaths annually.[8] Mortality rate is 30%. Many die before transport to the hospital.

The most significant effect of CO exposure is hypoxia. Toxicity is the result of hemoglobin's affinity for CO, altered oxygen-hemoglobin dissociation curve, and impaired cytochrome oxidase systems. Hemoglobin's affinity for CO is 200 times greater than for oxygen. Hemoglobin preferentially binds with CO, so oxygen-carrying capacity is diminished even when oxygen is available. Carboxyhemoglobin (HbCO), formed when hemoglobin binds with CO, can be measured to determine the severity of CO poisoning. HbCO is measured in parts per million, with concentration indicated by percentage (Table 43-7). CO also binds with myoglobin at a rate 40 times greater than oxygen. Consequently, hypoxia occurs at the tissue level as well as in the oxygen transport system. Pulse oximetry indicates adequate saturation despite the presence of hypoxia.

Generally, oxygen diffuses from the blood into the tissues. The oxygen-hemoglobin dissociation curve describes this process. Any event that shifts the curve to the left or right affects cellular oxygenation. Hypoxia that results from a shift in the HbCO dissociation curve is more significant than hypoxia that results from a simple reduction in functional hemoglobin. HbCO shifts the oxygen curve so that partial pressure needed to unload oxygen from blood to the tissue is lower than in normal tissue.

CO also interferes with cytochrome oxidase systems. Decreased function of these systems impairs cellular respiration by displacing oxygen, particularly in high-rate metabolic organs, that is, the brain and heart. Oxygen displacement is responsible for dysrhythmias and many CNS symptoms.

Symptoms may be initially vague but worsen with increased exposure. Variability of symptoms in individuals with identical exposure exists; the longer the time between exposure and presentation, the greater the variability. Chil-

Table **43-7**   **Signs and Symptoms of Carbon Monoxide Exposure**

Exposure level	Signs and symptoms	Treatment
Mild		
10% to 25% HbCO when no cardiac or neurologic involvement	Throbbing headache, nausea, impaired function for complex tasks	Maintain airway; administer IV fluids; cardiac monitor; oxygen administration by tight-fitting mask for 4 hours or until HbCO < 5%
Moderate		
20% to 30% HbCO; *less* if cardiac or neurologic involvement is present	Severe headache, irritability, weakness, visual problems, palpitations, loss of dexterity, nausea and vomiting, decreased mentation	Hyperbaric oxygen administration at 3 atmospheres for 46 minutes; repeat in 6 hours if full CNS recovery does not occur; maintain airway; administer IV fluids; cardiac monitor
Severe		
40% to 50% HbCO	Tachycardia, tachypnea, collapse, syncope	As above
Life-threatening		
50% to 60% HbCO	Coma, Cheyne-Stokes respirations, intermittent convulsions, cherry red mucous membranes	As above
Lethal		
Greater than 60% HbCO	Cardiac and respiratory depression, likely cardiac arrest	CPR and as above

dren may have increased susceptibility to CO toxicity. A child's higher metabolic rate may cause syncope and lethargy at HbCO levels of 25%. Specific signs and general management of CO poisoning are discussed in Table 43-7. The cornerstone for all treatment is high-flow oxygen to displace CO from hemoglobin. The half-life of CO is 5 to 6 hours on room air. Half-life is reduced to 1 hour with 100% oxygen and less than 20 minutes with hyperbaric oxygen therapy.

CO promotes dysrhythmias and myocardial ischemia. Alterations in the alveolar-capillary membrane may lead to pulmonary edema and hemorrhage. Neurologic deficits include seizures, cerebral edema, and coma. Renal failure occurs secondary to myoglobinuria. Patients with HbCO levels greater than 25% or signs of cardiac ischemia and neurologic deficits should be admitted for observation. If patients are discharged, instructions should include discussion of neurologic sequelae such as headache, loss of memory and concentration, irritability, personality changes, and excessive fatigue. Hyperbaric oxygen therapy may be required if symptoms return.

BITES AND STINGS

Specific environmental emergencies related to bites and stings include bites from snakes, animals, spiders, and ticks, and stings from scorpions and hymenopterans, that is, bees, wasps, hornets, and fire ants. Table 43-8 summarizes bites and stings. Lethality is the result of poisonous venom and stings or secondary to anaphylaxis. Anaphylactic shock and respiratory distress are discussed in Chapters 34 and 36.

Snakebites

There are 3000 species of snakes in the world. Of these, 375 species, from five different families, are venomous: Crotalidae, Elapidae, Viperidae, Colubridae, and Hydrophidae. Two families of poisonous snakes indigenous to the United States are Crotalidae, or pit vipers (rattlesnakes, copperheads, and cottonmouths), and Elapidae (coral snakes). Cobras and mambas belong to the Elapidae family but are not indigenous to the United States. Figure 43-4 summarizes the differences between poisonous and nonpoisonous snakes. More than 50,000 snakebites occur annually in the United States. Envenomation occurs in only 8000 cases. The most common poisonous snake in the United States is a pit viper (95%), usually the rattlesnake. Fortunately, fewer than 15 deaths occur per year.[3]

Venom is a complex substance containing enzymes, glycoproteins, peptides, and other substances capable of causing tissue destruction—cardiotoxic, neurotoxic, hemotoxic, or any combination of types. Pit viper venom is primarily hemotoxic, whereas coral snake venom is primarily neurotoxic. Venom is manufactured in salivary glands and stored in ducts in the fangs. Envenomation occurs when venom is injected into the victim through the fangs.

Signs and symptoms of snakebites depend on the type and size of the snake, size and age of the patient, location and depth of the bite, number of bites, and amount of venom injected. The patient may have a specific sensitivity to the venom that makes the reaction worse. The snake's teeth contain numerous microorganisms, so a bite can cause sec-

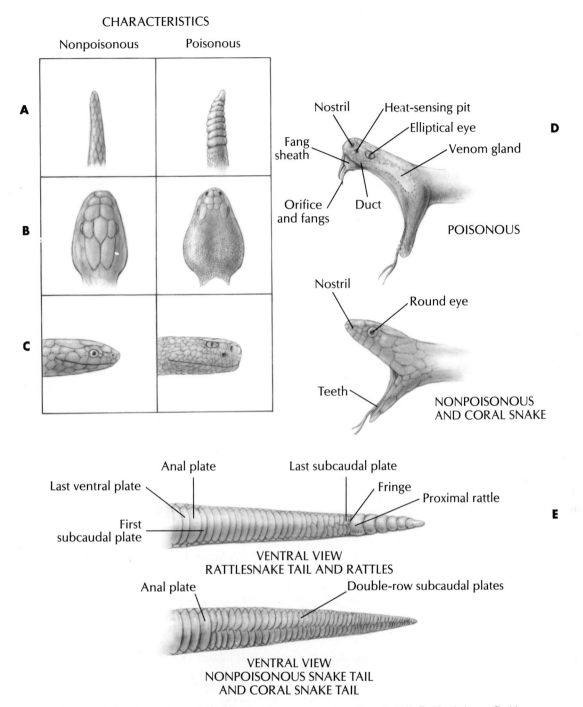

CHARACTERISTICS

Nonpoisonous   Poisonous

A

B

C

Nostril   Heat-sensing pit
Elliptical eye
Fang
sheath   Venom gland

Orifice   Duct
and fangs

POISONOUS   D

Nostril

Round eye

Teeth

NONPOISONOUS
AND CORAL SNAKE

Anal plate   Last subcaudal plate

Last ventral plate   Fringe
Proximal rattle

First
subcaudal plate   E

VENTRAL VIEW
RATTLESNAKE TAIL AND RATTLES

Anal plate   Double-row subcaudal plates

VENTRAL VIEW
NONPOISONOUS SNAKE TAIL
AND CORAL SNAKE TAIL

Figure **43-4** Comparison of venomous and nonvenomous snakes. **A,** Tail. **B,** Head shape. **C,** Absence or presence of heat-sensing facial pit between the eye and the nostril. **D,** Absence or presence of well-developed venom glands, duct, and fangs. **E,** Belly scales leading up to the tail. *(From Davis JH et al: Surgery: a problem solving approach, ed 2, vol 1, St. Louis, 1995, Mosby.)*

ondary infection. Major signs and symptoms are divided into local and systemic reactions. *Local reactions* have one or two fang marks, teeth marks, edema around the bite site 1 to 36 hours after the bite, pain at the site, petechiae, ecchymosis, loss of function of the limb, and necrosis 16 to 36 hours after the bite. *Systemic reactions* include nausea,

vomiting, diaphoresis, syncope, and a metallic or rubber taste. The patient may develop paralysis, excessive salivation, difficulty speaking, visual disturbances, muscle twitching, paresthesia, epistaxis, blood in the stool, vomitus or sputum, and ptosis. Neurologic symptoms include constricted pupils and seizures. Life-threatening systemic reac-

Table **43-8** **Bites and Stings**		
Type of arthropod	Signs and symptoms	Management
Stinging		
Honeybee *(Apis mellificus)* Bumblebee *(Bombus)*	Painful injection wound; stinger often visibly protruding. Edema and itching may be apparent.	Remove stinger by scraping with dull object. Do not grasp and pull; this contracts venom sac, releasing more toxin. Cleanse site and apply antiseptic. Apply ice and elevate part. Oral antihistamines and steroids may be indicated.
Yellow jacket *(Vespula maculifrons)* Wasp *(Chlorion ichneumonica)*	Painful injection wound. Does not leave stinger behind; stings repeatedly. Wheal formation, edema, and itching may be present.	See bee sting, *above*. Watch for anaphylaxis.
Hornet *(Vespula maculata)* Velvet ant *(Mutilla sacken)* Fire ant *(Solenopsis geminata)*	Painful injection wound with wheal that expands to large vesicle; as purulence develops, reddening of area occurs; scarring and crusting follow reabsorption of pustule.	See bee sting, *above*. Watch for anaphylaxis.
Scorpions *(Centruroides sculpturatus, Centruroides vittatus,* and *Centruroides gertschi)*	Lethal: No visible local effect. Sharp pain, hyperesthesia followed by hypoesthesia, itching, and speech disturbances are common. Jaw muscle spasms, nausea, vomiting, incontinence, and seizures follow. Death may occur from cardiovascular or respiratory failure.	Apply tourniquet as near to sting site as possible, and pack area in ice well beyond the tourniquet. After 5 minutes, loosen tourniquet and reapply.
	Nonlethal: Sharp burning pain at sting site with edema and discoloration; anaphylaxis is rare.	Caution: Morphine and opiates are contraindicated; they enhance toxic effects.
Biting and piercing		
Tick *(Dermacentor variabilis)*	Victim unaware of presence; local irritation and possible infection when body removed but head remains in tissue; some species (which transmit Rocky Mountain spotted fever) cause flaccid paralysis from neurotoxin. Initial symptoms are paresthesias and pain in lower extremity. Respiratory failure results from bulbar paralysis.	Remove offending ticks. Apply gasoline, ether, or hot (not burning) match to the tick body. Wait 10 minutes for disengagement. Do not manually remove; squeezing the body may inject more virus into victim. Paralysis will dramatically subside after removal.
Centipedes Eastern house centipede *(Scutigera cleoptratu)* Western house centipede *(Scolopendra heros)*	Wound site red, edematous, and painful; sometimes tissue necrosis occurs.	Cleanse wound. Employ analgesics and antibiotics if indicated.
Spiders Black widow *(Latrodectus mactans)* (hourglass spider, female)	Pricking sensation followed by dull, numbing pain. Edema and tiny red fang marks may become visible. Chest and abdomen pain may be evident adjacent to site of the bite. Pain and rigidity of muscles subside after 48 hours. Blood pressure, temperature, and white blood count may be elevated. Hematuria rarely develops. Spinal fluid may have increased pressure.	Use ice locally to slow absorption of toxins. Employ muscle relaxants and 10% calcium gluconate IV to reduce spasms. Use antivenin *(Latrodectus mactans)*. Do skin test before administration of the horse serum. Symptoms subside 1-3 hours after antivenin administration.

Table 43-8 Bites and Stings—cont'd

Type of arthropod	Signs and symptoms	Management
Biting and piercing—cont'd		
Brown recluse (*Loxosceles reclusa*) (fiddleback)	Local reaction begins 2-8 hours after bite with pain, edema, bleb formation, and ischemia. On third or fourth day after bite, central area turns dark and is firm to touch. In second week, central area becomes depressed and demarcated with open ulceration formation. Healing may take place in about 3 weeks. Fever, chills, malaise, weakness, nausea, vomiting, joint pain, and petechiae may also be noted. Blood dyscrasias such as hemolytic anemia and thrombocytopenia rarely occur.	Immediate excision of wound with toxins may be useful. Steroids, antihistamines, and antibiotics are to be employed as indicated. Skin grafting may be necessary if healing does not take place.
True bugs		
Kissing bug (*Conenose triatoma*)	Mild or no pain at wound site. Redness, edema, itching, or nodular hemorrhagic lesions, depending on sensitivity.	Cleanse wound with soap and water. Oral antihistamines may be indicated. Anaphylaxis has been reported.
Assassin bug (*Arilus christatus*) (wheel bug)	Intense pain at wound site. Usually lasts 2-5 hours. Localized edema, itching, and redness.	Cleanse wound with antiseptic solution. Anaphylaxis rare.
Vesicating or urticating		
Blister beetles	Clear amber fluid (cantharidin) released from the insects' knee joints, prothorax, and genitalia. Mild burning sensation may become apparent as a result of fluid released at site.	Cleanse area with soap and water as soon as possible.
Lepidoptera (larva) Lo caterpillar (*Automeris lo*) Puss caterpillar (*Megalopyge opercularis*) Saddle back caterpillar (*Sibine stimulea*) Range caterpillar (*Hemileuca oliviae*)	Distinct row of released spines may be seen at site of intense pain. Nausea, vomiting, headache, and fever may be present.	Remove spines with adhesive tape if possible. Apply ice to the wound; analgesics may be indicated. Unremoved spines could cause infection.
Aquatic organisms*		
Stingray	Wound contains venom sacs from furrowed spine of stingray tail. Fainting, nausea, vomiting, and diarrhea occur with occasional progression to muscle paralysis, respiratory distress, seizures, and even death.	Immediately irrigate wound with normal saline to remove venom sacs. Follow initial irrigation with immersion in hot water for 30 minutes (43.3°-45.5°C) to inactivate venom. Antibiotics recommended; antihistamines and steroids may also be indicated. For severe cases, have ventilatory support and resuscitation equipment at hand. Surgical closure of wounds may be necessary in some instances.
Catfish	Wound from dorsal spine causes pain and infection.	Use deep irrigations of hydrogen peroxide. Employ antibiotics as indicated.

*Antivenins for most aquatic bites and stings (e.g., stonefish, jellyfish, sea snake) are available from Commonwealth Serum Laboratories, Melbourne, Australia.

Continued

Table **43-8** **Bites and Stings—cont'd**

Type of arthropod	Signs and symptoms	Management
Vesicating or urticating—cont'd		
Portuguese man-of-war *(Physalia physalis)*	Tentacles become embedded in skin. Welts, burned areas, or streaks may be present. Pain may be intense enough to produce shock and collapse. Headache, cramps, and paralysis also noted.	Tourniquet may be tried. Remove tentacles with alcohol and sodium bicarbonate scrub (prevents further stinging and neutralizes acid). Leave alcohol on for 6-8 min. Follow with sodium bicarbonate, allowing it to dry. Employ antihistamines and steroids locally and systemically. General anesthesia may be necessary to control pain.
Stings (cone shell snails, sea anemones, corals, and jellyfish)	Acid wound produced.	Cleanse wound with alkali (ammonia, sodium bicarbonate).
Bites (sea snake and octopus)	Wounds contain neurotoxin. Muscle stiffness, paralysis, myoglobinuria, and death from respiratory arrest can occur.	Apply tourniquet. Control shock. Use indicated resuscitation measures.
Scorpion fish	Intense pain, edema, shock, and ECG changes.	See stingray injuries, *above,* for wound cleansing and heat application. Give antivenin.
Sea urchins	Painful injection site with erythema, edema, numbness, and paralysis. Respiratory distress and death may occur.	Use heat as described under stingray. Do not attempt to remove spines initially. Attempt to locate with x-ray films. Granulomatous lesions often develop from embedded spines.

ECG, electrocardiogram.

tions include severe hemorrhage, renal failure, and hypovolemic shock.

Initial assessment includes a history of the snakebite, that is, the size of the snake, location and depth of the injury, number of bites, and amount of venom injected (if known). Document the time of injury and all interventions employed prior to ED arrival. Prehospital interventions include stabilization of ABCs, keeping the patient calm and supine to minimize exertion. Immobilize the limb below the level of the heart to reduce blood flow. Do *not* apply ice or a tourniquet. Place a band 4 inches proximal to the bite to impede lymphatic flow while preserving arterial and venous flow. Remove potentially constrictive jewelry. Do *not* cut or attempt to suck venom from the wound.

Incision for venom suction is rarely indicated. If incision and suction are performed *immediately,* 25% to 30% of the venom may be removed; effectiveness drops dramatically 30 minutes after the bite. Ice has not proved beneficial and may impair absorption of antivenin and increase necrosis secondary to decreased circulation. The patient should not drink coffee or alcohol and should not smoke.

Hospital interventions begin with the ABCs. Initiate aggressive intravenous infusion of normal saline or Ringer's lactate to maintain renal blood flow and fluid volume. Obtain a complete blood count, coagulation studies, elec-

trolytes, blood urea nitrogen, creatinine, creatinine phosphokinase, blood type, and crossmatch. Clean the wound. Administer analgesics for pain, preferably acetaminophen, since hemorrhage can occur with aspirin or nonsteroidal antiinflammatory drugs. Avoid narcotics because of the risk of respiratory depression. Administer tetanus prophylaxis if the patient's immunization history is incomplete or outdated.

Antivenin therapy is reserved for life-threatening snakebites, since there is a high incidence of sensitivity reactions and anaphylaxis.[6] If antivenin is administered, the patient should be closely monitored. Resuscitation equipment and emergency medication should be readily available. Antivenin is prepared in horse serum; therefore the patient should be questioned carefully about allergies to horse serum. Perform a skin test for antivenin if the patient will receive the medication, has had no previous antivenin treatments, and is not allergic to horse serum. Inject 0.02 ml of a 1:10 dilution intradermally. Observe for 15 to 20 minutes, and then check for wheals. After a negative skin test, administer antivenin by slow IV drip (see Table 43-9 for dosage regimen). Insufficient dosage is the most common cause of treatment failure. Administer antivenin until symptoms subside.

The physician may elect to give the antivenin despite a positive skin reaction. Monitor closely for systemic reac-

Table **43-9** **Antivenin Dosage Regimen**		
Signs and symptoms	Degree of envenomation	Dose
Fang marks; no local swelling or paresthesia	None	No skin test or antivenin required
Fang marks; local swelling of hands or feet; pain; no systemic responses	Minimal	3-5 vials*
Fang marks; progressive swelling beyond site of bite; mild systemic symptoms	Moderate	8-10 vials*
Multiple fang marks; progressive swelling, pain, and ecchymosis; marked systemic symptoms, hypotension, fasciculations, or clotting deficits	Severe	15-20 vials*

*Dilute antivenin in half-normal saline at a 1:4 ratio. Infuse within 2 hours. Repeat dose every 2 hours until symptoms subside. Children generally require 50% more antivenin.

tions such as urticaria, wheezing, or other symptoms of progressing anaphylaxis. Meticulous patient observation and slow administration of the medication are essential. Explain the risks of treatment to the patient. A consent may be required in some areas. Administration of antivenin is not a common ED procedure in most areas of the country; therefore, consultation with a professional poison control center is advised.

Lizard Bites

The iguana is a member of the family Iguanidae. The bite is generally nontoxic, causing pain without systemic reactions. Two venomous varieties are the Gila monster *(Heloderma)* and the Mexican bearded lizard. Gila toxin is released in saliva. Symptoms may begin with pain and swelling, progressing to systemic symptoms of nausea, vomiting, weakness, hypotension, syncope, shock, and anaphylaxis. No antivenin is currently available for Gila toxin. Treatment includes wound care, tetanus prophylaxis, and analgesics. Meperidine enhances the effect of Gila toxin and should be avoided. Provide supportive care for systemic response.

Animal Bites

Approximately two million animal bites occur annually in the United States. The number of animal bites peak during the spring. Incidence is greater in urban areas than rural areas. Dogs and cats are the most frequent offenders, with wild rodents and pet rodents ranked second. Treatment of animal bites includes cleaning the wound, tetanus prophylaxis, copious irrigation with saline solution, and analgesics as necessary.

Dog bites

Dog bites account for 75% to 90% of all bites occurring to humans in the United States.[7] Most victims own the dogs that bite them, with children the population at greatest risk. The most common sites of injury are the extremities. Dog bite wounds may be simple punctures or major deforming lacerations, tears, avulsions, or soft tissue crush injuries. Tissue necrosis may occur with a crush injury. The type of injury usually depends on the size of the dog and the body area where the wound is inflicted.

Therapeutic intervention focuses on reducing the possibility of infection and neutralizing rabies virus. Potentially disfiguring wounds of the face, particularly eyelids, lips, and ears, should be cleansed gently before evaluation for repair by a reconstructive surgeon. Irrigate the wound with copious amounts of normal saline using a pressure irrigation set or 20-gauge intravenous catheter. Anticipate debridement of nonviable tissue. Puncture wounds are left open, whereas lacerations are loosely sutured. The extremity should be splinted and immobilized. Prophylactic antibiotic therapy is used with high-risk injuries such as hand and foot bites, puncture wounds, and wounds greater than 6 to 12 hours old. Report the incident to the local animal control or public health authorities. The dog should be quarantined for 10 days if immunization history is unknown or rabies is suspected.

Aftercare instructions for wound care should be given to the patient and family with a careful explanation of signs and symptoms of infection. If a bite is not treated, infection, cellulitis, osteomyelitis, and residual neurovascular damage may occur. Puncture wounds have a higher rate of infection because of the depth of the wound. An estimated 5% of all dog bites become infected. Other complications include rabies. Fortunately, rabies is not a routine outcome of dog bites because of effective canine immunization programs.

Cat bites and scratches

Cat bites account for 10% of all bites inflicted on humans in the United States each year. Cats are notorious for scratches because of their sharp claws. Cat scratches cause the same complications as bites and are treated in the same manner. Cat bites cause deep puncture wounds, which can involve tendons and joint capsules. There is little incidence of crush injury because cats' teeth are sharp, narrow, and long and the jaw lacks power. Incidence of wound infections from cat bites is greater than in dog bites. Cats are hunters and often come in contact with bacteria-infested rodents, which contaminate their mouths with *Pasteurella multocida*. Consequently, rapid onset of infection can occur after the bite. Cats also use their paws to groom themselves and may have considerable bacteria on their claws. Treatment for cat bites is the same as for dog bites. Osteomyelitis, septic arthritis, and tenosynovitis have been reported. Cat-scratch disease may cause lymphadenitis of the extremity days to weeks after the scratch. Because risk of infection is so great, thorough wound care instructions with clear instructions for follow-up are essential.

Human Bites

Human bites have the highest rate of infection and tissue damage of all bite injuries. The human mouth has great crushing ability and also harbors over 40 potential pathogens. The most common sites for bites are the fingers, hands, ears, and tip of the nose. A human bite may cause a laceration, puncture, crush injury, soft tissue tearing, or even amputation. Boxer's fractures are often associated with an open wound over the knuckles that may have occurred when the fist impacted another person's teeth. Treatment is similar to other bites with the exception that the patient always receives prophylactic antibiotics. If infection is already present, the patient is usually admitted for parenteral antibiotic therapy. Human bites have an increased risk of osteomyelitis, cellulitis, and septic arthritis. Human bites are reported to the local police in some states.

Spider (Arachnid) Bites

All spiders inject venom when they bite. Most venom causes itching, stinging, swelling, or a combination of symptoms in a local area. Despite the vast number of arthropod bites and stings occurring on a daily basis, systemic reactions occur in only 4% of the population, with anaphylaxis in only 0.4%. Tarantula bites usually cause only local reactions, that is, slight pain and stinging. Black widow spider venom and brown recluse spider venom may cause systemic reactions and anaphylaxis.

Black widow spider bites

Black widow spiders are usually found in damp, cool places, such as under rocks or in woodpiles. They are recognizable by their black body and the bright red hourglass marking on their abdomen (Figure 43-5). The black widow spider's venom is neurotoxic. A local reaction begins within minutes, including a painful sting out of proportion to the size of the bite. Tiny red marks appear at the point of venom entry. Systemic reactions develop within 24 to 48 hours and include nausea, vomiting, hypertension, hyperactive deep tendon reflexes, and elevated temperature. Patients may also have respiratory difficulty, headache, syncope, weakness, and chest and abdominal pain or spasms. Seizures and shock may also develop. Symptoms from envenomation peak 2 to 3 hours after onset and may last several days.

Reactions may be minor and require only local wound care. However, severe systemic responses can also occur. Interventions begin with stabilization of the ABCs. Apply ice to the bite area to slow the action of the neurotoxin. Apply steroid ointment for comfort. Administer muscle relaxants such as methocarbamol (Robaxin) or diazepam (Valium), and give calcium gluconate (10 ml of 10% solution) for muscle spasms, rigidity, and pain. Narcotic analgesic may be required for severe pain. Consider antivenin therapy for severe reactions or high-risk individuals (e.g., young children, adults with hypertension or cardiac disease). Contact a poison control center for further consultation. With aggressive, supportive therapy, symptoms usually subside within

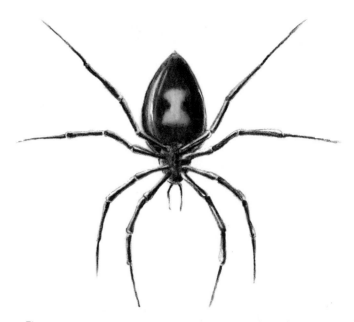

Figure **43-5** Female black widow spider *(Latrodectus mactans)* with typical hourglass marking on the abdomen. *(From Davis JH et al:* Surgery: a problem solving approach, *ed 2, vol 1, St. Louis, 1995, Mosby.)*

48 hours; however, hypertension and muscle spasms may recur for 12 to 24 hours.

Brown recluse spider bites

Brown recluse spiders, also known as fiddleback or violin spiders, have a light brown color with a dark brown fiddle-shaped mark that extends from the eyes down the back (Figure 43-6). These spiders are found in the southeastern, south central, and southwestern United States; however, they can appear anywhere in the country if the spider crawls into luggage or a car. They prefer dark areas such as basements, garages, closets, and boxes.

Venom is cytotoxic. Characteristic symptoms occur within minutes to several hours. A mild stinging occurs at the time of the bite and progresses to severe pain a few hours later. Local edema, a bluish ring around the bite, and a bleb develop. Erythema, local ischemia, and tissue necrosis appear on the third or fourth day. Eschar forms on the fourteenth day; however, the patient may have an open sore for days or even weeks. The wound should heal within 21 days. Systemic reactions rarely occur. If present, symptoms begin 24 to 48 hours after envenomation and include fever, chills, nausea, vomiting, weakness, general malaise, arthralgia, joint pain, and petechiae.

Management includes ice, elevation, and rest of the affected area. Consider antihistamines for itching. Systemic or local steroids may be used. Local debridement with skin grafting may be indicated. Recent studies have shown dapsone, a polymorphonuclear leukocyte inhibitor, to be highly effective in management of crater lesions in adults. The recommended oral dosage is 50 mg 2 times a day for 10 days.

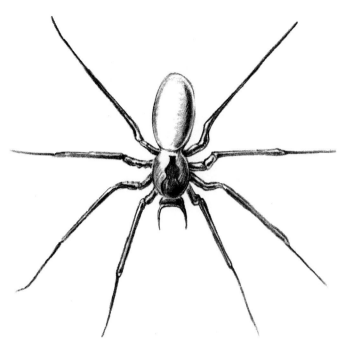

Figure **43-6** Brown recluse spider *(Loxosceles reclusa)* with typical dark violin-shaped marking on the cephalothorax. *(From Davis JH et al: Surgery: a problem solving approach, ed 2, vol 1, St. Louis, 1995, Mosby.)*

This drug should be used cautiously because of potential blood dyscrasias. Intolerance in patients with glucose-6-phosphate dehydrogenase (G6PD) deficiency has been reported; therefore, G6PD screening and complete blood count monitoring must accompany administration.

Scorpion Stings

Scorpions are found primarily in the warm southwestern states and exotic pet shops across the country. Stings occur most often in the early evening and night hours. Scorpions appear to sting in self-defense; they are not by nature aggressive creatures. There are several kinds of scorpions, but only one is considered lethal—*Centruroides sculpturatus,* also known as "bark scorpions" because they dwell in tree bark.

The tail of the scorpion contains a telson where venom is produced and stored. A stinger injects a neurotoxic venom, which produces immediate local pain at the sting site, edema, discoloration, hyperesthesia, numbness, and agitation. Drowsiness, itching, speech disturbances, tachycardia, hypertension, and tachypnea occur with extensive envenomation. Systemic reactions include wheezing, respiratory stridor, profuse salivation, visual disturbances, ataxic gait, incontinence, muscle spasms of the jaw muscles, nausea and vomiting, dysphagia, seizures, and anaphylaxis. Pain and numbness resolve without treatment in a few hours; however, systemic responses may last several days. Patients with severe envenomation may exhibit complicated neuromuscular and autonomic symptoms.

Support the ABCs. Apply ice or cool compresses to relieve pain. Immobilize the extremity to slow venom absorption. Antihistamines are indicated for some patients. Scorpion antivenin is available from the Antivenin Production Laboratories of Arizona State University; however, the antivenin is not approved by the Food and Drug Administration. The antivenin is effective only for stings from the *Centruroides exilcicauda* found in the United States. Specific antivenin for local species are available in other countries.

Hymenopteran Stings (Bee, Wasp, Hornet, and Fire Ant)

Hymenopterans are an insect family that includes the honeybee, wasp, hornet, and fire ant found in temperate regions. Stings are more common in the summer months. Hymenopteran venom varies among species and may be cytotoxic, hemolytic, allergenic, or vasoactive. Hymenopteran stings cause 40 to 150 deaths annually in the United States.

Hymenopteran stings cause a variety of reactions ranging from mild local reactions to anaphylactic shock depending on the type and amount of venom and the patient's sensitivity to the venom. Reactions can occur at the time of the sting and up to 48 hours later. Stings are usually cumulative. The greater the number of stings, the more severe the reaction. With the exception of the honeybee, most hymenopterans sting repeatedly. Fire ants have a painful sting that causes a wheal that expands to a large vesicle. The area then reddens, and a pustule forms. When the pustule is reabsorbed, crusting and scar formation occur.

Symptoms vary from mild stinging or burning sensations, swelling, and itching to severe local reactions such as edema of the entire extremity. The patient may also have severe systemic reactions, including urticaria, pruritus, edema, bronchospasm, laryngeal edema, and hypotension. Treatment begins with removal of the stinger to prevent absorption of the venom. Do not grasp or squeeze the stinger with tweezers, since this squeezes out more venom. Scrape the stinger away using a dull object such as the side of a credit card or needle. Further treatment is determined by the severity of the reaction. If the reaction is mild, minimal medications are required, usually oral antihistamines. If the reaction is severe, medications such as epinephrine may be required.

Tick Bites

Most tick bites are harmless; however, tick bites can cause Rocky Mountain spotted fever, Lyme borreliosis, and tick paralysis.[1] Regardless of the species and subsequent illness, principal management consists of tick removal followed by supportive therapy.

Rocky Mountain spotted fever

Rocky Mountain spotted fever is caused by *Rickettsia rickettsii.* Occurring across the country, the disease is most prevalent in the south Atlantic and south central states. Most cases have been reported when ticks are most active, from

April to September. Incubation period is 2 to 14 days. Major symptoms include fever, chills, malaise, myalgias, and headache. During the first 10 days, the patient develops a pink, macular, or petechial rash over the palms, wrists, hands, soles, feet, and ankles. However, the rash may involve any part of the body. Treatment includes antibiotic therapy.

Lyme disease

Lyme disease, the most widespread tick-borne disease, is transmitted via the *Ixodes* tick and caused by the spirochete *Borrelia burgdorferi*. Incubation is 3 to 32 days. In 1992, over 90% of reported cases occurred in the northeastern and midwestern states.[1] Most cases occur in the spring and summer.

Within days of the tick bite, symptoms develop in three distinct stages. During the first stage, erythema migrans, the patient experiences an expanding circular area of redness or rash at least 5 cm in diameter and flulike symptoms. This stage may last 2 months. Generally the rash disappears without treatment. The second stage occurs days to weeks after the tick bite. Patients may exhibit neurologic, cardiac, and musculoskeletal complications such as meningitis, hepatitis, cranial neuropathies, atrioventricular blocks, cardiomyopathies, and arthralgia. The third and final stage may last months or years. In this stage, the patient primarily manifests musculoskeletal and neurologic symptoms such as chronic arthritis and peripheral radiculoneuropathy. Lyme disease appears to respond to various medications; however, the most effective regimen remains controversial.

Tick paralysis

Tick paralysis is a neurotoxic disease transmitted by a bite from a female *Dermacentor andersoni* (wood tick) or *Dermacentor variabilis* (dog tick). Incubation is 5 to 7 days. Most cases occur in the southeastern and northwestern United States. Tick paralysis is primarily ascending motor paralysis occurring over 1 to 2 days. Symptoms include ataxia, lower extremity weakness progressing to upper extremities, paresthesia, decreased to absent reflexes, and eventually respiratory failure.

Treatment begins with tick removal. Gently grasp the tick with forceps at the point of entry, and pull upward in a steady motion. Other methods include covering the tick with alcohol, mineral oil, or petroleum jelly or killing the tick with ether or a hot match. Once the tick is removed, symptoms should gradually improve. Supportive care is necessary until symptoms resolve, usually within 48 to 72 hours.

SUMMARY

Environmental emergencies cover a broad spectrum of diseases arising from a variety of environmental factors. These emergencies can occur in any geographic area and at any time of the year. Morbidity and mortality are directly related to the magnitude and duration of the exposure, regard-

Box **43-8**

NURSING DIAGNOSES FOR ENVIRONMENTAL EMERGENCIES

Ineffective airway clearance
Impaired gas exchange
Altered tissue perfusion
Fluid volume deficit
Ineffective thermoregulation
Impaired skin integrity
Knowledge deficit

less of the source. Box 43-8 highlights nursing diagnoses for these patients. Prevention is the key to management of environmental emergencies. Those at greatest risk require information on protection against environmental dangers, use of good judgment, survival skills, and awareness of early signs and symptoms for specific emergencies.

REFERENCES

1. Gentile D: Tick-borne diseases. In Auerbach P, Geehr EC, editors: *Management of wilderness and environmental emergencies*, ed 3, St. Louis, 1995, Mosby.
2. Hector MG: Treatment of accidental hypothermia, *Am Fam Physician* 45(2):785, 1992.
3. Hodge D: Snake bites. In May HL, editor: *Emergency medicine*, ed 2, vol 2, Boston, 1992, Little, Brown.
4. Jerrard DA: Diving medicine, *Emerg Med Clin North Am* 10(2):329, 1992.
5. O'Connor N: Cold injuries. In May HL, editor: *Emergency medicine*, ed 2, vol 2, Boston, 1992, Little, Brown.
6. Soski JE: *Snakebite assessment and treatment in the eastern United States*, ed 2, Midway, Fla, 1994, Snakebite Publishing.
7. Strange G, Towns D: Environmental emergencies. In Strange GR et al, editors: *Pediatric emergency medicine: a comprehensive study guide*, New York, 1996, McGraw-Hill.
8. Thom SR, Keim LW: Carbon monoxide poisoning: a review of epidemiology, pathophysiology, clinical findings and treatment options including hyperbaric oxygen therapy, *Clin Toxicol* 27(141), 1989.
9. Uttrell PP: Care of the pediatric near-drowning victim, *Crit Care Nurs Clin North Am* 3(2):294, 1991.

SUGGESTED READING

Danz F, Ghezzi K: Hot tips on handling hypothermia, *Patient Care*, p 89, Dec 1991.
Kitt S, et al: *Emergency nursing: a physiologic and clinical perspective*, ed 2, Philadelphia, 1995, WB Saunders.
Saunders CE, Ho MT: *Current emergency diagnosis and treatment*, ed 4, Norwalk, Conn, 1992, Appleton & Lange.
Shields CP: Treatment of moderate-to-severe hypothermia in an urban setting, *Ann Emerg Med* 19(10):1093, 1990.
Stine R, Harding MH: Environmental emergencies. In Stine R, Chudnofsky CR, editors: *A practical approach to emergency medicine*, ed 2, Boston, 1994, Little, Brown.

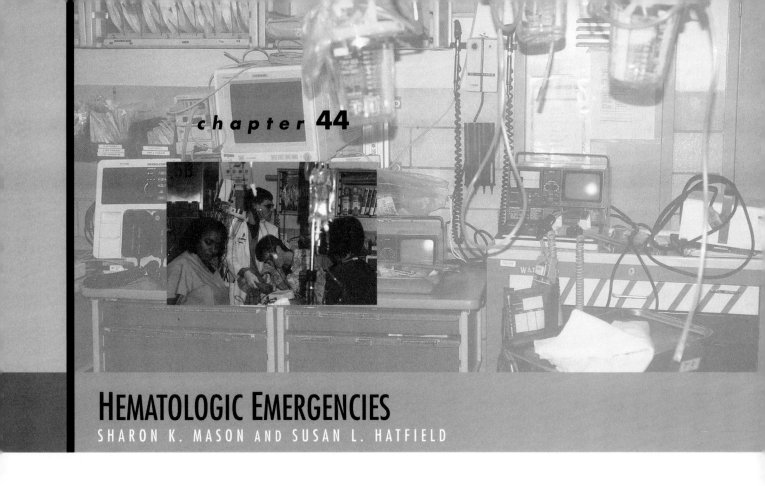

chapter 44

HEMATOLOGIC EMERGENCIES

SHARON K. MASON AND SUSAN L. HATFIELD

Hematologic emergencies may be the acute onset of a new condition or a sudden exacerbation of an existing disease. Knowledge of the disease process and astute assessment skills enhance the ability of the emergency nurse to care for individuals with a hematologic emergency. This chapter provides an overview of blood physiology, discusses general assessment of individuals with hematologic emergencies, and describes specific hematologic emergencies: anemia, hemophilia, sickle cell disease, disseminated intravascular coagulation (DIC), leukemia, and thrombocytopenia.

ANATOMY AND PHYSIOLOGY

Blood is a suspension of erythrocytes, leukocytes, platelets, and other particulate material in an aqueous colloid solution. It provides a medium for exchange between fixed cells in the body and the external environment. Nutrients such as oxygen are carried to each cell while cellular wastes such as nitrogen are removed. Other essential functions include regulation of pH, temperature, and cellular water; prevention of fluid loss through coagulation; and protection against toxins and foreign microbes. Table 44-1 summarizes the basic characteristics of blood.

Plasma

Plasma is a clear, yellow fluid containing blood cells, electrolytes, gases, amino acids, glucose, fats, and nonprotein nitrogens such as urea, creatine, and uric acid.[10] These and other substances may be dissolved in the plasma or may bind

with various plasma proteins for transport. Albumin is the major plasma protein. It maintains blood volume by providing colloid osmotic pressure, regulates pH and electrolyte balance, and transports substances such as drugs. Other major plasma proteins include globulins and fibrinogen.

Erythrocytes

Adults have approximately 5 million erythrocytes or red blood cells (RBCs) per microliter of blood. The number of RBCs is slightly higher in men. Natives living at altitudes greater than 14,000 feet may have as many as 7 million/μl. The primary role of RBCs is transport of oxygen and carbon dioxide. Erythrocytes have no nucleus and cannot reproduce. Their life span is only 120 days, so new cells must be constantly produced.[4] The normal rate of hematopoiesis, or RBC production, is 2 million RBCs per second. Production occurs in the bone marrow, but it is regulated by the kidneys. When oxygen levels drop, the kidneys release erythropoietin, which stimulates RBC production by the bone marrow. Reticulocytes are an erythrocyte precursor that mature within 24 to 48 hours of release into the circulation. Increased reticulocytes indicate increased bone marrow activity.

Erythrocytes are soft pliable cells that change shape easily, thereby increasing the cell's oxygen-carrying capability by increasing its surface area. The outer stroma of the cell contains antigens A, B, and Rh factor. The inner stroma contains hemoglobin, the primary vehicle for oxygen transport. Hemoglobin molecules are so small that they would leak across the blood vessel's endothelial membrane if left floating free in the plasma. There are 300 different types of genetically determined hemoglobin. With the exception of Hb F, Hb A, and Hb S, hemoglobins are identified by sequential letters of the alphabet. Abnormal hemoglobin molecules are produced in response to molecular abnormalities within blood. Tests such as hemoglobin electrophoresis are used to differentiate normal and abnormal hemoglobin. The most common hemoglobins are described in Table 44-2.

Red cell indices provide information about the size and weight of average red cells and are used in diagnosis differentiation of acute and chronic anemias (Table 44-3). Mean corpuscular volume (MCV), mean corpuscular hemoglobin (MCH), and mean corpuscular hemoglobin concentration (MCHC) values provide information on how well the red cells function.

Erythrocyte sedimentation rate (ESR) measures the time required for erythrocytes in a whole blood specimen to settle to the bottom of a vertical tube. ESR is a product of red cell volume, surface area, density, aggregation, and surface charge.[2] Increased ESR occurs with widespread inflammation, red cell aggregation, pregnancy, and some malignancies, whereas polycythemia, sickle cell disease, and decreased plasma proteins are associated with decreased ESR.

Leukocytes

The body's primary defense against infection is leukocytes, or white blood cells (WBCs). Six types of leukocytes normally occur in the blood: neutrophils, eosinophils, basophils, monocytes, lymphocytes, and occasionally plasma cells (Table 44-4).[7] The WBC count quantifies the total number of leukocytes in the circulation. The WBC differential count quantifies the percentage of each type. This count is based on 100 WBCs; therefore a differential count should always total 100%. The ratio of RBCs to WBCs is 700:1.

Neutrophils

Neutrophils are the primary defense against bacterial infection. Bone marrow contains a reserve approximately 10 times greater than daily neutrophil production. About one half of all mature neutrophils adhere to the vessel walls and are not measured by the traditional WBC count. The bone marrow reserve and the number of neutrophils on vessel walls account for sudden increases in the WBC count in response to stress or infection. Once released into the circulation, neutrophils live 4 to 8 hours. Immature neutrophils are called bands, and mature neutrophils are called polymorphonuclear neutrophil leukocytes. An increased number of bands indicates acute infection.

Eosinophils

Eosinophils accumulate at the site of allergic reactions. Increases also occur during asthma attacks, drug reactions, and parasitic infections. Eosinophils decrease in response to stressors such as trauma, shock, or burns. Cell half-life is approximately 4.5 to 5 hours after release into the circulation.

Basophils

Basophils contain histamine, heparin, bradykinin, serotonin, and lysosomal enzymes. During allergic reactions, basophils rupture and release these substances into surrounding tissue. This accounts for many of the typical manifestations of an allergic reaction. Numbers also increase in chronic inflammation and during times of stress.

Monocytes

Monocytes remain in the circulation less than 20 hours before moving into surrounding tissue to become macrophages. A macrophage acts as a "garbage collector," consuming bacteria and other debris in areas such as the spleen, lungs, and lymph nodes. Macrophages can live for months

Table **44-2**	**Types of Hemoglobin**
Type	Significance/occurrence
Hb A	92% adult hemoglobin
Hb A$_{1c}$	5% adult hemoglobin
Hb A$_2$	2% adult hemoglobin
Hb F	Fetal hemoglobin, thalassemia after 6 months
Hb C	Hemolytic anemia
Hb S	Sickle cell anemia
Hb M	Methemoglobinemia

Table **44-1**	**Characteristics of Blood**
Characteristic	Description/value
Color	
Arterial	Bright red
Venous	Dark red
pH	
Arterial	7.35-7.45
Venous	7.31-7.41
Specific gravity	
Plasma	1.026
RBCs	1.093
Viscosity	3.5-4.5 times thicker than water
Volume	5.5 L in the average adult

Table **44-3**	**Red Cell Indices in Adults**	
Component	Description	Normal value
MCV	Ratio of hematocrit (packed cell volume) to RBC count	80-95 μm^3
MCH	Hemoglobin/RBC ratio; gives weight of hemoglobin in average red cell	27-31 pg
MCHC	Ratio of hemoglobin weight to hematocrit; defines volume of hemoglobin in average red cell	32-36 g/dl

Table 44-4   Leukocytes: Functions and Characteristics

Name	Percent of total WBCs	Function	Circulatory life span
Neutrophils	62.0	Attack and destroy bacteria and viruses through phagocytosis	4-8 hr
Eosinophils	2.3	Attach to surface of parasites, then release substances that kill the organism; detoxify inflammatory substances that occur in allergic reactions	4-8 hr
Basophils	0.4	Prevent coagulation and speed fat removal from blood after a fatty meal	4-8 hr
Monocytes	5.3	Consume bacteria, viruses, necrotic tissue, and other foreign material	10-20 hr
Lymphocytes	30.0	Provide immunity against acquired infections; basis for antibody formation	2-3 hr
Plasma cells	—	Produce γ-globulin antibodies in response to specific antigens	Varies with need for antibodies

or even years. Monocytes are the body's second line of defense and are usually associated with chronic infection.

Lymphocytes

Lymphocytes play a major role in immunity against acquired infections. Their life span may be weeks, months, or even years, depending on the body's needs. Two types of lymphocytes provide essential protection against bacteria and viruses. B-cell lymphocytes become antibodies and are responsible for humoral immunity. T-cell lymphocytes are responsible for cell-mediated immunity. At least three major types of T-cell lymphocytes have been identified thus far: helper T cells, cytotoxic T cells, and suppressor T cells (Table 44-5).[4] Lymphocyte increases are associated with viral infection.

Plasma cells

Plasma cells produce γ-globulin antibodies in response to a specific antigen. Production continues until the plasma cells die from exhaustion days or even weeks later.

Platelets

Platelets, or thrombocytes, provide hemostasis at the site of injury. These granular, disk-shaped fragments form when a parent cell breaks into thousands of cell fragments. The parent cell has no nucleus, so it cannot divide. Platelet life span is 9 to 12 days. Approximately one third of the body's platelets are stored in the spleen as a reserve. Clotting factors V, VIII, and IX are found on the platelet's surface. Platelets provide hemostasis by clumping at the site of injury to form a platelet plug and seal bleeding capillaries. Substances such as ethanol and salicylates interfere with platelet aggregation by impairing their ability to clump. Decreased platelet aggregation leads to increased bleeding.

Hemostasis

Hemostasis refers to processes that prevent blood loss after vascular damage, that is, vascular spasm, platelet aggregation, coagulation, and fibrinolysis. When injury occurs,

Table 44-5   Types of T-Cell Lymphocytes

Name	Function
Helper T cells	Regulate immune functions by forming lymphokines or protein mediators such as interleukin and interferon; inactivated or destroyed by AIDS virus
Cytotoxic T cells	Also called killer T cells; capable of direct attack on microorganisms as well as the body's own cells; role in destroying cancer cells and heart transplant cells
Suppressor T cells	Protect from attack by the person's own immune system; suppress helper and cytotoxic T-cell functions

the initial response is reflex vasoconstriction. Arterioles contract, decreasing blood flow by decreasing vessel size and pressing endothelial surfaces together. Next, serotonin and histamine release cause immediate vasoconstriction and decrease blood flow to the injured area.[9] Vasoconstriction is followed by platelet aggregation at the injury site. This temporary measure prevents bleeding by sealing capillaries.

Platelet aggregation is followed by clot formation, which requires activation of the coagulation cascade (Figure 44-1). The coagulation cascade is a complex network of 12 different clotting factors (Table 44-6). A defect of any clotting factor or an injury that overwhelms the entire system can cause failure of the coagulation cascade and lead to life- or limb-threatening hemorrhage. The cascade may be activated by intrinsic factors, such as damage to a vessel wall, or extrinsic factors, such as damage to surrounding tissue. Regardless of the method of activation, the end result of the coagulation cascade is formation of a clot—a protein mesh made of fibrin strands.

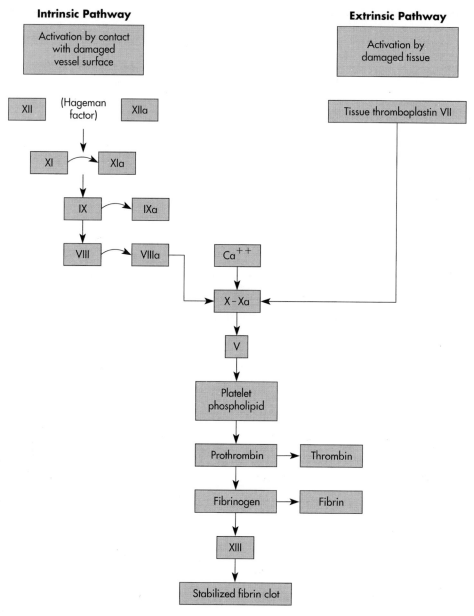

Intrinsic Pathway

Activation by contact with damaged vessel surface

Extrinsic Pathway

Activation by damaged tissue

XII   (Hageman factor)   XIIa

Tissue thromboplastin VII

XI → XIa

IX → IXa

VIII → VIIIa   Ca^{++}

X - Xa

V

Platelet phospholipid

Prothrombin → Thrombin

Fibrinogen → Fibrin

XIII

Stabilized fibrin clot

Figure **44-1** The coagulation cascade. *(From Huether SE, McCance KL:* Understanding pathophysiology, *St. Louis, 1996, Mosby.)*

The final step in hemostasis is clot resolution via the fibrinolytic system. Clot resolution maintains blood in a fluid state by removing clots that are no longer needed (Figure 44-2). Without this system, circulation to affected areas may be permanently lost because of obstructed blood vessels.

PATIENT ASSESSMENT

The type and severity of hematologic emergency depend on the individual's situation. Assessment is often complicated by vague complaints, for example, fatigue, headache, fever, syncope, and dyspnea on exertion. Therefore it is important to observe the patient for clues to hematologic problems, such as pale, jaundiced, or cyanotic skin. Ecchymosis,

purpura, petechia, and ulcerations may also be present. Evaluate skin for temperature, diaphoresis, warmth, coolness, texture, and turgor. Observe for joint deformity, edema, redness, limitation of movement, and difficulty or inability to ambulate. Obtain vital signs, including orthostatic blood pressure and pulse.

Note new onset of fever, weakness, cough, rash, dyspnea, and increased or unusual bruising. Does the patient complain of spontaneous bleeding, such as epistaxis or menorrhagia? Are bleeding gums, hematemesis, melena, dark urine, or hemoptysis present? These symptoms suggest a hematologic problem and indicate the need for more detailed evaluation.

Table **44-6**	**Coagulation Factors**	
Factor	Synonyms	Description/function
I	Fibrinogen	Fibrin precursor
II	Prothrombin	Thrombin precursor
III	Tissue thromboplastin	Activates prothrombin
IV	Calcium	Essential for prothrombin activation and fibrin formation
V	Labile factor, proaccelerin	Accelerates conversion of prothrombin to thrombin
VII	Prothrombin conversion accelerator	Accelerates conversion of prothrombin to thrombin
VIII	Antihemophilic factor A (AHF)	Associated with factors IX, XI, and XII; essential for thromboplastin formation
IX	Christmas factor, antihemophilic factor B	Associated with factors VIII, XI, and XII; essential for thromboplastin formation
X	Thrombokinase factor, Stuart-Prower factor	Triggers prothrombin conversion; requires vitamin K
XI	Plasma thromboplastin antecedent, antihemophilic factor C	Formation of thromboplastin in association with factors VIII, IX, and XII
XII	Contact factor, Hageman factor	Activates factor XI in thromboplastin formation
XIII	Fibrin stabilizing factor	Strengthens fibrin clot

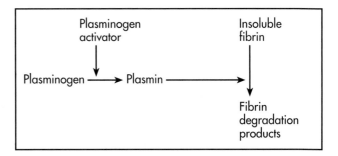

Figure **44-2** Fibrinolysis system.

uterine rupture. Response to blood loss depends on the patient's age, physical condition, and rapidity of blood loss. Signs and symptoms include cool, clammy skin, tachycardia, decreased blood pressure, narrowing pulse pressure, tachypnea, postural hypotension, and decreased urinary output. Thirst and complaints of "feeling cold" are early clues to acute blood loss. A decreased level of consciousness may also occur.

Treatment begins with stabilization of the patient's airway, breathing, and circulation (ABCs). Large-bore intravenous catheters and fluid resuscitation with normal saline or lactated Ringer's solution are used for volume replacement. Initial laboratory studies include complete blood count (CBC), type and crossmatch, prothrombin time (PT), partial thromboplastin time (PTT), and serum electrolytes. Supplemental oxygen is indicated because these patients have lost a source of oxygen. Blood replacement therapy may be necessary in severe anemia.

Other causes of anemia include sickle cell disease, massive burns, DIC, toxins, infections, ABO incompatibility, transfusion reactions, carbon monoxide poisoning, and medications. Sickle cell disease and DIC are discussed later in this chapter.

Chronic anemia

Chronic anemia is not considered life-threatening, has an insidious onset, and is often diagnosed prior to the emergency department (ED) visit. Patients complain of fatigue, headache, irritability, dizziness, and shortness of breath. Diagnosis is made by clinical assessment, history, and laboratory analysis, including a CBC with leukocyte differential, RBC indices, peripheral smear, and reticulocyte count. Patients are usually treated as outpatients unless they have acute shortness of breath, chest pain, severe dizziness, or altered level of consciousness.

Diminished RBC production occurs in iron deficiency anemia, thalassemia, lead poisoning, vitamin B_{12} deficiency, chronic liver disease, and hypothyroidism.[6] Decreased bone marrow production causes aplastic anemia. Other causes include increased destruction of RBCs due to enzyme defects (e.g., glucose-6-phosphate dehydrogenase deficiency), cell membrane abnormalities, or abnormalities of the hemoglobin molecule (e.g., sickle cell disease).

Identify existing hematologic diseases as well as family history of hematologic diseases. Obtain medication history, including the use of prescription and over-the-counter medications. Document allergies, exposure to toxic substances, and dietary history.

SPECIFIC HEMATOLOGIC EMERGENCIES
Anemia

Anemia is a reduction in the total number of RBCs or a deficiency in the cells' ability to transport oxygen. Anemia may be acute or chronic. Severity depends on the patient's ability to compensate for RBC loss and provide essential oxygen to the cells. Oxygenation depends on blood flow as well as hemoglobin's oxygen-carrying capacity and affinity for oxygen. A defect in any of these factors affects cellular oxygen.

Acute anemia

Acute anemia is usually due to blood loss. Causes include trauma, gastrointestinal hemorrhage, vaginal bleeding, and

Hemophilia

Hemophilia refers to a number of clotting disorders including hemophilia A, hemophilia B, and von Willebrand's disease.[5] Hemophilia is an inherited, sex-linked disorder that occurs almost always in males. Females carry the disease and pass it on to their children. Severity ranges from mild to severe. The primary defect in hemophilia is absence or dysfunction of a specific clotting factor.

Hemophilia A, or classic hemophilia, is due to a factor VIII disorder. In the majority of patients with hemophilia A, factor VIII is not missing. It may even be present in excess quantities; however, available factor VIII does not function adequately. Disease severity is directly related to the functional activity of factor VIII.

Hemophilia B, or Christmas disease, occurs less often than hemophilia A. It is caused by the absence or functional deficiency of factor IX.

Von Willebrand's disease is usually less acute than hemophilia A or B and occurs in both sexes. The specific coagulation defect in this type of hemophilia is defective platelet adherence and decreased levels of factor VIII.

Hemophilia A and hemophilia B have similar clinical presentations. Patients with von Willebrand's disease exhibit less severe symptoms, with a lower incidence of bleeding into joints and deeper tissues. When a patient has hemophilia, even minor trauma can cause major bruises, visceral bleeding, and subdural hematomas. With the exception of lacerations or major trauma, one of the worst features of hemophilia is hemarthrosis—bleeding into a joint. Hemarthrosis usually begins in adolescence and involves primarily the knees, ankles, and elbows. Patients almost always come to the ED because of severe pain associated with hemarthrosis rather than actual bleeding. Improperly managed hemarthrosis can lead to arthritis and ultimately joint destruction. Platelet-mediated hemostasis does not depend on factor VIII or factor IX; therefore the affected extremity should be elevated whenever possible. Identification of the specific type of hemophilia is crucial because hemophilia A and hemophilia B present the same clinical picture but require treatment with different clotting factors. A bleeding history should be obtained from all patients with abnormal bleeding. A screening coagulation panel should also be considered.

Fresh frozen plasma (FFP) has been used to treat hemophilia A and von Willebrand's disease. Unfortunately, FFP contains relatively small amounts of factor VIII per unit of volume, so large quantities are required for successful treatment. Cryoprecipitate is rich in factor VIII per unit of volume; however, it has been associated with transmission of hepatitis and the human immunodeficiency virus (HIV). Fortunately, recent product modifications have reduced this transmission risk and are also less expensive. Antibody-purified factor IX is the treatment for hemophilia B patients with limited prior exposure to cryoprecipitate who are HIV negative. Mild to moderate bleeding may be treated with FFP.

Sickle Cell Disease

Sickle cell disease is a genetically determined, inherited disorder that occurs in approximately 1 in 500 black Americans. RBCs contain Hb S, an abnormal hemoglobin that precipitates into long crystals when exposed to low oxygen concentrations. The resulting sickle shape of the cell gives the disorder its name. Sickle cell anemia occurs in persons whose parents have the Hb S gene. If only one parent has the Hb S gene, the offspring can have sickle cell trait and may pass the gene to their offspring. Hemoglobin electrophoresis shows a predominance of Hb S, variable amounts of Hb F, and no Hb A. In a person with sickle cell trait, Hb S and Hb A are both present.

As cells become hypoxic and sickling occurs, the cells clump in various parts of the body. The resulting ischemia causes a painful sickle cell crisis, occurring most often in long bones, large joints, and the spine. It may be precipitated by exposure to cold, infection, or acidosis. Prolonged ischemia leads to local tissue necrosis. Priapism may occur in males if sickling prevents exit of blood from the penis following normal erection. Treatment includes analgesia, oxygen, hydration with intravenous solutions, treatment of existing infections, local heat, and folic acid supplements.

Individuals with sickle cell disease rarely survive adolescence because of various physiologic sequelae and complications of their disease. These patients develop hepatomegaly, hepatic infarctions, and jaundice. There is a high risk for pneumonia, meningitis, salmonellosis, osteomyelitis, pulmonary emboli, cor pulmonale, and chronic skin ulcers. Complications include recurrent sickle cell crisis, hemolytic anemia, transient aplastic crisis, cholelithiasis, cholecystitis, delayed sexual maturation, renal disease, bone disease, cardiac failure, and autosplenectomy. There is also a high incidence of spontaneous abortion, prenatal mortality, and maternal mortality.

Disseminated Intravascular Coagulation

Disseminated intravascular coagulation (DIC) involves simultaneous clotting and bleeding. Associated conditions include infection, neoplasm, obstetric complications, thrombosis, trauma, hypoxia, and liver disease. In DIC, activation of the coagulation cascade leads to accelerated clotting, which triggers thrombosis as excessive fibrin is released in the circulation, especially in the small vessels. As coagulation continues at this accelerated rate, the fibrinolysis system also functions at an accelerated rate. Consequently platelets, clotting factors, and fibrinogen are consumed faster than the body can replace them. As the system becomes overwhelmed, simultaneous hemorrhage and clotting occur.

Patients with DIC may have acute bleeding or gradual blood loss, including epistaxis, hemoptysis, bleeding gums, menorrhagia, ecchymosis, purpura, and hematuria. Other signs associated with DIC are cough, dyspnea, confusion, fever, tachypnea, and cyanosis. Diagnostic laboratory studies include PT, PTT, fibrinogen levels, platelet levels, and fibrin split products.

Treatment focuses initially on the precipitating condition. Once that problem is controlled, the next step is restoration of depleted coagulation factors. Platelets, FFP, and cryoprecipitate are recommended. Heparin therapy is contraindicated in some types of DIC but is used when there is evidence of organ damage or loss of life or limb is imminent. PTT cannot be used to evaluate effectiveness of heparin therapy, since DIC is characterized by prolonged PTT. Fibrinogen levels are used to monitor effectiveness of heparin therapy. Hirudin therapy is considered experimental. Fluid replacement is used to maintain circulation, restore blood pressure, and ensure urinary output. The clinical picture of DIC can be further complicated by the development of renal failure, shock, cardiac tamponade, hemothorax, and gangrene.

Leukemia

Leukemia is a malignant disorder of blood and blood-forming organs characterized by excessive abnormal growth of leukocyte precursors in the bone marrow. An uncontrolled increase in immature leukocytes decreases the production and function of normal leukocytes.

Leukemia is classified as lymphogenous or myelogenous. Lymphogenous leukemias are caused by cancerous production of lymphoid cells, whereas myelogenous leukemias begin as cancerous growth of myelogenous cells in the bone marrow. Both types may be acute or chronic. Acute leukemia has an abrupt, rapid onset and is characterized by a massive number of immature leukocytes. Life expectancy for these patients may be as short as 6 months; however, life expectancy for all types of leukemia has increased. Chronic leukemia has a slower disease progression with longer life expectancy.

Regardless of type, leukemic cells invade the spleen, lymph nodes, liver, and other vascular regions. Clinical manifestations include fatigue, fever, and weight loss. The patient may also complain of bone pain. Elevated uric acid levels, lymph node enlargement, hepatomegaly, and splenomegaly are usually present. Neurologic findings include headache, vomiting, papilledema, and blurred vision.

Treatment includes chemotherapy, immunotherapy, and bone marrow transplants. Blood transfusions, antibiotics, antifungal agents, and antiviral agents are also used. These patients are at risk for infection as a result of their disease and their treatment; therefore, it is important to protect them against infection.

Thrombocytopenia

Normal platelet count is 150,000 to 450,000/µl. Thromobytopenia is an abnormal decrease in the number of platelets. The platelet count is affected by menses, nutrition, and severe deficiencies in iron, folic acid, or vitamin B_{12}. In-

Box **44-1**

NURSING DIAGNOSES FOR HEMATOLOGIC EMERGENCIES

Fluid volume deficit (actual or potential)
Altered tissue perfusion
Pain
Knowledge deficit
Potential for injury
Anxiety

fectious disorders (sepsis), tumors, medications (acetylsalicylic acid), and bleeding can also affect the platelet count.

Thrombocytopenia may be secondary to congenital or acquired disorders such as decreased bone marrow production, increased splenic sequestration, or accelerated destruction of platelets.[1] Idiopathic thrombocytopenic purpura (ITP), the most common form of thrombocytopenia, is an acquired disease caused by increased platelet destruction. Immune complexes containing viral antigens bind to iron receptors on the platelets, or antibodies produced against viral antigens react with the platelets.[1]

Acute ITP usually occurs in children several weeks after a viral infection such as rubella, rubeola, or chickenpox. It can also follow immunizations for these same viruses. Acute ITP occurs equally in males and females, is self-limiting, and resolves spontaneously within 6 months. Peak incidence is between the ages of 2 and 4 years.

Bruising and petechiae are considered universal presenting symptoms for ITP. Patients may also present with purpura, epistaxis, bleeding gums, gastrointestinal bleeding, and hematuria. A small percentage of the patients may have severe manifestations such as massive purpura, profuse epistaxis, and retinal hemorrhage. Differential diagnosis is based on clinical findings of isolated thrombocytopenia without evidence of another hematologic disorder. Bone marrow aspiration is used to rule out acute leukemia.

Observation may be all that is needed for acute ITP. Glucocorticoids are given if conservative measures prove ineffective. Intravenous immune globulins are used to rapidly increase the platelet count. Splenectomy is only recommended for children with severe bleeding symptoms related to their thrombocytopenia. In rare cases, plasmapheresis may be required.

SUMMARY

Hematologic emergencies cover an array of clinical conditions and represent a broad spectrum of patient acuity. Prioritization of patient care is essential to ensure optimal patient outcome. Box 44-1 identifies the most critical nursing diagnoses for the patient with a hematologic emergency.

REFERENCES

1. Alspach JG: *Instructors resource manual for the AACN core curriculum for critical care nursing teaching manual,* Philadelphia, 1992, WB Saunders.

2. Beutler E et al: *Williams hematology,* ed 5, New York, 1995, McGraw-Hill.

3. Erslew AJ, Gabusda TG: *Pathophysiology of blood,* ed 3, Philadelphia, 1985, WB Saunders.

4. Guyton AC, Hall JE: *Textbook of medical physiology,* ed 9, Philadelphia, 1996, WB Saunders.

5. Hoffbrand AV, Pettit JE: *Essential hematology,* ed 2, London, 1993, Blackwell Scientific Publications.

6. Isselbacher KJ et al: *Harrison's principles of internal medicine,* ed 13, vol 2, New York, 1994, McGraw-Hill.

7. Kitt S et al: *Emergency nursing: a physiologic and clinical perspective,* ed 2, Philadelphia, 1995, WB Saunders.

8. Kjeldsberg C et al: *Practical diagnosis of hematologic disorders,* 1989, ASCP Press.

9. McCance KL, Heuther SE: *Pathophysiology: the biologic basis for disease in adults and children,* ed 2, St. Louis, 1994, Mosby.

10. Rippe JM, et al: *Intensive care medicine,* ed 3, vol 1, Boston, 1996, Little, Brown.

11. Wyllie-Kajs M: Thrombotic thrombocytopenic purpura: pathophysiology, treatment, and related nursing care, *Crit Care Nurse,* 15(6):44, 1995.

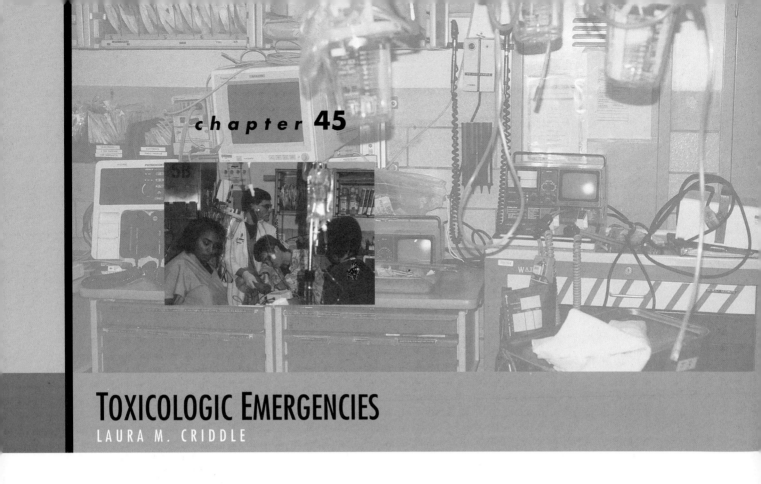

chapter **45**

TOXICOLOGIC EMERGENCIES

LAURA M. CRIDDLE

Toxic agents are manufactured or naturally occurring chemicals that have deleterious effects on humans. Toxins can enter the body through ingestion, inhalation, injection, ocular exposure, or dermal contact. The quantity of toxin required to produce symptoms varies widely among substances. Exposure may be accidental or intentional, related to recreation or occupation.

Management of the poisoned patient involves continued respiratory and hemodynamic support, careful assessment of toxicosis potential, interventions to reduce toxin absorption and promote excretion, and substance-specific therapy. An overview of assessment and management of the patient with a toxicologic emergency is followed by discussion of specific toxins.

PATIENT MANAGEMENT

Determining the precise agent or agents involved in a toxicologic emergency can be a daunting task because of the vast number of potentially toxic substances. Poison control centers are an excellent resource for information on various substances, potential toxicity, and patient management. Poison control centers, located across the nation, provide professionals and the public with 24-hour telephone advice on poisons.

Symptoms of toxic exposures range from subtle to dramatic and vary widely with the causative agent, dose, and extent of exposure. Toxins can affect every tissue in the body; therefore, effects can be seen in any body system (Table 45-1).

Assess the patient carefully. Obtain a detailed history from the patient, family, or prehospital care providers. Table 45-2 describes essential assessment information related to toxic exposure.

General Interventions

Stabilization of the airway, breathing, and circulation is the first priority when caring for an individual with a toxicologic emergency. Protect the airway, ensure adequate oxygenation and ventilation, and support the cardiovascular system while attempting to identify the specific toxin involved. Interventions may be as simple as positioning the patient, providing supplemental oxygen, and administering oral fluids. More significant exposures may require endotracheal intubation, mechanical ventilation, and vasoactive medications.

Significant substance-to-substance variations in toxicologic management exist; however, the need to ensure patient safety and provide psychologic support is common to all toxicologic emergencies (Table 45-3). Beyond issues of safety and psychologic support, medical management focuses on reduction of toxin absorption, enhanced drug elimination, and toxin-specific interventions (Box 45-1).

Reduce absorption

Options to reduce toxin absorption include emesis, gastric lavage, activated charcoal, dermal cleansing, and eye irrigation.[9] Specific interventions are determined by patient condition and the specific toxin.

Table **45-1**	**Potential Systemic Effects of Toxic Substances**
System	Potential effects
Neurologic	Altered level of consciousness, abnormal pupillary response, euphoria, depression, confusion, coma, hallucinations, agitation, violence, seizures
Pulmonary	Hyperventilation, hypoventilation, acid-base disturbances
Cardiovascular	Tachycardia, bradycardia, dysrhythmias, conduction abnormalities, decreased cardiac output, altered contractility, blood pressure instability
Gastrointestinal	Nausea, vomiting, diarrhea, abnormal liver function, coagulopathies
Renal/genitourinary	Renal failure, electrolyte disturbances

Induced emesis

Emesis is induced with syrup of ipecac, which causes gastric irritation and stimulates the emesis center in the brain.[10] Once the mainstay of poison management, ipecac has become increasingly less popular over the past decade. Ipecac is most useful when administered within 1 hour of oral toxin ingestion. The average adult dose is 15 to 45 ml followed by 250 to 500 ml of water. Emesis should occur within 20 minutes. Ipecac is not recommended in infants less than 6 months old.

There is a low overall rate of drug return with induced vomiting. Ipecac is not effective with drugs that are rapidly absorbed, such as alcohol. Ipecac has a delayed, unpredictable onset of action, so a repeat dose may be required for effective emesis. Violent, protracted vomiting caused by ipecac predisposes the patient to fluid loss, acid-base abnormalities, electrolyte disturbances, and Mallory-Weiss tears. Prolonged emesis, altered level of consciousness, and seizures place the patient at risk for aspiration; therefore ipecac should not be used in these situations. Use of ipecac for hydrocarbon or caustic ingestions places the patient at risk for oral, upper airway, and pulmonary injury.

Gastric lavage

Gastric lavage is used when gastric emptying is desirable but ipecac has failed or is contraindicated. As with induced emesis, gastric lavage produces the best results when performed as soon as possible after toxin ingestion. Place the patient in a left lateral position or elevate the head of the bed 30 to 45 degrees to decrease risk of aspiration. When the patient has a diminished gag reflex, protect the airway with endotracheal intubation prior to lavage. Monitor for bradycardia secondary to vagal stimulation. Insert a large-diameter

Table **45-2**	**Essential Assessment Information for Toxic Exposure**
Item	Description
Substance	Visually confirm medication involved. Family may say the patient ingested acetaminophen when the patient actually consumed salicylates. Ask what medications the patient takes at home.
Time of exposure	Time since exposure determines symptoms and treatment.
Acute or chronic	Acute exposures have different presenting symptoms and are managed differently than chronic exposures.
Amount of toxin	Determine maximal quantity possible. Count pills in the bottle, and confirm when prescription was filled.
Signs and symptoms	Assess for symptoms in all systems. Toxins can affect every tissue in the body.
Prior treatment	Assess for interventions from laypersons and prehospital personnel. Some home remedies can be detrimental.
Intentional or accidental	Poisoning is a popular form of suicide and suicidal gesture. Have there been previous suicide attempts? Does the patient have a history of depression or pre-existing mental health problem? Homicide may involve poisoning.

Table **45-3**	**Safety and Support in Toxic Emergencies**
Action	Discussion
Maintain patient safety	Individuals with an altered level of consciousness are predisposed to injury. Patients with intentional overdose or chronic substance abuse have an increased risk of self-destructive behavior.
Protect others	Confusion, agitation, aggressiveness, and violent behavior place others at risk for injury.
Support the patient and family	Provide basic emotional care, psychiatric intervention, referral to substance abuse programs, and information on self-help groups.

Box 45-1   Medical Management of Toxic Exposures

Reduce absorption

Induced emesis
Gastric lavage
Activated charcoal
Dermal decontamination
Ocular decontamination

Enhance elimination

Cathartic administration
Whole-bowel irrigation
Repeat-dose activated charcoal
Forced diuresis
Hemodialysis and hemoperfusion

Substance-specific interventions

Antidotes
Alkalinization

Box 45-2   Substances Effectively Absorbed by Charcoal

Alcohol	Nicotine
Antimony	Opium
Arsenic	Organophosphates
Atropine	Penicillin
Barbiturates	Phenol
Camphor	Phenothiazine
Chloroquine	Phenytoin
Chlorpheniramine	Primaquine
Cocaine	Probenecid
Colchicine	Propoxyphene
Dextroamphetamine	Quinacrine
Digitalis	Quinidine
Glutethimide	Quinine
Iodine	Salicylic acid
Ipecac	Selenium
Meprobamate	Silver
Mercuric chloride	Strychnine
Methyl salicylate	Sulfonamides
Morphine	Tricyclic antidepressants

From Rosen P et al: *Emergency medicine: concepts and clinical practice,* ed 2, vol 1, St. Louis, 1988, Mosby.

(36F to 40F) orogastric tube, using a bite-block to prevent the patient from occluding the tube. Repeatedly instill and remove 200- to 250-ml aliquots of normal saline until the return is clear. An adult may require 5 to 10 L. Administer 10 to 15 ml/kg in 50-ml boluses through a 24F to 28F tube for pediatric patients.[13]

Lavage is contraindicated in patients with caustic ingestions because of the potential for further injury as the caustic agent is removed. When large amounts of solution are required, serious fluid, electrolyte, and acid-base imbalances can occur. Other adverse effects include epistaxis, esophageal perforation, and aspiration. Lavage does not always remove all pill fragments. Only a small percentage of ingested material is retrieved through gastric lavage; even the largest tube cannot accommodate pill clumps or extremely large pill fragments. Another problem with gastric lavage is that fluid boluses can force pill fragments through the pylorus into the small intestine.

Activated charcoal

Activated charcoal appears to be the single most important therapeutic intervention for management of most toxic ingestions. Charcoal exposed to high temperatures has a dramatic increase in surface area, so particles can bind many times their weight in toxins. Binding prevents absorption into the portal circulation, so toxins can be eliminated in the feces.

Given orally or through a gastric tube in doses of 50 to 100 g for adults (1 g/kg for children), activated charcoal readily absorbs most poisons except heavy metals and toxic alcohols (Box 45-2). Some authors suggest administration of activated charcoal prior to gastric emptying, especially when more than 2 hours has elapsed since ingestion. Gastric emptying is associated with significant risks and a low rate of return, which becomes even less effective as time passes. Conversely, activated charcoal can still absorb toxins in the

intestines. Contraindications to charcoal administration are patients with diminished bowel sounds, ileus, or ingestion of a substance poorly absorbed by charcoal. Charcoal is not used when *N*-acetylcysteine (NAC) has been given because charcoal binds with and inactivates NAC. Adverse effects of activated charcoal include nausea, vomiting, gastrointestinal obstruction, and pulmonary aspiration.

Dermal decontamination

Dermal decontamination is indicated with dermal exposure of any toxin. Remove contaminated clothing and jewelry as soon as possible, and flush areas of contact for 10 to 15 minutes with copious amounts of water. Brush dry substances from the body prior to washing. Neutralizing agents should not be administered because the subsequent reaction produces heat and increases tissue damage. Depending on the substance and amount, the clothing and irrigant may be considered hazardous waste. Individuals with dermal toxic exposure also represent a risk to others, so health care workers should wear protective clothing (gloves, gowns, and goggles) to avoid secondary exposure.

Ocular decontamination

Ocular decontamination involves vigorous eye irrigation with copious amounts of normal saline. Prolonged flushing may be necessary with caustic substances, particularly alkalines. An ophthalmologist should be consulted if ocular complaints persist after irrigation. Refer to Chapter 48 for discussion of eye irrigation and ocular burns.

Enhance elimination

Techniques to enhance toxin elimination include cathartic administration, whole-bowel irrigation, repeat-dose activated charcoal, forced diuresis, hemodialysis, charcoal hemoperfusion, oxygen inhalation, surgical removal, and chelating agents.

Cathartic administration. Cathartic administration involves administration of sorbitol, magnesium citrate, or magnesium sulfate along with activated charcoal to enhance elimination of ingested toxins by stimulating intestinal motility. Without concomitant use of a cathartic, charcoal tends to cause constipation, which leaves charcoal and toxins in the gut and creates the potential for unbinding and systemic toxin absorption. Cathartics are contraindicated in corrosive ingestion and when vomiting, diarrhea, or an ileus is present. Multiple doses of cathartic agents should be avoided, since the subsequent diarrhea has been associated with fatal electrolyte imbalances, particularly in children. Occasionally, cathartics are used without activated charcoal to remove largely nontoxic materials or substances with poor affinity for charcoal, such as hydrocarbons. Sorbitol is not recommended for infants because of potential fluid and electrolyte abnormalities.

Whole-bowel irrigation

Whole-bowel irrigation can dramatically decrease gastrointestinal transit time by effectively emptying the entire large and small intestine. Whole-bowel irrigation is accomplished with an isotonic polyethylene glycol and electrolyte solution (GoLYTELY) administered by mouth or gastric tube in volumes of approximately 1 gal/hr. This process efficiently flushes heavy metals, enteric-coated medications, or slowly dissolving tablets. Swallowed foreign bodies such as cocaine-filled balloons or condoms have also been retrieved with this technique. Whole-bowel irrigation is not without problems. Despite use of electrolyte-balanced formulas, whole-bowel irrigation can cause fluid and electrolyte imbalances, particularly in pediatric patients.

Repeat-dose activated charcoal

Repeat-dose activated charcoal is used for theophylline, phenobarbital, cyclic antidepressants, salicylates, glutethimide, and carbamazepine toxicity.[5] When parenterally administered, these agents can be effectively removed with activated charcoal. Not only does the charcoal bind toxins in the intestines and prevent absorption, but charcoal also decreases serum concentration of some agents following absorption. Gastrointestinal dialysis occurs as a result of the concentration gradient between charcoal in the gut and the toxin in the blood. Because of the intestine's tremendous blood supply, activated charcoal can draw certain poisons from the circulation and bind them for elimination in the feces. This process is enhanced with repeated doses of charcoal every 2 to 4 hours.

Forced diuresis

Forced diuresis is useful for removal of alcohols, including ethanol, methanol, isopropyl alcohol, and ethylene glycol (Table 45-4). Large volumes of intravenous saline (3 to 6 ml/kg/hr) increase elimination of toxins that are primarily excreted by the kidneys. Adding mannitol or furosemide to the therapeutic regimen further enhances renal excretion.

Table **45-4** Drugs Eliminated by Forced Diuresis	
Agent	pH modification
Amphetamine	Acid
Bromide	N/A
Isoniazid	Alkaline
Lithium	N/A
Phencyclidine	Acid
Phenobarbital	Alkaline
Quinidine	Acid
Quinine	Acid
Salicylate	Alkaline
Strychnine	N/A
Sulfonamide	N/A

From Rosen P et al: *Emergency medicine: concepts and clinical practice*, ed 2, vol 1, St. Louis, 1988, Mosby.

Forced diuresis does carry a significant risk of fluid overload and electrolyte problems.

Hemodialysis and hemoperfusion

Hemodialysis and hemoperfusion not only remove toxins and their metabolites from the circulation but also rapidly and effectively correct acid-base and electrolyte disturbances. Substances such as alcohols, lithium, salicylates, and phenobarbital can be removed with dialysis (Box 45-3). Hemodialysis is generally reserved for poisonings associated with severe acidosis because of the requirements for vascular access, equipment, and skilled personnel. Charcoal hemoperfusion is similar to hemodialysis but binds toxins as blood moves across a charcoal filter rather than the traditional hemodialysis filter and dialysate. Hemoperfusion is particularly effective for severe cases of poisoning with paraquat, theophylline, and some sedative-hypnotic agents.

Additional Interventions

In addition to minimizing absorption and enhancing excretion, key interventions in management of toxic emergencies include intubation, mechanical ventilation, cardiovascular support, antidote administration, drug therapy, and supportive measures such as warming or cooling.

Antidote administration

Antidote administration is limited to a few select poisons because there are few true antidotes. Many recommended agents are minimally or moderately effective and often carry their own toxic potential. Antidotes such as oxygen, vitamin K, and naloxone are inexpensive, safe, and effective, whereas antidotes such as physostigmine, deferoxamine, and Fab fragments are costly, relatively ineffective, or dangerous. Table 45-5 summarizes antidotes currently used in most emergency departments.

Alkalinization

Alkalinization involves respiratory or metabolic manipulation. Toxins such as salicylates cause acidosis, which is

Box **45-3** **Poisons That Respond to Dialysis**	
Acetaminophen	Methanol
Alcohol	Paraldehyde
Amphetamine	Phenacetin
Antibiotics	Phenytoin
Arsenic	Potassium
Chloral hydrate	Quinidine
Ergotamine	Quinine
Ethylene glycol	Salicylate
Halides	Strychnine
Isoniazid	Sulfonamide
Meprobamate	Theophylline

From Rosen P et al: *Emergency medicine: concepts and clinical practice*, ed 2, vol 1, St. Louis, 1988, Mosby.

Table **45-5** **Recognized Antidotes**	
Antidote	**Indication**
Oxygen	Carbon monoxide
Ethanol	Ethylene glycol, methyl alcohol
Naloxone	Opiates
Atropine	Organophosphates
Pralidoxime (2-PAM)	Organophosphates
Methylene blue	Nitrites
Fab fragments	Digitalis
N-Acetylcysteine	Acetaminophen
Sodium nitrite	Cyanide
Flumazenil	Benzodiapines
Physostigmine	Atropine, tricyclic antidepressants

easily corrected with alkalinization. Many toxins are better excreted at a higher pH. Intubation and mechanical ventilation along with sodium bicarbonate administration are used to manipulate blood pH to 7.5 or greater for management of cyclic antidepressant overdose.[11] Urinary elimination of mildly acidic toxins, such as phenobarbital and salicylates, can be facilitated by addition of sodium bicarbonate to intravenous fluids. Alkalinization of urine (pH ≥ 7) is helpful in treatment of rhabdomyolysis secondary to drug toxicity.

SPECIFIC TOXIC EMERGENCIES
Salicylates

Salicylates have potent analgesic, antiinflammatory, and antipyretic properties, making them frequent components of prescription and nonprescription drugs (Box 45-4). Aspirin (acetylsalicylic acid) is the most readily available salicylate. Oil of wintergreen (methyl salicylate) is a liquid, highly toxic form of salicylate used in products such as Ben-Gay. Bismuth subsalicylate is an ingredient in Pepto-Bismol. Incidence of acute salicylate ingestion has decreased in the United States over the last two decades because of increased use of acetaminophen. However, acute and chronic accidental overdoses continue to occur.

Acute salicylate ingestions with serum salicylates greater than 150 mg/kg are associated with development of toxic clinical symptoms. Salicylates affect the brainstem, causing hyperventilation and respiratory alkalosis, and also decrease adenosine triphosphate (ATP) production, which leads to metabolic acidosis.[14] Direct gastrointestinal irritation causes nausea, protracted vomiting, and hematemesis. Effects on the clotting cascade increase prothrombin time (PT) and can lead to bleeding disorders. Other effects include ototoxicity (i.e., tinnitus).

Clinical findings vary significantly with patient age, amount of salicylate consumed, and whether ingestion was chronic or acute. Acidosis, electrolyte abnormalities, and impaired ATP lead to dysrhythmias and cardiac failure. Neural disturbances range from lethargy and confusion to

Box **45-4** **Products Containing Salicylates**	
Nonprescription products	**Prescription medications**
A.C.A. Caps	Allygesic
A.C.A. No. 2	APAC
Alka-Seltzer	Cordex
Anacin	Darvon with ASA
A.P.C.	Decagesic
Ascriptin	Empirin Compound with Codeine
Aspergum	Fiorinal
Asperin	Norgesic
Aspodyne	Percodan
Bayer	Phenaphen
Buffacetin	Predisal
Bufferin	Sedagesic
Congespirin	Synalgos
Cope	
Coricidin	
Counterpain	
Dristan	
Duragesic	
Empirin	
Excedrin	
Excedrin P.M.	
4-Way Cold Tabs	
Midol	
Novahistine with APC	
Quiet World	
Rhinex	
Sine-Aid	
Sine-Off	
St. Joseph	
Super Anahist	
Triaminicin	
Vanquish	

Modified from Rosen P et al: *Emergency medicine: concepts and clinical practice*, ed 3, St. Louis, 1992, Mosby.

seizures and cerebral edema. Signs of acute toxicity include vomiting, hyperventilation, upper gastrointestinal bleeding, diaphoresis, ketonuria, coagulopathies, hyperthermia, alkalemia, abdominal pain, and dysrhythmias. Chronic toxicity is associated with lethargy, confusion, dehydration, hallucinations, adult respiratory distress syndrome, elevated liver enzymes, and prolonged PT. The patient may also have hyperthermia, renal failure, tinnitus, and hypoglycemia.

Diagnostic studies include serial measurement of salicylate level, arterial blood gases, electrolytes (particularly potassium), PT, partial thromboplastin time (PTT), and urine pH. The Done nomogram aids in predicting salicylate toxicity; however, usefulness is limited to the patient with a recent, one-time, acute ingestion of nonenteric salicylates (Figure 45-1). The initial serum level should be drawn no less than 6 hours following ingestion. Serial measurements are required until values drop to asymptomatic levels (<40 mg/dl). In chronic ingestions, salicylates move from the blood to the tis-

sues, so serum levels do not accurately reflect total body content of salicylates.

Limit absorption of salicylates with gastric emptying using lavage or ipecac followed by administration of activated charcoal. Enhance elimination with multiple doses of activated charcoal, forced diuresis, and alkalinization. Consider hemodialysis in patients who do not respond to simpler measures. Patients are frequently dehydrated and require intravenous fluid replacement.

The kidneys release hydrogen ions only if ions can be exchanged for potassium ions. This places the patient at risk for hypokalemia as potassium is exchanged for hydrogen. Monitor serum potassium closely, and administer potassium as needed. Acidosis not only limits drug elimination but also can increase salicylate absorption by the brain. Correct metabolic acidosis with sodium bicarbonate. Use a short-acting benzodiazepine for emergency treatment of salicylate-induced seizures.

Acetaminophen

Like salicylates, acetaminophen is a common ingredient in many over-the-counter analgesics, antipyretics, and cold remedies (Box 45-5). Acetaminophen overdoses are usually accidental in the pediatric patient and intentional in adults. Although initial symptoms are mild, acetaminophen poisoning causes life-threatening hepatotoxicity.

Acetaminophen is rapidly absorbed from the gut and broken down by the liver, forming a toxic metabolite. In therapeutic doses, this intermediary product is rapidly detoxified by hepatic enzymes. However, toxic doses deplete these essential enzymes so that the liver is damaged as metabolites accumulate. Serum acetaminophen levels of 140 mg/kg or greater are considered toxic.[14] Individuals at risk for acetaminophen toxicity at lower doses are those with preexisting hepatic dysfunction secondary to ethanol abuse, hepatitis, or other liver disease. Signs and symptoms of acetaminophen toxicity develop slowly and can be overlooked until significant damage has occurred. Symptoms are divided into four phases according to elapsed time from ingestion (Table 45-6). Acetaminophen levels should be drawn 4 hours after acute ingestion. Plotting the 4-hour acetaminophen value on the Rumack-Matthew nomogram (Figure 45-2) determines if the patient has potential hepatic toxicity. This nomogram is only useful for acute, single-dose poisonings. Liver function studies, PT, PTT, complete blood count, blood urea nitrogen (BUN), and creatinine levels should be obtained on patients who present with clinical symptoms.

Limit acetaminophen absorption with syrup of ipecac if the patient is fully awake or gastric lavage for the patient with an altered level of consciousness or diminished gag reflex. Induced emesis or gastric lavage should be followed with activated charcoal, which effectively absorbs acetaminophen from the intestines. Some authors recommend charcoal administration in conjunction with a cathartic without prior gastric emptying.

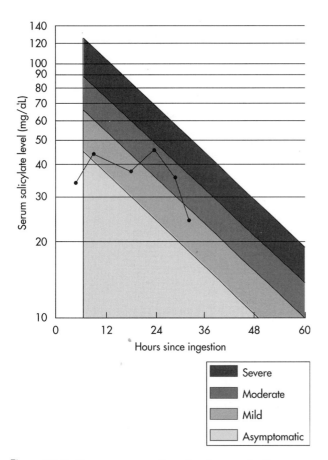

Figure **45-1** Done nomogram for estimating severity from serum salicylate level at varying intervals after ingestion of a single dose. Useful only if ingestion occurred in a single dose. This example shows levels in a patient who ingested a toxic dose of enteric-coated aspirin. *(From Pierce R, Gazewood J, Blake R: Salicylate poisoning from enteric coated aspirin: delayed absorption may complicate management,* Postgrad Med *89(5):62.)*

Box **45-5** **Products Containing Acetaminophen**	
Nonprescription medications	Sinarest
Acephen	Sine-Aid
Aceta	Sine-Off Extra Strength
Acetagesic	Sino-Aid
Amphenol	Sinugesic
Anacin-3	Sinutab
Arthralgen	St. Joseph Fever Reducer
Bowman Cold Tabs	Tempra
Bromo Quinine Cold Tabs	Tenol
Bromo-Seltzer	Triaminicin
Calm Aids	Triginc
Comtrex	Tylaprin
Congespirin Liquid Cold Medicine	Tylenol
Contac Jr.	Valadol
Datril	Valihist
Datril 500	Windolor
D-Sinus	**Prescription medications**
Excedrin	Aceta
Excedrin P.M.	Darvocet-N 50
Liquiprin	Darvocet-N 100
Mense	Demerol APAP
Midran Decongestant	Empracet With Codeine
Novahistine Sinus	Histogesic
Nyquil	Indogesic
Nyte Time Liquid	Percocet-5
Pamprin	Sinutab
Parafon Forte	Sinutab With Codeine
Percogesic	Tylenol and Codeine
Pertussin Plus Night-Time Cold Medicine	Tylox
Quiet Nite Liquid	Vicodin Tablets
Quiet World	Wygesic
Sinacon	

From Rosen P et al: *Emergency medicine: concepts and clinical practice,* ed 3, St. Louis, 1992, Mosby.

Multiple doses of charcoal do not decrease serum acetaminophen concentration but may be used to treat coingestions. NAC (Mucomyst) can be alternated with charcoal every 2 hours. Hemodialysis and hemoperfusion remove acetaminophen but do little to change the course of hepatic damage. Treat vomiting with antiemetics such as prochlorperazine and metoclopramide. All patients with a serum acetaminophen that falls in the range for possible hepatic toxicity should receive NAC.

NAC replenishes the liver's supply of essential enzymes and allows removal of acetaminophen metabolites. The earlier the therapy is initiated, the better the prognosis; however, NAC may still be effective up to 24 hours after ingestion. Activated charcoal absorbs NAC, but this effect does not appear to be clinically significant. Some authors do recommend lavaging out charcoal or waiting 1 to 2 hours after charcoal administration to begin NAC. The initial dose is 140 mg/kg, followed by half the calculated amount every 4 hours for 17 additional doses. NAC is usually given through the gastric tube or diluted in fruit juice or soft drinks because of the foul taste and odor. If the patient vomits within 1 hour of ingestion, the dose should be repeated. Intravenous NAC is available in Canada and Europe. Liver transplantation has been attempted in acetaminophen overdose patients when NAC therapy fails.

Central Nervous System Stimulants

Central nervous system (CNS) stimulants are a loosely related group of legal and illegal drugs that act by simulating or mimicking the sympathetic branch of the autonomic nervous system. Illicit CNS stimulants include cocaine and amphetamines (Table 45-7). Legitimate CNS stimulants such as caffeine, phenylpropanolamine, and pseudoephedrine are common ingredients in over-the-counter diet pills, cold remedies, and alertness aids. Legal CNS stimulants are less potent and produce fewer euphoric or psychotic effects than

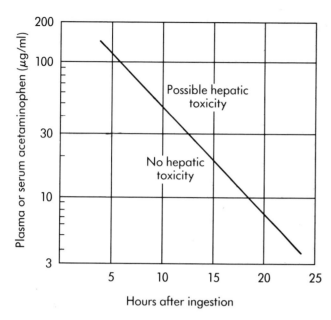

Figure **45-2** Rumack-Matthew nomogram. *(From American Academy of Pediatrics:* Pediatrics 55:871, 1975.)

Table 45-6		Acetaminophen Toxicity
Stage	Time frame	Symptoms
I	0-24 hr	May be asymptomatic or experience lethargy, diaphoresis, mild gastric upset including nausea, vomiting, anorexia
II	24-48 hr	May have no complaints or develop liver failure, abnormal liver function tests, prolonged PTT, increasing bilirubin levels, right upper quadrant pain, hepatomegaly, oliguria
III	72-96 hr	Massive hepatic dysfunction, liver enzymes ≥ 100 times normal, hypoglycemia, jaundice; patient appears acutely ill; can progress to hepatic failure, encephalopathy, and death
IV	4 days-2 weeks	If patient survives stage III, enters recovery phase characterized by slow resolution of hepatic dysfunction

their illegal counterparts; however, sufficient doses produce similar physiologic responses. CNS stimulants can be ingested, injected, inhaled, snorted transnasally, and absorbed rectally or vaginally.

Although CNS stimulants are not all the same, their actions, side effects, and hazards are similar. Street drugs, such as cocaine and amphetamines, are often diluted or "cut" with other CNS stimulants such as caffeine or phenylpropanolamine, making precise identification of specific agents difficult.[1] CNS stimulants are rapidly absorbed from the gut, with onset of action minutes after injection or inhalation. Stimulants have relatively short half-lives and produce varying degrees of sympathetic nervous system innervation of α-, β_1-, and β_2-adrenergic receptors.

Patients present with a wide range of responses and symptoms, usually related to the drug and quantity ingested (Table 45-8). The patient experiences a sense of omnipotence, excitement, hyperalertness, hyperactivity, hypersexuality, anxiety, agitation, aggression, hallucinations, mania, or paranoia.[2] Tachycardia, hypertension, cardiac dysrhythmias, cerebral vascular accidents, coronary artery spasms, and myocardial infarction also occur. Neurologic effects include pupil dilation, tremor, restlessness, seizures, and coma. Stimulation of the gastrointestinal tract produces nausea, vomiting, and diarrhea. Other effects include hyperpyrexia, rhabdomyolysis, piloerection, and coagulopathies.

Toxicologic screening of urine or blood provides a rapid qualitative test for common CNS stimulants; however, quantitative measures do not correlate well with the clinical status. Basic care addresses the airway, breathing, and circulation on a case-by-case basis. Because of increased metabolic rate, diaphoresis, and drug-induced diuresis, this popu-

lation is frequently dehydrated. Adequate fluid volume is essential to minimize complications such as tachycardia, hyperthermia, and myoglobinuric renal failure.

Orally ingested tablets or capsules may be removed by standard gastric emptying followed with activated charcoal. Gastric decontamination has no benefit if the drugs were inhaled, snorted, or injected. "Body-packers" who have ingested cocaine-filled balloons or condoms should receive activated charcoal. Charcoal absorbs cocaine in the gastrointestinal tract if the container ruptures.

No specific measures are used to enhance CNS stimulant elimination. Whole-bowel irrigation has been used successfully to remove swallowed body-packed or body-stuffed drugs. Endoscopic or surgical removal may be necessary if packets rupture.

Treatment of CNS stimulant toxicosis is largely symptomatic. Symptoms can progress rapidly, so close, diligent observation is necessary. Continuous cardiac and blood pressure monitoring will detect tachycardia, dysrhythmias, and hypertension. A 12-lead ECG is indicated for patients with chest pain or shock. Because of the potential for rapid development of severe hyperthermia, temperature should be checked frequently until symptoms subside.

The patient with a significant CNS stimulant overdose can be paranoid, incredibly strong, and anesthetized to pain. Prevent injury to the patient and others by sedating psychotic patients with benzodiazepines or haloperidol. Isolated use of physical restraints can cause extreme agitation and intense muscle activity, contributing to hyperthermia

Table **45-7** **Generic, Trade, and Street Names of Stimulants**		
Generic name	Trade name	Street name
Cocaine (alkaloid of coca plant; statutorily but not pharma-cologically a narcotic)		Bernice, bernies, big C, blow, burese, C, Carrie, Cecil, Charlie, Cholly, coke, Corine, dream, dust, flake, gin, girl, gold dust, GRS, happy dust, happy trails, heaven dust, her, jam, joy powder, lady, leaf, liquid lady, nose (candy, powder), Oz, paradise, rich man's drug, toot, whites
Amphetamines Phenylisopropylamine Sympathomimetic Synthetic agent	Delcobese Obetrol Benzedrine Biphetamine	A, beans, bennies, benz, black beauties, black mollies, bombido, browns, bumblebees, businessman's trip, chalk, Christmas tree, coast to coast, dexies, doublecross, drivers, eyeopeners, greenies, happies, hearts, jags, jelly babies, jelly beans, jugs, L.A. turn-abouts, lid poppers, nuggets, pep pills, roses, skyrockets, sweets, truck drivers, tens, ups, wake-ups, West Coast turnaround
Dextroamphetamines Dextroamphetamine sulfate Dextroamphetamine tannate	Dexamyl Dexedrine Eskatrol spansule Obotan tabs Obotan Forte	Blackies, copilots, dexies, dex, footballs, greens, oranges
Methamphetamine	Desoxyn Fetamin Methadrine Desbutal	Meth, STP, speed, dynamite, crystal meth, white cross, black hearty
Phenmetrazine	Preludin Phendimetrazine	
Diethylproprion	Tenuate Tepanil	
Methylphenidate	Ritalin	

From Rosen P et al: *Emergency medicine: concepts and clinical practice,* ed 2, vol 2, St. Louis, 1988, Mosby.

and rhabdomyolysis. Once the patient is under control, provide a minimal-stimulation environment.

CNS stimulants affect the sympathetic nervous system, so a β-blocker (e.g., propranolol) or combination α- and β-blocker (e.g., labetalol) may be used for treatment of significant overdoses. Intense muscle activity and increased metabolic rate can rapidly produce core temperatures greater than 104°F (40°C). Cool patients aggressively.

Intravenous benzodiazepines are the agents of choice for the treatment of seizures or impending seizures. Adequate control is essential, since seizure activity contributes significantly to hyperthermia. Phenytoin, phenobarbital, and even a neuromuscular blocking agent may be required.

Narcotics

Originally derived from the opium poppy, narcotics are among the oldest known analgesic agents. They have been used and abused for thousands of years. Today, opium is refined into many different drugs.[6] Numerous synthetic narcotics are also available. In the United States, single-agent and multidrug formula opiates can legally be obtained only by prescription. Narcotic toxicosis is often associated with intravenous abuse. Overdoses result from both pharmacologically prepared and "street drug" versions. Illicitly obtained narcotics may be cut with substances including caffeine,

Table **45-8** **Clinical Effects of CNS Stimulants**	
Degree of intoxication	Effects
Mild	Insomnia, talkativeness, restlessness, garrulousness, agitation, aggression, tremor, hyperactivity
Moderate	Mydriasis, headache, nystagmus, hypertension, tachycardia, chest pain, dysrhythmias, hallucinations
Severe	Paranoia, shock, hyperthermia, rhabdomyolysis, acute tubular necrosis, acidosis, hyperkalemia, seizures, coma, myocardial infarction
Late	Chronic abuser may be exhausted after a binge due to intense exertion and dopamine depletion; sleeps for hours and is difficult to arouse

amphetamines, mannitol, phencyclidine, strychnine, lactose, or powdered sugar. Cointoxicants may be responsible for many of the patient's symptoms.

Although there are significant differences among opiate agents, all act on the CNS, producing variable degrees of sedation, euphoria, analgesia, and amnesia. Psychic effects make opiates popular drugs of abuse. CNS depression sufficient to induce coma can occur with large drug doses or with relatively small amounts in those unaccustomed to narcotics, such as children. Tolerance and dependence are common phenomena with narcotic use; addiction may follow chronic use.

Opioids also act on the respiratory center in the brainstem, producing depression and apnea. The gastrointestinal system is slowed by narcotics, so constipation is a common side effect. Some opiates, such as paregoric and diphenoxylate hydrochloride with atropine (Lomotil), are prescribed specifically for this action. Signs and symptoms of opiate toxicity and abuse are related to the effects of the narcotics, substance abuse lifestyle, or withdrawal (Table 45-9).

A qualitative toxicologic screen documents recent opiate use, but levels do not correlate with clinical presentation because of the number of substances available and the wide range of individual tolerance. A naloxone (Narcan) challenge serves as a diagnostic tool and therapeutic intervention. A dose of 2 mg given intravenously, intramuscularly, subcutaneously, intratracheally, or injected under the tongue antagonizes opiate receptor sites in the CNS, reversing opioid effects and rapidly awakening patients with narcotic-induced CNS depression. Occasionally doses up to 10 mg are required.

Oral ingestions of opiates can be treated with induced emesis as long as the patient is alert, likely to remain so, and not otherwise at risk for aspiration. Gastric lavage may also be used to aid elimination of any drug remaining in the stomach. Since opioids decrease peristalsis, pill fragments may be retrieved after an extended period of time. Activated charcoal effectively binds narcotics and reduces absorption into the circulation.

Cathartic agents, in conjunction with activated charcoal, are particularly useful for enhancing drug elimination in

Table **45-9**	**Effects of Narcotic Abuse and Toxicity**
Etiology	Potential effects
Narcotic	Pinpoint pupils, respiratory depression, mental changes, hypotension, visual hallucinations, analgesia, amnesia, sleep, coma
Lifestyle	Skin abscesses, cellulitis, endocarditis, septicemia, track marks, malnutrition, dental disease, hepatitis, human immunodeficiency virus (HIV) infection, tuberculosis, pulmonary edema, fecal impaction, septic arthritis, frequent trauma
Withdrawal	Rhinorrhea, tearing, yawning, dilated pupils, abdominal pain, diarrhea, diaphoresis, nasal congestion, vomiting, headache, piloerection, chills, fever, joint pain, agitation, confusion, hyperactivity

narcotic toxicity because of opiate-induced intestinal hypomotility.

Naloxone is a specific narcotic antagonist that competes directly with opiates at their receptor sites. If the patient responds to an adequate naloxone challenge, the diagnosis of narcotic overdose is made, and treatment involves maintaining a desirable naloxone level until the opiate wears off. A narcotic's duration of action is very drug specific; sufentanil effects disappear within minutes, whereas methadone effects may last more than 24 hours. Naloxone lasts 2 to 3 hours, which may be considerably less than the duration of action for the particular narcotic involved. Repeat doses or continuous intravenous naloxone infusions are frequently indicated and should be titrated to clinical response. A newer narcotic antagonist, nalmefene hydrochloride (Revex), has a much longer half-life than naloxone (10.8 hours versus 1 hour), allowing patients to be treated with a single dose and safely discharged sooner than with naloxone therapy.

Clonidine

Although survival is possible following ingestions of much larger amounts, a dose as small as 0.1 mg of clonidine is considered a life-threatening emergency in the pediatric patient. Clinical effects seen with clonidine toxicity are similar to a narcotic overdose. Clonidine is an antihypertensive agent that acts centrally as an α-agonist, decreasing catecholamine release from the CNS, causing vasodilation and hypotension. Clonidine may also stimulate production of an opiatelike substance, creating other opioid characteristics.

In addition to profound cardiovascular effects, clonidine toxicity affects the respiratory and central nervous systems. While a qualitative toxicologic screen will confirm clonidine ingestion, quantitative levels are of no value, and therapy should be guided by clinical status. Bradycardia and hypotension are the usual findings, but paradoxical hypertension has also been reported. Respiratory depression, lethargy, ataxia, confusion, and coma are also seen with clonidine poisoning.

Induced emesis is contraindicated in clonidine overdose because of rapid onset of clinical effects. Gastric lavage and a single dose of activated charcoal are recommended to minimize absorption into the systemic circulation. No benefit is achieved with multidose charcoal therapy.

After immediate respiratory and cardiovascular needs are addressed, naloxone is administered. As with narcotic overdose, naloxone reverses the effects of clonidine toxicosis. Doses required for a therapeutic response are frequently higher than those used in narcotic toxicity. Continuous naloxone infusions are used to prevent recurrence of symptoms.

Benzodiazepines

Benzodiazepines are commonly prescribed anxiolytic and sedative-hypnotic agents (Table 45-10). Fortunately, the level of toxicity associated with these drugs is generally mild. In overdose situations, benzodiazepines ingested with

Table 45-10	Benzodiazepines
Generic name	Brand name
Lorazepam	Ativan
Prazepam	Centrax
Flurazepam	Dalmane
Quazepam	Doral
Triazolam	Halcion
Clonazepam	Klonopin
Chlordiazepoxide	Librium
Halazepam	Paxipam
Estazolam	ProSom
Temazepam	Restoril
Oxazepam	Serax
Clorazepate dipotassium	Tranxene
Diazepam	Valium
Midazolam	Versed

Table 45-11	Cyclic Antidepressants
Generic name	Brand name
Amitriptyline	Elavil, Endep
Amoxapine	Asendin
Clomipramine	Anafranil
Desipramine	Norpramin
Doxepin	Sinequan, Adapin
Fluoxetine	Prozac
Imipramine	Tofranil
Maprotiline	Ludiomil
Nortriptyline	Aventyl, Pamelor
Protriptyline	Vivactil
Trazodone	Desyrel
Trimipramine	Surmontil

other CNS depressants such as alcohol, cyclic antidepressants, and barbiturates produce more severe toxic effects.

Benzodiazepines potentiate effects of the inhibitory neurotransmitter γ-aminobutyric acid, producing CNS depression. Toxic effects of the benzodiazepines are an extension of their therapeutic effects. A milligram per kilogram toxic dose has not been established.

A qualitative serum benzodiazepine level confirms the presence of these agents; however, quantitative levels are not particularly useful because of significant individual variability. Interventions are dictated by the patient's clinical status rather than serum level.

Benzodiazepines cause drowsiness, lethargy, ataxia, and mild coma. Profound coma suggests involvement of other CNS depressants. Significant circulatory compromise after isolated benzodiazepine ingestion is rare, so other causes should be considered. Hypotension has been associated with rapid intravenous administration of diazepam (particularly in children) because of the propylene glycol base. With pure benzodiazepine ingestion, respiratory depression is not a common finding but has occasionally been associated with rapid administration of high-dose midazolam.

Emesis may be induced for recent or minor poisonings, but gastric lavage is indicated for large benzodiazepine ingestions, when toxic coingestants are involved, or when the patient has a decreased level of consciousness. Gastric emptying is followed by a single dose of activated charcoal.

Administer a cathartic agent along with charcoal to counteract gastrointestinal hypomotility and enhance fecal drug elimination. Hemodialysis and charcoal hemoperfusion have little benefit in benzodiazepine overdose.

Flumazenil (Romazicon) is an effective antagonist agent that competes directly with benzodiazepines at their receptor sites. Administering flumazenil produces a rapid change in level of consciousness in patients with benzodiazepine toxicosis, making it an effective diagnostic tool as well as a therapeutic agent.

Cyclic Antidepressants

There are a wide variety of unicyclic, bicyclic, tricyclic, and tetracyclic antidepressant drugs currently available, including amitriptyline (Elavil), imipramine (Tofranil), and fluoxetine (Prozac). Widely prescribed for depression, cyclic antidepressants (CAs) are the most commonly reported cause of death from overdose and are frequently associated with suicidal intent. Table 45-11 lists different cyclic antidepressant classes.

Each cyclic antidepressant has varying degrees of anticholinergic, adrenergic, and α-blocking properties. CAs are well absorbed from the gastrointestinal tract, highly tissue-bound with a large volume of distribution, and difficult to remove from the body once absorbed. Toxicity is not closely associated with milligram per kilogram ingested dose; therefore serum levels do not correlate well with clinical effects. A qualitative study is sufficient to confirm ingestion.

Since CAs produce neurotoxicity, cardiotoxicity, and anticholinergic effects, signs and symptoms of CA poisoning fall into three general categories. *Neurotoxicity* is characterized by both CNS depression and irritability. Common findings are lethargy, slurred speech, confusion, hallucinations, coma, myoclonus, and seizure activity. *Cardiac manifestations* include hypotension and numerous ECG changes including ST- and T-wave abnormalities, prolonged QT intervals, conduction blocks, tachycardia, bradycardia, ventricular dysrhythmias, and pulseless electrical activity. *Anticholinergic effects* include mydriasis, flushed skin, dry mucous membranes, anxiety or psychosis, tachycardia, elevated body temperature, and urinary retention. A mnemonic commonly used to recall signs of anticholinergic toxicity is "Blind as a bat. Red as a beet. Dry as a bone. Mad as a hatter, and hotter than Hades."

Aggressive gastric emptying is essential to minimize CA toxicity, since these drugs are difficult to eliminate once absorbed. CNS depression can develop rapidly; therefore the patient should be intubated and then lavaged. Do not induce emesis. Activated charcoal effectively binds CAs, dramatically reducing half-life. The first charcoal dose can be given prior to lavage.

Because of anticholinergic effects, intestinal transit time is significantly lengthened, making cathartic use an important adjunct for increasing drug elimination and preventing gastrointestinal obstruction. CAs are largely tissue-bound, so forced diuresis, hemodialysis, and charcoal hemoperfusion are not effective. CA toxicity is one of the few poisonings that clearly benefit from the "gastrointestinal dialysis" effect of repeat-dose charcoal.

Continuous cardiac monitoring is imperative for all significant CA ingestions. Dysrhythmias include sinus tachycardia secondary to anticholinergic effects and widened QRS complex, which can progress to ventricular irritability and conduction disturbances. Treat ventricular dysrhythmias with lidocaine or phenytoin. Serious conduction blocks may respond to an external pacemaker. Systemic alkalinization of serum with sodium bicarbonate can reverse life-threatening conduction disturbances and ventricular dysrhythmias associated with CAs. Sodium bicarbonate is administered initially at 1 mEq/kg and then titrated to maintain a systemic pH of 7.5. This can be accomplished by addition of sodium bicarbonate to IV fluids and guided by arterial blood gas values. Hypotension is initially managed with crystalloid boluses; however, catecholamine vasopressors (dopamine, norepinephrine, or phenylephrine) are necessary for refractory hypotension.

Treat seizures acutely with a short-acting benzodiazepine such as diazepam or lorazepam. Once seizure activity is controlled, a loading dose of phenytoin can be initiated, with subsequent maintenance doses as needed. Physostigmine, a cholinergic drug, is sometimes referred to as a CA antidote and may be considered for intractable hypotension; however, physostigmine has significant side effects. Hypotension can worsen and asystole develop. Therefore physostigmine should be used as an agent of last resort.[12]

Toxic Alcohols

In addition to ethanol, three other alcohols can cause severe poisoning. Toxic alcohols are found in common household products not generally considered dangerous. *Methanol,* also known as "wood alcohol," is found in antifreeze, canned fuel (Sterno), and solvents such as paint thinner. *Isopropanol,* which is the chief component of rubbing alcohol, is a common ingredient in disinfectants, cleansers, and nail polish remover. *Ethylene glycol* is a colorless, odorless substance contained in antifreeze, detergents, paints, polishes, and coolants. Many household products, such as lemon-scented nail polish remover and sweet, fluorescent antifreeze, are particularly appealing to children and pets. Toxic alcohol ingestion may be accidental or suicidal or occur in an alcoholic unable to obtain ethanol. In addition to oral ingestion, toxic alcohols may be inhaled or topically absorbed.

Toxic alcohols are relatively nonpoisonous prior to hepatic conversion by alcohol dehydrogenase to toxic metabolites. Glycolaldehyde (ethylene glycol), formaldehyde, formic acid (methanol), and acetone (isopropanol) produce widespread damage and metabolic dysfunction.

Clinical findings include CNS depression and respiratory depression. Methanol toxicity causes nausea, vomiting, abdominal pain, blindness, and coma. The patient with isopropanol ingestion has an acetone odor on the breath, is vomiting, and can present with renal failure. Ethylene glycol causes seizures, hallucinations, ataxia, coma, and ocular disturbances such as nystagmus and ophthalmoplegia. Profound acidosis may also occur.

Perform the appropriate laboratory studies to detect the following predicted abnormalities. For methanol, a pronounced metabolic acidosis results from the accumulation of formic acid. For isopropanol, serum acetone levels are elevated, and ketones are present in the blood and urine. Hyperglycemia may occur. For ethylene glycol, both an anion gap metabolic acidosis and a large osmolal gap are present with significant intoxication. Expect elevated BUN and creatinine levels and hypocalcemia.

Gastric lavage may be used in severe toxicity to remove any alcohol remaining in the stomach. Activated charcoal may also be used, as it decreases gastrointestinal absorption of ethylene glycol by about 50%. However, because of the rapid absorption of alcohols, there is limited indication for gastric lavage and activated charcoal. The lungs are responsible for significant excretion of toxic alcohols; therefore intubation and mechanical ventilation can be used to maximize respiratory excretion in severe poisoning. Hemodialysis effectively removes toxic metabolites and treats acidosis.

Ethanol and each of the toxic alcohols rely on enzyme alcohol dehydrogenase for metabolism. However, ethyl alcohol is preferentially metabolized by the liver. Therefore administration of intravenous ethanol (100 mg/kg/hr) slows methanol, isopropanol, and ethylene glycol degradation, preventing accumulation of toxic metabolites. Ethanol infusion must be continued during dialysis with the rate increased to 240 mg/kg/hr to reach a serum ethanol level of 100 mg/dl.

Organophosphates

Organophosphates are the major active ingredient in hundreds of insecticides found in most American homes, including ant and bug sprays and garden insect killers. Toxicity varies significantly among chemical formulations. Organophosphates can be ingested, inhaled, or absorbed topically. Mass poisoning occasionally occurs from ingestion of unwashed produce or airborne contamination during crop spraying.

Acetylcholine is released into synaptic junctions in response to parasympathetic and sympathetic impulses. Normally, cholinesterase enzymes rapidly break down acetylcholine, halting action until another stimulus is received. Organophosphates aggressively bind to cholinesterase molecules, blocking their effect and allowing acetylcholine to remain in the neural synapse with effects unopposed. Organophosphate-cholinesterase bonds do not spontaneously reverse. After 24 to 48 hours of continuous binding, cholinesterase molecules are destroyed. Complete regeneration of cholinesterase can take weeks or even months.

Two tests of cholinesterase, serum and red blood cell, should be performed; however, results may not be available for several days. Studies indicate the percent of cholinesterase that remains functional. Dermal exposures necessitate removal of all clothing and jewelry, followed by copious skin irrigation. Contaminated water should be considered hazardous waste. Suction or lavage ingested agents from the stomach; once absorbed, organophosphates are difficult to eliminate. Activated charcoal effectively reduces organophosphate absorption. Because of their toxin-induced diarrhea, patients seldom require concomitant cathartic administration.

Clinical findings depend on the specific organophosphate, the amount of poison involved, and patient size. Symptoms range from mild to severe and are usually evident within 12 hours of contact. A few lipophilic organophosphates may not produce significant distress for 24 to 36 hours. Effects include fatigue, lethargy, weakness, blurred vision, dizziness, headache, delirium, seizures, and coma. The patient is weak and presents with tremors, fasciculations, and inability to stand. Gastrointestinal effects include nausea, vomiting, anorexia, abdominal cramping, and diarrhea. Cough, bronchorrhea, and wheezing are also present. Classically, bradycardia is prominent, but tachycardia, atrioventricular blocks, dysrhythmias, and ST-wave abnormalities are not uncommon. Other effects include garlic odor, diaphoresis, pinpoint pupils, hypertension, and urinary incontinence.

Interventions are largely supportive. Effective antidote therapy exists to counteract organophosphate effects, although recovery requires synthesis of new cholinesterase, a process that may require several weeks. Organophosphates produce a cholinergic syndrome, so anticholinergics are the treatment of choice.[14] Immediate therapy includes administration of intravenous atropine titrated to clinical effect. Severe poisoning may necessitate up to 5 mg of atropine every 15 to 30 minutes. Continue boluses until signs of atropinization (dilated pupils, decreased secretions, tachycardia, and dry, flushed skin) appear. Once the patient is fully atropinized, initiate intravenous pralidoxime (2-PAM; Protopam) therapy. Pralidoxime has an anticholinergic effect like atropine but can actually rescue and reactivate

cholinesterase when administered within 24 to 36 hours of acute organophosphate poisoning. Pralidoxime doses are titrated to severity. An initial bolus is followed by additional boluses every 1 to 2 hours or a continuous infusion.

The organophosphate-intoxicated individual is at significant risk for contaminating others. Perform resuscitation and decontamination in a well-ventilated, isolated area. All persons coming in contact with the poisoned individual require full protective gear including gloves and goggles. Special decontamination gloves should be used if available; if not, wear two pairs of gloves. The patient's clothing is considered contaminated. Vomitus, gastric lavage material, and stool must be handled with caution, followed by careful disposal to avoid secondary contamination.

Hallucinogens

Phencyclidine (PCP), lysergic acid diethylamide (LSD), mescaline, jimsonweed, morning glory seeds, and tetrahydrocannabinol (THC, the active ingredient in marijuana and hashish) are among the most popular drugs in the hallucinogen category. Although some toxins are naturally occurring and have probably been used for thousands of years (e.g., psilocybin mushrooms, peyote), PCP and LSD are synthetic agents of recent invention. Table 45-12 compares PCP to other drug groups. Although not typically classed as hallucinogens, many medications and toxins can induce hallucinations when administered in sufficient quantities or to susceptible individuals.

Besides hallucinogenic effects, these drugs have other chemical properties that are responsible for a wide variety of sympathomimetic or anticholinergic responses. The vast majority of hallucinogen abusers have no reason to visit an emergency department. Patients who present are generally those with concomitant trauma, toxicity produced by coingestants, or psychotic reactions to the drug.

Hallucinogenic chemicals stimulate the brain, producing visual and auditory sensory-perceptual alterations with associated behavioral changes, cognitive disturbances, and even acute psychotic reactions. The environment, mood, and circumstances a patient is in at the time of ingestion greatly influence hallucinations, which vary from pleasant to terrifying.

The patient may be self-absorbed or exhibit self-absorbed inward-drawn behavior. Other symptoms include soliloquy, auditory and visual events experienced only by the drugged individual, paranoia, mood fluctuations, and attempts to perform superhuman feats. Physical findings are generally a product of sympathomimetic or anticholinergic properties associated with hallucinogens.

A urine or serum drug screen confirms the presence of certain common hallucinogenic substances (e.g., THC, PCP). Quantitative measurement has little clinical value. Some hallucinogens are smoked (e.g., marijuana) or ingested in such tiny quantities (e.g., LSD) that attempts at gastric emptying are unproductive. Toxicities secondary to

Table 45-12 PCP Comparison with Other Drug Groups

Classes of drugs	Similarities	Differences
CNS depressants	Coma Ataxia Nystagmus	Tachycardia Increased deep tendon reflexes Hypertension
Sympathomimetics	Tachycardia Hypertension	Coma Ataxia Muscle rigidity Increased secretions Nystagmus
Anticholinergics	Hypertension Tachycardia Hyperthermia Bizarre behavior Seizures Coma	Increased secretions Pupils usually normal or miotic Blank stare Muscle rigidity Nystagmus
Cholinergics	Increased secretions Meiosis Seizures	Tachycardia Hypertension Increased deep tendon reflex Muscle rigidity
Psychedelics	Bizarre behavior Tachycardia	Ataxia Muscle rigidity Increased secretions Coma Nystagmus
Opiates	Coma Meiosis Hyperventilation Apnea	No response to naloxone Increased deep tendon reflex Muscle rigidity Hypertension

From Rosen P et al: *Emergency medicine: concepts and clinical practice,* ed 3, St. Louis, 1992, Mosby.

ingestion of jimsonweed seeds or psychedelic mushrooms benefit from induced emesis and gastric lavage. Follow gastric emptying with activated charcoal. Cathartic administration also promotes fecal elimination of ingested agents. PCP and substances with concomitant anticholinergic effects should be treated with multiple doses of activated charcoal.

Many hallucinogen abusers are in a happy little world of their own. As long as the individual is safe, the effects of hallucinogens are not dangerous, are considered self-limiting, and require little intervention for uncomplicated toxicity. Agitation and violence can be controlled with benzodiazepines or haloperidol. Other supportive therapies are drug and patient specific.

Physostigmine has been suggested for reversal of anticholinergic effects frequently associated with hallucinogens; however, physostigmine's myriad side effects are often worse than the original toxicity. Administration should be limited to life-threatening emergencies.

Heavy Metals

Heavy metals involved in poisoning include lead, mercury, zinc, arsenic, and cadmium. Since heavy metals are a by-product of the industrial age, all inhabitants of developed countries have measurable heavy metal serum levels. Intoxication by these agents is often chronic and subtle, making diagnosis difficult. For example, lead exposure may be related to daily use of glazed ceramic dinnerware or occasional ingestion of paint chips by a small child. Industrial exposure to button batteries, dental cement, marine paints, solder, and countless other products and manufacturing processes puts individuals at risk for heavy metal poisoning. Water pollution has caused mercury toxicity from seafood ingestion.

Absorption of these metals can occur through inhalation and ingestion. Chronic toxicities have a very different presentation than acute poisonings. Exposures to an inorganic metal or organic metal salt also cause very different effects. Heavy metal toxicosis is frequently associated with other poisons such as hydrocarbons (leaded gasoline), organophosphates (arsenic-containing pesticides), and carbon monoxide (mercury released in fuel burning). Without careful assessment and diagnostic evaluation, such polytoxicities can be easily missed.

Heavy metals have no known physiologic activity in humans and are not metabolized, so they accumulate in the tissues. The metals bind with reactive protein groups and enzymes, disrupting enzymatic function. Excretion from the body is slow, so the effects are long-term. Although symptoms vary with the type of metal and extent of exposure, gastrointestinal disturbances ranging from nausea, vomiting, and diarrhea to gastrointestinal hemorrhage are frequently found. Central and peripheral nervous system effects include tremor, peripheral neuropathies, neuropsychiatric disturbances, and seizures. Table 45-13 summarizes toxin-specific findings.

Serum levels generally provide the best evaluation of heavy metal exposure, although urine and hair samples are sometimes tested. A plain film of the abdomen (KUB) may show recently ingested metals in the gastrointestinal tract. The need for therapeutic interventions is determined by extent of exposure and patient symptomatology. With certain chronic exposures, terminating contact with the offending agent or environment is all that is required. For recent ingestions, standard gastric emptying techniques can be employed; however, this is of no benefit for chronic ingestion or inhalation. Activated charcoal does not absorb metals.

Since heavy metals accumulate in the tissues and are not metabolized, chelation therapy is the best means of eliminating these substances from the body. Chelating agents, administered orally, intramuscularly, or intravenously, bind to the metals, facilitating excretion. Three chelating drugs are commonly used: dimercaprol (BAL), penicillamine, and edetate calcium disodium. The particular agent selected and route of administration vary with the toxin involved. Dosage is de-

Metal	Poisoning type	Findings
Lead	Acute	Lethargy, ataxia, constipation, colic, seizures, coma
	Chronic	Subtle behavioral changes, motor neuropathy, intellectual impairment
Mercury	Acute	Renal failure, gastrointestinal symptoms, irritation of the mucous membranes
	Chronic	Tremor, neuropsychiatric symptoms, irritability, memory loss
Arsenic	Acute	Garlic breath odor, tremor, seizures, severe gastrointestinal symptoms, hemolysis
	Chronic	Peripheral neuropathies, anemia, malaise, anorexia

Table **45-13** **Heavy Metal Poisoning**

pendent on patient size and severity of symptoms. Because of the highly individual circumstances surrounding each exposure, consultation with poison control personnel should be obtained before administering any chelating drug. Other supportive measures are largely determined on a patient-by-patient basis as symptoms dictate. Fluid volume deficits, anemia, and renal failure require intervention as appropriate.

Digitalis Glycosides

Digitalis glycosides are available in pharmaceutic preparations such as digoxin and digitoxin and can also be found in homes and yards in oleander, lily of the valley, and foxglove plants. At therapeutic and toxic doses, digitalis glycosides block the sodium-potassium pump. With high serum concentrations, vagal and sympathetic tone increases.

Clinical symptoms can be vague and difficult to diagnose, particularly with chronic overdose in elderly patients. Findings include drowsiness, lethargy, and coma. Cardiac conduction disturbances (first- second- and third- degree heart block), ventricular dysrhythmias (premature ventricular contractions, ventricular tachycardia, and ventricular fibrillation), asystole, and profound hypotension also occur. Visual changes include appearance of yellow or green halos around objects. The patient may experience anorexia, nausea, and vomiting, especially in cases of chronic poisoning.

Quantitative serum levels of digoxin can be useful for assessing individual degree of toxicity. Complete distribution of digoxin to the tissues requires at least 12 hours; therefore serum levels drawn prior to that time may not reflect a state of blood-tissue equilibrium. Concentrations greater than 10 ng/ml are an indication for treatment with digoxin immune Fab (Digibind).

Since toxicosis can occur at various serum concentrations, symptomatology must guide therapy. Asymptomatic patients can be treated with induced emesis for gastric emptying; lavage is indicated for those with signs of toxicity. Since gastric tube placement may increase vagal tone, atropine should be available for the management of significant bradycardia. Activated charcoal absorbs digitalis glycosides from the gastrointestinal tract, decreasing systemic absorption. Multiple doses of activated charcoal have been suggested for the treatment of digoxin and digitoxin overdose, although limited clinical experience with this treatment has been reported.

A digitalis glycoside antidote that consists of an ovine-derived antibody to digitalis glycosides is available. Digoxin immune Fab (Digibind) attaches to digitalis glycosides and renders them inactive. Indications for Digibind are the presence of two or more of the following: life-threatening dysrhythmias, serum potassium levels of 5 mEq/L, or serum digoxin concentration greater than 10 ng/ml. The Digibind manufacturer also suggests administration if a digitalis dose of more than 4 mg has been ingested by a child or more than 10 mg by an adult. An appropriate Digibind dosage is calculated based on pharmacokinetic determination of the total digoxin/digitoxin body load. One drawback to Digibind therapy is the high cost.

Hydrocarbons

Hydrocarbons are found in petroleum, natural gas, coal, and bitumen. Toxicity is related to viscosity—the more viscous the hydrocarbon, the less toxic the substance (Table 45-14). Exposure may be caused by inhalation, dermal contact, or ingestion. Intentional exposures are rare. Accidental exposure occurs in children less than 5 years old with access to kerosene, gasoline, or lighter fluid and in adolescents who sniff gasoline.

Clinical manifestations of hydrocarbon toxicity vary widely with substance and time from exposure. Inhaled hydrocarbons affect the nervous system, whereas ingested hydrocarbons affect the pulmonary system as a result of aspiration. Pulmonary edema is a frequent complication of significant exposure; pneumothorax and pneumomediastinum can also occur. Hydrocarbons affect the heart's conduction system, causing dysrhythmias such as complete heart block; asystole and ventricular fibrillation may also occur. Epinephrine may not be effective for dysrhythmia management in patients with hydrocarbon toxicity. Malaise and gastric discomfort including nausea, vomiting, and bloody diarrhea have also been reported. Significant fever (≥ 103° F) may continue for 48 hours because of neurologic irritation. Anaerobic metabolism secondary to damaged mitochondria leads to metabolic acidosis. Hepatic failure, liver failure, or hemolysis can occur days or weeks after exposure.

Continuous cardiac and pulse oximetry monitoring is recommended. Remove contaminated clothing, and flush skin with copious amounts of saline solution. Intravenous access should be established for emergency medications; however, fluids are limited because of potential development of pulmonary edema. Position the patient carefully to minimize

Table **45-14** **Hydrocarbon Ingestions**

Group	Type	Common forms	Toxicity†
I	Hydrocarbons of high viscosity (over 100 SSU*)	Lubricating oil, petroleum jelly, grease, diesel oil, tar, paraffin	Low (do not empty stomach)
II	Hydrocarbons of low viscosity (under 60 SSU)	Mineral seal oil, gasoline, turpentine, lighter fluid, kerosene, Stoddard solvent, petroleum ether	Moderate (empty stomach if more than 1 ml/kg)
III	Halogenated hydrocarbons	Vinyl chloride, carbon tetrachloride, trichloroethylene, 1,1,1 trichloroethane, halothane	High (empty stomach)
IV	Aromatic hydrocarbons	Benzene, toluene, xylene	High (empty stomach)

From Rosen P et al: *Emergency medicine: concepts and clinical practice,* ed 2, vol 2, St. Louis, 1988, Mosby.
*SSU, Saybolt seconds universal.
†Toxicity relative to risk of aspiration.

Table **45-15** **Poisonous Plants in the House and Garden**

Plant	Toxic components	Toxic effects
Aloe	Entire plant	Marked catharsis 6-12 hours after ingestion; alkaline urine may turn red; large doses cause nephritis
Bird-of-paradise	Pods and seeds	Vomiting, diarrhea, dizziness, vertigo, drowsiness
Castor bean	Leaves, pods, beans	Gastrointestinal distress, convulsions
Cherry	Pits	Dyspnea, vocal paralysis, convulsions, death
Dieffenbachia (dumbcane), philodendron, elephant ear	Entire plant	Mastication causes sudden pain followed by swelling of tongue and throat with dysphagia, blisters, and vocal cord paralysis; swallowing causes laryngeal edema
English ivy	Entire plant and berries	Skin irritation, nausea, vomiting, severe diarrhea, increased thirst and salivation, abdominal pain, dyspnea; can progress to coma
Holly	Berries and leaves	Vomiting, diarrhea, stupor, narcosis
Hunter's robe	Sap	Irritation of skin, lips, tongue; diarrhea can develop
Jack-in-the-pulpit	Leaves	Gastrointestinal irritation; swelling of tongue, lips, and palate
Jerusalem cherry	Entire plant	Stomach pain, low-grade fever, paralysis, dilated pupils, vomiting, diarrhea, depressed respiratory and circulatory function, loss of sensation, death
Lily of the valley, oleander	Entire plant	Gastrointestinal distress, conduction defects, sinus bradycardia, escape beats, hyperkalemia; digitalis-like toxicity depends on amount consumed
Mistletoe	Berries	Gastrointestinal irritation, diarrhea, bradycardia
Pencil tree	Spurges, milk sap	Severe irritation of mouth, throat, and stomach
Poinsettia	Milky sap, stem, leaves, flower bud	Irritation of mouth, throat, and stomach, skin; flower bud is a significant ocular threat
Rhododendron	Leaves and sap	Oropharyngeal burning followed hours later by salivation, diarrhea, vomiting, and paresthesias; weakness, decreased vision, bradycardia, coma, seizures
Rhubarb	Leaf blades	Stomach pains, nausea, vomiting, weakness, dyspnea, oropharyngeal burning, internal bleeding, death
Star of Bethlehem	Entire plant—fresh and dried	Nausea, gastrointestinal irritation
Yew	Entire plant	Diarrhea, vomiting, tremors, pupil dilation, facial pallor, circumoral cyanosis, rash, dyspnea, muscular weakness, seizures, coma, dysrhythmia, death

NURSING DIAGNOSES FOR TOXICOLOGIC EMERGENCIES

Ineffective airway clearance
Altered cardiac output
Impaired gas exchange
Ineffective breathing pattern
Ineffective thermoregulation
Altered tissue perfusion
Fluid volume deficit
Fluid volume excess
Ineffective individual coping
Risk for injury
Altered family processes
Risk for violence

risk of aspiration. Gastric emptying is indicated with recent ingestion of large quantities of a substance with low viscosity and high potential for toxicity. Use a cuffed endotracheal tube in conjunction with gastric lavage to protect the patient from aspiration. Obtain a chest radiograph to rule out early pulmonary alterations. All symptomatic patients should be observed for 24 hours for potential pulmonary and cardiac problems.

Toxic Plants

Many plants found in the home and surrounding environment contain toxic substances. There are approximately 100 toxic species of mushrooms, which usually produce gastrointestinal symptoms. Some mushrooms contain hallucinogenic or anticholinergic toxins. Jimsonweed found in the southwestern United States also contains anticholinergic agents. Other poisonous plants include lily of the valley, dieffenbachia, and poinsettia. Table 45-15 highlights some poisonous plants commonly found in the house and garden.

SUMMARY

Toxicologic emergencies are common events in the emergency department. This chapter highlights some of the more frequently seen poisonings. The initial focus of care in any poisoned patient is always stabilization of cardiopulmonary

or hemodynamic problems. Box 45-6 summarizes potential nursing diagnoses for these patients. Treatment priorities include limiting toxin absorption, enhancing drug elimination, and providing toxin- and patient-specific supportive interventions. The reader is referred to a detailed toxicology text for further information on any of the poisonings discussed in this chapter.

REFERENCES

1. Brent JA: Drugs of abuse, *Emerg Med* 27(7):56, 1995.
2. Dougherty J: Cocaine. In Hamilton GC et al, editors: *Emergency medicine: an approach to clinical problem-solving,* Philadelphia, 1991, WB Saunders.
3. Groleau G, Jotte R, Barish R: The electrocardiographic manifestations of cyclic antidepressant therapy and overdose: a review, *J Emerg Med* 8:597, 1990.
4. Hollander JE et al: Chest pain associated with cocaine: an assessment of prevalence in suburban and urban emergency departments, *An Emerg Med* 26(6):671, 1995.
5. Johnson D et al: Effect of multiple-dose activated charcoal on the clearance of high-dose intravenous aspirin in a porcine model, *An Emerg Med* 26(5):569, 1995.
6. Kitt S et al, editors: *Emergency nursing a physiologic and clinical perspective,* Philadelphia, 1995, WB Saunders.
7. Klein AR et al, editors: *Emergency nursing core curriculum,* Philadelphia, 1992, WB Saunders.
8. Ling LJ: Antidotes. In Barsan WG, Jastremski MS, Syverud SA, editors: *Emergency drug therapy,* Philadelphia, 1991, WB Saunders.
9. Olsen KR, Becker CE: Poisoning. In Ho MT, Saunders CE, editors: *Current emergency diagnosis and treatment,* Norwalk, Conn, 1990, Appleton & Lange.
10. Sheets CA: Emetics and antiemetics. In Barsan WG, Jastremski MS, Syverud SA, editors: *Emergency drug therapy,* Philadelphia, 1991, WB Saunders.
11. Singal B: Acidifying and alkalizing agents. In Barsan WG, Jastremski MS, Syverud SA, editors: *Emergency drug therapy,* Philadelphia, 1991, WB Saunders.
12. Talbot A et al: Plasma concentration of 2-pyridine aldoxime methiodide after bolus injection in organophosphate poisoning, *An Emerg Med* 26(6):116, 1995.
13. Tandberg D, GTW: Gastric lavage in the poisoned patient. In RJR, HJR, editors: *Clinical procedures in emergency medicine,* Philadelphia, 1991, WB Saunders.
14. Tintinalli JE, Krome RL, Ruiz E, editors: *Emergency medicine: a comprehensive study guide,* New York, 1996, McGraw-Hill.
15. Trunbull TL: The poisoned patient. In Hamilton GC et al, editors: *Emergency medicine: an approach to clinical problem solving,* Philadelphia, 1991, WB Saunders.
16. Weilemann LS, Besser R: Efficacy of obidoxime in human organophosphorus poisoning: determination by means of neuromuscular transmission studies, *An Emerg Med* 26(6):721, 1995.

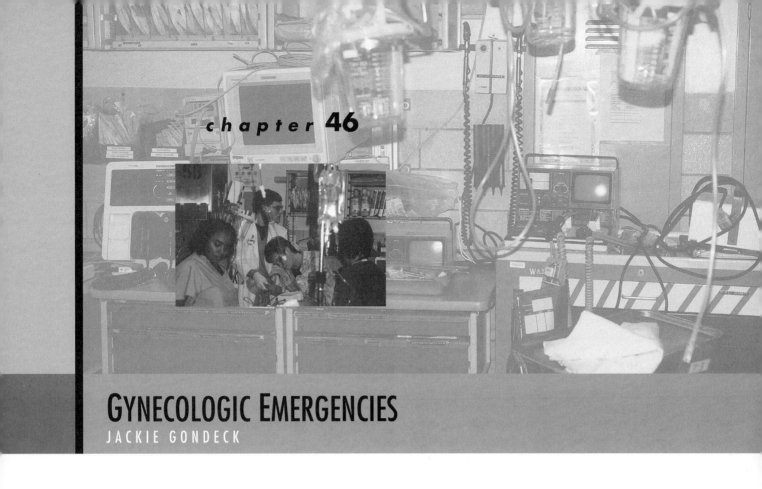

chapter 46

GYNECOLOGIC EMERGENCIES

JACKIE GONDECK

Each year a million American women seek health care for lower abdominal pain. Many come to the emergency department (ED).[1] Familiarity with a variety of gynecologic emergencies is essential to rapidly determine the severity of a patient's condition and intervene appropriately. This chapter focuses on gynecologic emergencies commonly seen in the ED. Sexual assault, obstetric emergencies, and genitourinary trauma are covered in separate chapters of this text.

ANATOMY AND PHYSIOLOGY

Gynecologic emergencies affect the nonpregnant female's reproductive organs: ovaries, fallopian tubes, uterus, vagina, and external genitalia. External genitalia include the mons pubis, labia majora and minora, clitoris, vestibular glands, hymen, urethral opening, and perineum (Figure 46-1). The vestibule is between the labia minora and contains the hymen, vaginal orifice, urethral orifice, ducts of the Bartholin's glands, and Skene's ducts. The Bartholin's glands secrete mucuslike fluid during sexual excitation. The perineum is a triangular area between the posterior portion of the vestibule and anus that supports portions of the urogenital and gastrointestinal tracts.

The ovaries, fallopian tubes, uterus, and vagina are located outside the peritoneal cavity (Figure 46-2). The ovaries are bilateral oval structures located between the uterus and lateral pelvic wall. During childbearing years, each ovary is 2.5 to 5.0 cm long, 1.5 to 3.0 cm wide, and 0.6 to 1.5 cm thick. Size diminishes significantly after meno-

pause. At birth, approximately 2 million ova are present in the ovaries. This number decreases to 300,000 to 400,000 by puberty. During ovulation, each ovary releases a single ovum, which is transported by muscular contractions down the fallopian tubes to the uterus. The fallopian tubes are approximately 10 cm long and transport the ovum to the uterus through muscle contractions. The fallopian tubes are not continuous with the ovaries; therefore the ovum can migrate into the peritoneal cavity.

The uterus is a pear-shaped, thick-walled organ located in the anterior pelvis. Suspended above the bladder and in front of the rectum, the uterus is 6 to 8 cm long in women who have never been pregnant and 9 to 10 cm in women who have been pregnant. A layer of peritoneum covers the superior portion of the uterus and forms the serous layer of the uterine wall. The middle layer of the uterine wall consists of smooth muscle with an inner mucous layer lining the uterine cavity known as the endometrium. The cervix is the lower portion of the uterus. The cervical os, the entrance to the uterine cavity, is located in the vagina between the bladder anteriorly and rectum posteriorly.

The female sexual cycle consists of ovulation and menstruation and is determined by changes in female hormone levels. Length of the cycle ranges from 20 to 45 days, with an average of 28 days for most women. Changes in hormone levels prepare the endometrium for implantation of the fertilized ovum. If the ovum is not fertilized, the endometrium sheds the inner lining as menstrual flow.

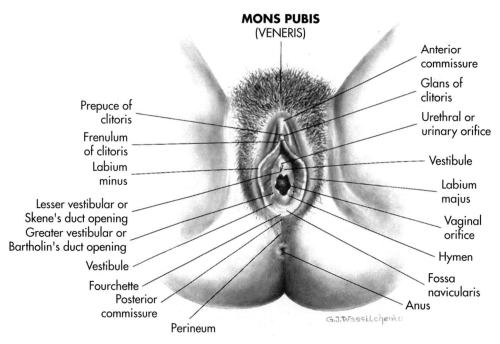

Figure **46-1** External female genitalia. *(From Lowdermilk DL, Perry SE, Bobak IM:* Maternity and women's health care, *ed 6, St. Louis, 1997, Mosby.)*

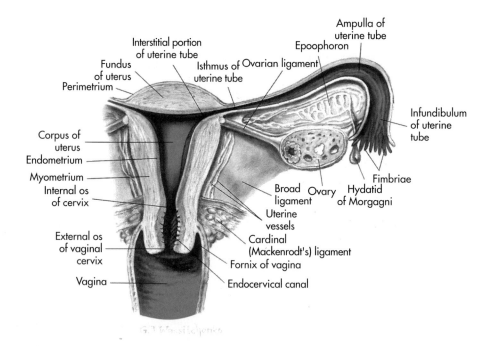

Figure **46-2** Female reproductive organs. *(From Lowdermilk DL, Perry SE, Bobak IM:* Maternity and women's health care, *ed 6, St. Louis, 1997, Mosby.)*

ASSESSMENT

A woman presenting to the ED with a gynecologic problem may be dealing with physical discomfort as well as emotional overtones related to sexuality. Public discussion of sexual activity and sexual history does not come easily to many people. The patient may be anxious and withdrawn. The emergency nurse should make every effort to reduce or alleviate anxiety by respecting the patient's privacy and personal dignity. Provide visual and auditory privacy while asking potentially embarrassing questions. Allow the patient to undress in private. Introductions of health care providers—physicians and nurses—should precede the pelvic examination! Box 46-1 summarizes essential interview questions for the patient with a gynecologic complaint.

Patients with gynecologic emergencies can develop hypovolemia secondary to blood loss. Assess carefully for clues to fluid volume deficits such as tachycardia, diaphoresis, narrowed pulse pressure, and orthostatic changes in blood pressure and pulse.

SPECIFIC GYNECOLOGIC EMERGENCIES
Menstrual Pain

Women may present to the ED with pain related to their menstrual cycle. Mittelschmerz is a benign pain associated with ovulation, usually localized to one side, which lasts a few hours but can persist for 24 to 48 hours. Etiology of mittelschmerz is unknown. Diagnosis is based on timing of the pain with the menstrual cycle as well as ruling out other sources for the pain. Mittelschmerz resolves without treatment.

Dysmenorrhea is pain caused by uterine spasms associated with menses. The patient also complains of breast tenderness, nausea, vomiting, headache, backache, abdominal distention, and loose stools. Approximately 50% of all women experience dysmenorrhea. As with mittelschmerz, diagnosis depends on ruling out other causes of the pain and correlating the pain with the patient's menstrual cycle. Treatment includes pain control with heating pads and nonsteroidal antiinflammatory drugs such as aspirin or ibuprofen. The emergency nurse may care for patients with mittelschmerz or dysmenorrhea; however, the focus of this chapter is gynecologic problems not associated with the normal menstrual cycle.

Vaginal Discharge

Normal vaginal discharge is composed of vaginal cells, lactic acid, and secretions from the cervical and Bartholin's glands.[5] Physiologic vaginal discharge is usually clear and usually odorless. Abnormal vaginal discharge may be caused by vaginitis, cervicitis, or sexually transmitted diseases (STDs). Changes in vaginal pH caused by pregnancy, antibiotics, oral contraceptives, vaginal creams or jellies, and douches also cause an abnormal vaginal discharge. Women usually seek care for a discharge that is abnormal for them, usually abnormal in color, consistency, or odor. Color abnormalitie ranges from white to yellow to green. A white discharge suggests *Candida albicans* (Figure 46-3), yellow discharge suggests *Neisseria gonorrhoeae,* and gray or greenish-gray color suggests *Trichomonas vaginalis* or *Gardnerella vaginalis.* Discharge may be thin and watery or have a cottage cheese consistency. *G. vaginalis* causes a fishy smell, whereas *T. vaginalis* makes the discharge malodorous. Related symptoms include vulvar swelling, itching, or redness. Urinary retention or dysuria related to pain may also occur.

During patient assessment, determine how long the patient has had the discharge, color and consistency of the discharge, and any associated foul odor. Sexual activity and possible STD exposure should also be evaluated. A pelvic examination is performed to obtain a Gram's stain and culture of the discharge. Urinalysis and culture are done if the patient has dysuria. Treatment of vaginal discharge includes antibiotics as well as general hygiene recommendations. Box 46-2 summarizes discharge instructions for the patient with a vaginal discharge.

Vaginal Bleeding

Abnormal vaginal bleeding is one of the most common gynecologic complaints treated in the ED. Dysfunctional vaginal bleeding can occur in both the pregnant and non-pregnant patient (see Chapter 49 for discussion of vaginal bleeding related to pregnancy). During assessment, determine when the bleeding began, the amount of bleeding, and associated symptoms such as pain. As a general rule of thumb, a saturated peripad equals 30 ml of blood loss. Irregular vaginal bleeding due to hormonal imbalances is not typically associated with pain. Vaginal bleeding in post-menopausal women suggests the possibility of benign or malignant uterine, ovarian, or cervical tumors. Patients on

---

Box **46-1**	**Interview Questions for Gynecologic Emergencies**

When was your last menstrual period?

Was your period normal?

How long does your period normally last?

Are you sexually active?

What type of birth control do you use? Do you consistently use it?

Is there a possibility you are pregnant?

Do you normally have a vaginal discharge? What is different about the discharge today?

How much are you bleeding? How many pads/tampons are you using per day/hour?

Do you have any swelling, itching, redness, or pain?

How many pregnancies have you had? How many children do you have?

Box **46-2**	**Discharge Instructions for Vaginal Discharge**

Cleanse the perineum from front to back using soap and water.

Wear cotton underwear.

Avoid tight-fitting clothes and pantyhose.

Avoid vaginal sprays and douches.

Change damp swimsuits and workout clothing as soon as possible.

Void before and after intercourse.

Use barrier protection during intercourse.

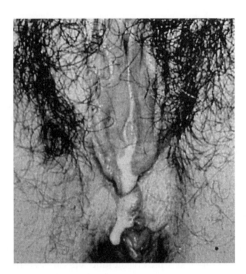

Figure **46-3** *Candida albicans. (From Zitelli BJ, Davis HW: Atlas of pediatric physical diagnosis, ed 2, London, 1992, Gower Medical Publishing. Courtesy Dr. Ellen Wald, Children's Hospital of Pittsburgh.)*

anticoagulant therapy may present with vaginal bleeding or hematuria even with therapeutic anticoagulant levels.

One of the most common causes of abnormal uterine bleeding in women of childbearing age is contraceptives. Breakthrough bleeding may occur with oral contraceptives if the patient's daily dose is too low. Increasing the dose should correct breakthrough bleeding. Depo-Provera, now approved for use as a contraceptive, may cause abnormal vaginal bleeding.[3]

Another cause of dysfunctional uterine bleeding is endometriosis—retrograde flow of endometrial tissue up the fallopian tubes. Endometrial tissue can attach to the fallopian tubes, ovaries, or anywhere in the pelvic cavity. Patients with endometriosis usually have abdominal pain approximately 2 weeks prior to menstruation. Treatment includes hormone therapy, surgery, or a combination of the two.

Ovarian Cyst

An ovarian cyst is a sac on the ovary, which contains fluid, semifluid, or solid material. The most common cause of an ovarian cyst is overgrowth of endometrial tissue. Hemorrhage of a mature corpus luteum into its cavity causes a blood-filled cyst in the wall of the ovary. Ovarian cysts differ in size, consistency, and development. Small cysts are usually asymptomatic. When small cysts rupture, the fluid is usually spontaneously reabsorbed. Surgical intervention is not required unless the patient exhibits signs of hypovolemia and shock. If the cyst enlarges, the patient may complain of a dull ache on the affected side and experience prolonged menstruation. Rupture of a blood-filled ovarian cyst is potentially life-threatening. The patient presents with signs of hypovolemia, ranging from mild tachycardia to severe hypotension and shock.

An extremely large ovarian cyst may actually twist around the vascular pedicle, causing an ovarian torsion. Symptoms include sudden onset of sharp, intermittent pain on the affected side. There is usually a history of similar episodes lasting hours or even days. The patient may also complain of continuous dull pain with periods of acute discomfort associated with nausea and vomiting. Temperature and heart rate are normal in most patients with an ovarian cyst.

The patient may seek care in the ED for pain related to the ovarian cyst or may present with obvious hemodynamic compromise. Treatment includes hemodynamic support as appropriate and pain control. Doppler ultrasonography is used to rule out ruptured ectopic pregnancy and appendicitis in stable patients, since these conditions present with similar symptomatology. If the patient has severe hemodynamic compromise, immediate surgical intervention may be required.

Sexually Transmitted Diseases

STDs include pelvic inflammatory disease (PID), gonorrhea, syphilis, genital herpes, genital warts, human immunodeficiency virus (HIV) infection, and hepatitis (see Chapter 42 for discussion of HIV infection and for discussion of hepatitis). When caring for the patient with an STD, discuss high-risk behaviors such as multiple partners, anal intercourse, and unprotected intercourse, and review safe sexual practices such as barrier protection. Sexual partners should be identified and referred for treatment. Information should be provided in a nonthreatening, nonjudgmental manner.

Pelvic inflammatory disease

PID is an acute or chronic infection of the fallopian tubes and surrounding structures. Infection may result from upward migration of genital infection or from contamination during gynecologic surgery or delivery. During assessment, question the patient about STD exposure, recent abortion or delivery, and use of an intrauterine device. The initial onset of PID is not considered an emergency situation; however, the condition is serious because of potential complications such as infertility, ectopic pregnancy, recurrent disease, and chronic pelvic pain.[1] The disease is very expensive for both the patient and the medical community. "Direct cost for PID and its associated sequelae of ectopic pregnancy and infertility approach three billion dollars a year. These costs are projected to approach ten billion dollars annually by the year 2000."[7]

The patient with PID presents with moderate to severe lower abdominal pain, hyperpyrexia, abnormal vaginal discharge, and occasionally vaginal bleeding. Pain increases with walking, urination, defecation, and intercourse. The patient walks stooped over or with a shuffling gait. There is a malodorous vaginal discharge, which is thick and cream colored. Pathogens most often responsible for PID are *N. gonorrhoeae* and *Chlamydia trachomatis*. *N. gonorrhoeae* causes the most dramatic display of symptoms. A patient with *C. trachomatis* has less severe symptoms. Pain may be diffuse rather than severe and the temperature normal, so the patient may not seek treatment or may delay treatment. One study reported that more than 50% of women with scarring of the fallopian tubes and subsequent infertility had no recollection of having PID.[7]

Treatment for PID includes positioning, pain control, and antibiotics. Elevating the patient's head 30 to 45 degrees facilitates pooling of secretions into the lower pelvic area. Pain control should be individualized for the patient's specific level of discomfort. The patient may be given intramuscular and/or oral antibiotics and then discharged or may be admitted for intravenous antibiotics. Criteria for admission and intravenous antibiotics are summarized in Box 46-3. Discuss with the patient the hazards of unprotected intercourse or intercourse with multiple partners, the use of barrier protection during intercourse, and the potential risk for HIV infection.

Genital herpes

An estimated 25 million Americans have genital herpes.[8] Genital herpes is a chronic, incurable STD caused by the herpes simplex virus type 2 (HSV-2). Herpes simplex virus type 1 (HSV-1) causes the cold sore. Clinically, lesions caused by these two viruses are identical. In general, HSV-1 is associated with skin lesions above the waist, whereas HSV-2 is associated with skin lesions below the waist.

The patient with genital herpes develops painful lesions in the genital area, buttocks, or thighs 2 to 12 days after exposure (Figure 46-4). In women, the most common site is the cervix and vulva. In men, the most common site is the glans and prepuce. Flulike symptoms such as fever, chills, headache, nausea, vomiting, and malaise occur during this initial period. The patient often has a stinging or burning sensation before blisters erupt. Inguinal lymphadenopathy may also be present. Urinary retention can occur because of pain when urine comes in contact with the ulcerated area. Symptoms normally subside 2 weeks after onset; however, about 50% of the patients will have a recurrence of symptoms every 2 months.

Treatment of genital herpes is palliative and includes acyclovir, warm baths, topical anesthetics, and mild analgesics.

Box 46-3   Criteria for Hospital Admission and Intravenous Antibiotics for PID

The patient is pregnant.
The patient is unable to comply with outpatient treatment.
The patient has not responded to outpatient treatment.
A pelvic abscess is present or suspected.
Underlying disease has lowered the patient's resistance to infections.
Other conditions such as appendicitis must be ruled out.

The patient should be encouraged to rest, eat a balanced diet, and reduce stress. Barrier protection should be used during intercourse. Sexual activity should not occur during infectious outbreaks or during the 24-hour prodromal period. Recommend that the patient avoid sexual activity until the lesions dry up. Make sure the patient understands that HSV-1 can cause HSV-2 if the patient has oral sex with an infected partner. Genital herpes increases the risk for cervical cancer; therefore discharge teaching should stress the importance of regular gynecologic examinations and an annual Pap smear.

Gonorrhea

Gonorrhea is caused by *N. gonorrhoeae* and is the most frequently reported communicable disease in the United States.[9] Some antibiotic-resistant strains have been reported. Concurrent infection with *C. trachomatis* is also common. Pharyngeal, vaginal, penile, and anal infections can occur. Ocular infections can result from transmission of the organisms by contaminated fingers. Symptoms usually occur within 1 week of exposure. Males present with a yellow or

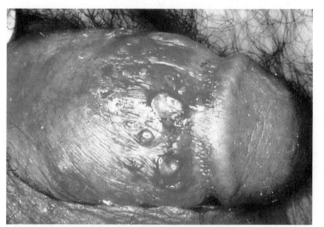

A

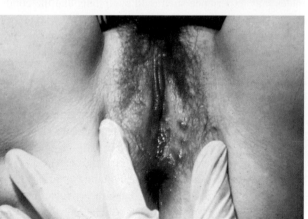

B

Figure **46-4**   Genital herpes in a male (**A**) and female (**B**) patient. (*From Lewis SM, Collier IC, Heitkemper MM: Medical-surgical nursing, ed 4, St. Louis, 1996, Mosby.*)

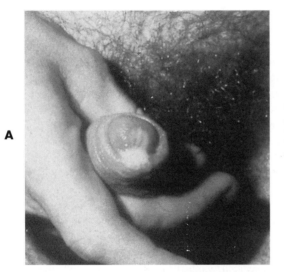

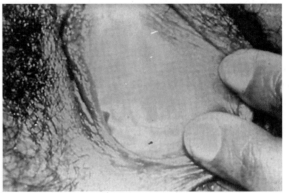

A

B

Figure **46-5** Gonorrhea in a male (**A**) and female (**B**) patient. *(From Morse SA:* Atlas of sexually transmitted diseases, *London, 1990, Gower Medical Publishing.)*

Table **46-1**   **Drug Therapy for Syphilis**

Stage	Benzathine penicillin G (IM)	Aqueous crystalline penicillin G (IV)	Other antibiotics*
Early syphilis (primary, secondary, and early latent)	At single visit		Doxycycline, tetracycline, erythromycin
Syphilis lasting >1 yr	Three weekly injections		
Symptomatic neurosyphilis		Daily for 14 days followed by penicillin G benzathine weekly for 3 doses	Doxycycline, tetracycline, erythromycin

Modified from Centers for Disease Control: *STD treatment guidelines of USPHS,* Atlanta, 1993, Centers for Disease Control.
IM, Intramuscular; *IV,* intravenous.
*Given when penicillin is contraindicated.

mucopurulent discharge and/or dysuria (Figure 46-5, *A*). Females may experience such mild symptoms that the condition is overlooked, or symptoms may occur in conjunction with symptoms of PID (Figure 46-5, *B*). Symptoms include vaginal discharge, lower abdominal pain, and abnormal menses. Five percent of all cases are asymptomatic.

Culture and Gram's stain are obtained to confirm the diagnosis and ensure appropriate antibiotic therapy. Treatment includes oral doxycycline or intramuscular ceftriaxone for the patient and the partner(s). Barrier protection should be encouraged. The patient should be sexually abstinent until treatment is completed. Untreated gonorrhea can lead to disseminated gonococcal infections including arthritis, tenosynovitis, dermatitis, and rarely hepatitis, myocarditis, endocarditis, and meningitis. Women with untreated gonorrhea often present with sudden-onset joint pain, swelling, and redness.

Syphilis
Syphilis is a systemic disease caused by *Treponema pallidum*. Although the incidence declined during the 1950s

with the advent of penicillin, there has been a resurgence of cases in the 1990s.[2] Incubation is 10 to 90 days.[4] Syphilis has three recognizable phases: primary, secondary, and tertiary.

Primary syphilis occurs approximately 3 weeks after exposure. The patient usually has one or two genital ulcers, which heal in approximately 3 weeks without any treatment (Figure 46-6). Primary syphilis progresses to *secondary syphilis* if the patient is not treated. During this phase, the patient develops a continuous or intermittent rash on the palms of the hand and the soles of the feet (Figure 46-7). Vague, flulike symptoms may also be present. Typically, secondary syphilis lasts 1 year. Without treatment during this stage, the infection progresses to the tertiary phase. *Tertiary syphilis* may cause symptoms in 3 to 4 years, or the patient may be asymptomatic for 10 to 15 years after the primary exposure. During this period, the patient experiences intermittent skin lesions and can develop cardiovascular or neurologic syphilis. Long-term sequelae of cardiovascular syphilis include aneurysms, narrowed coronary arteries, and

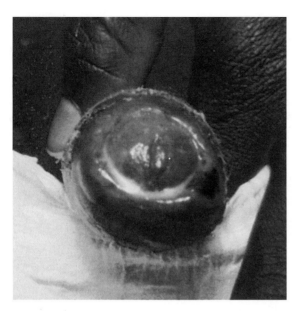

Figure **46-6** Primary syphilis in the male. *(From Greenberger NJ, Hinthorn DR:* History taking and physical examination: essentials and clinical correlates, *St. Louis, 1993, Mosby.)*

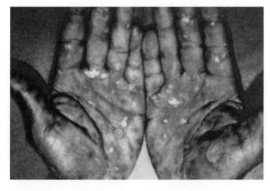

Figure **46-7** Secondary syphilis. *(From Goldstein BJ, Goldstein AO:* Practical dermatology, *St. Louis, 1992, Mosby.)*

aortic valve damage. Neurosyphilis causes gradual development of behavioral changes consistent with dementia. The patient may also have tremulous extremities and an abnormal gait.

Syphilis is a debilitating disease process that is increasing in frequency. Untreated, it will affect the patient's life forever. Treatment includes antibiotics for the patient and the partner(s) as well as barrier protection (Table 46-1).

Genital warts

Genital warts are caused by the human papillomavirus (HPV). Unlike other STDs, the incubation period for HPV has not been clearly identified. Incubation can vary from 1 to 6 months. Warts thrive in a warm, moist environment, so they occur most often on the vulva, perineum, and perianal regions. One third of women with vulvar warts have vaginal

Box **46-4**

NURSING DIAGNOSES FOR GYNECOLOGIC EMERGENCIES
High risk for fluid volume deficit
Potential for decreased cardiac output
Pain
Anxiety
Fear
Self-esteem disturbance
Body image disturbance
High risk for infection
Knowledge deficit

or cervical warts; therefore an internal examination with a speculum is always indicated.[4] Treatment consists of painting the affected area with 5% acetic acid. Multiple applications are required and may not totally eradicate the warts. In some instances, cauterization can be performed under local or general anesthesia. If this fails, surgical excision may be required.[4] Past and present partners should be evaluated and treated when appropriate. It is important for the patient to have follow-up care, since there is an increased risk of cervical cancer associated with some types of genital warts.

Bartholin's Cyst

The Bartholin's gland secretes fluid into a duct on the surface of the labium. Under normal circumstances, the gland cannot be palpated or visualized. If the duct becomes blocked, a small, painless lump can develop. If there is no infection, warm sitz baths are used to treat the blocked duct. Pathogens such as *N. gonorrhoeae, C. trachomatis,* or *Escherichia coli* can invade the duct and cause infection. The labium becomes extremely edematous and tender. The patient usually complains of extreme discomfort, which makes it difficult to walk or sit. Treatment for an infected Bartholin's gland is incision and drainage. A drain or wick may be inserted to facilitate drainage of the purulent fluid. The patient is placed on antibiotics and should be reevaluated in 24 to 72 hours for drain removal as appropriate.

CONCLUSION

The patient with a gynecologic emergency should be provided care without judging sexual practices or lifestyle. Lack of objectivity in the caregiver can interfere with identification of potentially life-threatening gynecologic conditions. Delayed identification and intervention can affect patients' sexuality, fertility, and even their life. Recognition of problems that require the most immediate attention is essential for the emergency nurse to minimize potential adverse outcomes for these patients. Box 46-4 identifies the most common nursing diagnoses for these patients.

REFERENCES

1. Apuzzio J, Hoegsberg B: PID: hard to find but essential to treat, *Contemp OB/GYN,* p 23, 1992.
2. Gilstrap L, Wendel G: Syphilis rise calls for accurate diagnosis, *Contemp OB/GYN,* p 56, 1992.
3. Kaunitz A: DMPA: a new contraceptive option, *Contemp OB/GYN,* p 19, 1993.
4. Martin D, Mroczkowski T: Dermatologic manifestations of sexually transmitted diseases other than HIV, *Infect Dis Clin North Am* 8(3):533, 1994.
5. *Mosby's medical encyclopedia for healthcare consumers,* St. Louis, 1995, Mosby.
6. Sanford JP: *The Sanford guide to antimicrobial therapy,* Dallas, 1995, Antimicrobial Therapy, pp 1-44.
7. Soper D: Pelvic inflammatory disease, *Infect Dis Clin North Am* 8(4):821, 1994.
8. Swanson J, Dibble S, Trocki K: A description of gender differences in risk behaviors in young adults with genital herpes, *Public Health Nurs* 12(2):99, 1995.
9. Zenilman JM: Gonorrhea in the 1990s, *Emerg Med,* p 101, July 1992.

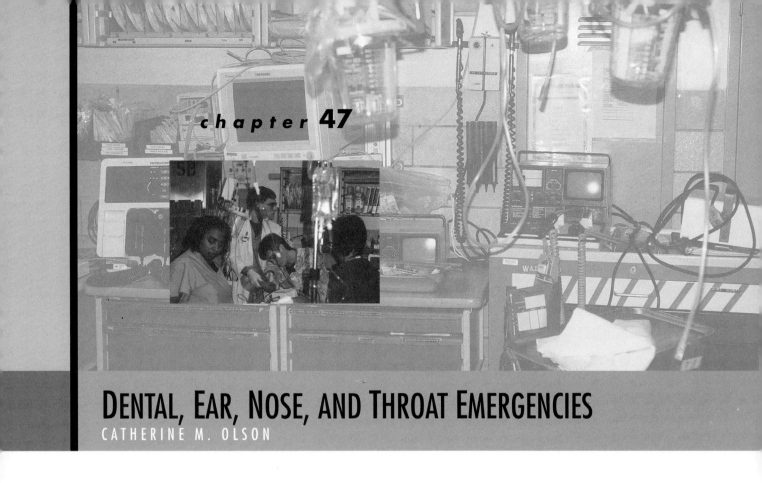

DENTAL, EAR, NOSE, AND THROAT EMERGENCIES

CATHERINE M. OLSON

Most emergencies involving the face, mouth, ears, nose, and throat involve discomfort and pain. However, certain conditions can become life-threatening if associated edema worsens to the point of airway compromise. Infectious processes in the mouth and face can spread to the brain, with potential systemic effects that may be fatal. Other concerns related to this area include loss of function and potential cosmetic deformities. This chapter describes conditions of the face, mouth, ears, nose, and throat that are frequently seen in the emergency department (ED). A brief review of anatomy is provided.

ANATOMY

Structures of the mouth, nose, ears, throat, and face are intimately connected. Injury to one area can affect the others, just as infection from one site can spread to adjacent areas.

Mouth

Dentition consists of two main structures: the teeth and periodontium. Teeth are composed of pulp, dentin, enamel, and root (Figure 47-1). The pulp, located at the center of the tooth, provides neurovascular supply and produces dentin. Dentin is a microtubular structure that overlays the pulp, provides hydration, and cushions teeth during mastication. Enamel, which covers the crown, is the visible part of the tooth and the hardest substance in the body. The root anchors the tooth into alveolar tissue and bone. The periodontium is made up of gingiva and the attachment apparatus. Gingiva, or gums, is a mucous membrane with supporting fibrous tissue encircling the teeth and also covering unerupted teeth. The attachment apparatus consists of the cementum, periodontal ligament, and alveolar bone.[1] Table 47-1 describes the function of each. In children, onset of primary and permanent teeth is important in determining management of injuries.[13] Normal primary dentition begins erupting at 6 months, with 20 teeth by 3 years. Permanent dentition begins at 5 to 6 years with eruption of the first molar and is usually completed by ages 16 to 18 for a total of 32 teeth.[1]

Ears

The ear is divided into three sections: external, middle, and inner ear (Figure 47-2). The external ear consists of the auricle (pinna), ear canal, and tympanic membrane (TM). The auricle is a cartilaginous appendage attached to each side of the head that collects and directs sound to sensory organs within the ear. The S-shaped ear canal is approximately 2.5 to 3.0 cm long in adults, terminating at the TM. The canal is lined with glands that secrete cerumen, a yellow, waxy material that lubricates and protects the ear.[8]

The TM, or eardrum, is a thin, translucent, pearly gray oval disk separating the external ear from the middle ear. It protects the middle ear and conducts sound vibrations to the ossicles.[3] On inspection with an otoscopic light, a cone of light at the anteroinferior aspect of the TM should normally be visible. Another landmark is the long process of the

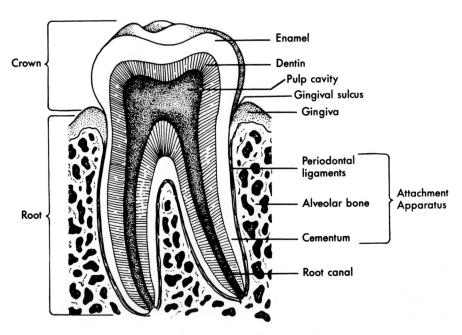

*Figure **47-1*** Dental anatomic unit and attachment apparatus. *(From Rosen P et al:* Emergency medicine: concepts and clinical practice, *ed 3, St. Louis, 1992, Mosby.)*

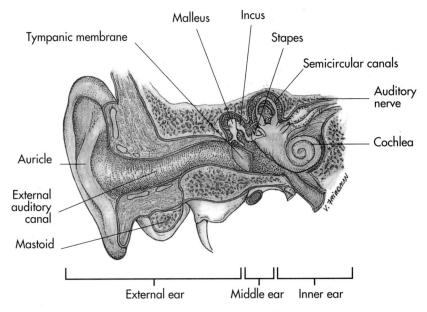

*Figure **47-2*** Ear structures. *(From Potter PA, Perry AG:* Fundamentals of nursing: concepts, process, and practice, *ed 4, St. Louis, 1997, Mosby.)*

malleus (manubrium) pointing posterior and inferior and terminating in the center of the TM (Figure 47-3).

The middle ear is an air-filled cavity inside the temporal bone, which consists of the ossicles, windows, and eustachian tube. Three tiny ear bones, or ossicles, are the malleus (hammer), incus (anvil), and stapes (stirrup), so named because of their appearance. Round and oval windows open into the inner ear, where sound vibrations enter.[3]

The eustachian tube connects the middle ear with the nasopharynx, allowing passage of air to equalize pressure on either side of the TM. The inner ear contains the bony labyrinth, which holds the sensory organs for equilibrium and hearing.[8]

Nose

Externally, the nose is a triangular, mostly cartilaginous structure that warms, filters, and moistens inhaled air, provides a sense of smell, and is the primary passageway for inhaled air to the lungs (Figure 47-4). The upper third of the nose where the frontal and maxillary bones form the bridge is bony. Two nares at the base of the triangle allow air to enter and pass into the nasopharynx. The internal nose is formed by the palatine (hard palate) bones inferiorly and superiorly by the cribriform plate of the ethmoid bone, through which branches of the olfactory nerve pass. The nasal cavity is separated by the septum, forming two anterior vestibules. The septum is usually deviated slightly to one side. Lateral walls are formed by three parallel bony projections—the su-

perior, middle, and inferior turbinates—which help increase surface area to warm inhaled air (Figure 47-5).

Blood supply to the nose originates from the internal and external carotid arteries. The internal maxillary artery branch of the external carotid supplies the posterior nasal septum and lateral wall of the nose. As a branch of the internal carotid artery, the anterior ethmoidal artery supplies blood to the anterior septum at Kiesselbach's plexus in Little's area.[20] This area is also supplied by the septal branches on the sphenopalatine and superior labial arteries (Figure 47-6).

Throat

The throat, or pharynx, consists of the nasopharynx, oropharynx, and laryngopharynx (Figure 47-7). The nasopharynx is positioned behind the nasal cavities and ex-

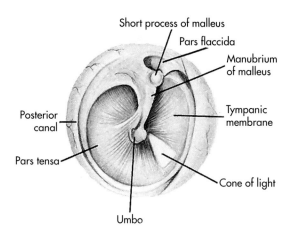

Figure **47-3** Normal tympanic membrane. *(From Bowers AC, Thompson JM: Clinical manual of health assessment, ed 4, St. Louis, 1992, Mosby.)*

Table **47-1**	**Dental Attachment Apparatus**
Component	**Function**
Cementum	Functions as connective tissue covering and supporting the root of the tooth
Periodontal ligament	Fibrous structure surrounds and anchors the root into alveolar bone
Alveolar bone	Anchors tooth to oral cavity and gives shape to dentition

Data from Amsterdam JT: Dental disorders. In Rosen P et al, editors: *Emergency medicine: concepts and clinical practice*, ed 3, St. Louis, 1992, Mosby.

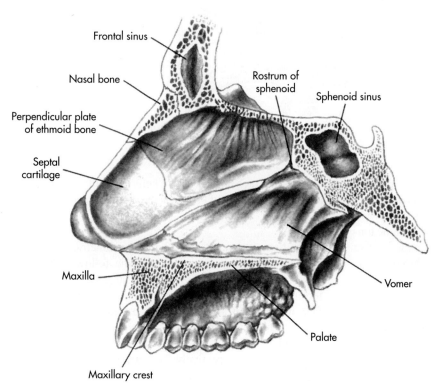

Figure **47-4** Nasal structures. *(From Thompson JM et al: Mosby's clinical nursing, ed 3, 1997, Mosby.)*

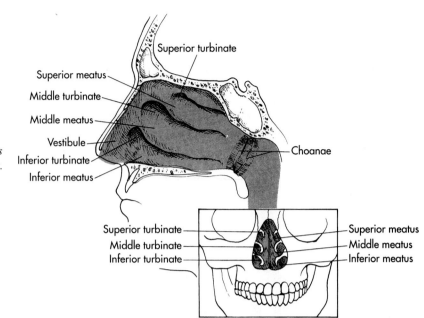

Figure **47-5** Nasal turbinates. *(From Barkauskas et al:* Health and physical assessment, *ed 4, St. Louis, 1994, Mosby.)*

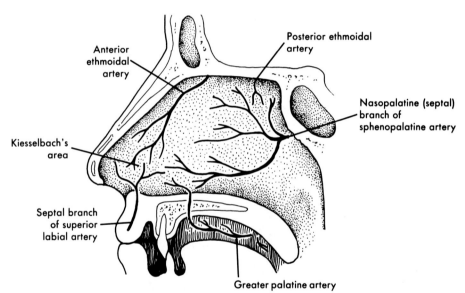

Figure **47-6** Arterial supply to nasal septum. *(From Rosen P et al:* Emergency medicine: concepts and clinical practice, *ed 3, St. Louis, 1992, Mosby.)*

tends from the posterior nares to the uvula.[19] The pharyngeal tonsils, or adenoids, and eustachian tube openings are located in this area.[8] The oropharynx extends downward from the uvula to the epiglottis and contains the palatine tonsils, lymphoid tissue that filters microorganisms to protect the respiratory and gastrointestinal tracts. The laryngopharynx extends from the epiglottis to the opening of the larynx.[19] The pharynx allows passage of air into the larynx. Pharyngeal constrictor muscles propel food or liquid into the esophagus.[10] These muscles are also responsible for the gag reflex, which is controlled by the cranial nerves.[19] The larynx is a tubular, mostly cartilaginous structure located between the trachea and pharynx; its main purpose is to allow air into the trachea. The larynx helps prevent aspiration, assists in coughing, and serves as the organ for speech.[19]

Face

The bony structures of the face are symmetric and consist of the vomer bone, mandible, and the following pairs of bones: maxillae, palatine, zygomatic, lacrimal, nasal, and inferior nasal conchae. The facial skull forms the shape of the face and provides attachment for muscles that move the jaw and control facial expressions.[19] Cranial nerves V (trigeminal) and VII (facial) are responsible for facial innervation and movement, respectively. The paranasal sinuses are sterile, air-filled pockets situated behind and around the nose, which lighten the weight of the skull, provide resonance for speech, and move secretions into the nasopharynx via ciliated mucous membranes.[8] Four pairs of sinuses are named for their craniofacial location (Figure 47-8). In children less than 6 years, the sinuses are not fully developed.[20] The ethmoidal and frontal sinuses are fairly well developed between 6 and 7 years and mature along with the maxillary and sphenoidal sinuses during adolescence.[8]

The temporomandibular joint (TMJ) is the point where

the mandible connects to the temporal bone of the skull; it can be palpated bilaterally just anterior to the tragus of the ear. The TMJ is a synovial joint that allows hinge action to open and close the jaws, gliding action for protrusion and retraction, and gliding for side to side movement of the lower jaw.[8]

DENTAL EMERGENCIES
Odontalgia

Dental caries are the most frequent cause of dental pain, or odontalgia (Figure 47-9).[1] Box 47-1 identifies other potential causes of dental pain. Dental caries are caused by poor oral hygiene, which allows bacterial plaque to develop, which forms acids that break down and calcify tooth enamel. Decay progresses and invades dentin and pulp, eventually producing a hyperemic response. The pulp becomes inflamed, leading to pulpitis and finally pulpal necrosis. Occasionally, pus leaks from the apex of the affected tooth as a periapical abscess forms. Toothaches accompanied by facial or neck swelling should be assessed and promptly treated to prevent spread of infection. Clinical management includes topical anesthetics, nerve blocks, and analgesics including parenteral narcotics to provide palliative treatment until the patient receives definitive care from the dentist.

Tooth Eruption

Between 6 months and 3 years of age, primary teeth erupt in children, causing a variety of symptoms including pain, irritability, disrupted sleep, nasal discharge, and crying. Increased salivary gland production causes diarrhea as well as significant drooling.[2] Decreased fluid intake related to den-

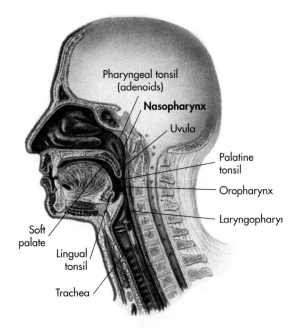

Figure **47-7** The pharynx. *(From Wilson SF, Thompson:* Respiratory disorders, *St. Louis, 1990, Mosby.)*

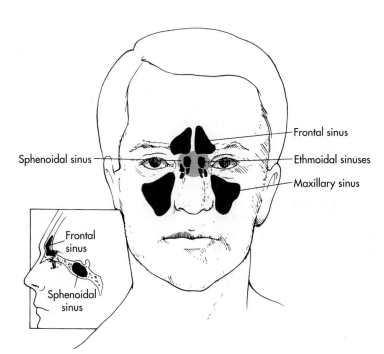

Figure **47-8** Paranasal sinuses. *(From Barkauskas et al:* Health and physical assessment, *St. Louis, 1994, Mosby.)*

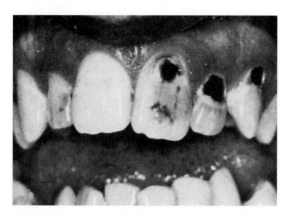

Figure **47-9** Dental caries. *(From Grundy JR, Jones JG: A color atlas of clinical operative dentistry crowns and bridges, ed 2, London, 1992, Wolfe Medical Publishing.)*

Box **47-1**	**Common Causes of Dental Pain**

Dry socket (postextraction pain)
Fractured teeth
Hematoma from anesthetic injection
Maxillary sinusitis
Pericoronitis secondary to erupting wisdom teeth
Periodontal (gum) disease
Post–root canal surgery
Prosthetic device pressure
Unerupted teeth—especially in children

tal pain may cause dehydration and low-grade fever of 37.9° C (100.6° F). Care must be taken not to attribute significant fevers (>37.9° C [100.6° F]) to this relatively benign process.[2] Tonsillar or throat infections, thrush, other oral lesions, and respiratory emergencies such as epiglottitis (especially with excessive drooling) should be considered. In the second decade of life, third molars, or wisdom teeth, begin erupting, causing pain in adolescents and adults. Gingival inflammation secondary to wisdom tooth eruption may cause pericoronitis.

Topical anesthetics such as benzocaine are used sparingly to prevent sterile abscess formation. Acetaminophen is useful for analgesia in young children. To maintain hydration, popsicles are usually well received and provide pain relief. When there is minimal oral intake, a bolus of intravenous fluids may be necessary. In adults, frequent saline irrigation may be used to remove debris from the affected tooth. Nonnarcotic analgesia is effective for pain relief in adult patients. Any consistent swelling or drainage from the eruption site requires referral to a dentist or oral surgeon.

Pericoronitis

If erupting molars become impacted or crowded, food and debris lodge under the pericoronal flap, causing gingival inflammation or pericoronitis. Pericoronitis is extremely painful, especially with opening and closing of the mouth. Earache on the affected side, sore throat, and fever may also occur.[9] Surrounding tissues appear red and inflamed, and submandibular lymphadenopathy and trismus may be noted.

Warm saline or peroxide irrigation and mouth rinses are helpful in early stages of pericoronitis. When pus is present, incision and drainage may be necessary. Antibiotic therapy, usually penicillin or erythromycin, is indicated. Follow-up with an oral-maxillofacial surgeon within 24 to 48 hours for removal of the affected third molar is highly recommended.[1]

Fractured Tooth

The most frequently seen dental emergency in the ED is a chipped or broken tooth, usually anterior maxillary teeth. Trauma to dentition occurs as a result of sports activity, motor vehicle collisions, physical assaults or abuse, propulsive objects, falls, and convulsive seizures.[9] The emergency nurse should assess for concurrent head injury or maxillofacial trauma. Aspiration of the tooth or fragment or an embedded tooth should also be considered. Management of fractures of the anterior teeth is determined by fracture relationship to the pulp and patient age.[1] The Ellis classification system is used to describe location of tooth fractures. Class I fractures are the most common, involving only enamel. Injured areas appear chalky white. Cosmetic restoration is possible with dental referral within 24 to 48 hours. Class II fractures pass through the enamel and expose dentin. The fracture area appears ivory-yellow. Fractures are urgent for children because there is little dentin to protect pulp. Bacteria pass easily into pulp, causing an infection or abscess if exposed more than 6 hours.[13] Adults may be treated up to 24 hours later because the pulp is protected by a thicker layer of dentin, which reduces potential for infection. Place warm, moist cotton covered by dry gauze to hold over the exposed area as needed for discomfort secondary to thermal sensitivity. Class III fractures are a dental emergency. Injury to the enamel, dentin, and pulp are affected, causing a pink or bloody tinge to the fractured area. When the pulp is exposed, the nerve is also exposed. Again, a dry gauze can be used to minimize discomfort from thermal sensitivity. The patient should be referred to a dentist for immediate intervention. Oral analgesics or nerve block is usually effective for pain control. Reassure the patient that cosmetic restoration is possible with enamel-bonding plastic materials.[1]

With facial trauma, assess the airway, breathing, and circulation (ABCs) before assessing the dental problem. History should include mechanism of injury, concomitant injuries, and tissue loss. Consider abuse in children, the elderly, or disabled adults when the history does not correlate to the injury. Assess for tooth pain, thermal sensitivity, stability of the tooth in the socket, and malocclusion. Complications of tooth fractures include infection (pulpitis), malocclusion, embedded tooth fragments, aspiration of tooth fragments, color change, or loss of affected teeth.

Tooth Avulsion

Tooth avulsion is a dental emergency. When the tooth has been torn from the socket, reimplantation within 30 minutes greatly increases chances for reimplantation and healing. Determine the mechanism and time of injury immediately on arrival. Handle the avulsed tooth by the crown to avoid damage to attached periodontal ligament fragments. Fragments aid healing of the reimplanted tooth.[13] Ideally, the tooth should be rinsed and placed back in the socket as soon as possible. Immediate reimplantation is not always possible because of lack of patient cooperation, life-threatening injuries, or other factors at the scene of injury. Transport the tooth in milk, saline, or under the tongue of an alert patient. Use discretion with children who may swallow or aspirate the tooth. Primary teeth (i.e., 6 months to 6 years) are not reimplanted because of fusion with the bone, which interferes with permanent tooth eruption and can cause cosmetic deformities.[1] If the tooth cannot be found, examine the oral cavity and face to ensure that the tooth is not embedded in soft tissue. A chest x-ray is recommended to rule out tooth aspiration.

Symptoms include pain and bleeding at the site of the avulsion. Assess for concomitant head, neck, or maxillofacial injuries. Moist saline gauze may be applied to exposed oral tissues for comfort and to control bleeding. Administer analgesics as prescribed. Instruct the patient not to bite into anything with the affected tooth and to avoid hot or cold substances.[9] Referral to a dentist or oral surgeon for definitive care is recommended.

Dental Abscess

Two primary dental abscesses are periapical, extension of pulpal necroses from a decayed tooth or traumatic injury, and periodontal, a pocket of plaque and food debris between the tooth and the gingiva that causes localized swelling at the apex of the tooth.[9] Normally abscesses are confined; however, certain infectious processes can spread to facial planes of the head and neck.[1] The upper half of the face is affected with extension of infection from the maxillary teeth. Cellulitis in the lower half of the face and neck extends from the infection of the mandibular teeth.[1] With localized abscesses, the patient may have severe pain unrelieved by analgesics, fever, malaise, foul breath odor, and slight facial swelling near the affected tooth. An extensive abscess causes facial and neck edema, trismus, dysphagia, difficulty handling secretions, and potential airway obstruction.

Oral or parenteral narcotics, antipyretics, and antibiotics such as penicillin or erythromycin are recommended.[9] If abscess fluctuance is present, incision and drainage with culture and sensitivity of the exudate are required. The patient should be instructed to take medications as directed, use warm saline rinses, and follow up with an oral-maxillofacial surgeon in 24 to 48 hours for definitive care.

Gingivitis

Gingivitis, or inflammation of the gums, is caused by accumulation of food debris and plaque in crevices between the gums and teeth.[9] Usually related to poor dental hygiene or vitamin C deficiency, gingivitis may also occur in pregnancy and puberty because of changing hormone levels.[8] If inflammation continues, alveolar bone is lost, leading to periodontitis and eventual loss of teeth. On inspection, gum margins appear red, swollen, and with possible bleeding. Pain unrelieved by over-the-counter analgesics, difficulty chewing, and low-grade fever also occur. Topical anesthetics, analgesics, and oral antibiotic therapy are indicated. Patient teaching regarding good oral hygiene, including brushing and flossing 3 to 4 times a day with peroxide–warm water rinses every hour, is extremely important to prevent extension of gingivitis. Figure 47-10 shows a severe form of gingivitis.

Ludwig's Angina

Ludwig's angina is spread of an existing, untreated dental infection or cellulitis into three mandibular spaces: submandibular, sublingual, and submental. Infection spreads downward from the jaws to the mediastinum and is characterized by bilateral, boardlike, brawny induration of involved tissues and elevation of the tongue.[9] The inherent danger with Ludwig's angina is respiratory distress and airway obstruction.

Symptoms include pain and tenderness, trismus, muffled voice, dysphagia, drooling, and fever or chills. Dyspnea and decreased PO_2 may occur secondary to edematous tissues. The patient may be anxious or restless. Offer reassurance, check the patient frequently, and explain all procedures to ease fears.[19]

Priorities in the ED include maintaining ABCs, pain relief, and intravenous antibiotics. Elevate the head of the bed to prevent aspiration of secretions. Administer supplemental oxygen in concert with continuous pulse oximetry monitoring. Respiratory and mental status should also be continuously monitored. Provide prescribed analgesics appropriate for the patient's degree of pain. Insert an intravenous catheter to prevent dehydration, to administer antibiotic therapy (usually high-dose penicillin), and as an access for

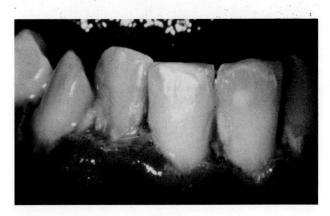

Figure **47-10** Acute necrotizing ulcerative gingivitis involving lower anterior teeth. *(From Rosen P et al: Emergency medicine: concepts and clinical practice, ed 3, St. Louis, 1992, Mosby.)*

emergency medications. Diagnostic procedures such as arterial blood gases, complete blood count (CBC) with differential, erythrocyte sedimentation rate, culture and sensitivity of exudate, and soft tissue x-rays of the neck may be ordered.[9] Definitive care by an oral-maxillofacial surgeon includes determining the site of the initial infection, surgical drainage of pus with removal of necrotic tissue, and continued antibiotic therapy.[1]

EAR EMERGENCIES

Ear emergencies may involve infection or a perforated TM. Most ear emergencies require instillation of some type of otic drops (Figure 47-11).

Otitis

Otitis, or inflammation of the ear, may occur in any section of the ear. Symptoms vary with location; however, almost all cases of acute otitis cause significant discomfort.

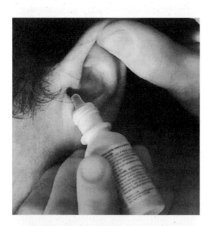

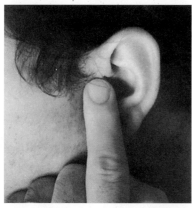

Figure **47-11** Ear drop instillation. Turn the head to the side so that the affected ear faces upward. The orifice is exposed, and the drops of medicine are directed toward the internal wall of the canal. The pinna is pulled up and back in a person over 3 years of age and down and back in a younger child. The tragus is then pushed against the ear canal to ensure that the drops stay in the canal. *(From Potter PA, Perry AG:* Fundamentals of nursing, *ed 4, St. Louis, 1997, Mosby.)*

Otitis externa is inflammation of the external ear canal and auricle. Also known as swimmer's ear, this condition is seen most often during the summer. Table 47-2 summarizes factors that predispose the patient to otitis externa. The infectious agent is usually bacteria such as *Pseudomonas* species, *Proteus vulgaris,* streptococci, and *Staphylococcus aureus.* Symptoms include pain, swelling, redness, and purulent drainage of the auricle and ear canal (Figure 47-12). Pain is usually worsened by chewing or movement of the tragus or pinna. Regional cellulitis, partial hearing loss, and lymphadenopathy may also be present. Treatment includes keeping the ear dry, applying heat with a heating pad, heating lamp, or warm, moist compresses, and providing analgesics and antibiotics. Topical or otic antibiotics are used unless the patient has a persistent fever or regional cellulitis. Otitis externa usually resolves in 7 days but frequently recurs.

Otitis media (OM), or infection of the middle ear, occurs most often children and is usually preceded by a viral upper respiratory infection (URI).[4] *Streptococcus pneumoniae* and *Haemophilus influenzae* are the most common causative organisms. Acute OM is characterized by rapid onset of ear pain, headache, tinnitus, hearing loss, and nausea or vomiting. Infants and young children may present with irritability, crying, rubbing or pulling the ears, restless sleep, and lethargy. Other symptoms such as fever, rhinitis, cough, otorrhea secondary to rupture of the TM, and conjunctivitis may occur at any age.[21] Visualization of the TM, necessary for diagnosis, usually reveals redness and a whitish-yellow opacity. Bulging may occur as the infection progresses.[11] Infants with a reddened TM may also be crying.[21]

Uncomplicated acute OM is treated with antibiotics, antipyretics, and analgesics such as acetaminophen or ibupro-

Table **47-2** Predisposing Factors for Otitis Externa	
Predisposing factor	**Description**
Swimming in contaminated water	Cerumen creates a culture medium for microorganisms found in the contaminated water.
Cleaning the ear canal with a foreign object	Objects such as hairpins can irritate the ear canal and introduce microorganisms.
Exposure to chemical irritants	Chemicals such as hair dye can cause an allergic irritation and inflammation.
Regular use of earphones, earplugs, or earmuffs	These devices trap moisture in the ear and create a culture medium for bacteria and other organisms.
Perforated TM	Chronic drainage from a ruptured TM can lead to infection.

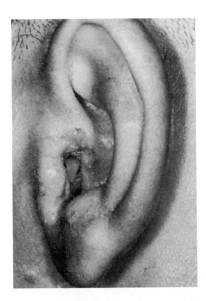

Figure **47-12** Acute external otitis. Note swelling of the ear canal and lymphadenopathy in front of the tragus. *(From Deweese DD et al: Otolaryngology: head and neck surgery, ed 8, St. Louis, 1994, Mosby.)*

fen. Topical anesthetic otic solutions (e.g., Auralgan) for pain relief should be warmed before instilling. If not treated promptly, acute OM can cause serious complications such as ruptured TM, meningitis, mastoiditis, intracranial abscess, neck abscess, facial nerve damage, or permanent hearing loss.[9] Patients should complete the full course of antibiotic therapy and be reevaluated if there is not improvement within 2 to 3 days.[21] Children should be reevaluated in 10 days to confirm that the infection has been eradicated or to determine if middle ear effusion (serous OM) persists. Chronic or persistent pediatric OM may require prophylactic antibiotics or referral to an otolaryngologist for myringotomy tube placement.[21]

Labyrinthitis, or inflammation of the inner ear, is rare. Causes include acute febrile illness and chronic otitis media. The inner ear is the body's center of balance. The patient usually develops severe vertigo with nausea and vomiting. Vertigo usually lasts 3 to 5 days but may persist for weeks. Treatment includes bed rest, meclizine to control vertigo, and fluids for dehydration secondary to vomiting. Antibiotics are indicated for purulent labyrinthitis.

Ruptured Tympanic Membrane

A ruptured TM is most often the painful result of a bacterial infection, acute or chronic OM. Trauma such as skull fracture, foreign body insertion (e.g., cotton swabs, hair pins), explosions, or blows to the ear may also rupture the TM. Perforation may be central or marginal. Marginal perforations have less chance of spontaneous closure.[19] Children, especially those with chronic ear infections, are most often victims of this disorder. Symptoms include pain,

bloody or purulent discharge, hearing loss, vertigo, and fever. Pain and pressure may be relieved with rupture. In trauma-related TM rupture, ear drainage should be checked for the presence of cerebrospinal fluid, indicative of basilar skull fracture.[4] Otoscopic examination reveals the TM as slit-shaped or irregular.[9] X-rays of the skull, temporal bone, and cervical spine may be indicated with trauma. Hearing loss of 35 dB may be present in the affected ear, so speak slowly and clearly toward the unaffected ear while facing the patient.[9] Large perforations require myringoplasty. If the middle ear is also involved, a tympanoplasty is performed.[3]

Management includes antibiotics, analgesics, and antipyretics. Carefully clean the ear canal of blood or debris with gentle suction, and obtain a culture and sensitivity of drainage. Irrigation is contraindicated with TM rupture. Instillation of antibiotic ear drops may be necessary to prevent otitis externa.[5] The patient should be instructed to keep water out of the ears, since this provides an environment conducive to bacterial or fungal growth.[19] A piece of cotton coated with petroleum jelly and placed in the affected ear helps repel water. The patient should follow up with an otolaryngologist for definitive care.

Foreign Body

Cerumen is the most common obstructive material seen in children's ears, often caused by cotton swabs pushing wax and cotton fibers deeper into the ear canal. Therefore, remind parents to put "nothing smaller than an elbow into the ear."[15] Cerumen is a brown, waxy material that obstructs view of the TM and must be removed. Adults, especially older patients, are also prone to impacted cerumen. In nursing home patients, the estimated incidence of cerumen impaction is almost 40%. Use of hearing aids is a contributing factor because of increased cerumen production and obstruction of natural outflow from the ear.[6]

The patient who presents with a foreign body in the ear is most often a child between 9 months and 4 years of age.[15] Beads, small stones, beans, corn, and dry cereal are common culprits. Parents, often unaware of the foreign body, bring the child to the ED with a purulent, foul-smelling ear discharge. Older children and adults may complain of decreased hearing and fullness in the affected ear. Insects, including roaches, can fly or crawl into the ear and become trapped, moving and buzzing in the ear, causing great distress and anxiety for the patient. Children with insects in the ear may be extremely frightened.

Before attempting removal of impacted cerumen or a foreign body, evaluate for a history of ruptured TM or current infection. Explain the procedure to the patient as appropriate for age. Cooperation is elicited from a child whose trust is not violated. Conscious sedation or restraints may be required in difficult situations.[11] Methods for foreign body removal include suctioning, irrigation, or use of special tools under direction visualization. A good light source such as an operating otoscope or head lamp is imperative for these procedures. To best expose the ear canal, pull the auricle up and back for adults, down and back for children. Vegetables or other soft materials that may absorb water should not be irrigated. Subsequent swelling caused by water absorption makes removal more difficult. Insects can be removed by placing a few drops of mineral oil in the ear, then shining a light in the ear canal to attract the insect out.[17] Another method is to fill the ear canal with 2% lidocaine or alcohol to kill the insect, allowing removal with direct instrumentation.[9]

Irrigation, often the safest[11] and most effective method for removal of impacted cerumen, is contraindicated with a history of TM rupture, with infection, with a soft or vegetable-like foreign body, or in children under age 5. Any

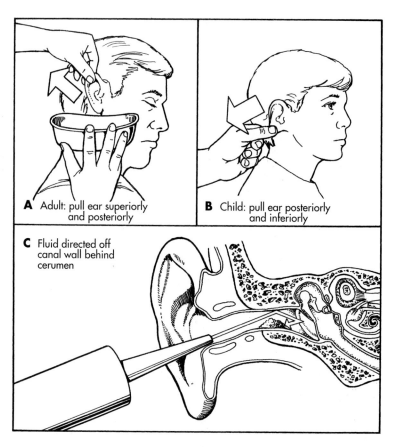

Figure **47-13** Ear irrigation. **A,** The external auditory canal in the adult can best be exposed by pulling the earlobe upward and backward. **B,** The same exposure can be achieved in the child by gently pulling the auricle of the ear downward and backward. **C,** An enlarged diagram showing the direction of irrigating fluid against the side of the canal. NOTE: This is more effective in dislodging cerumen than if the flow of solution were directed straight into the canal.

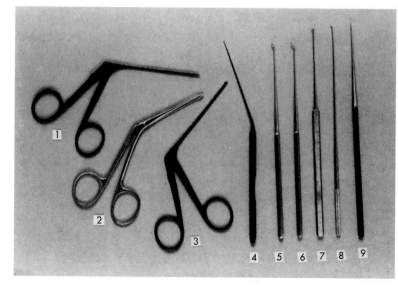

Figure **47-14** Useful ear foreign body tools. *1,* Alligator forceps; *2,* Hartman ear forceps; *3,* cupped forceps; *4,* Schuknecht pick; *5,* small Buck curette; *6,* large Buck curette; *7,* Sharpleigh curette; *8,* Day hook; *9,* Turner needle. *(From Cummings CW et al: Otolaryngology: head and neck surgery, ed 2, vol 4, St. Louis, 1993, Mosby.)*

solutions for the ear should be warmed to 37° C before instillation to prevent inner ear stimulation, causing dizziness, nausea, and vomiting.[6] Suggested guidelines for ear irrigation are described in Box 47-2 and illustrated in Figure 47-13.

Other methods of foreign body removal include use of an ear curette, right-angle hook, Frazier suction catheter, soft flexible catheter with funnel-shaped tip, and alligator forceps (Figure 47-14).[4] Surfactant ear drops (i.e., glycerin and peroxide) may soften cerumen.[21] If an impacted foreign body cannot be removed, refer the patient to an ENT specialist within 24 hours. Emergent referral is necessary with severe pain or the presence of a caustic foreign body substance.[11] Antibiotics may be prescribed to prevent or treat an existing infection. Complications include hearing loss, TM rupture, and acute OM or otitis externa from injury during attempted foreign body removal or from retained foreign body material.

Box 47-2   Irrigation of the Ear

Equipment

Warm tap water or 1:1 solution of hydrogen peroxide/warm H_2O
30 cc or 60 cc syringe
Large bore angiocath with needle removed or butterfly needle tubing cut about 3 cm from the hub
Basin to collect fluid
Towels and absorbent pad

Procedure

With patient in sitting position, protect clothing with towels/pads. Tilt head with affected ear up and provide a basin to hold under the ear to be irrigated.
Place *warmed* (37° C) solution in a sterile basin and put on gloves.
Straighten ear canal by method appropriate for age.
Using 30-60 cc's of solution at a time, direct stream superiorly against ear canal wall to exert back pressure on FB/cerumen, thus driving it outward, never directly against TM since rupture may occur. May require several attempts with frequent otoscopic exams to determine effectiveness of irrigation.
Discontinue procedure immediately if patient complains of dizziness, nausea, or pain.
Following irrigation, dry the external canal with a cotton ball. Have patient lie with the affected side down to drain excess fluid.
Alternatively, a Water-pik device designed for dental use may be used for irrigation; however, this practice is not recommended due to excessive uncontrolled fluid pressure on the TM.
(Commercial otic devices are also available.)

From Freeman FB: Impacted cerumen: how to safely remove earwax in an office visit, *Geriatrics* 50(6):52, 1995.
FB, Foreign body.

NASAL EMERGENCIES

Nasal emergencies involve infection, hemorrhage, or foreign bodies.

Rhinitis

Rhinitis is inflammation of nasal mucosa that usually accompanies the common cold. Acute rhinitis, the most prevalent disease among all age groups, is spread by droplet contact.[9] Upper respiratory viruses such as rhinovirus, adenovirus, or influenza virus are usually the causative organisms. Symptoms include copious, mucopurulent nasal secretions, red and swollen nasal mucosa, mild fever, and decreased sense of smell. Allergic rhinitis (hay fever) may be perennial or seasonal caused by pollens, grasses, trees, or flowers. Perennial allergic rhinitis is a chronic condition caused by environmental factors such as dust, animal dander, mold, and foods.[19] Perennial rhinitis is characterized by nasal mucosa that appears pale to bluish and swollen; tearing; periorbital edema; and thin, watery nasal discharge.

The single most effective treatment for all forms of rhinitis is warm saline irrigation; however, not all patients are willing to continue this treatment on their own.[21] Systemic or topical antihistamines are used to shrink swollen nasal tissues. Box 47-3 describes effective use of nasal spray. Analgesics and antipyretics are administered as prescribed. The patient should be instructed to drink plenty of clear fluids, humidify the home environment, avoid allergens, and rest. Complications associated with rhinitis include serous otitis media, nasal polyps, sinusitis, and exacerbation of asthma. Excessive use of topical medications and nose blowing may cause epistaxis.[21]

Epistaxis

Epistaxis, or nosebleed, is seen frequently in the ED and has many causes, including infection, trauma, local irritants, foreign bodies, anticoagulant drug therapy, hypertension, congenital or disease-induced coagulation disorders, and tumors. However, the most common cause is nose picking. The bleeding may occur anteriorly or posteriorly. Anterior bleeding is usually acute, almost always originating at Kiesselbach's plexus in Little's area, a highly vascularized area of the nose (Figure 47-6). Posterior epistaxis is usually chronic and is common in the elderly. Bleeding is more profuse, involving the posterior branches of the sphenopalatine artery. Hypertension as the cause of epistaxis may be unde-

---

Box 47-3   Using Nasal Sprays Effectively

Spray each nostril, and then lie supine for 2 minutes. Repeat the procedure.
The first dose shrinks nasal mucosa, which allows the second dose to reach the upper turbinates and sinus ostia.[4]
Using nasal sprays just prior to bedtime may enhance relief.[20]

tected if blood loss lowers blood pressure to normal.[21] In mild cases, bleeding may stop spontaneously within minutes or by simply pinching the nares. Bleeding may be profuse and continuous with a potential for hypovolemia, requiring aggressive management.

The patient usually presents clutching bloody tissues or towels to the nose and may be extremely anxious. A calm, reassuring systematic approach by the emergency nurse helps ease anxiety and allows efficient management. Obtain a quick history including duration, frequency, and amount of bleeding, recent trauma or surgery, nausea or vomiting, recreational drug use, and pertinent medical history. All staff caring for this patient should observe universal precautions including gloves, goggles, mask, and gown, since potential for blood splashing is high.

Maintain the patient in an upright seated position with the head tilted downward and nostrils pinched. Assess ABCs,

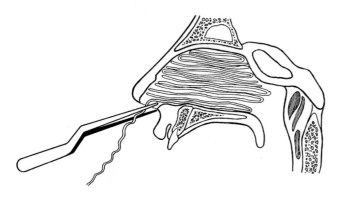

Figure **47-15**   Anterior nasal packing.

and initiate appropriate interventions such as suction, intravenous access, cardiac monitor, and oxygen saturation monitor. Obtain CBC, prothrombin time, partial thromboplastin time, and type and crossmatch as ordered. The bleeding site is determined after clearing the nose of clots by having the patient blow the nose or with suction using an 8F or 10F Frazier catheter. A nasal speculum is required to visualize the posterior nasal cavity. Treatment of anterior epistaxis consists of identification of the bleeding site, application of topical vasoconstrictors (i.e., 2% to 5% cocaine hydrochloride, Neo-Synephrine), direct pressure for 5 to 10 minutes, chemical (silver nitrate) or electrical cautery, and packing if necessary.[20] Nasal packing may be done with standard petrolatum-iodoform gauze (Figure 47-15) or newer commercial products such as the Merocel nasal sponge or Gelfoam, which eventually dissolve and do not require removal. Coat packing material with antibiotic ointment before insertion to help prevent sinusitis and toxic shock.[21]

Anterior nasal packing is left in place 24 to 72 hours. The patient should follow up with an otolaryngologist or return to the ED immediately for persistent bleeding or dislodged nasal packing.[17]

With posterior epistaxis, bleeding is much more difficult to control. Direct pressure is ineffective, and packing may be difficult. A posterior nasal pack should be inserted in anyone with posterior nasal hemorrhage[20] (Figure 47-16). Devices such as a Merocel nasal sponge, Nasostat epistaxis balloon (Figure 47-17), or 12F to 16F Foley catheter with the distal tip cut off can be used for posterior packing. These devices should be removed in 2 to 3 days. Posterior nasal packing predisposes the patient to respiratory obstruction, so

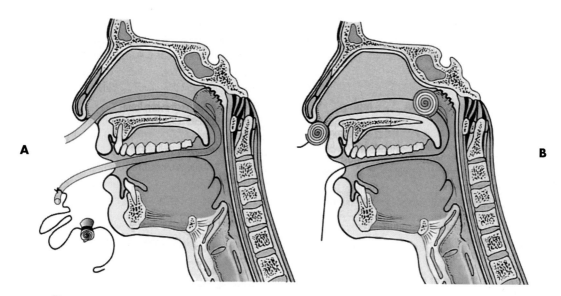

Figure **47-16**   Method for placing posterior nasal pack. **A,** Catheter is passed through the bleeding side of the nose and pulled out through the mouth with a hemostat. Strings are tied to the catheter and the pack is pulled up behind the soft palate and into the nasopharynx. **B,** Nasal pack in position in the posterior nasopharynx. Dental roll of the nose helps to maintain correct position. *(From Lewis SM, Collier IC, Heitkemper MM: Medical-surgical nursing: assessment and management of clinical problems, ed 4, St. Louis, 1996, Mosby.)*

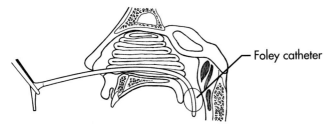

Figure **47-17** Nasal packing for severe epistaxis.

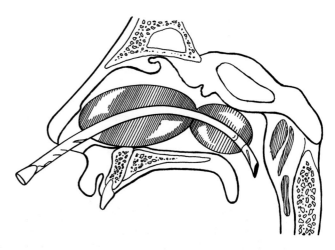

Figure **47-18** Anterior and posterior nasal balloon tamponade for control of both anterior and posterior epistaxis.

admission is necessary for airway monitoring, sedation, antibiotic therapy, and humidified oxygen. Surgical ligation of vessels may be required for control of severe posterior epistaxis.[21] Antihypertensives may be needed for patients whose blood pressure remains elevated.

Complications of anterior and posterior epistaxis include hypoxia, dislodged nasal packing, airway occlusion, hypovolemia, severe discomfort, sinusitis, toxic shock, cardiac arrhythmias, and respiratory or cardiac arrest. With severe blood loss, blood transfusion may be necessary. Figure 47-18 illustrates anterior and posterior nasal packing. Posterior epistaxis is often associated with significant atherosclerosis and may precipitate myocardial or cerebral infarction.[21]

Foreign Body

A foreign body in the nose usually occurs in children and is often discovered when a purulent nasal discharge is noticed.[17] Usually self-inserted, foreign bodies in the nose may also occur as a result of trauma. Nasal cavities are easily expanded, so unusual, large, or multiple retained foreign bodies are possible. The patient may present with pain and fullness from a recently placed foreign body or with purulent, foul-smelling nasal discharge, recurrent epistaxis, sinus pain, fever, and edematous nasal mucosa.[9] Care should be taken to prevent damage to the highly vascular nasal septum and mucosa during removal of a nasal foreign body. Children may require conscious sedation or a papoose board for restraint. Ask the cooperative patient to occlude the unobstructed nostril, close the mouth, and make a forceful nasal exhalation at least 15 times.[15] If unsuccessful, apply a topical anesthetic agent, and place the patient in Trendelenburg position. The object is then removed with alligator or ring forceps.[17] A Harman forceps, wire loop, or suction foreign body catheter may prove helpful. Extreme care must be taken not to dislodge or drive the foreign body deeper into the nasopharynx because aspiration may occur.[12] Complications such as epistaxis, septal hematoma or perforation, or inability to remove the foreign body should be referred to an otolaryngologist.

THROAT EMERGENCIES

Throat emergencies represent a threat to the patient's airway. The emergency nurse should evaluate the patient's ABCs carefully and monitor for significant changes in breathing and mentation.

Pharyngitis

Pharyngitis, inflammation of the pharynx, often accompanies the common cold. Symptoms include bright red throat, swollen tonsils, white or yellow exudate on tonsils and pharynx, swollen uvula, and enlarged tender cervical and tonsillar nodes.[8] The patient may complain of sore throat, fever, dysphagia, and halitosis (foul breath odor). Treatment for pharyngitis depends on the underlying pathology.[4] A throat culture and sensitivity should be obtained to distinguish bacterial or viral cause. Most sore throats in adults are viral and do not warrant antibiotics.[7] For bacterial pharyngitis, that is, streptococcal pharyngitis, treatment consists of antibiotics, antipyretics, and analgesics. Encourage the patient to gargle frequently with warm saline. Stress the importance of bed rest, increased fluid intake, and completing the full course of antibiotics. Tonsillectomy, or removal of tonsils, may be necessary in severe cases. Complications include retropharyngeal abscess, glomerular nephritis, and subacute bacterial endocarditis resulting from the invasion of group A β-hemolytic streptococci.[19]

Laryngitis

Acute laryngitis, inflammation of the vocal cords, may accompany URI or exist alone. Causes of acute laryngitis may be overuse, allergies, irritants, and viral or bacterial infections.[9] Tension in the vocal cords determines the amount of vibration produced when air flows upward through the glottis. Anything that alters this tension affects the ability to speak.[19] The patient presents with partial or complete voice loss, with or without URI symptoms. Dyspnea or stridor should be evaluated and treated immediately as potential airway obstruction. Throat culture and CBC are the usual diagnostic procedures. Treatment includes voice rest, steam inhalations to thin secretions and improve moisture, increased fluid intake, and topical anesthetic throat lozenges.[7] Patient teaching should emphasize preventive therapy, that is, avoiding airway irritants such as cigarette smoke and loud or excessive use of the voice. Gastroesophageal reflux due to excess acid production may also be responsible. This can be treated with diet, antacid, and H_2 inhibitors.[19] In the presence of infection, administer antibiotics, and instruct the patient to complete the entire course. Aspirin is contraindicated for analgesia because of its anticoagulant properties, which increase the risk of vocal cord hemorrhage and subsequent scarring and changes in voice quality.[16] Complications of laryngitis are aspiration pneumonia, decreased cough reflex, and airway compromise or obstruction.

Tonsillitis

Tonsillitis is inflammation of the palatine tonsils. Tonsils are lymphatic tissue that filters bacteria and other microorganisms to protect the respiratory and gastrointestinal tract.[7] Approximately 30% of tonsillitis cases are caused by group A β-hemolytic streptococci or staphylococci.[19] Viruses are also a leading cause of this contagious, airborne infection. Symptoms are similar to pharyngitis and may include a feeling of fullness in the throat, malaise, otalgia (ear pain), and swollen lymph nodes in the neck.[19] The patient may have difficulty speaking or swallowing. On examination, a white or yellow exudate may cover the tonsils, accompanied by foul breath odor. A throat culture and sensitivity, CBC, monospot test, and chest radiograph may be ordered.[7] As with pharyngitis, warm saline gargles, topical anesthetic lozenges, analgesics, antipyretics, and antibiotics (usually penicillin or erythromycin) are indicated. Surgery is recommended for recurrent streptococcal infections unresponsive to antibiotic therapy or tonsillar hypertrophy that predisposes the patient to respiratory obstruction or dysphagia. Retropharyngeal and peritonsillar abscess, glomerular nephritis, and subacute bacterial endocarditis are potential complications of tonsillitis.[19]

Peritonsillar Abscess

Untreated acute or chronic suppurative tonsillitis may evolve into a peritonsillar abscess, or quinsy, caused by a perforated tonsillar capsule and extension of the infection along deeper muscle planes.[18] The abscess is usually unilateral and causes dysphagia, drooling, muffled voice, painful swallowing, trismus, and anxiety.[9] Fever, malaise, and dehydration are usually present. In mild cases, needle aspiration relieves trismus and painful swallowing, so the patient is discharged on oral antibiotics with ENT follow-up.[11] In more severe cases with airway compromise, surgical incision and drainage or needle aspiration is followed by intravenous antibiotic therapy. Stability of the ABCs is a priority. Provide oxygen, monitor SaO_2 and respirations, and keep the head of the bed elevated at 80 to 90 degrees. Tonsillectomy may be required to prevent recurrence of the abscess.[19] Dangerous sequelae associated with peritonsillar abscess include aspiration, airway obstruction, parapharyngeal abscess, dehydration, glomerulonephritis, and subacute bacterial endocarditis. Fortunately complications can be avoided

with aggressive antibiotic treatment (penicillin based or erythromycin). Ice packs to the neck help decrease pain and edema. Encourage oral hygiene; however, gargling should be avoided to prevent inadvertent rupture of the abscess.[19]

FACIAL EMERGENCIES

Facial emergencies affect structures of the face such as the nerves, bones, and sinuses. These emergencies are secondary to infection or other disease processes.

Sinusitis

Acute sinusitis, inflammation of mucous membranes in any of the paranasal sinuses, generally occurs as a result of blockage and backup of secretions. The cause is usually attributed to URI or allergic rhinitis. Other causes include foreign bodies, trauma, dental disorders, inhalation of irritants (e.g., cigarette smoke, cocaine use), deviated nasal septum, polyps, and tumors. Secretions are retained in the sinus cavity as a result of altered ciliary activity and obstruction of the sinus ostia.[19] Negative pressure and air-fluid levels result from fluid accumulation and reabsorption of air in the sinus. Fluid accumulation forms a medium for bacteria to grow and multiply, resulting in bacterial sinusitis. *H. influenzae* and *S. pneumoniae* are common causative organisms.

In chronic sinusitis, the mucous membrane becomes permanently thickened from prolonged or repeated inflammation or infection.[7] The patient with sinusitis usually complains of a dull, achy pain over the affected sinus. In adults, frontal sinusitis with periorbital and forehead pain that worsens when bending over is common. Ethmoidal sinusitis, common in children, causes pain at the bridge of the nose and behind the eyes. A fever, decreased appetite, and nausea may also be present.[14] Ethmoidal sinusitis is especially serious in children because of a tendency to extend toward the retroorbital area and central nervous system.[20] The patient has tenderness to palpation over the involved sinus; swollen, erythematous mucosa with purulent nasal discharge; and diminished transillumination. X-rays are not always conclusive or reliable in diagnosis of sinusitis. Findings that are most reliable include sinus opacity, air-fluid level, or 6 mm of mucosal thickening. Absence of radiographic evidence does not exclude the diagnosis of sinusitis.[20] Other diagnostic methods include computed tomography scan, sinus endoscopy, and sinus cultures of the ostia via needle aspiration.

Over-the-counter nasal decongestant sprays (e.g., Afrin or Neo-Synephrine) may provide immediate relief; however, topical decongestants should not be used for more than 3 days because of a dangerous rebound effect.[4] Isotonic saline nose drops may also help. Encourage increased fluid intake and use of a humidifier in the home. Warm, moist compresses to the sinus areas promote drainage and comfort. Administer antibiotics and analgesics as prescribed. Instruct the patient to avoid environmental irritants and avoid bending over, since this increases sinus pressure and pain. If the condition worsens despite antibiotic therapy for 3 to 5 days, the patient should return to the ED immediately or see an ENT specialist. Complications of undertreated acute sinusitis are chronic sinusitis, orbital or periorbital cellulitis or abscess, cavernous sinus thrombosis, sepsis, brain abscess, meningitis, and osteomyelitis of the frontal bone.

Bell's Palsy

In Bell's palsy, a peripheral lower motor neuron lesion produces unilateral paralysis of the facial nerve (cranial nerve VII), which controls facial muscle movement (Figure 47-19). Bilateral paralysis rarely occurs. Although the cause is unknown, swelling of the facial nerve secondary to viral or immunodeficiency disease is a probable cause.[14] Bell's palsy can occur at any age but is most common in adults over 40 years, with men and women equally affected. Diagnosis is made by history and physical examination. Bell's palsy has a rapid onset that may begin with ear or facial pain; maximal paralysis occurs within 2 to 5 days. The patient cannot close the eye, wrinkle the forehead, smile, whistle, or grimace on the affected side.[7] Normal symmetry of the face is lost, with widening of palpebral fissures and flattening of the nasolabial folds on the affected side. Drooling may also be present.

Treatment includes steroids, analgesics, and artificial tears. Reassure the patient and family that this is not a stroke and that spontaneous recovery occurs in most cases within 3 weeks.[14] Instruct the patient to manually close the affected eye periodically and to keep the eye moist with prescribed eye drops. Frequent, small meals may be necessary if the patient experiences difficulty eating or drinking.[7] Moist heat, facial massage, active or passive range of motion exercises, and a facial sling are recommended to improve comfort. Complications include corneal abrasion, facial muscle atrophy, and residual weakness.

Temporomandibular Joint Dislocation

TMJ dislocation is anterior and superior bilateral displacement of the jaw. Unilateral dislocation rarely occurs. Jaw muscles attempt to close the mandible, but the resulting spasm prevents condyles from returning to normal position in the mandibular fossae.[1] TMJ dislocation usually occurs when opening the mouth too wide, as in yawning or laughing. Trauma or dystonic reaction to drugs may also be responsible. The patient will usually present with the chin protruding, the mouth open, drooling, and pain related to muscle spasms. The patient cannot close the mouth, talk, or swallow and may be extremely anxious.[4] Diagnostics include pre- and postreduction radiographs. Muscle relaxants may be administered to reduce muscle spasm and relax the patient.

To reduce the dislocation, seat the patient facing the emergency physician. The physician places the thumbs intraorally onto the lower molar ridge and applies a downward and backward pressure to return the condyle to the normal position.[1] The physician should pad the thumbs with a thick layer of gauze because the strong masseter muscles of the jaw con-

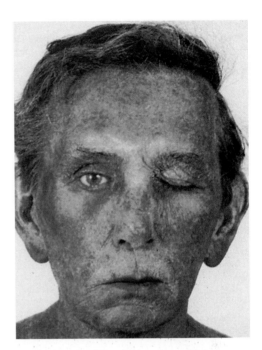

Figure **47-19** Bell's palsy. *(From Perkin GD et al:* Atlas of clinical neurology, *London, 1986, Gower Medical Publishing.)*

Box **47-4**

NURSING DIAGNOSES FOR DENTAL, EAR, NOSE, THROAT, AND FACIAL EMERGENCIES

Pain
Anxiety
Risk for infection
Ineffective airway clearance
Ineffective breathing pattern
Impaired gas exchange
Hypovolemia

tract with great force with reduction of the TMJ. Postreduction pain is rare and is minimal when present. Nonsteroidal antiinflammatory drugs and muscle relaxants may be helpful.[1] Instruct the patient to avoid stress on the TMJ by consuming a soft diet for 3 to 4 days.[14] Because patients with one episode of TMJ dislocation are predisposed to further dislocations, referral to an otolaryngologist is recommended.[4]

SUMMARY

Emergencies of the mouth, face, nose, and ears are a routine part of emergency nursing. Most are not life-threatening. However, the ability to discern problems that represent a potential threat to the patient's life is a requisite skill for the emergency nurse. Box 47-4 highlights nursing diagnoses for these patients.

REFERENCES

1. Amsterdam JT: Dental disorders. In Rosen P et al, editors: *Emergency medicine: concepts and clinical practice,* ed 3, St. Louis, 1992, Mosby.
2. Amsterdam, JT: General dental emergencies. In Tintinalli JE, Ruiz E, Krome RL, editors: *Emergency medicine: a comprehensive study guide,* ed 4, New York, 1996, McGraw-Hill.
3. Black JM, Matassarin-Jacobs E: In Black JM, Matassarin-Jacobs E, editors: *Luckmann & Sorensen's medical-surgical nursing: a psychophysiologic approach,* ed 4, Philadelphia, 1993, WB Saunders.
4. Criddle LM: Maxillofacial trauma and ear, nose, and throat emergencies. In Kitt S et al., editors: *Emergency nursing: a physiologic and clinical perspective,* ed 2, Philadelphia, 1995, WB Saunders.
5. Emergency Nurses Association: Eye, ear, nose, throat emergencies: orientation module. In *Orientation to emergency nursing: diversity in practice,* Chicago, 1993, Emergency Nurses Association.
6. Freeman FB: Impacted cerumen: how to safely remove earwax in an office visit, *Geriatrics* 50(6):52, 1995.
7. Ignatavicius DD, Workman ML, Mishler MA: *Medical-surgical nursing: a nursing process approach,* ed 2, Philadelphia, 1995, WB Saunders.
8. Jarvis C: *Physical examination and health assessment,* Philadelphia, 1992, WB Saunders.
9. Lee G: Dental, ear, nose, and throat emergencies. In Klein AR et al, editors: *Emergency nursing core curriculum,* ed 4, Philadelphia, 1994, WB Saunders.
10. McCaffrey TV: Physiological diagnosis and methodology to evaluate the anatomy and physiology of the esophagus. In Lee KJ, editor: *Textbook of otolaryngology and head and neck surgery,* New York, 1989, Elsevier Science.
11. Peacock WF: Otolaryngologic emergencies. In Tintinalli JE, Ruiz E, Krome RL, editors: *Emergency medicine: a comprehensive study guide,* ed 4, New York, 1996, McGraw-Hill.
12. Pons PT: Foreign bodies. In Rosen P et al, editors: *Emergency medicine: concepts and clinical practice,* ed 3, St. Louis, 1992, Mosby.
13. Rahman WM, O'Connor TJ: Facial trauma. In Barkin RM, editor: *Pediatric emergency medicine: concepts and clinical practice,* St. Louis, 1992, Mosby.
14. Revere CJ: Facial emergencies. In Klein AR et al, editors: *Emergency nursing core curriculum,* ed 4, Philadelphia, 1994, WB Saunders.
15. SantaMaria JP, Abrunzo TJ: Ear, nose, and throat. In Barkin RM, editor: *Pediatric emergency medicine: concepts and clinical practice.* St. Louis, 1992, Mosby.
16. Sataloff RT: Diagnosis and treatment of professional voice disorders. In Lee KJ, editor: *Textbook of otolaryngology and head and neck surgery.* New York, 1989, Elsevier Science.
17. Sheehy SB: Ear, nose, throat, facial, and dental emergencies. In Sheehy SB, editor: *Emergency nursing: principles and practice,* ed 3, St. Louis, 1992, Mosby.
18. Shemen LJ: Diseases of the oropharynx. In Lee KJ, editor: *Textbook of otolaryngology and head and neck surgery,* New York, 1989, Elsevier Science.
19. Sigler BA, Schuring LT: *Ear, nose, and throat disorders,* St. Louis, 1993, Mosby.
20. Smith JA: Nasal emergencies and sinusitis. In Tintinalli JE, Ruiz E, Krome RL, editors: *Emergency medicine: a comprehensive study guide,* ed 4, New York, 1996, McGraw-Hill.
21. Stair JA: Otolaryngologic disorders. In Rosen P et al, editors: *Emergency medicine: concepts and clinical practice,* ed 3, St. Louis, 1992, Mosby.

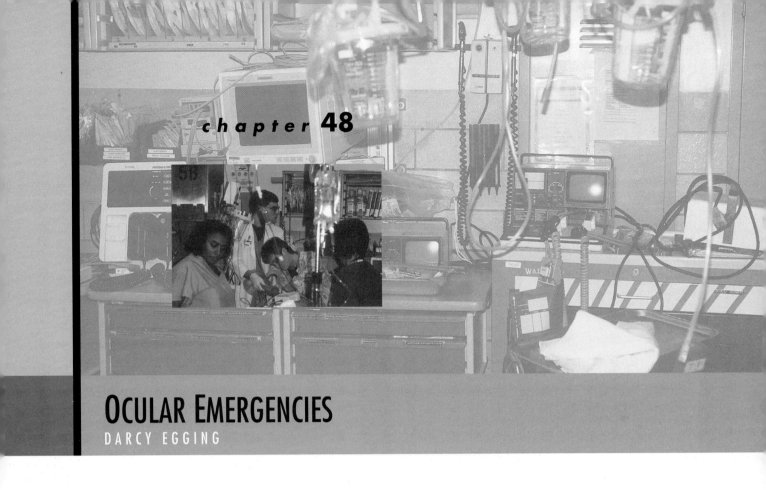

chapter 48

OCULAR EMERGENCIES

DARCY EGGING

Emergency nurses care for patients with eye problems on a regular basis; however, true ocular emergencies are not an everyday occurrence. Ability to identify conditions that represent a threat to the patient's vision is essential to protect the patient's vision. This chapter provides a brief description of anatomy, ocular assessment, and common ocular emergencies encountered in the emergency department (ED).

Quantifying ocular conditions seen in EDs and primary care settings is difficult if not impossible, since a single clearinghouse for ocular injuries and other conditions of the eye does not exist. Children are more likely to sustain eye trauma than adults.[6,18] True ocular emergencies, such as angle-closure glaucoma and retinal artery occlusion, usually occur in the older patient. The National Eye Trauma System Registry, established by ophthalmologists from 48 regional eye trauma centers, collects standardized information on penetrating ocular trauma. This voluntary system has increased reporting of eye trauma, but not all eye trauma is treated at eye trauma centers, so data are somewhat unreliable. Therefore, description of the prevalence of eye trauma in the United States is varied and inconsistent.

Typical ocular emergencies treated in the ED include corneal or conjunctival foreign body, conjunctivitis, and corneal abrasion. These conditions do not cause significant morbidity; however, the patient does experience discomfort and disruption of routine.

ANATOMY AND PHYSIOLOGY

The eyes are truly a window to the world. Vision is often considered the most important of the five senses. Basic understanding of ocular structures facilitates assessment and treatment of ocular problems. Figure 48-1 illustrates these ocular structures. The eyes are protected by surrounding bony structures, eyelids, and *sclera,* a tough, protective white covering over the eye.[18] Lacrimal glands secrete tears, which continuously bathe the eye to decrease friction and remove minor irritants (Figure 48-2). Tears are distributed by the eyelids and exit by lacrimal ducts and the nasolacrimal duct. Meibomian glands secrete oil, which lines eyelid margins and prevents tears from running out of the conjunctival sacs.

Light enters the eye through the cornea, passes through the lens, and is reflected off the retina. The amount of light entering the posterior chamber is controlled by the iris as it expands and contracts to open and close the pupil. Movement of the eye itself is controlled by six oculomotor muscles (Figure 48-3).

PATIENT ASSESSMENT

Assessment of the patient with an ocular problem begins with triage and continues into the treatment area. Triage acuity for patients with an ocular condition that is a potential threat to vision is emergent, preceded only by those patients with a threat to life.[21]

Following brief assessment to ensure that the airway, breathing, and circulation (ABCs) are stable, the patient is

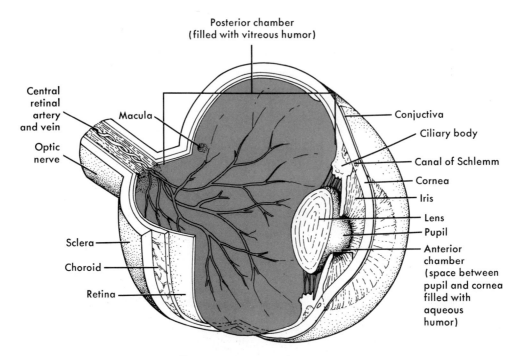

Figure **48-1** Anatomy of the eye.

evaluated to identify potential threats to vision. Ocular emergencies that represent a threat to the patient's vision and require immediate attention include *globe penetration, retinal artery occlusion, chemical burn,* and *acute angle-closure glaucoma.*

Focused assessment includes determination of precipitating events, duration of symptoms, and identification of anything that worsens or improves symptoms. When the patient verbalizes discomfort, a description of the discomfort helps clarify the patient's problem. Does the patient describe itching, burning, or the sensation of something in the eye? Determine the degree of pain and where the pain occurs. Clarify reported vision changes to determine if loss is partial or complete, in one or both eyes. Biocular changes suggest a neurologic condition rather than an ocular condition, whereas the presence of floaters suggests retinal tear.[13]

When the patient has a history of trauma, clarify the mechanism of injury and tetanus immunization status. Determine if the injury occurred during a motor vehicle crash, if the vehicle had an air bag, and if the air bag deployed. Alkaline powder in air bags can cause significant eye injury. Question the patient regarding use of protective eyewear, glasses, or contact lens. Evaluate past medical history including ocular history, use of corrective lenses, ocular medications, past ocular surgery, and disease such as diabetes.

The primary elements of the ocular examination are visual acuity, pupillary reactions, external examination, and ocular motility. A slit-lamp examination, intraocular pressure (IOP) measurement, and direct ophthalmoscopy may be done on some patients.

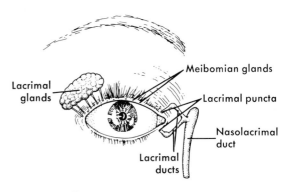

Figure **48-2** Lacrimal glands.

Visual Acuity

Visual acuity is a vital sign for patients with an ocular emergency. Physical examination begins with visual acuity unless the patient has been exposed to a chemical. In these situations, irrigation takes priority over determination of visual acuity. Measure visual acuity with the patient wearing corrective lenses and when the patient is not wearing corrective lenses.[15] When corrective lenses are not available, the pinhole test can be utilized for measurement of visual acuity. Punch a hole in a note card with an 18-gauge needle. Looking through the pinhole usually corrects any refractory error to at least 20/30. Test the affected eye first, then the unaffected eye, and finally both eyes together. The Snellen chart is the standard method for determination of visual acuity. Figure 48-4 shows two types of Snellen charts. Box 48-1 identifies alternate techniques for visual acuity when a Snellen chart is not available. Table 48-1 describes docu-

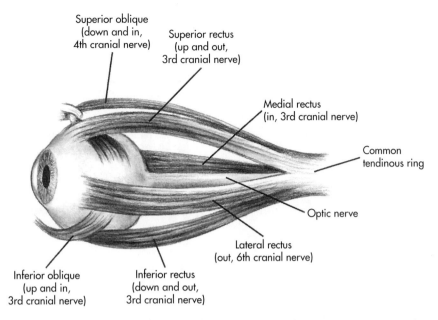

Figure **48-3** Extrinsic muscles of the eye. *(From Rudy EB:* Advanced neurological and neurosurgical nursing, *St. Louis, 1984, Mosby.)*

Box **48-1**	**Methods for Determining Visual Acuity**

Have patient read Rosenbaum Pocket Vision Screener 14 inches from the nose.

Have patient read newsprint, and record the distance at which the paper must be held for the patient to read it.

Hold up a specific number of fingers, and record the distance at which the patient can see your fingers; then ask the patient how many fingers you are holding up.

Record the distance at which the patient perceives hand motion, that is, when the patient cannot see fingers moving.

Record the distance at which the patient perceives light (when the patient cannot see hand motion).

Document inability to perceive light.

Table **48-1**	**Examples of Visual Acuity Examination**
20/20	Standing at 20 feet, patient can read what the normal eye can read at 20 feet.
20/20 2	Standing at 20 feet, patient can read what the normal eye can read at 20 feet; however, missed two letters.
20/200	At 20 feet, patient can read what the normal eye can read at 200 feet. Patient is considered legally blind if reading is obtained while wearing glasses or contact lenses.
10/200	When the patient cannot read letters on the Snellen chart, have patient stand half the distance to the chart. Record findings at the distance the patient is standing from the chart over the smallest line he or she can read.
CF/3 ft	Patient can count fingers at a maximum distance of 3 feet.
HM/4	Patient can see hand motion at a maximum distance of 4 feet.
LP/position	Patient can perceive light and determine the direction from which it is coming.
LP/no position	Patient can perceive light but is unable to tell the direction from which it is coming.
NLP	Patient is unable to perceive light.

mentation of visual acuity for the Snellen chart as well as alternate techniques for visual acuity. Visual acuity in children or illiterate patients can be determined using a chart with E shapes that become progressively smaller and rotate in different directions. Tell the patient the E is a table and ask in what direction the legs point. For verbal children, use a chart with pictures the child can identify. Be sure to name the objects before the test.

Pupil Examination

Pupil evaluation includes assessment of shape, size, and reaction. Pupils are normally round; therefore an irregular shape should be carefully evaluated. An irregular shape may result from injury or be secondary to ocular surgery. The pupil assumes a teardrop shape with globe rupture, with the teardrop pointing to the rupture site.[12] Pupil size is measured in millimeters. Assess and document the size change that occurs in each pupil in response to direct and consensual light stimulation (i.e., pupils equally round and reactive to light and accommodation [PERRLA], pupil constricts from 5 mm to 2 mm in response to light [5→2]). Specify in which eye

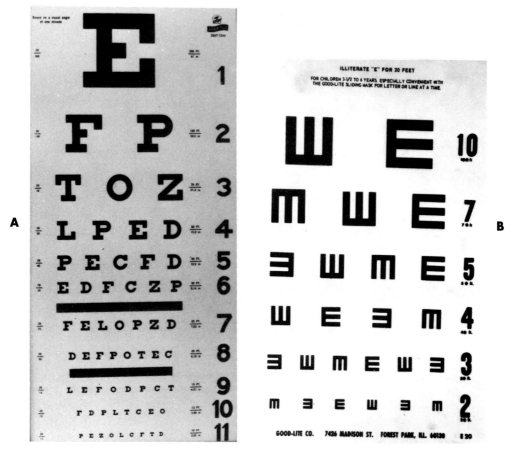

Figure **48-4** **A,** Snellen and **B,** E chart for assessment of visual acuity. *(From Beare PG, Myers JL: Principles and practice of adult health nursing, ed 2, St. Louis, 1994, Mosby.)*

Figure **48-5** Innervation and movement of extraocular muscles. *CN,* Cranial nerve. *(From Thompson JM et al: Mosby's manual of clinical nursing, ed 4, St. Louis, 1997, Mosby.)*

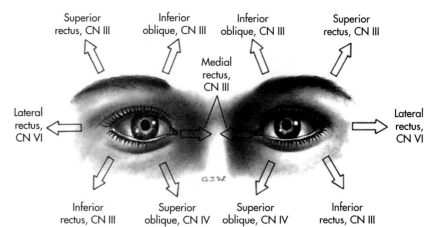

assessment findings occurred: right eye (OD), left eye (OS), or both eyes (OU).

External Examination

External examination for ocular injury begins away from the eye and gradually moves closer. Observe for bruising, lacerations, lesions, and other differences between the eyes. Assess eyelids, lashes, and how the eyes rest in the socket.

Examine the conjunctiva and sclera for abnormal color. Do not palpate the globe when globe rupture is suspected.

Ocular Motility

Evaluate the patient's ability to move the eyes through six cardinal positions of gaze by asking the patient to follow your finger as you move it through these positions. Ocular movement is controlled by the cranial nerves that regulate the oculomotor muscles.[3] Figure 48-5 shows these positions of gaze and identifies the specific oculomotor muscles and cranial nerves involved. Impaired ocular motility may occur with an entrapped muscle secondary to a blowout fracture, muscular injury, orbital cellulitis, or underlying central nervous system problem.[14] Evaluation of ocular motility in children requires patience and creativity. Hold toys, keys, or lights in different areas so the child glances in that direction. Children become easily bored with the same object, so a general rule of thumb is to use a different toy for each position.

Other Examinations

Other techniques used to evaluate ocular function include fluorescein staining, measurement of IOP, and funduscopic examination. Fluorescein is used to determine if the corneal epithelium is intact. Figure 48-6 and Box 48-2 illustrate this procedure. Remove any contact lens prior to staining because fluorescein permanently stains soft contact lenses. Figure 48-7 illustrates removal of hard contacts; Figure 48-8 illustrates soft contact removal. Following fluorescein application, flush the eye with normal saline and instruct the patient not to replace a soft contact lens for at least 1 hour.

IOP is measured with a Schiøtz tonometer or a tonopen (Figure 48-9). This procedure is contraindicated in patients with possible ruptured globe. Normal IOP is 12 mm Hg with a normal increase of 1 mm Hg per decade after age 40.[4] The Schiøtz tonometer is the most commonly used tonometer for measurement of IOP. A plunger measures indentation pressure when the tonometer is placed on the cornea. Normal indentation pressure is 12 to 18 mm Hg. A lower reading indicates increased IOP, whereas a higher reading indicates decreased IOP. A Schiøtz tonometer reads low when IOP is high because the plunger cannot indent the cornea. Box 48-3 describes the procedure for the Schiøtz tonometer.

Box 48-2 Fluorescein Staining

Explain the procedure to the patient.
Moisten end of sterile fluorescein strip with normal saline solution.
Pull down on lower lid.
Ask the patient to blink so tears distribute solution over the cornea.
Examine cornea with cobalt blue light. Disruptions appear as a bright yellow spot.

Box 48-3 Intraocular Pressure Measurement with a Schiøtz Tonometer

Explain the procedure to the patient prior to the test.
Assess visual acuity before the examination.
Place two drops of anesthetic in each eye.
Place the patient in a supine position.
Calibrate the tonometer prior to use.
Place sterile tonometer point directly on the eye and obtain reading.

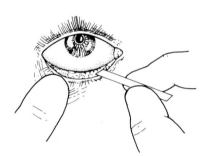

Figure **48-6** Fluorescein staining. Touch moistened fluorescein strip to inner canthus of lower lid.

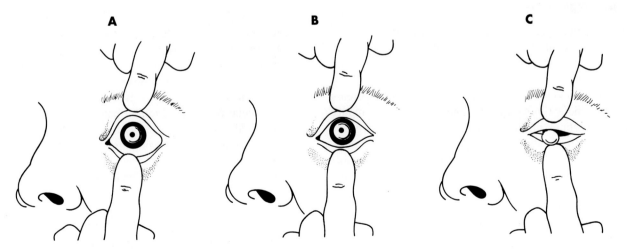

Figure **48-7** Technique for removing hard corneal contact lens from eye. **A,** Spread eyelids apart.
B, Push lids toward center of eye under contact lens. **C,** Remove lens.

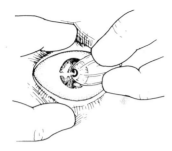

Figure **48-8** Soft contact lens removal. Lift soft lens off cornea.

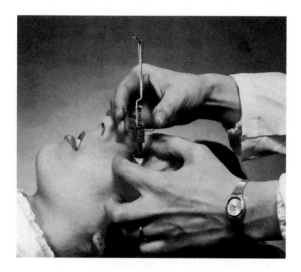

Figure **48-9** Measurement of ocular tension with Schiøtz tonometer. *(From Newell FW: Ophthalmology: principles and concepts, ed 8, St. Louis, 1996, Mosby.)*

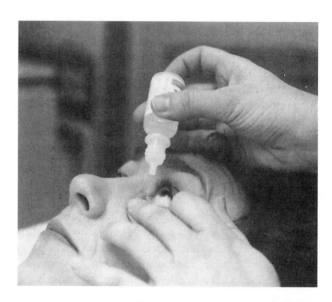

Figure **48-10** Eyedrop administration. *(From Phipps WJ et al: Medical-surgical nursing: concepts and clinical practice, ed 5, St. Louis, 1995, Mosby.)*

Table **48-2**	Color Codes for Ophthalmic Medications	
Cap color	Drug action	Examples
Red	Pupil dilation (mydriasis)	Epinephrine, atropine, neostigmine
Green	Pupil constriction (miosis)	Pilocarpine
Clear or white	Topical anesthesia	Proparacaine (Alcaine, Opthaine)
Blue	Irrigation, lubrication	Liquid tears
Yellow	Decrease aqueous humor production	Timolol

Adapted from Barish RA, Naradzay JF: Ophthalmologic therapeutics, *Emerg Med Clin North Am* 13(3):652, 1995.

Direct ophthalmoscopy, or funduscopic evaluation, is used to evaluate the posterior chamber of the eye using a light beam directed through the pupil.[19] Ophthalmoscopes provide different shapes and colored light beams to detect various conditions.

PATIENT MANAGEMENT

General management of ocular emergencies includes removal of any contact lens, instillation of ocular medications, irrigation, and eye patching. These techniques apply to almost all ocular emergencies.

Eyedrops and ophthalmic ointments are used to decrease pain, provide antibiotic therapy, change pupil size, reduce allergic reactions in the eye, and cleanse the eye. Topical ophthalmic medications are prepared under sterile conditions and distributed in single-dose containers. Container caps are color coded by the medication's effect on the pupil. Table 48-2 highlights this coding system. Various ophthalmic medications are described in Table 48-3.[1]

Instilling eyedrops or ointments requires attention to detail to prevent contamination and minimize systemic effects of the medication. Prior to instillation of eyedrops or oint-

ments, explain the procedure to the patient, and place the patient in the supine position. Instruct the patient not to roll the eyes, since this can worsen injury, particularly when anesthetic drops have been used. Box 48-4 and Figure 48-10 describe instillation of eyedrops; Box 48-5 discusses instillation of ocular ointments. Monitor patients carefully following instillation of eyedrops. Systemic effects of eyedrops may have an adverse effect on patients with cardiovascular disease.[22]

Irrigation is used to remove chemicals, small foreign bodies, and other substances. Isotonic saline is the fluid of choice for ocular irrigation; however, lactated Ringer's is also used.[17] Dextrose solutions should not be used. Irrigation is contraindicated in a patient with a possible ruptured globe. Box 48-6 describes the procedure for eye irrigation. A

Table **48-3**   **Ophthalmologic Medications**

Generic name	Common brand names	Action and use
Miotics		Constrict pupils; primarily used to treat glaucoma
Pilocarpine	Pilocar	Acts on myoneural junction
	Isopto Carpine	
	P.V. Carpine Liquifilm	
Carbachol	Carcholin	Acts on myoneural junction
	Carbamycholine	
	Isopto Carbachol	
	Doryl	
	P.V. Carbachol	
Echothiophate iodide	Phospholine	Cholinesterase inhibitor
Isoflurophate (diisopropyl flurophosphate)	DFP	Cholinesterase inhibitor
	Floropryl	
Acetazolamide	Diamox	Carbonic anhydrase inhibitor; decreases aqueous humor production
Mydriatics		Dilate pupils
Sympathomimetics		
Epinephrine	Adrenalin	Mydriasis and vasoconstriction
	Epitrate	
Phenylephrine	Neo-Synephrine	Mydriasis and vasoconstriction
Ephedrine	Epinedrine	Adrenergic vasoconstrictor and antiallergenic
Hydroxyamphetamine	Paredrine	Mydriasis
Parasympatholytic		Paralyze ciliary muscles; accommodation; dilate pupils
Atropine sulfate	Isopto Atropine	Mydriasis and cycloplegia
Cyclopentolate	Cyclogyl	Mydriasis and cycloplegia
Homatropine	Homatrocel	Mydriasis and cycloplegia
	Isopto Homatropine	Anticholinergic and sedative
Scopolamine		Mydriasis and cycloplegia
Tropicamide	Mydriacyl	
	Mydriaticum	
Physostigmine	Physostol	Mydriasis and cycloplegia
Neostigmine		
Cycloplegics		Paralyze ciliary muscles; accommodation
Cyclopentolate	Cyclogyl	Mydriasis and cycloplegia
Anesthetics		Surface anesthesia
Proparacaine	Ophthaine	Local anesthesia
Tetracaine	Pontocaine	Local anesthesia
Antibiotics		
Tetracycline	Achromycin	Antimicrobial
Chloramphenicol	Chloromycetin	Broad-spectrum antibiotic
Plymyxin B with neomycin	Cortisporin	To treat nonpurulent, bacterial infections
	Neo-Polycin	
Gentamicin	Garamycin	To treat gram-positive bacteria
Erythromycin	Ilotycin	For superficial topical infections
	Dista	
Sulfisoxazole	Gantrisin	Bacteriostatic
Sulfacetamide sodium	Sulamyd	Gram-negative and gram-positive bacteriostatic
Steroids		Decrease inflammatory response
Dexamethasone	Decadron	Decreases inflammatory response

Continued

Table **48-3** Ophthalmologic Medications—cont'd		
Generic name	Common brand names	Action and use
Combination steroid-antibiotics		
Prednisolone acetate	Metimyd	Antiinflammatory, antibacterial
Prednisolone sodium phosphate with sodium sulfacet-omide	Optimyd	Antiinflammatory, antibacterial
Neomycin sulfate and hydrocortisone acetate	Neo-Cortef	Antiinflammatory, antibacterial
Oxytetracycline with hydrocortisone acetate	Terra-Cortril	Antiinflammatory, antibacterial
Neomycin sulfate with methyl prednisolone	Neo-Delta-Cortef Neo-Medrol	Antiinflammatory, antibacterial
Herpes simplex virus inhibitors		
Idoxuridine	Stoxil	Inhibits herpes simplex virus
Vidarabine	Vira-A	Inhibits herpes simplex virus when nonresponsive to idoxuridine or if there is an allergic reaction to idoxuridine
Combination eyedrops		
Various combinations of phenylephrine hydrochloride, methylcellulose, boric acid, sodium borate, sodium chloride, ethylene diamine tetraacetate, and benzal-konium chloride	Ocusol Murine Visine Prefrin	Soothes tired eyes and decreases redness

---

Box **48-4**   **Instilling Eyedrops**

Pull the lower eyelid downward, and have the patient gaze upward.

Instill 1-2 drops of the intended solution into the cul-de-sac (the center of the inner lower lid).

Direct the patient to blink to distribute the solution.

Apply pressure to the medial canthus for several minutes to close the nasolacrimal duct and minimize systemic effects.

Instruct the patient *not* to squeeze eyelids together because this causes medication to leak out.

If more than one type of drop is ordered, wait several minutes between applications to allow maximal exposure.

Box **48-5**   **Instilling Ophthalmic Ointment**

Pull the lower eyelid downward while the patient gazes upward.

Apply ointment in a thin line from the inner aspect of the lower lid to the outer canthus.

Have the patient slowly close and rotate the eye to expose all surfaces to the medication.

Press the medial canthus gently for several minutes to decrease rapid drainage.

Instruct the patient *not* to squeeze eyelids together, since this repels the ointment.

Morgan lens can also be used for irrigation. The irrigating solution flows through the lens directly onto the eye. A separate lens should be used for each eye. When both eyes require irrigation, a nasal cannula placed across the bridge of the nose allows simultaneous irrigation of both eyes.

The eye is patched to minimize ocular stimulation by reducing movement and limiting light exposure. Patching both eyes simulates total blindness; patching one eye alters depth perception. Box 48-7 describes the procedure for patching the eyes. Figure 48-11 shows an appropriately applied eye patch. When the patient is discharged with an eye patch, discharge instruction must include discussion of altered vision and the hazards of driving or using machinery.

SPECIFIC OCULAR EMERGENCIES

Ocular emergencies may be caused by injury or disease. Comprehensive discussion of every disease process is beyond the scope of this text; however, those situations encountered most often by the emergency nurse are described.

Contact Lens Problems

Common problems associated with wearing contact lenses include removal, search for a lost contact, and chemicals or dirt particles under the lens that irritate the cornea. When hard or soft contacts are worn too long, the lens adheres to the cornea and is difficult to remove.

Contacts should be removed when the patient has ocular trauma or a change in mental status. Removal is contraindicated in globe perforation, since pressure on the globe can worsen leakage of vitreous humor. When a contact lens is lost, evert the upper lid to remove the lens (Figure 48-12). If lid eversion fails to reveal the contact, sweep the cul-de-sac with a moistened swab. If the lens is still not found, examine the eye with fluorescein. A corneal abrasion caused by the

contact lens may give the patient the sensation that the lens is still in the eye.

When there is a foreign body beneath the contact lens, the lens should be removed and cleaned before being returned to the eye. When the lens has been left in place too long, lubricating drops can be used to loosen the contact and facilitate removal. Prior to removal of the lens, fill two sterile containers with sterile saline and mark *left* and *right*. To remove a hard contact lens, use a suction cup designed specifically for removing contact lenses. Slide the contact off the cornea onto the sclera, and then gently lift. A two-handed method may also be used (Figure 48-7). With soft contact lenses, locate the lens, grasp be-

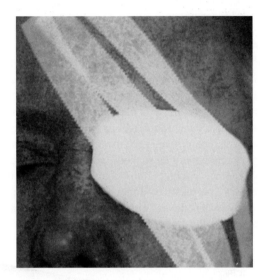

Figure **48-11**   Eye patch. *(From Grossman JA:* Atlas of minor injuries, *St. Louis, 1993, Gower Medical Publishing.)*

Box 48-6   Eye Irrigation

Cleanse the entire area around the eye and eyelid.
Prepare irrigation setup and solution.
Place patient supine, or adjust the examining chair to a reclining position.
Turn the head to the affected side, and pull the eyelid down.
Run solution directly over the eye and lower lid from the inner to the outer canthus.
Direct the patient to occasionally blink and look from side to side to distribute solution.
Irrigate for a minimum of 30 minutes with chemical exposure.
Evert and swab beneath the eyelid to remove residual particles.

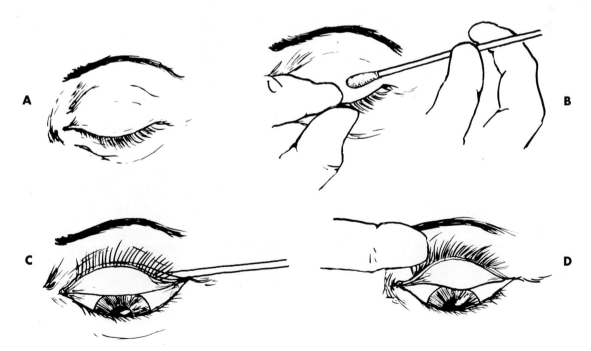

Figure **48-12**   Steps in everting eyelid. **A,** Eyelid. **B,** Placement of cotton swab (eyelashes are pulled down and back over swab). **C,** Eyelid everted over swab. **D,** Examination of inside of eyelid and eye.

tween the thumb and index finger, and lift the lens off the cornea (Figure 48-8).

Ocular Trauma

General principles pertaining to ocular examination are essentially the same for the patient with an eye injury; however, the patient's ABCs should be evaluated and stabilized prior to interventions for the ocular problem. Ocular injury often occurs in conjunction with head and facial trauma; therefore, the patient should be carefully evaluated for an associated eye injury. Check for contact lenses in the unconscious patient and remove as soon as possible. Do not instill eye drops before evaluation of ocular injury. Severe pain associated with ocular trauma can be minimized without medication by patching both eyes. When the patient cannot blink, protect the cornea from drying with ophthalmic ointment or artificial tears. The eyes may be taped shut when ointment is used.

Obtain pertinent details of history including mechanism of injury, time of injury, energy source, material involved when there is ocular penetration, and use of protective eyewear. If the foreign material is organic, there is increased risk of infection, whereas metallic materials cause vitreous and ocular reactions.

Box 48-7   Eye Patching

Administer antibiotic ointment or solution as directed.
Ask the patient to close both eyes.
Place a folded eye patch over the affected lid followed by an unfolded eye patch.
Tape the eye patch obliquely with paper tape. Avoid nasolabial folds.

Blunt trauma

Blunt trauma to the eye may be caused by a motor vehicle collision, assault with various weapons, or a fall. The most commonly seen ocular injury is *periorbital contusion,* or black eye. This injury is usually benign; however, the patient should be assessed for more serious injuries, such as a blowout fracture or basilar skull fracture. Therapeutic intervention includes ice, head elevation, and reassurance. Resolution of noncomplicated periorbital ecchymosis usually occurs within 2 to 3 weeks.

Orbital fractures

Orbital fractures involve the orbital floor and the orbital rim. Fractures of the orbital floor are serious and usually result from direct blunt trauma to the eye. A blowout fracture occurs when direct trauma increases IOP to the point where the orbital floor fractures (Figure 48-13).[20] Orbital contents may herniate into the maxillary or ethmoidal sinuses and trap the inferior rectus muscle in the defect. A blowout fracture is diagnosed by history and observation of periorbital hematoma, subconjunctival hemorrhage, periorbital edema, enophthalmos (sunken eye), an upward gaze, and a complaint of diplopia. The latter three conditions occur when the inferior rectus and oblique muscles are trapped in the fracture. Facial radiographs are used to assist with diagnosis. Computed tomography (CT) scan is more helpful in identification of the fracture than plain radiographs.

Orbital fractures are not considered an ocular emergency unless visual impairment or globe injury is present. Surgical intervention is usually delayed until swelling resolves in 10 to 14 days. Symptoms resolve without surgery in almost 85% of patients. Discharge instructions should include ice and cautions about Valsalva's maneuvers and nose blowing. The physician may also prescribe antibiotics to prevent orbital cellulitis.

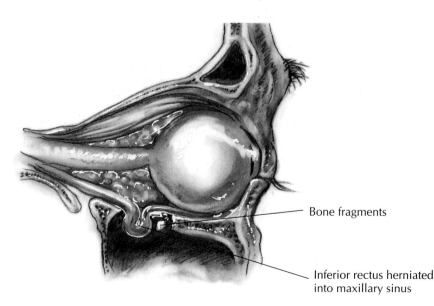

Figure **48-13** Mechanism of entrapment of inferior rectus muscle through an orbital floor defect. *(From Davis JH et al: Surgery: a problem-solving approach, ed 2, vol 2, St. Louis, 1995, Mosby.)*

Bone fragments

Inferior rectus herniated into maxillary sinus

Hyphema

Hyphema refers to bleeding into the anterior chamber of the eye, usually secondary to blunt trauma (Figure 48-14). Depression of the diaphragm of the iris or ciliary bodies causes bleeding. Hyphema size varies from microscopic to total involvement of the anterior chamber. The term *eightball hyphema* describes a total hyphema that has begun to clot.[9] Any patient with a hyphema requires evaluation by an ophthalmologist.

Symptoms of hyphema include pain, photophobia, and blurred vision. Blood in the anterior chamber may be easily seen in patients with lighter-colored eyes but may be extremely difficult to see in dark-eyed patients. Suspect concurrent head injury if the patient has an altered level of consciousness. Patients with bleeding disorders, anticoagulant therapy, kidney disease, liver disease, or sickle cell disease have an increased risk of complications; therefore these patients should be monitored carefully for increased bleeding. The most common complication of hyphema is rebleeding, usually within 2 to 5 days, but it can occur up to 14 days after the initial injury. Other complications include corneal blood staining, secondary glaucoma, loss of vision, and loss of the eye.

Management of hyphema is variable and controversial, particularly related to activity, that is, whether the patient should be allowed quiet activity or placed on strict bed rest. There is also disagreement regarding hospitalization and eye patching. Conservative therapy should be considered for those patients at risk for complications, children, and the elderly. Hospitalization should be considered when noncompliance with treatment is an issue. Pharmacologic management includes β-blockers to control elevated IOP, mydriatic agents to increase patient comfort, steroids to decrease inflammation in the anterior chamber, and an antifibrinolytic agent to delay clot dissolution and decrease the rate of rebleed. Analgesics may also be utilized; however, aspirin and nonsteroidal antiinflammatory medications should be avoided.

Iris injury

Iris injury is characterized by pain, photophobia, perilimbal conjunctival redness, and asymmetry in pupil size. Differentiation of iris injury from a microhyphema is often difficult. Hyphema is characterized by red blood cells in the anterior chamber, whereas iritis is characterized by white blood cells in the anterior chamber. Traumatic iridocyclitis is an inflammation of the iris and ciliary body following contusion of the eye. The affected pupil does not constrict as briskly as the unaffected one. Therapeutic intervention includes topical administration of cycloplegic agents and topical or systemic administration of corticosteroids. Complications include enophthalmos and loss of the eye.

Lens injury

Lens injury includes partial dislocation, total dislocation, and opacification or cataracts. Therapeutic intervention for each type of injury is surgery. Repair is not emergent unless obstructed outflow of aqueous humor is causing acute angle-closure glaucoma.

Subconjunctival hemorrhage

Subconjunctival hemorrhage is a very dramatic condition that is usually benign, painless, and heals spontaneously. Bleeding beneath the conjunctiva, caused by blunt trauma, sneezing, coughing episodes, or Valsalva's maneuver, makes the conjunctiva bright red (Figure 48-15). The hemorrhage may be limited to one area or involve the entire conjunctiva. With blunt trauma, the patient should be evaluated for other injuries to ocular structures. On rare occasions, hyphema can develop secondary to subconjunctival hemorrhage. When other ocular injuries have been ruled out, reassure the patient that this condition disappears within 2 to 3 weeks.

Penetrating trauma

Penetrating injury to the eye may occur during work or play and is often associated with lack of protective eyewear.[7] Injury may affect surface structures such as the cornea or damage the globe.

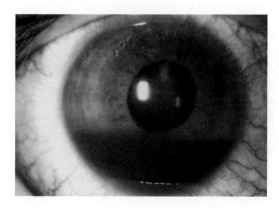

Figure **48-14** Traumatic hyphema. *(From Abrams D: Ophthalmology in medicine: an illustrated clinical guide, St. Louis, 1990, Mosby.)*

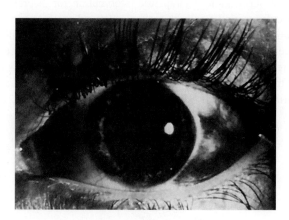

Figure **48-15** Subconjunctival hemorrhage. *(From Stein HA, Slatt BJ, Stein RM: The ophthalmic assistant, ed 6, St. Louis, 1994, Mosby.)*

Conjunctival laceration

Conjunctival laceration causes swelling and bleeding from the conjunctiva. The most common cause of this injury is a fingernail. If the laceration is less than 5 mm, treatment is antibiotics, patching, and observation. Lacerations greater than 5 mm usually require suturing by the ophthalmologist.

Corneal abrasion

Corneal abrasion is an extremely common injury (Figure 48-16). The cornea is damaged when a foreign body such as a contact lens scratches, abrades, or denudes the epithelium. Damage to the cornea exposes superficial corneal nerves, causing tearing, eyelid spasms, and pain.[10] Diagnosis is made with fluorescein staining after administration of local anesthetic. Antibiotic ointments are applied, and the eye is patched for 24 hours. Patching prevents eyelid movement, which can worsen the pain of the abrasion. The injury should be reevaluated in 24 hours.

Corneal laceration

Corneal laceration may be small or large. Small lacerations are treated as corneal abrasions. Larger corneal lacerations may require surgery to preserve the integrity of intraocular contents. An ophthalmology consult is indicated for these patients.

Corneal ulcer

Corneal ulcer usually occurs in the unconscious patient or the patient who leaves contact lenses in for an inordinate period of time. The ulcer appears as a white spot on the cornea. Symptoms include significant pain, photophobia, profuse tearing, and vascular congestion. Fluorescein staining causes a blue-green cast over the ulcer. Invasion of the ulcer by *Pseudomonas aeruginosa* can lead to eye loss within 48 hours. Therapeutic interventions include administration of systemic antibiotics, warm compresses, and an eye patch. Corneal ulcers are usually treated by an ophthalmologist.

Periorbital wounds

Periorbital wounds involve injury to the eyelids and surrounding periorbital tissue. Tissues lie in close proximity to the globe, so wounds should be examined carefully for globe penetration. Therapeutic intervention for lacerations includes wound care with early closure and careful approximation of wound edges before edema develops. For major lacerations or injuries with missing tissue, a plastic surgeon is recommended. The eyelid has an excellent blood supply, so trauma to the eyelid has a low incidence of infection and antibiotic treatment is rarely required.

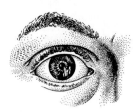

Figure **48-16** Corneal abrasion.

Globe rupture

Globe rupture is a major ocular emergency that results from blunt or penetrating forces. Rupture occurs at a point of weakness in the ocular structures, usually the insertion of the extraocular muscles or the corneoscleral junction (limbus). Penetrating injuries to the globe are caused by perforation with a sharp object such as a knife, stick, or dart. Blunt forces cause globe rupture secondary to an abrupt rise in IOP. The elderly are at greatest risk for globe rupture.

Signs and symptoms of globe rupture include an unusually deep or shallow anterior chamber, altered light perception, hyphema, and occasionally vitreous hemorrhage.[16] The pupil assumes a teardrop shape with the point toward the rupture site. When globe rupture is suspected, further eye manipulation should be avoided. If an impaled object is present, secure the object and patch both eyes to decrease eye movement and prevent further damage. A detailed examination is not performed until the ophthalmologist arrives. General anesthesia may be necessary to perform an adequate examination. Eye drops should not be used when globe rupture is suspected.

If the eye tissue has not eviscerated, the ophthalmologist usually removes the object during surgery and sutures the eye. With loss of vitreous humor and damage to the lens and ciliary body, enucleation may be required. Other therapeutic intervention includes keeping the patient NPO, antibiotics, tetanus prophylaxis, and corticosteroids.

Foreign body

The most common foreign body in the eye is a small object such as a dust particle. The patient usually presents with hypersensitivity to light, excessive tearing, or pain, especially when opening or closing the eye. Foreign bodies and corneal abrasions feel similar to the patient. With a foreign body, the first step is to locate the object. Local anesthesia may be required to examine the eye adequately. General anesthesia may be required for children. Good lighting and a magnification source are essential to locate and safely remove a foreign body from the eye.

With a foreign body in the conjunctiva and cornea, determine the identity of the foreign body, that is, what the patient believes is in the eye. A history of high-speed projectiles should increase the index of suspicion for an intraocular foreign body. Organic foreign bodies have a higher incidence of infection, whereas metallic objects leave a rust ring unless the object is removed within 12 hours. Inert foreign bodies do not cause infection but have a greater risk of penetration.

Therapeutic intervention includes everting the upper eyelid with a cotton-tipped swab, irrigating with normal saline solution, and gently removing the foreign body with a moistened cotton-tipped swab. If the foreign body adheres to the cornea, a 25- or 27-gauge needle is used at a tangential angle to remove the object. Larger embedded objects are referred to the ophthalmologist for removal or follow-up. Once the foreign body is removed, the cornea should be carefully examined for other objects, rust ring, or corneal abrasion. Ocular burr drills are also used to remove rust rings and may be used to free foreign bodies stuck to the cornea. Antibiotic ointment is applied, and the eye is patched and reevaluated in 24 hours. Patching is not recommended if the foreign object is organic. Broad-spectrum antibiotics are recommended because of the increased risk of infection. Bacterial flora of the eye is altered with contact lens use, so patching in these patients may increase the risk of infection caused by pathogenic bacteria. When the patient has one eye patched, depth perception is altered; therefore the patient should be instructed not to drive or operate heavy equipment. Topical anesthetics are used for initial evaluation but are not used for long-term management of pain, since these substances retard corneal healing. Oral analgesia is recommended. Mydriatics may be used to decrease pain secondary to ciliary spasm.

Intraocular foreign bodies

Intraocular foreign bodies are usually small and easily overlooked. Metal fragments and other small projectiles enter the eye at a high rate of speed and come to rest within the posterior chamber. The entry site may be small and difficult to locate. A high index of suspicion is required to prompt vigorous evaluation for this type of injury. Many patients experience only slight discomfort. Visual acuity may be significantly decreased or may be normal. The pupil may assume the shape of a cat's eye.

An intraocular foreign body is an ocular emergency. Early therapeutic intervention is essential to preserve vision. The amount of damage to the eye depends on the size, shape, and composition of the foreign body. All foreign bodies in the eye are considered contaminated, so the patient is treated with antibiotics and tetanus prophylaxis as appropriate. Plain radiographs are used to identify the number and position of foreign bodies. A CT scan may be used to delineate subtle intraocular injuries within the globe and orbit. Surgery is indicated for most patients to prevent further damage to the eye secondary to hemorrhage, infection, or a detached retina.

Ocular burns

Ocular burns are an immediate threat to the patient's vision. Burns of the eye may result from a chemical, a heat source such as a curling iron, or radiation. Regardless of etiology, these injuries cause significant discomfort.

Chemical burns

Chemical burns occur at home and at work. A chemical burn is the most urgent of all ocular emergencies. Burns may be caused by an alkaline, acid, or other irritant. These substances, particularly alkalines, have a devastating effect on the eye. Acid burns cause immediate damage to the cornea by denaturing the tissue, so the cornea appears white and opaque. No further damage occurs after the initial impact because the acid is neutralized on impact. Alkalines such as concrete, lye, and drain cleaners also cause the cornea to opacify; however, alkalines continue to damage the cornea until the substance is removed.

Treatment for chemical burns takes priority over assessment of visual acuity. Copious irrigation with normal saline should be initiated as soon as possible, preferably before the patient arrives in the ED. With alkaline burns, irrigation should continue until the ocular pH reaches 7.4. Irrigation for a minimum of 30 minutes with 2 L of fluid is the norm. With severe cases, irrigation for 2 to 4 hours may be necessary. Once the pH reaches the desired level, the eyelid should be everted and then the cul-de-sac swabbed and irrigated to remove any remaining particles. Patients should receive topical antibiotics, cycloplegic agents, and steroids. Parenteral or oral narcotic analgesia is also recommended.

Thermal burns

Thermal burns affect the eyelids as well as the surface of the eye. Facial burns are often associated with eyelid burns. Globe burns are rare except with burns caused by hot metal, steam, or gasoline. Burns to the eyelids may cause lid contracture, which is disfiguring and affects vision. Therapeutic interventions include analgesia, sedation, eye irrigation, antibiotics, cycloplegics, and bilateral eye patches.

Radiation burns

Radiation burns may be ultraviolet or infrared. Severity of the burn depends on wavelength and degree of exposure. Ultraviolet radiation burns occur in welders, snow skiers, ice climbers, people who read on the beach, and those who use a sunlamp. Ultraviolet radiation is absorbed by the cornea and produces keratitis, conjunctivitis, or both. Symptoms usually begin 6 to 10 hours after exposure and include severe pain, photophobia, and corneal irregularity. Ultraviolet burns are considered the most painful of all ocular burns. Visual acuity is usually decreased. Therapeutic interventions include topical antibiotics, cycloplegics, systemic analgesics, topical antibiotic ointment, and patching for 24 hours. The cornea usually heals within 24 hours without residual scarring.

Infrared radiation burns are more severe than ultraviolet radiation burns. Fortunately, infrared radiation injuries are rare since development of protective eyewear. Infrared radiation burns cause permanent loss of vision secondary to absorption of infrared rays by the iris and increased lens temperature, which leads to cataract formation. Table 48-4 describes common infrared burns.

Medical Problems Involving the Eye

Many ocular problems that present to the ED are not related to trauma. Problems may be a minor annoyance or represent a significant threat to the patient's vision. The most common medical conditions seen in the ED are described in the following sections.

Eyelid infections and inflammations

Hordeolum

A hordeolum, or stye, is an infection of the upper or lower eyelid at the accessory glands of Zeis or Moll caused by *Staphylococcus aureus*. The patient develops a small external abscess, pain, redness, and swelling (Figure 48-17).

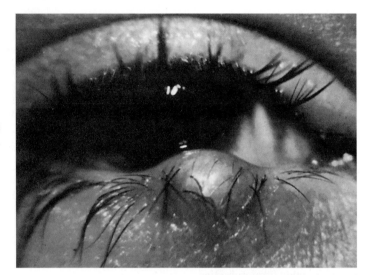

Figure **48-17** Acute hordeolum of the lower eyelid. *(From Newell FW:* Ophthalmology: principles and concepts, *ed 8, St. Louis, 1996, Mosby.)*

Table **48-4**	**Infrared burns**
Name	Description
Glassblower's cataracts	Caused by prolonged exposure to intense heat during production of glass.
Focal retinitis	Also called eclipse blindness; occurs during exposure to an eclipse or an atomic bomb.
X-ray burns	Injury proportional to penetration of rays. Soft rays produce superficial keratoconjunctivitis and dermatitis, whereas hard rays, such as gamma rays, produce retinal damage and cataracts.

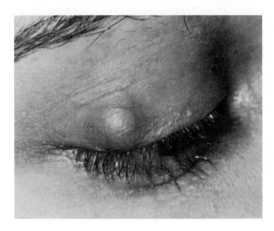

Figure **48-18** Chronic chalazion of meibomian gland of the upper eyelid. *(From Newell FW:* Ophthalmology: principles and concepts, *ed 8, St. Louis, 1996, Mosby.)*

Therapeutic intervention includes application of warm compresses 4 times a day until the abscess comes to a point. A hordeolum may rupture spontaneously or require incision to drain the abscess. If the abscess points to the conjunctiva, a vertical incision is made by the physician; if the abscess points toward the skin, a horizontal incision is made. Ophthalmic antibiotic ointment should be applied every 4 hours. The patient should be instructed not to squeeze the abscess because this spreads the infection and worsens the condition.

Chalazion

A chalazion is an internal hordeolum caused by chronic granulomatous inflammation of a meibomian gland (Figure 48-18). The patient presents with several weeks of painless, localized swelling. A chalazion is differentiated from a hordeolum by absence of acute inflammation. Treatment in the early stages includes topical antibiotic ointment and incision and drainage when the chalazion affects vision.

Blepharitis

Blepharitis is an ulcerative inflammation of the lid margin, usually with *S. aureus.* Symptoms include burning, stinging, and itching of the lids. The eye appears rimmed with red, and scales may appear on the lashes. Treatment consists of removing the crusts and cleaning lid margins twice daily with baby shampoo and antibiotic ophthalmic ointment.

Corneal infections

Keratitis

Keratitis is a generic term for inflammation of the cornea. The cornea becomes light sensitive, red, and painful, with profuse tearing. Keratitis may be caused by a corneal ulcer, bacteria, or fungus. The patient presents with a "white spot" on the cornea, an epithelial defect, or a corneal ulcer (Figure 48-19). Risk factors for bacterial keratitis include traumatic corneal injury and corneal injury secondary to contact lens use. Pus in the anterior chamber (hypopyon) may be present.

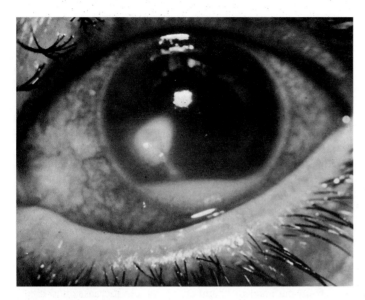

Figure **48-19** An acute hypopyon ulcerative keratitis caused by a *Streptococcus* infection in a 69-year-old patient with facial nerve paralysis that prevented adequate closure of the eyelid. Leukocytes in the anterior chamber form a hypopyon. *(From Newell FW: Ophthalmology: principles and concepts, ed 8, St. Louis, 1996, Mosby.)*

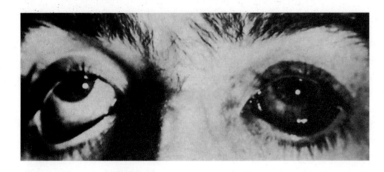

Figure **48-20** Acute conjunctivitis. *(From Stein HA, Slatt BJ, Stein RM: The ophthalmic assistant, ed 6, St. Louis, 1994, Mosby.)*

Culture and sensitivity should be obtained to determine the specific cause of the infection. Therapeutic interventions include warm compresses, broad-spectrum antibiotics, and possibly fungal drops.

Viral keratoconjunctivitis

Viral keratoconjunctivitis is acute conjunctivitis and keratitis usually caused by adenovirus. The patient complains of redness of the eye, tearing, and pain. Photophobia usually begins several days later. Eyelids and conjunctiva also become swollen. In adults, this condition is confined to the eye; however, children may have fever, pharyngitis, and diarrhea. Therapeutic intervention is usually symptomatic. Topical antibiotics may be started while awaiting laboratory results. Infection spreads easily; therefore scrupulous hand washing is critical. All instruments utilized on the patient should be sterilized.

Herpes simplex

Herpes simplex infection presents primarily with corneal ulcers. Treatment consists of topical trifluridine (Viroptic) 9 times a day for 2 to 3 weeks. Steroids should not be utilized when herpes simplex is suspected.

Herpes zoster

Herpes zoster dermatitis usually involves the trigeminal nerve; however, all parts of the eye can be affected. Oral acyclovir (800 mg 5 times a day for 10 days) decreases the severity of ocular complications. Topical steroids are used to treat associated iritis. Prophylactic topical antibiotics may be utilized. Treatment for herpes simplex is not effective for herpes zoster.

Conjunctivitis

Conjunctivitis is a bacterial infection of the conjunctiva characterized by the eyelids sticking together when the patient wakes in the morning (Figure 48-20). Infection may be caused by staphylococcal, gonococcal, pneumococcal, *Haemophilus,* or *Pseudomonas* organisms.[3] Therapeutic interventions include antibiotic ophthalmic ointment or drops. Warm soaks are used to keep the lids and lashes free of debris. Culture and sensitivity are obtained before antibiotic therapy is initiated.

Acute conjunctivitis is contagious. Detailed aftercare instructions should include how to prevent the disease from spreading. Teaching should include discussion of cross-contamination through eye makeup, pillows, washcloths, towels, and pillowcases. Appropriate hand-washing techniques should also be reviewed.

Conjunctivitis secondary to *Neisseria gonorrhoeae* causes copious purulent discharge with extremely red and swollen conjunctiva. Therapeutic intervention is application of penicillin G drops, tetracycline, or bacitracin ophthalmic ointment. Intramuscular ceftriaxone (Rocephin) should also be given. Home treatment includes frequent ocular saline irrigations. Other potential contacts, including sexual contacts, should be treated.

Uveitis

Uveitis, or iritis, is inflammation of the uveal tract including the iris, ciliary body, and choroid. Uveal inflammation usually affects the anterior portion of the uveal tract and is categorized as iritis. Severe inflammation may decrease the patient's vision. Symptoms include blurred vision, deep aching, photophobia, tearing, and redness of the eye. The more posterior the inflammation, the less redness is observed. Therapeutic interventions include warm compresses, systemic analgesia, topical corticosteroids, and mydriatics to dilate the pupil and prevent adhesions of the iris and lens. Antibiotic ophthalmic ointment may also be used.

Orbital cellulitis

Acute infection of the orbital tissue is commonly caused by *Streptococcus pneumoniae, S. aureus,* and *Haemophilus influenzae.* The patient presents with recent or concurrent sinusitis or periorbital injury. Symptoms include pain in and around the eye, decreased visual acuity, swelling and redness of the eyelids and periorbital tissues, conjunctival redness, and varying degrees of exophthalmos. Therapeutic interventions include blood and periorbital fluid cultures and intravenous cefuroxime (Zinacef). A CT scan may be obtained to rule out orbital abscess and intracranial involvement. The patient should be hospitalized.

Cavernous sinus thrombosis is an infection that has spread from an infected sinus to the orbital area. Signs and symptoms include chills, headache, lethargy, nausea, pain, and decreased vision. The patient may also have fever, vomiting, and other signs of systemic involvement. Therapeutic interventions include hospitalization, blood cultures, and CT of the head and orbit. Intravenous antibiotic such as nafcillin (Unipen) are required. Evaluation by an ophthalmologist and neurologist and a medical consultation are recommended.

Retinal emergencies

Retinal emergencies may be due to a congenital defect in the retina or secondary to an inherited condition. Evaluate the patient's ocular history carefully.

Central retinal artery occlusion

Central retinal artery occlusion produces sudden, painless blindness and is usually limited to one eye. This is a true ocular emergency. Retinal circulation must be reestablished within 60 to 90 minutes to prevent permanent loss of vision. Occlusion occurs most often in the elderly and has a poor prognosis. Therapeutic interventions are directed at increasing retinal circulation and include gentle ocular pressure on the globe, breathing into a paper bag, or surgical decompression by an ophthalmologist. The patient should be hospitalized.

Retinal detachment

Retinal detachment occurs when the retina tears and allows vitreous humor to seep between the retina and the choroid. When the retina is torn, loss of blood and oxygen supply renders the retina unable to perceive light. Normal function of the retina is to perceive light and send an impulse to the optic nerve. With retinal detachment, the patient complains of flashes of light (photopsia), veil or curtain effect in the visual field, and dark spots or floaters. Therapeutic interventions include hospitalization, bed rest, and bilateral eye patches. Ophthalmologic consultation for laser repair or a scleral buckling procedure is indicated.

Glaucoma

An estimated 1.5 million Americans have some degree of blindness caused by glaucoma. *Acute glaucoma is an emergency situation;* blindness may occur in a matter of hours. Acute glaucoma occurs when aqueous humor cannot escape from the anterior chamber, so volume increases and chamber pressure rises (Figure 48-21). Normally, aqueous humor leaves the anterior chamber and enters the vascular system via the Schlemm's canal at the junction of the iris and the cornea (Figure 48-22). With glaucoma, increased anterior chamber pressure decreases circulation to the retina and increases pressure on the optic nerve. Untreated, these high pressures may eventually cause blindness.

Acute glaucoma

Acute or angle-closure glaucoma occurs with blockage of the anterior chamber angle near the root of the iris. The patient presents with severe eye pain, a fixed and slightly dilated pupil, hard globe, foggy-appearing cornea, severe

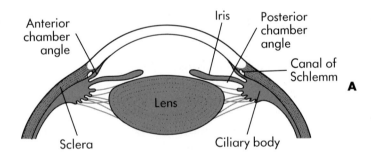

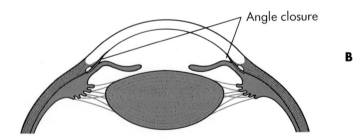

Figure **48-21** Comparison of, **A,** normal angle of eye with, **B,** closed angle in angle-closure glaucoma.

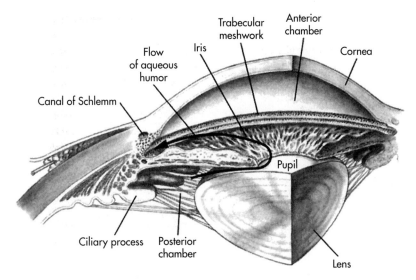

Figure **48-22** Close view of trabecular meshwork and flow of aqueous humor. *(From Thompson JM et al:* Mosby's clinical nursing, *ed 4, St. Louis, 1997, Mosby.)*

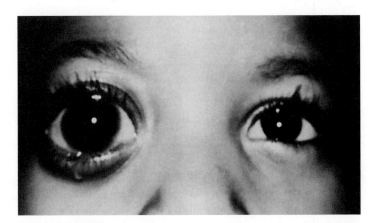

Figure **48-23** Marked enlargement of the right eye of a 3-year-old girl with infantile glaucoma. *(From Newell FW:* Ophthalmology: principles and concepts, *ed 8, St. Louis, 1996, Mosby.)*

headache, halos around lights, diminished peripheral vision, and occasionally nausea and vomiting. Diagnosis may be difficult because symptoms can mimic cardiovascular or gastrointestinal processes. IOP greater than 60 to 70 mm Hg damages the corneal endothelium, lens, iris, optical nerve, and retina.

Therapeutic intervention focuses on decreasing IOP by decreasing aqueous humor production, reducing vitreous humor volume, and facilitating aqueous flow. Topical β-adrenergic antagonists, such as timolol, decrease aqueous production. Intravenous acetazolamide also decreases aqueous production. Agents such as oral glycerol or intravenous mannitol draw water from the globe and reduce the volume of vitreous humor. Aqueous humor outflow is enhanced with 2% to 4% pilocarpine drops every 15 minutes for the first 1

to 2 hours. Once the acute attack is broken and IOP is reduced, surgery is required.

Open-angle glaucoma

Open-angle glaucoma is a chronic condition. Obstruction of the Schlemm's canal develops gradually, so the condition progresses slowly. The patient may be unaware of its presence. Therapeutic interventions include miotic eye drops and surgery.

Congenital glaucoma

Congenital glaucoma is also known as infantile or juvenile glaucoma (Figure 48-23). Failure of the anterior chamber angle to develop normally is the causative event. Early signs and symptoms are copious tearing and photophobia, which causes the baby to keep the eyelids closed more than usual. Therapeutic intervention is surgery.

Box **48-8**

NURSING DIAGNOSES FOR OCULAR EMERGENCIES
Anxiety
Pain
Sensory-perceptual alteration
Risk for infection
Risk for injury
Knowledge deficit

Secondary glaucoma

Secondary glaucoma is caused by increased IOP secondary to surgery, trauma, hemorrhage, inflammation, tumors, or various other conditions that may interfere with humor drainage. Therapeutic intervention varies with etiology.

SUMMARY

Ocular emergencies do not represent a threat to the patient's life. However, these conditions represent a great threat to the patient's well-being. Once lost, vision cannot be replaced. The emergency nurse should assess patients who present with various ocular problems and identify those patients with actual or potential threats to vision. Early recognition of true ocular emergencies is essential for preservation of sight. Box 48-8 summarizes nursing diagnoses for patients with an ocular problem.

REFERENCES

1. Barish RA, Naradzay JF: Ophthalmologic therapeutics, *Emerg Med Clin North Am* 13(3):649, 1995.
2. Bertolini J, Pelucio M: The red eye, *Emerg Med Clin North Am* 13(3):561, 1995.
3. Biswell R: Cornea. In Vaughn DG, Asbury T, Riordan-Eva P, editors: *General ophthalmology,* ed 13, Norwalk, Conn, 1992, Appleton & Lange.
4. Boltri JM: Tonometry. In Pfenninger JL, Fowler GC, editors: *Procedures for primary care physicians,* St. Louis, 1994, Mosby.
5. Catalano RA: *Ocular emergencies,* Philadelphia, 1992, WB Saunders.
6. Catalano RA: Eye injuries and prevention, *Pediatr Clin North Am* 40(4):827, 1993.
7. Dannenberg AL, Parver LM, Fowler CJ: Penetrating eye injuries related to assault: the National Eye Trauma System Registry, *Arch Ophthalmol* 110(6):849, 1992.
8. Datner EM, Jolly BT: Pediatric ophthalmology, *Emerg Med Clin North Am* 13(3):669, 1995.
9. Epifanio PC: Ocular emergencies. In Emergency Nurses Association: *Emergency nursing core curriculum,* ed 4, Philadelphia, 1994, WB Saunders.
10. Fowler GC: Corneal abrasions and removal of corneal or conjunctival foreign bodies. In Pfenninger JL, Fowler GC, editors: *Procedures for primary care physicians,* St. Louis, 1994, Mosby.
11. Greenberg MD: Emergency care for acute visual loss, *Emerg Med* 24(8):112, 1992.
12. Handler JA, Ghezzi KT: General ophthalmologic examination, *Emerg Med Clin North Am* 13(3):521, 1995.
13. Handysides G: Neurologic and head and neck problems. In Handysides G, editor: *Triage in emergency practice,* St. Louis, 1996, Mosby.
14. Janda AM: Eye, ear, nose, throat, and oral surgery. In Tintinalli JE, Ruiz E, Krome RL, editors: *Emergency medicine: a comprehensive study guide,* ed 14, New York, 1996, McGraw-Hill.
15. Jarvis C: Eyes and visual status. In Jarvis C, editor: *Physical examination and health assessment,* Philadelphia, 1992, WB Saunders.
16. Linden JA, Genner GS: Trauma to the globe, *Emerg Med Clin North Am* 13(3):581, 1995.
17. Ocular irrigation: normal saline is not the only choice, *Emerg Med* 23(18):60, 1991.
18. Rubin S, Hallagan L: Lids, lacrimals, and lashes, *Emerg Med Clin North Am* 13(3):631, 1995.
19. Santen SA, Scott JL: Ophthalmologic procedures, *Emerg Med Clin North Am* 13(3):681, 1995.
20. Snell RS, Smith MS: The eye and orbit. In Snell RS, Smith MS, editors: *Clinical anatomy for emergency medicine,* St. Louis, 1993, Mosby.
21. Tabbara KF: Eye emergencies. In Saunders CE, Ho MT, editors: *Emergency diagnosis and treatment,* ed 4, Norwalk, Conn, 1992, Appleton & Lange.
22. Whelan AJ: Patient care in internal medicine. In Ewald GA, McKenzie CR, editors: *Manual of medical therapeutics,* ed 28, Boston, 1995, Little, Brown.

unit VI

SPECIAL PATIENT SITUATIONS

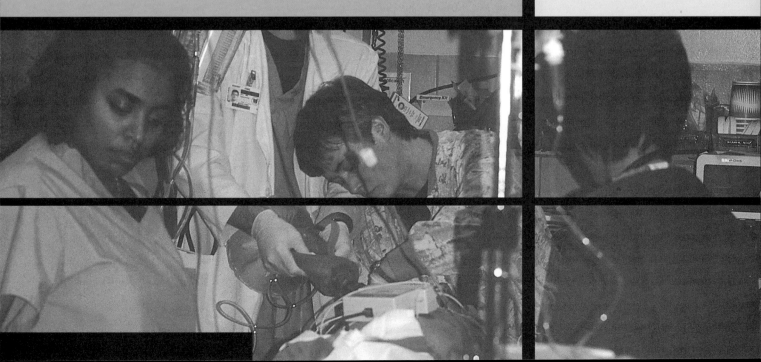

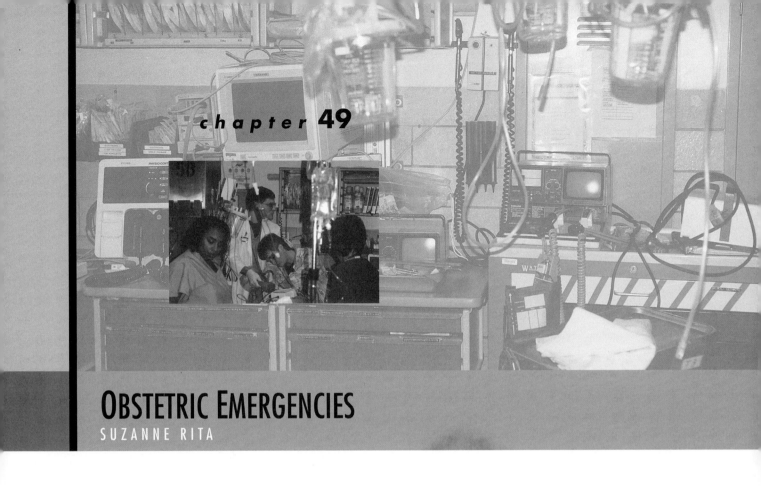

chapter 49

OBSTETRIC EMERGENCIES
SUZANNE RITA

Pregnant women can present to the emergency department (ED) with a variety of complaints related to the pregnancy. These may occur prior to delivery, during delivery, or after delivery. Management of obstetric emergencies requires acute assessment skills to identify life-threatening conditions and intervene quickly to prevent adverse outcomes for the mother and baby. This chapter describes changes in pathophysiology related to pregnancy, assessment of the pregnant patient, and management of emergencies commonly associated with pregnancy.

ANATOMY AND PHYSIOLOGY

The female reproductive system consists of the fallopian tubes, ovaries, uterus, vagina, and external genitalia (Figure 49-1). The cervical os, the opening to the uterus, is located within the vagina. The vagina serves as the exit route for menstrual blood flow, the entry point for sperm, and the birth canal. Physiologic activity of the reproductive system is cyclic. Each month the uterus prepares for implantation of a fertilized egg through proliferation of the uterine endometrium. The eggs are stored in the ovaries and released in a cyclic pattern. If the egg is not fertilized, the uterine lining sloughs and is shed as menstrual blood flow. If the egg is fertilized, it begins to reproduce and replicate. The embryo is formed, transported through the fallopian tube, and embedded in the uterine wall to continue its growth.

As the pregnancy progresses, it is characterized by increasing size of the embryo and various sexual organs. Uter-

ine size goes from about 50 g to about 1100 g.[4] Concurrently, the breasts double in size, and the vagina enlarges. Total weight gain during pregnancy is about 25 pounds. Other body systems affected by pregnancy include the cardiovascular system, respiratory system, gastrointestinal system, and genitourinary system. Changes in these systems are summarized in Table 49-1.

PATIENT ASSESSMENT

Many EDs care for pregnant patients throughout the pregnancy, while others provide care only for complaints not related to the pregnancy: colds, flu, sprains, and so on. Each pregnant patient should be carefully assessed (Box 49-1).

Regardless of gestation, the first priority for assessment of women with an obstetric emergency is airway, breathing, and circulation (ABCs). The age of fetal viability is considered 24 weeks' gestation. Management of obstetric emergencies after onset of fetal viability involves two patients, mother and fetus. See Chapter 50 for a discussion of neonatal resuscitation. After assessment of the patient's ABCs, the next priority is determination of gestation and evaluation of impending delivery.

FIRST TRIMESTER EMERGENCIES
Ectopic Pregnancy

Ectopic pregnancy occurs when the fertilized ovum implants anywhere other than the endometrium of the uterus, such as the fallopian tube, ovary, or abdominal cavity.

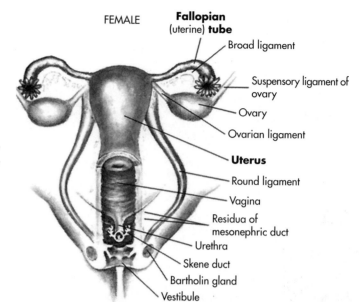

Figure **49-1** Female reproductive system. *(From Huether SE, McCance KL:* Understanding pathophysiology, *St. Louis, 1996, Mosby.)*

Table 49-1	Physiologic Changes Related to Pregnancy
Body system	Changes
Cardiovascular	Cardiac output increases 30-40% by week 27.
	Placental blood flow is 625-650 ml/min.
	Blood volume increases by 30%.
	Heart rate increases throughout pregnancy.
Respiratory	Respiratory rate increases.
	Oxygen consumption increases by 20%.
	Minute volume increases by 50%.
	Arterial PCO_2 decreases secondary to hyperventilation.
Urinary	Rate of urine formation increases slightly.
	Sodium, chloride, and water reabsorption increases as much as 50%.
	Glomerular filtration rate increases about 50%.
Gastrointestinal	Smooth muscle relaxes, which increases gastric emptying time.
	Intestines are relocated to the upper abdomen.
Other	Anemia develops because of increased iron requirements by mother and fetus.

Box 49-1 Assessment Guidelines for the Pregnant Patient

Last normal menstrual period
Birth control method
Gravida, parity, and abortion history
Bleeding, discharge, or tissue present
Nausea and/or vomiting
Urinary symptoms
Abdominal pain—location, duration, description
Estimated date of confinement
Prenatal care
Problems with present or previous pregnancies
Medications and allergies
Maternal medical and surgical history
Blood type and Rh factor if known

Ninety-five percent of all ectopic pregnancies occur in one of the fallopian tubes. The most common site for implantation is the ampulla, followed by the isthmus (Figure 49-2). The ovum begins to grow but may rupture, usually after the twelfth week of pregnancy. Ectopic pregnancy is one of the major causes of maternal death, usually as a result of hemorrhage.

On assessment, the patient gives a history of being pregnant (at least 12 weeks). However, 15% of patients with ectopic pregnancy are symptomatic before the first missed period. Complaints include pelvic pain and/or vaginal bleeding. Pain, if present, may be mild to severe. If the ectopic pregnancy is leaking or has ruptured, the diaphragm becomes irritated from blood in the peritoneum, causing referred pain to the shoulder (Kehr's sign).

Pelvic pain and vaginal bleeding or spotting in a woman of childbearing years should be treated as an ectopic pregnancy until this life-threatening condition is ruled out.[2] Predisposing factors for ectopic pregnancy include previous ectopic pregnancy, adhesions from previous pregnancies and surgeries, history of pelvic infections, and possibly the presence of an intrauterine device.

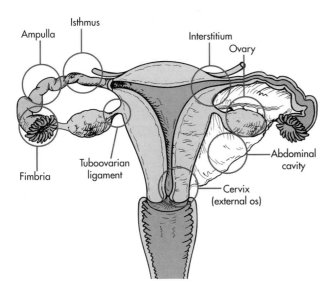

Figure **49-2** Sites of implantation of ectopic pregnancies. Order of frequency of occurrence is ampulla, isthmus, interstitium, fimbria, tuboovarian ligament, ovary, abdominal cavity, and cervix (external os). *(From Lewis SM, Collier IC, Heitkemper MM: Medical-surgical nursing, ed 4, St. Louis, 1996, Mosby.)*

Table 49-2	Types of Abortion
Type	Signs and symptoms
Threatened	Vaginal bleeding
	Mild abdominal cramping
	Closed or slightly open os
Inevitable	Heavy vaginal bleeding
	Severe abdominal cramping
	Open os
Incomplete	Heavy vaginal bleeding
	Abdominal cramping
	Some products of conception retained
Complete	Slight vaginal bleeding
	No abdominal cramping
	All products of conception passed
Missed	Usually no maternal symptoms
	Discrepancy in fetal size when compared to dates
Septic	Severe abdominal pain
	High temperature
	Malodorous vaginal discharge

A pregnancy test should be obtained on all women presenting with pelvic pain and vaginal bleeding or spotting. A pelvic examination should be done to evaluate the cervical os and identify the amount and source of bleeding. Bimanual pelvic examination defines uterine size and allows palpation of masses outside the uterus.

If an ectopic pregnancy is suspected, intravenous access should be established with a large-bore catheter in anticipation of potential life-threatening hemorrhage. A quantitative serum β-human chorionic gonadotropin (β-hCG) level, complete blood count (CBC), and type and screen should be obtained. An abdominal ultrasound is done to identify an ectopic pregnancy.

Methotrexate and misoprostol can be used up to 8 weeks of pregnancy if rupture is not present. This procedure has not been approved by the Food and Drug Administration but is being trialed at some centers.[1] The combination of these drugs is 96% effective in inducing nonsurgical abortion. An injection of methotrexate is administered on an outpatient basis, eliminating further duplication of the embryonic cells. Five to seven days later, a misoprostol suppository inserted into the vagina produces a miscarriage.

Treatment for ectopic pregnancy includes operative and nonoperative interventions. Operative interventions are indicated when the ectopic pregnancy has ruptured, the patient is in shock, or nonoperative interventions are not available.

In addition to assessment and intervention of the patient's physiologic needs, the emergency nurse must recognize the patient's and family's need for emotional support. The patient may fear for her life as well as her future childbearing ability, feel concern the pregnancy is not normal, or experience personal guilt related to the pregnancy.

Abortion

Abortion is the number one cause of vaginal bleeding in women of childbearing years, with an estimated 15% to 20% of all pregnancies resulting in spontaneous abortion.[5] Abortion should be considered a possibility in any woman of childbearing years with vaginal bleeding. Abortion is defined as termination of pregnancy at any time before the fetus has achieved viability (24 weeks' gestation). Table 49-2 summarizes the types of abortion.

The patient presents to the ED complaining of vaginal bleeding and may also have abdominal pain. She may or may not report a missed period. A good gynecologic history should be elicited from the patient, including the amount of bleeding. Ask the patient how many pads she has used in an hour; a general rule of thumb is a saturated pad equals 30 ml of blood loss.

Obtain a urine pregnancy test or a serum β-hCG level. Palpate the patient's abdomen for pain or tenderness, which may indicate ectopic pregnancy. A pelvic examination determines the source of bleeding, visualizes any products of conception, and determines dilatation of the cervical os. Observe for vaginal discharge. A bimanual examination is performed to determine size of the uterus and other reproductive organs. Palpation of the adnexa is performed to determine tenderness. Consider a pelvic ultrasound to exclude ectopic pregnancy.

Therapeutic interventions depend on the type of abortion. Fifty percent of threatened abortions may result in a complete or incomplete abortion within a few hours. A patient with threatened abortion should be observed closely for changes in her hemodynamic status. Document the amount of blood loss. If the patient exhibits signs of shock, replace blood loss with fluids or blood. Provide emotional support to the patient, significant other, and family.

If the abortion is inevitable or incomplete, obtain blood for Rh type, CBC, and type and screen. Start at least one IV line with a large-bore catheter, and administer fluids (normal saline or Ringer's lactate). Prepare for suction curettage.

If the patient will be discharged, aftercare instructions should include information on bed rest and instructions to return to the ED or call the primary caregiver for increased vaginal bleeding, increasing abdominal pain, passage of tissue, or fever or chills. The patient should also be told to avoid douching and intercourse while on bed rest because these can increase vaginal bleeding or cramping or cause infection if the cervical os begins to open. The patient should be instructed to follow up with the appropriate referral caregiver.

ANTEPARTUM EMERGENCIES
Pregnancy-Induced Hypertension

The term *pregnancy induced hypertension* (PIH) refers to toxemia of pregnancy and includes preeclampsia and eclampsia. It is characterized by hypertension, proteinuria, and edema. Systolic blood pressure increases 30 mm Hg over the nonpregnant level. This condition usually occurs in the last few months of pregnancy (after 20 weeks' gestation), can appear up to 72 hours after delivery, and has been reported weeks after delivery. This syndrome occurs most often in women who are primigravida, younger than 20 years, or older than 35 years. PIH is a leading cause of maternal morbidity and death. Fetal mortality is five times higher in the woman with PIH.

Preeclampsia and eclampsia are phases of the syndrome. Preeclampsia is characterized by hypertension, edema, proteinuria, headaches, and decreased urinary output. In eclampsia, symptoms are magnified and worsened. The patient presents with seizures or may be in a coma. Pulmonary edema may be present. This situation is an immediate threat to the mother and fetus.

Treatment includes oxygen, intravenous access, and fetal monitoring (Figure 49-3). If the fetus is in distress, an emergency cesarean section is indicated. Pharmacologic interventions to lower the blood pressure include hydralazine and magnesium (Boxes 49-2 and 49-3). Hydralazine is effective because it lowers the blood pressure slowly and effectively. This prevents sudden reduction in blood flow to the fetus. If hydralazine is ineffective, magnesium is used. In some centers, magnesium may be used as the first medication. Diazepam or midazolam can be used to control seizures. Fetal monitoring is essential. Any drop in fetal heart rate or deceleration of heart rate during contractions indicates the need for immediate emergency cesarean section.

THIRD TRIMESTER EMERGENCIES
Placenta Previa

Previa means "in front of"; therefore placenta previa occurs when the placenta will present before the fetus. Pla-

---

Box 49-2 Hydralazine (Apresoline) in PIH

Parameters
Give when SBP > 180 mm Hg and/or DBP > 110 mm Hg.

Dosage
May be given as bolus or IV drip
Bolus: 5 mg hydralazine IV, 10 mg given 15 minutes later if BP remains above 150/90-100 mm Hg; 10 mg bolus may be repeated as needed to maintain blood pressure at 150/90-100 mm Hg
IV drip: 80 mg hydralazine in 500 ml D₅W solution infused at 30 to 32 ml/hr (5 mg/hr); titrate infusion rate every 15 minutes until BP is 150/90-100 mm Hg

Caution
Pay close attention to hypotension. Remember that hypotension decreases blood flow to the placenta.

Side effects
Flushing, tachycardia

Modified from Farrell RG, editor: *OB/GYN emergencies: the first 60 minutes*, Rockville, Md, 1986, Aspen.
SBP, Systolic blood pressure; *DBP*, diastolic blood pressure; *BP*, blood pressure; *D₅W*, 5% dextrose in water.

Box 49-3 Magnesium Sulfate in Eclampsia

Loading dose
4 g 10% magnesium sulfate in 250 ml D₅W solution, given IV over 15 minutes

Maintenance dose
1-3 g 10% magnesium sulfate per hour

Therapeutic serum magnesium level
4.8-8.4 mg/dl

Monitoring parameters
Cardiac monitor

Urinary output
30 ml/hr

Deep-tendon reflexes
Loss means toxicity

Cautions
Respiratory rate must be greater than 12 breaths/min.
Antidote for decreased respirations is calcium gluconate 1 g (10 ml in 10% solution) given slowly IV.

Modified from Farrell RG, editor: *OB/GYN emergencies: the first 60 minutes*, Rockville, Md, 1986, Aspen.

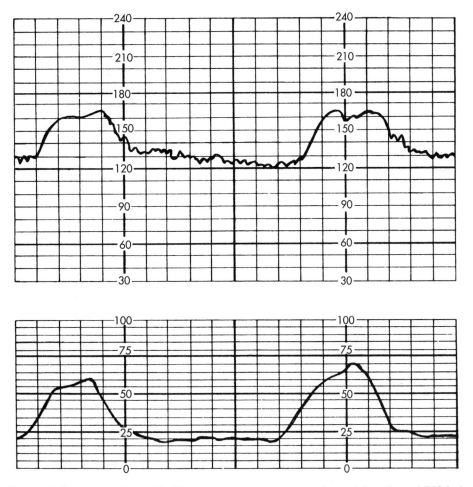

Figure **49-3** Acceleration of fetal heart rate in response to uterine activity. *(From* AJN/Mosby nursing boards review for NCLEX-RN, *ed 10, St. Louis, 1997, Mosby.)*

centa previa is caused by implantation and development of the placenta in the lower uterine segment rather than the normal implantation site in the upper uterine wall. Implanting in the lower segment of the uterus puts the placenta in the zone of effacement and dilation, which causes the placenta to partially or completely cover the internal cervical os. There are three types of placenta previa based on how much the os is covered (Figure 49-4):

- Total—the placenta completely covers the os.
- Partial—the placenta partially covers the os.
- Marginal or low implantation—the placenta is adjacent to but does not extend beyond the margin of the os.

Although total placenta previa is rare, marginal or partial placenta previa occurs in 1 of every 200 pregnancies. Seventy-five percent of cases of placenta previa occur in multiparous women. Multiparity with advancing age and a rapid succession of pregnancies are believed to be predisposing factors for placenta previa.

Hemorrhage, the first and most commonly seen sign of placenta previa, is not accompanied by contractions, so there is no associated pain. Because the cervix begins to di-

late and efface in the eighth month, maternal vessels tear when the patient is asleep. Bleeding may cease spontaneously or continue, depending on how large the torn vessels are. After two or three hemorrhages, labor usually begins. Membranes may rupture prematurely, which can lead to infection. Premature labor and an abnormal presenting part can further complicate the delivery. In total placenta previa, bleeding occurs earlier and is more profuse. Placenta previa should always be suspected when painless uterine bleeding occurs in the last half of the pregnancy.

Diagnostic studies include ultrasonography for specific determination of position of the placenta. A CBC type and crossmatch for several units of blood and clotting studies should be immediately performed. Establish a large-bore IV line, administer a crystalloid solution such as Ringer's lactate, and transfer the patient to labor and delivery for monitoring and, if indicated, immediate cesarean section. Pelvic examination is contraindicated because of potential perforation of the placenta and catastrophic hemorrhage.

Assessment of vital signs should always include assessment of fetal heart rate. If fetal heart tones are not heard, this

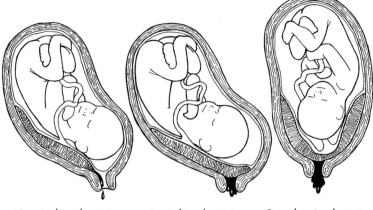

Figure **49-4** Placenta previa. *(Modified from AJN/Mosby nursing boards review for NCLEX-RN, ed 10, St. Louis, 1997, Mosby.)*

Marginal implantation   Partial implantation   Complete implantation

finding should be reported immediately. Normal fetal heart rate is 120 to 160 beats/min. Stay with the patient, and encourage her to talk. Provide necessary assistance for her husband or significant other with admitting procedures and calling family.

Abruptio Placentae

Another major complication of pregnancy in the last trimester is premature separation of the placenta from the uterus, or abruptio placentae. The primary cause is unknown, but theories include that abruptio placentae is related to PIH. Another suspected cause is increased venous pressure when the vena cava is compressed in the supine position by the gravid uterus. Contributing factors such as advanced maternal age (35 years and over), multiparity, a short cord, and trauma also play a large part. A partial separation can cause occult or frank hemorrhage. Although frank hemorrhage is always an emergency because of blood loss and the associated hypotension and hypoxia, the more dangerous of the two is occult hemorrhage.

Abruptio placentae should be considered in any woman in the third trimester who presents to the ED complaining of vaginal bleeding and abdominal pain or contractions. This is an emergency requiring immediate intervention.

Maternal assessment and assessment of vital signs and fetal heart rate are essential. At least one IV line should be started with a large-bore catheter and lactated Ringer's solution. A CBC and type and crossmatch for blood should be sent to the laboratory. Fetal monitoring is essential. The patient should be sent to labor and delivery for monitoring and, if indicated, immediate cesarean section.

DELIVERY

With decreasing access to a dwindling number of obstetricians, the probability of deliveries occurring in prehospital care settings and the ED is high. If a patient in labor arrives in the ED and time permits, a rapid obstetric examination should be performed and a brief obstetric history obtained.

An in-depth, rapid maternal assessment should be completed, and always remember that when the mother states, "The baby is coming," she is always right.

The first stage of labor is the time from onset of regular contractions until complete cervical dilation. This is generally the longest of the three stages of labor. The second stage of labor is the time from full cervical dilation until delivery of the baby. The mother may have the urge to push in this stage. The average time for stage two is 20 minutes to 1 hour. The third stage of labor is from delivery of the baby until delivery of the placenta. This stage usually lasts from 5 to 15 minutes. In cases in which the placenta fails to detach from the uterine wall, it may be necessary to manually remove the placenta.

When a woman in labor arrives at the ED, if time permits, a brief physical examination should be performed. First check fetal heart tones. Normal fetal heart tones are 120 to 160 beats/min. Prolonged bradycardia or tachycardia may indicate fetal distress. When this occurs, place the mother on her left side, and give supplemental oxygen at high flow. Arrange for immediate obstetric consultation for possible emergency delivery by cesarean section.

Once it has been determined that the fetus is well, examine the mother's abdomen. Measure the uterine height. A full-term fetus elevates the uterus to the xiphoid level. Palpate contractions as they occur. Help the mother to relax between contractions. As an emergency nurse involved in delivery, you need to remember that the mother does most of the work. Your basic role is to provide psychologic support, "coach" the mother, and ensure the infant, once delivered, is breathing adequately, has a good pulse, and is kept warm.

If crowning (Figure 49-5) is not present, perform a manual vaginal examination to determine dilation, effacement, and the station of the fetus. Use sterile technique. If fluid is present, check to see if it is amniotic fluid by determining the acidity of the fluid. Amniotic fluid is neutral, whereas normal vaginal secretions are acidic. If the test is equivocal because of the presence of blood, assume the membranes have ruptured and that amniotic fluid is present.

A rapid decision should be made as to whether delivery is imminent and the baby will be delivered in the ED or whether time permits transport to labor and delivery. If there is any indication that the mother will deliver imminently (i.e., crowning), she should be kept in the ED for delivery.

In an emergency situation, place the mother on a stretcher. Equipment for an imminent delivery should be readily available. Sterile disposable delivery kits usually have most equipment necessary for the delivery. Do not place the equipment between the mother's legs but rather on a surface beside the stretcher.

After donning appropriate attire, cover one hand with a sterile towel or a 4 × 4 inch dressing. Apply gentle pressure to the infant's head as it crowns to prevent an explosive delivery and possible tearing of the perineum. When the head is delivered, quickly suction the infant's mouth and then nose to prevent aspiration. At this point, check for the umbilical cord around the infant's neck. If the cord is loose, carefully slip it over the infant's head. If it is tight, clamp it in two places and cut the cord. Once the head is delivered and has rotated, hold it gently in both hands (Figure 49-6). Apply a gentle downward pressure to assist with delivery of the anterior shoulder and gentle upward traction to assist with delivery of the posterior shoulder. Carefully support the infant's head (Figure 49-7). Once the shoulders are delivered, delivery of the rest of the infant's body usually occurs quite rapidly (Figure 49-8).

Keep the infant in a head-dependent position at the level of the introitus to prevent aspiration. Once again, suction the mouth and nose. If spontaneous breathing or crying does not occur, gently rub the infant's back with a towel to stimulate breathing.

Clamp the umbilical cord in two places at least 6 inches from the umbilicus. The cord can be cut as soon as it is convenient, usually when the cord has stopped pulsating.

Place the infant in a warmed environment. Assess airway, breathing, and circulation. If necessary, open the infant's airway with a slight chin lift, being careful not to overextend the neck. If breathing is absent or the heart rate is less than 80 beats/min, begin resuscitation measures. A useful pneumonic, "TABS," is described in Box 49-4. For additional information on neonatal resuscitation, see Chapter 50.

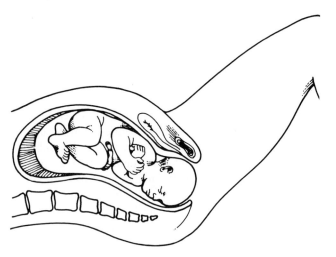

Figure **49-5**   Cross-sectional view of crowning.

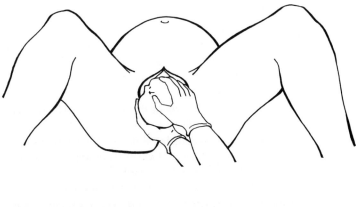

Figure **49-6**   Hold infant's head gently in both hands.

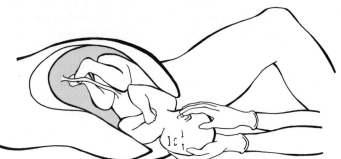

Figure **49-7**   Carefully support infant's head as it is born.

Figure **49-8** Once anterior shoulder is delivered, remainder of delivery occurs quite rapidly.

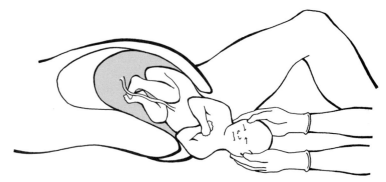

| Box **49-4** | **TABS Procedure for Newborn Resuscitation** |

T (temperature)

Dry and cover the neonate as soon as possible to prevent heat loss. Place in a heated environment as soon as possible.

A (airway)

Suction the mouth first and then the nose. A neonate with fetal distress in utero may have meconium present. Suction early, when the head is delivered, with a suction trap. If the airway cannot be cleared, the neonate should be endotracheally intubated and suctioned.

B (beats [heart rate])

If significant bradycardia is present (<80 beats/min) and does not improve with ventilation, initiate chest compressions. A brachial pulse should be palpable with compressions. Continue ventilating the neonate.

Consider pharmacologic support with drugs such as epinephrine, atropine, naloxone, dextrose, and sodium bicarbonate.

S (sugar)

A blood glucose level < 40 mg/dl is a critical level in a neonate. When glucose is given, administer a 25% solution at 0.5 g/kg (or 2 ml/kg of a 25% solution).

Determine the infant's Apgar score at delivery, then again 5 minutes after delivery (Table 49-3). The Apgar score is a system used to predict health outcomes by scoring and totaling five key factors. Each factor is scored from 0 to 2. Zero is a poor response or absence of the factor being measured, 1 indicates some response, and 2 indicates a normal finding. A total high score of 10 is possible, with 7 to 10 being considered very good. A score of 4 to 6 indicates a moderately depressed infant, and a score of 0 to 3 indicates a severely depressed infant.

After ensuring the health of the infant and its continued warmth, place the infant on the mother's abdomen and encourage the mother to breastfeed the infant. Suckling stimulates the uterus to contract. It also reassures the mother that the infant is fine and helps to keep the infant warm. Put an identification band on the infant's wrist and ankle.

After delivery of the infant, stage three labor begins. At this point, unclamp the cord and obtain laboratory specimens from the cord for determinations of hematocrit, hemoglobin level, blood type, Rh factor, and bilirubin level. Reclamp the cord, and palpate the uterus through the abdominal wall. Prepare for delivery of the placenta, usually 5 to 10 minutes after the infant is born. A sudden gush of blood occurs when the placenta separates from the uterine wall; the uterus rises into the abdomen, and the umbilical cord protruding from the vagina lengthens. Do not pull on the umbilical cord; this could cause uterine inversion.

When the placenta has separated, apply slight traction on the umbilical cord, and place your hand on the dome of the uterus, pressing downward slightly toward the suprapubic area. As the placenta enters the vaginal area, continue applying gentle traction to the umbilical cord, and carefully remove the placenta.

Unusual Deliveries

Prolapsed cord

A prolapsed umbilical cord constitutes an obstetric emergency. The umbilical cord precedes the fetus through the birth canal, becomes entrapped when the fetus passes through the birth canal, and obstructs fetal circulation (Figure 49-9).

There are three variations of this condition. The first is a situation in which uterine membranes are intact and the cord is compressed by fetal parts but is not visible externally. This variation should be suspected when there are signs of fetal distress, most prominently bradycardia.[7] This variation is actually called "cord presentation" rather than a true prolapse.

In the second variation, the cord may not be visible but can be felt in the vagina or cervix. In the third and most extreme variation, the umbilical cord actually protrudes from the vagina.

Cord compression can be determined in two ways. On examination, the cord can be felt as the presenting part. Most often, cord compression is determined when the fetus suddenly exhibits symptoms of distress identified through decreasing fetal heart beat or deceleration on the fetal monitor.

Therapeutic intervention is aimed at relieving pressure on the cord and minimizing fetal anoxia. Place the mother lying

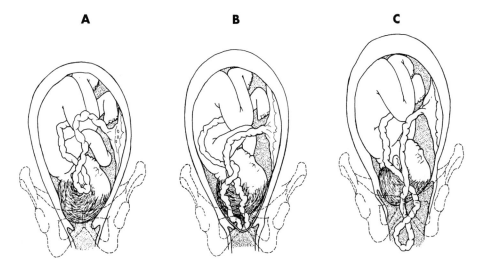

Figure **49-9** Prolapse of the umbilical cord. Note pressure of presenting part on umbilical cord, which endangers fetal circulation. **A,** Occult (hidden) prolapse of cord. **B,** Complete prolapse of cord. Note membranes are intact. **C,** Cord presenting in front of fetal head may be seen in vagina. *(Modified from Lowdermilk DL, Perry SE, Bobak IM:* Maternity and women's health care, *ed 6, St. Louis, 1997, Mosby.)*

Table **49-3** **Apgar Score**

Factor	Score		
	0	1	2
A = Appearance (color)	Blue	Blue limbs, pink body	Pink
P = Pulse (heart rate)	Absent	<100 beats/min	>100 beats/min
G = Grimace (muscle tone)	Limp	Some flexion	Good flexion
A = Activity (reflexes irritable)	Absent	Some motion	Good motion
R = Respiratory effort	Absent	Weak cry	Strong cry

on her left side. This position removes some of the pressure of the huge gravid uterus on the abdominal aorta. Administer oxygen via nonrebreather mask at 100%. If the cord is exposed, it will dry out. Place saline-moistened sterile gauze on the cord to prevent this complication. If the cervix is dilated completely, the physician may choose to rapidly deliver the baby with the use of forceps. If the cervix is not fully dilated, emergency cesarean section is performed.

Breech delivery

With breech delivery, the head, the largest fetal body part, is delivered last. A woman whose fetus is a breech presentation is often scheduled for cesarean section. Unfortunately, in the emergency setting when a woman arrives in labor with delivery imminent, even if the fetus is in a breech position, there may not be time to arrange for cesarean section. Delivery must be completed in the ED, especially if the fetus has been delivered to the level of the umbilicus.

Categories of breech presentation are (1) a complete breech, in which the fetus has both knees and hips flexed; (2) an incomplete breech, in which one or both feet or knees present first; and (3) a front breech, in which the fetus's hips are flexed and the legs extend in front of the fetus.

With any breech presentation, call for obstetric support, if possible. It is usually best to allow the fetus to deliver spontaneously to the level of the umbilicus. If the fetus is in a front breech presentation, after the buttocks are delivered, one may have to extract the legs down into the introitus. Once the umbilicus is visualized, gently extract a generous amount of umbilical cord. Rotate the fetus to align the shoulders in an anterior-posterior position. Place gentle traction on the fetus until you see the axilla. Pull upward gently on the feet to allow delivery of the posterior shoulder. Carefully extract the posterior arm. Then gently pull downward on the feet to deliver the anterior shoulder. Rotate the fetus's buttocks to the mother's front. Using a Mauriceau maneuver, rest the fetus on your arm, and place your index and middle finger in the fetus's mouth, gently flexing the head. Do not apply traction with this hand. Grasp the fetus at the base of the neck and tip of the shoulders with your other hand, and apply gentle traction. If assistance is available, have the other person apply firm, steady pressure to the top of the fundus toward the suprapubic area. The neonate should then be suctioned and the cord clamped.

Multiple fetuses

With delivery of twins or other multiple births, there are additional concerns. Often multiple birth neonates are premature or have a host of other problems. The initial and most important objective is to ensure safe delivery of all fetuses. The best advice is to take one at a time "as they come." The first may present vertex or breech. Follow the information given previously for the type of presentation seen. The second fetus usually has membranes intact. If the second fetus is in the head-first position, you may rupture the membranes and allow the mother to deliver the fetus by pushing when she has a contraction. If the second fetus is breech, the feet should be delivered, and then the membranes should be ruptured. Both neonates should be suctioned as they are delivered. Both cords should be clamped, and both neonates should receive identification bands.

Amniotic fluid embolism

Amniotic fluid embolism is a catastrophic event with maternal mortality as amniotic fluid leaks into the mother's venous circulation during labor or delivery. This "embolus," composed of squamous epithelial cells, lanugo, and vasoactive chemicals, travels to the pulmonary circulation, causing sudden, severe obstruction, followed by respiratory arrest and then cardiac arrest.

Amniotic fluid emboli are seen most commonly with placenta previa, with abruptio placentae, with precipitate labor, in the multiparous woman, and in cases of intrauterine fetal death.[5]

Initially, the mother may demonstrate profound hypotension, tachycardia, tachypnea, cyanosis, and hypoxia followed by cardiopulmonary arrest. Coagulopathies are also seen.[5]

Therapeutic intervention must be rapid and aggressive. Administer oxygen at high flow via nonrebreather mask. Consider rapid endotracheal intubation and mechanical ventilation with positive end-expiratory pressure. Crystalloid solutions and blood products should be administered. Fresh frozen plasma may be used in anticipation of coagulopathies.

POSTPARTUM EMERGENCIES
Disseminated Intravascular Coagulation

Disseminated intravascular coagulation (DIC) is characterized by acceleration and hyperactivity of clotting mechanisms in pregnancy. It is most often seen in severe cases of abruptio placentae in the form of hypofibrinogenemia, but it can also occur secondary to excessive blood loss after amniotic fluid embolus or after fetal death in utero. In this hypercoagulatory state, clotting factors are consumed before the liver has time to replace them. See Chapter 44 for additional discussion of DIC.

Postpartum Hemorrhage

Excessive bleeding in the postpartum period is an emergency. Bleeding can occur immediately after delivery, or it can be delayed for 7 to 14 days. The main causes of postpartum bleeding are subinvolution of the uterus, retained products of conception (pieces of placenta or membranes present in the uterus), and vaginal or cervical tears incurred during delivery. Postpartum hemorrhage is usually described as blood loss in excess of 1000 ml within 24 hours of delivery.

Subinvolution usually occurs 7 to 14 days after delivery, when thrombi detach from the placental sites and the sites begin to bleed. If the involutional process is not returning the gravid uterus to its nonpregnant state, bleeding may become excessive. Retention of membranes or placental fragments can also cause sudden hemorrhage because they interfere with the involutional process. The emergency nurse should also be aware of a condition known as placenta accreta. When the placenta fails to separate from the uterine wall after delivery because it has grown into the uterine muscle itself, postpartum bleeding results, and immediate surgery is indicated. Cervical tears and vaginal lacerations can also cause postpartum hemorrhage.

When assessing the patient with postpartum bleeding, survey the patient's general condition, and note the presence or absence of pain, the color of the skin, and the patient's posture, gait, motor activity, and facial expression. In obtaining a history of the present problem, the following information should be elicited:

- Quantity, character, and duration of bleeding. How does it compare with the patient's normal menstrual period? How many pads has she used? How does it compare with the number she normally requires during a period?
- Menstrual history. When was the date of her last period?
- Does she have pain? What is the nature of the pain—dull, achy, cramping, constant, or radiating? Where is the pain? How long has she had it? Was its onset gradual or sudden?
- Is there any history of trauma?
- When did she deliver? Has she ever had any infections of the reproductive system? Has she had previous episodes of bleeding?

Continued assessment should include vital signs, fundal palpation for firmness, and evaluation of vaginal bleeding. Check the pad the patient is wearing to objectively evaluate the amount of bleeding. Note the presence or absence of clots or odor. Examine and save any clots or tissue that the patient may have brought with her for laboratory examination. Note the condition of the fundus. If the fundus is boggy and relaxed, it should be massaged gently until firm.

Evaluate the patient's condition, and institute appropriate measures for stabilization. If bleeding is profuse, two IV lines with large-bore needles for warmed crystalloids and blood should be established. If respirations are labored, administer oxygen. For all patients, a CBC with sedimentation rate and a clot tube for type and crossmatch should be obtained.

While collecting data and stabilizing the patient, prepare for a vaginal examination. Explain each procedure, and reassure her of your concern for her feelings by allowing her to express them.

Postpartum bleeding generally responds to the administration of intravenous oxytocin (Pitocin), bed rest, and fundal massage. If bleeding continues, prepare the patient for operative evaluation of bleeding.

Treatment of retained products of conception includes removal of the offending piece by dilation and curettage and thorough exploration of the uterus after the patient has received general anesthesia. Suturing of vaginal lacerations can be performed in the ED. However, with the possibility of damage at the cervix, suturing is best performed after the patient has received general anesthesia. A complete pelvic examination can also be performed after anesthesia.

Postpartum Infection

Vaginal lacerations, cervical tears, episiotomy sites, placental implant sites, and retained tissue may be host sites for infection. Patients usually have fever, abdominal or pelvic pain, and occasionally foul-smelling lochia. Therapeutic intervention includes culture of drainage and treatment with antibiotics as indicated.

OTHER EMERGENCIES
Hydatidiform Mole

Hydatidiform mole, or molar pregnancy, occurs when the trophoblast villi grow very rapidly and then die. If an embryo is formed, it dies very early. As the trophoblast cells degenerate, they fill with a jellylike fluid. The cells become vesicles that look like grapes filled with fluid. It is essential to diagnosis hydatiform mole early because of the high incidence of association with choriocarcinoma, a rapidly growing carcinoma.

Hydatidiform mole occurs in 1 in 100 pregnancies. It is noticed most often in women of poor socioeconomic status with lack of protein in their diet, mothers younger than 18 years or older than 35 years, and women of Asian background.

Because the trophoblast secretes hCG and grows very rapidly, the uterus grows larger than expected for the due date. At about 16 weeks' gestation, the woman presents to the ED complaining of vaginal bleeding. She gives a history of a positive pregnancy test and enlarging uterus. Bleeding may be mixed with clear fluid as the vesicles begin to rup-

Box **49-5**

> ### NURSING DIAGNOSES ASSOCIATED WITH OBSTETRIC EMERGENCIES
>
> Fluid volume deficit related to vaginal bleeding
> Fear related to threatened loss of pregnancy
> Anxiety related to threat of premature labor
> Fetal risk related to hypoxia
> Altered tissue perfusion related to elevated pressure and vasoconstriction
> Fear related to mother's own health state and that of the fetus
> Knowledge deficit related to nutrition

ture. No fetal heart tones can be auscultated. With pelvic ultrasound, no viable fetus is found.

Intervention for hydatidiform mole is removal of the mole. The patient should be prepared for a suction and curettage. The patient and family need much emotional support. They now know this is an abnormal pregnancy and must also worry about the possibility of a tumor.

SUMMARY

The emergency nurse will use the nursing process and pertinent nursing diagnoses to assess and prioritize care for women with obstetric complaints (Box 49-5). Through this process, the emergency nurse can identify life-threatening problems and intervene quickly. The ability to do this while providing emotional support for the mother and family is the hallmark of emergency care for the obstetric patient in the ED.

REFERENCES

1. ACOG technical bulletin number 150—December 1990: Ectopic pregnancy, *Int J Gynecol Obstet* 37:213, 1992.
2. Cahill S, Balskus M, editors: *Intervention in emergency nursing: the first 60 minutes,* Rockville, Md, 1986, Aspen.
3. Farrell RG, editor: *OB GYN emergencies: the first 60 minutes,* Rockville, Md, 1986, Aspen.
4. Guyton AC, Hall GE: *Textbook of medical physiology,* Philadelphia, 1996, Saunders.
5. Jones HW, Jones GS: *Novak's textbook of gynecology,* ed 10, Baltimore, 1981, Williams & Wilkins.
6. Pillitteri A: *Maternal and child health nursing,* Philadelphia, 1992, Lippincott.
7. Scanlon VC, Sanders T: *Essentials of anatomy and physiology,* ed 2, Philadelphia, 1995, FA Davis.

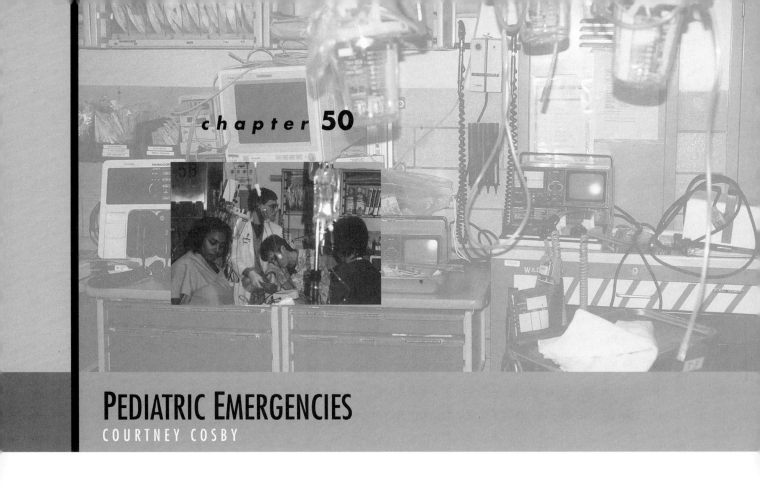

chapter 50

PEDIATRIC EMERGENCIES

COURTNEY COSBY

Sick children present unique challenges to health care professionals. Assessment and treatment of sick children are unique because children's perceptions may be radically different from those of adults. In a busy emergency department (ED), nurses may not always take the time to realize that children brought in for care are likely to be scared at the sight of strangers and the unknown "hurts" that lie ahead. Furthermore, depending on age, children may or may not be able to say what is bothering them. Patience and understanding are the key to overcoming or averting these problems.

Communicating with a child and the family is a three-way process involving the nurse, child, and parent. For the most part, information about the child is acquired by direct observation or is communicated to the nurse by parents. Usually, it can be assumed that close contact with the child makes information imparted by the parent reliable. Assessment requires input from the child (verbal and nonverbal), information from parents, and the nurse's own observations of the child and interpretation of the relationship between the child and parent. Box 50-1 outlines guidelines for communicating with children. In most cases, parents should stay with the child during all phases of the visit (Figure 50-1).

Most emergency nurses, regardless of practice area, will encounter a sick child at some stage in their career. Interaction with sick children requires patience and the ability to interpret subtle assessment clues.[9] The ability to intervene in critical situations requires a strong foundation of knowledge and assessment skills. This chapter provides an overview of pediatric assessment and common emergencies. Pediatric trauma and child abuse are discussed in Chapters 31 and 51, respectively.

TRIAGE

Pediatric patients account for approximately 25% to 35% of annual ED visits nationally.[7] Children require careful triage for rapid identification of serious illness or injury. The triage nurse must have excellent assessment, communication, and organization skills.

A sick child in the ED usually makes nurses not used to dealing with children uneasy, just as an adult with chest pain causes alarm in a pediatric nurse. Triage of a child does not require familiarity with every childhood disease, medication, and neurologic reflex or a bevy of specialized equipment. Pediatric triage does require understanding of concepts related to pediatric emergencies including the following:

- Anatomic, physiologic, and developmental differences between children and adults
- Recognition of conditions leading to pediatric arrest (hypoxia and shock) and appropriate interventions
- Dealing with parents
- "Rules" of pediatric triage

Children are difficult to evaluate compared to adults for several reasons. Children often have nonspecific symptoms, such as fever. Communication can be difficult because of limited vocabulary and verbal skills, so nurses must depend on the parent for history. A child's response to illness or in-

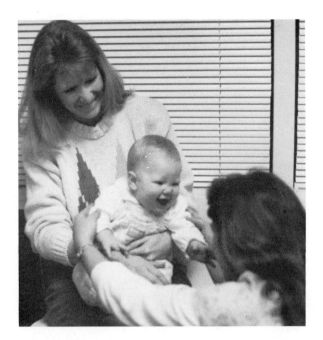

Figure **50-1** Take time to gain child's and parent's trust.

jury depends on current developmental stage. Toddlers cling to parents, whereas adolescents are independent. Children compensate for longer periods of time in the face of illness; therefore they may not be outwardly symptomatic even though they have a life-threatening condition. Normal vital signs do not always indicate a stable condition.[3]

Special Pediatric Considerations

The most important differences between children and adults lie in the respiratory and circulatory systems, that is, airway, breathing, and circulation (ABCs). Respiratory disorders are a common cause of illness in infants and children and are the third most common cause of death in the 1- to 12-year-old age-group, following cancer and congenital malformations. Respiratory distress is the preceding event in most pediatric cardiac arrests. Pediatric differences in ABCs and nursing implications are listed in Table 50-1.

"Rules" of Pediatric Triage

The following unofficial "rules" of pediatric triage may assist triage nurses in evaluating children.
1. Parents know their children better than you—listen to them. Parent history can give clues to the cause of illness or injury and help triage nurses determine urgency (Figure 50-2).
2. Remember the ABCs—children are different. Do not focus on the obvious; a subtle, more serious problem can be overlooked.
3. Some children can talk, walk, and still be in shock. You cannot always depend on appearance. Consider history and vital signs; however, normal vital signs should not give a false sense of security.

4. Never tell parents their child cannot be evaluated in the ED, no matter what the chief complaint. With the development of preferred provider and health maintenance organizations, authorization for payment may be refused. Make sure parents realize authorization for *payment* is being denied, not authorization for *care*. A triage assessment must still be performed to evaluate whether immediate care is needed before referral elsewhere.

Pediatric Triage Examination

Depending on the facility, triage examination may be brief, determining the chief complaint and looking at the child, or may include obtaining vital signs and providing treatment such as antipyretics, splinting, or ice packs. Whatever triage protocols or critical pathways exist, the most important aspect is prompt assessment with observation and history.

History is an important part of the pediatric triage assessment. With small infants, history may be vague, nonspecific, and limited by the parent's ability to communicate. Past medical history is important in determining if the child has a prior condition that may affect assessment, such as congenital heart disease or a chronic respiratory condition. Ask the parent, "What does your child normally look like?" or "Does your child look normal to you?"

Observation variables such as playfulness, eye contact, and attention to environment are also important. The triage nurse can usually observe the child while obtaining the history or performing the assessment. Observation may have to be performed as a separate part of the examination to allow the child to feel comfortable.

Observation scales and scoring systems have been developed to assist in identifying sick children. These scoring systems are general and do not apply to a specific organ system but may be a useful tool for the triage nurse. An example of an observation scoring system is shown in Table 50-2.

Pediatric primary assessment

Primary assessment consists of evaluation of ABCs and neurologic status. ABCs may be the only part of the assessment performed in triage if the child has an emergent condition. The primary survey should include assessment of level of

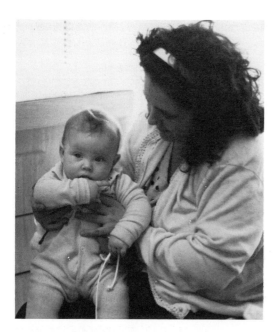

Figure **50-2** Listen to the parent's concerns and assessment of child's condition.

consciousness; respiratory effort, rate, and quality; skin color and temperature; and pulse rate and quality.

Secondary assessment

Secondary assessment consists of vital signs and head-to-toe survey. During triage, the secondary assessment is usually limited to evaluating the area of chief complaint. The rest of the examination is performed later in a treatment room. Secondary assessment is summarized in Table 50-3. When performing secondary assessment on a child, do not focus on the obvious injury. Don't be fooled by a known patient with a chronic condition. Listen to the parent's concerns. Consider child abuse in suspect circumstances. Know your responsibility in reporting possible abuse. Communicate your findings to other personnel, and document your assessment. Often parents offer information to the triage nurse and then assume they don't have to mention it again.

Vital signs

All triage systems should include vital signs in the initial assessment, including temperature, pulse rate, respiration rate, blood pressure, and weight (Figure 50-3). Weight, considered the "fifth vital sign," is necessary because all medications and fluids are based on the child's weight.

Pulse and respirations can be measured while the nurse is evaluating airway and breathing. Temperatures are easily

Table 50-1   Pediatric Differences in Airway, Breathing, and Circulation

Factor	Nursing considerations
Airway	
Large tongue	Airway easily obstructed by tongue; proper positioning is often all that is necessary to open the airway.
Smaller diameter of all airways (in a 1-year-old child, tracheal diameter is less than child's little finger)	Small amounts of mucus or swelling easily obstructs the airways; child normally has increased airway resistance.
Cartilage of larynx is softer than in adults; cricoid cartilage is narrowest portion of larynx.	Airway of infant can be compressed if neck is flexed or hyperextended; provides a natural seal for endotracheal tube; cuffed tubes are not necessary in children less than 8-10 years of age.
Breathing	
Sternum and ribs are cartilaginous; chest wall is soft; intercostal muscles are poorly developed; infants are obligate nose breathers for first 4 weeks of life; increased metabolic rate (about twice that of an adult); increased respiratory demand for oxygen consumption and carbon dioxide elimination.	Infant's chest wall may move inward instead of outward during inspiration (retractions) when lung compliance is decreased; greater intrathoracic pressure generated during inspiration; anything causing nasal obstruction can produce respiratory distress; respiratory distress increases oxygen demand, as does any condition that increases metabolic rate, i.e., fever.
Circulation	
Child's circulating blood volume is larger per unit of body weight, but absolute volume is relatively small; 70%-80% of newborn's body weight is water (compared to 50%-60% of adult body weight); about one half of this volume is extracellular.	Blood loss considered minor in an adult may lead to shock in child; decreased fluid intake or increased fluid loss quickly leads to dehydration.
Increased heart rate, decreased stroke volume; cardiac output is higher per unit of body weight.	Tachycardia is the child's most efficient method of increasing cardiac output if heart rate is greater than 180-200 beats/min.

Table 50-2 Predictive Model for Pediatric Illness

Observation item	Normal	Moderate impairment	Severe impairment
Quality of cry	Strong with normal tone; content and not crying	Whimpering or sobbing	Weak, moaning, or high-pitched
Reaction to parenteral stimulation	Cries briefly, then stops; content and not crying	Cries off and on	Continual cry or hardly responds
State variation	If awake, stays awake; if asleep and stimulated, wakes up quickly	Eyes close briefly; awake or awakes after prolonged stimulation	Falls asleep or will not rouse
Skin color	Pink	Pale extremities or acrocyanosis	Pale, cyanotic, mottled, or ashen
Hydration	Skin normal; eyes normal; mucous membranes moist	Skin normal; eyes normal; mouth slightly dry	Skin doughy or tented; dry mucous membranes; sunken eyes
Response (talk, smile) to social overtures	Smiles or alert (less than or equal to 2 months of age)	Brief smile or alert briefly (less than or equal to 2 months of age)	No smile; face anxious, dull, expressionless, no alerting (less than or equal to 2 months of age)

From McCarthy PL et al: Predictive values: observation scales to identify serious illness in febrile children, *Pediatrics* 70(5):802, 1982.

Table 50-3 Pediatric Secondary Assessment

Body area	Condition to be assessed
Head	Presence of injuries, pain, or tenderness; anterior fontanelle—depressed, flat, bulging (most infants have an open anterior fontanelle until 18 months)
Eyes	Pupil size and reaction; tears; movement of eyes; drainage or periorbital swelling; presence of injuries; visual acuity (if appropriate)
Ears	Drainage; presence of pain, bruising behind ears
Nose	Nasal flaring, odor, mucus crusting
Throat	Do not attempt to examine if child is in severe respiratory distress, swelling or exudates in pharynx; swelling of cervical lymph nodes
Mouth	Color of oral mucosa; presence of lesions; moistness of lips and mucous membranes; odor of breath
Chest	Respiratory status as indicated during primary assessment; presence of rashes or bruising
Abdomen	Distention; bowel sounds; tenderness
Genitalia and rectum	Diaper rash; vaginal discharge or irritation; odor; rectal bleeding or tears; discharge from penis; trauma
Skin, extremities, and bilateral comparison	Presence of swelling, deformity; pain; movement; sensation; color; pulse rates; presence of rashes, bruising
Vital signs	Temperature, pulse rate, respiration rate, blood pressure, weight

Table 50-4 Average Vital Signs by Age

	Pulse rate (beats/min)	Respiration rate (breaths/min)	Blood pressure (mm Hg)
Newborn	120 to 160	40 to 60	70/40
1 year	80 to 130	30 to 40	82/44
3 years	80 to 120	25 to 30	86/50
5 years	70 to 115	20 to 25	90/52
7 years	70 to 115	20 to 25	94/54
10 years	70 to 115	15 to 20	100/60
15 years	70 to 100	15 to 20	110/64

obtained, especially with availability of thermometers that measure temperature of the tympanic membrane. Tympanic measurement in infants less than 2 years may not be accurate because of anatomic considerations. Blood pressure measurements are often deferred because a cuff the right size is not available or because the child resists the procedure. The cuff must cover two thirds of the upper arm. A cuff that is too small gives a false high reading, whereas an oversized cuff gives a false low reading.

Weight can be obtained at triage or a recent value obtained from the parent. Weight is important for calculating medication doses, assessing dehydration, and comparing the child's growth and development to normal growth and development for that age group.

Vital signs vary with age (Table 50-4). Alterations from normal must be viewed along with the child's history and other signs and symptoms. Some causes of alterations in vital signs are listed in Table 50-5. Infants localize infections poorly; therefore any child less than 3 months old should be evaluated for possible bacterial infection. Infants cannot regulate body temperature effectively for several months af-

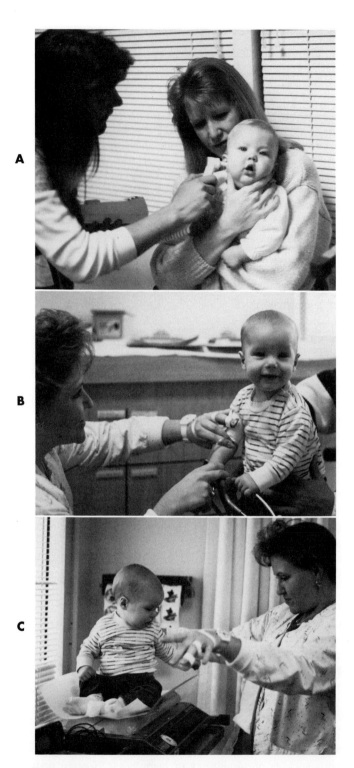

Figure **50-3** **A,** Tympanic thermometer. **B,** Blood pressure. **C,** Weight.

ter birth; therefore every attempt should be made to keep the infant warm.

RESPIRATORY EMERGENCIES

Recognition of respiratory distress and failure in the pediatric patient is crucial because respiratory arrest is almost al-

ways the precursor to cardiac arrest in children.[5] The dyspneic child is apprehensive and restless and has expiratory stridor with wheezing and intercostal and sternal retractions. Airway obstruction in children results from a myriad of causes including congenital anomalies, peritonsillar abscess, laryngeal obstruction, elevated diaphragm, cardiac failure, cystic fibrosis, drug intoxication, pneumothorax, and foreign bodies such as coins or toy parts.

Sudden onset of respiratory distress suggests foreign body obstruction or spasms. Gradual onset of respiratory distress with coughing and perhaps hemoptysis indicates pulmonary or cardiac insufficiency. Allergies and exposure to disease processes are also considerations. When the child breathes through the mouth, has heavy nasal secretions, or both, consider adenoid infection or a foreign body. Pharyngeal infections can produce dysphagia.

When a child first arrives in the ED with any respiratory problem, rapid assessment must be completed using a systematic approach with the least intrusive methods first. Observation is the simplest assessment tool, providing the nurse with vital information. Inspect the child's bare chest for structural abnormalities, symmetry of movement, and use of accessory muscles. Any movement of the head in association with respiratory effort indicates severe distress.

Assessment

Observe the child's position. A child in respiratory distress finds a position of comfort with the body leaning slightly forward and the head in the "sniffing" position, as if smelling a flower. This position allows maximum airway opening.

Respiratory rate and pattern

The young child's respiratory muscles are not well developed, so the diaphragm plays an essential role in breathing. Chest auscultation and observation of rise and fall of the abdomen are the best methods for assessing respiratory rate in patients less than 2 years old. Respiratory rates are often irregular in small children, so the rate should be carefully assessed for a full minute.

Normal respiratory rates vary by age. A neonate has a normal respiratory rate from 30 to 40 breaths/min, which slows as the child grows older. With respiratory distress, the child's respiratory rate initially increases. *A resting respiratory rate faster than 60 breaths/min is a sign of respiratory distress in a child, regardless of age.* Box 50-2 lists common causes of respiratory distress in children. As respiratory failure progresses and the child becomes more acidotic, mental status changes and respiratory rate slows. Bradypnea is therefore a serious sign in a pediatric patient. An adult respiratory rate (12 to 16 breaths/min) is an unusually slow rate for any preadolescent child.

Work of breathing

Children in respiratory distress have increased work of breathing and use of accessory muscles (intercostal, spinal extensor, and neck muscles) for breathing. As work of breathing increases, intercostal, substernal, and supraclavicular retractions are observed.

Table 50-5 Some Causes of Abnormal Vital Signs in Children

Vital sign and variation	Causes and nursing considerations
Temperature	
Hyperthermia (fever)	Viral infections (upper respiratory, gastrointestinal); bacterial infections (pneumonia, otitis media, urinary tract infections, bacteremia, meningitis, epiglottitis); collagen vascular diseases (rheumatic fever, Schönlein-Henoch purpura) drug intoxications (salicylates, atropine, amphetamines); malignancies; hyperthermia can lead to febrile seizures
Hypothermia	Sepsis; shock; exposure; infants have an unstable temperature-regulating mechanism and can become hypothermic as a result of exposure; hypothermia can lead to metabolic acidosis, decreased respiration rates, bradycardia, and cardiopulmonary arrest
Pulse rate	
Bradycardia	Most common cause is hypoxia (bradycardia equals hypoxia until proved otherwise,); other causes include hypotension, acidosis, drug ingestions (narcotics, sedatives); bradycardia in children is always an emergency condition, possibly signaling impending arrest; supplemental oxygen should always be provided immediately, as well as any other interventions to support ABCs
Tachycardia	Earliest sign of shock is supraventricular tachycardia, the most common dysrhythmia in children[2]; other common causes include anxiety, fever, ingestions (anticholinergics, tricyclic antidepressants)
Respiration rate	
Tachypnea	"Quiet" tachypnea (occurs with no other signs of respiratory distress): diabetes, ketoacidosis, poisonings, or dehydration Other causes of tachypnea: respiratory distress, fever, and congestive heart failure in the child who has congenital heart disease
Bradypnea	Respiratory failure; shock; acidosis; hypothermia; ingestions (narcotics)
Blood pressure	
Hypertension	Increased intracranial pressure; renal disease; cardiovascular disease (children with coarctation of the aorta have increased blood pressure in upper extremities, as compared with blood pressure in lower extremities); endocrinologic disorders; drugs (pressor agents, corticosteroids, amphetamines)
Hypotension	Shock (late sign); drug ingestions (tricyclic antidepressants, narcotics, clonidine)

Box 50-2 Causes of Respiratory Distress in Children

Upper airway
Croup
Epiglottitis
Foreign body aspiration
Other infections (bacterial tracheitis, retropharyngeal abscesses)
Congenital anomalies

Lower airway
Asthma
Bronchiolitis
Pneumonia
Foreign body
Trauma

Inspiration is an active process in which muscles expand the chest. Exhalation is passive, relying on elasticity of the lungs and chest wall. Under normal circumstances, these two processes are balanced; expiration takes roughly the same amount of time as inspiration (inspiration/expiration ratio 1:1). When air passages are narrowed by inflammation or obstruction, time required for inhalation may remain the same with an increase in effort; however, exhalation takes substantially longer than inspiration (inspiration/expiration ratio 1:2 or 1:3).

Alertness, willingness to play, and consolability are important observations in assessing mental status with children. Irritability is often a sign of hypoxia; however, a restless child who becomes progressively quieter should be carefully assessed to make certain improved oxygenation rather than respiratory failure or exhaustion is causing restlessness to abate.

Quality of breathing

Quality of breathing includes depth and sound of breathing. A child's chest should expand symmetrically; therefore asymmetry or inadequate expansion indicates serious problems such as pneumothorax or hemothorax, foreign body obstruction, or flail chest. To auscultate a child's chest, place the stethoscope at the anterior axillary line on the level of the second intercostal space on either side. This helps identify the location of any abnormal breath sounds. The small size of the child's chest and thinness of the chest wall allow sounds on one side of the chest to resonate throughout the thorax (and even into the abdomen); therefore listening to the anterior and posterior aspects of the

Table 50-6 Abnormal Breath Sounds and Their Significance in Children*

Breath sounds	Significance
Stridor, inspiratory crowing sound	Caused by upper airway obstruction; high-pitched in croup and foreign body aspiration, low-pitched and muffled in epiglottitis
Wheezing, usually inspiratory but may be expiratory	Caused by lower airway obstruction; bilateral wheezing suggests asthma or bronchiolitis; unilateral wheezing suggests foreign body aspiration
Decreased or unequal breath sounds	Airway obstruction, pneumothorax, pleural effusion, pneumonia
Grunting	Caused by early closure of the glottis during exhalation with active chest wall contraction; increases expiratory airway pressure, preventing airway collapse; creates positive end expiratory pressure (PEEP); seen in diseases with diminished lung compliance such as pulmonary edema; also occurs as a result of pain

From American Academy of Pediatrics and American College of Emergency Physicians: *Advanced pediatric life support*, Elk Grove Village, Ill, and Dallas, 1989, The Academy and College.

*Breath sounds should be assessed over the lateral chest wall and over the anterior chest. Breath sounds heard only over the anterior chest may be misleading, because the child's thin chest wall allows transmission of central airway breath sounds.

chest may not be as useful for pediatric assessment as it is for an adult.

Breath sounds

Various pulmonary abnormalities produce adventitious sounds that are not normally heard over the chest. Crackles result from passage of air through moisture or fluid. Wheezes are produced as air passes through airways narrowed by exudate, inflammation, spasm, or tumor. Other abnormal breath sounds include rales and rhonchi. Table 50-6 lists abnormal breath sounds and their possible significance.

Monitoring

The child with a respiratory problem should be monitored carefully for changes in level of consciousness, work of breathing, and level of fatigue. Respiratory rate monitors should be used when available.

Arterial blood gas (ABG) analysis gives the clearest picture of the respiratory status of a patient. For pediatric patients, ABG values must be carefully considered because additional stress brought on by the procedure is likely to cause further deterioration in patient condition.[5]

Pulse oximetry is a useful, noninvasive means of continuously measuring oxygen saturation. Oxygen saturation correlates well with ABG measurement of this variable (Figure 50-4). Oxygen saturation of 90% to 93% is the lowest acceptable range in children. Pulse oximetry's major limitation is that carbon dioxide and acid-base balance are not evaluated. Pulse oximetry relies on analysis of hemoglobin color and may not be useful when extremity perfusion is diminished from trauma, cold ambient temperature, or vasopressors or when the number of erythocytes is decreased, as in anemia.

A   **B**

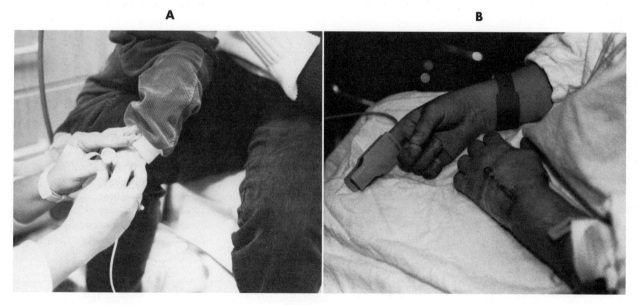

Figure **50-4** Use of pulse oximeter can help determine degree of respiratory distress. Different probes are available. **A,** For infants, finger or toe probes. **B,** For older, more cooperative children, finger probe.

Bronchiolitis

Bronchiolitis is a viral infection commonly found in infants less than 18 months of age and can be a life-threatening illness. The most common causative organism of bronchiolitis is the respiratory syncytial virus. An inflammatory process causes edema in the bronchial mucosa with resultant expiratory obstruction and air trapping. Bronchiolitis has a broad spectrum of severity. Determination of when dyspnea began helps predict the course of the illness because the critical period of bronchiolitis usually occurs during the first 24 to 72 hours after onset of dyspnea. History typically includes symptoms of a cold, cough, and coryza for a few days before the onset of dyspnea. Bronchiolitis is often difficult to differentiate from bronchial asthma; therefore careful evaluation should be made in the ED including oxygen saturation, ABGs, complete blood count (CBC), and cultures from the nasopharynx. Chest radiograph may demonstrate air trapping. Hospitalization is necessary for infants less than 2 months old and those with an apneic episode.

Aerosolized bronchodilators provide symptomatic relief of wheezing in these infants. Albuterol is the drug of choice, although isoetharine is still occasionally used.

Asthma

Asthma, a recurrent reactive airway disease, affects 5% of all American children.[8] Wheezing, the most obvious sign of asthma, may range from mild to severe and is accompanied by tachycardia, chest retractions, and anxiety. Expiration may be prolonged because of narrowed airways. Obtaining a thorough history may be useful in trying to determine the cause and severity of the attack. Repeated asthma attacks are a dangerous sign because of increasing fatigue and potential complications. Recent hospitalization is likely to be an indication of a seriously ill child.

When assessing a child with asthma, evaluate respiratory rate, quality, and effort to determine the degree of respiratory distress. The child may require supplemental oxygen if saturation on room air is less than 95% and tachypnea and tachycardia are present.

Treatment of a child in the ED with moderate to severe distress involves inhaled β-adrenergic agents with oxygen (Table 50-7). Nebulized albuterol treatments are usually given every 20 minutes for three doses. Terbutaline nebulized with normal saline solution is frequently used when the child does not respond to albuterol treatments. Subcutaneous epinephrine is reserved for severe attacks. Use of intravenous

---

Table 50-7 Medications Used for Asthma

Medication	Dosage	Age dosage	Method	Comments
Albuterol 5% solution	0.01-0.03 ml/kg in 2 ml NS (0.5-0.15 mg/kg); maximum 0.5 ml (2.5 mg)	<2 yr, 0.15-0.3 ml; 2-5 yr, 0.3-0.4 ml; 5-10 yr, 0.4 ml	Nebulizer	Peak onset 30-60 min; duration 4-6 hr
Aminophylline				
Epinephrine 1:1000 solution	0.01 ml/kg; maximum 0.35 ml		Subcutaneous	May cause tremors, restlessness, tachycardia
Hydrocortisone	4 mg/kg		IV	
Isoproterenol, 0.2 mg/ml	0.5-5.0 mg/min; 5 ml (1 mg) in 250 ml NS	0.1 mg/kg/min	IV infusion	
Ipratropium bromide	Pediatric dose not established; 2 puffs 4 times daily	Pediatric dose not established	Nebulizer	Peak onset 1-2 hr; duration 3-4 hr
Isoetharine	0.3 ml/kg up to 0.5 ml (0.03 mg/kg); dilute in 2 ml NS		Nebulizer	Peak onset 15-30 min; duration 2-4 hr; contains sulfites
Methylprednisolone	1-2 mg/kg/dose every 6 hr		IV	
Metaproterenol 5% solution (50 mg/ml)	0.01 ml/kg (0.5 mg/kg) in 2.5 ml NS; maximum 0.4 ml/dose	<3 yr, 0.1 ml; 3-7 yr, 0.2 ml; >7 yr, 0.3 ml	Nebulizer	Peak onset 30-60 min; duration 4-6 hr
Epinephrine (Sus-Phrine), 5 mg/ml	0.005 ml/kg; maximum 0.015 ml/kg	1 mo-12 yr, 0.005 ml/kg	Subcutaneous	May cause tremor, restlessness, tachycardia
Terbutaline 0.1% solution	0.03-0.5 ml/kg (0.03-0.05 mg/kg); dilute in 2 ml NS	<2 yr, 0.15-0.2 ml; 2-5 yr, 0.3 ml; 5-10 yr, 0.5 ml	Nebulizer	Peak onset 30 min; duration 3-4 hr
Aminophylline	0.9 mg/kg/hr (adjusted by blood level)	Child, 1.1 mg/kg/hr; adolescent, 0.9 mg/kg/hr	IV	Toxicity: nausea, vomiting, tachycardia, seizures

NS, Normal saline solution.

aminophylline has declined because of belief that the drug is not as effective in patients treated with β-agonists. Concerns over increased mortality related to β-agonists have increased the use of glucocorticoids. Another factor contributing to steroid management is understanding of the inflammatory process of asthma.[8]

Good hydration for children with asthma is important. They are prone to fluid loss during hyperventilation. Intravenous fluids may be necessary in some patients.

Croup

Croup, or laryngotracheobronchitis, is viral inflammation of the subglottic area, including the trachea and bronchi. Croup occurs most frequently in infants and children 6 months to 3 years of age but may occur in older children. It is slightly more prevalent in boys. Croup is seen most frequently in cooler months.

The inflammatory process of viral croup produces edema of the trachea and surrounding structures. Edematous airways secrete tenacious mucus, which leads to problematic removal of secretions. The child's effort to inspire air through edematous structures produces characteristic stridor.

History usually includes an upper respiratory infection for a few days followed by nocturnal onset of the characteristic barking cough. The child may have a hoarse voice or cry. Nursing assessment should be performed carefully to keep the child calm. The stress of crying increases the work of breathing, so both stridor and retractions markedly increase. Assessment should focus on cardiorespiratory status, hydration, anxiety, or fatigue level as well as parental anxiety.

Nursing interventions in croup focus on relieving anxiety and reducing work of breathing. Cool humidified oxygen should be provided in a manner comfortable for the child. Many times this is done with the child sitting on the parent's lap, where humidified oxygen is delivered close to the nose and mouth. Most anxious children become more anxious if forced to wear a face mask. Racemic epinephrine is used in severe cases to reduce mucosal edema and laryngospasm. Steroids are used with severe cases, usually methylprednisolone sodium succinate or dexamethasone. Cross-table soft tissue radiograph of the neck may be used to rule out epiglottitis.

Croup responds well to mist treatments, and children may improve sufficiently to be able to go home. The decision for hospital admission rests on the degree of respiratory distress, ability to maintain adequate hydration, ability to rest, and degree of parental apprehension. When a child with croup is discharged, parents should be provided instructions for home care of croup including use of a cool mist vaporizer, keeping windows open at night, fever control, and offering frequent cool fluids. Parents often require considerable reassurance. Table 50-8 shows some of the differences between croup and epiglottitis (supraglottitis) and identifies emergent treatment of both.

Epiglottitis

Epiglottitis, or supraglottic laryngitis, is the most emergent acute airway obstruction of childhood. This disease produces rapid onset of inflammatory edema of the epiglottis. Epiglottitis occurs throughout the year, is seen in boys and girls with equal frequency, and usually affects children aged 2 to 5 years. However, the advent of *Haemophilus influenzae* type B vaccine has led to an increase in older children.[8]

A child with epiglottitis typically presents in an anxious state, with respiratory distress, drooling because of difficulty swallowing, and sitting forward with the neck extended. The child may have audible respiratory sounds and generally appears flushed and toxic with a high temperature. The epiglottis becomes swollen and cherry red, and it can cause total airway obstruction if manipulated during examination. Many children with acute epiglottitis require intubation, cricothyroidotomy, or tracheostomy. Therefore necessary

Table **50-8**	**Comparison of Epiglottitis and Croup**	
	Epiglottitis (supraglottitis)	Laryngotracheitis (croup)
Age	1 to 6 years	6 months to 3 years
Onset	Rapid	Preceded by several days of upper respiratory infection, cough, or both
Usual cause	Bacteria, i.e., *Haemophilus influenzae*	Parainfluenza or other virus
Fever	>39.4° C (103° F)	Varies; often low grade
Clinical assessment	Appears ill; dyspnea, drooling, dysphagia	Upper respiratory infection, barking cough, stridor
Complications	Asphyxia caused by inflammation and obstruction in *supraglottic* area	Asphyxia caused by inflammation and obstruction in *subglottic* area
Field treatment	Oxygen; rapid transport to health care facility	Oxygen; rapid transport to health care facility
ED treatment	Calm environment; oxygen; defer IV line; prepare resuscitation equipment; possible need for ventilatory support with bag-valve-mask device, intubation, or surgical airway	Varies with severity; oxygen, mist treatment, epinephrine, racemic epinephrine; hospitalization if severe, if racemic ephinephrine is given, or if caretakers are unable to treat patient at home

equipment should be on hand and ready before an examination is done.

Once epiglottitis is suspected, keep the child calm and quiet. The primary focus is to maintain a patent airway. If the child is quiet in the parent's lap, let the child stay there during a brief assessment. A lateral soft tissue radiograph of the neck is taken if the patient is stable, to identify the swollen epiglottis.

Most patients with severe respiratory distress from supraglottitis go directly to the operating room for intubation or tracheostomy. Oxygenation is provided as passively as possible to prevent agitation and increased edema of the epiglottis. Hospital admission is always necessary for known or suspected epiglottitis. Intravenous fluids are necessary until oral fluids can be swallowed. The preferred route for antibiotics is intravenous.

Peritonsillar and Retropharyngeal Abscess

Other diseases with signs and symptoms similar to supraglottitis include peritonsillar abscess and retropharyngeal abscess. Peritonsillar abscess on rare occasions can compromise the child's airway. Retropharyngeal abscess has a less abrupt onset than supraglottitis but also poses substantial risk to airway patency. A child with peritonsillar or retropharyngeal abscess needs attention to and support of respiratory and circulatory function. Retropharyngeal abscesses require drainage in the operating room, whereas peritonsillar abscess may sometimes be drained in the ED if there is danger of airway compromise. Both conditions are treated with intravenous antibiotics.

Pneumonia

Pneumonia is inflammation of the pulmonary parenchyma. It is common throughout childhood but occurs more frequently in infancy and early childhood. Clinically, pneumonia may occur as a primary disease or complication of other illnesses. A majority of pneumonias in children are caused by viruses, although bacterial pneumonia, usually caused by group B streptococci and gram-negative bacilli, is more likely to occur in the first weeks of life. Whether viral or bacterial, pathogens reach the lung and cause an inflammatory response that leads to accumulation of fluid in the lungs, tachypnea, cough, and fever. Bacterial pneumonia tends to have abrupt onset with high fever, 38.5° to 41° C (101.3° to 105.8° F). In viral pneumonia, fever is usually less than 39° C (102.2° F). With bacterial pneumonia, there is an increase in the number of granulocytes and bands on the white cell differential count.

Treatment varies with the child's age, suspected causative agent, severity of symptoms, and immune status of the child. Infants younger than 2 months old usually require hospitalization for intravenous antibiotic treatment. Children with minimum distress who are tolerating oral fluids well can usually be treated at home with oral antibiotic therapy. Aerosolized bronchodilators may be helpful at any age.

Foreign Body Airway Obstruction

Small children spend a good deal of time exploring their world. Small objects hold a special fascination for children and are likely to end up in their mouths. Foreign body aspiration can occur at any age but is most commonly seen in children under 3 years old. A child brought to the ED with sudden onset of respiratory distress should be evaluated for foreign body aspiration if no other cause is apparent. Initially, a foreign body obstruction produces choking, gagging, wheezing, or coughing. Once the object is lodged in the larynx, the child cannot speak or breathe. After the initial period, there may be an interval of hours, days, or even weeks without symptoms. Secondary symptoms relate to the anatomic area in which the object is lodged and are usually caused by a persistent respiratory infection.

Foreign body obstruction that completely occludes the airway is an acute emergency. Initial treatment is immediate removal of the object using age-appropriate maneuvers, that is, finger sweeps and chest or abdominal thrusts. If these maneuvers fail, forceps may be used to remove the foreign body. Immediate tracheostomy must be performed to open the airway if the airway remains obstructed. Cardiopulmonary resuscitation must be initiated if the child is not breathing and has no heartbeat.

If ventilation appears adequate, allow the child to assume whatever position is most comfortable. Unless the object is observed high in the upper airway, its exact location must be determined by radiograph. Bronchoscopy may be necessary for removal. A swallowed object is allowed to pass normally through the gastrointestinal tract, unless it is long and sharp. The danger of intestinal perforation is significant. Nickel-cadmium batteries must be removed because of the danger of toxic leakage.

Carbon Monoxide Poisoning

Carbon monoxide (CO) is a colorless, odorless gas resulting from incomplete burning of organic substances, such as gasoline, coal products, tobacco, and building materials. CO causes injury and death by interfering with or inhibiting cellular respiration. When CO enters the bloodstream, it readily combines with hemoglobin to form carboxyhemoglobin, but it is released less easily. Tissue hypoxia can reach dangerous levels before oxygen is available to meet tissue needs.

Accidental poisoning is often the result of fumes from heaters or smoke from structural fires. Signs and symptoms of CO poisoning are the result of tissue hypoxia. Severity varies with the level of carboxyhemoglobin. Mild manifestations produce irritability, headache, visual disturbances, and nausea, whereas more severe cases cause confusion, hallucinations, ataxia, and coma. Bright, cherry-red lips and skin, described as classic signs of poisoning, occur less often then pallor and cyanosis.

Primary treatment is administration of 100% oxygen with a nonrebreather mask or bag-valve mask. Efforts should be made to reduce the child's metabolic demand for oxygen by keeping the child quiet and calm. Severe cases may require intubation or hyperbaric oxygen therapy. Children with suspected or known inhalation of CO are admitted for close observation and oxygen therapy. Because CO has a half-life of approximately 2 hours, oxygen therapy is needed for a prolonged period.

Pertussis

Pertussis, or whooping cough, is an acute respiratory infection caused by *Bordetella pertussis.* Whooping cough usually occurs in children younger than 4 years who have not been immunized. Highly contagious, whooping cough is particularly threatening to young infants, in whom there are higher morbidity and mortality rates. Incidence is highest in the spring and summer.

Pertussis is usually indistinguishable from a common cold until the paroxysmal stage. During this stage, the child has a fever, hypoxia, and cough. Petechiae above the nipple line, otitis media, atelectasis, pneumothorax, and vomiting may also be present. Hernias may appear suddenly as a result of exertion during coughing.

Excitement and crying tend to worsen the coughing paroxysms, so care should be taken to keep the child as calm as possible. Airway clearance is important in management of pertussis and may require gentle suctioning. Humidified oxygen should be used. The child should be isolated from other patients. Caregivers should utilize universal precautions, wear masks, and handle secretions carefully. Antibiotic therapy should be initiated as soon as possible. Hospitalization is recommended for those infants who exhibited respiratory distress in association with the coughing paroxysms. Infants may also require intravenous fluids for dehydration secondary to inability to feed caused by coughing.[8]

Pneumothorax

A pneumothorax is collection of air in the pleural space caused by rupture of an alveolar bleb on the surface of the pleura that results in partial collapse of one or both lungs. A pneumothorax may occur spontaneously or secondary to obstruction, trauma, cancer, or tuberculosis. A history of a previous pneumothorax increases the likelihood of recurrence.

Symptoms depend on how much air escapes into the pleural space. Small amounts may be asymptomatic. A large amount of air prevents full expansion of the affected lung, which causes tachypnea, dyspnea, grunting, hypoxia, and cyanosis. Contrary to most respiratory problems, which cause retraction of the chest wall musculature, a pneumothorax may cause bulging of these muscles, especially intercostal muscles over the affected area. Bilateral breath sounds are usually heard in infants and small children.

Hospital admission is almost always recommended. Oxygen administration and bed rest are used in mild cases. Children with more than 40% pneumothorax usually require a chest tube with closed drainage to evacuate air from the pleural space and reexpand the lung. The child must be continually assessed for development of tension pneumothorax, a life-threatening problem.

CARDIOVASCULAR EMERGENCIES

Causes of cardiovascular emergencies in the pediatric age-group differ from those in adults, but the three basic categories of cardiovascular compromise are the same: inadequate heart function, inadequate volume for circulation, and problems of fluid distribution. Table 50-9 summarizes common causes of cardiovascular emergencies in children.

Most pediatric cardiac arrests are related to respiratory arrest rather than primary cardiac arrest. Support the child's respiratory efforts and intervene early to prevent potential cardiac problems.

Cardiovascular Assessment

Blood volume in a child is 80 ml/kg, with total blood volume much less than in an adult. Loss of 1 cup of blood in a 10-kg child is equivalent to blood loss of 1 quart in an adult. With infants and children, immaturity of the sympathetic innervation of the ventricles keeps stroke volume at a relatively fixed rate. A child responds to the need for increased cardiac output with tachycardia. Tachycardia may initially increase cardiac output during periods of distress; however, prolonged tachycardia more than 200 beats/min for infants and 170 beats/min for children causes decompensation and decreased cardiac output. Close attention to heart rate, skin signs, and mental status is the key to early recognition of "compensated" shock. Capillary refill time is also recommended as a sensitive indicator of perfusion in the pediatric patient. Use of this parameter has not been studied extensively; however, normal capillary refill time is considered to be about 2 seconds. More than 3 seconds may indicate poor perfusion in a normothermic child.

Cardiovascular assessment should identify shock or conditions leading to shock that require the emergency nurse to in-

Table **50-9**	**Causes of Cardiovascular Collapse in Children**
Problem	Etiology
Inadequate heart function	Cardiac dysrhythmia
	Congestive heart failure
	Congenital heart disease
Inadequate volume	Dehydration
	Burns
	Trauma
Maldistribution of fluid	Septic shock
	Anaphylaxis
	Drug ingestion
	Sickle cell disease

tervene. A history of illness or injury is important in interpreting signs and symptoms. Observing the child plays a major role. Important elements to assess include the following:

- *Color of the child.* Pallor may indicate decreased perfusion caused by diminished cardiac output.
- *Capillary refill.* A delay of 3 seconds or more is abnormal.
- *Level of consciousness.* Decreased perfusion to the brain may cause lethargy and confusion.
- *Skin turgor.* Check mucous membranes for moistness.
- *Anterior fontanelle.* A bulging fontanelle may indicate increased intracranial pressure, whereas a sunken fontanelle suggests dehydration.
- *Peripheral pulse rates.* Decreased perfusion to extremities results in weak peripheral pulse(s).
- *Vital signs.* Temperature, pulse rate, respiration rate, and blood pressure. Average vital signs for the pediatric patient are listed in Table 50-4.

Vital signs should be documented as part of the baseline assessment. Children in early shock may have a normal blood pressure reading initially because of their ability to compensate. A dropping blood pressure is a serious sign warranting immediate intervention. A child can lose a significant amount of blood before the blood pressure decreases.[3] Table 50-4 lists average blood pressures by age. Another method of estimating normal blood pressure is to use the following formula:

$$\text{Systolic pressure} = 80 + (\text{age in years} \times 2)$$

Inadequate Heart Function
Rhythm disturbances

Children have young, strong hearts, so rhythm disturbances are seldom primary events. Dysrhythmias usually result from hypoxia or metabolic disturbances. Pediatric patients with rhythm disturbances from congenital cardiac problems are seen with increasing frequency in the ED, probably because of increased survival rates. The most common congenital problems causing rhythm disturbances are

Table 50-10   Rhythm Disturbances in Children

Rhythm	Cause	Characteristics	Treatment
Fast rhythms			
Sinus tachycardia	Fever, anxiety, pain, hypovolemia	Rapid sinus rhythm; rate 140-220 beats/min	Treat underlying cause
Supraventricular tachycardia	Reentry mechanism	Paroxysmal sinus rhythm; P waves often undetectable; rate ≤230 beats/min	*Unstable:* cardioversion, 0.2-1.0 J/kg; *persistent:* cardioversion, 2.0 J/kg; *stable:* vagal maneuvers Adenosine, 0.05-0.1 mg/kg rapid IV infusion; maximum dose 2 mg
Ventricular tachycardia	Structural disease, hypoxia, acidosis, electrolyte imbalance, toxic ingestion	Rate ≤120 beats/min; wide QRS; no P waves	Oxygen If unstable, synchronized cardioversion, 0.5-1.0 J/kg Lidocaine IV bolus, 1 mg/kg, followed by lidocaine infusion, 20-50 mg/kg/min
Slow rhythms			
Sinus bradycardia	Hypoxemia, hypotension, shock	Sinus rhythm; slow rate (<80 beats/min in infants, <60 beats/min in children)	Ventilation, oxygenation, cardiopulmonary resuscitation Epinephrine (1:10,000), 0.01 mg/kg IV/IO Atropine, 0.02 mg/kg; minimum dose 0.1 mg
Junctional rhythm, heart blocks	Hypoxemia, hypotension, acidosis	Rare in children; slow rate; P waves may or may not be present	Ventilation, oxygenation, CPR Atropine, 0.02 mg/kg; minimum dose 0.1 mg Epinephrine (1:10,000), 0.1 ml/kg
Absent/disorganized/nonperfusing rhythms			
Asystole	Hypoxia, hypovolemia, acidosis	Flat line on ECG; absent pulse; absent respirations	CPR, ALS procedures
Ventricular fibrillation	Rare in infants and children; hypoxia, acidosis	No identifiable P, QRS, or T waves; wavy line on ECG	CPR, ALS procedures (defibrillate 2 J/kg, then 4 J/kg)
Pulseless electrical activity	Hypoxia, acidosis, tension pneumothorax, hypovolemia	Pulselessness, with organized electrical activity on ECG	CPR; treat underlying cause

CPR, Cardiopulmonary resuscitation; *ECG*, electrocardiogram; *ALS*, advanced life support.

transposition of the great vessels and congenital mitral stenosis. Acquired cardiac diseases such as cardiomyopathies, rheumatic heart disease, and viral myocarditis may also cause rhythm disturbances.

Abnormal rhythms in this age-group are divided into three categories: fast, slow, and absent (Table 50-10). Absent rhythms are disorganized or nonperfusing rhythms. Sinus tachycardia and supraventricular tachycardia are two major rhythm disturbances found in children. Sinus tachycardia in children is a rate of 140 to 220 beats/min, whereas supraventricular tachycardia is usually higher than 220 beats/min. Bradycardia is an ominous sign in a pediatric patient. Sinus bradycardia is frequently caused by hypoxia and should be treated aggressively with ventilation and oxygenation. An infant with a rate less than 80 beats/min requires immediate cardiac compressions. Junctional and idioventricular rhythms are usually terminal rhythms. Absent, disorganized, and nonperfusing rhythms require cardiopulmonary resuscitation and advanced life support procedures.

Congestive heart failure

Congenital heart disease accounts for the majority of children seen in the ED with congestive heart failure (CHF), Preload, afterload, and myocardial contractility are major factors in determining the amount of blood pumped through the circulatory system. When the heart is not able to pump effectively because of chronic disease, rhythm disturbance, pressure on the heart, or excessive fluid volume, fluid backs up in the system, causing signs of overload such as pulmonary edema, jugular vein distention, and enlarged liver.

Signs of CHF include tachycardia, tachypnea, cough, wheezes, cyanosis, pallor, poor appetite, and failure to thrive. Many times infants with CHF have a very rapid respiratory rate (60-100 breaths per minute) but do not appear in distress. Lack of distress is evidence of the infant's ability to compensate. Observe for presence and degree of other indicators of respiratory effort such as nasal flaring, intercostal retractions, head bobbing, and expiratory grunting.

Primary treatment of CHF is aimed at decreasing heart rate while improving myocardial contractility with digoxin and reducing preload with diuretics. Furosemide (Lasix), 1 mg/kg, is usually the first medication given. If dyspnea is present, the child may benefit from cool, humidified oxygen. Hospitalization is required to determine the cause of CHF and develop a treatment plan with the family.

Inadequate Volume

The major medical cause of hypovolemia in children is dehydration. A child who has been sick for even a short time with vomiting and diarrhea is at risk, as is a child who has been ill for several days with fever and decreased fluid intake. When output exceeds intake over a period of time, dehydration becomes clinically significant and electrolyte imbalances occur. Electrolyte disturbances cause more nausea and vomiting, starting a downward spiral that can be reversed only with medical intervention. A dehydrated child looks sick, with sunken eyes, pale skin, and lethargy. When

5% or more of the child's body mass (weight) is lost, skin and mucous membranes appear dry. It is often helpful to ask the parent about intake and output, that is, the number of bottles the child has taken and the number of stools or wet diapers per day for small children. Unless fluid volume is replaced and balance between intake and output restored, the condition will progress to hypovolemic shock.

Heart rate, skin signs, and capillary refill provide the most useful information about the child's cardiovascular status. If the patient shows signs of shock, ensure adequate ventilation and oxygenation, and then give 20 ml/kg of normal saline solution, repeated until improvement is seen.[1] If vascular access cannot be obtained, intraosseous access should be obtained in children 6 years of age and younger. Intraosseous vascular access is a quick, safe, and dependable route for administering fluids, medications, and blood products.

Diagnostic tests, usually CBC, electrolytes, glucose, blood urea nitrogen (BUN), and urinalysis, are needed to assess hydration status, guide treatment, and determine the cause of the dehydration. Patients requiring admission are those who are more than 5% to 10% dehydrated as evidenced by weight loss, dry mucous membranes, tachycardia, oliguria, urine specific gravity greater than 1.030, and elevated BUN or those who are unable to retain oral fluids. Patients who are only slightly dehydrated with laboratory results within normal limits are discharged with home care instructions unless there are other reasons for admission.

Septic shock

Sepsis, or septicemia, is a profound, life-threatening bacterial infection in the bloodstream. Septic shock occurs in patients with septicemia when inadequate tissue perfusion occurs as a result of vasodilation. The ABCs should be rapidly assessed and supported. The nurse must keep in mind that hypotension is a late sign of shock in infants and young children. When present, it indicates severe shock. The skin is often cool, especially the extremities, but can also be warm and pink because of early vasodilation. Capillary refill time may be delayed longer than 2 seconds. Skin should be inspected for petechia or purpura, jaundice, pallor, cyanosis, or mottling.

Management in the ED focuses on preservation of vital functions. Adequate ventilation and oxygenation are the first priority. Administer oxygen and assist with breathing if ventilation is inadequate. Institute nursing interventions to decrease oxygen demand, that is, thermoregulation, alleviation of pain, and reassurance. Allow the parent to remain with the child as much as possible. Diagnostic studies include blood culture, CBC with white cell differential, chest radiograph, and urinalysis.

Isotonic crystalloids such as normal saline are usually given for volume replacement. An indwelling urinary catheter is inserted to monitor urinary output. Once the diagnosis of sepsis or septic shock is made, intravenous antibiotic therapy should be instituted immediately. The antibiotics administered vary with the child's age and the presumed source of infection. Once culture results are available, antibiotic therapy can be more specific. Severe metabolic acidosis should be corrected with sodium bicarbonate (0.5-1.0 mg/kg). Sympathomimetic and inotropic drugs such as epinephrine (0.05-0.15 mg/kg/min) and dopamine (2-5 mg/kg/min) may be used to increase heart rate and cardiac output in patients with poor myocardial function and systemic perfusion despite adequate oxygenation and fluid resuscitation. Serum glucose should be carefully monitored. In younger infants and children, there are limited glycogen stores in the liver, so the child is at risk for hypoglycemia. The child is admitted, usually to the intensive care unit for continued intravenous antibiotics and monitoring.

Anaphylaxis

Anaphylaxis is an acute clinical syndrome resulting from the interaction of an allergen with a patient who is hypersensitive. Severe reactions are immediate, often life-threatening, and frequently involve multiple systems. Skin flushing and urticaria are common early signs, followed by angioedema, most notable in the eyelids, lips, and tongue. Bronchiolar constriction may follow significant narrowing of the airway.

Recovery from anaphylactic reactions depends on rapid recognition and institution of treatment. The goal of treatment is to provide ventilation, restore adequate circulation, and prevent further exposure by identifying and removing the cause. A mild reaction with no evidence of respiratory distress is managed with subcutaneous epinephrine, H_2 blockers, and antihistamines. Moderate or severe distress represents a potentially life-threatening emergency. Establishing an airway is the first concern. Epinephrine is given subcutaneously or intravenously as an antihistamine to support the cardiovascular system and increase blood pressure. Fluids are given to restore blood volume. Children with severe anaphylaxis should be hospitalized and monitored for at least 24 hours.

Sickle cell disease

Sickle cell disease is a hereditary blood disorder found mostly in the black population. Sickled hemoglobin molecules are produced, causing irregularly shaped red blood cells. Sickle cells clump together, occluding small blood vessels, causing tissue ischemia.

There are three major categories of sickle cell crisis. *Vasoocclusive crisis* occurs when small vessels in bone, soft tissue, and organs (i.e., liver, spleen, brain, lungs, penis) are occluded, which leads to ischemia, pain, and swelling. The first presentation of vasoocclusive crisis, usually after 2 or 3 months of age, is precipitated by infection, exposure, dehydration, or other stress. Initial signs of vasoocclusive crisis in the very young child may be warmth and swelling of one or both hands or feet. Older patients have pain in affected organs, visual disturbances, respiratory distress, and priapism.

Another problem resulting from sickle cell disease is *aplastic crisis,* caused by red blood cell destruction coupled with impaired red blood cell production in bone marrow. Aplastic crisis worsens anemia and leads to high-output CHF.

Sequestration crisis is the most fulminant manifestation of sickle cell disease but is less common than other crises and can be rapidly fatal. Incidence is greater in young children, months to 6 years of age. Blood suddenly pools in the spleen and other visceral organs, causing severe anemia and hypovolemic shock.

Because of the need for close monitoring, most patients with sickle cell disease are cared for by specialists. However, a first crisis or severe crisis may lead to treatment in the ED. Medical management is usually directed at supportive, symptomatic treatment. The main objectives are oxygenation, hydration with oral or intravenous solutions, electrolyte replacement, rest, analgesics, and blood replacement as needed and antibiotics as required.

NEUROLOGIC EMERGENCIES

Head trauma is the most common cause of neurologic emergency in children; however, seizures, shunt malfunction, and rarely brain tumors and congenital vascular malformations can also affect mental status in the pediatric agegroup. Infectious processes such as meningitis and sepsis are another cause for neurologic changes in children.

Neurologic Assessment

When a child has altered mental status, it is important to remember the first priority is the airway and ventilation. Neurologic assessment of pediatric patients presents special challenges, especially for the preverbal child. When parents say their child is "not acting normal," this should be taken seriously. Early signs and symptoms of increased intracranial pressure include altered mental status, restlessness, irritability, headache, and vomiting. Constricted or dilated pupils and decorticate or decerebrate posturing are late signs of increased intracranial pressure.

Numerous methods of assessing neurologic function in children have been proposed, including various adaptations of the Glasgow coma scale. The simplest and probably the most useful in the emergency setting is the mnemonic AVPU:

A (*a*lert)
V (responds to *v*erbal stimuli)
P (responds to *p*ainful stimuli)
U (*u*nresponsive)

Serial assessment with this mnemonic, together with a description of the patient's behavior, is the clearest means for documenting changes. An accurate history from parents is also helpful. When a child has altered mental status, ask about trauma, previous medical problems, ingestions, headache, and signs and symptoms of infection. Box 50-3 presents a mini neurologic examination for the pediatric patient.

Evaluating history and level of consciousness can be enough to classify the child's condition as an emergency. An altered level of consciousness in any child is an emergent condition.

Box 50-3 Mini Neurologic Examination

History

1. Time and mechanism of injury
2. Neurologic status immediately after injury; elapsed time between time of injury and arrival in hospital
3. Any neurologic change that may have occurred

Level of consciousness

1. Aware: may be disoriented or confused but still awake
2. Lethargic: can be aroused to follow commands
3. Stuporous: cannot be aroused to follow commands; purposeful withdrawal in response to deep painful stimuli
4. Semicomatose: only reflex responses to pain, i.e., decorticate or decerebrate
5. Comatose: no response to pain

Pupils

1. Size: equal or unequal
2. Reaction to light

Response to pain

1. Purposeful
2. Semipurposeful
3. Decorticate
4. Decerebrate
5. No response

Movement of extremities

1. Spontaneous
2. Response to pain
3. Equal strength and movement

Plantar responses

1. Upgoing
2. Downgoing
3. Equivocal

Facial movements

Central or peripheral weakness may be present.

Fundi

Describe hemorrhages. Rare to see papilledema sooner than 12-24 hours after injury.

Cerebrospinal fluid otorrhea or rhinorrhea

Usually blood with or without cerebrospinal fluid in acute phase

Vital signs

Obtain baseline; monitor closely.

Table 50-11 AEIOU TIPS Mnemonic for Evaluating Altered Level of Consciousness

Cause	Comments
*A*lcohol	More common in adolescents than younger pediatric patients
*E*ncephalopathy	Hypertension, hepatic, Reye's syndrome
*E*ndocrinology	Thyroid, adrenal
*E*lectrolytes	Alterations in sodium, potassium, calcium, or magnesium levels
*I*nsulin	Hypoglycemia or hyperglycemia
*I*ntussusception	Decreased level of consciousness may be the first manifestation of intussusception before abdominal symptoms appear
*O*verdose	Opiates and other toxins, ingested, inhaled, or transferred to the fetus before birth
*U*remia	Hemolytic uremic syndrome, chronic renal impairment
*T*rauma	One of the major causes; usually, head injuries and chest injuries leading to hypoxia
*I*nfection	More common in children than in adults; meningitis, encephalitis, Reye's syndrome, and sepsis
*P*sychiatric	Rare in children; should be considered only after other factors are ruled out
*S*eizure	Postictal states, syncope

From American Academy of Pediatrics and American College of Emergency Physicians: *Advanced pediatric life support,* Elk Grove Village, Ill, and Dallas, 1989, The Academy and College.

---

be evaluated for symptoms of increased intracranial pressure to prevent central nervous system injury. Laboratory studies may be ordered to detect toxins or electrolyte abnormalities.

Seizures

Seizures are involuntary movements and/or alteration in sensation, behavior, or consciousness caused by abnormal electrical activity in the brain. In young children, seizures associated with fever are one of the most common neurologic disorders of childhood, affecting 3% to 5% of children.[8] Most febrile seizures occur after 6 months of age and usually before 3 years with increased frequency in children younger than 18 months.

The cause of febrile seizures is still uncertain. In most children, height and rapidity of temperature elevation seem to be important factors. Temperature usually exceeds 38.8° C (101.8° F). Seizures usually occur during temperature rise rather than after prolonged elevation. Febrile seizures may accompany upper respiratory infection, gastrointestinal infection, or otitis. Twenty-five to thirty percent of children with simple febrile seizures have a recurrence with subsequent infections.[8]

Treatment for febrile seizures consists of ensuring the safety of the child during the seizure, controlling the seizure, and

---

A commonly used mnemonic, AEIOU TIPS, is useful for identification of causes for altered level of consciousness (Table 50-11). Intussusception as a cause of altered consciousness in the infant has been added to this mnemonic, since lethargy has been found to be a common symptom of this condition. Treatment of children who arrive in the ED with an altered level of consciousness includes assessment of ABCs along with assessment for injury or illnesses. The child must

reducing the temperature. Parents need reassurance of the benign nature of febrile seizures.

Other seizure disorders have numerous and varied causes. Seizure disorders are idiopathic if the cause is unknown and organic or symptomatic if the cause is identifiable.

Epilepsy is the diagnosis when seizures are recurrent with no apparent cause for the seizures. Seizure patients may exhibit a wide range of behaviors, from lip smacking and staring to violent muscular contractions or sudden loss of consciousness. Urinary and bowel incontinence also occur. Status epilepticus occurs when seizure activity is prolonged or the patient has sequential seizures without regaining consciousness between each seizure. Airway management, prevention of injury, and cessation of seizure activity with drug therapy are indicated for management of seizures (Table 50-12).

Whether the patient is admitted to the hospital or discharged home depends on the patient's history, laboratory findings, and physical findings. Children with first-time febrile seizures are often admitted for further observation and diagnostic testing. Children with previously undiagnosed febrile seizures are often admitted for further evaluation and anticonvulsant therapy. Children with previously diagnosed seizure disorders whose condition has stabilized are often discharged home with a referral to their neurologist.

Status epilepticus

Prolonged continuous seizure activity, or status epilepticus, may be a manifestation of anoxia, infection, trauma, ingestion, or metabolic disorder. In about half the children in whom status epilepticus develops, the cause is not identified. Sustained seizure activity produces cerebral anoxia and possible ischemic brain damage, so airway maintenance, oxygenation, and rapid termination of convulsive activity are priorities. Ensure the child's safety, and insert an oral air-

way to keep the airway open. Do not attempt insertion of the airway, tongue blade, or bite-block if the child's teeth are clenched. If the child is in severe respiratory distress or stops breathing, bag-valve-mask ventilation should be used until intubation is possible. A large-bore IV catheter should be inserted for administration of fluids and medication. Anticonvulsant medications are usually given IV until seizure activity ceases. Laboratory tests include CBC; electrolyte, glucose, calcium, magnesium, and BUN levels; urinalysis; and toxicology screening.

GASTROINTESTINAL AND GENITOURINARY EMERGENCIES
Dehydration

Dehydration is a common disturbance in children that occurs when total output of fluids exceeds total intake, regardless of underlying cause. Dehydration can result from lack of oral intake but is more often a result of abnormal fluid losses, such as vomiting or diarrhea.

Innumerable children are brought to the ED with nausea, vomiting, diarrhea, and poor feeding. Most often the problem is viral gastroenteritis or viral syndrome, so the patient is discharged. If the child has abdominal pain, an acute abdominal condition must be ruled out, so the child should not be allowed to drink any fluid until evaluation is complete. CBC, electrolyte, glucose, and BUN levels, and urinalysis are usually obtained. Patients whose laboratory analyses are within normal limits, who are only mildly dehydrated, and who are able to take fluids by mouth can be discharged. Instruct the parents to give the child small amounts of clear liquids frequently (a teaspoon at a time), progressing to the BRAT (bananas, rice, applesauce, and tea and toast) diet. Apple juice should not be used because it is hyperosmolar and may worsen diarrhea. Also instruct parents to return to

Table **50-12** **Seizure Medications**			
Medication	Dosage	Method	Side effects
Lorazepam*	0.03-0.05 mg/kg; status epilepticus, 0.1 mg/kg; has longer half-life and faster onset than diazepam	IV	Respiratory depression
Diazepam*	0.2-0.5 mg/kg	IV, intramuscular, endotracheal, rectal	Respiratory depression
Paraldehyde*	0.1-0.25 mg/kg	Usually rectal (when given rectally must be mixed with equal amounts of mineral oil); may be given IV, IM, NG	Respiratory depression
Phenytoin*	18-20 mg/kg	Slow IV push, 50 mg/min; mix only with normal saline solution; monitor heart rate and rhythm	Hypotension, respiratory depression, cardiac rhythm disturbance (prolonged QT interval)
Phenobarbital*	12-20 mg/kg; maximum dose 300 mg	Slow IV push, 50 mg/min; only in normal saline solution	Hypotension, drowsiness, respiratory depression

*Lorazepam, diazepam, and paraldehyde are used in emergency situations to treat status epilepticus. Phenytoin and phenobarbital have more long-term use in preventing recurrence.

their physician or the ED if the patient does not improve within 24 hours, there is increasing abdominal pain, or the child is acting strangely in any way. Severe dehydration is treated with crystalloid solutions, 20 ml/kg.

Abdominal Pain

Other illnesses causing gastrointestinal upset and/or abdominal pain are infection with bacterial agents and parasites; surgical emergencies such as appendicitis, strangulated hernia, intussusception, testicular torsion, and bowel obstruction; urinary tract infection; and toxic ingestion. Frequencies of these various causes of abdominal pain are listed by age in Table 50-13.

For the most part, ED treatment of the stable patient with abdominal pain focuses on assessing the patient, including history and vital signs; deciding whether the patient can be discharged or requires hospitalization; and determining if the problem needs medical or surgical management. In general, the possibility of a surgical abdomen should be considered for any patient with abdominal pain associated with palpation or movement. Basic diagnostic tests include CBC, urinalysis, and chest and abdominal radiographs. Adolescent female patients should be asked about pregnancy before radiographs are obtained. Assume that a female of childbearing age is pregnant until proven otherwise, so a serum pregnancy test should be obtained.

Appendicitis

Appendicitis is inflammation of the vermiform appendix or blind sac of the cecum. It is the most common condition requiring surgical intervention during childhood. Primarily an acute condition, appendicitis can progress to perforation and peritonitis without appropriate treatment. Signs and symptoms of appendicitis vary greatly but may include epigastric or lower right quadrant pain with rebound tenderness, nausea, and vomiting. The most important diagnostic test is a white blood cell count with differential. With appendicitis, total white blood cell count is usually 15,000 to 20,000 cells/μl with bands present. Fever is usually present, varying from 37.5° to 38.5° C. If the temperature is greater than 39° C, viral illness or perforation is likely.

Definitive treatment for appendicitis before perforation is surgical removal of the appendix, or appendectomy. However, fluid and electrolyte imbalance should be corrected before the child goes to surgery. The child should be NPO until surgery. Prophylactic antibiotics may be started prior to surgery for patients with evidence of perforation. Recovery from this surgery is rapid; the child may be discharged within a matter of days.

Incarcerated Hernia

A hernia is a protrusion of a portion of an organ through an abdominal opening. Classic presentation is an asymptomatic bulge that becomes more prominent with crying, defecation, coughing, or laughing.[8] Danger from herniation arises when the organ protruding through the opening is constricted to the extent that circulation is impaired. Hernias can often be manually reduced in the ED. Giving pain medication, placing the patient in Trendelenburg's position, and applying ice to the area may assist in this process. Surgical intervention is eventually required for most patients.

Intussusception

Intussusception occurs when a proximal portion of intestine telescopes into a more distal portion of intestine. This occurs in infancy, most often between 3 months and 1 year. Telescoping prevents passage of intestinal contents beyond the defect. Fecal material is unable to move beyond the obstruction. Stools contain primarily blood and mucus, which

Table **50-13** **Causes of Pediatric Abdominal Pain by Age**		
Under 2 years	2 to 5 years	5 to 16 years
Common		
Gasteroenteritis, viral syndrome, bowel obstruction	Gastroenteritis, appendicitis, urinary tract infection, pneumonia, asthma, viral syndrome, otitis, trauma or abuse	Gastroenteritis, appendicitis, urinary tract infection, constipation, viral syndrome, otitis, pelvic inflammatory disease, sickle cell crisis
Less common		
Sickle cell crisis, strangulated hernia, trauma or abuse, lead poisoning	Strangulated hernia, intussusception, pyelonephritis, Meckel's diverticulum, hepatitis, diabetic ketoacidosis, bowel obstruction, lead poisoning	Pneumonia, asthma, ectopic pregnancy, ovarian cyst, cholecystitis, diabetic ketoacidosis, gastritis
Least common		
Appendicitis, volvulus, ovarian torsion	Strangulated hernia, rheumatic fever, myocarditis, pericarditis	Rheumatic fever, ovarian or testicular torsion

Jaffe D: Quick triage of children with abdominal pain, *Emerg Med* 22(14):39, 1988.

results in the "currant jelly" stools characteristic of intussusception.

In most cases, initial treatment is nonsurgical hydrostatic reduction by barium enema concurrent with diagnostic testing. If this does not reduce the obstruction, surgical intervention is necessary.

Testicular Torsion

A prepubertal male with sudden onset of severe scrotal pain radiating to the abdomen may have testicular torsion. Twisting of spermatic vessels causes ischemia, swelling, and a high-lying testis. The duration of pain is usually less than 24 hours. Testicular salvage is approximately 20% with more than 12 hours of pain.[8] Patients may complain of nausea and vomiting. Scrotal edema is present, and blood pressure may be elevated because of pain and anxiety. Fever is rarely present. If the torsion has been present less than 3 or 4 hours, manual reduction by the ED physician or urologist may be possible. If surgery is indicated, keep the patient NPO, and administer analgesics as ordered.

Other Genitourinary Problems

Other genitourinary problems seen in the ED include urinary tract infection, phimosis, dysmenorrhea, and pregnancy-related problems. Treatment for these illnesses is essentially the same as for adults.

INFECTIOUS DISEASE EMERGENCIES

Children with upper respiratory infections such as colds, sore throats, sinuitis, and otitis are often brought to the ED. For the most part, they are rapidly discharged and followed by their private physicians. Some of the more serious infectious diseases are described in this section.

AIDS

Infants and children with acquired immunodeficiency syndrome (AIDS) or infected with the human immunodeficiency virus (HIV) present to the ED with numerous physical problems requiring supportive nursing care, both physiologic and psychologic. HIV has created a whole new population of chronically ill and disabled children. The virus has been found in blood and almost all body fluids, including semen, saliva, vaginal secretions, urine, breast milk, and tears. Evidence to date indicates the virus is transmitted primarily through direct contact with blood or blood products. There is no evidence that casual contact between affected and unaffected individuals can spread the virus.[2]

In the pediatric population, three age-groups are primarily affected. These are children exposed in utero to an infected mother, children who received blood products infected with the virus, and adolescents infected through high-risk behaviors. The majority of children with AIDS are less than 2 years old and constitute a small percentage of the total AIDS population.

Children, like adults, have a wide range of signs and symptoms related to this infection. Most children with AIDS have recurrent bacterial and fungal infections, chronic diarrhea, chronic anemia, renal disease, cardiomyopathy, neurologic deterioration, or general failure to thrive. Infection with HIV is a multisystem problem; therefore ED presentation can vary greatly. Diagnosis of AIDS in children is suspected on the basis of the clinical presentation and the presence of risk factors associated with AIDS. Clinical presentation may be failure to thrive, chronic pneumonia, respiratory distress due to pneumonia, liver or spleen enlargement, oral lesions, or recurrent bacterial infections. Currently no cure for pediatric HIV or AIDS exists. Treatment is primarily supportive, aimed at prevention of infections and complications, early recognition of complications, and support of optimal general health. Current drug therapy includes zidovudine (AZT) and dideoxyinosine (DDI), which have been shown to increase life expectancy.

In the ED, the child and family need support dealing with this terminal disease. Family reaction to the disease may include shock, anger, fear, or guilt. Family members should be encouraged to express their feelings. Emergency nurses should listen and provide support. The emergency nurse can play a part in family education concerning the disease. Teaching in the ED should focus on the presenting problem and discussion of resources available for follow-up care.

Bacteremia

The effects of bacterial invasion of the bloodstream may range from relatively mild symptoms of infection (bacteremia) to overwhelming, life-threatening infection (sepsis or septicemia). Bacteremia and septicemia represent the two extremes on a continuum of severity rather than disparate entities.

Bacteremia may occur in association with meningitis, cellulitis, or kidney infection. It may also occur without localized findings (occult bacteremia). Bacteremia is most common in children younger than 2 years and may be difficult to detect in the child less than 2 months of age. Any child less than 2 years old should be suspected of bacteremia when there is fever and documented infection (white blood cell count greater than 15,000 cells/μl) without an observable focus of infection. Bacteremia rarely occurs in infancy and may be especially difficult to detect at this age because infants do not always respond to infection with fever. Bacteremia should be suspected when a child has a fever with malaise, poor feeding, and irritability and is not playful or easily consoled. Diagnostic workup includes CBC, blood cultures, a chest radiograph, urinalysis, and complete septic workup, including lumbar puncture if indicated.

In the ED, the child with fever more than 38.4° C may be given acetaminophen (10 to 15 mg/kg) to lower temperature. Frequently, oral antibiotics are prescribed. If the patient is discharged, careful attention should be given to the parent's ability to give medication on schedule as well as clear directions concerning danger signs of sepsis. The child should be reevaluated within 24 to 48 hours. Bacteremia can progress to sepsis if the patient is not adequately treated.

Sepsis

Sepsis is an overwhelming, life-threatening infection of the bloodstream with an overall mortality rate of 15% to 50%, depending on infectious agent. The younger the child, the higher the risk. The child with sepsis appears very ill. A child less than 3 months may be afebrile. Older children often have a high fever with tachycardia, abnormal skin signs, altered mental status, and sometimes petechiae or purpura. Sepsis requires immediate assessment and intervention for shock and determination of the cause of infection by laboratory analysis. CBC, electrolyte, glucose, BUN, and creatinine levels, blood cultures, prothrombin time, partial thromboplastin time, aspartate transaminase, alanine transaminase, urinalysis, and chest radiograph are recommended. Intravenous antibiotics are indicated. The patient with sepsis requires a high level of care, namely, the intensive care unit.

Meningitis

Meningitis, an acute inflammation of the meninges, is a common cause of death and disability in children. Annual incidence of meningitis is 1 case per 2000 children with a peak in children 2 months to 5 years.[8] Causative organism is often bacterial, but viral meningitis also occurs. With bacterial meningitis, organisms enter the bloodstream through focal infection or by routes such as open wounds, skull fractures, and surgical procedures and spreads the infection through the subarachnoid space, causing swelling and pain. Recognition and treatment are essential to prevent death and residual damage.

Increased intracranial pressure is a major concern in meningitis. As inflammation increases, expansion within the rigid skull causes direct pressure on the brain. Narrow passageways to the ventricles are occluded and cerebrospinal fluid outflow is obstructed, which produces an altered sensorium.

Many children present with headache, nausea, vomiting, or poor feeding. Most children have an elevated temperature; however, infants may have normal temperature or even hypothermia. A classic sign of meningitis is nuchal rigidity, which is rarely seen in infancy. Common signs and symptoms of increased intracranial pressure may be evident, including irritability, restlessness, altered mental status, and seizures. Bulging fontanelles are a late sign. A severely ill child may be in respiratory distress, exhibit cyanosis, and have a rash or petechiae.

In the late stages, meningitis requires aggressive intervention including airway management, hyperventilation to prevent increased intracranial pressure, intravenous medication (mannitol, steroids, diuretics, antibiotics), and admission to the intensive care unit. Strict isolation is required. Seizures are treated with anticonvulsant medication until seizure activity stops. Definitive diagnosis requires a lumber puncture and laboratory analysis of cerebrospinal fluid for protein, white cells, and Gram's stain. Other laboratory tests include serum electrolyte and glucose determinations obtained before the lumbar puncture because stress of the procedure may raise the glucose level.

Meningococcemia

Meningococcemia, caused by invasion of the bloodstream with *Neisseria meningitidis,* can occur with or without meningitis. The child with meningococcemia has fever, headache, and rash, usually maculopapular rash, petechiae, and purpura. Shock and disseminated intravascular coagulation occur very quickly. Meningococcemia can be rapidly fatal. Rapid assessment and intervention are critical. Diagnostic tests include CBC, electrolytes, glucose, and urinalysis. Lumbar puncture, blood cultures, and clotting studies are also necessary.

Encephalitis

Acute encephalitis, or inflammation of the brain parenchyma, may be caused by direct viral invasion or may follow an infection such as measles. Symptoms and treatment of encephalopathy vary by cause. Associated symptoms include but are not limited to headache, fever, altered sensorium, and nuchal rigidity. Supportive measures with fluid restriction and monitoring of electrolytes may be all that are required for acute encephalitis. Herpes encephalitis is a life-threatening disease requiring aggressive intervention.

Reye's Syndrome

Reye's syndrome, encephalopathy associated with fatty infiltration in the liver, is rarely seen today. This illness develops a few days after what appears to be a mild viral illness. The cause is unknown, but genetic predisposition, use of aspirin during the viral illness, and an intrinsic toxin affecting mitochondrial metabolism have all been proposed. Symptoms of Reye's syndrome are recurrent vomiting and altered mental status, progressing rapidly to coma. Reye's syndrome requires rapid diagnosis and aggressive, complex intervention to prevent death or devastating sequelae. Standard diagnostic tests as well as aspartate transaminase and alanine transaminase determinations are required, but presumptive diagnosis is initially made by elevated blood ammonia level, usually with a normal bilirubin level.

Skin Rashes (Measles, Chickenpox, Scarlet Fever, Roseola, and Meningitis with Petechiae)

Children are brought to the ED with various rashes. Most rashes, such as neonatal acne, diaper dermatitis, and viral exanthem, are not life-threatening. Other diseases have long-term consequences and should be taken seriously.

Table **50-14** **Infections with Skin Rashes**					
Characteristic	Measles (rubeola)	Chickenpox (varicella)	Scarlet fever	Roseola (exanthema subitum)	Petechial rash (from meningitis)
Incubation Signs and symptoms	10-11 days 3-5 days fever, cough, coryza, toxic appearance, conjunctivitis; Koplik's spots (mucosal lesions) appear 2 days	10-20 days Fever and cough, simultaneously with rash; headache; malaise	2-4 days Fever for 1-2 days, sore throat, strawberry tongue, vomiting, chills, malaise	10-15 days Rapid rise of high fever lasting 3-4 days in otherwise well child	None May be sudden onset or preceded by fever and malaise; if sudden onset and accompanied by fever, may indicate sepsis
Exanthem (rash)	Reddish brown; begins on face, spreads downward; confluent high on body, discrete lesions in lower portions; lasts 7-10 days	Vesicles appearing in crops; trunk, scalp, face, extremities; lesions in all stages of development	Punctate, sandpaper texture; blanches on pressure; appears first in flexor areas; rash lasts 7 days	Appears discrete, rose-colored; appears after fever; begins on chest and spreads to face	Reddish purple vascular, *non-blanching* rash
Complications	Pneumonia, encephalitis, otitis media	Pneumonia, encephalitis, Reye's syndrome	Rheumatic heart disease	None	Sepsis, septic shock, long-term sequelae from increased intracranial pressure

Some infectious diseases that present with a skin rash are shown in Table 50-14.

Kawasaki Disease

Kawasaki disease is acute systemic vasculitis occuring mainly in children under the age of 5 years. The acute disease is self-limiting; however, without treatment, one in five children can develop cardiac sequelae. Kawasaki disease is the leading cause of acquired heart disease in children in the United States. The etiology remains a mystery.

Children present with fever and irritability. Parents should be asked about any rash or erythema. The child may present dehydrated with nausea and vomiting.

Treatment is geared toward prevention of complications. High-dose γ-globulin (2 g/kg) has been useful in reducing the risk of coronary artery disease. High doses of aspirin, 30 to 100 mg/kg/24 hr, are often given simultaneously. Beyond these two treatments, treatment is largely supportive. Intravenous fluids should be given to correct dehydration.

Tuberculosis

Tuberculosis (TB) is a disease that is controlled in most developed countries but still remains a health hazard and a leading cause of death in many parts of the world. It is caused by *Mycobacterium tuberculosis*. The source of infection in most situations is usually a member of the household.

A steady increase in new cases has occurred during the past several years. This increasing incidence is attributed, in part, to the influx of foreign-born persons as well as recognition of the disease in the native-born population.

The clinical manifestations of TB are extremely variable. Fever, malaise, anorexia, weight loss, or cough may be present. Coinfection with HIV is also common. Most children with pulmonary TB have noninfectious disease; therefore they seldom require isolation. Hospitalization is seldom necessary; most children can be managed at home. Antimicrobial agents cure most cases of TB, the limiting factor being patient compliance with drug administration. Drug therapy usually lasts 6 to 9 months. Historically, TB has been regarded with fear of infection, so it is important to clarify any misconceptions parents may have regarding this disease.

Lyme Disease

Lyme disease is a systemic, tick-borne illness. A skin lesion, known as erythema chronicum migrans, is present in a majority of cases. Lyme disease, caused by the spirochete *Borrelia burgdorferi,* is carried by a tick that lives primarily on white-tailed deer and white-footed field mice. The multisystem nature and slow evolution of the illness make diagnosis difficult. In a child with suspected Lyme disease, a history of tick bite or being in a wooded area is important. The small size of the tick may prevent the patient from realizing its presence. General malaise, achiness, sore throat, or fever may cause the patient to seek treatment.

Treatment is doxycycline, 100 mg bid, for children 9 years or older or ampicillin, 50 mg/kg/day, for children younger than 9 years. Prevention of the disease involves awareness and taking precautions before and after being in areas where the ticks are. Parents should check the child's entire body after being in a wooded area.

OTHER DISEASES WITH SKIN LESIONS
Scabies

The major symptom of scabies is severe itching. Scabies is caused by the itch mite *Sarcoptes scabiei*. Infestation results in eruption of wheals, papules, vesicles, and often visible threadlike burrows. Scabies is transmitted by direct contact. Application of lindane or crotamiton is the treatment for children over 1 year old. Oral antihistamines may be required to control itching. All bedding and clothing should be removed and washed.

Impetigo

Impetigo is a skin infection caused by group A streptococci. It is typically found in children less than 6 years old. The patient has skin lesions that ooze serous fluid and crust when dry. Most cases of impetigo can be treated on an outpatient basis with oral or intramuscular antibiotics.

Cellulitis

An injury that breaks the skin barrier, such as insect bite, abrasion, laceration, or surgical procedure, may allow entry of organisms that cause cellulitis, that is, *Staphyloccoccus aureus* or group A streptococci. Inflammatory response causes edema and swelling, usually without fever. Most patients are treated on an outpatient basis. Children less than 3 years old with facial cellulitis are more likely to have bacteremia and may require intravenous antimicrobial therapy.

SUMMARY

Most children seen in the ED are not critically ill or severely injured. Those who are can cause great anxiety for the emergency nurse. Developing expertise in pediatric triage, assessment, and care requires the emergency nurse to develop a system that is comfortable, systematic, thorough,

Box **50-4**

NURSING DIAGNOSES FOR THE PEDIATRIC PATIENT

Altered nutrition
Ineffective thermoregulation
High risk for fluid volume deficit
Impaired verbal communication
Ineffective breathing pattern

---

and adaptable. Box 50-4 gives just a few nursing diagnoses pertinent for the pediatric patient.

This chapter provides a brief review of medical emergencies seen in the pediatric population. In caring for pediatric illnesses, it is important to remember that the child's medical care is only one aspect of treatment. Recognition of the fundamental importance of the parent-child relationship is essential for both parent and child. This can be difficult in an emergency; however, this does not negate its importance. Showing concern and offering support for the family, including the family in the child's care whenever possible, and giving thorough clear discharge instructions lay the groundwork for ongoing care of the child once the emergency is over.

REFERENCES

1. American Academy of Pediatrics and American College of Emergency Physicians: *Advanced pediatric life support,* Elk Grove, Ill, and Dallas, 1989, The Academy and College.
2. Caldwell M, Rogers M: Epidemiology of pediatric HIV infection, *Pediatr Clin North Am* 38(1):1, 1991.
3. Hazinski M: *Nursing care of the critically ill child,* ed 2, St. Louis, 1992, Mosby.
4. Jaffe D: Quick triage of children with abdominal pain, *Emerg Med* 22(14):39, 1988.
5. Luten R: *Problems in pediatric emergency medicine,* New York, 1988, Churchill Livingstone.
6. McCarthy P et al: History and observation variable in assessing febrile children, *Pediatrics* 65:6, 1980.
7. Seidel J, Hendersonn D, editors: *Emergency medical services for children: a report to the nation,* Washington, DC, 1991, National Center for Education in Maternal & Child Health.
8. Strange GR et al: *Pediatric emergency medicine,* New York, 1996, McGraw-Hill.
9. Weinerman E et al: Yale studies in ambulatory medical care: use of hospital emergency services, *Am J Public Health* 56:1037, 1966.

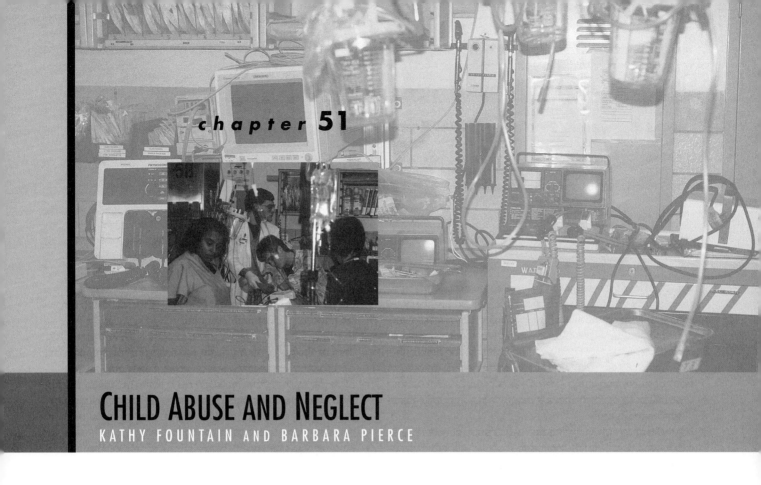

chapter **51**

CHILD ABUSE AND NEGLECT

KATHY FOUNTAIN AND BARBARA PIERCE

Child abuse and neglect are problems more prevalent today than ever before. In 1994, over 3 million incidents of suspected child abuse and neglect were reported to child protection services; nearly half the victims were less than 1 year old. Reports of violence against children have almost tripled since 1976. The National Clearinghouse on Child Abuse and Neglect estimates that 9 of 10 children are maltreated by parents or family friends in some manner.[23]

In Chicago, a 35-year-old mother kicks and throws her 16-month-old baby out a window because he would not stop crying; an Alabama couple shackles their twin daughters above the knees and locks them in a room to live in their own excrement; a Detroit drug addict sells her son to settle a $1000 crack cocaine debt; a trusted priest is sentenced to over 30 years for sexually abusing children during his reign as youth leader; in California, a teenage girl is abducted from her home and later found raped, beaten, and dead; a 4-year-old is beaten to death by her father while a neighbor reports she had to walk to another part of the house and turn up the television volume to drown out the child's screams; a 3-year-old raped by a trusted family friend is left infected with *Neisseria gonorrhoeae* and human immunodeficiency virus (HIV); and in North Carolina, the drowning of two young boys at the hand of their mother mortifies the nation. Our country is in a state of national emergency.[18]

NEGLECT

Although there may be no visible bruises or broken bones, ongoing child neglect is a silent, serious attack on children that can leave lasting mental and physical problems (Table 51-1). Neglect, defined as intentional or unintentional omission of needed care and support, may appear to the emergency nurse as a child who is unkempt, left unattended, not dressed appropriately for the weather, malnourished, or diagnosed as "failure to thrive." Identification of neglect must consider whether parents attempt to provide essentials despite limited resources. Failure to provide adequate physical protection, nutrition, or health care is generally considered neglect, but neglect can also include lack of human contact and love. "Neglect slowly and persistently eats away at children's spirits until they have little will to connect with others or explore the world."[3] Currently, 45% of all abuse cases involve neglect.[3] Recognizing neglect is often difficult in the emergency department (ED) because of limited, one-time contact with most patients. However, the emergency nurse should be alert for behaviors that suggest neglect (Box 51-1).

Failure to Thrive

Failure to thrive is defined as the condition in children under 5 years old whose growth persistently and significantly deviates from norms for age and sex based on national growth charts. Measurements for height, weight, and head circumference are plotted against normal childhood growth patterns. Failure to thrive children generally fall below aver-

743

Table **51-1**	**Types of Child Neglect**
Type	Description
Medical	Caregiver fails to provide medical treatment, immunizations, recommended surgery, or other interventions necessary in a serious health problem. Often occurs when parent's religious beliefs conflict with the medical community. Issue is often resolved in court.
Physical	Failure to protect from harm or danger; failure to provide basic physical needs such as food, clothing, and shelter. Most widely recognized and reported type of neglect.
Emotional	Difficult to recognize and diagnose due to lack of physical evidence. Occurs in the home unobserved by professionals and child is often too young to speak out. Extreme forms of emotional abuse can lead to physical illness, failure to thrive, and death. Definition of emotional abuse includes inability to meet the child's emotional needs; however, there is no universal agreement on what those needs are. Emotional abuse is often typified by child behaviors such as depression, habit disorders (sucking, biting, rocking, enuresis), conduct and learning disorders such as antisocial behaviors, i.e., cruelty.
Educational	Caregivers fail to comply with state requirements for schooling and school attendance. Can also be parental resistance to essential specialized education programs.
Mental health	Similar to medical neglect in that parent refuses to comply with recommended corrective or therapeutic measures in cases where child has serious emotional or behavioral problems.

From American Professional Society on the Abuse of Children.

Box **51-1**	**Potential Indicators of Child Neglect**
Behavioral	**Physical**
Begs or steals food	Height and weight significantly below normal for age level
Falls asleep in school, lethargic	Inappropriate clothing for weather
Poor school attendance, frequent tardiness	Poor hygiene, including lice, body odor, scaly skin
Chronic hunger	Child abandoned and left with inadequate supervision
Dull, apathetic appearance	Untreated illness or injury
Runs away from home	Lack of safe, warm, and sanitary shelter
Reports no caregiver in the home	Lack of necessary medical and dental care
Assumes adult responsibilities	

From *For kids sake: a child abuse prevention and reporting kit,* rev ed, Oklahoma City, 1992, Oklahoma State Department of Health.

age in all three areas. The cause of failure to thrive may be medical (e.g., *Giardia* infection, celiac disease, lead poisoning, or malabsorption) or psychosocial.

Psychosocial causes are often linked to and reported as child neglect. Maladaptive parenting practices, chronic family illnesses, parental depression, and substance abuse among caregivers are recognized causes. Failure to thrive does not necessarily imply abuse or neglect but does require aggressive treatment and follow-up by appropriate health care professionals. Untreated, failure to thrive can lead to developmental and behavioral difficulties resulting from nutritional deprivation of the nervous system and other systems. A multidisciplinary approach in treating failure to thrive has the best opportunity for success. Family assessment, nutritional counseling, medical intervention, and fam-

ily support are needed to correct failure to thrive. Table 51-2 describes medical evaluation for suspected neglect and failure to thrive.

PHYSICAL ABUSE

Physical abuse is nonaccidental injury to a child under age 18 years by a parent or caregiver. Typically a pattern of behavior repeated over time, child abuse can also be a single attack. Child abuse is characterized by injury, torture, maiming, or use of unreasonable force. Abuse may result from harsh discipline or severe punishment. Box 51-2 identifies behavioral and physical indicators found in physical abuse. Children rarely tell anyone about physical abuse because of feelings of shame or confusion. The emergency nurse should be cognizant of reasons for failure to communicate potential abuse situations (Box 51-3).

Specific Abuse Patterns

Children can experience a multitude of insults and injuries at the hands of primary caregivers or other adults. Two patterns seen with increasing frequency are shaken baby syndrome and Munchausen syndrome by proxy.

Shaken baby syndrome occurs when infants are shaken vigorously. Acceleration-deceleration of the head creates a triad of injuries: subdural hemorrhage, retinal hemorrhage, and altered level of consciousness. There are often no external signs of trauma.[8]

Munchausen syndrome by proxy is a complex condition exhibited when a child is knowingly kept ill by a caretaker to get secondary gain or attention through the child's illness. The child is subjected to illnesses perpetuated by caregivers, who may give ipecac or other drugs, introduce pathogens, or otherwise contribute to a child's illness. Caretakers also falsify medical histories and symptoms. Munchausen syndrome, often undetected by caregivers, can lead to death in extreme cases.[6]

One difficulty in identification of abuse is the number of conditions that mimic physical abuse. Physiologic or pathologic causes for physical findings should always be considered.

Table **51-2**	**Medical Evaluation of Suspected Neglect and Failure to Thrive**
Component	Description
History	Lack of parental concern about physical illness, delayed development, or failure to thrive
	Bizarre dietary or feeding history
	Isolated or depressed parent
	Financial or social crisis
	Alcohol or drug abuse in parent
	Any evidence of organic failure to thrive
	Possible physical abuse
Physical examination	Lack of subcutaneous tissue
	Developmental delay
	Evidence of organic disease
	Signs of physical abuse
Laboratory tests	Complete blood cell count
	Renal assessment, including measurement of electrolytes and urinalysis
	Does baby gain weight when adequate intake of a regular diet is established?

Courtesy Helen Britton, MD, Primary Children's Medical Center, Salt Lake City, Utah.

- *Sudden infant death syndrome* can appear as child abuse because of pooling of blood, mottling, and other discoloration associated with death. The definitive cause of death should be determined by autopsy.
- *Clotting disorders* such as Wiskott-Aldrich syndrome, hemophilia, and thrombocytopenia purpura cause bruises in varying stages of healing.
- *Mongolian spots* are birthmarks found predominantly in Spanish Americans, southeast Asians, southern Europeans, Native American Indians, or anyone with dark pigmentation. Mongolian spots do not change coloration or size over time and have a grayer appearance than bruises.
- *Multiple petechiae and purpura of the face* can result when vigorous crying, retching, or coughing increases vena cava pressure. Unlike intentional choking, there are no marks around the neck.
- *Bullous impetigo* may appear as an infected wound or burn. This condition may reflect neglect if caregivers are apathetic about care of lesions.
- *Cultural or ethnic practices* such as coining or cupping are used to treat pain, fever, or poor appetite. Coining—rubbing a coin over bony prominences—causes a striated "pseudoburn." Cupping refers to warming a cup, spoon, or shot glass in oil and then placing it on the neck, back, or ribs, which results in a petechial or purpuric rash over the affected area.[24]
- *Osteogenesis imperfecta* is an inherited disease that can result in multiple fractures with minimal trauma and causes a tendency to bleed easily.

Interviewing Caregivers

When abuse is suspected, the caregiver should be carefully interviewed to obtain as much as information as possi-

Box **51-2** **Physical Abuse Findings**	
Behavioral findings	**Physical findings**
Requests or feels deserving of punishment	Unexplained bruises or welts found most frequent, usually on face, torso, buttocks, back, or thighs; can reflect shape of object used, i.e., electric cord, hand, belt buckle; may be in various stages of healing
Afraid to go home, and/or requests to stay in school or daycare	
Overly shy, tends to avoid physical contact with adults especially parents	Unexplained burns often on palms, soles of feet, buttocks, or back; can reflect pattern of cigarette burn, electrical appliance, or rope burn
Displays behavioral extremes (withdrawal or aggressiveness)	
Cries excessively or sits and stares	Unexplained fractures/dislocation involving skull, ribs, and bones around joints; may include multiple fractures or spiral fractures
Reports injury by parent or caretaker	
Gives unbelievable explanations for injuries	Other unexplained injuries such as lacerations, abrasions, human bite, or pinch marks; loss of hair/bald patches; retinal hemorrhages; abdominal injuries
Clings to health care worker rather than parent	

From *For kids sake: a child abuse prevention and reporting kit,* rev ed, Oklahoma City, 1992, Oklahoma State Department of Health.

Box **51-3**	**Reasons Children Do Not Discuss Physical Abuse**

Feelings of shame
Low value of self
Fear of breaking up family
Isolation
Confusion
Ill-equipped to deal with outside world
Loss of trust
Unaware that activity is inappropriate
Alienation of family member
Threats
Dependency needs of victim
Chaotic lifestyle

From *Educators' resource manual on child abuse*, Montgomery, Alabama.

ble. Make every effort to establish rapport, conveying genuine concern and understanding. A nonjudgmental, noncritical attitude is essential. Judgmental attitudes hinder communication and limit information. Tactfully determine issues of concern to the caretaker. The person may feel desperate and inadequate. Use reflective statements, such as "You sound really frustrated right now." Do not agree or condone, merely listen and reflect, using critical listening skills.

Parents often feel intense neediness and helplessness about their inability to meet their own needs, so a child who is needy, demanding, or misbehaves proves extremely stressful. Parents may also feel intensely negative about themselves and dwell on their own worthlessness, helplessness, and incompetence. Support the caregiver, but do not convey pity. Emphasize anything positive; for example, the parent sought help. Reinforce the decision to seek help; normal behavior is to withdraw without seeking help. Help parents draw on personal strengths. Helplessness and worthlessness are self-destructive, so effort should be made to draw parents away from negative feelings. Parents may be agitated, embarrassed, or tearful, so work to make them feel valued as individuals.

Parents are often distressed because of isolation and lack of a social network. Discuss places for support such as church, family, and friends. Talk about stressors the person is experiencing, including economic worries, unemployment, poverty, illness, divorce, and single-parenting concerns.[22]

Allegations of abuse

Allegations of child abuse sometimes arise during separation, divorce, and child custody proceedings. Perceptions exist that false allegations can be made during divorce or custody proceedings in an attempt to place one parent in a "favored" position for child custody. False accusations are sometimes made; however, all allegations of abuse or neglect during divorce proceedings deserve serious consideration because of the increased risk for abuse during this time.

Sexual allegations in divorce (SAID)[24] syndrome occurs when allegations of sexual abuse arise during pre- or post-divorce periods. A higher index of suspicion for abuse and neglect is required with divorcing families because families are experiencing increased stress and are dysfunctional as a result of the divorce process. Separation of parents increases the opportunity for sexual and physical victimization but also can provide an opportunity for a child to disclose that abuse has taken place if the abuser is out of the home. Risk for extrafamilial abuse is higher because of changes in caregivers or the presence of a nonbiologic caregiver in a home.

Reporting Abuse

When suspicion of nonaccidental trauma or sexual abuse is raised, appropriate agencies must be notified immediately. Each state defines child neglect and abuse differently; however, the ultimate goal, regardless of geographic location, is prevention of further injury through prompt intervention. If child endangerment is a concern, the child should be taken into protective custody. State statutes regarding protective custody vary, so become familiar with local requirements. State statutes designate specific individuals, that is, law enforcement, physicians, health care professionals, and educators, who must report suspected child abuse and neglect. Over 20 states require anyone who suspects neglect or abuse to notify appropriate authorities. State reporting laws grant immunity for good-faith reporting. In most states, liability exists only if the reporter knows the allegations are false or the individual acted with malicious purpose.

Reasonable judgment should be exercised when disclosing to caregivers that police agencies or child protective services have been contacted. Avoid inflammatory statements when relaying information to caregivers. When it is near the arrival time for outside agencies, simply state the legal responsibility to report suspicions.

Treatment

Care of injury is the primary medical concern. Once immediate physical needs are resolved, further assessment is then initiated. Query the child and caregivers, avoiding judgments of possible perpetrators or reasons the injury occurred. Health care providers must remember that investigation of child abuse allegations are the responsibility of police or the appropriate division of family services. Emergency nurses who *suspect child abuse or neglect must report specific concerns* and the reasons for those concerns.

Reassure the child and caregiver that you are there to help. Establish trust, allay fears, and lay groundwork for expression of concerns. Give the child some degree of control by providing choices. "Which color gown do you want—blue or green?" "May I listen to your heart, or do you want to listen to it first?" Be clear and explain what you are doing. Be honest; if something will hurt, say so.

Obtain a detailed history, paying close attention to the sequence of events. Is the history consistent with the child's age and nature of injury? Interview the child and parent(s) separately if the child is old enough to talk. Is the parent at high risk for abuse—isolated, abused as a child, low self-esteem? Is the child at high risk for abuse—difficult child, difficult developmental age, premature infant? Is the family experiencing a crisis—financial, social? Are other children at home at risk for abuse? Is alcohol or drug abuse present?

Physical examination

Identify and document all injuries, old and new, comparing historical information to clinical evidence. Measure, draw, and describe location, color, induration, and scarring. Assess for limited range of motion, which may indicate old fractures. Look for pattern injuries such as cigarette burns or spiral femur fractures in a nonambulatory child. Measure height, weight, and head circumference and then compare to standard growth charts. Assess developmental level of function. An ocular and funduscopic examination is required to identify any retinal hemorrhages. Skeletal surveys are obtained on children under 2 years to rule out existing or healed fractures. Prothrombin time, partial thromboplastin time, factor XIII, fibrinogen level, platelet count, and bleeding time are recommended to rule out existing blood dyscrasia.

SEXUAL ABUSE

Child sexual abuse, involvement of children in sexual activities that violate social taboos, is usually done for gratification or profit of a significantly older person. Children do not understand these acts and are not able to give informed consent.[17] Types of sexual abuse include, but are not limited to, fondling, digital manipulation, exhibitionism, pornography, and actual or attempted oral, vaginal, or anal intercourse. In 1995, over 300,000 cases of suspected child sexual abuse were reported to child protective services.[27] Unfortunately, the definition of child sexual abuse varies from state to state, and there is no national reporting system, so determination of actual incidence and prevalence rates is difficult. During anonymous surveys of adults, 20% of women and 10% to 15% of men reported sexual abuse before reaching adulthood.[4]

The primary portal of entry into the health care system for children with sexual abuse is the ED. One study showed 46% of children with suspected sexual abuse were first evaluated in the ED.[12] Without appropriate intervention, there is a 50% chance of further abuse and a 10% chance for death.[28] Physicians historically hesitate to become involved because they lack confidence in the medical examination, fear testifying in court, and are uncomfortable handling social problems that accompany a diagnosis of sexual abuse.[13,19] However, legal and social systems depend heavily on medical examination to provide evidence that can withstand intense scrutiny when used to protect children from further abuse and prosecute the offender.[13] Consequently, emergency care professionals must recognize sexual abuse and be skilled in examinations with medical and forensic strength. Treatment protocols specifically addressing child sexual abuse are recommended for all EDs.

Clinical Presentation

Most children are brought by their mothers for evaluation of complaints directly related to the anogenital region such as discharge, bleeding, pain, swelling, dysuria, or difficulty stooling as well as nonspecific symptoms such as headache, abdominal pain, or fatigue.[4,9,12,15] Behavioral symptoms such as excessive masturbation, depression, inappropriate sexual expression (verbal or physical), suicidal gestures, delinquency, fearfulness, anxiety, decline in school performance, sleep disturbances, and/or drug and alcohol abuse may also be identified.[10] Abel et al[1] state that the majority of pedophiles molest boys; however, most reported victims are girls. Male victims abused by males may be reluctant to report sexual abuse because of fear of being labeled a homosexual. Most children are sexually molested by individuals they know, a family member or close family friend. In most cases, abuse has been ongoing for many years.[4]

Urgency for medical evaluation depends on timing of the last abuse episode and presenting symptoms. Immediate examination is required if abuse occurred within 72 hours or there is bleeding, pain, or discharge. Evidence may still be present, so specimens for a rape kit are collected for law enforcement. Genital examination may be deferred when there is no history of acute trauma and the child is asymptomatic and considered safe. A general physical examination should be performed prior to patient discharge to ensure that no acute problems exist.[14]

Emergency personnel should ascertain the safety of the child and of the home environment and treat current conditions (e.g., pelvic inflammatory disease, sexually transmitted diseases [STDs]). Prophylaxis against pregnancy should be given for the pubescent female. Other responsibilities include emotional support, reporting suspected abuse to child protection authorities (including law enforcement), and involving the hospital-based child protection team or medical social worker.[24]

The most important component of sexual abuse evaluation is obtaining the patient history.[14,24,26] Physical findings or behavioral indicators rarely stand alone; they are most valuable in supporting the history given by the child.[24] The type and extent of interview are contingent on many factors. If a multidisciplinary forensic interviewing team is available, emergency health care providers should collect just enough information to complete the medical examination and make recommendations.[12] When a team is not available, a social worker may be helpful in coordinating care. History taking requires a quiet, child-friendly environment. A health care professional should begin by interviewing the adult who accompanied the child—without the child present. A careful, comprehensive medical history should document previous traumas to the anogenital area and attempt to gain an understanding of the adult's perception and emotional response to what has occurred.[20]

Although children may not exhibit external trauma, a mental health emergency may develop, since victim and family are in a state of crisis.[24] Ideally, child and caregivers should be interviewed separately. Obtaining a child's statement requires an interviewer who is sensitive, nonjudgmental, nonthreatening, and trained in forensic interviewing of children. Interviewers must respond to the child's developmental and cognitive level and ask questions accordingly, using the child's terminology for body parts. Allow time for the child to ask questions. General questions should include inquiries about the caregiver, where the child lives, sleeping arrangements, school habits, friends, names for body parts, and primary care provider. Focus on specific questions by addressing hurtful touches, pain, bleeding, or other

"ouches."[4,11,20,24,29] Health care professionals should not be overzealous; however, interviewers should attempt to determine what abuse occurred, who was involved, when the last abuse occurred, and where it occurred.[11] If the child becomes uncomfortable at any time, stop the interview. Children should not be further traumatized in an attempt to collect history. Always close the interview with praise for the child and reassurance that they have done nothing wrong and are not at blame for someone else's actions.

Physical Examination

Health care providers must be confident in their ability to correctly identify anatomy and detect acute injuries, nonspecific findings, scars, and healed tissue of genital trauma.[11] One study found 59% of 110 participating doctors correctly labeled the hymen.[19] Physical findings in the genital area are communicated using the face of a clock. The clitoris is always at 12 o'clock with the posterior fourchette at 6 o'clock. The area of the anus closest to the posterior fourchette is always at 12 o'clock. Tanner staging determines a child's outward sexual development and helps communicate level of sexual maturity (Box 51-4). The effect of estrogen on female genitalia is described by Huffman stages (Table 51-3).[11]

Preparing the child for medical evaluation is extremely important (Table 51-4). Give the child lots of decisions to make, such as what color of gown to wear, who they want in the examination room, and if they want to sit on the right or left side of the table. Always tell the truth and promise only what you can control. While the child is fully clothed, explain the purpose of the examination. Most experts in the

---

Box 51-4   Secondary Sex Characteristics (Tanner Stages)

Breast development

Stage I	Preadolescent; elevation of papilla only
Stage II	Breast and papilla elevated as small mound; areolar diameter increased
Stage III	Breast and areola enlarged; no contour separation
Stage IV	Areola and papilla form secondary mound
Stage V	Mature; nipple projects; areolar part of general breast contour

Note: Stages IV and V may not be distinct in some patients.

Genital development (male)

Stage I	Penis, testes, and scrotum preadolescent
Stage II	Enlargement of scrotum and testes, texture alteration; scrotal sac reddens; penis usually does not enlarge
Stage III	Further growth of testes and scrotum; penis enlarges and becomes longer
Stage IV	Continued growth of testes and scrotum; scrotum becomes darker; penis becomes longer; glans and breadth increase in size
Stage V	Genitalia adult in size and shape

Pubic hair (male and female)

Stage I	None; preadolescent
Stage II	Sparse growth of long, slightly pigmented downy hair, straight or only slightly curled, chiefly at base of penis or along labia
Stage III	Considerably darker, coarser and more curled; hair spreads sparsely over junction of pubes
Stage IV	Hair resembles adult in type; distribution still considerably smaller than in adult. No spread to medial surface of thighs.
Stage V	Adult in quantity and type with distribution of the horizontal pattern
Stage VI	Spread up linea alba: "male escutcheon"

Modified from Tanner JM: *Growth at adolescence*, ed 2, 1962, Blackwell Scientific Publications.

Table 51-3   Huffman Stages

Stage	Description
Stage 1 (0 to 2 months)	Post-neonatal regression—external genitalia is highly estrogenized due to mother's hormones; hymen pink, thick, and moist.
Stage 2 (2 months to 7 years)	Early childhood—little estrogen evident; hymen thin; wispy, lacelike vascular pattern; sticky and painful to touch.
Stage 3 (7 to 11 years)	Late childhood—estrogen increase begins; changes in hymen directly correlated to increase in estrogen; hymen begins to thicken and take on a scalloped edge.
Stage 4 (11 to 12 years)	Premenarche—rapid pubertal changes occurring; hymen thickens, is redundant, pinkish-white, and not as sensitive to touch; physiologic white discharge.

From Giardino AP, et al: *A practical guide to the evaluation of sexual abuse in the prepubertal child*, Newberry Park, Calif, 1992, Sage.

Table 51-4 **Preparing the Child for Medical Examination**

Questions/concerns	Helpful responses
Do you know why you're here today?	To make sure your body is okay. We are going to look in your eyes, ears, nose, throat, mouth, where you go tee-tee (private area), and your skin all over. (Justify why they must undress.)
What is that big machine?	That is called a colposcope or big flashlight. It helps us see little bitsy things. The camera lets us take pictures. Do you think you could take some pictures for us? (Let child use long shutter cord to take pictures.)
Explain culture collection.	We all have germs on our hands. They are also all over your body. I'm going to use a "bug-collector" (Dacron swab) to see if we can catch some germs, and if we do, let's feed them this chocolate bug food (modified Thayer-Martin culture medium for *N. gonorrhoeae*) and give them some orange bug drink (*Chlamydia* culture medium).

field use a colposcope, which allows magnification of the genital area up to 25 times, serves as an excellent light source, and is capable of photographing physical evidence. A colposcope can be frightening to a small child and should be fully explained prior to use. Demonstrate the colposcope, saline, and culture swabs. Use this time to assess the developmental, behavioral, and emotional status of the child. Allow the child as much control as possible. Let the child take pictures or hold swabs.[8,20]

When the child appears comfortable, begin with a general head-to-toe examination to deemphasize the anogenital examination and look for other medical conditions.[3] In males, the penis, testes, and scrotum are examined in the standing position. Look for urethral discharge, bleeding, swelling, bruising, or bite marks. Females are placed in the supine frog-leg position (Figure 51-1) on a pelvic table, flat examination table, or mother's lap. With legs open, identify external genitalia and assess Tanner stage of development. Assess for ecchymoses, bleeding, lacerations, or abrasion. Use gloved hands to grasp the labia majora with thumb and forefinger, and apply gentle traction in a lateral, downward, and outward motion (toward the examiner). Gentle traction can best be explained as "opening double doors so we can look where you go pee-pee and make sure everything is okay." A normal hymen can exist in many shapes and forms: crescentic, annular, septated, redundant, cribriform, or rarely imperforate. If the hymen does not visualize well, saline solution may be squirted on the hymen, and then a moist Dacron swab is used to tease the hymenal edge up for better view. If

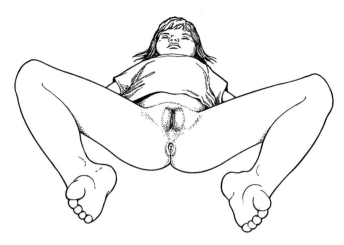

Figure **51-1**   Frog-leg position for evaluation.

the edge is still difficult to visualize, place the child in the knee-chest position. The knee-chest position is often the position in which abuse occurs and may be very uncomfortable for the child. The knee-chest position uses gravity to help redundant hymenal tissue fall downward for inspection. Assess for loss of tissue, lesions, transections, tears, notches, or bumps (Table 51-5).[24] Look for discharge or signs of foreign body. Table 51-6 depicts conditions that can be mistaken for sexual abuse.[3] Speculum examination is not required for the prepubertal child unless there is vaginal bleeding, laceration requiring suturing, or strong suspicion of a foreign body. The child should be sedated if such examination is required.

Multiple studies have shown that a high percentage of children with documented sexual abuse have no physical findings.[25] For example, oral-genital contact and fondling do not cause physical trauma.[6] The anus is made to allow large objects to easily pass with care and lubrication, so signs of abuse may not be evident. Physical findings are usually nonspecific and require a good history to determine significance. Legal and social systems are often unwilling to protect children unless evidence exists of physical trauma.[13]

Anorectal examination is performed with the child in a lateral decubitus position. Observe for rugae symmetry of verge tissue. Gently separate the buttocks and inspect for tears, fissures, bruising, or abrasions as well as sphincter tone. Holding traction can prevent blood flow from the anus, resulting in venous pooling, which can be mistaken for bruising.

Explain actions with a soft reassuring voice throughout the examination to keep children informed and to decrease anxiety. Remind children that they are in charge so if anything hurts the examiner will stop and together they will decide a different way to do things. When the examination is over, reassure them that their "bottom is okay," and then give them a chance to ask questions.

Specimen Collection

For prepubertal females, use saline-moistened Dacron swabs to obtain cultures from the vagina, pharynx, and rec-

Table **51-5**	**Classification of Sexual Abuse Physical Findings**
Category	Findings
Category 1, Normal appearing exam *Majority (60% or more) of abused children fall into this category*	Mounds, clefts, bands, septal remnants, bumps, and mild urethral dilation
Category 2, Nonspecific findings of sexual abuse *Often seen in children who have not been sexually abused*	Condylomata (children < 2 years), hymenal thickening, erythema, increased vascularity, rounding of hymenal edges, labial adhesions, narrowing of hymen, enlargement of hymenal opening, increased pigmentation, venous pooling in anus
Category 3, Specific (suspicious/highly suspicious) for sexual abuse	Hymenal/vaginal tears or scars, herpes type 2, *Chlamydia trachomatis* (outside the newborn period), reflex anal dilatation > 2 cm with no stool in the vault, hymenal attenuation (narrowing <2 mm or flat), perianal skin tags outside the midline, PID
Category 4, Conclusive of sexual abuse *For children under 12 years, as older children may be sexually active*	*Neisseria gonorrhoeae* (nonneonatal), *Treponema pallidum* (syphilis—nonneonatal), sperm, pregnancy, HIV (nonneonatal and no history to explain)

From Monteleone JA, Brouder AE: *Child maltreatment: a clinical guide and reference,* St. Louis, 1994, GW Medical Publishing.
PID, Pelvic inflammatory disease; *HIV,* human immunodeficiency virus.

Table **51-6**	**Conditions Mistaken for Sexual Abuse**
Findings	Possible causes
Genital	
Accidental trauma	Straddle injury with labia majora/minora affected; hymen unaffected
Lichen sclerosis	Dermal condition, skin is atrophic and easily traumatized; hymen not affected
Urethral prolapse	Often associated with bleeding; seen in African-American females aged 4 to 8 years old
Congenital malformations	Midline failure to fuse; along median raphe
Hemangioma	May bleed and be mistaken for trauma
Anus	
Inflammatory bowel disease	Crohn's disease may be accompanied by fissures, fistulas, tags, or abscess; usually older children and accompanied by fever, weight loss, and stooling problems
Hemorrhoids	Rare; question intra-abdominal venous congestion
Anal abscess associated with neutropenia	Possible leukemia
Perianal streptococcal infection	Painful erythematous rash

From Berkowitz CD: Child sexual abuse, *Pediatr Rev* 13(12):443, 1992.

tum for *N. gonorrhoeae* and the endocervix and rectum for *Chlamydia trachomatis.* Obtain wet prepation, KOH slide, and Gram's stain for vaginal discharge as well as viral cultures if herpes is suspected. If there is a history of penilegenital contact, obtain a serum pregnancy test. If the patient can tolerate a speculum, obtain a Pap smear.

In males, culture the urethra, rectum, and pharynx for *N. gonorrhoeae,* and the rectum and urethra (if there is a discharge) for *C. trachomatis.* Obtain a Gram's stain of any discharge from male or female victims of acute assault or where the perpetrator has a high risk for sexually transmitted diseases. Obtain hepatitis B surface antigen, VDRL or rapid plasma reagin test (repeat in 12 weeks), and HIV antibody test (repeat in 6 months). See Table 51-7 for medical management of STDs.[2]

Documentation

Child protection services rely heavily on the medical record; however, many child protective service workers admit they cannot read the writing, understand the terminology, or discern the significance of findings or lack of findings in these records. Health care providers have a responsibility to disseminate information in an understandable manner to law enforcement, child protective service workers, and the judicial system. Document findings accurately and precisely. Use quotation marks, draw pictures, and write clearly and legibly. Avoid statements like "hymen intact" or "has not been sexually abused," since they are ambiguous and children with normal examinations may have been sexually abused. Samples of documentation are provided in Figure 51-2. Opening paragraphs should describe the examination, and the last paragraph provides significance of the examination. This format communicates findings and allows

Table **51-7**	**Treatment of Sexually Transmitted Diseases**
STD	Treatment
N. gonorrhoeae	Single dose ceftriaxone 125 mg IM
Chlamydia trachomatis	Erythromycin: 2 grams/day × 7 days, **OR**
	Doxycycline (for children older than 8 years) 200 mg/day BID × 7 days, **OR**
	Azithromycin 1 gram PO single dose
Herpes genitalis	Acyclovir 1200 mg/day TID × 7-10 days
Trichomonas	Metronidazole:
	Prepubertal—15 mg/kg/day (max 250 mg) TID × 7 days
	Pubertal—2 grams PO single dose
Condyloma acuminata	May spontaneously resolve; podophyllin is often initial therapy of choice; relapses may occur
Bacterial vaginosis	Metronidazole: 1 gram/day BID PO × 7 days

Data from American Academy of Pediatrics: *1994 Red Book: Report of the Committee on Infectious Diseases,* ed 23, Elk Grove Village, Ill, 1994, The Academy.

better understanding of the medical report and facilitates more informed decisions. Monteleone[24] classified sexual abuse physical findings into categories along with their significance (Table 51-5). No "gold standard" for true significance of physical findings exists; however, this classification has approval of many experts in the field.

OTHER ISSUES RELATED TO CHILD ABUSE AND NEGLECT
Multidisciplinary Teams

Child abuse and neglect issues are complex and require the expertise of many professionals. Many hospitals and communities have adopted a multidisciplinary approach, using a core team with a health care provider (physician or nurse practitioner), social worker, and team coordinator. A consulting team may include a child psychiatrist, developmental specialist, psychologist, public health coordinator, adult psychiatrist, and attorney. Professionals who can offer opinions on a case-by-case basis include family physicians, public health nurses, child protection workers, police officers, mental health therapists, guardians ad litem, foster parents, county attorneys, and teachers.

A cooperative approach has decreased the incidence of re-abuse, serious injury, and child death while consistently ensuring that hospitals fulfill the legal mandate to report suspected abuse. Consistent use of trained experts increases case findings and reporting within the community while focusing treatment on the entire family. A team approach also provides expert collection of forensic evidence and court testimony,

ensures continuing education across disciplines, and decreases burnout for professionals in this field. An interdisciplinary approach appears to be extremely successful but does have drawbacks, such as high salaries and communication. Without effective communication among team members, there is a chance for conflict. However, strong direction and coordination can overcome these and other obstacles.[16]

Testifying for Child Abuse and Neglect Cases

Health care providers are often the first professionals who become aware of child abuse, so the quality of documentation is critical to future prosecutorial decisions. The medical record and the health care professional who examined the child will almost certainly be involved if the case goes to court. Consequently, effective communication skills are essential for charting, obtaining history, handling parents, and interacting with investigators and attorneys. Physician testimony is not considered hearsay, so doctors are allowed to testify as to what the child told them during a medical exam.[21]

If you do receive a subpoena and have never testified, contact the attorney. Find out what is expected from your testimony and discuss what you can and cannot say. If you are called as material witness, there is an expectation to "tell what you observed." An "expert" witness is required to prepare and support expert knowledge with current scientific literature.[5] The National Center for Prosecution of Child Abuse provides a hotline for more information on how to focus the examination for children who have been sexually abused (contact number is 703-739-0321).[21]

Child Death Review Teams

The past 5 years have seen an increased focus on child deaths due to abuse and neglect. The National Center on Child Abuse and Neglect found a 49% increase in reports of child death since 1985. In 1992, more than 1200 deaths from abuse were reported: over 90% of children less than 5 years and greater than 40% infants less than 1 year.[22] Children vulnerable to serious or fatal abuse are those least visible to the community, educational programs, and protective services.

Child death review teams grew from an effort to determine how and why children were dying. In 1983, a tiny infant was beaten and eventually starved to death. A Los Angeles deputy sheriff mapped over 52 contacts with 10 agencies. Investigations of drug abuse, domestic violence, reports of suspicious injuries, and drunken brawls were conducted; however, no agency knew the other was involved, and no one saw a need to remove the infant. From that meeting, a small group of professionals began to meet, share records, and make team decisions. Teams stood together, faced judges returning children to abusive settings, and started asking questions about siblings. Michael Durfee, a child psychiatrist, pressed for child death review teams across the country. Because of Durfee's efforts, most states have designated teams to review all child deaths. For more information, call Durfee at 213-240-8146.[30]

Clinic Note

NAME: Female Child   DOB: 00/00/00
MR#   000000   DOV: 00/00/00

This child was examined in the frog leg supine position. This is a Tanner stage 1 female with unestrogenized female genitalia. The labia majora and minora are well formed and without acute or chronic signs of trauma. The hymen has a crescentic orifice, with a thin velamentous border. The vestibular surface and posterior fourchette do not demonstrate any acute or chronic signs of injury. There is no abnormal degree of redness.

A

The external anal verge tissues have a symmetric rugal pattern, normal sphincter tone, normal response to traction, and no post-inflammatory pigment change.

IMPRESSION: <u>Class 1 - Normal</u> These are findings which have been noted in non-abused, prepubertal children. These physical findings do not preclude the possibility of sexual abuse.

_____   _____
Health Care Examiner   Date

_____   _____
Exam Assistant   Date

Clinic Note

NAME: Female Child   DOB: 00/00/00
MR#   000000   DOV: 00/00/00

This child was examined in the frog leg supine position. This is a Tanner stage 1-2 female with unestrogenized female genitalia. The labia majora and labia minora are well formed and without acute signs of trauma. Posterior labial adhesions are present. The hymen is poorly visualized due to the labial adhesions. The vestibular surface and posterior fourchette do not demonstrate any acute or chronic signs of injury. There is no abnormal degree of redness. We did not obtain cultures at this time.

B

IMPRESSION: <u>Class 2 - Nonspecific</u> Labial Adhesions - These findings are nonspecific and may be seen in both abused and non-abused children. We prescribed premarin cream and will re-examine this child in approximately one month.

_____   _____
Health Care Examiner   Date

_____   _____
Exam Assistant   Date

Clinic Note

NAME: Female Child   DOB: 00/00/00
MR#   000000   DOV: 00/00/00

This child was examined in the frog leg supine position. This is a Tanner stage 1 female with unestrogenized female genitalia. The labia majora and minora are well formed and without acute or chronic signs of trauma. The hymen has a crescentic orifice, with a thin velamentous border. There are intravaginal ridges at 3, 4, and 6 o'clock. The area of hymen adjacent to the intravaginal ridge at 6 o'clock has a diameter which is less than 1 mm. This does not appear to be a deformation associated with the intravaginal ridge. The vestibular surface and posterior fourchette do not demonstrate any acute or chronic signs of injury. There is no abnormal degree of redness.

C

The external anal verge tissues have a symmetric rugal pattern, normal sphincter tone, normal response to traction, and no post-inflammatory pigment change.

IMPRESSION: <u>Class 3 - Specific for Sexual Abuse</u>
There is a minimal amount of hymenal tissue adjacent to the intravaginal ridge at 6 o'clock. This is abnormal and suggestive of penetrating injury.

_____   _____
Health Care Examiner   Date

_____   _____
Exam Assistant   Date

Clinic Note

NAME: Female Child   DOB: 00/00/00
MR#   000000   DOV: 00/00/00

This child was examined in the frog leg supine position. This is a Tanner stage 1 female with unestrogenized female genitalia. The labia majora and minora are well formed and without acute or chronic signs of trauma. The hymen has a crescentic orifice, with a thin velamentous border. There is a complete transection of the hymen at 5:30. This extends to the vaginal floor, and no hymenal tissue is present in this area. The vestibular surface and posterior fourchette do not demonstrate any acute or chronic signs of injury. There is no abnormal degree of redness. Microscopic exam of wet prep found sperm to be present.

D

The external anal verge tissues have a symmetric rugal pattern, normal sphincter tone, normal response to traction, and no post-inflammatory pigment change. A small fissure is present at 12 o'clock.

IMPRESSION: <u>Class 4 - Conclusive of Sexual Abuse</u>
These findings are diagnostic of blunt force penetrating trauma to the hymen. The most common cause of this type of blunt force penetrating trauma in pre-pubertal girls is sexual abuse. The small anal fissure is a nonspecific finding and may or may not be associated with sexual abuse.

_____   _____
Health Care Examiner   Date

_____   _____
Exam Assistant   Date

Figure **51-2** Documentation samples. **A,** Class 1—normal. **B,** Class 2—nonspecific. **C,** Class 3—specific for sexual abuse. **D,** Class 4—conclusive of sexual abuse.

Prevention

Precursors to physical maltreatment include excessive parental physical discipline, failure to provide basic necessities such as food and a safe home, and unobtainable goals set by parents. Programs for prevention of child abuse and neglect typically focus on physical abuse, centering on the parent, parenting skills, and damaging practices. Pilot programs such as home visiting and increased public awareness have decreased physical abuse of children in some areas. Changing attitudes and modifying behaviors require 6 to 12 months. To successfully reduce physical abuse and neglect within diverse populations, preventive services should begin before or shortly after birth of the first child to support effective child-rearing skills.[6] Prevention efforts should tie the child's developmental level to parent enhancement education. Parents must observe and be able to model desired parental behaviors. Child safety can depend on the parent's ability to take advantage of social programs and obtain assistance as needed. All prevention programs must recognize and accept cultural differences.

Sexual abuse prevention focuses on the child. The child is given the responsibility for saying "no." Classroom education teaches "good touches" and "bad touches" and who to tell if someone tries to hurt you. But what if the abuser is mom or dad? Sexual abuse is convoluted; secrecy is a large component of manipulation. Effective prevention programs should stress community involvement, self-confidence, and the child's cognitive abilities.[6]

SUMMARY

Child abuse and neglect are complex, life-threatening situations. Medical professionals who work with children must speak out for abused children. No one agency or discipline can be solely responsible for protection of children. The community, law enforcement, child protection workers, mental health counselors, legislators, educators, health care providers, and the judicial system must work together to remove barriers to identification, treatment, and prevention of child abuse and neglect.

REFERENCES

1. Abel G et al: Self reported sex crimes of nonincarcerated paraphiliacs, *J Interpersonal Violence* 2:3, 1987.
2. American Academy of Pediatrics: *1994 Red Book: Report of the Committee on Infectious Diseases,* ed 23, Elk Grove Village, Ill, 1994, American Academy of Pediatrics.
3. Berkowitz CD: Child sexual abuse, *Pediatr Rev* 13(12):443, 1992.
4. Berkowitz CD: *Pediatrics: a primary care approach,* Philadelphia, 1996, WB Saunders.
5. Berliner L, Roe RJ: Tips for experts when testifying, *National resource center on child sexual abuse* 4(5):3, 1992.
6. Briere J et al, editors: *The APSAC handbook on child maltreatment,* London, 1996, Sage.
7. CHIPS: *Children's hospital intervention and preventions services,* Birmingham, Ala, 1996.
8. Coody D, et al: Shaken baby syndrome: identification and prevention for nurse practitioners, *J Pediatr Health Care* 8:50, 1994.
9. De Jong AR, Hervada AR, Emmett GA: Epidemiologic variations in child sexual abuse, *Child Abuse Neglect* 7:155, 1983.
10. For Kids Sake: *A child abuse prevention and reporting kit,* rev ed, Oklahoma City, 1992, Oklahoma State Department of Health.
11. Giardino AP et al: *A practical guide to the evaluation of sexual abuse in the prepubertal child,* Newberry Park, Calif, 1992, Sage.
12. Grant LJ: Assessment of child sexual abuse: eighteen months experience at the child protection center, *Am J Obstet Gynecol* 148:617, 1984.
13. Heger A, Emans SJ: *Evaluation of the sexually abused child: a medical textbook and photographic atlas,* New York, 1992, Oxford.
14. Hyden PW, Gallagher TA: Child abuse intervention in the emergency room, *Pediatr Clin North Am* 39(5):1053, 1992.
15. Kahn M, Sexton M: Sexual abuse of young children, *Clin Pediatr* 22:369, 1983.
16. Krugman RD: The multidisciplinary treatment of abusive and neglectful families, *Pediatr Ann* 13(10):761, 1984.
17. Krugman RD: Recognition of sexual abuse in children, *Pediatr Rev* 8:25, 1986.
18. Krugman RD: Child abuse and neglect: critical first steps in response to a national emergency. The report of the US advisory board on child abuse and neglect, *Am J Dis Child,* 145:513, 1991.
19. Ladson S, Johnson CF, Soty RE: Do physicians recognize sexual abuse? *Am J Dis Child* 141:411, 1987.
20. Levitt CJ: Medical evaluation of the sexually abused child, *Family Violence Abusive Relation* 20(2):343, 1993.
21. Marx SP, DeJong A: When you suspect sexual abuse, *Pediatr Manage* 3:24, 1994.
22. McClain PW et al: Geographic patterns of fatal abuse or neglect in children younger than 5 years old, United States, 1979 to 1988, *Arch Pediatr Adolesc Med* 148(1):82, 1994.
23. McCurdy K, Daro D: Current trends in child abuse reporting and fatalities, *J Interpersonal Violence* 9(4):75, 1994.
24. Monteleone JA, Brodeur AE: *Child maltreatment: a clinical guide and reference,* St. Louis, 1994, GW Medical Publishing.
25. Muram D: Child sexual abuse: relationship between sexual acts and genital findings, *Child Abuse Neglect* 13:211, 1989.
26. Myers JEB: Role of physician in preserving verbal evidence of child abuse, *J Pediatr* 109:409, 1986.
27. National Committee to Prevent Child Abuse: *1995 child abuse report,* Chicago, 1996, NCPCA.
28. Orr DP: Limitations of emergency room evaluations of sexually abused children, *Am J Dis Child* 132:873, 1978.
29. Ricci LR: Child sexual abuse: the emergency department response, *Ann Emerg Med* 15:711, 1986.
30. Stewart J: They have the world's worst job, *Los Angeles Times Magazine,* p 9, July 16, 1995.

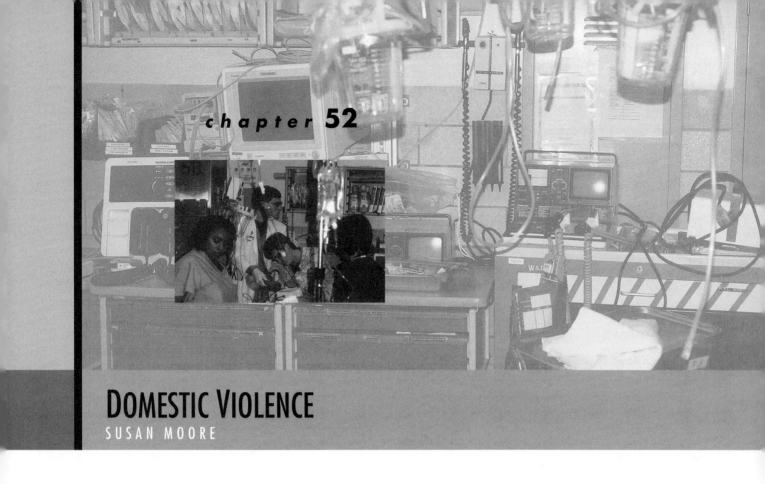

chapter**52**

DOMESTIC VIOLENCE

SUSAN MOORE

Domestic violence is a term that refers to violence within a household. The term encompasses child abuse, sexual abuse, and elder abuse; however, it is used primarily as a reference to partner or spouse abuse. *Partner abuse* is defined as the use of physical force in intimate relationships among adults.[6] Legally, domestic abuse includes various nonphysical actions in addition to actual physical violence. Most state laws define specific acts that constitute domestic violence (Box 52-1). Victims of partner abuse in heterosexual relationships are almost always female. The defining factor in these relationships is fear. While women may strike men or threaten them in some way, rarely is the man afraid of the woman. Women who live with chronic partner abuse live in chronic fear. The focus of this chapter is spousal or partner abuse. Sexual assault is discussed in more detail in Chapter 56, child abuse in Chapter 51, and elder abuse in Chapter 53.

HISTORY

The United States has a violent history. The pioneer fought for his family, protecting his wife and children. Until recently, laws implied that a man owned his family. The wife and children were his possessions, and what he did with them was a private matter. He protected his family; therefore, the family should be grateful and subservient.

Our society has a high tolerance for violence. This is dramatically illustrated in a multitude of violent scenes on television and in the movies. Acceptance of certain forms of violent behavior is ingrained in the American value system.[22]

Cultural beliefs that lead to partner abuse do exist in the United States today. Many men and women believe a woman should be subservient to a man. They may believe the man suffers so much stress in his work life or from various personal events that he is justified in "taking it out" on his wife. Many are unwilling to invade the privacy of the home, even though what occurs is against the law.

Only in the past few years has domestic violence become a societal issue. Sadly, many people still do not believe that it is a problem. A number of judges continue to sentence men to "a slap on the wrist" for beating their wives. Many people, men and women, blame the victim, by believing she did something to warrant the abuse or by asking, "Well, why doesn't she just leave?"

INCIDENCE

An estimate of the number of domestic violence incidents is difficult because many are never reported. Domestic violence is one of the most underreported crimes in the United States.[8] What is known is that 2000 to 4000 women die each year at the hands of men who say they love them.[4] More women die from domestic violence than automobile crashes, rapes, and muggings combined.[4] Most women are not killed by strangers. At every age in the life span, females are more likely to be sexually or physically assaulted by their father, brother, family member, neighbor, boyfriend, husband, partner, or ex-partner than by a stranger or anonymous assailant. Warning signs include increasing violence, substance abuse,

Box **52-1** **Acts of Domestic Violence**[17]

Battery or actual physical violence

Assault or the threat of violence

Compelling the other person by force or threat of force to perform an act from which he or she has a right to refrain or to refrain from an act that he or she has a right to perform

Sexual assault

Knowing, purposeful, or reckless course of conduct to harass the other

False imprisonment

Unlawful entry of the other's residence, or forcible entry against the other's will if there is a reasonable, foreseeable risk of harm to the other from the entry

Box **52-2** **Reasons Women Remain in an Abusive Situation**[4]

When a woman leaves, she leaves her house, neighbors, and frequently her friends because they are probably also his friends. If the abuser has behaved in a typical manner, he has narrowed her circle of friends to those he considers acceptable, who will not accept her if she leaves.

If she has children, her husband, even though convicted of spouse abuse, can gain custody of the children. He is often the one with a job and the house and is frequently very charming in court. If the woman leaves her children with the abuser, he may turn his anger toward them, and she will not be there to protect them.

The victim's family may not support her decision. Because of religious beliefs, they may insist she stay and make the marriage work. More commonly, they do not want to be in a position where they have to support and protect her. Family members may simply not believe her.

She loves the abuser. Typically, after an explosive episode of abuse, the perpetrator is repentant and treats the victim very kindly. She finds herself forgiving him and believing him when he says it will not happen again.

The abuser becomes more violent if she threatens to leave or actually does so. Most murders related to domestic abuse happen after the partner has tried to leave the relationship. Some abusers do not become physically violent until the victim leaves; then he begins stalking her. As many as half of all batterers threaten to retaliate, and more than 30% inflict further assaults while they are under prosecution.

and a family history of violence. Intrafamily homicide generally occurs after previous assaults have been reported.[10]

Surveys of women who visit emergency departments (EDs) show quite a range in the incidence of domestic violence. Studies show that 6% to 28% of women who visit EDs have suffered some form of partner abuse. The number of women currently in abusive relationships is 11% to 14%.* Between 1% and 6% of women who come to EDs present with complaints directly related to domestic violence.[1,4,12]

THE VICTIM

The question health care providers ask most frequently is "Why does she stay?" The most common reasons why a woman stays are described in Box 52-2. The victim lives every day with a degree of fear. After years of such conditions, self-esteem suffers, and the woman develops a "learned helplessness." The woman may reach a point where saving herself or her children is no longer conceivable. Fortunately, most women do not get to that point; many do eventually leave.

Signs Indicating a Woman Is Ready to Leave

Women who fight back during the assault and those who develop a consistently uncaring attitude toward their partners are more likely to leave. As with quitting an addiction, the victim rehearses many times before she is successful. She may experiment, packing up and leaving while her spouse is at work, only to return and put everything away before he returns home. She may actually move out of the home several times, only to return when the abuser apologizes and begs her to return or threatens increased violence toward her or her children.

Not all victims are pleasant people who easily gain our feelings of pity. Many are substance abusers, who can be hostile toward emergency staff and their significant others.

They may have come to the relationship with personality disorders or developed them in the fearful environment. The bottom line, however, is that no one deserves to be hit. Every victim of domestic violence deserves information that can help her save herself.

THE BATTERER

The abuser creates a web of power and possessiveness. His response to challenge or disappointment is to blame someone else[4]: if he is driven to beat his partner, she made him do it through her thoughtlessness, infidelity, sloppiness, stupidity, or any other negative descriptor. If the batterer does enter therapy, he may spend his first sessions explaining why his partner made him abuse her.

Counseling is not enormously effective. More than 25% of convicted batterers engage in physical violence within 1 or 2 years of counseling.[16] Arrest does stop the violence, at least while the batterer is incarcerated. Some batterers say that arrest is what finally caught their attention.

The typical picture of an abuser is the man who will not allow his wife to answer any questions in the ED and will not allow her to be alone with a nurse. The batterer may also be very charming toward nursing staff and appear very com-

*References 1, 3, 4, 11, 12, 20.

passionate toward his spouse. He may communicate his control to the spouse with very subtle gestures and expressions that only the victim, after years of living in fear, can perceive.

Alcohol and other drugs of abuse play a large role in domestic violence. In some cases, both partners may be substance abusers. Alcohol eliminates inhibitions. A person inclined to violence finds it easier to commit aggressive acts while intoxicated. Methamphetamines and, to a lesser degree, cocaine can alter thought processes and cause paranoia, which may be aimed at the partner. Despite this, mind-altering substances are not an excuse for violent behavior. There are many people who use drugs who do not beat their spouses. The tendency for violence must already exist.

Spouse abuse is not a disease or addiction. The batterer abuses because he thinks he has the right to do so and because he can get away with it.[4] He must first see the need to change his behavior and then learn alternative ways to deal with frustration.

THE ROLE OF THE EMERGENCY NURSE

A large number of patients are in violent relationships; therefore, the emergency nurse must have a high index of suspicion and be alert for physical and behavioral clues. Which patients are most at risk for partner abuse? Though domestic violence can happen in any household, higher rates of physical violence were reported by women who had fewer than 12 years of education, lived in crowded conditions, participated in the Special Supplemental Food program for Women, Infants, and Children, received delayed or no prenatal care, were of races other than white, were under 20 years old, or were not married.[22] Domestic violence is associated with poverty and unemployment. Violence is more prevalent in relationships between people who believe in the traditional roles of women and among partners who abuse drugs, including alcohol.[5]

Many women do not experience physical violence in a relationship until they become pregnant. The unborn child may be perceived as a threat to the abuser, as someone coming between the partners who takes away the woman's attention. Many spontaneous abortions and preterm deliveries are related to physical abuse.

Women in violent relationships may come to the ED with complaints related to depression or gastrointestinal disorders. All "frequent flyer" patients should be viewed through a filter of domestic violence. They may be using the ED as an escape from the home or may unconsciously develop physical complaints as legitimate reasons for requesting help.

Many behavioral clues related to domestic violence are the same as those for child abuse. The patient may wait several hours or days before seeking help for her injuries. She may hope to avoid embarrassment or the need to lie about her injuries, or the perpetrator may prevent her from leaving home. The patient may have a history of several old injuries,

telling the nurse that she is clumsy or stupid and frequently falls or bumps into things. She may bypass closer EDs so personnel do not get suspicious of her frequent visits. The given mechanism of injury may not fit physical findings.

Physical Findings Related to Battery

As with child abuse, the victim may have bruises, fractures, and other injuries in various stages of healing. Most victims of domestic violence do not present for treatment of their injuries. The emergency nurse must be alert for injuries unrelated to the chief complaint. Box 52-3 describes injuries suggestive of domestic violence.

The first step in assessment of a case of domestic violence is acknowledgment that it actually occurs. Many nurses are uncomfortable asking about domestic violence and fear invading the patient's privacy or offending the patient. Surveys of patients in violent relationships and those not in violent relationships show that most patients are grateful to health care providers who inquire about violence and abuse in relationships and do not consider this line of inquiry offensive or intrusive.[2]

Privacy is essential for the patient interview. Questions should not be asked in a public place, such as a centrally located triage desk or the waiting room. The patient should not be questioned in the presence of a possible abuser. Separating the victim from the abuser may be difficult, since neither the patient nor the partner may be willing to part. Sending the patient to the radiology department for x-rays may be the only opportunity to separate them, since you can explain that visitors cannot be exposed to unnecessary radiation. The patient may then be approached while in the x-ray room.

If a patient presents with a chief complaint of battery, the first pieces of information to obtain are the current location of the batterer, whether he has access to a weapon, and whether he is under the influence of drugs or alcohol. Ask if law enforcement personnel have been notified and if the

---

Box 52-3 **Injuries Suggesting Domestic Violence**[5,18]

Bruises or fractures of the ulnar surfaces of the forearms and fingers, sustained when the victim holds up her arms to protect her face

Injuries to various planes of the body; falls are likely to injure one side or the other

Injuries to the face, neck, throat, chest, abdomen, or genitals; a sober person tends to protect these areas in a fall, whereas perpetrators tend to aim for these areas

Injuries that show the shape or pattern of a specific instrument that is used as a weapon

Punch or kick injuries to the pregnant abdomen

Clumps of hair pulled from the scalp

Dental and mandibular fractures

abuser has been apprehended. If the abuser is not in custody, determine if he knows that the patient was coming to the ED. It is important to maintain safety for the patient, nurse, and others in the ED. If it is possible that the perpetrator will follow the victim, notify security, and move the patient to a safe place.

Most patients in violent relationships will not present with partner abuse as their chief complaint. The emergency nurse may become suspicious because of physical and behavioral findings. These findings should be the basis for a more focused assessment. Suggested questions include "I notice you have bruises on your face. Has someone hit you?" or "Your husband seems very anxious. Did he hurt you?" As with all patient communication, the emergency nurse should assess the patient's level of education, trust, sobriety, and anxiety and then plan the approach accordingly.

Most patients who do not say they have been battered will deny it when asked. If the patient does deny it or becomes angry, the emergency nurse should let the patient know that the door is always open and that if the patient changes her mind she can always return to the ED for help.

Provide the patient with information about domestic violence resources in the community. Local domestic violence support groups can provide a great deal of information for emergency nurses. If local groups are not available, two national organizations (Box 52-4) can provide information regarding state and local resources, as well as posters and leaflets for the ED.

Most patients are aware that battering one's partner is against the law. They may not be aware that more subtle acts such as threats of bodily harm, false imprisonment, harassment, or forcing someone to perform acts against her will are also against the law. Frequently, discussion of these issues is the first step in providing the patient information on domestic violence.

The patient should be given a phone number she can call 24 hours a day to get help. The nurse may offer pamphlets or cards with phone numbers. Patients may refuse cards or phone numbers because it may not be safe to bring home material that deals with domestic violence. If the patient will not take any material, give her the number of the ED or the name of a local domestic violence organization that she can look up in the phone book.

Reassure the patient that she is not to blame for the battering. Many patients assume they have done something to incite the beating and are sure they can prevent further beatings if they simply behave in the appropriate manner. This is absolutely untrue. Studies have not identified any behaviors of the wife that can stop domestic violence.[14] The pattern of abuse will continue until an outside intervention stops it.

If the patient is receptive, discuss the effect partner abuse has on children. Many women may not be motivated to leave for themselves but may be willing to leave for the sake of their children. Much research has shown that violence travels in family lines. If children witness abuse or are victims of abuse, they are much more likely to become abusers.[9,24] Partner abusers are frequently child and animal abusers. If the abuser is not already hitting the children, chances are very good that he will soon do so.

The best place to display posters and provide pamphlets on domestic violence is in the treatment room.[19] The waiting room is too public, and the victim may have to walk in front of several people, including the perpetrator, to get the information. Treatment rooms provide the patient a chance to read a pamphlet in private, even if she is not able to take it home.

Once the patient decides to seek treatment for her injuries, the next decision she faces is whether to report the crime. In a few states, reporting is mandatory. Be sure you tell the patient that the crime will be reported. If the choice belongs to the patient, the emergency nurse can help the patient decide whether to report the crime by discussing the consequences if it is reported and if it is not.

Rarely does a patient immediately decide to leave the batterer. This is one of the most common reasons nurses give for not getting involved. When intervening in domestic violence, the nurse must not use the "did she leave him" factor as a determinant of effectiveness. Most patients do not leave after the first few episodes. Years later, the patient may use the information the nurse provided. Survivors report that simple acknowledgment and a nonjudgmental attitude helped them enormously in the emergency setting.

If the patient has decided not to go home, the nurse should help her explore resources. Most shelters do not automatically accept all comers if they have safe alternatives. Does the patient have relatives or friends who will accept her? Does she have financial resources for traveling to friends or relatives out of town? Are there children still at home who must be protected?

The immediate plan usually involves protection for the patient and her children. Once the patient has formed a plan, she needs access to a phone to implement it. Long-term needs center around legal assistance, employment, and housing.[23] The ED is not the best place to make plans for meeting these needs.

If the patient decides to return home, the nurse can help her make an emergency action plan. Encourage her to pack a suitcase with the essential items for rapid escape (Box 52-5). The suitcase should be kept at a neighbor's or relative's home. Make sure the patient does not keep it at her house, where the batterer can find it.

Box **52-4**	**National Resources on Domestic Violence**
National Resource Center on Domestic Violence	(800) 537-2238
Health Resource Center on Domestic Violence	(800) 313-1310

LEGAL ISSUES

Mandatory reporting laws specifically for domestic violence have been enacted in just a few states. There is a great deal of controversy associated with mandatory reporting. Many advocates for victims of domestic violence do not want mandatory reporting because they fear that mandatory reporting will deter visits to the ED for necessary medical care. The first question many victims of domestic violence ask is "Will you have to call the police?" At the least, victims want to avoid the shame. At the worst, victims are placed at risk for retribution.[13]

Supporters of mandatory reporting feel that domestic violence is a crime, like child abuse, and that perpetrators should be dealt with like other violent criminals. They feel mandatory reporting can relieve the victim from the onus of reporting. The victim has no choice; therefore, she cannot be blamed.

Many episodes of domestic violence are already reported, even in states with no mandatory reporting law. Unfortunately, these are usually the most serious episodes, since all states require reporting any injuries secondary to firearms, knives, or other weapons as well as "grave injuries" incurred as a result of criminal acts.

A controversial area of law surrounds the ED's responsibility to protect the patient. Should a victim, even at her request, be discharged home when emergency care providers know that domestic violence, in most cases, escalates and therefore the patient may be in serious danger? Unfortunately, there is no clear answer to this dilemma.

Patients in abusive situations who present with communicable diseases that must be reported to the health department may be put in danger when the health department contacts her partner(s).[21] The patient should always be told when a reportable disease has been diagnosed, so she can take protective action, if necessary.

If they decide to leave, most victims should obtain civil protective orders.[15] Local domestic violence organizations are usually well informed regarding the process and can help the woman through the legal steps. Protection orders in themselves tend to be fairly useless, since they are difficult to enforce and batterers routinely ignore them. Their most effective use is in court. If a victim can show her abuser violated a protective order, she has a better case against him.

Documentation on the medical record can be very helpful to a victim when it can be used as evidence in court. The nurse who practices in a state with mandatory reporting must report any documented suspicions. Documentation should note that the crime was reported to the appropriate law enforcement authority.

The nurse who practices in a state where there is no mandatory reporting of domestic violence is still free to chart any suspicions. Documentation should include that the patient was asked if she wanted to report the crime and what the patient said in reply. Even if a patient denies physical abuse, the nurse should chart findings and the suspicion that the findings do not fit the history and may indicate battery. If the victim changes her mind later, a chart in evidence that says her injuries indicated abuse will go a long way to help her case.

The nurse should also document any referrals or resources given to the patient and the patient's reaction to the information.

SUMMARY

Domestic violence is prevalent in today's society and is frequently seen in the ED. About 15% of all female patients seen in the ED are in abusive relationships. Emergency nurses have an obligation to provide these patients useful information should they decide to leave the relationship at that time or later. Most patients do not immediately leave. Patients are best served by acknowledging the problem and supporting their decisions in a nonjudgmental manner.

REFERENCES

1. Abbott J, et al: Domestic violence against women: incidence and prevalence in an emergency department population, *JAMA* 273 (22):1763, 1995.
2. Alpert EJ: Violence in intimate relationships and the practicing internist: new "disease" or new agenda? *Ann Intern Med* 123(10): 775, 1995.
3. Bates L, et al: Domestic violence experienced by women attending an accident and emergency department, *Aust J Public Health* 19(3): 293, 1995.
4. Bicehouse T, Hawker L: Domestic violence: myths and safety issues, *J Holistic Nurs* 13(1):83, 1995.
5. Butler MJ: Domestic violence: a nursing imperative, *J Holistic Nurs* 13(1):54, 1995.
6. Campbell JC, Harris MJ, Lee RK: Violence research: an overview, *Scholarly Inquiry Nurs Practice* 9(2):105, 1995.
7. Chez N: Helping the victim of domestic violence, *AJN* 94(7):32, 1994.
8. Denham S: Confronting the monster of family violence, *Nurs Forum* 30(3):12, 1995.
9. Dutton DG, Golant S: *The batterer: a psychological profile*, New York, 1995, Basic Books.
10. From public health to personal health: violence against women across the life span, *Ann Intern Med* 123(10):800, 1995 (editorial).
11. Gin NE, et al: Prevalence of domestic violence among patients in three ambulatory care internal medicine clinics, *J Gen Intern Med* 6(4): 317, 1991.
12. Grunfeld AF, et al: Detecting domestic violence against women in the emergency department: a nursing triage model, *J Emerg Nurs* 20(4):271, 1994.

13. Hyman A, Schillinger D, Lo B: Laws mandating reporting of domestic violence: do they promote patient well-being? *JAMA* 273(22): 1781, 1995.

14. Jacobsen NS, et al: Affect, verbal content, and psychophysiology in the arguments of couples with a violent husband, *J Consult Clin Psychol* 62(5):982, 1994.

15. Keilitz SL: Civil protection orders: a viable justice system tool for deterring domestic violence, *Violence Victim* 9(1):79, 1994.

16. Murphy CM: Treating perpetrators of adult domestic violence, *Md Med J* 43(10):877, 1994.

17. Nevada *Revised Statutes* 33.018.

18. Nevada State Council of the Emergency Nurses Association, Nevada Office of the Attorney General, and the Nevada Network Against Domestic Violence: *Suggested health care protocols for assisting victims of domestic violence in Nevada,* 1994.

19. Randall T: Tools available for health care providers whose patients are at risk for domestic violence, *JAMA* 266(9):1179, 1991.

20. Roberts GL, et al: Domestic violence victims in a hospital emergency department, *Med J Aust* 159(5):307, 1993.

21. Rothenberg KH, et al: Domestic violence and partner notification: implications for treatment and counseling of women with HIV, *J Am Med Women's Assoc* 50(3-4):87, 1995.

22. Sigler RT: The cost of tolerance for violence, *J Health Care Poor Underserved* 6(2):124, 1995.

23. Sullivan CM, et al: After the crisis: a needs assessment of women leaving a domestic violence shelter, *Violence Victim* 7(3):267, 1992.

24. Wolfe DA, Korsch B: Witnessing domestic violence during childhood and adolescence: implication for pediatric practice, *Pediatrics* 94(4):594, 1994.

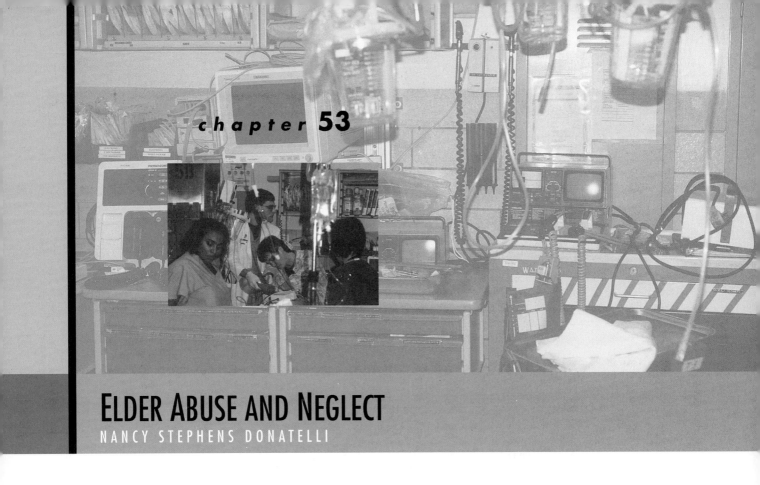

chapter 53

ELDER ABUSE AND NEGLECT

NANCY STEPHENS DONATELLI

Elder abuse and neglect take different forms. However, the common denominator is harm or threatened harm to the health or welfare of the elderly. Abuse and neglect of the elderly have increased steadily as the number of older adults requiring care has increased. Caregivers for this group are sandwiched between careers, families, and changing health care insurance that does not provide custodial care. Abuse is found among all racial, ethnic, and socioeconomic backgrounds. Women are victims more often than men.

The incidence of elder abuse in the United States is reported to be between 4% and 10%, or 1.5 to 3.2 million abused individuals.[3] Between 1980 and 1985, the number of people 65 years and older increased from 25 million to 28 million, and the cases of elder abuse increased by 100,000 per year.[4] Researchers estimate that by 2020 the number of elderly people in the United States will exceed 64 million.[4] The life span of the average American is increasing, whereas the U.S. birth rate has declined. More people require care, and fewer people are available to provide care; therefore elder abuse is expected to increase at an alarming rate.

Elder abuse and neglect have been defined by the American Medical Association as "actions or the omission of actions that result in harm or threatened harm to the health or welfare of the elderly."[5] Five primary categories of elder mistreatment—physical abuse, neglect, psychologic abuse, violation of personal rights, and financial abuse—are described in Table 53-1.

Obtaining a clear, accurate picture of demographics surrounding elder abuse is difficult. There is significant shame and embarrassment associated with this problem, so abused individuals may keep the problem within the family to decrease further embarrassment. Abuse is found among people of all racial, ethnic, and socioeconomic backgrounds. Most studies show that women are more likely than men to be victims of elder abuse. Female victims tend to suffer abuse at the hands of their children, whereas men suffer neglect from their wives.[3] Box 53-1 describes risk factors associated with elder abuse.

ORIGIN OF THE PROBLEM

Four main theories may explain elder abuse: role theory, transgenerational theory, psychopathology theory, and stressed caregiver theory.

Role Theory

As the parent ages and becomes more childlike, the child must assume a parental role. The elder who once helped the child must now take orders from that child. The psychologic impact of this role reversal is significant for both generations. When role conflicts are present, the potential for abuse increases substantially.[6]

Transgenerational Theory

The underlying philosophy of transgenerational theory is that violence is a learned behavior. If a child grows up in a

Table 53-1	Primary Categories of Elder Mistreatment
Category	Description
Physical abuse	Pain, injury, and/or physical confinement; an act of violence that results in bodily harm or mental distress; includes sexual abuse
Neglect	The most common form of abuse[4]; deliberate refusal to meet basic needs; withholding assistance vital to performance of activities of daily living or behavior that causes mental anguish
Psychologic abuse	Verbal aggression, intimidation, and humiliation; threats to deprive the elder of property or services, place in a nursing home, or remove financial support; unreasonable demands; deliberately ignoring the person
Violation of personal rights	Deprivation of inalienable rights, i.e., personal liberty, personal property, free speech, privacy, and/or voting
Financial abuse	Unauthorized use of money and/or goods for personal gain; includes petty theft or declaration of the elder as incompetent to confiscate property; failure to pay bills

Box 53-1	Risk Factors Associated With Elder Abuse

Advanced age
Greater dependency on the caregiver increases the risk for abuse
Alcohol abuse in the elder or caregiver
Child abuse by the parent may lead to a role reversal where the child now abuses the parent
Past history of abuse is a great risk for future abuse in the same setting
Caregiver inexperience
Economic stress
Caregiver mental illness
Caregiver stress from effects of "the sandwich generation," i.e., being squeezed between demands of dependent parents and dependent children
Lack of support systems or practical help for the caregiver
Sudden, unwanted, or unexpected dependency of the elder on the caregiver
Cramped living conditions

family where aggressive behavior is a part of life, the child exhibits similar behavior. If the parent abused the child, then the child as the caregiver abuses the parent in retribution.

Psychopathology Theory

Altered impulse control caused by psychologic problems such as mental illness or drug or alcohol dependence places the elder at greater risk for abuse. The typical abuser is a middle-aged, white woman who lives with the victim, is an alcohol or drug addict, and has long-term financial problems and high stress levels. The abuser perceives the victim as the source of this stress.[4]

Stressed Caregiver Theory

This is one area where the nurse providing long-term care for the elderly can abuse the elderly as easily as the family caregiver. Caregivers under stress have limited amounts of internal resources. Stress associated with the health care environment as well as stress in the individual's personal and family life may lead the caregiver to express stress through mistreatment of the elderly. Women may also find themselves in the caretaker role for their spouse's parents.

SIGNS AND SYMPTOMS

Abuse of the elderly occurs slightly less often than child abuse; however, it is important for the emergency nurse to

remember that despite rising concerns about elder abuse, there are no uniform comprehensive definitions of the term. Identification of elder abuse is easy only in cases where outright battering is visible.[1]

Elder abuse cannot be assessed quickly or easily from a cluster of signs and vague presenting symptoms. Keen awareness when performing the physical examination is essential to identify elder abuse. Potential indicators of abuse are described in Box 53-2.[1]

Each category of abuse or neglect is associated with distinct diagnostic and clinical findings (Table 53-2). The typical victim is a white woman over 75 years old who lives with a relative and has a physical or mental impairment.[1] The elder person's history should be obtained from several sources whenever possible. Interactions between the caregiver and the elder should be carefully observed. The patient may be fearful or agitated in the presence of the caregiver or may appear passive and compliant. The caregiver may use harsh words and tone when speaking to the patient or say demeaning things to the elder. Assess the patient's mental status carefully.

When assessing the patient, observe carefully for signs of malnourishment. Note the presence of old and new bruises. Bruises on both the upper arms may indicate the patient has been held tightly and shaken. Bruises on the trunk suggest beating with fists. Bruises on the wrists or ankles occur when the patient has been tied down. Cigarette burns on the skin may be present. Old, healed burns appear as skin discoloration. Alopecia secondary to repeated pulling and tugging of the person's hair is another significant finding. Blows to the eyes can cause dislocation of the lens, subconjunctival hemorrhage, or retinal detachment. Whiplash injuries are seen after repeated, violent shaking. Consider the possibility of sexual abuse. Difficulty walking or sitting may be a subtle sign, whereas bruises or lacerations of the inner thighs or genitalia are more overt signs. Pain or itching in the genital area may indicate a sexually transmitted disease.

Box 53-2   Clues to Elder Abuse

Pattern of "health care shopping"
Series of missed appointments
Previous unexplained injuries
Presence of old and new bruises
Poor personal hygiene
Sexually transmitted diseases
Extreme mood changes
Depression
Fearfulness
Excessive concern with health care cost

Table 53-2   Clinical Findings with Elder Abuse

Type of abuse	Clinical findings
Physical	Bruises, welts, lacerations, fractures, burns, rope marks; medication overdose, inadequate medication; unexplained venereal disease or genital infection
Neglect	Dehydration, malnutrition, decubitus ulcers, poor personal hygiene, lack of compliance with medication regimens
Psychologic abuse	Berated verbally, harassed, intimidated, threatened punishment or deprivation; elder treated like an infant; isolated from family, friends, or activities
Psychologic neglect	Elder left alone for long periods; ignored or given the silent treatment; failure to provide companionship, changes in routine, news, or information
Financial or material abuse	Denial of a home for the elder; stolen money or possessions; coercion of the elder to sign contracts, assign durable power of attorney, purchase goods, or change the elder's will
Financial or material neglect	Lack of substantial care in the home despite adequate financial resources; patient confused about or unaware of financial situation or suddenly transfers assets to a family member

INTERVENTION

Access is a major issue in assessment and intervention of alleged abuse or neglect of the elderly. The competent elder has the right to make his or her own personal care decisions. The elder may choose to stay in the abusive situation despite all efforts to effect a change. Victims of abuse often have both positive and negative feelings toward their abusers. Such ambivalence makes separation from the abuser difficult for the abuse victim.[7]

The Older Americans Act of 1965 and the 1987 Amendment required each state to identify agencies involved in recognizing and treating abused, neglected, and exploited elders and to determine the need for appropriate services. Although all 50 states have adult protection legislation, mandatory reporting laws vary from state to state. Emergency nurses should be familiar with the reporting requirements for their specific state.

The primary goal of intervention is to protect the patient from immediate and future harm. A secondary and equally important goal of intervention is to break the cycle of mistreatment. The well-being of the abused individual must be considered as well as the coping ability of the abuser.

Elder abuse is divided into two broad categories with regard to intervention in family-mediated abuse and neglect.[1] First are cases in which the elder has physical or mental impairment and is dependent on the family for daily care needs. The second group comprises individuals with minimal needs or care needs overshadowed by pathologic behavior of the caregiver. Potential intervention strategies include referrals to community agencies for continual monitoring of the situation, support services to decrease caregiver stress, close health care follow-up to prevent switching to another health care provider, reports to adult protective services with removal of the individual from a harmful environment, or use of 24-hour supervision from a home health agency.

Care needs of the elder in the home increase over time; however, the resources of the family in terms of psychosocial and financial reserves do not always increase at the same rate. Intervention requires a multidisciplinary team approach. Such a team is able to assess aspects of the situation such as physical injury, mental status, competency, financial irregularities, legality, treatment, assistance, protection, or prosecution. When there is a high degree of suspicion for elder abuse, consult social services or the appropriate agency within your area. When appropriate, contact a home health agency to make an initial home assessment. In acute situations, the elder may require shelter or protective care.

SUMMARY

The American population is living longer. As the baby boomer generation enters their senior years, there are more and more seniors with increasing health problems who require assistance to perform simple activities of daily living. Caregivers remain trapped between the demands of a young family, career, and aging parents. Until emergency departments and other sources of health care have accurate records of the types of victims and the services they receive, a major part of epidemiologic information is unavailable to frame public health policy.[2]

As children we are taught to honor our mothers and fathers and to respect and care for the elderly. The notion of frail elderly human beings facing a life of fear and pain caused by someone they love and trust is beyond our comprehension. Likewise, understanding the frustration, fear, and sadness of the person who has gone from being a child cared for and nurtured by a parent to being the adult caring for that parent as one would a small child is also difficult to accept. For health care professionals to successfully diagnose and treat elder abuse, a nonjudgmental, open, and caring attitude toward all those involved is essential.

REFERENCES

1. All AC: A literature review: assessment and intervention in elder abuse, *J Gerontol Nurs*, p 25, July 1994.
2. Bell CC, et al: Response of emergency rooms to victims of interpersonal violence, *Hosp Community Psychiatry* 45(2):142, 1994.
3. Costa AJ: Elder abuse, *Prim Care* 20(2):375, 1993.
4. Criner JA: The nurse's role in preventing abuse of elderly patients, *Rehabil Nurs* 19(5):277, 1994.
5. Jones JS: Elder abuse and neglect: responding to a national problem, *Ann Emerg Med* 23(4):845, 1994.
6. Lay T: The flourishing problem of elder abuse in our society, *AACN Clin Issues* 5(4):507, 1994.
7. Paris BE, et al: Elder abuse and neglect: how to recognize warning signs and intervene, *Geriatrics* 50(4):47, 1995.

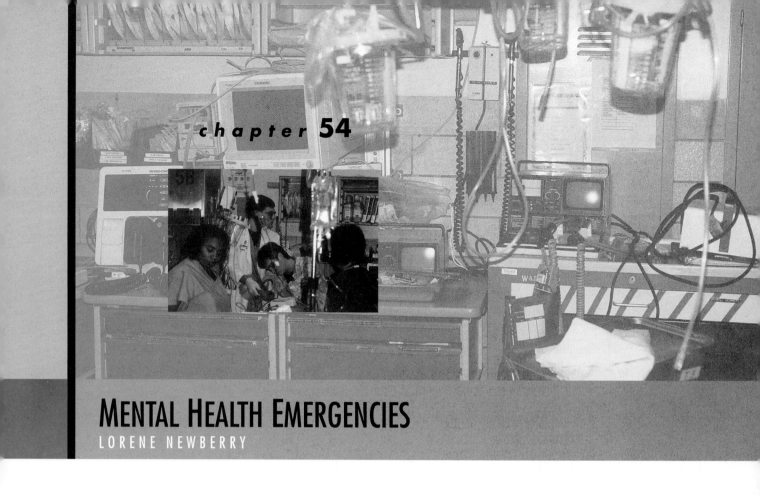

chapter **54**

MENTAL HEALTH EMERGENCIES

LORENE NEWBERRY

The patient with a psychiatric emergency arrives at the emergency department (ED) with a severe dysfunction of behavior, mood, thinking, or perception that may create a threat to life, adequate functioning, or psychologic integrity. Severity is related to the patient's ability to function and adapt as well as the available support system, regardless of the presence of mental illness.[21]

The term *psychosocial* usually denotes understanding that internal (psychologic) and interpersonal (social) factors determine a person's emotional state. In emergency situations, the term *psychosocial* is frequently used to describe conditions that arise from situational causes, whereas the term *psychiatric* is used to describe conditions attributed to mental illness.

Working with this type of patient requires many skills. Three approaches may be used for comprehensive assessment of patients with a psychiatric emergency.

Aguilera and Messick[1] present a model for *crisis intervention* that includes assessment and resolution components. The *stress-adaptation* approach emphasizes the role of stress in the increased incidence of illness. Illness is viewed as a pattern of human reactions to stress or as maladaptation. The *human needs* theory is basic to the nursing process. When an individual is unable to meet a need, a problem exists. Maslow[30] outlined individual needs in a hierarchy from basic to complex.

CRISIS INTERVENTION MODEL

Since patients who enter the ED in a state of crisis exhibit many behavioral problems, the emergency nurse must adapt to change readily and view each patient as a unique individual with special immediate needs. Emergency nurses must be able to correctly assess immediate problems in a systematic manner.

The crisis intervention model incorporates a problem-solving approach designed by Aguilera and Messick.[1] This model views human beings as organisms that exist in a state of equilibrium until a stressful event occurs, which changes a human being's state to one of disequilibrium. For the problem to be resolved, specific balancing factors must be present: (1) realistic perception of the event by the patient, (2) availability of adequate situational support, and (3) adequate coping skills with which to address the problems. If these balancing factors are present, there is potential for resolution of the problem, return to equilibrium, and prevention of crisis. This model postulates that when one or more balancing factors are absent, the problem is unresolved, disequilibrium increases, and crisis occurs or is imminent (Figure 54-1). Figure 54-2 shows this paradigm as it applies to a specific patient.

Steps in the crisis intervention model correlate with the first step in the nursing process, assessment of the crisis and identification of the problem. This assessment gives the nurse direction for measures including planning and therapeutic intervention to prevent increased maladaptive behav-

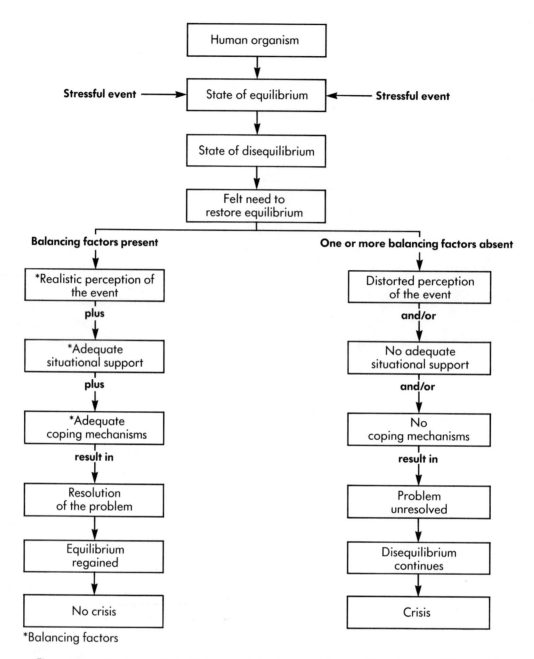

Figure **54-1**   Paradigm: effect of balancing factors in stressful event. *(From Aguilera DC, Messick JM: Crisis intervention: theory and methodology, ed 7, St. Louis, 1994, Mosby.)*

iors and evaluation and anticipatory planning for admission, discharge, or referral.

Resolution of crisis, usually within 6 weeks, may result in adaptive or maladaptive behaviors. Immediate action taken by the emergency nurse is imperative, since this is a time of increased vulnerability for the patient. Crisis intervention may lead to a return to the original level of functioning, increased personal growth, or a less effective level of functioning.[9]

Stress-Adaptation

Emotions can cause physical changes, as with response to rage or fear when the body prepares for aggression or flight

(fight-or-flight response). Swanson[35] identified stress as an actual cause of physical disorders. Emotional arousal triggers the sympathetic branch of the autonomic nervous system and the endocrine system. The physiologic response to stress is more predictable than behavioral responses.[28] The response remains the same whether the stress is physical, psychologic, or social. When the fight-or-flight response is sustained, pathophysiologic changes may ensue, such as high blood pressure, ulcers, or cardiac problems.[6]

In contrast to the fight-or-flight response, the relaxation response[8] is synonymous with functioning of the parasympathetic branch of the autonomic nervous system. This re-

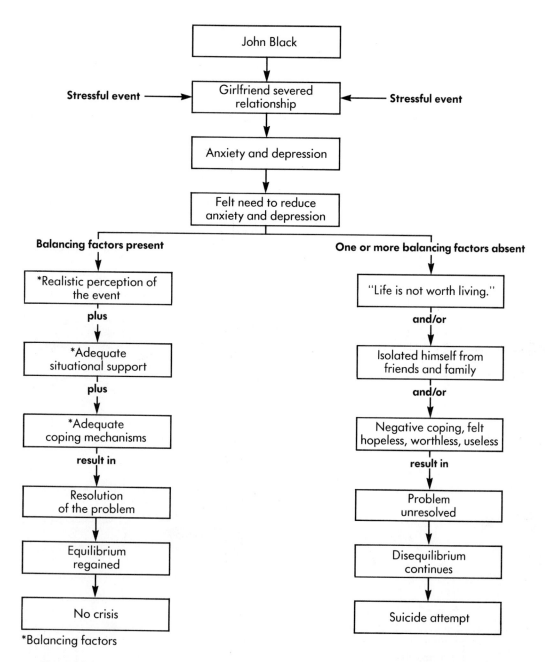

Figure **54-2** Paradigm: effect of balancing factors in stressful event. *(From Aguilera DC, Messick JM: Crisis intervention: theory and methodology, ed 7, St. Louis, 1994, Mosby.)*

sponse has a stabilizing effect on the nervous system that is directly opposite to the fight-or-flight response. Selye[33] further demonstrated the body's organized response to stress. In his general adaptation syndrome, response progresses through three stages: alarm, resistance, and exhaustion.

The alarm stage is an immediate life-preserving reaction by the sympathetic nervous system. During this stage, the flight-or-fight response is activated, which increases epinephrine and norepinephrine release.

Resistance occurs when the body adapts through changes in the adrenocortical response that sustain the body's fight for preservation. If the body adapts psychologically, physio-logically, or behaviorally, or if stressors have decreased, the body returns to a normal level of function. If the stressors continue over time, exhaustion occurs. When physical, emotional, and social resources are depleted (exhaustion), physical or emotional disorders ensue, occasionally to the point of death.

Figure 54-3 and Table 54-1 demonstrate an intermingling of stress-adaptation and human needs theories in the assessment of a patient with a stress-related or psychiatric complaint. Table 54-1 outlines stages of adaptation and physical and psychologic changes that occur in each as outlined in Selye's model of the general adaptation syndrome. Figure

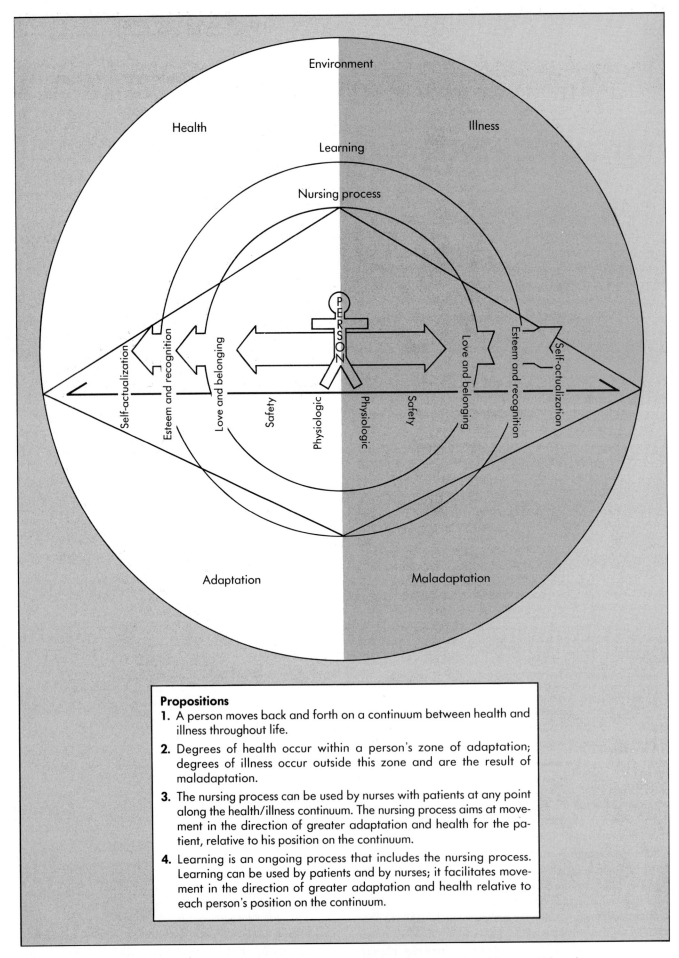

Propositions
1. A person moves back and forth on a continuum between health and illness throughout life.
2. Degrees of health occur within a person's zone of adaptation; degrees of illness occur outside this zone and are the result of maladaptation.
3. The nursing process can be used by nurses with patients at any point along the health/illness continuum. The nursing process aims at movement in the direction of greater adaptation and health for the patient, relative to his position on the continuum.
4. Learning is an ongoing process that includes the nursing process. Learning can be used by patients and by nurses; it facilitates movement in the direction of greater adaptation and health relative to each person's position on the continuum.

Figure **54-3** Model demonstrates adaptive and maladaptive routes for coping with stress. *(Adapted from Husson College and Eastern Maine Medical Center Baccalaureate Nursing Program.)*

Table **54-1**   **General Adaptation Syndrome**

Stage	Physical changes	Psychologic changes
Stage I		
Alarm reaction: immobilization of defense forces and activation of fight-or-flight mechanism	Norepinephrine and epinephrine release cause vasoconstriction, increased blood pressure, and increased rate and force of cardiac contractions.	Level of alertness increases.
Stage II		
Stage of resistance: optimal adaptation to stress within the person's capabilities	Hormone levels readjust; activity and size of adrenal cortex decrease; lymph glands return to normal size; weight returns to normal.	Use of coping mechanisms increases and intensifies; patient has tendency to rely on defense-oriented behavior.
Stage III		
Stage of exhaustion: loss of ability to resist stress because of depletion of body resources	Immune response decreases with suppression of T cells and atrophy of thymus; production of hormones by adrenal glands is depleted; weight loss, enlargement of lymph nodes, and dysfunction of lymphatic system occur; if exposure to the stressor continues, cardiac failure, renal failure, or death may occur.	Defense-oriented behaviors are exaggerated; disorganization of thinking and disorganization of personality become apparent; sensory stimuli may be misperceived with appearance of illusions; reality contact may be reduced with appearance of delusions or hallucinations; if exposure to the stressor continues, stupor or violence may occur.

Adapted from Kneisl CR, Ames SW: *Adult health nursing: a biopsychosocial approach,* Menlo Park, Calif, 1986, Addison-Wesley.

54-3 demonstrates both adaptive and maladaptive routes for coping with stress.

Abraham Maslow's hierarchy of needs theory[30] is one of the most popular and widely known theories of motivation. According to Maslow, individuals are motivated to satisfy specific needs (Table 54-2).

Maslow[30] believed these needs were arranged in a hierarchy of ascending importance with lower-level needs satisfied before the next level could motivate behavior. A person can descend as well as ascend the hierarchy. For example, if an individual's life is threatened, the need for safety becomes the dominant need, replacing the need for personal recognition. For patients in the ED in states of crisis, recognition of unmet needs is made evident from information gathered during assessment. An unmet need constitutes a problem. Problems are formulated into nursing diagnoses and prioritized.[12] An acceptable alternative for dealing with the unmet need is found by means of assessment, planning, interventions, and evaluation.[2]

ASSESSMENT OF PATIENTS WITH PSYCHOSOCIAL STRESSORS

Five to fifteen percent of patients who seek emergency care have a primary psychiatric diagnosis; 33% have a psychologic problem in addition to a physical problem.[42] The holistic view of a patient as a biopsychosocial interactive system reinforces the belief that any insult to the patient's overall system has the potential to cause psychosocial as well as biologic problems.[5,11] Therefore trauma patients ad-

Table **54-2**   **Maslow's Hierarchy of Needs**

Category	Example
Physiologic	Food, water, air, sex
Safety/security	Stability, self-preservation, freedom from fear of threat
Social	Friendship, affection, acceptance, interaction with others, love
Esteem	Personal feelings of achievement and self-respect; respect and recognition from others
Self-actualization	Self-fulfillment, reaching for one's potential

mitted to the ED need interventions for psychologic stressors as well as for biologic stressors.

Additionally, the increasing number of mentally ill patients who live in the community and the growing number of young, unemployed homeless persons with emotional problems make the ED the primary "port of entry" for health care problems of this patient population.

When a patient with psychosocial stressors enters the ED, the practitioner must be aware the patient is usually extremely anxious because of maladaptive responses to stressors or to a crisis situation.

The nursing process, an interactive, systematic, problem-solving approach, gives the ED practitioner direction to facilitate the patient's speedy return to a state of equilibrium.[38] Accurate assessment is essential for determining the patient's problem and involves an in-depth multidimensional interview. The psychiatric interview is an important means of collecting pertinent data from the patient and significant others. The interview should be structured and goal oriented so that both the practitioner and the patient feel comfortable. The interview is conducted to answer three questions: (1) Is something wrong? (2) How urgent is the situation? and (3) Must I, as the practitioner, take action?[15] Table 54-3 identifies nursing actions and theoretic rationales for the interview.[40]

For the interview to progress in a proficient, concise manner, the practitioner must apply specific principles and skills, with the most important initial step to establish rapport and trust. The nurse needs to be aware of his or her own thoughts and feelings regarding mental health patients and to use effective communication skills. A quiet, safe environment for the patient and nurse facilitates open communi-

---

Table 54-3 Nursing Actions and Theoretic Rationales When Interviewing

Nursing actions	Theoretic rationales
Introduce by name, title, and role. Address the patient by name and ask how he or she prefers to be addressed.	Addressing the client by name and introducing self by name and title is a way to convey respect for the patient.
Provide an interview room that is private and quiet and does not contain distracting objects. When a room is unavailable, provide some measure of privacy with curtains and screens. Keep interruptions and interference by other staff members to a minimum.	Privacy encourages the reticent, embarrassed patient to disclose personal problems and feelings and eliminates some concerns about confidentiality. Distracting objects may prove disturbing to a confused, disoriented, or psychotic patient. The psychiatric interview is demanding for the patient and the nurse and requires concentration.
Provide two chairs of equal size, comfort and choice of seating. Additional seating should be available for family interviews and consultations.	The choice of where patient sits provides clues to the patient's need for personal space, fears of interpersonal closeness, and possible suspiciousness.
Make prior arrangements and establish protocol to provide safety and security for the patient and self. This is particularly important in the ED.	Medical paraphernalia is potentially dangerous and may also frighten the patient. Help is sometimes needed to manage the confused, assaultive, or suicidal patient. Prior arrangement for this help can allay the nurse's anxiety. Limit setting is also reassuring to the disturbed or impulsive client.
Begin with an open-ended question that indicates general inquiry, defines area of interest, but leaves wide range of interpretation possible. Example: "What brought you here today?"	Open-ended questions are broad and allow the patient to verbalize views, thoughts, and feelings. Closed questions tend to elicit facts only. Direct, more specific questions are asked to get additional information after the patient has told his or her story. This response is nonrestrictive and does not sharply define the answer for the patient, but rather elicits spontaneous and individualistic responses that describe how the patient sees the problem.
Use verbal or nonverbal response that encourages the patient to say more. The response may be anything from an expectant look to a request to "tell me more about that."	
Communicate with the patient through use of silences. Silences, on the part of the patient and the nurse, are accompanied by facial and body expression, gestures, or postures that convey meaning. For example, when the patient transmits feelings of anger, the nurse might state something about the anger and ask the patient to put it into words.	The nurse's silence can convey concern and interest and facilitate continued communication. The nurse can determine possible meaning of the patient's silences by observing nonverbal communication and by examining his or her own empathic response.
Use responses that convey support, empathy, and understanding. Example: "You seem to feel guilty about being unable to work."	Affirms that the nurse accepts feelings and information the client has offered with concern but without criticism.
Use confrontation and interpretation to make explicit connection between feeling or symptom and the patient's interpersonal or intrapsychic life. Example: "You seem to have these headaches at times when you are most angry."	Encourages the patient to make his or her own additional connections and to explore matters further.
Pay attention to interview content (words spoken), as well as the process (what is happening) between the patient and the nurse. Example: The patient states he or she feels relaxed but fidgets in his or her chair and cannot make eye contact.	By attending to both levels of a message (content and process), the nurse may more accurately assess the patient, what is occurring in the interview, and what may be occurring in the patient's life.

Adapted from Webster M: Psychiatric nursing assessment. In Lego S, editor: *The American handbook of psychiatric nursing*, Philadelphia, 1984, JB Lippincott.

cation and exploration of the precipitating event. When possible, the nurse should obtain information from the family and available members of the patient's support system after the initial interview with the patient. Additional data collected include developmental stage, medical history, medication assessment, mental status examination, life changes, and risk for suicide or homicide. After data have been collected and analyzed, the nurse formulates a nursing diagnosis.[12] Table 54-4 identifies necessary assessment skills with corresponding examples of a verbal statement or query to elicit information from the patient. Table 54-5 identifies predictors for suicide, and Table 54-6 presents a lethality scale for suicide attempts. Table 54-7 reviews developmental stages identified by Erikson.

ANXIETY

Some individuals view stress as a challenge and are able to cope positively by learning adaptive behaviors, which reduces stress to a manageable level. Others view common, everyday occurrences as negative, stressful events, use maladaptive coping mechanisms, and have ongoing, unrelenting anxiety. This state of overwhelming anxiety may cause functional impairment and subjective distress; over time a pathologic neurotic disorder may develop in the anxious person.

Conditions that occur when anxiety is not relieved by ordinary use of defense mechanisms include anxiety disorders, somatoform disorders, and dissociative disorders.

Behaviors and symptoms observed in persons with these disorders include overt anxiety, phobias, obsessions, compulsions, changes in consciousness, and alterations in identity.[13]

Anxiety Disorders

Anxiety disorders, originally called neurotic diseases, are considered some of the most common psychiatric problems that cause a patient to seek professional help. The person with an anxiety disorder responds maladaptively to stressors that do not ordinarily cause discomfort for the average person. Anxiety disorders include panic disorder, phobias, generalized anxiety, and somatoform disorders.

Panic disorder. Panic disorders are recurrent attacks of severe anxiety characterized by sudden onset of intense, apprehensive dread and at least four of the following symptoms: dyspnea, palpitations, chest discomfort, syncope or dizziness, trembling or shaking, sweating, choking, nausea or abdominal distress, depersonalization, numbness or tingling sensations, flushes (hot flashes) or chills, fear of dying, and fear of going crazy or losing control.[4]

Panic attacks usually last for several minutes; however, persons with panic disorders are typically plagued by anticipatory anxiety or constant dread of the next attack. Because the psychologic terror experienced during a panic attack can be so compelling, many people begin to doubt their sanity. A person who has panic attacks over a long period may develop symptoms of agoraphobia.

Phobias. Phobia is an irrational, persistent fear related to one or several specific objects in the environment. Phobias are divided into three categories: agoraphobia, simple phobia, and social phobia.

Agoraphobia is a fear of becoming terrified in situations from which there is no easy escape or in which no help can be found. Persons with agoraphobia may be fearful in any situation away from their homes and may become homebound. Others may avoid open spaces, standing in a line, or being in a crowd. Many people with agoraphobia also have panic disorder.

Simple phobia is fear of becoming terrified and needing to escape from a single, specific situation such as driving on bridges or through tunnels, flying, elevators, closed spaces, or heights.

Social phobia is fear of embarrassing oneself in public (for example, eating in public). The person with social phobia may become preoccupied with the risks of choking on food

Table **54-4**	**Psychiatric and Mental Health Nursing Skills Necessary in the ED**
Skill	Communication
Determine self-awareness (autognosis)	"What are my thoughts and feelings?"
Maintain safe environment	"Let's sit in this safe, quiet place."
Establish rapport; build trust	"I want to help you."
Explore precipitating event	"Tell me about the present problem."
Observe and validate patient's feelings (verbal and nonverbal cues)	"You look sad; tell me how you're feeling."
Set priorities (determine risk for suicide or homicide)	"Have you considered harming yourself or others?"
Assess developmental stage	"Tell me some important events that have occurred during your life."
Explore life changes	"What changes have you had recently? What changes have occurred within the past year?"
Assess health history (medication assessment)	"Has anything like this happened to you in the past? What medications have you taken?"
Mental status examination	"Tell me the meaning of this proverb: 'A rolling stone gathers no moss.'"
Collect data from support system	"How does this problem affect the whole family?"

Table 54-5	Predictors of Suicide Risk: Comparison of Persons Who Complete or Attempt Suicide With the General Population		
Signs	Suicide	Suicide attempt	General population
Suicide plan*	Specific, with available, highly lethal method; does not include possibility of rescue	Less lethal method, including plan for rescue; risk increases if lethality of method increases	None or vague ideas only
History of suicide attempts*	65% have history of highly lethal attempts; if rescued it was probably accidental	Previous attempts are usually low lethal; rescue plan included; risk increases if there is a change from many attempts that are low lethal attempts to one that is highly lethal	None or low lethal with definite rescue plan
Resources* (psychologic, social)	Very limited or nonexistent; or, person *perceives* self as having no resources	Moderate, or in psychological and/or social turmoil	Either intact or able to restore them through nonsuicidal means
Communication*	Feels cut off from resources and unable to communicate effectively	Ambiguously attached to resources; may use self-injury as a method of communicating with significant others when other methods fail	Able to communicate need fulfillment directly and nondestructively
Recent loss	Increases risk	May increase risk	Is widespread but is resolved nonsuicidally through grief work, etc.
Physical illness	Increases risk	May increase risk	Is common but responded to through effective crisis management (natural and/or formal)
Drinking and other drug abuse	Increases risk	May increase risk	Is widespread but does not lead to suicide of itself
Isolation	Increases risk	May increase risk	Many well-adjusted persons live alone; they handle physical isolation through satisfactory social contacts
Unexplained change in behavior	A possible clue to suicidal intent, especially in teenagers	A cry for help and possible clue to suicidal ideas	Does not apply in absence of other predictive signs
Depression	65% have a history of depression	A large percentage are depressed	A large percentage are depressed
Social factors or problems	May be present	Often are present	Widespread but do not of themselves lead to suicide
Mental illness	May be present	May be present	May be present
Age, sex, race, marital status	These are statistical predictors that are most useful for identifying whether an individual belongs to a high-risk group, not for clinical assessment of individuals	May be present	May be present

From Hoff LS: *People in crisis*, ed 3, Redwood City, Calif, 1989, Addison-Wesley.
*If all four of these signs exist in a particular person, the risk for suicide is very high, regardless of all other factors. If other signs also apply, the risk is further increased.

and vomiting in front of others or with fear of public speaking. Extreme shyness is a generalized form of social phobia.

Generalized anxiety. Unrealistic or excessive anxiety and worry that persists for 6 months characterizes generalized anxiety. At least six of the following symptoms are present. Symptoms of *motor tension* include trembling, twitching, or feeling shaky; muscle tension, aches, or soreness; restlessness; and easy fatigability. Symptoms of *autonomic hyperactivity* include shortness of breath, smothering sensations; palpitations or accelerated heart rate; sweating; cold, clammy hands; dry mouth; dizziness, light-headedness; nausea, diarrhea, other abdominal distress; flushes; chills; fre-

Table **54-6**	**Lethality Assessment Scale**	
Key to scale	Danger to self	Typical indicators
1	No predictable risk of immediate suicide	Has no notion of suicide or history of attempts, has satisfactory social support network, and is in close contact with significant others
2	Low risk of immediate suicide	Has considered suicide with low lethal method; has no history of attempts or recent serious loss; has satisfactory support network; has no problems with alcohol; basically wants to live
3	Moderate risk of immediate suicide	Has considered suicide with highly lethal method but has made no specific plan or threats; or, has plan with low lethal method, history of low lethal attempts, with tumultuous family history and reliance on Valium or other drugs for stress relief; is weighing the odds between life and death
4	High risk of immediate suicide	Has current highly lethal plan, obtainable means, or history of previous attempts; has a close friend but is unable to communicate with him or her; has a problem with alcohol; is depressed and wants to die
5	Very high risk of immediate suicide	Has current, highly lethal plan with available means or history of highly lethal suicide attempts; is cut off from resources; is depressed and uses alcohol to excess; is threatened with a serious loss such as unemployment, divorce, or failure in school

From Hoff LA: *People in crisis*, ed 3, Redwood City, Calif, 1989, Addison-Wesley.

Table **54-7**	**Erikson's Eight Stages of Development***		
Age	Stage of development	Task and area of resolution	Concepts and basic attitudes
Birth to 18 months	Infancy	Trust versus mistrust	Ability to trust others and a sense of one's own trustworthiness; a sense of hope
18 months to 3 years	Early childhood	Autonomy versus shame and doubt	Self-control without loss of self-esteem; ability to cooperate and express one's self
3 to 5 years	Late childhood	Initiative versus guilt	Realistic sense of purpose; some ability to evaluate one's own behavior versus self-denial and self-restriction
6 to 12 years	School age	Industry versus inferiority	Realization of competence; perseverance versus feeling that one will never be "any good"; withdrawal from school and peers
12 to 20 years	Adolescence	Identity versus role diffusion	Coherent sense of self; plans to actualize one's abilities versus feelings of confusion, indecisiveness, possibly antisocial behavior
18 to 25 years	Young adulthood	Intimacy versus isolation	Capacity for love as mutual devotion; commitment to work and relationships versus impersonal relationships, prejudice
25 to 65 years	Adulthood	Generativity versus stagnation	Creativity, productivity, concern for others versus self-indulgence, impoverishment of self
65 years to death	Old age	Integrity versus despair	Acceptance of the worth and uniqueness of one's life versus sense of loss, contempt for others

*Erikson E: *Childhood and Society*, ed 2, New York, 1963, WW Norton.

quent urination; and trouble with swallowing. Symptoms of *vigilance and scanning* include feeling "keyed up" or on edge; exaggerated startle response; difficulty concentrating or "mind going blank" because of anxiety; trouble with falling or staying asleep; and irritability.[4]

Obsessive-compulsive disorder consists of preoccupation with persistent, intrusive thoughts that cannot be dismissed (obsessive) or repeated performance of rituals, designed to produce or prevent some event (compulsive).

Posttraumatic stress disorder (PTSD) occurs after a psychologically traumatic event outside the range of usual experience, such as military combat, rape, natural disasters, or disasters of human origin. The individual with PTSD has experiences such as recurrent dreams or thoughts about the event; feelings of numbness, detachment, or estrangement from the environment or people in it; and at least two of the following: sleep disturbance, hyperalertness, guilt about surviving, difficulty concentrating, memory impairment, and avoidance of activities that trigger memory of the event.[4]

Most patients with anxiety disorders do not seek help from the ED; however, the patient with a panic attack does come to the ED. A patient who enters the ED with panic disorder appears agitated and terrified. The patient may have cardiac-related symptoms such as palpitations, precordial pain, and shortness of breath, disturbances of respiration, gastrointestinal distress, trembling, diaphoresis, and paresthesias. The characteristic psychologic symptom is a feeling of apprehension that something terrible is going to happen. Attacks may last from a few minutes to a few hours.

Anxiety is a form of fearful reaction that is without a tangible object or reason for fear. Anxiety differs from object-related fear in the following ways:

- Anxiety is "free floating" and not restricted to definite situations or objects.
- Anxiety is not accompanied by any degree of insight into its immediate cause.
- Anxiety is usually experienced in terms of physical manifestations, although the individual does not recognize them as such.
- Anxiety is prompted by anticipation of future threats against which current avoidance responses would not be effective.
- Anxiety is not controlled by specific psychologic defense mechanisms.

Immediate interventions for the patient with extreme stress resulting from a panic attack include the following medications, communication, and encouraging the patient to verbalize feelings[7]:

- Medications may include alprazolam (benzodiazepine), imipramine (tricyclic antidepressant), and phenelzine (monoamine oxidase inhibitor).
- Relieve fight-or-flight symptoms by moving the patient to a quiet, safe space.
- Communicate in short, single statements: "I will stay with you." "You are safe here."
- Allow the patient to pace around the room to expend energy.
- Be aware that touching the patient may cause increased fear and anxiety; however, once rapport and trust are established, touching the patient on the arm, shoulder, or hand may be comforting.
- Encourage the patient to vent feelings and verbalize fears.
- Reassure the patient that symptoms subside with time.
- Initiate and teach relaxation and visualization exercises.
- Encourage the patient to reduce use of caffeine.
- Identify adaptive coping behaviors and reinforce positive behaviors.

Panic attacks may occur without an identifiable precipitant, or attacks may develop in response to sudden loss.

Therefore the patient should be encouraged to express feelings when losses occur to reduce exacerbation of the panic attack. Additional treatment for panic disorders includes drug therapy, supportive therapy, and behavioral therapy.

Somatoform Disorders

Somatoform disorders are a group of disorders characterized by physical symptoms with no apparent organic or physiologic basis. Distinct diagnostic groups include somatization disorder, conversion disorder, hypochondriasis, and somatoform pain disorders.

In these disorders, anxiety is transformed into physical symptoms that may involve sensory and motor function. Symptoms cannot be explained by physical findings but can be linked to psychologic factors such as stress at the time of onset and secondary gain. Physical symptoms are the primary gain, since they provide temporary relief from anxiety. Physical symptoms are experienced as real and are not under voluntary control of the individual.[10]

Somatization disorder. Somatization disorder is characterized by expression of emotional turmoil or conflict through physical symptoms. Patients with somatization disorder have multiple somatic complaints with 15 or more symptoms persisting for several years. After medical workup, no physiologic disorder is found. These patients frequently consult with numerous doctors and have exploratory surgery and many diagnostic tests performed. Abuse of alcohol or medications is often associated with this disorder.

Conversion disorder. Conversion disorder, originally known as hysterical neurosis, describes the loss of physical functioning for which no organic basis exists, such as blindness that occurs without cause. Conversion disorder is an expression of psychologic conflict or need. One of the following psychologic factors must always be present for this diagnosis: (1) a close relationship exists between time of symptom onset and occurrence of a conflict-producing event, (2) presence of the symptom allows the individual to avoid some activity that is personally unpleasant, and (3) the symptom enables the patient to get support from the environment. Primary gain is achieved by avoiding the conflict, with secondary gain achieved by avoiding unpleasant activity and receiving support from the environment. An important outward appearance that the patient maintains is *la belle indifference,* an attitude of unconcern about the symptom, which reaffirms that primary gain has been achieved.

Hypochondriasis. Hypochondriasis is a disorder in which patients have an abnormal preoccupation with the belief that they have a serious illness or illnesses. These individuals continually seek medical care for physical signs and vague symptoms. These patients are commonly seen hopping from one physician to another and frequently seek care from EDs. They also frequently overuse medications. Symptoms help control anxiety. Impaired social and occupational functioning is always present.

Somatoform pain disorder. Somatoform pain disorder is characterized by severe, prolonged pain related to psychophysiologic factors. Pain is psychogenic; however, health care providers must be aware that the patient experiences real pain. Secondary gain may be prevalent because of attention received when painful sensations are expressed.

When the patient with a somatoform disorder enters the ED, the nurse should treat the patient with respect and in a caring manner. Health care professionals may have difficulty being objective with these patients. However, extreme anxiety is present but has been repressed by use of physical problems to "hide" it. Repression is not a conscious process; therefore the nurse needs to help the patient to identify connections between anxiety, stress, and physical symptoms. A teaching model may be beneficial for explaining the effects of stress on the body. Additionally, urge the patient to verbalize perceived positive and negative feelings, as well as fears and concerns. Decrease the amount of time and attention given to the patient's physical complaints. Discuss the concept of secondary gain with the patient and family; set limits and develop a mutual plan to reduce secondary gains. When the patient does not readily comply, the nurse should not get discouraged because these behaviors usually have been part of this person's life for a long time and change is a difficult process. Maintain a positive, hopeful posture: change can occur.

Dissociative Disorders

Dissociative disorders, like somatoform disorders, provide the patient a means to avoid anxiety by use of dissociation, a defense mechanism. In the dissociative process, there is splitting off from awareness of an idea, emotion, or experience that is too difficult to handle. Anxiety-producing material is then repressed and remains in the unconscious where it has a life of its own, separate from what is known to the individual.[37]

Dissociative disorders include psychogenic amnesia, fugue disorder, depersonalization disorder, and multiple personality disorder.

A patient who exhibits characteristics of dissociative disorder may be brought to the ED by law enforcement officials or may seek help for physical problems brought on by abuse, homelessness, or exposure to multiple biopsychosocial stressors.

Psychogenic amnesia. An individual with psychogenic amnesia is unable to remember important personal information, usually following psychologic stress. Stressors include a broken love affair, financial ruin, extreme marital difficulties, and combat duty in wartime. The patient may appear calm, with other areas of memory intact. Amnesia is adaptive and allows the patient relief from anxiety (primary gain). *La belle indifference,* a relaxed state, may be present. Hypnosis may assist in uncovering repressed information. Brief therapy focuses on building trust and supporting the patient until memory returns and conflicts can be explored.

Fugue disorder. A fugue state is an abrupt, massive amnesia with sudden temporary alteration in consciousness. A new identity is assumed. During this process, individuals have amnesia about their old identity, assume a new one, and travel away from home or customary place of work. Stress and major disruption of significant relationships are precipitators. There may be a history of heavy drug or alcohol use before onset of symptoms. Recovery from a fugue state leaves these individuals able to remember their former life but not time spent in the fugue state. Therapy focuses on identifying adaptive coping styles after uncovering the conflict.

Depersonalization. In depersonalization, sense of self is altered so individuals perceive parts of their body as increased or decreased in size or altered in form. A sensation of being outside one's own body as an observer is a prominent symptom. This process can serve as a defense mechanism, protecting an individual's sense of self through "splitting off." Therapy aims at assisting the patient to recognize anxiety and the role that splitting plays in the avoidance of stressful events. The patient should be assisted in developing new coping strategies for dealing with anxiety.

Multiple personality disorder. The essential feature of multiple personality disorder is existence within the person of two or more distinct personalities or personality states. At least two personalities or personality states recurrently take full control of the person's behavior.[4] Physical and emotional abuse and sexual trauma during childhood are common factors in most cases. Transition from one personality to another often occurs during times of extreme stress. Hypnosis is used to explore the existence and characteristics of other personalities. The aim of this long-term therapy is to unite the personalities and form a whole, integrated personality.

Patients with dissociative disorders may enter the ED seeking relief from deep-seated anxiety and express feelings of loss of "real self." A calm, empathetic posture focusing on encouraging verbalization of anxious feelings assists these patients in maintaining some control in their out-of-control, "split" environment.

PERSONALITY DISORDERS

Personality disorders are a group of psychiatric disorders characterized by lifelong patterns of maladaptive responses to stress, problems in developing work behaviors and intimate relationship behaviors, and the capacity to perpetuate interpersonal problems and annoy others, often with little or no anxiety or guilt.[31] Table 54-8 summarizes personality disorders.

Personality disorders are present in about 15% of the adult population. Not much is known about etiology, but genetic factors and disturbances in early childhood may be the root cause. Early childhood disturbances could be faulty or arrested emotional development that interferes with adequate social control or "conscience" formation, deprivation of basic needs during early childhood, and physical or emotional trauma or both during childhood or adolescence.

Table 54-8	**Personality Disorders**
Type	Description
Paranoid personality	History of mistrust of others
Schizoid personality	Withdrawal from society
Histrionic personality	Dramatic displays of emotions, including temper tantrums and suicide threats, attention-seeking behaviors, a desire for activity, and brief relationships with others
Antisocial personality	Antisocial behavior involving courts, prisons, and health and welfare agencies
Borderline personality	Affect, instability, impulsivity, periods of intense anger; intense, clinging relationships; unpredictable, self-destructive acts; involves use of primitive defenses (splitting: people and the world are viewed as good or bad), projective identification, and denial; accounts for only 1% to 5% of cases, but patient is remembered because of management problems and the intense feelings they arouse in staff members
Compulsive personality	Orderliness, obstinateness, parsimony, emotional constriction, rigidity, indecisiveness, devotion to a task; overly concerned with rules and morals
Passive-aggressive personality	Resistance to most expectations involved in social and work settings and by procrastination, forgetfulness, and inefficiency
Avoidant personality	Hypersensitivity to potential humiliation, rejection, or shame; unwillingness to develop relationships unless there is a guarantee of uncritical acceptance; usually isolated and low in self-esteem
Schizotypal personality	Oddness in thought, perception, speech, and behavior, but not enough to meet the criteria for schizophrenia; multiple features may be present in this disorder
Narcissistic personality	Inflated sense of esteem with extreme self-centeredness; the individual shows deficient empathy for others in spite of a wish for their admiration; these individuals feel entitled to special treatment without reciprocity and have little capacity for warmth or mutual interpersonal relationships
Dependent personality	Passively allowing others to assume responsibility for major areas of person's life because of lack of self-confidence and an inability to function independently

Characteristics of personality disorders include common use of fantasy, isolation, dissociation, projection, somatization, and splitting. These individuals perceive themselves as extremely important and powerful. Dependent, demanding, and entangled interpersonal relationships are used to achieve specific need gratification. There is a low tolerance for frustration and stress without apparent anxiety, but the individual rarely seeks help. Pathologic behavior is directed toward and against others, and there are frequent confrontations with society's mores, norms, and laws.

Nursing care of individuals with personality disorders rests heavily on nurses' abilities to deal with their own emotional reactions to the patient's character traits. Nurses must be able to set firm, consistent limits on behavior, communicate expectations for change in behavior, and maintain a consistent team approach in understanding dynamics of the behavior.[31]

Treatment is difficult because anxiety is generated in therapists and staff members when a patient responds with anger, defensiveness, and authoritarianism. In addition, patients with these disorders do not perceive themselves as sick. The key to initial management of demanding patients (including those with personality disorders) is to determine the exact nature of their demands and to find a way to meet the demands or find acceptable substitutes. Excessive demands are usually symptoms of fears or sense of being overwhelmed by anxiety and other painful feelings. Satisfying demands reduces the patient's fears and also reduces the chance of more primitive behaviors.

Psychotherapy is helpful and can be *long-term,* with focus on personality change, or *short-term,* with focus on adaptation—involving support and guidance with problems of living, assistance in limiting contact with situations that provoke problems, and help with developing personal assets. Self-help groups are useful because patients usually require more support than any one person can provide.

Drug therapy involves use of antianxiety agents, antipsychotics during psychotic episodes, and antidepressants; there is no one specific medication for the treatment of personality disorders.

PSYCHOSES

Psychoses are psychogenic reactions in which severe personality disorganization and disintegration occur along with marked distortions of perception of reality, thought, affect, and motivation. Types of psychoses are schizophrenia, major affective disorders, and organic brain syndrome. These disorders involve loss of ego boundaries, denial of reality, severe regression, threatened security and identity, superficial interpersonal relationships, and failure or inability to trust self or others.

Schizophrenia is characterized by varied symptoms of disordered simple thinking and bizarre social behaviors. Table 54-9 summarizes types of schizophrenia.

Table 54-9	Types of Schizophrenia
Type	**Description**
Hebephrenic or disorganized	Characterized by incoherence, foolishness, and regressive behavior
Catatonic	Stuporous state in which the patient is mute, immobile, and displays waxy flexibility; may retain urine and feces; or characterized by an excited state in which the patient is negative, assaultive, aggressive, hyperactive, or agitated; may complain about or refuse to respond to a request
Paranoid	Characterized by delusions of persecution and grandeur
Schizoaffective	Characterized by disturbances in affect and thought association; some autistic and ambivalent behaviors, but not to the degree of severity associated with acute paranoid schizophrenia
Chronic undifferentiated	Characterized by variety of symptoms found in several types of psychosis
Childhood	Occurs in childhood; often described as autism

Manic-depressive, or bipolar disorder, and involutional melancholia are examples of *major affective disorders*.

Organic or acute brain syndrome is caused by a combination of biochemical, social, and psychologic factors. Characteristics include major personality disorganization and marked interference with ability to function personally and interpersonally. Significant discrepancies between thoughts or feelings and behavior are also present. Substitution of fantasy for reality often occurs. Delusional and hallucinatory systems, disorientation, and regression are commonly present.

Attitudes of staff members can make or break the possibility of recovery for the patient with psychosis. Care must be directed toward maintenance of "reality" relationships. Genuine interest, honesty, warmth, and optimism are essential for establishing contact with persons who have psychoses. Physical and psychologic needs merit equal attention. Familiar routines and familiar persons contribute to security. As a social being, a human being's psychologic equilibrium needs to be maintained through satisfying relationships with others, both individually and in groups.[18]

Psychosis occurs when persons' mental capacity, affective response, and capacity to recognize reality, communicate, and relate to others are impaired enough to interfere with their capacity to deal with ordinary daily life. Patients with a psychosis are often brought to the ED by concerned family members or police officers. Occasionally these patients appear alone, with minor, vague, or no complaints. They may be or may become out of control to the point of hurting themselves or others.

When disturbed patients first come in, they should be immediately brought to a quiet, sparsely furnished room, preferably one that includes just a sturdy stretcher and heavy desk, with perhaps one chair. Nothing should be left in the room that can be thrown or could prove to be dangerous. Police officers and family members should quickly be asked for a brief account of the behavior that preceded arrival to determine how much protection is needed and whether presence of a family member helps or hinders.

Two dangerous types of patients are the patient with paranoid psychosis and the patient in a toxic condition. When persons are intensely paranoid, they may feel as if they are fighting for their lives so any behavior is rationalized as self-defense. When patients are in toxic conditions, emotionality is increased at the same time that normal inhibitions to aggressive or self-destructive behavior are stripped away.

If there is any reason to think a patient may be dangerous, a locked room or restraints should be available. Create an environment that is controlled and safe for the time-consuming tasks of evaluating, treating, planning, and implementing hospitalization or other disposition for such patients. The patient should be advised of what is being done to allay any fears. Emergency nurses should pay attention to their "gut" reactions to a patient and never underestimate or disregard their intuition. Because a patient can be carrying any number of dangerous objects, from a nail file to a concealed razor blade, all patients should be undressed and placed in hospital clothing. Personal effects should be gathered and put into safekeeping. Patients should be told matter-of-factly that this procedure is hospital policy followed for all patients so that physicians can examine them. They should be reminded they are in a hospital and that they are safe. Patients should be told that the restraints provide some of the control that they will regain soon. Patients should also be told that as long as they are having difficult, frightening, extremely painful feelings, they will be confused about making decisions. Patients should be reminded that staff members are there to help make decisions for them until they can make decisions for themselves. This information is sometimes reassuring and lifts some of the burden of decision making from patients who may feel ambivalent about any decision. Optimally, a family member, aide, or security guard should stand by and watch each patient.

If the legality of detaining patients against their will is a concern, ED staff members should be guided by the knowledge that courts are less concerned with the absolute "right or wrong" of an action than with how justifiable it is. If the nurse can justify such precautions in light of a patient's past or present behavior and the reasonable possibility of harm to self or others, the action is usually well advised. Nurses might ask themselves if it would be more difficult to justify why they did not treat the patient and allowed the patient to leave. Safety is the foremost concern for the patient and others.

Every patient whose behavior seems bizarre deserves to have as complete a medical workup as possible. Unwillingness to cooperate and refusal of treatment are usually symptoms of illness, not reasons to dispense with examination or allow the patient to leave. The ED has just as much responsibility to treat someone who is not competent to refuse that treatment and who is in need of it as to treat a pleasant, cooperative patient. A psychiatrist, psychiatric clinical nurse specialist, or mental health professional should be consulted to assist with evaluation and treatment of the patient.

As soon as the patient is brought under control and is as comfortable as possible, diagnostic detective work begins. The first task is to decide whether there is any question that the behavior is organic, that is, caused by chemical or physiologic sources. It is often helpful for the nurse to gather information and become knowledgeable about the situation before speaking with these patients. If they deny any problem, the nurse can gently remind them of the reasons that others are concerned. The nurse should ask them about how they perceive certain events that others have told the nurse about. When patients are unaccompanied or unable to communicate, names and telephone numbers are especially helpful and may be furnished by police officers or ambulance attendants or may be found in the patient's wallet or address book. Neighbors and landlords may help, if relatives are not available. To predict the patient's course, it is important to know how acute the patient's condition is and what the progression of symptoms has been. When no information but a name is available, calling nearby state and private psychiatric hospitals may be helpful. The patient may have left a facility or wandered away from a group of patients on an outing in the area. In the aftermath of "deinstitutionalization," many former patients from "closed wards" are without structure and may decompensate or wander from ED to ED. Without resources, these patients seem to fall in the cracks between inpatient and outpatient facilities. The nurse should ask about previous hospitalizations and medications and try to learn about the pattern of illness characteristic for this patient.

When any patient is interviewed, there should be only one anxious person in the room. Therefore the nurse should begin by arranging the environment to be as safe and comfortable as possible. The patient may exhibit pressured speech, the content of which may be tangential or a "word salad." If the nurse listens well, themes such as fear and vulnerability may become apparent. Patients are often very sensitive and alert to feelings and actions of others around them and may quickly sense negative feelings or insecurity in staff members. Nurses should appear calm, competent, and genuinely interested. They should not become angry if the patient's behavior is disagreeable. Patients may overreact to perceived anger. The nurse may instead appear disappointed and convey to these patients a respect for them and the clue that more is expected from them. People often live up to others' expectations; if patients overhear that they are being called crazy, they may be more likely to act that way. The nurse should not directly challenge what delusional patients are saying but should ask more questions about their thoughts and should explore them further in conversation. If the patient demands to know whether the nurses agree, nurses can honestly answer by saying that they are trying to understand and are sure that the patient realizes how difficult it is and ask for further explanation. They may tell the patient they do believe that the patient would not mislead others intentionally.

Sometimes anxiety may be reduced by offering the patient coffee, a cigarette, or drink of water, although this should be done only if the nurse feels comfortable. (Matches should be kept, coffee should be cooled, and water and cigarettes held for the patient as needed.)

Some type of mental status examination should always be performed. The patient should be asked about frightening voices: auditory hallucinations are common in functional psychosis. Men report voices saying they are homosexual, women say they are being called prostitutes, and both describe voices that tell them to kill themselves or tell them they are better off dead. Patients with acute schizophrenic psychosis usually have a flat or shallow affect, accompanied by ambivalent, constricted, and inappropriate responsiveness and loss of empathy with others. They may exhibit forced speech, lack of speech, or blocking. Thinking may be disturbed, and these patients may misinterpret reality. Disordered thought with clear sensorium is common. Schizophrenic patients commonly say their mind is being controlled, either electronically or in some other way. They may be combative, withdrawn, regressive, or catatonic. These patients may be late adolescents, young adults having their first psychotic episode, or chronic schizophrenics having a stressful experience.

Careful observation of these patients provides clues to their history. For example, the nurse may notice that an incoherent male patient, who appears not to have shaved for a few days, has a bank deposit receipt dated 1 week ago. If the person's condition has deteriorated to this extent in 1 week, his condition may be acute.

Acute paranoid schizophrenia is characterized by persecutory or grandiose delusions and occasionally by hallucinations or excessive religiosity. A patient with this type of schizophrenia is often hostile. A systematized delusion, sometimes built on actual situations but carried to outlandish lengths, may be present. The patient may carry a notebook with handwritten, loosely associated themes. Some patients carry religious objects on their persons. The patient with paranoid psychosis should be managed with the utmost care because of the high risk for aggression or violence.

Hypomania and manic psychosis are occasionally encountered in the ED. Hypomania involves a classic triad of symptoms: elated but unstable mood, incessant speech, and increased motor activity. Patients with hypomania talk easily, humorously, and endlessly. They are friendly, then uninvitedly personal. Beneath this thin veneer of well-being is an intolerance for frustration, impulsive, ill-considered actions, and blatant disregard of obvious difficulties.

In acute mania, all these characteristics are present but are more intense and more disturbing. Propriety and discretion are painfully absent. Content of the patient's conversation is frequently sexual and often loud. Manic patients may have recurrent episodes of mood elevation and may also have periods of depression. Lithium is a specific drug used in treatment of manic-depressive illness. The manic patient should not be encouraged to talk and should be asked to provide a succinct history in the interest of effecting the best care. Physical restraints are often agitating so use of them should be avoided. These patients should be given a private room or area in which they can pace if they feel the need.

Whatever the type of psychosis, appropriate disposition should be determined. If the family is willing and patients are able, relatively undisturbed persons may go home with medication, solid follow-up care, and the option of returning to the ED or a more appropriate place if they become worse or worry the family. If patients are clearly unmanageable in another setting, hospitalization must be arranged. Determination of where patients should be hospitalized depends on such factors as willingness to be admitted, insurance status, and availability of beds. If patients are extremely agitated and self-destructive, even when restrained, some medication may be required. If patients are going to be hospitalized, particularly if they are to be committed to another hospital where concurrence of the accepting physician determines whether they will be admitted, staff members in the ED should use drugs sparingly, if at all. Ideally, the person at the accepting facility should clearly observe the pathologic condition or trust the judgment of the referring agency. Medication may miraculously "cure" these patients or make them so sleepy as to preclude an interview. Family or friends should accompany these patients to enhance transition and facilitate further history taking. Even if patients are willing to go to the hospital, the ED may want to send them with a commitment paper, in the event they change their mind en route and ambulance drivers are left without the legal right to restrain them.

Schizophrenia

Schizophrenia, as discussed earlier, encompasses a group of mental disorders with varied symptoms of disordered thinking and bizarre social behaviors. Clinical manifestations include blocking or cutting off conversation, not responding as usual to friends, and appearing aloof. Blackouts or other spells may be reported with consistent expression of concerns about body symptoms. The individual forgets and abandons plans or life goals. Social customs are disregarded, with ideas such as love, creation, and equality frequently included in conversation.

Schizophrenia may occur after experience involving loss, separation, rejection, or use of lysergic acid diethylamide (LSD), marijuana, alcohol, or amphetamines. Hallucinations, especially auditory hallucinations, may be present during the acute phase. The patient hears voices making general comments, making obscene or threatening remarks, or commanding the patient to perform a violent act. Tactile and olfactory hallucinations may indicate temporal lobe epilepsy or presence of a tumor. Cocaine abuse may also cause tactile hallucinations. Visual hallucinations occur in both hysteria and schizophrenia, but they can also be indicators of organic disorders. Patients have sensory disturbances, especially optical, seeing changing shapes and figures during the acute phase. Delusions of persecution, grandeur, or impending destruction are also present. Thinking is autistic and characterized by being highly personal and not logical, with perseveration, blocking, concretization, and loosening of associations. Speech is characterized by incoherence, use of symbols, and concrete responses; also possible are echolalia, flight of ideas, neologisms, and inability or unwillingness to speak. Patients exhibit inappropriate behavior such as grimacing, negativism, low energy (state of inaction), suggestibility, poor personal hygiene, and few social manners. Blunting, ambivalence, and inappropriateness of affect are also indicators of the acute phase.

Paranoid Disorders

Paranoid disorders represent a group of mental disorders manifested by delusions of jealousy and persecution unexplained by the presence of other psychiatric disorders.

No specific cause of paranoid disorders is known, but research suggests several factors. The psychodynamic theory postulates that delusions are based on use of denial and projection as defenses against homosexual wishes. Other possible causes are childhood developmental deficits or failure to develop basic trust, which may be related to physical abuse, single-parent families, unpredictable parental behavior, or other forms of rejection. Parental expectations of perfection and high achievement and stressful situations involving lowering of self-esteem, increasing distrust, envy, isolation, and other factors may lead to a delusional system that is frightening but partially comforting.

Paranoia is characterized by a clear, logical, lasting delusional system. Interpersonal relationships are poor because the person with a paranoid disorder mistrusts everyone.

Hospitalization is generally not indicated because the person with paranoia seldom seeks treatment. The community develops a tolerance for odd behaviors. If delusions cause a person to behave in ways that are dangerous to self or others, hospitalization is indicated. Drug therapy consists of antipsychotic medications. Psychotherapy initially deals with the problem of establishing a trusting relationship and with immediate, concrete problems; later, delusions and mistrust of others are discussed.

Affective Disorders

Affective disorders are a group of mental disorders characterized by symptoms of mood disturbance and associated changes in thinking and behavior. Major depression, bipolar disorder, and dysthymic disorders are all affective disorders.

Major depression. Symptoms of major depression include sadness, apathy, feelings of worthlessness, self-blame, thoughts of suicide, desire to escape, avoidance of simple problems, anorexia, weight loss, decreased interest in sex, sleeplessness, and either reduction in activity or ceaseless activity. In infants and older children, symptoms include refusal to eat, listlessness, lack of activity, fear of death of a parent, and fear of separation from parents. In adolescents, symptoms include social isolation, negative attitude, sulkiness, feelings of being unappreciated, and acting in antisocial ways.

Bipolar disorder. In a bipolar disorder, periods of depression alternate with periods of mania. In a manic episode of bipolar disorder, symptoms include hyperactivity, grandiosity, manipulativeness, irritability, euphoria, mood lability, hypersexuality, delusions, aggression, and sleeplessness. In a depressive episode, symptoms are the same as those of major depression.

Dysthymic disorder. Dysthymic disorder is a disorder in which a person has a depressed mood for at least 2 years, no pleasure in activities of daily living, impairment in social skills, and numerous bodily complaints.

Therapeutic interventions for affective disorders include hospitalization, electroconvulsive therapy, drug therapy, psychotherapy, cognitive psychotherapy, behavioral therapy, maintenance of social supports, prevention of suicide, and vigorous exercise.

Organic Disorders

Organic disorders represent a group of disorders with a variety of symptoms, especially disturbance of cognition. ED personnel tend to view bizarre behavior negatively. Such behavior is often considered functional rather than organic in cause until proven otherwise. In many instances, organic (or functional) illness is such that patients are not capable of good judgment or decision making. Whether patients have a history of psychiatric problems or not, they deserve to have ED staff members search out, methodically and logically, all possible causes for their illness. The rationale for thorough investigation of causes of abnormal behavior is that in many cases, such as acute organic brain syndrome (AOBS), the pathologic condition is transient and reversible.

Acute Organic Brain Syndrome

In AOBS, biochemical or structural impairment is usually present. Characteristics include a disturbed level of consciousness and cognition, clouding of sensorium, physical abnormalities that include changes in pulse rate and focal re-

flexes, and presence of delirium. Symptoms include behavioral changes; altered appearance, speech, and affect; and visual hallucinations. The ability to identify behavioral changes depends on knowledge of the premorbid personality. Vacillating symptomatology can sometimes lead the health professional to think the patient is "fooling" or that the patient is better and can be released. Affect may be vacant and appearance disheveled and preoccupied. The patient may exhibit inappropriate and weird responses, purposeless movements, general agitation, or lethargy. Eyes may be darting and either glossy or dull. Speech may be slurred with perseveration and echolalia.

Affect may be variable, that is, labile. Thought content is a major diagnostic differentiator between organic and functional illness and includes a continuum of wakefulness or somnolence, inability to focus attention, distractibility by exogenous or endogenous things, inability to grasp meanings, and disorientation that depends on the severity and progression of illness. The patient is disoriented first to time, then to place, then to person. Many patients with AOBS are disoriented. Visual hallucinations are sometimes mere distortions of what the patient actually sees; visual hallucinations are more common than auditory ones.[34]

Probably most common in AOBS are cases associated with drug or poison intoxication. Other cases are associated with circulatory disturbances producing cerebrovascular insufficiency; disturbances in metabolism or nutrition, such as hypoglycemia or hypokalemia; brain trauma, such as a concussion; infections, such as meningitis, syphilis, or hepatitis; intracranial neoplasms, such as gliomas, metastatic carcinomas, and meningiomas; and epilepsy, including grand mal, petit mal, and focal seizures.

Many cases of AOBS have psychiatric symptomatology. Classic catatonic states are sometimes encountered in patients with AOBS; such states may be produced by frontal lobe lesions, tumors, vascular lesions, encephalitis, and degenerative states of toxicosis. Most often, multiple, possibly interacting etiologic factors influence a particular case of AOBS, with response dependent on the degree of the insult and the person's premorbid ego strengths. Thus, differential diagnosis can sometimes be difficult and confusing but certainly worth the effort, given the treatable and potentially harmful nature of the illness. Medical management is dictated by the cause of symptoms. Nursing management, in general, includes simplifying and familiarizing the patient with the environment. The nurse should attempt to decrease the number of objects or shadows in the room, which can be misinterpreted by the patient, keep the same staff members or family members in the room, orient the patient to reality with simple statements, and keep lights on. Avoiding physical restraints is optimal if available personnel can stay with the patient; restraints only increase confusion and agitation. It is often helpful to reassure these patients that this state of confusion is temporary by telling them that even though they do not remember something at that particular moment, they need not worry because the nurse will remember for them until their memory improves.[7]

Violence

Violence is not necessarily the product of a particular disorder, but is usually associated with functional illnesses, such as character disorders and paranoid schizophrenia, or organic disorders, such as toxicity and temporal lobe epilepsy. Psychodynamically, violent behavior can be seen as a defense mechanism by which the individuals protect themselves from unbearable and overwhelming feelings of helplessness. Organically, violence can be seen as the result of a disorder, specific cerebral anatomic structural, electrical or metabolic function, or combination of these.

If psychologic or functional causes induce the behavior, the nurse should look for events, feelings, and conflicts that may help explain outbursts. If the root of the behavior is organic, it may involve such sources as electrical disturbances of the brain or metabolic abnormalities such as those caused by barbiturate or alcohol use or withdrawal, electrolyte imbalance, or hypoxia.

In the ED, it is often necessary to decide quickly what to do when a patient has or escalates to violent behavior. If the patient is so out of control that there seems to be imminent danger to self or others, restraints may be required. Attempts to subdue a patient with inadequate staff should not be attempted. Usually no fewer than five strong persons should approach the patient, one staff member for each limb, plus one more. The restrainers should plan their actions beforehand and act quickly and decisively. If the patient requires restraints, they should remain on the patient. Staff members may tend to watch patients less after they are restrained (they should actually watch them more closely). Experienced ED personnel know that a patient who gets partially or fully out of restraints represents a high-risk situation. If leather or specifically designed restraints are not available, soft material such as Kerlix or stockinette may be used but should be knotted as securely as possible without interfering with blood supply and neural pathways. A securely tied restraint defies quick, easy extrication by determined patients, which often occurs when "loops" are used. (Looping restraints around extremities may be more useful for the senile, mildly disoriented, and combative patient.) If the patient is extremely intoxicated, supine positioning should not be considered because of potential for aspiration. Side rails should be up and the stretcher locked. The stretcher should be positioned so that tipping it over by rocking is less likely. Many patients with severe psychosis seem to feel relieved after being restrained, perhaps because they feel they are being given the control they lack, and decisions (even the smallest of which are often difficult for these patients) are being made for them. Patients who are restrained should be reassured that it is primarily for their own safety, that no one will harm them in any way, and that restraints will be used for a short time, until they regain their own control.

Even with the restraints, some patients may still present a significant danger to themselves. Patients may hit their heads or bite or pull dangerously at restraints. In such cases benefits of chemical intervention may outweigh risks of confusing the toxicologic picture, potentiating effects of other drugs, or clouding the clinical picture.

Abusive, angry patient

The abusive, angry patient is a more frequent problem in the ED than the violent patient. Although prevention is the best means to alleviate the problem of the angry patient, the key to secondary prevention is to remain calm and professional. Nurses should refuse to become embroiled in a personal struggle. Because nurses are professionals, they should keep the patients focused on the substance of the issues or point out objectively how they see the situation. Nurses should also listen to what patients are saying and allow them to vent angry feelings. Ventilation relieves pressure of an anger drive. If patients are not talking but are acting out their anger, the nurse should try to understand the need that prompts the behavior, what the patients are trying to express, and how the environment and the nurse may be influencing their behavior. The nurse may explain that it would be more helpful for patients to explain what they need rather than merely showing anger, since it is impossible for the nurse to know everything a person is feeling and thinking.

Anger being expressed may actually be displaced (misdirected), that is, the object of that anger may not be the ED or the nurse. The patient may be feeling rage at a terminal diagnosis or the tension and frustration of a lifetime. The nurse may ask if it is the ED or the staff toward which the patient's anger is really directed. It is important not to feed into the patient's "angry system" by fueling potential fires. The nurse should do nothing toward which patients can direct their ready anger and should be a "reality tester" for these patients, asking whether their anger is really appropriate in its intensity, in spite of the legitimacy of their complaint.

PSYCHIATRIC MEDICATIONS

The best advice concerning use of psychiatric drugs in the ED is to avoid using them. Whenever possible, medicating patients or dispensing prescriptions from such a transient and episodic area as the ED should be avoided. Often, interpersonal intervention can accomplish much more good and do far less harm than drugs. However, medications to manage a condition and afford relief to the severely disturbed patient in the ED are sometimes necessary. When and whether to medicate are often difficult decisions, especially since diagnoses are seldom clear-cut and reliable. If diagnostic certainty is not possible, the risk of medicating the patient must be carefully weighed against consequences of not medicating the patient.

Haloperidol (Haldol) is, in many ED situations, the drug of choice for attenuation of common problems of severe agitation, psychomotor hyperactivity, assaultiveness, mania, and extreme mental anguish that accompany an acute psychosis. Haloperidol seems to be the safest medication for these purposes and is seldom accompanied by instances of hypotension, which are more common occurrences with chlorpromazine (Thorazine), an effective antipsychotic that has a greater sedative effect. Because haloperidol does not cause pronounced sedation, it seems to be less threatening to the patient with paranoid psychosis, who may be afraid of being "put to sleep." Dystonic reactions are infrequent and seem to occur more often and become problematic when the patient is given the lowest oral doses rather than intramuscular doses. If possible, the nurse should check for vital signs, in particular blood pressure, and determine and report suspicion of any other drugs or alcohol that the patient may have ingested, even days or weeks before admission, giving special attention to any history of use of central nervous system depressants. Blood pressure and general physical condition should be monitored carefully and frequently after administration of medication to any patient but particularly in those patients whose mental or emotional status is compromised.

Patients with compromised mental status may not be able to give feedback regarding the effect of the medication or to understand its purpose. Initial intramuscular dose of haloperidol is 0.5 to 5 mg, with subsequent doses in the same range administered every 30 to 60 minutes. A 40-minute interval between doses prevents unnecessary somnolence caused by rapid administration of additional doses; such an interval should be maintained unless patient safety demands a dose be administered sooner. Infrequent side effects of lowered seizure threshold and cholinergic blocking can occur.

Contraindications to the use of haloperidol are pregnancy, hypersensitivity, narrow-angle glaucoma, central nervous system depression, and severe cardiac disease with dysrhythmia. Haloperidol is commonly used in the ED for acute schizophrenia, alcoholic hallucinosis, and emergency sedation with uncertain diagnosis. Results with patients for whom the drug is appropriately used are often dramatic. Thought disorders improve significantly, and few and minimal side effects occur. The danger involved with this drug is that it often works so well that ED staff perceive patients as cured and may be more inclined to discharge patients who do not have social supports or the ability to continue with medication on their own and who will probably again become sick when the medication wears off.

Two commonly used minor tranquilizers, or antianxiety agents, are *chlordiazepoxide (Librium)* and *diazepam (Valium)*. The initial intramuscular adult dose of chlordiazepoxide is 25 to 50 mg, with subsequent doses of 25 to 100 mg every 1 to 2 hours. Doses given orally range from 5 to 25 mg, with subsequent doses of 5 to 25 mg and total doses of up to 100 mg daily. Initial intramuscular doses of diazepam range from 5 to 10 mg, with doses of 5 to 10 mg every 1 to 2 hours. Oral doses range from 2 to 10 mg, up to 40 mg daily. When chlordiazepoxide or diazepam is used for management of acute withdrawal from alcohol, higher doses may be required, depending on the severity of withdrawal. Doses of chlordiazepoxide (50 to 100 mg) may be followed by re-

peated doses as needed, until agitation is controlled; up to 300 mg/day may be administered. Diazepam, 10 mg administered 3 to 4 times daily during the first 24 hours, is also recommended. With both medications, drowsiness and ataxia are frequently encountered side effects. Confusion, hypotension, prolonged sedation, and paradoxic excitement are less common. The last side effect, called "Valium rage" when induced by that drug, is a distinct ED management problem.

Oxazepam (Serax) has been found to be efficacious in the treatment of a wide variety of disorders: anxiety, tension, agitation and irritability, and anxiety associated with depression. An oral medication, oxazepam seems to be safer in terms of tolerance and toxicity than other related compounds such as chlordiazepoxide and diazepam. Doses of 10 to 30 mg, up to 120 mg per day, are suggested. Oxazepam may be considered when a prescription is being given to a patient in the ED. As with all prescriptions given in the ED, the number of pills should be limited to less than the number that would produce serious consequences if taken at one time. Before patients are given a sizable prescription, they should be asked honestly and with concern if they have had any suicidal ideation or if self-destructive behavior is a possibility. The patient should then be referred to a resource that can provide long-term therapy, including further medication and other support, if necessary.

CHEMICAL TOXIC REACTIONS

When a chemical toxic reaction has occurred, a comprehensive history is vital. If the patient is an unreliable historian, gather as much data as possible from a friend or family member with the patient.

Alcohol-Related Emergencies

Alcohol-related emergencies are common in most EDs and have become more so with recognition that alcoholism is a disease rather than a criminal offense. Police officers in many parts of the country are currently mandated to bring an alcoholic to an emergency care unit or detoxification center rather than to jail. Although alcoholism is considered a psychiatric illness from one vantage point, in the ED it should always be first considered a medical emergency. Acute alcohol intoxication can result in death. An acutely intoxicated person is more likely to sustain a head injury and less likely to provide accurate history or present a clear-cut diagnostic picture. Chronically intoxicated persons often have chronic illnesses and many medical problems. Nutritional deficiencies with mental sequelae, such as Wernicke-Korsakoff syndrome and Korsakoff's syndrome, seizure disorders, tuberculosis, hepatic coma, alcoholic hallucinosis, and delirium tremens are frequently observed.

Obtaining telephone numbers of relatives, friends, landlord, and so on is particularly helpful. These persons may be able to tell the nurse what and how much the patients drink, what their behavior baseline is, whether they have currently stopped drinking, and what their behavior is like when they drink, when they stop, and when they involuntarily withdraw. Occurrence of blackouts (periods during which patients are drinking and continue to function but later do not recall what they did) is particularly indicative of chronic alcoholism. A particularly helpful question is one that asks whether patients have been "sick" lately. In particular, have they been vomiting for the past couple of days, and consequently been unable to keep down the normal amount of liquor? These patient may be in withdrawal, although they may deny that drinking has stopped. The possibility that drugs have been taken in combination with alcohol should always be suspected at the beginning of the patient's visit to the ED, not 5 hours later when the patient is obtunded as a result of a serious overdose that went unrecognized.

While emergency nurses are assessing the alcohol-affected patient, they must consider the possibility that immediate management of potentially disruptive and possibly dangerous behavior may be necessary. Intoxication produces confusion, moroseness, combativeness, regression, and general lack of inhibitions.

While patients are being evaluated and detoxified, a safe environment must be provided. They should be positioned on the stomach or side, especially if restraints are required, to prevent aspiration. The possibility of vomiting or seizure activity should always be considered. Accordingly, patient restraints should be kept loose, to prevent injuries to soft tissue or bones in the event of seizure.

After initial evaluation, watchful waiting while the patient has some restorative sleep is the safest and most desirable approach. Caffeine in any form may precipitate seizures, and sedatives may potentiate the effects of alcohol. The patient's behavior may present imminent danger to self or others. Occasionally a patient is extremely agitated, suicidal, and self-destructive. Avoid unnecessary active intervention. If the patient does not respond to the structure and intervention of the ED after a reasonable time, a small, almost subtherapeutic dose of haloperidol may be effective. With haloperidol, as with other medications, desired effects must be weighed against the possibilities of respiratory depression and coma in the situation of excessive alcohol intoxication. Haloperidol seems to have much less central nervous system depression than other tranquilizers.

An objective, sympathetic approach should be used with every intoxicated person. A punitive approach is counterproductive and may result in a greater management problem. Nurses' responses to verbal abuse from an intoxicated patient are indicative not only of their maturity, self-confidence, and level of professionalism but also of their understanding of the disease of alcoholism and appreciation of the alcoholic's past and present psychic pain.

The nurse should remain kind and supportive, indicating belief in the patient's basic worthiness and expecting the best behavior possible from the patient. Serious consideration should be given to what the patient says while intoxi-cated, whether it be suicidal ideation or information about situational stresses. However, it is not productive to spend long periods talking with patients who are intoxicated. Although they may feel uninhibited enough to divulge painful information, extremely intoxicated individuals may not remember what was said and may feel differently when sober. A case in point is patients who arrive in an agitated, suicidal state lamenting that there is nothing to live for, only to leave 4 hours later wondering what happened and quite surprised when asked if they would like to talk to someone about the way they are feeling.

Ideally, every intoxicated patient should have at least some evaluation of the circumstances that led to the intoxication and the overall pattern of alcohol use. A good way to begin evaluation with a patient who may dismiss, understate, or deny the incident is to gently, positively, and in the least threatening way say the following:

- "Although the ED is glad to help you, there may be something that could be done to prevent similar visits."
- "It is important for you to understand the connection between your drinking and your presence in the ED today."
- "I'm concerned that during your period of intoxication you could have been seriously hurt because of reports I have had of your activity."
- "This worries me and should worry you."

Persons with an alcohol problem may be more likely to return for follow-up treatment to the institution with which they have become familiar through the visit to the ED and which they see as "knowing their situation" more than another. The first and biggest step for any person with alcoholism is to admit the problem exists. It may be easier to do this if a foundation and tone of trust and help are set during the ED visit, often the patient's only contact with helping professionals.

If what patients say is at variance with what others have said about their drinking, they should be confronted, but the nurse should be careful not to engage in a battle about whether they had three or four drinks or whether they have a problem. This kind of confrontation only puts the patient on the defensive and increases denial. The important message to send is that there is genuine concern on the nurse's part, not an effort to get the patient out of the ED as quickly as possible. Depending on the patient, referrals to Alcoholics Anonymous, clinics for the treatment of alcoholism, individual therapists, detoxification centers, or halfway houses may be in order. Families of such patients may need support, ventilation, reality testing, and referral for themselves. An alcoholism information and referral source is usually available if making a referral for someone is a problem.

If there is alcoholism within the patient's family, there is greater likelihood, whether because of genetic or environmental factors, that the patient will have alcoholism. This information should be presented in a matter-of-fact way, much as you would caution patients with a history of diabetes in their family.

Alcohol-induced states that may be confused with psychiatric illness are delirium tremens, alcoholic hallucinosis, alcohol paranoid state, Wernicke-Korsakoff syndrome, and Korsakoff's syndrome.

Delirium tremens is an acute, potentially fatal medical emergency. Although the patient's behavior is psychotic, the differential diagnosis can be made quickly on the basis of history, physical appearance, and behavior. Patients are often anxious, extremely agitated, and diaphoretic; they also exhibit fine tremors, visual hallucinations, a "picking motion" of the fingers, and elevated vital signs. Delirium is usually preceded by restlessness, irritability, aversion to food, tremulousness, and disturbed sleep.

Alcoholic hallucinosis exists on a continuum with delirium tremens. The patient is often oriented to time, place, and person and may not be tremulous. This particular condition may resemble schizophrenia. Differential diagnosis is important, since the patient requires prompt and careful medical evaluation and hospitalization rather than psychiatric hospitalization. Medical admission is necessary because many psychiatric facilities are ill-equipped and unable to deliver medical care, even though many physicians are reluctant to hospitalize someone whom they see as a psychiatric case and who presents many potential management problems. The patient may have threatening auditory hallucinations accompanied by an elaborate delusional system.

These patients are likely to respond to their hallucinations and ideas, conversing with and acting on them. Symptoms may wax and wane in the ED, which provides a clue to the intoxication. Wernicke-Korsakoff syndrome and Korsakoff's syndrome are caused by nutritional deficit, especially of thiamine and niacin, often accompanying alcoholism. Wernicke-Korsakoff syndrome involves brainstem destruction, whereas in Korsakoff's syndrome, degeneration is mainly in the cerebrum and peripheral nerves.

Signs and symptoms of Wernicke-Korsakoff syndrome include ophthalmoplegia, apathy or apprehension, clouding of consciousness, and even coma. Korsakoff's syndrome involves disorientation to time and place and peripheral neuropathy. An especially helpful diagnostic clue in both conditions is presence of memory impairment (especially recent memory) and confabulation (covering up for memory deficit by "filling in false details").

Drug-Related Problems

Theories and postulations about drug dependence are beyond the scope of this chapter. In dealing with this type of patient, two important points must be remembered. These patients are usually emotionally needy and vulnerable and have suffered, or feel that they have suffered, to the point that they feel they deserve help and these patients may be emotionally draining or manipulative or both and may evoke mixed feelings from the ED practitioner. The practitioner, therefore, must combine self-confidence with kindness and set reasonable but firm limits with such patients.

Addicted patients commonly seek drugs in the ED, especially in large urban hospitals. Patients may request paregoric for a teething child or mimic symptoms of kidney stones, even by pricking a finger to drop blood in the urine sample. They may say they are allergic to codeine and pentazocine (Talwin) and ask specifically for oxycodone (Percodan) or meperidine (Demerol) when being treated for "whiplash." They may be desperate enough to steal prescription blanks from the hospital or change a prescription given to them.

ED practitioners should be alert, although not suspicious or punitive, when treating patients with possible drug addictions. Needle marks can be observed while taking blood pressure measurements. Take these measurements in the arm that the patient does *not* offer. Yawning, pinpoint or enlarged pupils, sneezing, nervousness, reddened nose from scratching or rubbing, unusual thirst, slurred speech, and general physically rundown appearance (weight loss, unkempt appearance, dental caries) may point to drug dependence.

Heroin and methadone. With the popularity of heroin and the number of methadone-dependent persons maintained at outpatient clinics, the ED encounters many patients who specifically request relief from withdrawal symptoms or the possibility thereof. It has been the policy of many large hospitals confronted with this problem to be firm in not giving anything but medications to provide relief from symptoms, that is, prochlorperazine (Compazine) for nausea and vomiting, Kaopectate for diarrhea, diazepam (Valium) for agitation, and referral to other facilities for maintenance or detoxification. Often patients may be more afraid of possibly withdrawing than having actual withdrawal symptoms. They may have acute anxiety about their need for drugs. Methadone or heroin users may come to the ED on a weekend evening saying that they are on a program in another state and in need of a methadone dose. The following considerations should be kept in mind in such situations:

1. Drug-dependent persons did not become dependent overnight; in spite of the urgency and anxiety they feel, these patients may not belong in an ED.
2. Most maintenance programs have rules, regulations, and contingency plans (such as planning for patients to get their medication in another state if they are traveling or in another center in the area if necessary) with which patients are familiar.
3. Methadone stays in the patient's system for approximately 48 hours. Withdrawal symptoms do not begin until 24 to 36 hours after that time, so there is a sufficient "grace period" to allow a patient to skip a day if unavoidable.

Patients who are taking methadone usually do not know their doses, and the history of how many bags of heroin were used per day is unreliable for many reasons.

In planning for referral or individual or family counseling in the ED, nurses should keep in mind individual needs of the particular types of patients. Needs of the young include peer support, a sense of identity, self-esteem, purpose, involvement, a place to go, people to fit in with, and a positive role in society. Needs of the elderly patient may include company, purpose, activity, and better medical care. Women may need the means to obtain a life outside the home and assistance obtaining day care and transportation and in acquiring vocational skills. Homosexuals may need social acceptance, self-understanding, acceptance of their sexual orientation, and perhaps counselor support from a homosexual resource group. Veterans may need help with the social,

economic, and mental adjustment of leaving the service or help with an addiction that developed during military service. Referrals and advice, then, differ according to the individuals and their situations.[17] Therefore individual and symptomatic treatments in the ED are best. Patients exhibiting withdrawal usually manifest symptoms of pupil dilation, increased blood pressure, pulse rate, and respiratory rate (greater than 24 breaths per minute), restlessness, stomach cramps, nausea and vomiting, diaphoresis, low back pain, yawning, and tearing eyes. If significant withdrawal is present and need to treat the patient is apparent, it may be best to

Table **54-10** **Side Effects of Antipsychotic Drugs**

Side effects	Comments
Dry mouth, blurred vision, constipation, urinary hesitance, paralytic ileus	Effects result from interference with acetylcholine. First three should be treated symptomatically and patient should be reassured. In instances of urinary hesitance and paralytic ileus, medication should be withheld until medical evaluation is obtained.
Orthostatic hypotension	Drug should be used with caution if cardiovascular disease is present and in elderly patients. Patient should be warned about possible occurrences and taught to rise slowly and dangle legs before standing.
Photosensitivity	Protect patient from exposure to ultraviolet light. Have patient use sunscreen. Effect occurs most frequently with chlorpromazine. Examine skin often.
Endocrine changes	Endocrine changes include weight gain, edema, lactation, and menstrual irregularities. Treat symptomatically. Reassure patient.
Extrapyramidal reactions	Such reactions are related to dose and duration. Manage by adjusting dose of drug or adding antiparkinsonian drug.
Pseudoparkinsonism	Typical shuffling gait, masklike facies, tremor, muscular rigidity, slowing of movements, and other symptoms mimicking those seen in Parkinson's disease
Akathisia, dystonia	Continuous restlessness, fidgeting, and pacing occur. Spasm of neck muscles, extensor rigidity of back muscles, carpopedal spasm, swallowing difficulties occur; eyes roll back. Onset is acute, but condition is reversible with appropriate medication. Provide reassurance until symptoms subside.
Akinesia	Lethargy and feelings of fatigue and muscle weakness occur; must be differentiated from withdrawal.
Skin reactions	Urticarial, maculopapular, edematous, or petechial responses may occur 1 to 5 weeks after initiation of treatment. Withhold drug until after medical evaluation.
Jaundice	Jaundice develops in about 4% of patients and is a dangerous complication; drug should be discontinued.
Agranulocytosis and leukopenia	Chlorpromazine depresses production of leukocytes. Initial symptoms of sore throat, high temperature, and lesions in mouth indicate that drug should be stopped immediately. Rarely, outcome may be lethal.
Ocular changes	Corneal and lenticular changes and pigmentary retinopathy may occur with high dosages over long periods. Periodic ocular examinations are recommended.
Convulsions	Antipsychotic agents lower seizure threshold, making seizures more likely in seizure-prone persons. Persons with a history of seizures or organic conditions associated with seizures require an increased dosage of anticonvulsant medication if antipsychotics are used.
Tardive dyskinesia	Insidious onset of fine vermicular movements of tongue occurs, which is reversible if drug is discontinued at this time; can progress to rhythmic involuntary movements of the tongue, face, mouth, or jaw, with protrusion of tongue, puffing of cheeks, and chewing movements; no known treatment is available; often irreversible. Prevention is imperative. Women more than 50 years of age who have taken prolonged doses are particularly at risk. Do not withhold drug until after medical evaluation; symptoms will increase.[37]

give methadone rather than meperidine or another such drug. Meperidine or morphine is needed in fairly large doses every 4 hours, whereas methadone may be given in increments of 5 or 10 mg, titrating the medication while closely watching the pupil size become smaller, the vital signs decrease, and the other symptoms abate.

Dystonic reactions to phenothiazines. Dystonic reactions can be easily mistaken for tetanus, calcium deficiency, seizures, and a host of other conditions. Most often, however, dystonic reaction is seen as hysterical conversion or posturing in the psychiatric patient or as malingering for drugs or other secondary benefit by a drug abuser. The psychiatric patient is often unable to articulate history and symptomatology and may even regress under stress of the interview and the frightening and painful effects of the antipsychotic medication (e.g., haloperidol). Vacillating symptoms are typical but often cause staff members to dismiss the symptoms. Young persons who bought a pill on the street they believed to be Valium or a hallucinogenic may be unwilling to tell the staff what has happened for fear that their family or the police will be notified, or they may have taken the pill 4 or 5 days before and not even associate the pill with the reaction. In a large percentage of cases, symptoms do not appear for 4 to 5 days after an oral dose. Thus history often makes diagnosis of a relatively clear-cut reaction confusing.

Treatment should be considered for oculogyric crisis, buccolingual crisis, torticollic crisis, opisthotonic crisis, or tortipelvic crisis.[5] Results of treatment are usually fast and dramatic; diphenhydramine (Benadryl), benztropine (Cogentin), or trihexyphenidyl (Artane) may be used. Since half-life of phenothiazines is 24 hours, the patient must be given medication orally to prevent return of symptoms for the next 2 or 3 days.

Nursing considerations include reduction of early anxiety to facilitate accurate initial history. Drug abusers may be reminded that personnel will not divulge their story to anyone else. Patients should be assured that symptoms are easily and completely reversible. The nurse should convey his or her ability to handle the situation to the patients and let them know this happens to many people. Symptoms are terrifying, especially to patients normally unable to cope who are susceptible to delusions. The temptation to tell a psychiatric patient to stop taking the medication should be considered carefully. The particular medication may be the drug of choice for the patient, who may become psychotic without it. Ideally, the patient's physician should be notified and the patient

Table 54-11	**Psychotropic Medications: Medical Contraindications and Precautions**	
Drug group	Contraindications	Precautions
Antipsychotics	Comatose states, central nervous system depression, bone-marrow depression, impaired liver function, epilepsy, and hypersensitivity to these medications	Use cautiously in pregnant patients and in patients with depression, respiratory disease, cardiovascular disease, hypotension, allergy history. Use lower doses in elderly patients.
Antidepressants Tricyclics	Acute myocardial infarction, hypersensitivity to these medications, concurrent administration of a monoamine oxidase inhibitor	Use cautiously in patients with urinary retention, benign prostatic hypertrophy, narrow-angle glaucoma, increased ocular pressure, convulsive disorders, cardiovascular disorders, thyroid disease, organic mental disorders in children under 12 years of age, and pregnant patients.
Monoamine oxidase inhibitors	Hypertension, cardiovascular disease, headaches, pheochromocytoma, liver or advanced renal disease, quiescent schizophrenia, concurrent administration of a tricyclic antidepressant	Safe use in pregnancy is not established.
Lithium	Significant renal disease, dietary salt restriction, cardiovascular disease, brain damage	Use cautiously in pregnant patients, children under the age of 12, elderly patients, patients who are breastfeeding, and patients with thyroid disease, mild kidney or heart disease, or epilepsy.
Antianxiety medications	Glaucoma, hypersensitivity to these medications	Use cautiously in patients who have a history of allergies, dependency on these drugs, hepatic disorder, or renal impairment. Use lower doses with the elderly patients or breastfeeding mothers.
Carbamazepine	Severe renal disease, cardiovascular disease, liver disease	Use cautiously in patients with cardiovascular disease, renal or liver disease, or blood dyscrasias.

Adapted from Birkhimer LJ, DeVane CL: The neuroleptic malignant syndrome: presentation and treatment, *Drug Intell Clin Pharm* 18(6):462, 1989 and Jann MW et al: Alternative drug therapies for mania: a literature review, *Drug Intell Clin Pharm* 18(7,8):577, 1984.

should be told to contact that physician for advice as soon as possible. These patients should be told that their medication is a good one with controllable side effects, which many medications have. This information reassures these patients and reinforces their faith in their physician and the prescribed medications.

Table 54-10 presents side effects of antipsychotic drugs, and psychotropic medications are presented in Table 54-11.

SUMMARY

Nursing skills, including self-awareness, maintaining a safe environment, establishing rapport and building trust, exploring the precipitating event, observing, validating and setting priorities, and assessment of health history, developmental state, mental status, and support systems are vital for a comprehensive psychiatric interview. The interview is the main tool by which the practitioner gains knowledge of the patient, interprets what is wrong, and identifies a nursing diagnosis. This process facilitates establishment of a therapeutic alliance that allows effective interventions leading to adaptive coping behaviors and resolution of the crisis or problem.

REFERENCES

1. Aguilera DC, Messick JM: *Crisis intervention: theory and methodology,* ed 7, St. Louis, 1994, Mosby.
2. American Nurses' Association Division on Psychiatric and Mental Health Nursing Practice: *Standards of psychiatric and mental health nursing practice,* Kansas City, Mo, 1982, The Association.
3. American Psychiatric Association: *Diagnostic and statistical manual of mental disorders,* ed 2, Washington, DC, 1968, American Psychiatric Association.
4. American Psychiatric Association: *Diagnostic and statistical manual of mental disorders,* ed 3, Washington, DC, 1987, American Psychiatric Association.
5. Baker LJ: Psychophysiological disorders. In Gary F, Kavanaugh CK, editors: *Psychiatric mental health nursing,* Philadelphia, 1991, JB Lippincott.
6. Barkauskas VH et al: *Neurological system including mental status,* St. Louis, 1994, Mosby.
7. Benfer BA, Schroder PJ: Dissociative disorders. In Gary F, Kavanaugh CK, editors: *Psychiatric mental health nursing,* Philadelphia, 1991, JB Lippincott.
8. Benson H: *The relaxation response,* New York, 1975, William Morrow.
9. Benter SE: Crisis intervention. In Stuart GW, Sundeen SJ, editors: *Principles and practice of psychiatric nursing,* ed 5, St. Louis, 1995, Mosby.
10. Braverman BG: Calming a patient with panic disorder, *Nursing 90* 20(1):32C, 1990.
11. Burgess A, Holstrom L: *Rape: victims of crisis,* Bowie, Md, 1975, Prentice-Hall.
12. Carpenito LJ: *Nursing diagnosis: applications to clinical practice,* ed 2, Philadelphia, 1987, JB Lippincott.
13. Charran HS: Repetitive and ineffective neurotic defenses. In Varcarolis EM, editor: *Foundations of psychiatric mental health nursing,* Philadelphia, 1990, WB Saunders.
14. Erikson E: *Childhood and society,* ed 2, New York, 1963, WW Norton.
15. Folstein M et al: Mini-mental state: a method for grading the cognitive state of patients for clinicians, *J Psychiatr Res* 12:189, 1975.
16. Reference deleted in proofs.
17. Germain CP: Sheltering abused women: a nursing perspective, *J Psychosoc Nurs* 22:24, 1984.
18. Grimes J, Burns E: Mental health assessment. In *Health assessment in nursing practice,* ed 2, Boston, 1987, Jones & Bartlett.
19. Hansen PA, Rhode JM, Wolf-Wilets V: Stress management. In McFarland GK, Thomas MD, editors: *Psychiatric mental health nursing,* Philadelphia, 1991, JB Lippincott.
20. Henry G: Neurologic emergencies, *Emerg Med Clin North Am* 209(5):22, 1988.
21. Herman S: *Handbook of emergency nursing: the nursing process approach,* Norwalk, Conn, 1988, Appleton-Lange.
22. Hoff LE: *People in crisis,* ed 3, Menlo Park, Calif, 1989, Addison-Wesley.
23. Reference deleted in proofs.
24. Horowitz JA: Human growth and development across the life span. In Wilson HS, Kneisl CR, editors: *Psychiatric nursing,* ed 3, Menlo Park, Calif, 1988, Addison-Wesley.
25. Reference deleted in proofs.
26. Reference deleted in proofs.
27. Reference deleted in proofs.
28. Lesse S: Relationship of anxiety to depression, *J Psychother* 36:332, 1982.
29. Reference deleted in proofs.
30. Maslow AH: *Toward a psychology of being,* ed 2, New York, 1982, D. Van Nostrand.
31. McFarland, GK, Wasli EL: *Nursing diagnoses and process in psychiatric mental health nursing,* ed 3, Philadelphia, 1996, JB Lippincott.
32. Reference deleted in proofs.
33. Selye H: *Stress without distress,* New York, 1974, JB Lippincott.
34. Siegel BS: *Love, medicine and miracles,* New York, 1986, Harper & Row.
35. Swanson AR: Psychophysiological disorders. In Varcarolis EM, editor: *Foundations of psychiatric nursing,* ed 1, Philadelphia, 1990, WB Saunders.
36. Reference deleted in proofs.
37. Taylor M: *Mereness' essentials of psychiatric nursing,* St. Louis, 1990, Mosby.
38. Varcarolis EM: The nursing process in psychiatric settings. In Varcarolis EM, editor: *Foundations of psychiatric mental health nursing,* Philadelphia, 1990, WB Saunders.
39. Reference deleted in proofs.
40. Webster M: Psychiatric nursing assessment. In Lego S, editor: *The American handbook of psychiatric nursing,* Philadelphia, 1984, JB Lippincott.
41. Reference deleted in proofs.
42. Yoder L, Jones SL: Changing emergency department use: nurses' perception and attitudes, *JEN* 7:156, 1986.

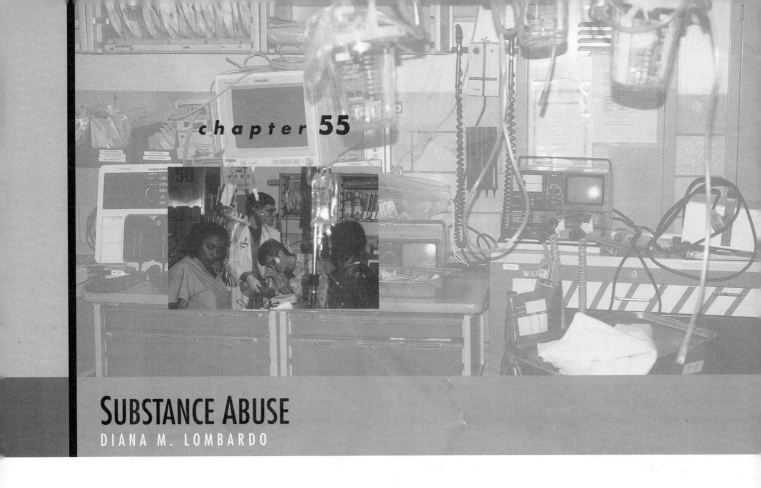

chapter **55**

SUBSTANCE ABUSE

DIANA M. LOMBARDO

Substance abuse has reached crisis proportions in the United States, and the reality is that the problem will only get worse.[14] Drugs have invaded every social level and stratus of our society, including schools and the workplace. According to Drug Abuse Resistance Education (DARE), almost one in five workers uses dangerous drugs regularly on the job, including health care workers. The effects of drugs in the workplace center around three key areas: absenteeism, work habits, and interpersonal relations.[29] Box 55-1 identifies characteristics of drug users in the workplace. Law enforcement authorities estimate that two thirds of all serious crimes can be linked to drug abuse.[14] The National Institute on Drug Abuse estimates that one quarter of the 4 million babies born annually in the United States are drug and alcohol affected. The National Association for Families and Addiction Research and Education estimates that 15% of all babies born in the United States in 1995 will test positive for illicit drugs. In the face of such overwhelming data, society, particularly health care providers, must learn the facts about drugs and substance abuse.

Substance abuse refers to inappropriate use of prescription drugs or use of illicit substances. Regardless of legal status, these substances generally fall into five categories (Table 55-1). For the purposes of this chapter, specific information is presented on alcohol, cocaine, designer drugs, and heroin. The reader is encouraged to seek other sources for a more comprehensive discussion of prescription drug abuse.

ADDICTION

Researchers have discovered evidence that some alcoholics are genetically predisposed to alcoholism[21]; however, scientists have not been able to determine if drug abusers have a genetic predisposition. Some drug abusers say they feel normal after substance abuse rather than euphoric. This may indicate that drug abuse has a biologic basis in certain individuals.

Drugs exert a powerful control on behavior because they act directly on the primitive brainstem and the limbic structure.[17,22] If you do something pleasurable, the message received reinforces the behavior responsible for the pleasure.[16] Understanding this process makes it easier to understand addiction.

Drug addiction is a biologically-based disease that alters the pleasure center and other aspects of the brain via the neurotransmitter dopamine. Dopamine connects neurons through the dendrite synaptic junction to a receptor site. When a neurotransmitter couples to a receptor, like a key fitting into a lock, the biochemical process in that neuron is activated. This process, called chemical neurotransmission, allows a receptor neuron to connect with other neurons. Heroin mimics the effects of the natural neurotransmitter, whereas substances like lysergic acid diethylamide (LSD) block receptors and prevent natural transmission. Cocaine interferes with the process of neurotransmission by preventing release of the neurotransmitter. Phencyclidine (PCP) interferes with the way messages proceed from the surface receptors into the cell interior.[16]

Box 55-1   **Characteristics of Drug Users in 12 Major Companies**

Late three times as often as their fellow workers
Ask for early dismissal or other time off 2.2 times as frequently as their fellow workers
Have 2.5 times as many absences totaling eight days or more per year
Five times more likely to file a worker's compensation claim
Involved in accidents 3.5 times more than their fellow workers

Data from Tanner J et al: Substance abuse and mandatory drug testing in health care institutions, *Health Care Manage Rev* 13(4):33, 1988.

Table 55-1   **Substances of Abuse**

Category	Examples/common names
Cannabis	Marijuana, pot
Stimulants	Crack, amphetamines, cocaine
Depressants	Sedatives, hypnotics, tranquilizers, alcohol
Narcotics	Morphine, heroin, meperidine (Demerol)
Hallucinogens	Psychedelic drugs, PCP, LSD

The biologic basis for addiction is the repeated process of altering chemical neurotransmission. Repeated use of these drugs can and will affect the brain on a permanent basis. Addiction begins when the pleasure circuit is repeatedly stimulated. The pleasure circuit is activated in a variety of ways depending on the drug of choice. Heroin activates the opiate receptors, whereas cocaine allows dopamine to accumulate in the synapses, where it is released. Increasing amounts of dopamine at the synapses lead to euphoria.

SPECIFIC SUBSTANCES

Emergencies related to substance abuse may be acute or chronic. The patient may come to the emergency department (ED) in acute withdrawal, with severe drug intoxication, or seeking help for the addiction. This chapter focuses on addiction rather than acute drug intoxication. Refer to Chapter 45 for comprehensive discussion of drug overdose, intoxication, and other toxicologic emergencies.

In addition to the previously mentioned substances of abuse, many individuals abuse alcohol, tobacco, steroids, and some natural stimulants available in health food stores. It is beyond the scope of this text to describe all potential substances of abuse; however, the use of alcohol and tobacco does warrant brief discussion.

Sixty percent of the American population has a drink at least once a month. There are 10.5 million alcoholics in America; 17.5 million others abuse alcohol. Accidents involving drunk drivers account for 45.1% of all traffic deaths. This translates to 1 death every 30 minutes, more than

---

Box 55-2   **Facts about Tobacco Abuse**

In 1992, 418,690 people died prematurely from the effects of smoking.
Smoking is linked to 30% of chronic heart disease deaths and 21% of other cardiovascular disease deaths.
Smoking a cigarette shortens life expectancy by seven minutes.
Three million teenagers smoke tobacco on a regular basis. In 1994, 10.8% of 12- to 17-year-old teens reported cigarette use in the last month.
Adolescents who smoke are 30 times more likely to try illicit drugs, 45 times more likely to smoke marijuana, 10 times more likely to use inhalants, and 75 times more likely to use cocaine.

Data from Drug Awareness Resistance Education America: *1995 drugs awareness resistance education facts: drugs and addiction*, 1995.

100,000 deaths per year. Two out of five Americans will be involved in an alcohol-related car accident in their lifetime.[14, 15]

Tobacco abuse is related to a multitude of health care problems, including cardiovascular disease, lung cancer, bronchitis, and many more. Box 55-2 highlights a few facts about this common addiction. Ironically, tobacco abuse is also common in the health care community. The emergency nurse should recognize the broad effects of tobacco abuse and provide pertinent education to the patient and family.

Tobacco

In 1992, 418,690 people died prematurely from the effects of smoking. Smoking is linked to 30% of chronic heart disease deaths and 21% of other cardiovascular disease deaths. Every cigarette smoked shortens life expectancy by 7 minutes. Three million teenagers smoke tobacco on a regular basis. In 1994, 10.8% of 12- to 17-year-old teens reported cigarette use in the past month. Adolescents who smoke are 30 times more likely to try illicit drugs, 45 times more likely to smoke marijuana, 10 times more likely to use inhalants, and 75 times more likely to use cocaine.[14]

Cocaine

Almost 2 million Americans use cocaine; more than 20 million Americans have tried cocaine once.[34] In 1993, 2.9% of all eighth graders had tried cocaine. In 1994, 6.9% of all high school seniors had tried cocaine, with 3.8% reporting annual use. Teens become addicted to cocaine in 15.5 months, whereas adults take more than 4 years to develop a serious cocaine problem. Crack, the smokable form of cocaine, was introduced to the drug scene in 1986. The high is 10 times more powerful than that caused by snorting the drug.[18] The associated rush or euphoria lasts only 5 to 10 minutes, which encourages more frequent use, so greater dependency develops.[14]

Cocaine can be snorted through the nose, smoked, or injected.[19] Injecting cocaine and other drugs carries the added risk of contracting human immunodeficiency virus (HIV). According to Murdock,[31] the effects of cocaine on the cardiovascular system include chest pain, myocarditis, cardiomyopathy, endocarditis, ventricular arrhythmias, aortic dissection, hypertension, cerebrovascular accident, and myocardial infarction (MI).[6,7] The literature is limited: only 19 published studies since 1982 with a total of 63 patients. MI is the most commonly reported cardiovascular consequence of cocaine use.[31] The first reported MI related to recreational/illegal drugs occurred in 1982.[31] Other effects of cocaine are excitation, increased alertness, increased heart rate, increased blood pressure, loss of appetite, insomnia, dilated pupils, runny nose, and nasal congestion.[30] In some situations, cocaine can trigger paranoia. Cocaine is an extremely strong stimulant, which may lead to seizures, cardiac and respiratory arrest, and even stroke. Long-term use of cocaine causes mucous membranes of the nose to disintegrate. Heavy cocaine use can actually cause the nasal septum to collapse.[10,11,12] Despite views to the contrary, cocaine does not improve performance. Use can lead to loss of concentration, irritability, loss of memory, loss of energy, anxiety, and a loss of interest in sex.

In 1990, Brody, Slovis, and Wrenn[3] found that 216 cocaine-using patients had 233 visits to EDs over a 6-month period. The majority (56.2%) of complaints were cardiopul-

monary. Short-term pharmacologic intervention was necessary in only 24% of the patients; only 9.9% required admission. Acute mortality was less than 1%. The authors concluded that most complications of cocaine are short-term; therefore, the major focus in the treatment of cocaine emergencies should be medical detoxification followed by referral for treatment of the addiction.

Cocaine is also an issue in pregnancy. Literature supports the fact that cocaine, like other drugs, can increase the risk of prematurity, stillbirth, low birth weight, central nervous system damage, and uterine rupture.[26] Concomitant use of alcohol increases these risks and contributes to long-term development problems.[4] Claire Coles, a clinical psychologist who studied "crack kids," states, "There is not evidence of genetic damage. Additionally, many 'crack kids' were born prematurely to mothers who had little or no prenatal care."[27] Chasnoff believes the environment may have a greater role than drug exposure in utero. Researchers found IQ scores of children exposed to crack the same as those not exposed to crack.[27] Table 55-2 summarizes effects of maternal cocaine use on mothers and fetuses/babies.

It is not uncommon for a substance abuser to use more than one drug. This polysubstance abuse creates additional problems and often jeopardizes the health of the user. The

Table **55-2**   **Effects of Maternal Cocaine Use on Mothers and Fetuses/Babies**

System	Effects on mother	Effects on fetus/baby
Neurologic	Seizures Neural damage* Insomnia	Increased irritability Increased startle response Difficult to console Tremors Jittery
Eyes	Retinal crystals causing flashes of light called snow lights	Eye defects*
Respiratory	Shortness of breath Lung damage, if smoked Nasal membrane burns and lesions Respiratory paralysis in overdose	Increased respiratory rate Abnormal ventilatory patterns Increased risk for sudden infant death syndrome*
Cardiovascular	Acute hypertension Angina Arrhythmias Tachycardia Palpitations Cerebral artery injury/cerebrovascular accident Cardiac failure	Intrauterine growth retardation Tachycardia Cerebral artery injury/infarction* Acute hypertension*
Gastrointestinal	Sore throat Hoarseness Anorexia leading to weight loss and malnutrition	Diarrhea Poor tolerance for oral feeding Prune-belly syndrome*
Renal		Hydronephrosis*
Reproductive	Increased uterine contractility Abruptio placentae Spontaneous abortion Premature labor Stillbirth	Cryptorchidism*

*Suspected but not established.

most frequently used substance in association with cocaine or crack is alcohol; however, barbiturates, marijuana, and tranquilizers are often taken with or immediately after cocaine or crack. Combining cocaine or crack with heroin, called "speedballing," can be deadly. Recent reports from the National Institute on Drug Abuse indicate increasing use of cocaine or crack with a hallucinogenic drug such as PCP to form a preparation called "space ball." Another combination that is extremely deadly is called "freebase." Freebasing is the process of converting street cocaine to pure form by removing some of the cutting agents. The result is the drug is more powerful, reaching the brain in seconds. The high occurs rapidly, but the euphoria disappears quickly, so the user still has a craving to freebase again and again.[8]

Life-threatening emergencies related to cocaine include chest pain, MI, seizures, severe hypertension, and stroke. Management of these life-threatening emergencies is no different in the patient who uses cocaine than in other patients with these problems. Recognition of cocaine as a causative agent is not essential to manage these patients in the ED; however, long-term management must address the issue of substance abuse. Other cocaine-related problems include agitation, paranoia, and epistaxis. There is an increased risk for injury to self and others with these patients. Decrease stimulation, and monitor them carefully.

Designer Drugs

Designer drugs are synthetically produced from a mixture of substances. Examples include PCP, methamphetamine, LSD, mescaline, psilocybin, and many others. Table 55-3 lists some designer drugs and their most common street names. Crystallized methamphetamine has been tried by 1% to 3% of all high school students. Honolulu police estimate that methamphetamine may be involved in almost 70% of spousal abuse cases within their jurisdiction. Over 100 deaths

on the West Coast have been linked to MPPP. One drop of MPPP is strong enough to kill 50 people. Dimethyltryptamine is a hallucinogen used to soak tobacco or marijuana.

Phencyclidine

PCP is a hallucinogen that alters reality, touch, hearing, smell, taste, and visual perceptions. These effects may lead to serious bodily injury to the user. Chronic and long-term use can cause permanent changes in cognitive ability, memory, and fine motor function.[9] Pregnant women who use PCP often deliver babies with visual, auditory, and motor disturbances.

The patient under the influence of PCP may be extremely violent with an increased risk for harm to self and others. Decrease stimulation in these patients, and monitor carefully for escalating violence.

Heroin

Over 500,000 Americans are addicted to heroin,[14] and nearly 2.5 million have used heroin at least once.[34] Intravenous heroin use increases risk of HIV, hepatitis, skin abscesses, phlebitis, and bacterial endocarditis. Heroin may be intentionally used with cocaine to enhance the rush or high. The heroin dealer may also cut the heroin with other substances such as strychnine, PCP, and others.

Heroin is an opiate that affects the pleasure center, causing physical dependence. Any attempt to stop using the drug causes severe painful withdrawal symptoms including watery eyes, runny nose, yawning, loss of appetite, tremors, panic, chills, sweating, nausea, muscle cramps, and insomnia. Elevated blood pressure, pulse, respiratory rate, and temperature occur as withdrawal progresses.[9] Heroin causes shallow breathing, pinpoint pupils, nausea, panic, insomnia, and a need for increasingly higher doses of the drug.[9]

The heroin addict may present to the ED in acute withdrawal, after an overdose, or with problems related to intravenous drug injection. The patient in acute withdrawal is

Table **55-3**	**Designer Drugs**
Chemical name	Street name
Phencyclidine	Angel dust, dust, peace pill, Captain Crunch
Methamphetamine	Ice, meth, crank, speed, crystal
1-Methyl-4-phenyl-4-propionoxy-piperidine	MPPP
Methylenedioxyamphetamine	Ecstasy, MDA
Lysergic acid diethylamide	LSD, acid, Mickey Mouse, paper acid, blotter acid
Mescaline	Peyote
Psilocybin	Magic mushrooms
Dimethyltryptamine	DMT

Box **55-3**	**Federal Drug-Free Workplace Act Requirements**

Publish a policy statement prohibiting unlawful manufacture, distribution, dispensing, possession, or use of controlled substances in the workplace. Policy must specify actions that will be taken for those who violate these policies. A copy of the policy must be given to each employee.
Establish a drug-free awareness program.
Inform employees they are required to report any criminal convictions for drug-related activities in the workplace.
Notify the federal contracting or granting agency of any criminal activity.
Take appropriate action, from discharge to rehabilitation.
Make a good faith effort to maintain a drug-free workplace.

From Employers get broader power to fight drug use, *Hospitals*, p 44, Aug 1989.

treated symptomatically with antianxiety agents, antihypertensive agents, and in some cases, administration of methadone. Acute heroin intoxication is treated with administration of naloxone, ventilatory support, and intravenous fluids when appropriate. Naloxone administration can precipitate severe withdrawal in some patients, so careful monitoring is essential.

ECONOMIC IMPACT

The overall economic impact of substance abuse exceeds $140 billion.[2] A study in *Nursing Administration Quarterly* concluded that health professionals are 30 to 100 times more likely to be addicted than the general population. According to a 1984 *Journal of Occupational Medicine* report, 15% of all American physicians are drug dependent. Reported cases of drug abuse among nurses indicate that 7 out of 100 registered nurses abuse drugs; however, the actual percentage may be higher.[2]

Drug abuse costs American industries $36.6 billion in lost productivity, medical expenses, theft, and damage.[13] The problem drinker uses eight times more medical care, is absent 2.5 times more often, and has 3.6 times more accidents on and off the job.[24] The cost of a single incident of nursing

Table **55-4** **Illegal Drugs and Their Effects**

Drugs	Street name	Signs of use	Overdose	Route taken
Cocaine	Coke Crack Snow	Excitation Increased alertness Increased heart rate Increased blood pressure Insomnia Runny nose Nasal congestion Dilated pupils	Agitation Increase in body temperature Hallucinations Seizures Possible death	Snorted Smoked (freebased) Injected
Amphetamines	Crank Ice Meth Speed Crystal	Excitation Increased alertness Increased heart rate Increased blood pressure Insomnia Runny nose Nasal congestion Dilated pupils	Agitation Increase in body temperature Hallucinations Seizures Possible death	Swallowed Snorted Smoked Injected
Heroin	Smack Stuff Horse Dope Boy	Excitation Drowsiness Respiratory depression Constricted pupils Nausea	Respiratory depression Seizures Coma Clammy skin Possible death	Injected Smoked Snorted
Phencyclidine	PCP Angel dust Hog	Illusions and hallucinations Poor perception of time and distance	Psychosis Longer, more intense "trip" episodes "Awake" coma Bizarre behavior Violence Possible death	Oral Injected Snorted Smoked
Lysergic acid diethylamide	LSD Acid Mickey Mouse Paper acid Blotter acid	Illusions and hallucinations Poor perception of time and distance	Psychosis Longer, more intense "trip" episodes Violence Possible death	Oral
Marijuana	Weed Grass Pot THC Acapulco gold	Difficulty concentrating Euphoria Short-term memory loss Dilated pupils Loss of depth perception Disciplinary problems Increased appetite Disoriented	Fatigue Paranoia Possible psychosis	Oral Smoked

impairment is extremely expensive. According to the *Journal of Nursing Administration,* costs through the course of the disease are estimated at $54,120, with the impaired nurse assuming an additional $31,953 from lost income and treatment. The employer loses $17,867 for overtime and recruitment costs, and the state board of nursing spends $4300 to pull a nursing license.[2]

In 1988, the federal government enacted the Federal Drug-Free Workplace Act. The law requires all employers who apply to federal agencies for contracts of $25,000 and more or who receive federal grants of any amount to certify they maintain a drug-free workplace.[25] The Federal Drug-Free Workplace Act requirements are summarized in Box 55-3. Today, many hospitals, businesses, and other industries have implemented preemployment drug testing. Many companies require drug screening when an accident occurs or there is a behavioral indication for such testing.[33] These tests are often done in the ED. The financial and emotional costs of replacing valuable employees have led many employers to institute Employee Assistance Programs (EAPs). EAP is a system to motivate and assist personnel with drug abuse or personal problems so they may remain productive at work.[5]

NURSING CONSIDERATIONS

Emergency nurses should continue to educate themselves and others about the effects of substance abuse. Drug abuse knows no social boundaries; therefore emergency nurses should be meticulous in assessment of patients seen in the ED. Obtain a detailed history, and observe the patient for behaviors or physical symptoms that indicate drug use or abuse. Table 55-4 summarizes the effects of the most common legal drugs. If you suspect the patient is abusing drugs, report your findings to the physician managing the patient's care so that appropriate testing or screening can be initiated. Ensure a safe environment for the patient, visitors, and personnel working in the ED.

The potential for violence increases in individuals under the influence of drugs. Increased injury severity and increased length of hospital stay occur in the presence of drug abuse.[28] Patients often present for treatment of injuries associated with high-risk behavior such as assaults, penetrating trauma, or blunt trauma rather than the drug abuse. Treat potentially life-threatening injuries, and then evaluate the patient for drug-related problems. Patients with acute signs and symptoms of abuse need medical intervention for the effects of the drug(s) taken.[20] Consultation or referral to a drug treatment center is indicated for substance abuse treatment after the patient is medically cleared.[1]

SUMMARY

Every day, ambulances and police cars race through neighborhoods because someone has been injured in a drug-related incident. Drugs in schools and the workplace will significantly affect the future of our society. Violence and crime have increased tremendously in the past decade. The most powerful weapon in the war on drug abuse is knowledge. Be an informed citizen.

REFERENCES

1. Arcidiacono A, Saum CA: Substance abuse treatment options: a federal initiative, *J Psychoactive Drugs* 27:105, 1995.
2. Brice J: Confronting drug abuse on the job, *Healthcare For J,* p 25, Jan-Feb 1995.
3. Brody SL, Slovis CM, Wrenn KD: Cocaine-related medical problems, *Am J Med* 88(4):325, 1990.
4. Buehler BA: Cocaine: how dangerous is it during pregnancy? *Nebr Med J* 80:116, 1995.
5. Callery YC: Chemical abuse rehabilitation for hospital employees, *AAORN J* 42(2):67, 1994.
6. Cohen P, Arjan S: *Ten years of cocaine,* Drug Research, Department of Human Geography, University of Amsterdam, 1993.
7. Department of Justice, Drug Enforcement Administration: *Controlled substances: uses and effects,* March 1995.
8. Department of Health and Human Services: *Cocaine/crack: the big lie,* 1991.
9. Department of Health and Human Services: *What you can do about drug use in America,* 1991.
10. Department of Health and Human Services: *When cocaine affects someone you love,* 1989.
11. Division of Alcohol and Drug Abuse: *As a matter of fact: cocaine,* 1994.
12. Drug Awareness Resistance Education: *Drugs of abuse,* Las Vegas Metropolitan Police Department, 1995.
13. Drug Awareness Resistance Education: *Workers at risk: drugs and alcohol on the job,* 1995.
14. Drug Awareness Resistance Education America: *1995 drugs awareness resistance education facts: drugs and addiction,* 1995.
15. Fuller MG et al: The role of a substance abuse consultation team in a trauma center, *J Stud Alcohol* 56:267, 1995.
16. Health Responsibility System, Inc: *Substance abuse,* 1995.
17. Health Responsibility System, Inc: *Addiction or dependency?* 1993.
18. Health Responsibility System, Inc: *Cocaine and stimulants,* 1993.
19. Health Responsibility System, Inc: *Collective works and database on substance abuse,* 1995.
20. Health Responsibility System, Inc: *Drug addiction treatment,* 1993.
21. Health Responsibility System, Inc: *Genetics and addiction,* 1993.
22. Health Responsibility System, Inc: *Impact on the brain,* 1993.
23. Health Responsibility System, Inc: *Marijuana and hallucinogens,* 1993.
24. Substance abuse in the workplace, *Hospitals,* p 68, June 1987.
25. Employers get broader power to fight drug use, *Hospitals,* p 44, Aug 1989.
26. Kearney MH et al: Salvaging self: a grounded theory of pregnancy on crack cocaine, *Nurs Res* 44:208, 1995.
27. Kennedy D: "Crack babies" catch up, *Associated Press,* Dec 1992.
28. Mackersie RC et al: High risk behavior and the public burden for funding the cost of acute injury, *Arch Surg Abstr* 130:844, 1995.
29. Mazzoni J: Management of drug abuse in the hospital environment, *Top Health Rev Manage* 9(1):54, 1988.
30. Mirchandani HG et al: Cocaine-induced agitated delirium, forceful struggle, and minor head injury: a further definition of sudden death. *Am J Forensic Med Pathol* 15(2):95, 1994.
31. Murdock M: *Cocaine-induced myocardial infarctions,* 1994.
32. Roberts TC: *Built for speed?* 1995.
33. Tanner J et al: Substance abuse and mandatory drug testing in health care institutions. *Health Care Manage Rev* 13(4):33, 1988.
34. Tintinalli JE, Ruiz E, Krome RL: *Emergency medicine: a comprehensive study guide,* ed 4, New York, 1996, McGraw-Hill.

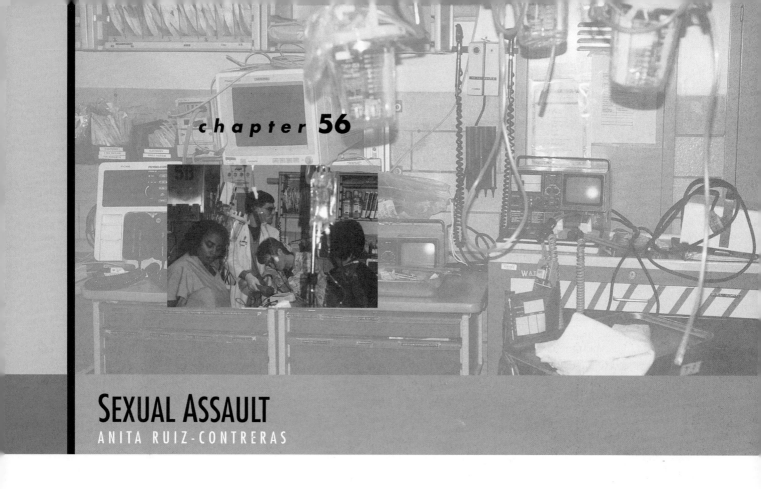

chapter 56

SEXUAL ASSAULT
ANITA RUIZ-CONTRERAS

One of four women will be sexually assaulted in their lifetime.[5] The Uniform Crime Reports of the Federal Bureau of Investigation (1994) do not maintain statistics on the sexual assault of males, although the numbers of reported assaults on males are increasing.[8]

Sexual assault is one of the most feared and least understood crimes. Of all the choices made in our lives, the most intimate choices are sexual. In a sexual assault, this choice is taken away. Sexual assault is not a crime of passion. In a classic study of more than 600 sex offenders, Amir[1] was one of the first to describe rape as a crime of power and control. Groth[6] interviewed more than 500 sexual "aggressors" and found power and anger described as motivating factors. Sex is used by the rapist as a tool to control and humiliate the victim. Slaughter and Brown[11] define *rape* as a forensic term characterizing sexual activity perpetrated against the will of a victim.

Survivor is a common term used for sexual assault patients. The patient who has experienced sexual assault has lived through a life-threatening event. Use of the term *victim* denotes helplessness and hopelessness. The term *survivor* has more of a positive, empowering connotation. Some professionals working in the area of sexual assault treatment do not use the term because it may minimize or take away from the devastation of the actual event.

The patient may arrive with expectations about the hospital and the staff that may be based on misconceptions. The patient, the law enforcement officer, and the emergency nurse may all have long-held beliefs. It is important for health care professionals to examine their own attitudes regarding survivors of sexual assault.[9] Myths and misconceptions surrounding sexual assault harm the patient and hamper development of a trusting relationship with the emergency nurse.

Common myths such as "victims are women wearing suggestive clothing" or "a woman cannot be raped by an acquaintance" have long ago been dispelled. Regrettably, other myths continue to remain prevalent. The media often portray women as secretly wanting to be raped; this is described as a "rape fantasy." When an individual fantasizes, he or she selects the players, the setting, and the sexual acts. In a sexual assault, all choice is taken away. This myth confuses sex and rape. Sex becomes the tool used by the rapist to degrade and humiliate the victim. Emergency nurses can use their knowledge regarding myths and misconceptions when counseling patients and families to dispel these beliefs and help to begin the process of healing.

RAPE-TRAUMA SYNDROME

In a landmark study of 94 rape victims, Burgess and Holmstrom[4] first identified *rape-trauma syndrome,* a cluster of symptoms experienced by survivors of sexual assault. Symptoms include somatic, behavioral, and psychologic reactions. The framework of rape-trauma syndrome includes recognition of the long-term reorganization a survivor goes through when recovering from the assault.[12] Reorganization may take weeks or even years. There is recognition of the differences in lifestyle choices made by individuals, where lifestyles are not judged but accepted as normal for that person. Prostitutes who normally charge for sexual services can be raped. An individual who enjoys a "one-night stand" can be raped. The wife can be raped.

It is also important to remember that men can be the victims of sexual assault. Male sexual assault may be one of the most underreported of all groups. Myths surrounding male sexual assault include a belief that it only happens in prison or that homosexuality is a causative factor. Lipscomb et al.[7], in a study of 99 adult male victims of sexual assault, found no statistically significant difference between incarcerated and nonincarcerated victims. All men are potential victims regardless of sexual orientation. Men are raped for the same reasons women are raped: power, control, and humiliation.

Rape-trauma syndrome is an approved nursing diagnosis and can be used to plan nursing care. The initial hospital interaction can have a major impact on the acute phase of the sexual assault survivor's recovery. When interacting with the sexual victim, it is essential for the emergency nurse to develop a trusting relationship. As with any patient, a calm, confident approach facilitates this process. Listen to the patient. Show concern for the patient's experience. Specific questions that require the patient to relive the assault are not needed. Determining the presence of physical trauma that requires immediate treatment is the priority. The extent of emotional injury cannot be estimated. Each person's response to a sexual assault is different. Individuals may laugh, cry, tell a joke, or become catatonic. Patients may blame themselves for fighting back or for not fighting back. Tell these patients that their actions helped get them through the ordeal, regardless of what those actions were. Patients may believe they caused the rape by accepting the ride or opening the door. Remind these patients that they did not cause the assault. These patients need to hear that they have the right to decide what to do with their own bodies and that no one has the right to hurt them.

THE SEXUAL ASSAULT SURVIVOR IN THE EMERGENCY DEPARTMENT

Evaluation of the sexual assault survivor in the emergency department (ED) requires planning, development of specific policies and procedures, and staff education. The goal is to provide sensitive, individualized care for each person in a manner that ensures adherence to legal and regulatory requirements. Each hospital should be knowledgeable of its state's laws and regulations regarding sexual assault. If a standard form or protocol is required, the hospital should be in compliance. For example, the *California State Medical Protocol for the Examination and Treatment of Sexual Assault Victims,* a 125-page document, must be used by all California hospitals and health care practitioners who perform examinations on survivors of sexual assault. If hospitals do not wish to comply, they must develop a referral protocol with a hospital that does comply. For each case, a standard form is used. The protocol outlines the steps of examination including evidence collection, laboratory testing, medications, and follow-up care.

For more than 15 years, specialized teams of nonphysician medical providers have been utilized,[3] for example, sexual assault response teams (SART) or suspected abuse response teams. The team consists of a nurse examiner, rape crisis advocate, and law enforcement personnel. Nurses with specialized training are identified as sexual assault/abuse nurse examiners (SANE). The SART program trains registered nurses to obtain the patient history, conduct evidentiary exams, provide sexually transmitted disease (STD) prophylaxis and pregnancy prevention, and ensure follow-up care. The SANE personnel are usually on call and respond when a sexual assault victim arrives at an identified hospital. In a policy statement, the American College of Emergency Physicians[2] stated that specially trained, nonphysician medical personnel should be allowed to perform evidentiary examinations in which evidence collected in such a manner is admissible in criminal cases. Offices of the district attorney in areas with established programs have found the SANE personnel to be competent, well-informed witnesses.

Development of a specialized team should be the ideal; however, hospitals without specialized programs have conducted effective sexual assault treatment programs. Specialized programs generally include training all ED nurses or an identified number of nurses to care for sexual assault survivors during their work hours. The SANE personnel may conduct the complete evidentiary examination independently in conjunction with a physician. The nurse acts as a patient care coordinator, ensuring adherence to established procedures.

Patient Assessment

Sexual assault survivors should be an emergent priority behind patients experiencing an acute life-threatening event. The patient should be immediately placed in a safe, secure room. A nurse should be identified to remain with the patient throughout the ED visit. The patient should be allowed to have a support person such as a family member, friend, or representative from a rape crisis center. Asking "Whom can I call for you?" makes the patient think of a name, whereas asking "Is there someone I can call for you?" is often followed by a "No" answer. Rape crisis advocates are an integral part of any sexual assault treatment program. If available, it should be hospital policy to contact the local rape crisis center when the patient arrives.

Consent

The examination of a sexual assault survivor has often been called a "re-rape." All interactions should be handled with sensitivity and understanding. Every effort should be made to ensure that the patient has the opportunity to make informed choices about medical care. By obtaining consent, the nurse begins to develop a therapeutic relationship with the patient. Most states require law enforcement notification when patients seek treatment after sexual assault. Sexual assault is a crime, and any injury incurred during the commission of a crime is reportable. The hospital may be required to report; however, the patient has the right to decide whether they wish to speak with law enforcement. Law enforcement officers today have special training and are better able to deal sensitively with survivors of sexual assault. The nurse needs to ensure that the patient is well informed and understands the examination process. Consent should be obtained for medical treatment including evidentiary examination. The patient must understand that the evidence collected will be used for prosecution of the accused rapist. Consent for any photographs is also required.

History

A consistent form should be used to gather the patient's history. The history helps the nurse decide on the manner of evidence collection. Examinations performed within 72 hours of the assault are more likely to yield evidence of assault. When questioning the patient, the nurse does not need the patient to describe the assault in specific minute by minute detail. Pertinent areas for questioning are summarized in Box 56-1. Ask questions in a manner understood by the patient. Translate medical terms into everyday language. The history taking can be delayed depending on the patient's emotional response to questioning. Documentation should be completed legibly and clearly. If this case is called to court, the nurse may be asked to discuss what was written in the record.

Physical Examination and Evidence Collection

Laboratory testing should be accomplished early to allow for pregnancy test results. A test for syphilis can be obtained at the same time. The patient's clothing is collected and placed in paper rather than plastic bags for evaluation at the local crime laboratory. A head-to-toe physical assessment is completed to look for injuries. Documentation of injury should include color and size of injuries such as bruises and abrasions. Use of body figures on the documentation tool can assist in recording injury. A Wood's lamp or other ultraviolet light is used to look for semen on the patient's skin. Semen may fluoresce an orange or blue-green color on the skin. The fluorescent area should be swabbed with a moistened cotton-tipped applicator, which is then swabbed over a slide. A control swab should then be taken from an area of the body near the area of fluorescence. Oral swabs are taken for evidence of semen and as a reference sample. Reference samples are saliva, blood, semen, pubic hair, and body hair that are taken from the survivor. The reference samples are compared to specimens from potential suspects. Table 56-1 lists essential evidentiary requirements.

For the female patient, the next part of the examination is a pelvic examination. Some institutions may use colposcopic photographs as the first part of the pelvic or genital evaluation. Photographs are used to detect and document genital trauma.[11] Examine external genitalia for signs of injury or foreign materials. Documentation should indicate if the injury is apparent without use of the colposcope. Injuries should be described by size, appearance, and location. Pubic hair is combed to look for foreign hair. A representative number of the patient's pubic hairs are then cut for comparison. During the pelvic examination, swabs and slides are taken from the vaginal pool. Testing for chlamydia and gonorrhea is done on these specimens. Rectal examination includes colposcopy, swabs, slides, and baseline testing for STDs. Obtain rectal swabs before vaginal swabs to avoid contamination from vaginal fluid. Table 56-2 summarizes laboratory testing for sexual assault. All swabs and slides must be labeled to identify the patient and the source. Once collected, swabs or slides should be placed in a drying box with cool air flow. Drying prevents deterioration of evidence and helps maintain genetic marker enzymes. Genetic marker enzymes can be identified by the crime laboratory and linked to potential suspects.

Chain of custody

To maintain validity of evidence collected, the nurse must be able to verify the whereabouts of all evidence. A chart can be used to indicate that evidence was taken from the patient by the nurse and then given to the law enforcement officer. All transfers of the evidence need to be logged to show that evidence was transferred from one person to another. The transfer should be dated and timed. The best practice is to keep transfers of evidence to a minimum. If a drying box is used, it must have a lock that is closed and opened only by the nurse.

Postexamination

A shower and clean clothing should be available for the patient after the sexual assault examination. Ideally, the hospital maintains a closet with clean, used, donated clothing. Medication should be provided for prevention of pregnancy and STDs (Table 56-3). Consent for pregnancy prevention should be obtained after a negative pregnancy test result and after the patient is informed of associated risks. A specific postcoital consent form should be used.

Box **56-1**	**Areas for Patient Questions Related to Sexual Assault**

Time and date of assault
Surroundings
Body orifices penetrated
Use of any foreign objects
Other sexual acts
Injuries incurred during the assault
Activities after assault such as urination, showering, or douching
Recent gynecologic treatment or surgery
History of consensual intercourse within the last 72 hours

Table 56-1	**Evidentiary Requirements for Sexual Assault**
Item	Description
Clothing	Note condition of the clothing. Place each piece of clothing in a separate paper bag.
Fingernail scrapings	Collect when indicated. Hold each hand over a piece of paper. Using wooden sticks, scrape under each nail.
Skin	Scan body with Wood's lamp. Collect dried and moist secretions using cotton-tipped swabs. Collect a control swab from same area of the body.
Oral cavity	Collect if oral penetration occurred within the last 6 hours. Collect 2 swabs from oral cavity and 1 swab from area around the mouth.
Reference sample—oral	With clean forceps, place clean gauze or cotton pledget under the tongue.
External genitalia	Examine with Wood's lamp. Collect dried material and matted hair. Swab areas of fluorescence with a moistened cotton-tipped applicator.
Pubic hair	Local requirements may include samples of body and facial hair or head hair. Comb pubic hair and then place in evidence envelope. Cut up to 40 pubic hairs from different perineal areas per local guidelines.
Vagina	Collect 3 separate swabs/slides from the vaginal pool. Do 1 wet mount slide and 2 dry mount slides. Examine wet mount for motile or nonmotile sperm.
Penis	Collect dried secretions using 2 swabs. Collect 1 swab from the urethral meatus and 1 swab from the glans and shaft. Examine the penis and scrotum for injury.
Rectum	Collect dried secretions using 2 rectal swabs. Collect 2 separate swabs/slides. Do 2 dry mount swabs. Examine buttocks, perianal skin, and anal folds for injury. Anoscopic or proctoscopic exam may be indicated.
Other evidence such as foreign material or dried secretions	When dried secretions are collected using a moistened cotton-tipped swab, a control sample should be taken from the same area of the body.

Adapted from the Office of Criminal Justice Planning: *California state medical protocol for examination of sexual assault and child sexual abuse victims,* State of California, 1987.

Table 56-2	**Laboratory Testing for Sexual Assault**
Area of body penetrated	Recommended tests
Oral	Culture for gonorrhea; blood test for syphilis
Vaginal	Culture for gonorrhea, chlamydia; blood test for syphilis; pregnancy testing
Penile	Culture for gonorrhea, chlamydia; blood test for syphilis
Rectal	Culture for gonorrhea, chlamydia; blood test for syphilis

Table 56-3	**Medication Prophylaxis in Sexual Assault**		
Potential problem	No penicillin allergy	Penicillin allergy
Gonorrhea, chlamydia, syphilis* in non-pregnant patient	Cefixime 400 mg PO as stat dose, then doxycycline 100 mg PO BID for 7 days	Spectinomycin 2 gm IM, then doxycycline 100 mg PO BID for 7 days
Gonorrhea, chlamydia, syphilis* in pregnant patient	Cefixime 400 mg PO stat dose, then erythromycin 500 mg PO QID for 7 days	Spectinomycin 2 gm IM, then erythromycin 500 mg PO QID for 7 days
Pregnancy**	Ovral 2 tablets PO and 2 tablets in 12 hours	

From Sexual Assault Response Team: *Standardized procedure: medication administration, sexual assault victims,* San Jose, 1996, Santa Clara Valley Medical Center.
*Efficacy against syphilis not proven.
**Give only after obtaining negative pregnancy test.

Follow-up care

Patients should be rechecked in 10 days to 2 weeks. Referral to a gynecologist or nearby clinic is essential, since cultures should be repeated. Testing for human immunodeficiency virus (HIV) may occur during the initial laboratory screening or may be deferred until the first follow-up appointment. Many established specialized teams include follow-up care as part of their overall program.

Legal aspects

When the case goes to court, the nurse may be called as a witness to describe what the nurse did and saw. Each encounter with a sexual assault patient is a potential court case. The nurse does not represent one side or the other.

The nurse is there to report or give an opinion, not to offer judgment. The nurse may receive a subpoena from the district attorney's office or a defense attorney representing the accused. In preparation for court, the nurse should review the patient's medical record. Box 56-2 pro-

Box 56-2	**Tips for Being a Witness**

Listen to the complete question.
Respond to the question by facing the jury.
Tell the truth.
Remain calm.
Be objective.
Avoid becoming defensive or angry.
Be prepared to spell and define medical terms.
Ask for clarification of any questions you do not understand.
Answer only the question you are asked.
Ask the judge for permission to speak if you feel an explanation is needed.
Wait to answer until the judge has ruled on an objection.
Say "I don't know" confidently if you don't know.

vides clues to answering questions while on the witness stand.

SUMMARY

In an expanded role, emergency nurses are uniquely suited to act as sexual assault nurse examiners or as coordinators of the care of a sexual assault survivor. However, if this role is not accepted in the nurse's institution or state, it is still vital that the emergency nurse be knowledgeable about the local or state protocol. The emergency nurse should care for the patient in a supportive, nonthreatening, nonjudgmental manner. The ED visit can significantly affect the emotional recovery of the sexual assault survivor.

REFERENCES

1. Amir M: *Patterns of forcible rape,* Chicago, 1971, University of Chicago Press.
2. American College of Emergency Physicians: Management of the patient with the complaint of sexual assault, *Ann Emerg Med,* May 1995.
3. Antognoli-Toland P: Comprehensive program for examination of sexual assault victims by nurses: a hospital-based project in Texas, *J Emerg Nurs* 11(3):132, 1985.
4. Burgess AW, Holmstrom LL: Rape trauma syndrome, *Am J Psychiatry* 131:981, 1974.
5. Emergency Nurses Association: *Position statement: treatment of sexual assault victims,* Chicago, 1995.
6. Groth AN: *Men who rape: the psychology of the offender,* New York, 1979, Plenum Press.
7. Lipscomb GH et al: Male victims of sexual assault, *JAMA* 267(22):3064, 1992.
8. Office of Criminal Justice Planning: *The California state medical protocol for the examination and treatment of sexual assault victims,* State of California, 1987.
9. Piercy M: *Living in the open,* New York, 1976, Knopf.
10. Ruiz-Contreras A: Emergency nurses' attitudes toward victims of sexual assault, Unpublished thesis, 1992, San Jose State University.
11. Slaughter L, Brown CRV: Colposcopy to establish physical findings in rape victims, *Am J Obstet Gynecol* 166(1):83, 1992.
12. Warner CG: *Rape & sexual assault: Management & intervention.* Germantown, Colo, 1980, Aspen Publications.

INDEX